The Johns Hopkins
Internal Medicine
Board Review

The Johns Hopkins
Internal Medicine
Board Review
Certification and Recertification
Fifth Edition

Bimal H. Ashar, MD, MBA
Associate Professor of Medicine
The Johns Hopkins University School of Medicine
Baltimore, Maryland

Redonda G. Miller, MD, MBA
Associate Professor of Medicine
The Johns Hopkins University School of Medicine
Baltimore, Maryland

Stephen D. Sisson, MD
Professor of Medicine
The Johns Hopkins University School of Medicine
Baltimore, Maryland

ELSEVIER

ELSEVIER

1600 John F. Kennedy Blvd.
Ste 1800
Philadelphia, PA 19103-2899

Notices

Knowledge and best practice in this field are constantly changing. As new research and experience
broaden our understanding, changes in research methods, professional practices, or medical treatment
may become necessary.

Practitioners and researchers must always rely on their own experience and knowledge in evaluating and
using any information, methods, compounds, or experiments described herein. In using such information
or methods they should be mindful of their own safety and the safety of others, including parties for whom
they have a professional responsibility.

With respect to any drug or pharmaceutical products identified, readers are advised to check the most
current information provided (i) on procedures featured or (ii) by the manufacturer of each product to be
administered, to verify the recommended dose or formula, the method and duration of administration, and
contraindications. It is the responsibility of practitioners, relying on their own experience and knowledge
of their patients, to make diagnoses, to determine dosages and the best treatment for each individual
patient, and to take all appropriate safety precautions.

To the fullest extent of the law, neither the Publisher nor the authors, contributors, or editors, assume
any liability for any injury and/or damage to persons or property as a matter of products liability, negligence
or otherwise, or from any use or operation of any methods, products, instructions, or ideas contained in the
material herein.

Library of Congress Cataloging-in-Publication Data

The Johns Hopkins internal medicine board review : certification and
recertification / [edited by] Bimal H. Ashar, Redonda G. Miller,
Stephen D. Sisson.—Fifth edition.
    p. ; cm.
    Internal medicine board review
    Includes bibliographical references and index.
    ISBN 978-0-323-37733-1 (pbk. : alk. paper)
    I. Ashar, Bimal H., editor.   II. Miller, Redonda G., editor.
III. Sisson, Stephen D., editor.   IV. Johns Hopkins University.
V. Title: Internal medicine board review.
    [DNLM: 1. Internal Medicine—Examination Questions.   2. Internal
Medicine—Outlines. WB 18.2]
    RC46
    616.0076—dc23
                                        2015031188

Executive Content Strategist: Kate Dimock
Content Development Manager: Stacy Eastman
Publishing Services Manager: Patricia Tannian
Project Manager: Amanda Mincher
Book Designer: XiaoPei Chen

Gram stain cover image from Haslett C, Chilvers ER, Boon NA,
Colledge NR, eds. *Davidson's Principles and Practice of Medicine.* 19th ed.
Edinburgh: Elsevier Science; 2002: Fig. 13.30. Neurofibromatosis type 1
Lisch nodules cover image from Habif TP. *Clinical Dermatology: A Color
Guide to Diagnosis and Therapy.* 4th ed. Philadelphia: Mosby; 2004: Fig.
26-13A. Left-shifted myelopoiesis cover image reused with permission
from Klatt EC. Hematopathology. In: *Robbins and Cotran Atlas of
Pathology.* Philadelphia: Saunders; 2010:63-91: Fig. 3-53.

Printed in India

Last digit is the print number: 10 9

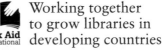

Working together
to grow libraries in
developing countries

www.elsevier.com • www.bookaid.org

SECTION EDITORS

Natasha Mubeen Chida, MD, MSPH
Clinical Fellow in Infectious Diseases
The Johns Hopkins University School of Medicine
Baltimore, Maryland
Section 2: Infectious Disease

David Cosgrove, MB, BCh
Assistant Professor of Medical Oncology
The Johns Hopkins University School of Medicine
Baltimore, Maryland
Section 8: Hematology
Section 9: Oncology

Brian Thomas Garibaldi, MD
Assistant Professor
The Johns Hopkins University School of Medicine
Baltimore, Maryland
Section 3: Pulmonary and Critical Care Medicine

Uzma Haque, MD
Assistant Professor of Medicine
The Johns Hopkins University School of Medicine
Baltimore, Maryland
Section 7: Rheumatology

Nestoras N. Mathioudakis, MD
Assistant Professor of Medicine
Associate Director, Inpatient Diabetes Management
   Service
The Johns Hopkins University School of Medicine
Baltimore, Maryland
Section 6: Endocrinology

Michael T. Melia, MD
Assistant Professor of Medicine
The Johns Hopkins University School of Medicine
Baltimore, Maryland
Section 2: Infectious Disease

Justin James Roesch, BS, MD
Assistant Professor
Division of Hospital Medicine
University of New Mexico
Albuquerque, New Mexico
Section 11: Selected Topics in General and Internal Medicine

Eun Ji Shin, MD, PhD
Assistant Professor
The Johns Hopkins University School of Medicine
Baltimore, Maryland
Section 4: Gastroenterology

C. John Sperati, MD, MHS
Assistant Professor of Medicine
The Johns Hopkins University School of Medicine
Baltimore, Maryland
Section 5: Nephrology

Sammy Zakaria, MD, MPH
Assistant Professor of Medicine
The Johns Hopkins University School of Medicine
Baltimore, Maryland
Section 1: Cardiology

CONTRIBUTORS

Thura T. Abd, MD, MPH
Cardiology Fellow
The Johns Hopkins Ciccarone Center for the Prevention
  of Heart Disease
Baltimore, Maryland
Lipid Disorders

D'Jahna Akinyemi, MD, MS
Assistant Professor
The Johns Hopkins University School of Medicine
Baltimore, Maryland
Allergy and Immunology for the Internist

Deborah K. Armstrong, MD
Associate Professor of Oncology
Associate Professor of Gynecology and Obstetrics
The Johns Hopkins University School of Medicine
Baltimore, Maryland
Breast and Ovarian Cancer

Bimal H. Ashar, MD, MBA
Associate Professor of Medicine
The Johns Hopkins University School of Medicine
Baltimore, Maryland
Anemia
Complementary and Alternative Medicine
Immunization and Prevention

John N. Aucott, MD
Assistant Professor of Medicine
The Johns Hopkins University School of Medicine
Baltimore, Maryland
Selected Topics in Infectious Disease II

Paul G. Auwaerter, MD
Sherrilyn and Ken Fisher Professor of Medicine
The Johns Hopkins University School of Medicine
Baltimore, Maryland
Respiratory Infections

Wendy L. Bennett, MD, MPH
Assistant Professor
The Johns Hopkins University School of Medicine
Baltimore, Maryland
Selected Topics in Women's Health

Gail Berkenblit, MD, PhD
Assistant Professor
The Johns Hopkins University School of Medicine
Baltimore, Maryland
Human Immunodeficiency Virus Infection

Adam R. Berliner, MD
Instructor
The Johns Hopkins University School of Medicine
Nephrology Center of Maryland
Baltimore, Maryland
Acute Kidney Injury

O. Joseph Bienvenu, MD, PhD
Associate Professor
The Johns Hopkins University School of Medicine
Baltimore, Maryland
Psychiatry for the Internist

Dionne Blackman, AB, MD
Associate Professor of Medicine
University of Chicago
Chicago, Illinois
*Maximizing Test Performance: Effective Study and Test-
  Taking Strategies*

Roger S. Blumenthal, MD
Professor of Medicine
The Johns Hopkins University School of Medicine
Baltimore, Maryland
Lipid Disorders

Todd T. Brown, MD, PhD
Associate Professor of Medicine and Epidemiology
The Johns Hopkins University School of Medicine
Baltimore, Maryland
Reproductive Endocrinology

Michael A. Carducci, MD
AEGON Professor in Prostate Cancer Research
The Johns Hopkins University School of Medicine
Baltimore, Maryland
Genitourinary Cancer

Michael A. Chattergoon, MD, PhD
Robert Meyerhoff Assistant Professor of Medicine
The Johns Hopkins University School of Medicine
Baltimore, Maryland
Selected Topics in Infectious Disease II

Po-Hung Chen, MD
Fellow in Transplant Hepatology
The Johns Hopkins University School of Medicine
Baltimore, Maryland
Acute and Chronic Liver Disease
Complications of Liver Disease

Michael J. Choi, MD
Associate Professor of Medicine and Clinical Director
The Johns Hopkins University School of Medicine
Baltimore, Maryland
Selected Topics in Nephrology

Grant V. Chow, MD
Electrophysiology Fellow
The Johns Hopkins University School of Medicine
Baltimore, Maryland
Arrhythmias

Colleen Christmas, MD
Associate Professor
The Johns Hopkins University School of Medicine
Baltimore, Maryland
Selected Topics in Geriatric Medicine

John O. Clarke, MD
Associate Professor of Medicine
The Johns Hopkins University School of Medicine
Baltimore, Maryland
Peptic Ulcer Disease and Gastrointestinal Bleeding
Esophageal Disease

David S. Cooper, MD
Professor of Medicine
The Johns Hopkins University School of Medicine
Baltimore, Maryland
Thyroid Disease

Mary Corretti, MD
Associate Professor of Medicine
Director, Adult Echocardiography Lab
The Johns Hopkins University School of Medicine
Baltimore, Maryland
Pericardial Disease

David Cosgrove, MB, BCh
Assistant Professor of Medical Oncology
The Johns Hopkins University School of Medicine
Baltimore, Maryland
Colorectal Cancer
Selected Topics in Oncology

Kelly E. Dooley, MD, PhD
Assistant Professor
The Johns Hopkins University School of Medicine
Baltimore, Maryland
Mycobacterial Infections

M. Bradley Drummond, MD, MHS
Assistant Professor of Medicine
The Johns Hopkins University School of Medicine
Baltimore, Maryland
Obstructive Lung Disease

James P. Dunn, MD
Professor of Ophthalmology
The Sidney Kimmel Medical College
Director, Uveitis Unit/Retina Division
Wills Eye Hospital
Philadelphia, Pennsylvania
Ophthalmology for the Internist

Michelle M. Estrella, MD, MHS
Assistant Professor of Medicine
The Johns Hopkins University School of Medicine
Baltimore, Maryland
Selected Topics in Nephrology

Derek M. Fine, MD
Associate Professor of Medicine and Fellowship Director
The Johns Hopkins University School of Medicine
Baltimore, Maryland
Glomerular Disease
Chronic Kidney Disease and End-Stage Renal Disease

April S. Fitzgerald, MD
Assistant Professor
The Johns Hopkins University School of Medicine
Baltimore, Maryland
Headaches

John A. Flynn, MD, MBA, Med
Professor
The Johns Hopkins University School of Medicine
Baltimore, Maryland
Office Orthopedics

Patrick Forde, MD
Assistant Professor of Oncology
The Johns Hopkins University School of Medicine
Baltimore, Maryland
Lung Cancer and Head and Neck Cancer

Allan C. Gelber, MD, MPH, PhD
Associate Professor of Medicine
The Johns Hopkins University School of Medicine
Baltimore, Maryland
Arthritis

Khalil G. Ghanem, MD, PhD
Associate Professor of Medicine
The Johns Hopkins University School of Medicine
Genitourinary Infections

Gabriel Ghiaur, MD, PhD
Assistant Professor of Medicine and Oncology
The Johns Hopkins University School of Medicine
Baltimore, Maryland
Blood Smear and Bone Marrow Review

Sherita H. Golden, MD, MHS
Professor of Medicine
Executive Vice-Chair, Department of Medicine
The Johns Hopkins University School of Medicine
Baltimore, Maryland
Diabetes Mellitus

Eduardo J. Gonzalez-Velez, MD
Assistant Professor
The Johns Hopkins University School of Medicine
Baltimore, Maryland
Peptic Ulcer Disease and Gastrointestinal Bleeding

Thomas B. Habif, MD
Adjunct Professor of Medicine
Dartmouth Medical School
Hanover, New Hampshire
Dermatology for the Internist

David N. Hager, MD, PhD
Assistant Professor
The Johns Hopkins University School of Medicine
Baltimore, Maryland
Critical Care Medicine

Noah M. Hahn, MD
Associate Professor
The Johns Hopkins University School of Medicine
Baltimore, Maryland
Genitourinary Cancer

James P. Hamilton, MD
Assistant Professor
The Johns Hopkins University School of Medicine
Baltimore, Maryland
Acute and Chronic Liver Disease
Complications of Liver Disease

Hans Hammers, MD, PhD
Assistant Professor of Oncology
The Johns Hopkins University School of Medicine
Baltimore, Maryland
Genitourinary Cancer

Ashley M. Harris, MD, MHS
Fellow
The Johns Hopkins University School of Medicine
Baltimore, Maryland
Selected Topics in Women's Health

Maureen R. Horton, MD
Associate Professor of Medicine and Environmental
    Health Sciences
The Johns Hopkins University School of Medicine
Baltimore, Maryland
Interstitial Lung Disease

Carol Ann Huff, MD
Associate Professor of Medicine and Oncology
The Johns Hopkins University School of Medicine
Baltimore, Maryland
Plasma Cell Dyscrasias

Mark T. Hughes, MD, MA
Assistant Professor of Medicine
The Johns Hopkins University School of Medicine
Baltimore, Maryland
Medical Ethics

Parag H. Joshi, MD, MHS
Clinical Fellow in Cardiology
The Johns Hopkins University School of Medicine
Baltimore, Maryland
Lipid Disorders

Yvette L. Kasamon, MD
Associate Professor of Oncology
The Johns Hopkins University School of Medicine
Baltimore, Maryland
Lymphoma and Chronic Lymphocytic Leukemia

Rebecca A. Kazin, MD
Assistant Professor of Dermatology
The Johns Hopkins University School of Medicine
Baltimore, Maryland
Dermatology for the Internist

Ali Reza Keramati, MD
Postdoctoral Fellow
The Johns Hopkins University School of Medicine
Baltimore, Maryland
Lipid Disorders

Thomas W. Koenig, MD
Assistant Professor
The Johns Hopkins University School of Medicine
Baltimore, Maryland
Psychiatry for the Internist

Klitos Konstantinidis, MD
Postdoctoral Fellow
The Johns Hopkins University School of Medicine
Baltimore, Maryland
Coronary Artery Disease

Sophie M. Lanzkron, MD, MHS
Associate Professor of Medicine
The Johns Hopkins University School of Medicine
Baltimore, Maryland
Platelet Disorders

Howard P. Levy, MD, PhD
Assistant Professor
The Johns Hopkins University School of Medicine
Baltimore, Maryland
Genetics for the Internist

Rafael H. Llinás, MD
Associate Professor
The Johns Hopkins University School of Medicine
Baltimore, Maryland
Cerebrovascular Disease and Seizure Disorders
Selected Topics in Neurology

Kristle L. Lynch, MD
Gastroenterology Fellow
The Johns Hopkins University School of Medicine
Baltimore, Maryland
Esophageal Disease

Joseph E. Marine, MD
Associate Professor of Medicine
The Johns Hopkins University School of Medicine
Baltimore, Maryland
Arrhythmias

Karim R. Masri, MD
Rheumatology Fellow
The Johns Hopkins University School of Medicine
Baltimore, Maryland
Office Orthopedics

Meredith C. McCormack, MD, MHS
Assistant Professor of Medicine
The Johns Hopkins University School of Medicine
Baltimore, Maryland
Pulmonary Function Testing

Christian A. Merlo, MD, MPH
Assistant Professor of Medicine and Epidemiology
The Johns Hopkins University School of Medicine
Baltimore, Maryland
Chest Radiograph Review

Redonda G. Miller, MD, MBA
Associate Professor of Medicine
The Johns Hopkins University School of Medicine
Baltimore, Maryland
Selected Topics in Women's Health

Paul S. Nestadt, MD
Psychiatry Resident
The Johns Hopkins University School of Medicine
Baltimore, Maryland
Psychiatry for the Internist

Kelly Norsworthy, MD
Clinical Hematology and Oncology Fellow
The Johns Hopkins University School of Medicine
Baltimore, Maryland
Acute and Chronic Leukemias
Myelodysplastic Syndrome

Roy Anthony Orden, MD
Clinical Fellow
The Johns Hopkins University School of Medicine
Baltimore, Maryland
Allergy and Immunology for the Internist

David B. Pearse, MD
Professor of Medicine
The Johns Hopkins University School of Medicine
Baltimore, Maryland
Venous Thromboembolic Disease

Brent G. Petty, MD
Associate Professor of Medicine
The Johns Hopkins University School of Medicine
Baltimore, Maryland
Electrocardiogram Review

Albert J. Polito, MD
Assistant Professor of Medicine
The Johns Hopkins University School of Medicine
Baltimore, Maryland
Selected Topics in Pulmonary Medicine
Pleural Disease

Craig Pollack, MD, MHS
Associate Professor of Medicine
The Johns Hopkins University School of Medicine
Baltimore, Maryland
Clinical Epidemiology

Gregory P. Prokopowicz, MD, MPH
Assistant Professor
The Johns Hopkins University School of Medicine
Baltimore, Maryland
Hypertension

Darius A. Rastegar, MD
Associate Professor of Medicine
The Johns Hopkins University School of Medicine
Baltimore, Maryland
Substance Use Disorders

Rosanne Rouf, MD
Assistant Professor
The Johns Hopkins University School of Medicine
Baltimore, Maryland
Heart Failure

Sarbjit S. Saini, MD
Associate Professor
The Johns Hopkins University School of Medicine
Baltimore, Maryland
Allergy and Immunology for the Internist

Roberto Salvatori, MD
Professor
The Johns Hopkins University School of Medicine
Baltimore, Maryland
Neuroendocrine and Adrenal Disease

Joseph M. Savitt, MD, PhD
Assistant Professor
The Johns Hopkins University School of Medicine
Baltimore, Maryland
Movement Disorders

Paul J. Scheel Jr., MD
Director
The Johns Hopkins University School of Medicine
Baltimore, Maryland
Chronic Kidney Disease and End-Stage Renal Disease

Cynthia L. Sears, MD
Professor of Medicine
The Johns Hopkins University School of Medicine
Baltimore, Maryland
Infectious Diarrhea

Deborah E. Sellmeyer, MD
Associate Professor of Medicine
The Johns Hopkins University School of Medicine
Baltimore, Maryland
Calcium Disorders and Metabolic Bone Disease

Philip Seo, MD, MHS
Director, The Johns Hopkins Vasculitis Center
Director, Johns Hopkins Rheumatology Fellowship
Associate Professor
The Johns Hopkins University School of Medicine
Baltimore, Maryland
Vasculitis

Tariq Shafi, MBBS, MHS
Assistant Professor of Medicine
The Johns Hopkins University School of Medicine
Baltimore, Maryland
Glomerular Disease
Chronic Kidney Disease and End-Stage Renal Disease

Satish Shanbhag, MBBS, MPH
Assistant Professor of Medicine and Oncology
The Johns Hopkins University School of Medicine
Baltimore, Maryland
Anemia

Mary Sheu, MD
Assistant Professor
The Johns Hopkins University School of Medicine
Baltimore, Maryland
Dermatology for the Internist

Eun Ji Shin, MD, PhD
Assistant Professor
The Johns Hopkins University School of Medicine
Baltimore, Maryland
Pancreatic and Biliary Disease

Stephen D. Sisson, MD
Professor of Medicine
The Johns Hopkins University School of Medicine
Baltimore, Maryland
Acid-Base Disorders and Renal Tubular Acidosis
Preoperative Evaluation

B. Douglas Smith, MD
Associate Professor
The Johns Hopkins University School of Medicine
Baltimore, Maryland
Acute and Chronic Leukemias
Myelodysplastic Syndrome

Shawn F. Smyth, MD
Neurologist
The Johns Hopkins University School of Medicine
Baltimore, Maryland
Movement Disorders

C. John Sperati, MD, MHS
Assistant Professor of Medicine
The Johns Hopkins University School of Medicine
Baltimore, Maryland
Electrolyte Disorders

Ellen Stein, MD
Assistant Professor of Medicine
The Johns Hopkins University School of Medicine
Baltimore, Maryland
Disorders of the Small and Large Intestine

Neil J. Stone, MD, MACP, FACC, FAHA
Bonow Professor of Medicine
Northwestern's Feinberg School of Medicine
Chicago, Illinois
Lipid Disorders

Michael B. Streiff, MD
Associate Professor of Medicine
The Johns Hopkins University School of Medicine
Baltimore, Maryland
Coagulation Disorders

Laila S. Tabatabai, MD
Assistant Professor of Clinical Medicine
Houston Methodist Hospital
Houston, Texas
Calcium Disorders and Metabolic Bone Disease

Peter B. Terry, MD, MA
Professor of Medicine
The Johns Hopkins University School of Medicine
Baltimore, Maryland
Chest Radiograph Review

Sumeska Thavarajah, MD
Assistant Professor
The Johns Hopkins University School of Medicine
Baltimore, Maryland
Selected Topics in Nephrology

Thomas A. Traill, FRCP
Professor of Medicine
The Johns Hopkins University School of Medicine
Baltimore, Maryland
Valvular Heart Disease

Julie B. Trivedi, MD
Clinical Associate in Medicine
The Johns Hopkins University School of Medicine
Baltimore, Maryland
Selected Topics in Infectious Disease I

Christine L. Vigeland, MD
Fellow
The Johns Hopkins University School of Medicine
Baltimore, Maryland
Interstitial Lung Disease

Rainer von Coelln, DR MED
Assistant Professor
University of Maryland School of Medicine
Baltimore, Maryland
Movement Disorders

Robert A. Wise, MD
Professor of Medicine
The Johns Hopkins University School of Medicine
Baltimore, Maryland
Obstructive Lung Disease
Pulmonary Function Testing

Swaytha V. Yalamanchi, MD
Endocrinology, Diabetes, and Metabolism
The Johns Hopkins University School of Medicine
Baltimore, Maryland
Thyroid Disease

Mia Yang, MD
Geriatric Fellow
The Johns Hopkins University School of Medicine
Baltimore, Maryland
Selected Topics in Geriatric Medicine

Sammy Zakaria, MD, MPH
Assistant Professor of Medicine
The Johns Hopkins University School of Medicine
Baltimore, Maryland
Coronary Artery Disease

Carol M. Ziminski, MD
Associate Professor of Medicine
The Johns Hopkins University School of Medicine
Baltimore, Maryland
Selected Topics in Rheumatology

PREFACE

With the assistance of our publisher, Elsevier, we are pleased to offer the fifth edition of *The Johns Hopkins Internal Medicine Board Review*. The strength of any book of this type ultimately hinges on the quality of its contributors; in this regard, we are quite fortunate because each chapter has been written by an accomplished faculty member with extensive knowledge of the topic discussed. The book is divided into sections that are weighted according to the level of emphasis they are given on the American Board of Internal Medicine certifying examination, with additional coverage of the related (and also tested) fields of psychiatry, dermatology, and ophthalmology. Our format is unique in that it features comparative tables, figures, and decision algorithms, which lend themselves to ease of study and quick review. The book also includes a link to an exclusive website that provides practice questions and answers that are patterned after those seen on the actual board examination and that stress important "take home" points and allow self-assessment of knowledge retention.

For this edition we have added specialty section editors to our team to ensure the inclusion and emphasis of high-value material in each chapter and in the online questions. We would like to thank Drs. Chida, Cosgrove, Garibaldi, Haque, Mathioudiakas, Melia, Roesch, Shin, Sperati, and Zakaria for their hard work and commitment toward making this book an invaluable resource for internists.

In many ways, this book is the product of more than a century of medical teaching at Johns Hopkins. In the late nineteenth century, Sir William Osler developed the modern concept of an internal medicine training program during his tenure as the first Chair of Medicine at The Johns Hopkins Hospital. He became famous for his bedside teaching and instituted the practice of "rounds," which remains the principal method of clinical instruction used today. Among Dr. Osler's many achievements during his remarkable life was the completion of his magnum opus, *The Principles and Practice of Medicine*, which was the first textbook to systematically categorize and describe disease with a measure of precision and clarity that had not previously been seen. In the words of Osler, "Books are tools, doctors are craftsmen, and so truly as one can measure the development of any particular handicraft by the variety and complexity of its tools, so we have no better means of judging the intelligence of a profession than by its general collection of books."

We hope you find the text to be a worthy addition to your preparation materials.

Bimal H. Ashar, MD, MBA
Redonda G. Miller, MD, MBA
Stephen D. Sisson, MD

CONTENTS

Maximizing Test Performance: Effective Study and Test-Taking Strategies

DIONNE BLACKMAN, AB, MD

Research has identified a number of factors that affect test performance:

- Study skills
- Content knowledge
- Practice of questions in the same format as the test
- Test-taking skills
- Anxiety
- Fatigue and sleep deprivation

By reading this book, the exam taker will improve content knowledge and have the opportunity to test this knowledge with many case-based practice questions. This chapter, however, addresses the three topics not related to content knowledge: study skills, test-taking skills, and anxiety. The strategies provided will make studying for the Board Examination more effective and optimize test performance on the exam.

Strategies for More Effective Studying

Anticipate Test Content

A strategic approach to studying has been found to lead to better performance on examinations:

- Review the examination blueprint to understand the percentage of questions derived from each content area (available on the website for the American Board of Internal Medicine [ABIM] at www.abim.org)
- Complete the tutorial on taking the computer-based exam, which you can download from the ABIM website. The tutorial sample questions will explain how to use exam functions and provide a practice test to help you familiarize yourself with the different types of exam questions and format. Specifically, you will preview how to:
  - Answer questions
  - Change answers
  - Make notes electronically
  - Access the table of normal laboratory values, calculator, and electronic calipers
  - View figures and video clips
  - Mark questions for review

- Use the Progress Indicator and Time Remaining functions to keep track of item completion and time remaining for the test session
- Use the Navigation button or Review screen to view item completion status, items you have marked for review, or items with an electronic note, and to move quickly to items within the test
- Board Examination questions are derived using the following criteria and will:
  - Be focused on patient care
  - Address important clinical problems for which medical intervention has a significant effect on patient outcomes
  - Address commonly overlooked or mismanaged clinical problems
  - Pose a challenging management decision
  - Assess ability to make optimal clinical decisions
- Maintenance of Certification examination questions will not address clinical problems that are typically referred to specialists or recent clinical advances before they are widely used in practice
- Clinical decision making can be broken down into different tasks; the Board Examination is meant to test your ability to perform these tasks:
  - Identify characteristic clinical features of diseases
  - Identify characteristic pathophysiologic features of diseases
  - Choose the most appropriate diagnostic tests
  - Determine the diagnosis
  - Determine the prognosis or natural history of diseases
  - Select the best treatment or management strategy
  - Choose risk-appropriate prevention strategies
- **Board Examination questions will never address an area in which there is no consensus of opinion among experts in the field**
- Carefully review visual information because this is frequently used in Board Examination questions regarding disorders with characteristic skin lesions or findings on blood smear, bone marrow, electrocardiogram, radiograph, and other visual diagnostic tests

Time Management

- **Use the Residency In-Training Examination or a full-length practice test (such as the practice test**

TABLE 1-1	SQ3R Study Method
Step	**Description**
Survey	Survey section headings and summaries first
Question	Convert headings, legends, and board examination tasks into "questions"
Read	Read to answer your "questions"
Recite	Recite answers and write down key phrases and cues
Review	Review notes, paraphrase major points, draw diagrams, and make flashcards for material that is difficult to recall

on the website accompanying this book) to identify your areas of weakness
- Complete practice tests in your weaker subjects first to identify specific gaps in content knowledge to address a focused review of these subjects
- Use a "question drill-to-content" review ratio of 2 : 1 or greater to review subjects because this has been shown to be more successful than traditional review using the reverse ratio
- After addressing your weaker subjects, conduct a focused review of other subjects as discussed earlier
- Create a realistic study schedule and stick to it
- Using the examination blueprint, budget your study time to cover all of the examination content areas without last-minute cramming
- **Plan to complete your study several days before the examination**
- **Plan a question drill period for the last few days before the examination; use answers to incorrectly answered practice questions for targeted content review**

Effective Approaches to Studying

- The Survey, Question, Read, Recite, Review (SQ3R) study method has proven effective in improving reading efficiency, comprehension, and material retention
  - It provides a useful way to study for the Board Examination, regardless of the study resource used
  - Steps in the method are outlined in Table 1-1
- Similar to the SQ3R method, students performing repeated cycles of studying, followed by writing down as much as they can recall, then restudying material and recalling again improved learning and retention of material and test performance
- Studying with a small group can enhance study effectiveness by providing social support and increased confidence as individuals assume responsibility to review and teach particular areas to the group

Strategies for More Effective Test Taking

The following strategies will only be effective if practiced, so plan to practice them in your question drill sessions; the website accompanying this book allows exam takers to practice answering questions in a timed test format.

Strategies for Time Use

- Know the examination schedule for the computer-based examination (see www.abim.org)
- **Return from breaks 10 minutes early; you must check in after breaks, and the examination clock restarts at the end of the break regardless of your return time**
- Know the time allotted per exam question (i.e., exam time in minutes divided by number of exam questions); this is about 2 minutes per question based on the maximum 60 questions allowed per 2-hour board exam session
- Budget your time; unfinished questions are lost scoring opportunities
- Keep track of your use of time by checking time targets at each quarter of the total exam time
- To fully use other test-taking strategies, use less than the allotted time per question (we suggest 15 to 30 seconds less per question)
- **To focus on pertinent data, read the question and the answer options before reading the question stem; the stem is the part of the test item that precedes the question and answer options and is usually case-based**
- Answer questions you know first and quickly guess on those you do not know

Strategies for Guessing and Reasoning

- Identify key words or phrases that affect the question's intent (e.g., *at this time, now, initially, most, always, never, except, usually, least*)
- Determine whether the following factors limit your thinking to certain disease categories:
  - Patient factors
    - Age, sex, race, or ethnicity
    - Habits (e.g., smoking, alcohol or illicit drug use)
    - Exposures caused by occupation, travel, or residence
    - Immune status
  - Factors related to illness presentation
    - Time course of illness (i.e., acute, subacute, or chronic)
    - Symptoms or findings present or stated to be absent
    - Pattern of diagnostic data (e.g., presence of a known symptom triad, pathognomic finding)
- Eliminate answer options likely to be incorrect. Remember that incorrect options are usually written to be plausible or even partially correct.
- Examine similarities and differences between answer options (e.g., mutually exclusive options)
- Answer questions based on established standards of care, not anecdotal experiences (many current guidelines are available at the National Guideline Clearinghouse at www.guideline.gov)
- Do not be afraid to use partial knowledge to eliminate answers
- When unsure of an answer, enter your best guess (research shows it is often correct) and flag the question on the computer for later review

- **Answer all questions—there is no penalty for wrong answers**
  - **Please note that, once you click the End Session button, you cannot go back to review or change responses for that test session**
  - **Check that you have completed any answer review of changes and have entered a response for all questions before you click the End Session button**

Strategies for Changing Answers

- Spending less than the allotted time per exam question allows you to finish exams early; this extra time allows you to benefit from answer changing
- **Despite conventional wisdom, research shows most test takers benefit from answer changing**
- You are more likely to change from a wrong to a right answer if you
  - Reread and better understand the test item
  - Rethink and conceptualize a better answer
  - Gain information from another test item
  - Remember more information
  - Correct a clerical error (e.g., the intended answer was not the entered answer)

Strategies for Error Avoidance

- Read each question and all answer options carefully; be certain you understand the intent of the question before answering (e.g., questions stating "all of the following are correct except …")
- Do not "read into a question" information or interpretations that are not there
- Check that the answer entered is the answer you intended

Strategies for Anxiety Reduction

- Anxiety is a natural part of taking an examination, but high test anxiety will adversely affect test performance
- Consider formal counseling if you have had problems with high test anxiety in the past
- Consider writing about your negative thoughts and worries about the examination for 10 minutes on the day of the test; this has been found to significantly improve test performance for those with high test anxiety
- Actively manage anxiety by decreasing the effect of unknowns on your anxiety level. Use the following methods:

- Review "Exam Day: What to Expect" section of the ABIM's guide to the certification exam (see www.abim.org)
- **Test-drive the travel route and determine time to the test site;** locate parking and the site itself if it is in a building with other businesses
- **Bring a sweater or dress in layers to prepare for examination room temperature variations**
- **Bring a snack for unexpected hunger and medications for potential illness symptoms**
- Allow a minimum of 30 minutes before your test appointment for check-in procedures (see www.abim.org for details regarding check-in)
- Avoid overly anxious test takers; they heighten your anxiety level, which can hurt your test performance
- Use relaxation techniques:
  - Deep muscle relaxation is an effective relaxation technique; it involves tensing and relaxing each muscle group until all muscles are relaxed
  - To reduce anxiety further, engage in exercise during the period when you are preparing for the examination
- Being well-rested is imperative

SUGGESTED READINGS

Frierson HT, Hoband D. Effect of test anxiety on performance on the NBME Part I Examination. *J Med Educ.* 1987;62:431-433.

Frierson HT, Malone B, Shelton P. Enhancing NCLEX-RN performance: assessing a three-pronged intervention approach. *J Nurs Educ.* 1993;32:222-224.

Harvill LM, Davis G III. Test-taking behaviors and their impact on performance: medical students' reasons for changing answers on multiple choice tests. *Acad Med.* 1997;72:S97-S99.

Hembree R. Correlates, causes, effects, and treatment of test anxiety. *Rev Educ Res.* 1988;58:47-77.

Karpicke JD, Blunt JR. Retrieval practice produces more learning than elaborative studying with concept mapping. *Science.* 2011;331:772-775.

McDowell BM. KATTS: a framework for maximizing NCLEX-RN performance. *J Nurs Educ.* 2008;47:183-186.

McManus IC, Richards P, Winder BC, Sproston KA. Clinical experience, performance in final examinations, and learning style in medical students: prospective study. *BMJ.* 1998;316:345-350.

Ramirez G, Beilock SL. Writing about testing worries boosts exam performance in classroom. *Science.* 2011;331:211-213.

Robinson FP. *Effective Study.* Rev ed. New York: Harper & Row; 1961.

Seipp B. Anxiety and academic performance: a meta-analysis of findings. *Anxiety Res.* 1991;4:27-41.

Waddell DL, Blankenship JC. Answer changing: a meta-analysis of the prevalence and patterns. *J Cont Educ Nurs.* 1994;25:155-158.

Ward PJ. First year medical students' approaches to study and their outcomes in a gross anatomy course. *Clin Anat.* 2011;24:120-127.

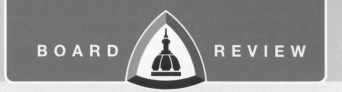
Cardiology

Hypertension

GREGORY P. PROKOPOWICZ, MD, MPH

Hypertension is present in nearly 30% of the general population, and with the aging of the population and the increase in obesity, its prevalence is expected to increase. Hypertension is an important risk factor for many common diseases including stroke, end-stage renal disease, heart failure, and myocardial infarction, and is the most common modifiable cardiovascular disease risk factor. Aggressive control of elevated blood pressure (BP) results in a significant decline in morbidity and mortality.

Basic Information

- Hypertension definition
  - **BP 140/90 mm Hg or higher (i.e., a systolic BP ≥140 mm Hg, a diastolic BP ≥90 mm Hg, or both) (Table 2-1).**
    - The classification of BP applies to patients not taking antihypertensives and without acute illness (which may raise or lower BP); patients taking antihypertensive medication are considered to have hypertension
  - BP of 140 to 159/90 to 99 mm Hg is designated as Stage 1 hypertension, and BP 160/100 mm Hg or higher as Stage 2 hypertension
    - If the systolic and diastolic BPs fall in different stages, the higher stage is used (e.g., a BP of 182/95 mm Hg is categorized as Stage 2)
  - **BP of 120 to 139/80 to 89 mm Hg is designated as prehypertension**
    - Prehypertension is a risk category, not a disease; patients with prehypertension are at high risk of progressing to actual hypertension and should be targeted for lifestyle modification
  - **Hypertensive urgency refers to severe hypertension without acute end-organ dysfunction**
    - There is no agreed-upon BP that defines hypertensive urgency, although some sources use 180/120 mm Hg
    - Headache, anxiety, or medication nonadherence often contribute to elevated BP in patients with hypertensive urgency
  - **Hypertensive emergency implies elevated BP with acute end-organ dysfunction (Table 2-2)**
    - Although hypertensive emergency is not defined by any specific level of BP, most patients have BPs 180/120 mm Hg or higher
- Epidemiology
  - Hypertension affects more than 60 million Americans and is the most common modifiable cardiovascular disease risk factor
  - Hypertension is more prevalent among African Americans, who also experience more end-organ damage
  - There is a graded relationship between BP level and the incidence of stroke, end-stage renal disease, heart failure, and ischemic heart disease
    - **Younger than age 50, diastolic BP is the most important predictor of adverse cardiovascular outcomes; older than age 50, systolic BP is the most important predictor**
  - The prevalence of hypertension rises with age (Fig. 2-1).
    - Systolic BP rises continuously; diastolic BP rises until approximately age 50 years and then declines
    - Isolated systolic hypertension (i.e., systolic BP >140 mm Hg and diastolic BP <90 mm Hg) is common among the elderly and is an important cardiovascular risk factor
    - Patients with prehypertension have an increased risk of progression to hypertension
- Pathophysiology
  - **Most patients (>90%) do not have an identifiable cause of hypertension; this is commonly referred to as essential hypertension**
  - BP is the product of cardiac output and peripheral vascular resistance; increased cardiac output can play a role in the initiation of hypertension; however, most patients with long-standing hypertension have increased peripheral resistance with normal or diminished cardiac output
  - In some "salt sensitive" patients, BP responds strongly to changes in sodium intake and extracellular fluid; salt sensitivity occurs more commonly among African Americans and the elderly
  - End-organ damage from hypertension can affect the kidneys, heart, vasculature, brain, and eyes (Table 2-3)

Clinical Presentation

- Most patients are asymptomatic
- Some have evidence of target organ damage at first presentation (see Table 2-3)
- Occasionally, patients may present with hypertensive urgencies or emergencies (see Table 2-2)

Diagnosis and Evaluation

- Measurement of BP
  - Allow patient to relax and sit quietly for more than 5 minutes

TABLE 2-1	Classification of Blood Pressure			
Category	**Systolic BP (mm Hg)**		**Diastolic BP (mm Hg)**	
Normal	<120	and	<80	
Prehypertension	120 to 139	or	80 to 89	
Hypertension				
Stage 1	140 to 159	or	90 to 99	
Stage 2	≥160	or	>100	

BP, Blood pressure.
Modified from The Seventh Report of the Joint National Committee on Prevention, Detection, Evaluation, and Treatment of High Blood Pressure. *JAMA.* 2003;289:2560–2572.

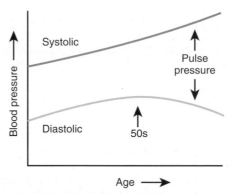

FIGURE 2-1 Blood pressure and age.

TABLE 2-2	Manifestations of Acute End-Organ Damage in Hypertensive Emergency
Hypertensive encephalopathy	Headache Altered mental status Seizures Nausea, vomiting Papilledema (see Fig. 2-2) Abnormalities on brain imaging
Intracranial hemorrhage	Headache Altered mental status Focal neurologic abnormalities Hemorrhage on brain imaging
Unstable angina	Chest pain ECG abnormalities
Acute myocardial infarction	Chest pain ECG abnormalities Cardiac enzyme elevation
LV failure with pulmonary edema	Dyspnea Hypoxia Pulmonary congestion on chest imaging
Acute aortic dissection	Chest pain Syncope End-organ ischemia
Eclampsia	Proteinuria Seizures

ECG, Electrocardiographic; LV, left ventricular.

TABLE 2-3	Clinical Manifestations of Chronic Target Organ Damage in Hypertension
Heart	Left ventricular hypertrophy 1) Enlarged PMI or S₄ gallop 2) Evidence of LVH on ECG or ECHO Left ventricular dysfunction 1) Signs/symptoms of CHF 2) Enlarged PMI or S₃ gallop 3) Systolic or diastolic dysfunction on ECHO Coronary artery disease 1) Angina 2) History of MI, PCI, or CABG
Brain	Cerebrovascular disease 1) History of stroke 2) Carotid bruit
Eyes	Retinovascular disease 1) Arteriolar narrowing 2) Arteriovenous nicking 3) Hemorrhage 4) Exudates
Vasculature	Atherosclerosis 1) Claudication 2) Diminished or absent pulses 3) Renal or femoral bruits
Kidneys	Hypertensive nephrosclerosis, ESRD 1) Proteinuria or microalbuminuria 2) Elevated serum creatinine

CABG, Coronary artery bypass graft; CHF, congestive heart failure; ECG, electrocardiography; ECHO, echocardiography; ESRD, end-stage renal disease; LVH, left ventricular hypertrophy; MI, myocardial infarction; PMI, point of maximum impulse; PCI, percutaneous coronary intervention.

- The patient should also refrain from smoking or consuming caffeine for more than 30 minutes before BP measurement
- **Use an appropriate sphygmomanometer cuff size; the bladder of the cuff should encircle 80% or more of the arm without overlapping; using a smaller cuff may yield falsely elevated readings**
- The arm in which BP is being measured should be supported and relaxed at the level of the heart
- BP should be measured in both arms, and the higher of the two readings used
- At each clinical visit, the BP preferably should be taken at least twice in the arm with the higher BP measurement
  - The average BP should guide management

- Two methods to assess BP:
  - Auscultatory method: Systolic BP is defined as the first appearance of Korotkoff sounds, and diastolic pressure is defined as the disappearance of Korotkoff sounds
  - Oscillometric method: used by electronic BP measuring devices, which detect pressure fluctuations in the cuff. This method is often preferred over the auscultatory method because it is not subject to human bias or error.
- Elevated BP readings on two separate clinical visits should be obtained before classifying a patient as hypertensive; however, if BP is very high (systolic BP >180 mm Hg) on multiple readings at the initial

visit, it is reasonable to start antihypertensive medications at that time
- In elderly patients, or when orthostatic hypotension is suggested, standing BP measurements should be taken
- Some patients may have a marked discrepancy between BP measurements obtained at home and in the clinic
  - **Elevated BP in clinic with normal out-of-office readings is referred to as white-coat hypertension**
  - **Elevated out-of-office BP with normal clinic readings is referred to as masked hypertension**
  - In either case, home BP readings and/or 24-hour ambulatory BP monitoring should be obtained and used to guide management.
- For daytime home BP monitoring, hypertension is defined as an average BP greater than 135/85 mm Hg
- For 24-hour BP monitoring (which includes readings taken during sleep), an average BP greater than130/80 mm Hg is considered hypertensive
- Goals in initial evaluation of the hypertensive patient:
  - Assess for target organ damage (Fig. 2-2; see also Table 2-3)
    - Requires comprehensive physical examination, including assessing vital signs, body mass index, and cardiopulmonary systems, and auscultation of the major blood vessels to identify bruits in the eyes, neurologic system, and limbs

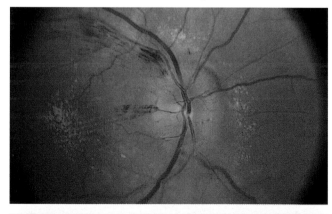

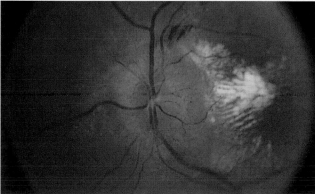

FIGURE 2-2 Papilledema in hypertension. (From Yanoff M. *Ophthalmology.* 2nd ed. Philadelphia: Mosby; 2004, Fig. 113-7.)

- Identify comorbidities
  - Diabetes mellitus (DM)
  - Chronic kidney disease (CKD)
  - Ischemic heart disease and cardiomyopathy
- Identify other cardiovascular disease risk factors: cigarette smoking, dyslipidemia, older age, obesity, physical inactivity, family history
  - Assess for identifiable (secondary) causes of hypertension (see later discussion)
- Recommended laboratory tests for initial evaluation
  - Serum creatinine, sodium, potassium, fasting glucose
  - Urinalysis with microscopic examination
  - Electrocardiogram (or echocardiogram)
  - Fasting lipid profile
  - Optional: serum calcium, thyroid-stimulating hormone
  - Screen for identifiable (secondary) causes of hypertension (Table 2-4)
- **Consider secondary hypertension in the following scenarios:**
  - **Sudden onset of hypertension in a previously normotensive patient**
  - **Age, history, physical examination, severity of hypertension, or initial laboratory findings suggestive of a specific cause (see Table 2-4)**
  - **Recurrence of hypertension in a previously well-controlled patient (nonadherence should also be considered)**
  - **Hypertension resistant to three or more drugs, including a diuretic**
- Substances that may cause or worsen hypertension
  - Alcohol (use or withdrawal)
  - Amphetamines, cocaine
  - Over-the-counter medications (decongestants, diet pills, nonsteroidal antiinflammatory drugs [NSAIDs])
  - Prescription medications (NSAIDs, oral contraceptives, cyclosporine, erythropoietin)
  - Supplements (ephedra)
  - Licorice (inhibits metabolism of endogenous cortisol to cortisone)
- Other correctable causes of hypertension
  - Acute pain or stress in hospitalized or institutionalized patients
  - Obstructive sleep apnea
  - Hyperthyroidism or hypothyroidism
  - CKD (caused by renin oversecretion and impaired sodium excretion)
  - Co-arctation of the aorta (very uncommon in adults)
    - Delayed femoral pulses, diminished leg BP, and rib notching on chest radiograph suggest this diagnosis, which is confirmed with computed tomography or magnetic resonance imaging
    - Treatment is either surgery or angioplasty

Treatment (Essential Hypertension):

- Management requires close BP follow-up:
  - Table 2-5 suggests follow-up intervals, depending on the degree of elevation
  - Suggested follow-up intervals should be shorter if important risk factors (e.g., DM) or target organ damage is present

TABLE 2-4	*Major Causes of Secondary Hypertension*		
Pathophysiology	**Clinical Presentation**	**Diagnosis**	**Treatment**
Renal Artery Stenosis			
Underperfused kidney produces excess renin, which increases angiotensin II (vasoconstriction) and aldosterone (sodium retention and volume expansion) Usually caused by atherosclerosis, especially in older patients May also be caused by FMD, which usually occurs in young female patients	Sudden onset of significant hypertension at older (>55 years) or younger (<30 years) age Abdominal bruits Patient with peripheral vascular disease Unexplained deterioration in renal function Consider FMD in young females Unusually large drop in BP with ACEI or ARB treatment	Magnetic resonance angiography: highly sensitive, no contrast required CT angiography: highly sensitive, contrast required Doppler ultrasound: sensitivity dependent on operator skill, no contrast required Captopril radionuclide scan: less sensitive, requires discontinuation of antihypertensive medications before test Renal artery angiography: gold standard, invasive, may be performed with CO_2 to avoid use of iodinated contrast	Goal is to improve HTN control and measures to preserve renal function Revascularized patients usually still require medication for BP control Statin therapy decreases progression The longer stenosis has been present, the less likely intervention will help (kidney becomes atrophic) Interventional options: (1) Angioplasty ± stent (lesions at ostia of renal arteries are often not amenable to angioplasty) (2) Surgical bypass (3) Surgical excision of kidney if size <8 cm Medical therapy usually best if recovery of renal function is unlikely
Pheochromocytoma			
Tumors that originate in the adrenal medulla or sympathetic ganglia and release catecholamines periodically Most are sporadic Familial forms (20% to 35%) are associated with: (1) Multiple endocrine neoplasia IIA and IIB (2) Neurofibromatosis (3) von Hippel-Lindau disease (with retinal angiomas, cerebellar hemangioblastomas, and renal cell carcinoma)	Headache Sweating Palpitations Pallor Anxiety Weight loss Orthostatic hypotension HTN may be episodic or sustained	Screen with plasma free-metanephrines, confirm with 24-hour urine collection for catecholamines, VMA, metanephrines Certain drugs may cause false-positive or false-negative screens If screen is positive, localize with MRI (or MIBG scan if MRI negative)	Surgical resection Preoperatively, patients should receive phentolamine or phenoxybenzamine to prevent crisis
Hyperaldosteronism (see Chapter 42)			
Most common cause of secondary hypertension Can be caused by an adenoma that produces aldosterone (Conn syndrome) or bilateral adrenal hyperplasia (zona granulosae) Rarely can be caused by an aldosterone-producing carcinoma	Spontaneous hypokalemia in a hypertensive patient (may cause cramps and muscle weakness) Severe hypokalemia induced by diuretics Mild metabolic alkalosis	Screen with plasma aldosterone and renin serum: ratio of aldosterone to renin >20 suggests disease Confirm by measuring 24-h urine aldosterone after 3 days of salt loading: >12 µg confirms disease If screen positive, localize with CT or MRI; adrenal vein sampling	Surgical resection of adenoma Treat with spironolactone for patients with hyperplasia
Hypercortisolism (see Chapter 42)			
Several possible causes: (1) ACTH-secreting pituitary tumor (Cushing disease) (2) Adrenal adenomas (3) Ectopic ACTH secretion (4) Iatrogenic steroid administration	Truncal obesity Moon facies Purple striae Proximal weakness Hirsutism Hyperglycemia Osteoporosis	Screen with 24-h urinary free cortisol, salivary cortisol, or 1 mg overnight dexamethasone suppression test If positive, perform high-dose dexamethasone suppression test and measure plasma ACTH Localize with imaging of adrenals or pituitary	Surgical resection of tumor or discontinuation of steroid therapy

ACTH, Adrenocorticotropic hormone; ACEIs, angiotensin-converting enzyme inhibitors; ARB, angiotensin receptor blocker; BP, blood pressure; CO_2, carbon dioxide; CT, computed tomography; HTN, hypertension; FMD, fibromuscular dysplasia; MIBG, iodine-131 metaiodobenzylguanidine; MRI, magnetic resonance imaging; VMA, vanillylmandelic acid.

- **Target BP goal is 140/90 mm Hg for all patients (including those with DM or CKD), except patients aged 60 or older without DM or CKD, who should be treated to a goal BP of 150/90 mm Hg**
- Therapy choice depends on hypertension stage and the presence of risk factors or target organ damage (Table 2-6)
- Management recommendations:
  - **Always start with lifestyle modification even if drug therapy is also needed**
    - Recommend weight reduction of 10 pounds or more
    - Encourage 30 minutes or more of moderately intense physical activity (e.g., brisk walking) four or more times a week
  - Counsel moderate alcohol intake (1 ounce or less per day in men, ½ ounce in women)
  - Recommend diet modifications:
    - Advise low sodium intake (100 mmol/day, i.e., 6 g NaCl or 2.4 g Na⁺, or less)
    - Recommend a diet high in fruits, vegetables, and low-fat dairy products: Dietary Approaches to Stop Hypertension (DASH) eating plan
  - Recommend smoking cessation, although not demonstrated to cause chronic hypertension
  - No strong recommendations for altering caffeine intake; chronic caffeine intake not shown to correlate with elevated BP
  - Relaxation therapy and stress management are of uncertain benefit
- Drug therapy:
  - See Figure 2-3 for suggested therapeutic algorithm and Table 2-7 for a list of medications
  - **General principles: initial therapy**
    - **In the general population, including those with DM, start either a thiazide-type diuretic, calcium channel blocker (CCB), angiotensin-converting enzyme inhibitor (ACEI), or angiotensin receptor blocker (ARB), either alone or in combination (exception: do not use ACEIs and ARBs in combination)**
    - **In the general black population, including patients with DM, start either a thiazide-type diuretic or CCB**
    - **In patients with CKD, start either an ACEI or ARB**
    - In most cases, choose agents with 24-hour duration of action and once-daily dosing
  - General principles: subsequent therapy
    - Monotherapy is successful in approximately 40% of patients; in approximately 60%, consider using two or more drugs to attain goal BP, especially in patients with a BP higher than 160/100 mm Hg
    - If there is a partial but inadequate response to the first antihypertensive drug, either increase the dose or add a second agent from a different class

TABLE 2-5	Initial Management of Blood Pressure

INITIAL BLOOD PRESSURE (mm Hg)		Recommended Follow-up
Systolic	**Diastolic**	
<120	<80	Recheck in 2 years
120 to 139	80 to 89	Recheck in 1 year*
140 to 159	90 to 99	Confirm within 2 months*
160 to 179	100 to 109	Evaluate or refer within 1 month
≥180	≥110	Evaluate and treat immediately or within 1 week, depending on clinical situation and complications

*Provide advice about lifestyle modification.
Modified from Chobanian AV, Bakris GL, Black HR, et al. The seventh report of the Joint National Committee on Prevention, Detection, Evaluation, and Treatment of High Blood Pressure. *JAMA.* 2003;289:2560-2571.

TABLE 2-6	Treatment Recommendations by Risk Group

Blood Pressure (BP) Classification	Lifestyle Modification	INITIAL DRUG THERAPY	
		No Compelling Indication	**Compelling Indication(s) Present**
Normal (<120/80 mm Hg)	Encourage	None	None
Prehypertension (120 to 139/80 to 89 mm Hg)	Yes	None	Appropriate drug(s) for DM, CKD, or CAD if BP >130/80 mm Hg, for HF if BP >120/80 mm Hg
Stage 1 (140 to 159/90 to 99 mm Hg)	Yes	Thiazide diuretic for most; may consider other drug classes	Appropriate drug(s) for compelling indication
Stage 2 (≥160/>100 mm Hg)	Yes	Two-drug combination for most, including thiazide diuretic	Two-drug combination for most, usually including appropriate drug(s) for compelling indication

CAD, Coronary artery disease; HF, heart failure; CKD, chronic kidney disease; DM, diabetes mellitus.
Modified from The Seventh Report of the Joint National Committee on Prevention, Detection, Evaluation, and Treatment of High Blood Pressure. *JAMA.* 2003;289:2561.

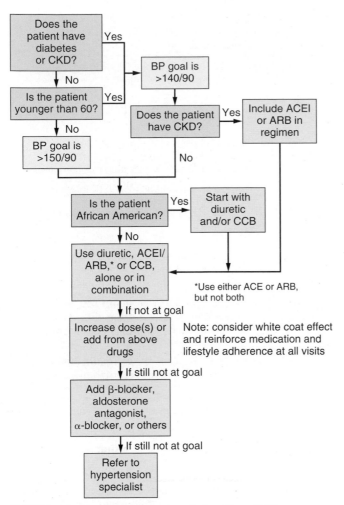

FIGURE 2-3 Hypertension treatment algorithm. ACEI, Angiotensin-converting enzyme inhibitor; ARB, angiotensin receptor blocker; BP, blood pressure; CCB, calcium channel blocker; CKD, chronic kidney disease. (Modified from James PA, Oparil S, Carter BL, et al. 2014 evidence-based guideline for the management of high blood pressure in adults: report from the panel members appointed to the Eighth Joint National Committee [JNC 8]. *JAMA.* 2014;311:507-520.)

- If there is no response to the first drug or if the drug is not tolerated, substitute a drug from a different class
- **Always consider a diuretic in any patient needing three or more drugs**
- Consider using low-dose combination therapy instead of higher doses of a single agent, to minimize dose-dependent side effects
  - Formulations combining two or more drugs may offer improved convenience or lower cost, examples include:
    - Low-dose diuretics and ACEIs, ARBs, or β-blockers
    - Thiazides with potassium-sparing diuretics
    - CCBs with ACEIs or ARBs
    - Three-drug combinations containing a CCB, an ACEI or ARB, and a diuretic
- Comorbidities can help guide choice of antihypertensive medication:
  - CKD: ACEI or ARB

- Heart failure: ACEI or ARB, β-blocker, aldosterone antagonist, diuretics
- Myocardial infarction: β-blocker, ACEI, aldosterone antagonist
- Migraines: β-blockers, CCBs
- Benign prostatic hypertrophy: α-blockers
- Essential tremor: β-blockers
- Hyperthyroidism: β-blockers (nonselective)
- Contraindications to certain antihypertensives with conditions/disease states:
  - **Pregnancy: ACEIs and ARBs are absolutely contraindicated**
  - Asthma, chronic obstructive pulmonary disease, peripheral vascular disease: use caution with β-blockers
  - Gout: avoid or minimize dose of diuretics
  - First- or second-degree heart block: avoid β-blockers, verapamil, and diltiazem
  - Uncomplicated hypertension:
    - β-Blockers: Unless there is a specific indication, such as coronary artery disease or heart failure, avoid β-blockers unless diuretic, CCB, and ACEI or ARB therapy have all been tried
    - Loop diuretics: Should be used only when thiazide diuretics are likely to be inadequate (i.e., congestive heart failure or Stage 4 CKD). Short-acting loop diuretics (furosemide, bumetanide) should be taken twice daily, or replaced with a long-acting diuretic (e.g., torsemide).

Treatment (Hypertensive Urgency and Emergency)

- Hypertensive urgency (severely elevated BP without acutely progressive end-organ damage):
  - Need prompt but gradual control of BP using oral agents
  - Outpatient follow-up is appropriate, but needs BP assessment at least weekly
  - Rapidly acting oral agents, such as clonidine, are not usually needed
- Hypertensive emergency (severely elevated BP with acutely progressive end-organ damage):
  - BP must be brought down rapidly but in a controlled fashion in an intensive care unit by administering intravenous antihypertensive medications, which have a rapid effect and are easily titratable (Table 2-8)
  - **Initial goal is to lower mean arterial BP by approximately 25%, but not more, within 2 hours**
  - Subsequent goal is to lower BP to approximately 160/100 mm Hg over the next 2 to 24 hours (if aortic dissection is also present, reduce BP further as tolerated)

Prevention

- Provide counseling to patients with prehypertension (BP <140/90 mm Hg and >120/80 mm Hg) on lifestyle modifications to decrease their risk of progression to hypertension

TABLE 2-7	*Antihypertensive Agents*		
Class	**Examples**	**Side Effects**	**Comments**
Thiazide diuretics	Hydrochlorothiazide Chlorthalidone Indapamide	Hypokalemia Hyponatremia Alkalosis Hyperuricemia Dehydration Hypercalcemia	Thiazides not effective if GFR <30 mL/min Side effects rarely a problem at low doses

Loop diuretics	Furosemide
	Torsemide
	Bumetanide
		As for thiazide diuretics,
		  except for hypercalcemia
			Furosemide and bumetanide have short
			  half-lives; dose twice a day for HTN
			Sodium restriction should accompany diuretics

Potassium-sparing
diuretics
	Distal tubule sodium
	  channel blockers:
	  triamterene, amiloride
	Aldosterone antagonists:
	  spironolactone,
	  eplerenone
		Hyperkalemia
		Hyponatremia
		Dehydration
			Often given in combination with thiazides (to
			  prevent hypokalemia)
			Avoid or use with caution in renal insufficiency

β-Adrenergic
antagonists
(β-blockers)
	β_1-selective: atenolol,
	  metoprolol
	Non–β_1-selective:
	  propranolol, nadolol
	α_1 and β_1 blockade:
	  carvedilol, labetalol
		Bradycardia
		Fatigue
		Insomnia
		Erectile dysfunction
		Bronchospasm in asthma and
		  COPD patients
			May mask hypoglycemic symptoms in
			  diabetics
			Do not use alone in cases of catecholamine
			  excess (cocaine intoxication,
			  pheochromocytoma) as unopposed α_1
			  vasoconstriction without β_2 vasodilation may
			  increase BP precipitously

ACEIs	Benazepril
	Captopril
	Enalapril
	Fosinopril
	Lisinopril
	Moexipril
	Perindopril
	Quinapril
	Ramipril
	Trandolapril
		Cough
		Angioedema
		Hyperkalemia
		Use cautiously if CKD,
		  renovascular disease, CHF,
		  or dehydration is present
			Inhibit the renin-angiotensin-aldosterone
			  system by blocking conversion of
			  angiotensin I to angiotensin II
			Dilate renal efferent arterioles
			Also inhibit degradation of bradykinin, which
			  may lead to cough
			Do not use in pregnant patients; teratogenic

ARBs	Azilsartan
	Candesartan
	Eprosartan
	Irbesartan
	Losartan
	Olmesartan
	Telmisartan
	Valsartan
		Hyperkalemia	Inhibit the renin-angiotensin-aldosterone
			  system by blocking the angiotensin II
			  receptor
			Do not use in pregnant patients; teratogenic

α-Adrenergic
antagonists
	Doxazosin
	Prazosin
	Terazosin
		Orthostatic hypotension	Block postsynaptic α_1 receptors, causing
			  vasodilation
			Favorable effect on lipid profile and glucose
			  level
			May increase CHD mortality if used as a single
			  agent

Nondihydropyri- dine CCBs	Verapamil Diltiazem	Bradycardia, heart block Decreased cardiac contractility Constipation	Verapamil may increase cyclosporine and digoxin levels

Dihydropyridine
CCBs
	Amlodipine
	Felodipine
	Isradipine
	Nicardipine
	Nifedipine
	Nisoldipine
		Headache
		Flushing
		Tachycardia
		Pedal edema
			Dilate arterioles
			Possibly increase heart rate
			Short-acting nifedipine and nicardipine cause
			  marked reflex tachycardia and are *not*
			  recommended for HTN
			Nifedipine increases cyclosporine levels

Direct
vasodilators
	Minoxidil
	Hydralazine
		Headache
		Tachycardia
		Fluid retention
		Minoxidil: hirsutism,
		  pericardial effusion
		Hydralazine: drug-induced
		  lupus
			Considered third-line agents

TABLE 2-7	*Antihypertensive Agents* (Continued)		
Class	**Examples**	**Side Effects**	**Comments**
Central adrenergic inhibitors	Clonidine Guanfacine Methyldopa Reserpine	Clonidine, guanfacine: Sedation, dry mouth, Withdrawal hypertension Methyldopa: Coombs-positive hemolytic anemia Liver toxicity	Inhibit sympathetic outflow from CNS Clonidine also available in patch Methyldopa safe in pregnancy

ACEIs, Angiotensin-converting enzyme inhibitors; ARBs, angiotensin receptor blockers; BP, blood pressure; CCBs, calcium channel blockers; CHD, coronary heart disease; CHF, congestive heart failure; CKD, chronic kidney disease; CNS, central nervous system; COPD, chronic obstructive pulmonary disease; GFR, glomerular filtration rate; HTN, hypertension.

TABLE 2-8	*Drugs Used in Treatment of Hypertensive Emergency*	
Drug	**Indication**	**Precaution**
Nitroprusside	Most emergencies	Thiocyanate toxicity
Nitroglycerin	Angina, MI	Headache, tolerance
Nicardipine	Most emergencies	Tachycardia
Labetalol	Most emergencies	CHF, bradycardia
Fenoldopam	Most emergencies	Tachycardia
Enalaprilat	CHF	Rapid, unpredictable BP drop
Esmolol	Perioperative, aortic dissection	Nausea

BP, Blood pressure; CHF, congestive heart failure; MI, myocardial infarction.

Review Questions

For review questions, please go to ExpertConsult.com.

SUGGESTED READINGS

James PA, Oparil S, Carter BL, et al. 2014 evidence-based guideline for the management of high blood pressure in adults: report from the panel members appointed to the Eighth Joint National Committee (JNC 8). JAMA. 2014;311:507-520.

Kaplan NM. *Clinical Hypertension*. 11th ed. Baltimore: Lippincott Williams & Wilkins; 2014.

Weber MA, Schiffrin EL, White WB, et al. Clinical practice guidelines for the management of hypertension in the community: a statement by the American Society of Hypertension and the International Society of Hypertension. *J Clin Hypertension*. 2014;16:14-26.

CHAPTER 3

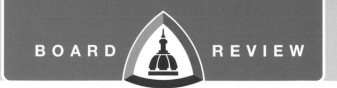

Lipid Disorders

ALI REZA KERAMATI, MD; THURA T. ABD, MD; ROGER S. BLUMENTHAL, MD;
PARAG H. JOSHI, MD, MHS; and NEIL J. STONE, MD, MACP, FACC, FAHA

Lipid disorders (dyslipidemias) increase the risk of atherosclerotic vascular disease. Many are a result of both genetic and environmental factors. In 2013, the American College of Cardiology/American Heart Association (ACC/AHA) released new guidelines for the evaluation and management of dyslipidemias, which provide a useful resource for clinicians.

Basic Information

- Cholesterol
  - Vital for cell membrane biogenesis, steroid synthesis, and bile acid formation
  - The liver is the primary producer of endogenous cholesterol and is the main processor of dietary cholesterol
  - Cholesterol is produced when 3-hydroxy-3-methylglutaryl coenzyme A (HMG-CoA) is converted to mevalonic acid by HMG-CoA reductase
- Lipoproteins
  - Spherical complexes consisting of a lipid core and an outer protein monolayer that transport lipids, such as cholesterol and triglyceride, in the circulation
  - Lipoprotein particles are classified according to increasing density; a patient's cholesterol levels are most commonly expressed as the concentration of cholesterol in each of the listed individual lipoprotein particle groups:
    - Chylomicrons
    - Very-low-density lipoprotein (VLDL)
    - Intermediate-density lipoprotein (IDL)
    - Low-density lipoprotein (LDL)
    - High-density lipoprotein (HDL)
- Chylomicrons
  - Triglyceride-rich lipoproteins responsible for transporting dietary fat and cholesterol into the body
  - Synthesized by intestinal epithelial cells from dietary fatty acids absorbed via the NPC1L1 transporter
  - Increased fat consumption leads to increased chylomicrons in the blood
  - Lipoprotein lipase releases free fatty acids from chylomicrons, leaving chylomicron remnants
- VLDL
  - Synthesized in the liver from free fatty acids (obtained from chylomicrons [dietary fat]) and from endogenously produced triglycerides (generated from excess dietary protein and carbohydrates)
  - Hydrolyzed by lipoprotein lipase and converted to smaller particles (IDL) and then into LDL
- LDL
  - **Principal cholesterol-containing lipoprotein and a major atherogenic lipoprotein**
  - The peripheral tissues clear 25%, and the liver takes up 75% of serum LDL, primarily via LDL receptors. LDL transports cholesterol to peripheral tissues
  - Cholesterol homeostasis is regulated by hepatic LDL receptor expression:
    - Decreased hepatocyte cholesterol levels leads to an increase in LDL receptor expression, causing a greater clearance of serum LDL
    - Increased dietary saturated fatty acids decreases hepatic LDL receptors and leads to increased serum LDL levels. Dietary cholesterol inhibits the production of endogenous cholesterol, but once endogenous cholesterol production is fully suppressed, additional dietary cholesterol may also result in increased serum cholesterol
- HDL
  - Small lipoprotein that transports cholesterol from the arteries back to the liver (reverse cholesterol transport)
  - **Increased HDL is generally inversely associated with atherosclerotic vascular disease**
  - HDL is potentially atheroprotective because it is instrumental in reverse cholesterol transport and has intrinsic antiinflammatory, antithrombotic, antiapoptotic, antioxidative, and endothelial function-enhancing properties
- Apolipoproteins
  - Major component embedded in the lipoprotein surface monolayer
  - Affect lipoprotein metabolism by activating different enzymes and mediating cellular uptake through interactions with cell-surface receptors
  - Apoproteins are divided into five classes (apo A–apo E):
    - Apo A-containing lipoproteins are associated with reduced atherosclerosis (major protein component of mature HDL)
    - Apo B-containing lipoproteins are associated with increased atherosclerosis (and major protein component of LDL)
    - Apo CII-containing lipoproteins are on the surface of VLDL and activate lipoprotein lipase to

promote triglyceride hydrolysis, although apo CIII inhibits lipoprotein lipase

- Lipoprotein(a) [Lp(a)]
  - Lp(a) is an LDL-like particle with apo B covalently linked to apo A
  - Elevated Lp(a) levels are associated with an increased risk of atherosclerotic events, especially in those with a personal or family history of premature atherosclerotic cardiovascular disease (ASCVD)
  - In a large prospective study of women older than 45 years of age, increased Lp(a) levels correlated with higher coronary events when LDL-cholesterol (C) levels were above average levels

Clinical Presentation

- Most patients are asymptomatic until the development of ASCVD
- Physical signs
  - A few patients with lipid disorders have associated physical signs (Table 3-1 and Figures 3-1 and 3-2), including:

- Tendinous xanthoma
  - Nontender, firm nodules on the extensor surfaces of various tendons, including Achilles, hand extensor, and patellar tendons
  - Highly suggestive of familial hypercholesterolemia (if LDL-C ≥190 mg/dL)
- Xanthelasma (palpebral xanthomas)
  - Soft, off-white plaques near the eyelids
  - Associated with any type of hyperlipidemia; not specific to familial hypercholesterolemia (FH)
- Corneal arcus (arcus cornealis)
  - White circumferential peripheral corneal rings
  - Increased prevalence with advanced age
  - Diagnostic for FH when seen in white individuals younger than age 45 (along with tendon xanthomas); it is not diagnostic in older adults
- Tuberous xanthomas
  - Raised, yellowish nodules about 0.5 to 1 cm in diameter
  - Found in areas susceptible to pressure, such as elbows and knees

TABLE 3-1	*Characteristics of Various Lipid Disorders*				
Name	**Group**	**Abnormal Lipid**	**Defect**	**Possible Clinical Findings**	**Risk of CHD**
Familial lipoprotein lipase deficiency	I	↑ Chylomicrons	Lipoprotein lipase deficiency	Eruptive xanthomas, Lipemia retinalis, Abdominal pain, Hepatosplenomegaly	0
Familial hypercholesterolemia	IIa	↑ LDL	Defective LDL receptor or apo B-100	Tendinous xanthomas Xanthelasma planar Xanthomas Corneal arcus	↑↑
Combined hyperlipidemia	IIb	↑ VLDL, LDL	↑ Secretion of apo B-containing particles	Often asymptomatic except for CHD	↑↑
Familial dysbetalipoproteinemia	III	↑ VLDL, IDL	Apo E polymorphism	Tuberoeruptive xanthomas Hyperuricemia Glucose intolerance Corneal opacities Yellow-orange discoloration of palmar creases	↑↑
Familial hypertriglyceridemia	IV	↑ VLDL	↓ Activity of lipoprotein lipase	Often asymptomatic	↑
	V	↑ VLDL, chylomicrons	Acquired lipoprotein lipase dysfunction, and chylomicronemia	Often asymptomatic	↑
Tangier disease	N/A	↓ HDL	↓ Ability to esterify cholesterol	Corneal opacities Polyneuropathy Orange tonsils	↑
Gain of function of proprotein convertase subtilisin-like kexin type 9 (PSCK9)	N/A	↑ LDL	↑ LDL receptor degradation	None	0

Apo, Apolipoprotein; CHD, coronary heart disease; HDL, high-density lipoprotein; IDL, intermediate-density lipoprotein; LDL, low-density lipoprotein; N/A, not available; VLDL, very low-density lipoprotein; ↑, increase; ↓, decrease.

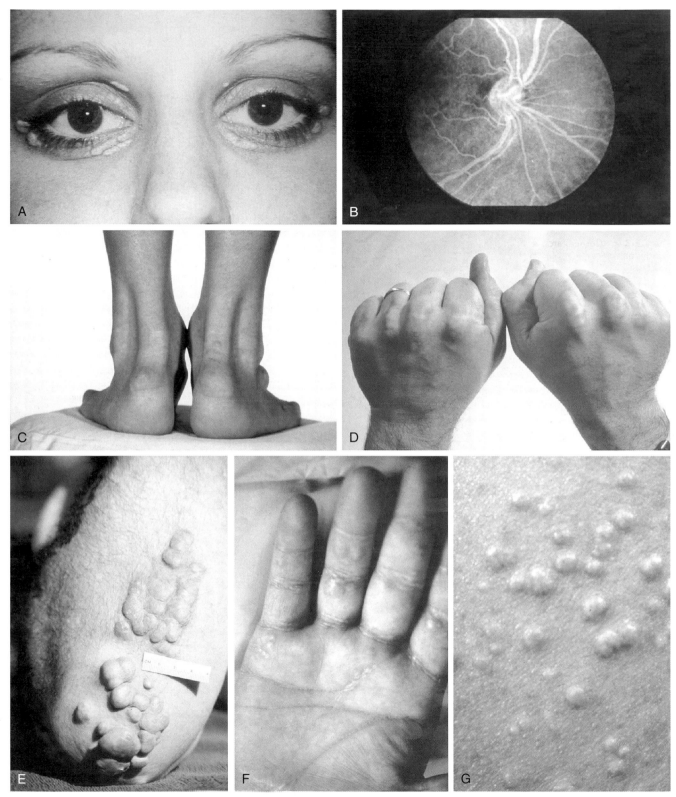

FIGURE 3-1 Physical findings of hyperlipidemia. **A,** Xanthelasma. **B,** Lipemia retinalis. **C,** Achilles tendon xanthomas. Note the marked thickening of the tendons. **D,** Tendon xanthomas. **E,** Tuberous xanthomas. **F,** Palmar xanthomas. **G,** Eruptive xanthomas. (**A** and **B,** Courtesy of Dr. Mark Dresner and *Hospital Practice* [May 1990, p 15]. **C** to **F,** Courtesy of Dr. Tom Bersot. **G,** Courtesy of Dr. Alan Chait. From Larsen PR, Kronenberg HM, Melmed S, et al: *Williams Textbook of Endocrinology.* 10th ed. Philadelphia: Saunders; 2003 [Fig. 34-26].)

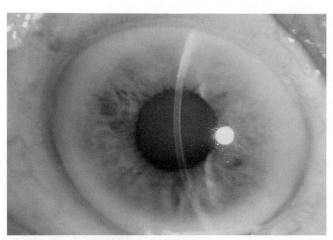

FIGURE 3-2 Corneal arcus (arcus senilis). Corneal arcus in an elderly man. (From Yanoff M, Fine BS: *Ocular Pathology.* 5th ed. St. Louis: Mosby; 2002 [Fig. 60-4].)

- Lipemia retinalis
  - Creamy and/or pink discoloration of both arterioles and venules in the retina
  - Seen on fundoscopic examination in patients with severe hypertriglyceridemia
- Eruptive xanthomas
  - Small, light yellow papules on a reddish base
  - May be present on arms, thighs, dorsal neck, and buttocks; can be missed if a patient is examined when supine
  - May occur diffusely in those with severe hypertriglyceridemia

Diagnosis and Evaluation

- Phenotypes: describing the clinical lipid profile
  - Primary dyslipidemias can be classified into Fredrickson types I through V based on levels of LDL, normal and abnormal VLDL, and fasting chylomicrons (see Table 3-1)
  - Secondary dyslipidemias are caused by a concomitant disorder; for example, severe hypertriglyceridemia is associated with an underlying genetic lipid disorder exacerbated by excessive alcohol consumption, diabetes, or pregnancy
  - The most common cause of dyslipidemia in industrialized countries is caused by a sedentary lifestyle, caloric excess, excessive consumption of saturated and trans–fatty acids, and low consumption of foods rich in fiber and nutrients (fruits, vegetables, whole grains) and monounsaturated and polyunsaturated fatty acids (fish, nuts, seeds, olive and canola oil)
  - Elevated LDL-C differential diagnosis: hypothyroidism, chronic liver disease, cholestasis, nephrotic syndrome, and pregnancy
  - Hypertriglyceridemia differential diagnosis: alcohol consumption, obesity, pregnancy, diabetes mellitus, hypothyroidism, chronic renal failure, and medications (nonselective β-blockers, high-dose diuretics, oral estrogen replacement therapy, and oral contraceptives)

- Low HDL-C differential diagnosis: tobacco use, diabetes mellitus, obesity, sedentary lifestyle, hypertriglyceridemia, medications (progestins, anabolic steroids, corticosteroids)
- Type B pattern
  - Apo B numerically nearly equal to or greater than LDL-C, indicating the presence of small, dense atherogenic particles
  - Associated with impaired fibrinolysis, endothelial dysfunction, and accelerated ASCVD
  - Associated with metabolic syndrome (see later)
- ASCVD risk assessment
  - Clinical ASCVD is diagnosed when patients have had acute coronary syndrome, myocardial infarction (MI), stable or unstable angina, coronary or other arterial revascularizations, stroke, transient ischemic attack, or peripheral arterial disease
  - **In patients older than age 20 years and without clinical ASCVD, fasting lipoprotein levels (total cholesterol [TC], LDL-C, HDL-C, and triglycerides) should be checked at least once every 5 years**
  - **In nonfasting samples, only TC, HDL-C, and non–HDL-C (total cholesterol/HDL-C) levels are accurate. Both TC and HDL-C (not LDL-C) levels are used in the 2013 ACC/AHA risk estimator; hence, nonfasting lipid levels are acceptable in determining 10-year (ages 40 to 79 years) and lifetime (ages 20 to 59 years) global ASCVD risk**
  - 2013 ACC/AHA guidelines emphasize lifestyle modification for ASCVD risk reduction, before and in conjunction with medications. For patients aged 20 to 59 years, the lifetime risk estimator should be primarily used to emphasize lifestyle modification to reduce ASCVD risk
  - 2013 ACC/AHA guidelines identify four major groups who have favorable risk/benefit ratios when treated with statin medications in preventing ASCVD events
    - **The four high-risk groups include patients with:**
      - Clinical ASCVD
      - Primary elevation of LDL 190 mg/dL or higher
      - Diabetics aged 40 to 75 years with an LDL of 70 to 189 mg/dL
      - LDL of 70 to 189 mg/dL and an estimated 10-year ASCVD risk greater than 7.5% (see later for risk calculation). (This category is at lower risk for ASCVD events compared with the first three groups.)
  - Group 4 patients at lower risk should not be treated with a statin without a clinician–patient risk discussion, addressing other risk factors such as cigarette smoking and hypertension, lifestyle, potential benefits and adverse effects of drug–drug interactions, and informed patient preference
  - Of note, previous guidelines (Adult Treatment Panel III) used the modified Framingham risk score (FRS) to set thresholds for lipid management. The new guideline uses a different global risk equation derived from pooled National Heart, Lung, and Blood

Institute (NHLBI) cohorts larger than the Framingham original cohort.

- NHLBI Pooled Cohort Equations (PCEs):
  - PCEs identify the risk of fatal and nonfatal coronary heart disease (CHD) and strokes
  - PCE risk factors include age, sex, race (African American vs non-African American), TC, HDL-C, systolic blood pressure, treatment for hypertension, and cigarette smoking status
  - PCE lipid risk factors include untreated cholesterol and HDL-C, and are used for both short-term (10 years) and long-term (30 years or lifetime) risk estimations; thus, the 2013 AHA/ACC guidelines emphasize non–HDL-C (TC minus HDL-C) and do not use LDL-C in risk estimation. Non–HDL-C correlates much more strongly than LDL-C with atherogenic apo B and other LDL particles.
  - **The PCE 10-year risk calculation should be performed every 4 to 6 years in individuals aged 40 to 75 years without diabetes or ASCVD with LDL-C 70 to 189 mg/dL**
  - Other factors should be considered in evaluating the need for drug therapy:
    - **Family history of premature ASCVD:** onset at younger than 55 years of age in a first-degree male relative or younger than 65 years of age in a first-degree female relative
    - **LDL-C 160 mg/dL or higher:** especially useful in younger patients when the 10-year risk score is low and there is FH
    - **High-sensitivity C-reactive protein (hsCRP) 2 mg/dL or higher:** Associated with a 30% to 40% increase in predicted risk (JUPITER trial). If elevated, statin therapy can be considered in men older than 50 years of age or women older than 60 years of age with a LDL-C greater than 130 mg/dL who are not on lipid-lowering, hormone replacement, or immunosuppressant therapy, and who do not have clinical CHD, diabetes, chronic kidney disease, severe inflammatory conditions, or contraindications to statins
    - **Coronary artery calcium (CAC) score greater than 300 Agatston units or greater than the 74th percentile for age, sex, and ethnicity:** CAC is highly specific for atherosclerosis. A high score is associated with higher ASCVD rates, and can be used to reclassify risk upward. 2013 ACC/AHA guidelines specifically favor CAC greater than or equal to 300 as the cutoff for high-risk status, but there is strong observational data that supports a cutoff of CAC greater than or equal to 100. In contrast, a CAC score of 0 is associated with low short-term event rates and reclassifies risk downwards
    - **Ankle to brachial index greater than 0.9**
  - The following risk factors are of uncertain benefit in assessing the risk for future ASCVD:
    - Carotid artery intimal-medial thickness without assessment of the presence of carotid plaque: no longer considered reasonable
    - Lipoproteins, apolipoproteins, and particle size and density measurements: not recommended in

TABLE 3-2	*Metabolic Syndrome Criteria**
Risk Factor	**Defining Level**
1) Abdominal obesity (waist circumference)	
In men	>40 inches
In women	>35 inches
2) Triglycerides	≥150 mg/dL
3) High-density lipoprotein	
In men	<40 mg/dL
In women	<50 mg/dL
4) Blood pressure	≥130/85 mm Hg
5) Fasting glucose	≥100 mg/dL

*Three or more risk factors are required for the diagnosis.

asymptomatic patients. Can be used to follow non–HDL-C in those with metabolic syndrome. Of note, lifestyle changes can improve non–HDL-C
  - Glomerular filtration rate, albuminuria, or cardiorespiratory fitness measurements: No data show improvement in net ASCVD risk reclassification. In clinical practice, these parameters are important for other reasons
- Metabolic Syndrome (Table 3-2)
  - Associated with a constellation of factors related to insulin resistance, including:
    - Abdominal obesity
    - Atherogenic/type B dyslipidemia (low HDL, elevated triglycerides, non–HDL-C, or small LDL particles)
    - Increased blood pressure
    - Glucose intolerance
  - Metabolic syndrome is not as good as a global risk score for predicting ASCVD risk, but it does indicate a group who are prone to develop diabetes as well as cardiovascular disease; all these factors improve with adherence to a healthy lifestyle that leads to modest weight loss
  - Developing metabolic syndrome should warrant reevaluation of a person's 10-year risk of ASCVD; the PCE results can guide a discussion emphasizing lifestyle modification to improve waist circumference, TG, HDL, and treatment of individual metabolic risk factors with medications, if necessary
- Dyslipidemia treatment (to decrease ASCVD risk)
  - Statins
    - Inhibit HMG-CoA enzyme and up-regulate hepatic surface LDL receptors
    - Options: atorvastatin, fluvastatin, lovastatin, pitavastatin, pravastatin, simvastatin, and rosuvastatin; all are generic except rosuvastatin and pitavastatin
    - Lower LDL-C by 20% to 60% (more than most other agents), raise HDL-C by 3% to 12%, and lower triglyceride levels by 10% to 35%.
    - **2013 AHA/ACC guidelines emphasize the use of statin therapy for ASCVD prevention; compared with previous guidelines, nonstatin**

therapies for the initial management of hypercholesterolemia are no longer recommended

- The 2013 guidelines classify statins into high-, moderate- and low-intensity groups (see Table 3-3)
  - High-intensity statin therapy on average lowers LDL by approximately greater than 50%
  - Moderate-intensity statin therapy lowers LDL by approximately 30% to less than 50%
  - Lower-intensity statin therapy lowers LDL by less than 30%
- Figure 3-3 suggests an algorithm for considering moderate- versus high-intensity statin therapy
- **2013 cholesterol treatment guidelines no longer recommend treating to defined LDL targets; rather, they recommend globally lowering LDL and non-HDL with proven therapy to reduce ASCVD**

TABLE 3-3	*High Intensity vs Moderate Intensity Statin Therapy**

High-Intensity Statin Therapy

Daily dose lowers LDL cholesterol level by approximately ≥50% on average
Recommended: atorvastatin, 40 to 80 mg; rosuvastatin, 20 to 40 mg

Moderate-Intensity Statin Therapy

Daily dose lowers LDL cholesterol level by approximately 30% to 50% or less on average
Recommended: atorvastatin, 10 to 20 mg; rosuvastatin, 5 to 10 mg; simvastatin, 20 to 40 mg; pravastatin, 40 to 80 mg; lovastatin, 40 mg; extended-release fluvastatin, 80 mg; fluvastatin, 40 mg twice a day; pitavastatin, 2 to 4 mg

*According to 2013 American College of Cardiology-American Heart Association Cholesterol Guidelines.
From Keaney JF, Curfman GD, Jarcho JA. A pragmatic view of the new cholesterol treatment guidelines. *N Engl J Med.* 2014;370:275–278.

- This is controversial: Some experts recommend aiming therapy to an LDL goal
- The 2013 guideline recommends considering nonstatin therapy for certain "high-risk" patients if they are unable to tolerate statin therapy. In addition, nonstatin therapy should be considered for those with a suboptimal response (i.e., less than the expected LDL-C response to that prescribed statin). Also, greatly elevated triglycerides (500 mg/dL or higher) should be treated with nonstatins such as fibrates, omega 3 fatty acids, and/or niacin to prevent pancreatitis.
- Side effects:
  - Less than 3% risk of myositis or increased liver enzymes; often resolve without intervention or dose reduction
  - Myalgias are more common (as high as 15%); the risk depends on a person's age and the number of and type of concomitant medications
  - Very modest risk of new-onset diabetes (i.e., 0.1 excess cases per 100 individuals treated for 1 year with moderate-intensity statin therapy and approximately 0.3 excess cases per 100 individuals treated for 1 year with high-intensity therapy); the benefits of statin therapy are believed to outweigh the risks of new-onset diabetes
  - Rhabdomyolysis is very rare (<1%) but potentially fatal; there is increased risk when statins are used in combination with gemfibrozil and macrolide antibiotics (e.g., erythromycin or clarithromycin)
  - Increased adverse effects in patients with:
    - Multiple or serious comorbidities, including impaired renal or hepatic function
    - History of statin intolerance or muscle disorders
    - Genetic polymorphisms (e.g., SLCO1B1) or concomitant use of drugs affecting statin metabolism
    - Age older than 75 years
    - Asian ancestry

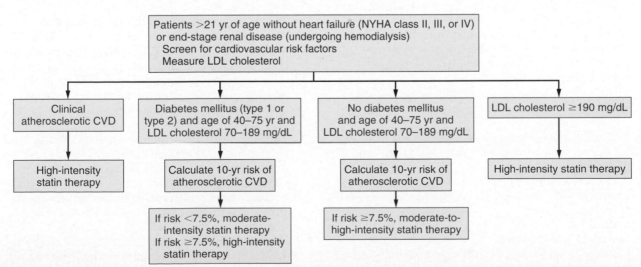

FIGURE 3-3 Approach to the patient. CVD, Cardiovascular disease; LDL, low-density lipoprotein; NYHA, New York Heart Association. (From Keaney JF, Curfman GD, Jarcho JA. A pragmatic view of the new cholesterol treatment guidelines. *N Engl J Med.* 2014;370:275–278.)

- History of hemorrhagic stroke
- Monitoring
  - Initial fasting lipid panel, followed by a repeat lipid panel 4 to 12 weeks after statin initiation to determine patient's response and adherence. Repeat testing should be considered every 3 to 12 months. Beneficial changes in values could be because of statin therapy and lifestyle modifications. Conversely, a 10% increase in LDL may be caused by statin nonadherence or weight gain.
  - Baseline hepatic function panel. No need to monitor hepatic function after initiating therapy; however, it should be rechecked if symptoms suggesting hepatotoxicity develop.
  - Creatine kinase (CK). This should not be routinely measured; however, baseline measurement is reasonable for individuals at increased risk for adverse muscle events because of a personal or family history of statin intolerance or muscle disease, or in whom concomitant drug therapy that might increase the risk of myopathy. It is also reasonable to measure CK in those who develop muscle symptoms, including pain, tenderness, stiffness, cramping, weakness, or generalized fatigue
- Bile acid sequestrants (BASs) (e.g., cholestyramine, colestipol, and colesevelam)
  - This medication group binds to certain bile components within the gastrointestinal tract to disrupt enterohepatic cholesterol circulation
  - Lower LDL by 10% to 25%
  - Can decrease the absorption of other drugs, which should be taken at least 90 minutes before or 4 hours after BAS administration
  - Can raise triglycerides; 2013 ACC/AHA guidelines discourage BAS therapy in patients with TG 300 mg/dL or higher and caution if TG is greater than or equal to 250 mg/dL
  - Absolute contraindications: TG greater than 500 mg/dL, history of TG-induced pancreatitis, history of bowel obstruction
  - Side effects: gastrointestinal symptoms (bloating, cramping, flatulence)
  - BASs are useful in lowering LDL in individuals with FH at highest dose statin therapy, as well as in individuals with ASCVD and partial or complete statin intolerance. Colesevelam is especially useful in those with diabetes because it helps control blood glucose via improved β-cell function.
- Ezetimibe
  - Inhibits cholesterol absorption in the small intestine through inhibition of the NPC1L1 transporter
    - Decreases delivery of cholesterol to the liver, thereby reducing hepatic cholesterol stores and increasing hepatic LDL receptors and serum LDL uptake by the liver
  - Lowers LDL by 15% to 25%
  - Given as monotherapy or in conjunction with a statin to lower LDL
  - Side effects (uncommon): transaminitis, abdominal and back pain, diarrhea, fatigue

- A recent study showed a modest decrease in CVD events in patients with acute coronary syndrome when ezetimibe was added to simvastatin
- Fibrates (gemfibrozil, fenofibrate)
  - **Lower triglycerides by 25% to 50% (more than most other agents)**
  - Raise HDL-C by 10% to 20%
  - Lower LDL-C by 5% to 20%
  - **Reduce CHD events but do not reduce CHD mortality rates; especially useful in patients with type 2 diabetes**
  - Not a substitute for statins to lower LDL-C (statins lower mortality rates)
  - **Gemfibrozil should not be used with atorvastatin, simvastatin, or lovastatin** as all compete for the glucuronidation pathway, leading to supratherapeutic levels and increased risk for muscle symptoms and rhabdomyolysis. Of note, fenofibrate can be used in conjunction with statins.
  - Side effects: dyspepsia, myalgias, gallstones
  - Unclear role for fibrates in the management of hyperlipidemia and ASCVD risk management. The 2013 guidelines recommend use in high-risk patients who are either intolerant or have a suboptimal response to statins. Some experts, however, favor fibrate therapy in addition to statin therapy in diabetic patients with low HDL and high triglycerides levels.
- Nicotinic acid (niacin)
  - Lowers LDL by 5% to 25%
  - **Raises HDL by 15% to 35%**
  - Lowers triglyceride levels by 20% to 40%
  - Modest long-term decrease in mortality rates in post-MI patients in the prestatin era
  - No benefits when used with concomitant statin therapy. Extended-release niacin has been shown to slow carotid intimal-medial thickness progression but has no ASCVD benefits and is associated with possible higher risks compared with statin therapy
  - Side effects: flushing, hyperuricemia, hyperglycemia (in high doses), gastrointestinal distress, and hepatotoxicity
    - Flushing ameliorated with aspirin premedication
  - Uncertain role for niacin therapy in management of hyperlipidemia and ASCVD risk management. The 2013 guidelines recommend use in high-risk patients who are either intolerant or have a suboptimal response to statins. Patients treated with statins should not also be given niacin because two large scale clinical trials have documented no incremental benefits in patients with low levels of LDL. This is despite further decreases in already low baseline levels of LDL and non-HDL and elevations in HDL. Some experts recommend niacin therapy if there are residual elevations in non-HDL despite maximum dose statin therapy; however, this has not been confirmed yet in a clinical trial.
- Lifestyle modification
  - Critically important in lipid and cardiovascular risk management
  - Comprises diet and physical activity recommendations and management of obesity

- **Diet: Emphasize vegetables, fruits, and whole grains; include low-fat dairy products, poultry, fish, legumes, nontropical vegetable oils, and nuts, while limiting sweets and sugar-sweetened beverages**
  - This dietary pattern can be achieved by plans such as the Dietary Approaches to Stop Hypertension (DASH) diet, the United States Department of Agriculture (USDA) Food Pattern, or the AHA Diet.
- Physical activity: can consist of 150 minutes per week of moderate-intensity physical activity or 75 minutes per week of vigorous-intensity aerobic physical activity, or an equivalent combination of moderate-and vigorous-intensity aerobic physical activity. Aerobic activity should be performed in episodes of at least 10 minutes, preferably spread throughout the week
- Obesity management: Weight and body mass index (BMI) should be measured at every clinic visit
  - Definitions: overweight (BMI 25.0 to 29.9 kg/m^2), class I obesity (BMI 30 to 34.9 kg/m^2), class II obesity (35.9 to 39.9 kg/m^2), and class III obesity (≥40 kg/m^2)
  - Modest sustained weight loss of 3% to 5% in overweight or obese adults with cardiovascular risk factors (high blood pressure, hyperlipidemia, and hyperglycemia) can result in meaningful health benefits (greater weight losses can produce even greater benefits)

Approach to the Patient

- Measurement of lipids
  - Fasting lipid profile beginning at age 21 years
  - If nonfasting, TC and HDL values remain accurate and are adequate for ASCVD risk estimation with the ACC/AHA PCE risk estimator
  - If normal, repeat measurement at approximately every 5 years
  - If abnormal, pursue intensive lifestyle modification therapy first
  - **All patients hospitalized for an ASCVD event should have a lipid profile checked within 24 hours**
  - Do not routinely measure emerging risk factors: Lp(a), hs-CRP, apo B, LDL particle number, and other prothrombotic and proinflammatory factors
  - Consider recommending diet therapy for 4 to 6 months in most patients with moderately elevated LDL and no known ASCVD. In patients at higher risk (as determined by PCE calculation), consider medication therapy.
- Management of triglyceride disorders
  - Classification
    - Normal triglycerides: greater than 150 mg/dL
    - Borderline high: 150 to 199 mg/dL
    - High: 200 to 499 mg/dL
    - Very high: greater than 500 mg/dL
  - Treatment
    - Lifestyle modification: weight reduction, increased physical activity, and decreased alcohol intake
    - Medications:
      - Omega-3 fatty acids: can lower TG, not LDL, and can help reduce markedly elevated TG and help prevent pancreatitis
      - Fibrate therapy: Initial therapy if TG levels are greater than 500 mg/dL
- Management of low HDL
  - Defined as less than 40 mg/dL
  - Exercise, weight loss, and tobacco cessation may raise HD
  - **Niacin is the most effective drug for raising HDL, but the 2013 ACC/AHA Guidelines do not recommend niacin therapy; instead, statin therapy should be used in patients with low HDL and an ASCVD risk greater than 7.5%**
  - The pharmacologic raising of HDL has not been shown to reduce ASCVD events to date

Acknowledgment

We are grateful to Drs. J. Gabriel Schneider, Lori Tam, and Andrew DeFilippis for their help in preparing previous drafts of this chapter for previous editions of this textbook.

Review Questions

For review questions, please go to ExpertConsult.com.

SUGGESTED READINGS

ACCORD Study Group, Ginsberg HN, Elam MB, et al. Effects of combination lipid therapy in type 2 diabetes mellitus. *N Engl J Med.* 2010;362:1563-1574.

Amin NP, Martin SS, Blaha MJ, et al. Headed in the right direction but at risk for miscalculation: a critical appraisal of the 2013 ACC/AHA Risk Assessment Guidelines. *J Am Coll Cardiol.* 2014;63:2789-2794.

American College of Cardiology (ACC). *2013 prevention guidelines ASCVD risk estimator.* ACC; 2013. Available at: <http://www.acc.org/tools-and-practice-support/mobile-resources/features/2013-prevention-guidelines-ascvd-risk-estimator>.

American Heart Association (AHA), ACC. *2013 prevention guidelines tools: CV risk calculator. A companion to the 2013 ACC/AHA guideline on the assessment of cardiovascular risk.* AHA/ACC; 2013. Available at: <http://my.americanheart.org/cvriskcalculator>.

Ashen MD, Blumenthal RS. Clinical practice: low HDL cholesterol levels. *N Engl J Med.* 2005;353:1252-1260.

Cui Y, Blumenthal RS, Flaws JA, et al. Non-high-density lipoprotein cholesterol level as a predictor of cardiovascular disease mortality. *Arch Intern Med.* 2001;161:1413-1419.

Eckel RH, Jakicic JM, Ard JD, et al. 2013 AHA/ACC Guideline on Lifestyle Management to Reduce Cardiovascular Risk. A report of the American College of Cardiology/American Heart Association Task Force on Practice Guidelines. *J Am Coll Cardiol.* 2014;63:2960-2984.

Gluckman TJ, Baranowski B, Ashen MD, et al. A practical and evidence-based approach to cardiovascular disease risk reduction. *Arch Intern Med.* 2004;164:1490-1500.

Goff DC Jr, Lloyd-Jones DM, Bennett G, et al. 2013 ACC/AHA Guideline on the Assessment of Cardiovascular Risk. A report of the American College of Cardiology/American Heart Association Task Force on Practice Guidelines. *J Am Coll Cardiol.* 2014;63:2935-2959.

Greenland P, Alpert JS, Beller GA, et al. 2010 ACCF/AHA Guideline for the assessment of cardiovascular risk in asymptomatic adults: a report of the American College of Cardiology Foundation/American

3

Heart Association Task Force on Practice Guidelines. *Circulation.* 2010;122:e584-e636.

Jensen MD, Ryan DH, Apovian CM, et al. 2013 AHA/ACC/TOS Guideline for the Management of Overweight and Obesity in Adults. 2013. A Report of the American College of Cardiology/American Heart Association Task Force on Practice Guidelines and The Obesity Society. *J Am Coll Cardiol.* 2014;63:2985-3023.

Lakoski SG, Greenland P, Wong ND, et al. Coronary artery calcium scores and risk for cardiovascular events in women classified as "low risk" based on Framingham risk score: the Multi-Ethnic Study of Atherosclerosis (MESA). *Arch Intern Med.* 2007;167:2437-2442.

Martin SS, Abd TT, Jones SR, et al. 2013 ACC/AHA Cholesterol Treatment Guideline: what was done well and what could be done better. *J Am Coll Cardiol.* 2014;63:2674-2678.

Mudd JO, Borlaug BA, Johnston PV, et al. Beyond low-density lipoprotein cholesterol: defining the role of low-density lipoprotein heterogeneity in coronary artery disease. *J Am Coll Cardiol.* 2007;50:1735-1741.

Ridker PM, Danielson E, Fonseca FA, et al. Rosuvastatin to prevent vascular events in men and women with elevated C-reactive protein. *N Engl J Med.* 2008;359:2195-2207.

Stone NJ, Robinson J, Lichtenstein AH, et al. 2013 ACC/AHA Guideline on the treatment of blood cholesterol to reduce atherosclerotic cardiovascular risk in adults. A Report of the American College of Cardiology/American Heart Association Task Force on Practice Guidelines. *J Am Coll Cardiol.* 2014;63:2889-2934.

Coronary Artery Disease

KLITOS KONSTANTINIDIS, MD; and SAMMY ZAKARIA, MD, MPH

In the United States, over 17 million people have coronary artery disease (CAD), and the cost of caring for these patients is over $150 billion per year. Despite great advances in treatment, CAD remains the leading cause of death for both men and women, affecting approximately 1 million per year; roughly 25% of these deaths occur suddenly.

Chronic Coronary Artery Disease

Basic Information

- Atherogenesis
  - The endothelial cells lining the coronary arteries have two major roles:
    - Regulate vascular tone: vasodilation (e.g., nitric oxide) and vasoconstriction (e.g., endothelin, angiotensin-converting enzyme [ACE])
    - Prevent intravascular thrombosis (e.g., prostacyclin, plasminogen)
  - Factors that can impair endothelial function (in both epicardial vessels and microvessels) include:
    - Hemodynamic (e.g., shear stress, hypertension [HTN])
    - Chemical (e.g., low-density lipoprotein [LDL], modified LDL, homocysteine)
    - Biologic (e.g., viruses, bacteria, immune complexes)
  - Atherosclerotic plaque formation
    - Begins with disruption of endothelial cell integrity
    - Leukocytes, mostly macrophages, are then attracted to the site of disruption, where they collect lipids and coalesce to form a fatty streak
    - Fatty streaks mostly consist of lipid-laden macrophages containing cholesterol ester droplets (atheroma)
    - Chemoattractants (e.g., platelet-derived growth factor) then cause smooth muscle cells to migrate to the atheroma, where they produce collagen and fibrous tissue that contribute to plaque formation, covered by a layer of connective tissue called the fibrous cap
    - Most acute coronary syndromes (ACSs) occur when the fibrous cap ruptures, leading to thrombus formation (see later section on Acute Coronary Syndromes)
    - **Note: Plaque characteristics, not size, determine its vulnerability to rupture; a large, fibrotic plaque with a thick cap is more stable and less prone to rupture than a small plaque with a soft lipid core and a thin fibrous cap**

- Pathophysiology of chronic CAD and chronic stable angina
  - **The fundamental problem is an imbalance between myocardial oxygen supply and demand**
  - Anginal symptoms occur during periods of exercise or stress when increased myocardial oxygen demand (e.g., from an increase in heart rate, contractility, afterload, or wall stress) is not met because of impaired coronary blood flow
  - Insufficient coronary blood flow occurs when:
    - A plaque leads to arterial stenosis
    - There is endothelial dysfunction preventing adequate vasodilation during exercise, which can occur in the absence of severe luminal narrowing

Clinical Presentation

- **Risk factors for coronary atherosclerosis (Table 4-1)**
- **Special considerations**
  - **A low high-density lipoprotein (HDL) level is an independent risk factor for CAD (see Chapter 3)**
  - **Small, dense LDL has the lowest affinity for the LDL receptor and is therefore cleared to the least degree from plasma by the liver; it may be the most atherogenic type of LDL**
  - Homocysteinuria: rare homozygous genetic disorder impairing homocysteine metabolism, leading to severe premature atherosclerosis
    - 1% to 2% of population are heterozygous, which may account for up to 30% of cases of premature atherosclerosis
    - Treatment of elevated homocysteine levels with folate, vitamin B_6, and vitamin B_{12} does not reduce the risk of myocardial infarction (MI) or death
  - Elevated lipoprotein(a) [Lp(a)]: Increased number of LDL particles that contain the large glycoprotein apoprotein (a), which has a higher density than LDL and is more atherogenic
    - Higher levels are associated with CAD
    - Niacin, estrogen, fenofibrate, and bezafibrate all reduce Lp(a) levels; however, none of these treatments have been shown to reduce cardiovascular events
  - Elevated C-reactive protein (CRP) and fibrinogen levels: associated with MIs and CAD. Unclear if they cause CAD or are simply markers of an associated inflammatory process.
  - *Chlamydia pneumonia*: This bacterium has been isolated from atheromas and may contribute to

TABLE 4-1	*Risk Factors for Coronary Artery Disease*		
Strong Epidemiologic Evidence	**Moderate Epidemiologic Evidence**	**Mild Epidemiologic Evidence**	
Older age	High triglycerides	Lipoprotein(a)	
Male	Small dense LDL	*Chlamydia*	
Postmenopausal females	Elevated homocysteine	*pneumoniae*	
Elevated LDL	Stress or depression		
Low HDL	Inflammatory markers (C-reactive protein, fibrinogen)		
Cigarette smoking			
Hypertension			
Diabetes mellitus			
Obesity or sedentary lifestyle			
Family history of early CAD			

CAD; Coronary artery disease; HDL, high-density lipoprotein; LDL, low-density lipoprotein.

plaque inflammation. However, patients hospitalized with an ACS had no reduction in cardiovascular events when treated with long-term gatifloxacin.
- Clinical symptoms
  - Symptoms typically occur during physical exertion and gradually resolve with exercise cessation
  - Symptoms can also occur in conditions that increase oxygen demand (e.g., anemia, fever, sepsis, thyrotoxicosis)
  - Typical symptoms:
    - Substernal chest pressure or burning (less common to have sharp pain)
    - Pain may radiate to the upper extremities (left arm more often than right arm), neck, jaw, or face
    - Associated symptoms include dyspnea, diaphoresis, palpitations, and lightheadedness
    - Women, diabetics, and the elderly are more likely to have atypical symptoms

Diagnosis and Evaluation

- **The Framingham Risk Score**
  - **Scoring system used to calculate a patient's risk for having a coronary event**
  - Uses the following risk factors to assess cumulative risk: age, smoking status, systolic blood pressure (BP), treatment for HTN, total cholesterol, and HDL cholesterol
  - **The cumulative score classifies patients as:**
    - **Low risk (<10% coronary heart disease [CHD] risk at 10 years)**
    - **Intermediate risk (10% to 20% risk of coronary event at 10 years)**
    - **High risk (>20% risk of coronary event at 10 years)**
- The Pooled Cohort Equations (PCEs)
  - A new risk estimator that assesses 10-year and lifetime risk of cardiovascular events using multiple risk factors (race, sex, systolic BP, total cholesterol, HDL, presence of diabetes, smoking status)

- **The most recent ACC/AHA guidelines use this risk score to guide lipid-lowering treatment for primary and secondary cardiovascular disease prevention (see Chapter 3)**
- Resting electrocardiogram (ECG)
  - Approximately 50% of patients with chronic stable angina have a normal resting ECG
  - Pathologic Q waves and conduction system abnormalities (e.g., left bundle branch block [LBBB], left anterior fascicular block) increase the likelihood of having CAD
- Stress tests
  - The presence of CAD can never be definitively ruled in or out through stress testing alone, because stress testing can yield both false-negative and false-positive results (the sensitivity of an exercise treadmill test is approximately 70%, the specificity is approximately 80%)
  - **Stress testing can help risk-stratify patients: The information obtained from the test can help determine the patient's risk for future cardiovascular events and death (see the following examples):**
- Need to know pretest probability for having CAD
  - The likelihood of a patient having CAD increases with age, having CAD risk factors (e.g., diabetes mellitus [DM]), and presenting with a history typical for exertional angina
    - The clinician should be able to determine from history and physical examination alone whether a patient has a low, medium, or high pretest probability of CAD:
      - Example 1: A 25-year-old woman with atypical symptoms and no risk factors for CAD has a very low pretest probability
      - Example 2: A 75-year-old man with exertional angina and a history of HTN, DM, high cholesterol, and cigarette use has a high pretest probability
  - Pretest probability helps stress test result interpretation:
    - Example 1: A healthy 25-year-old woman presents with atypical symptoms of chest pain and no CAD risk factors. She exercises for 15 minutes on a Bruce protocol and has no symptoms, but her stress ECG shows 1- to 2-mm ST-segment depression in some leads, and the test is read as positive.
      - *Interpretation:* This patient has a very low pretest probability of having CAD. This is reinforced by her high treadmill performance without symptoms. The ECG changes almost certainly represent a false-positive result.
    - Example 2: For the past several months, a 75-year-old man with DM, HTN, and high cholesterol has been having substernal chest pain when he walks up a hill. His symptoms resolve quickly with rest. On a treadmill, he exercises for 6 minutes on a Bruce protocol and develops chest pain at peak exercise. The ECG shows only nonspecific changes, and the test is read as negative.

- *Interpretation:* This man is older, has a classic story for exertional angina, and has several major risk factors. His pretest probability is very high, and it is almost a certainty that he has CAD. The stress test is likely a false-negative result.
  - **Stress tests add little diagnostic information for patients with either high or low pretest probabilities for CAD**
  - **Stress tests are most useful for diagnosing CAD in patients with intermediate pretest probability**
- Determining risk with stress testing
  - Stress test results should be categorized as:
    - Inadequate
    - Negative
    - Positive low risk
    - Positive high risk
  - **Features of a stress test that make it high risk (Box 4-1):**
  - Duke Treadmill Score (a scoring system that can be used to assess long-term risk)
    - Score = (duration of exercise in minutes) − (5 × maximal ST-segment depression in millimeters) − (4 × treadmill angina index)
      - Treadmill angina index: 0 = no symptoms, 1 = angina that does not limit exercise, 2 = angina that limits exercise
    - Score: less than −10: 79% 4-year survival; −10 to +4: 95% 4-year survival; +5 or greater: greater than 99% 4-year survival
  - **Patients with positive stress tests without high-risk features are often treated medically**
  - **Patients with positive tests and high-risk features are more likely to have high-risk coronary anatomy (e.g., left main disease, proximal left anterior descending [LAD] artery disease, three-vessel disease); the best approach usually requires cardiac catheterization and revascularization**
- Types of stress tests (Table 4-2):
  - To decide which stress test is best for a given patient, ask two questions:
    - Can the patient exercise?
      - If yes, a treadmill test is the best choice; allows for assessment of a patient's functional capacity, which correlates with overall long-term survival.

- If the patient cannot exercise (e.g., severe chronic obstructive pulmonary disease [COPD], peripheral vascular disease, arthritis), pursue pharmacologic stress (e.g., regadenoson, dobutamine) with accompanying imaging modality.
- Does the resting ECG have ST-segment abnormalities?
  - If there are baseline ST-segment abnormalities (e.g., left ventricular hypertrophy with strain, paced rhythm, LBBB, ST-segment depression on resting ECG, accessory pathways), the ECG alone may not permit an accurate diagnosis of ischemia, and an imaging modality will be required.
- Stress testing is very safe
  - 1 to 2 deaths per 10,000 tests
  - **Should be avoided in patients with active symptoms of unstable angina (UA), severe aortic stenosis, possible aortic dissection, severe HTN, tachyarrhythmias or bradyarrhythmias, hypertrophic cardiomyopathy, and other forms of outflow tract obstruction**
  - **Pharmacologic testing with adenosine agonists should be avoided in patients with severe COPD and active wheezing**
- Computed tomography (CT)
  - Noninvasive assessment of coronary arteries
  - Calcium score screening CT
    - Noninvasive and quantitative assessment of coronary artery calcification
    - Higher coronary artery calcium scores are associated with increased risk of MI and death
    - **Only obtain in asymptomatic patients:**
      - **Coronary artery calcium scores >75th percentile for age and sex identify higher risk patients who would benefit from aggressive lipid-lowering therapy**
      - **A coronary artery calcium score of 0 is associated with excellent survival, with all-cause, 10-year mortality risk less than 1% or less than 0.1% per year)**
  - Calcium scoring, when added to PCE risk score, further risk stratifies patients; coronary artery calcium greater than 300 or greater than 75th percentile for age, sex, and ethnicity is associated with higher risk for cardiovascular events and can identify patients who would most benefit from aggressive risk reduction/statin treatment
  - **Coronary CT angiography (CCTA)**
    - **Can also measure coronary calcification**
    - CCTA allows for direct coronary artery visualization of a beating heart with little motion artifact
    - Most accurate noninvasive modality in ruling out CAD with a very high negative predictive value (>95%)
    - Less accurate in differentiating degrees of coronary artery stenosis greater than 50%; the positive predictive value varies between 60 and 90

| BOX 4-1 | *Features of a High-Risk Stress Test* |

Exercise-induced hypotension
Angina or ischemic ECG changes at a low workload (<6 min or <4 METS on Bruce protocol)
ST-segment depression >2 mm
ST-segment depression persisting >6 min into recovery period
Any ST-segment elevation
Ventricular arrhythmias
Imaging reveals reversible defects in multiple territories or left ventricular cavity dilation

ECG, Electrocardiogram; METS, metabolic equivalents.

TABLE 4-2	*Types of Stress Tests*		
	Agent	**Advantages**	**Disadvantages**
Options for Stress			
Exercise	N/A	Mimics physiologic increases in O_2 demand Provides useful clinical information (e.g., exercise capacity) Inexpensive	Not all patients can exercise adequately ECG alone without imaging modality has higher rates of false positives and false negatives
Pharmacologic	Dobutamine: β-agonist that ↑ heart rate and myocardial contractility (and thus O_2 demand) Adenosine agonists: (adenosine, dipyridamole and regadenoson) vasodilate coronary vascular bed and ↑ myocardial blood flow; dilation greater in normal arteries than diseased arteries resulting in steal phenomenon from diseased vascular beds	Helpful in patients who cannot exercise	More expensive Drugs can cause chest pain, nausea, and hypotension, making test interpretation more difficult
Options for Imaging			
Nuclear isotope	Thallium-201: potassium analogue taken up by myocardial cells; hypoperfused myocardium initially shows decreased uptake; tracer redistributes over several hours Technetium-99m (sestamibi): also taken up by myocardial cells but binds irreversibly; no late washout makes it ideal for imaging MI and unstable angina	Helpful in distinguishing ischemia from infarcted myocardium Technetium-99m has higher proton energy; better agent for imaging obese patients Increases sensitivity and specificity of test	More expensive More invasive Requires radiation
Echocardiography	N/A	Direct visualization of ventricular function Can quantify and localize ischemia Noninvasive Increases sensitivity and specificity of test	More expensive Imaging may be limited in obese patients Can yield false positives in patients with LBBB

ECG, Electrocardiogram; LBBB, left bundle branch block; MI, myocardial infarction; N/A, not available.

- Coronary angiography
  - Considered the gold standard for diagnosing CAD
  - Refer for cardiac catheterization if:
    - Need to confirm or exclude CAD
    - Medical therapy fails to relieve anginal symptoms
    - History and noninvasive testing suggest high-risk coronary anatomy

TREATMENT OF CHRONIC CAD

- Address modifiable risk factors (e.g., lipid lowering, cigarette cessation)
- Correct illnesses that can precipitate or exacerbate angina (e.g., anemia, infection, thyroid disease)
- Consider the following medications that can relieve angina:
  - **β-Blockers**
    - **First-line therapy**
    - Reduce myocardial oxygen (O_2) demand by decreasing heart rate, BP, and contractility
    - Does not reduce MI or death in patients with chronic stable angina without history of MI or HF; in patients with recent MI or HF with CAD, β-blockers reduce both morbidity and mortality
  - **Nitrates**
    - **First-line therapy**
    - Major effect stems from venodilation, which decreases cardiac preload, thereby decreasing wall stress and O_2 demand
    - Very good at relieving angina and improving exercise tolerance but does not affect mortality
    - Contraindicated in patients using sildenafil
  - Calcium channel blockers
    - Second-line therapy
    - Improve myocardial oxygen supply by decreasing coronary vascular resistance and augmenting epicardial conduit vessel and systemic arterial blood flow; myocardial demand is decreased by a reduction in myocardial contractility, systemic vascular resistance, and arterial pressure
    - Do not use short-acting dihydropyridines, which increase mortality rates in patients with ACS (see later discussion); however, long-acting agents are safe and effective in treating patients with chronic stable angina

- Ranolazine
  - Second-line agent
  - Inhibits the late inward sodium current, indirectly reducing the sodium-dependent calcium current during ischemic conditions and leading to improvement in ventricular diastolic tension and O_2 consumption
  - Reduces the frequency of angina, improves exercise performance, and delays the development of exercise-induced angina and ST-segment depression
- Medications that decrease morbidity and mortality
  - Aspirin
    - Reduces risk of MI and death
    - **All patients with CAD should be on aspirin unless there is a clear contraindication**
  - Lipid-lowering agents
    - **3-Hydroxy-3-methylglutaryl coenzyme A (HMG-CoA) reductase inhibitors (statins) reduce risk of MI and death**
    - The 2013 AHA/ACC guidelines recommend high-intensity statin therapy in patients with CAD if age older than 75 years and moderate-intensity therapy in patients older than 75 years or patients who are not candidates for high-intensity therapy (see Chapter 3)
    - If statins are not tolerated, other agents (e.g., ezetimibe, fibrates) could be used but they are without strong evidence in the literature
  - ACE inhibitors
    - **Clear decrease in mortality and morbidity rates in patients with left ventricular (LV) dysfunction (ejection fraction [EF] <40%)**
- Revascularization of chronic CAD
  - The major indication for revascularization in chronic CAD is for relief of angina symptoms in patients on optimal medical management.
  - Two methods of revascularization:
    - Percutaneous coronary intervention (PCI)
      - Two components: Percutaneous transluminal coronary angioplasty (PTCA), in which a balloon is used to split the atheromatous plaque and stretch the artery, and stent deployment, which provides a metal scaffold to help maintain artery patency
      - There are two types of stents:
        - Bare metal stents (BMSs)
        - Drug-eluting stents (DESs): Stents are coated with a drug that blocks cell proliferation, thus decreasing prolific neointimal hyperplasia and restenosis
          - The drug also inhibits reendothelialization of the stent, so there is increased risk of metallic material being exposed to thrombotic factors, leading to an increased risk of in-stent thrombosis
          - To decrease this risk, patients should be treated with lifetime aspirin and at least 1 year of thienopyridine therapy
      - Major benefits: highly successful (>90%); decreases the need for coronary artery bypass surgery

- Deciding between a BMS and a DES:
  - No survival differences, but a DES reduces risk of repeat target-vessel revascularization and reinfarctions
  - BMS should be used in patients who cannot tolerate long-term dual-antiplatelet therapies
- Antiplatelet agents commonly used during PCI
  - Aspirin: An irreversible cyclooxygenase inhibitor
  - Thienopyridines:
    - Clopidogrel: Inhibits adenosine diphosphate (ADP)-mediated platelet activation; helps to prevent acute stent thrombosis; side effects include rash and gastrointestinal (GI) upset; can rarely cause thrombotic thrombocytopenic purpura
    - Prasugrel: Mechanism of action is similar to clopidogrel but has a more rapid onset of action and more effective inhibition of platelet activation; lower rate of death and reinfarction in patients treated with prasugrel compared with clopidogrel but a slightly higher rate of bleeding (risk of bleeding is higher in patients with previous stroke/transient ischemic attack [TIA], body weight less than 60 kg, and age older than 75 years)
    - Ticagrelor: Similar to clopidogrel and prasugrel but does not require activation by CYP enzymes in the liver; compared with clopidogrel, it is a more effective and faster inhibitor of platelet activation, leading to lower rates of death and ischemic events, with a slightly higher rate of bleeding
    - Ticlopidine: Rarely used, because of association with thrombotic thrombocytopenic purpura and neutropenia
  - Glycoprotein IIb/IIIa inhibitors: Abciximab and eptifibatide; reduce cardiovascular complications of PCI in the acute setting
- Risks and complications
  - Restenosis: Narrowing of the arterial lumen following PCI; mechanism incompletely understood but likely involves neointimal thickening caused by smooth muscle cell proliferation
    - Also, the dilated segment can shrink because of elastic recoil
    - Incidence peaks between 3 and 6 months after PCI but has significantly decreased with DES use
  - Other: 1% to 2% risk of emergent bypass, 2% to 4% risk of MI (i.e., thrombosis), 1% risk of death; risks increase with complicated lesions, which are often long, tubular, and eccentric, as well as calcified lesions
- **In patients with stable CAD, PCI is quite effective in reducing angina, but it does not reduce the risk of death or MI**

- Coronary artery bypass grafting (CABG)
  - Excellent for relieving anginal symptoms
  - Benefits: decreased repeated revascularization procedures compared with PCI
  - Complications: sternal wound infection, MI, stroke, postoperative arrhythmias, and death
  - **Characteristics of patients with stable CAD who have lower mortality rates after CABG:**
    - **Left main disease**
    - **Three-vessel CAD and decreased LV function**
      - This is a weaker recommendation: A recent study suggests no significant difference in all-cause mortality between medical management and CABG
    - **Three-vessel CAD and ischemia at low workload**
    - **Two-vessel or three-vessel disease with proximal LAD involvement**
    - **Patients with DM: higher 5-year survival with CABG than with PTCA**
  - Following CABG, use statin therapy, which can help decrease graft vessel disease (even in patients with only mild LDL elevation)
  - How does multivessel PCI compare with CABG in patients with left main or three-vessel CAD?
    - At 1 year, major adverse cardiac events rates are higher in the PCI group, largely caused by an increased rate of repeat revascularization
    - At 1 year, rates of death and MI are the same in both groups, but stroke is more likely to occur with CABG
  - Can consider calculating the SYNTAX score to determine if CABG or PCI is preferable
    - SYNTAX is an angiographic scoring system that uses various angiographic parameters to assess the multivessel CAD complexity
    - Patients with low SYNTAX scores have no differences in outcomes when treated with either multivessel PCI or CABG
    - Patients with a high SYNTAX score derive greater benefit from CABG, which is associated with less major cardiac events (cardiac death and MI)

PRIMARY PREVENTION OF CORONARY ARTERY DISEASE AND MYOCARDIAL INFARCTION

- Risk factor modification
  - Smoking cessation
    - Cessation decreases CHD event risk by 60% within 3 years
    - Both behavior and pharmacologic interventions should be considered
  - Blood pressure control
    - A 5- to 6-mm Hg reduction in BP results in a 16% reduction in cardiovascular events
    - Management should include lifestyle changes, weight loss, exercise, and medical therapy

- Cholesterol reduction
  - Reduction in serum cholesterol by 10% reduces cardiovascular events by 18% and cardiovascular death by 10%
  - Management should include dietary modification, exercise, and lipid-lowering therapy (based on ACC/AHA 2013 guidelines)
- DM management
  - DM increases risk of heart disease by twofold to fourfold in men and threefold to sevenfold in women
  - Tight glycemic control reduces microvascular disease and may reduce risk of cardiovascular events
  - Patients with metabolic syndrome are at increased risk of cardiovascular disease; aggressive risk factor modification is warranted in these patients (diet, exercise, weight loss, and lipid and glucose management)
- Weight loss
  - Obesity and physical inactivity are risk factors for CAD
  - Though data are limited, maintaining ideal body weight and staying physically active may reduce risk of MI by 50%
- Pharmacologic therapy
  - Aspirin
    - In men, pooled data suggest a 33% reduction in first MI
    - In women, aspirin reduces the risk of stroke in those 65 years or older but has no effect on risk of MI or death from cardiovascular causes
  - Statins
    - Statins reduce the risk of first MI, even in patients with only moderately elevated cholesterol
  - Hormone therapy
    - Hormone therapy increases the risk of cardiovascular disease in the first 2 years of use; routine use for primary prevention of ASCVD events should be avoided
- Diet
  - Fish consumption and omega-3 fatty acids are associated with reduced CAD risk in both men and women
  - Moderate alcohol intake (one drink per day) decreases risk of MI by 30% to 50%; decision to recommend moderate intake should be based on risk/benefit ratio in setting of comorbidities (e.g., liver disease, peptic ulcer disease)
  - Antioxidants do not decrease risk; in a large study of patients with vascular disease, administration of folic acid and vitamins B_6 and B_{12} did not reduce the risk of cardiovascular death, MI, or all-cause mortality

Acute Coronary Syndromes

BASIC INFORMATION

- Epidemiology
  - More than 1 million people experience an MI in the United States annually.

- Leads to death in one third of patients, with 50% occurring within the first hour of a MI
- Pathophysiology
  - ACSs include unstable angina (UA), non–ST-segment elevation MI (NSTEMI), and ST-segment elevation MI (STEMI)
  - **All three syndromes occur when a vulnerable plaque ruptures, leading to platelet activation and aggregation, resulting in the formation of intracoronary thrombus (Fig. 4-1)**
  - The vulnerable plaque
    - Larger, fibrotic plaques with thicker caps are less prone to rupture than smaller plaques, which have softer atherogenic lipid cores and thinner caps
  - Inflammation can lead to plaque instability and rupture; elevated serum levels of certain inflammatory markers (e.g., CRP, fibrinogen, interleukin-6, tumor necrosis factor) correlate with increased ACS risk
  - Other factors can contribute to plaque vulnerability, including shear stress and enzymatic degradation, which both weaken the plaque cap
  - Formation of thrombus
    - Following plaque rupture, thrombotic factors from within the lipid core are exposed to the bloodstream
    - Activated platelets then adhere to the vessel wall when platelet glycoprotein binds to the von Willebrand factor

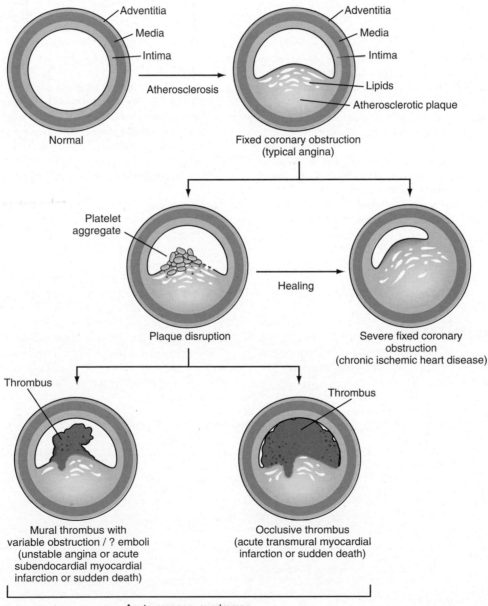

FIGURE 4-1 Schematic representation of sequential progression of coronary artery lesion morphology, beginning with stable chronic plaque responsible for typical angina and leading to the various acute coronary syndromes. (Modified from Schoen FJ. *Interventional and Surgical Cardiovascular Pathology: Clinical Correlations and Basic Principles.* Philadelphia: WB Saunders; 1989: 63; and from Zipes DP, Libby P, Bonow RO, Braunwald E, eds. *Braunwald's Heart Disease: A Textbook of Cardiovascular Medicine.* 7th ed. Philadelphia: Saunders; 2005: Fig. 12-12.)

- Tissue factor is also released from the lipid core, activating the coagulation cascade and leading to thrombin formation, the most potent platelet activator
- Platelets stick to one another during the final common pathway of platelet activation, when platelets expose glycoprotein IIb/IIIa receptors that bind to fibrinogen

- Definitions
  - *UA:* Characterized by angina at rest (usually prolonged more than 20 minutes), new-onset exertional angina of at least class III in severity (i.e., angina with only mild exertion), or preexisting angina that has increased in frequency or duration or that is now brought on with less exertion than before
  - *NSTEMI:* Clinically similar to UA, but distinguished by evidence of myocardial necrosis (i.e., an elevation in serum cardiac enzymes); ECG does not show ST-segment elevation
  - *STEMI:* Defined by the presence of elevated cardiac enzymes and ECG criteria that include greater than 1-mm ST-segment elevation in two or more contiguous limb leads, or greater than 2-mm ST-segment elevation in two or more contiguous precordial leads.
    - **ST-segment elevation suggests total occlusion of the infarcted artery by thrombus; in contrast, most patients presenting with UA or NSTEMI do not have a totally occluded infarct artery**
    - Of note, a new or presumed new LBBB is no longer considered a STEMI equivalent, based on the most recent 2013 AHA/ACC guidelines; must employ other ECG criteria to diagnose MI in these cases
  - Other differences between NSTEMI and STEMI are shown in Table 4-3

CLINICAL PRESENTATION

- Unlike chronic stable angina, in which symptoms occur with exertion, ACS is often characterized by abrupt onset of symptoms while at rest

- Symptoms can include chest pain or pressure (radiating to the left arm, neck, or jaw), dyspnea, nausea, vomiting, and diaphoresis
- Symptoms can be atypical, particularly in women, diabetics, and the elderly
- Of note, 20% to 30% of ACSs are clinically silent

DIAGNOSIS AND EVALUATION

- ECG findings
  - UA and NSTEMI
    - Variable ECG findings, including having no abnormalities, ST-segment depression, T-wave inversions, or nonspecific ST-segment and T-wave changes
  - STEMI
    - Characterized by greater than 1-mm ST-segment elevation in two or more contiguous limb leads, or greater than 2-mm ST-segment elevation in two or more contiguous precordial leads
- Cardiac enzymes used to diagnose NSTEMI and STEMI
  - ***Troponin T and I:* highest sensitivity and specificity for detecting MI; appear within 4 hours; peak at 24 to 48 hours and decline slowly; remain detectable for up to 7 to 10 days**
  - *Creatine phosphokinase myocardial band (CPK-MB):* first measurable in the bloodstream at 6 to 10 hours; peaks at 24 hours; baseline by 48 to 72 hours
  - *Lactate dehydrogenase:* obsolete; increases at 24 to 48 hours and remains elevated for 10 days
  - *Myoglobin:* one of the earliest enzymes released in the circulation during MI (2 to 3 hours), returns to normal within 24 hours; very low specificity
- UA/NSTEMI risk stratification
  - Determine if patient is at low, intermediate, or high risk for adverse cardiac events
    - Adverse risk factors:
      - ECG: ST-segment depression greater than 1 mm in two or more contiguous limb leads (or >2 mm in two or more contiguous precordial leads)
      - Troponins: elevated levels

TABLE 4-3	*Comparison of Non–ST-Segment Elevation MI and ST-Segment Elevation MI*	
	NSTEMI	**STEMI**
ECG findings	ST-segment depressions; T-wave inversions; nonspecific ST-T changes	ST-segment elevation
Vessel at time of catheterization	Only 30%–40% totally occluded	>80% totally occluded
Type of clot	Rich in platelets (white)	Rich in fibrin (red)
Extent of disease	More likely multivessel with collateral formation	More commonly single vessel
Treatment	Thrombolysis not recommended; GP IIb/IIIa inhibitors can be useful	Thrombolysis beneficial; GP IIb/IIIa inhibitors usually not indicated (unless PCI performed)
Hospital mortality	Lower	Higher
Reinfarction rate	Higher after hospital discharge	Lower after hospital discharge
Long-term prognosis	Higher 1-year mortality rate after discharge	Lower 1-year mortality rate after discharge

GP, Glycoprotein; MI, myocardial infarction; NSTEMI, non–ST-segment elevation myocardial infarction; PCI, percutaneous coronary intervention; STEMI, ST-segment elevation myocardial infarction; ST-T, ST segment and T wave.

BOX 4-2	*TIMI Risk Score for Unstable Angina and Non–ST-Segment Elevation MI*

Risk Factors

1. Age >65 years
2. Three or more coronary artery risk factors
3. Prior coronary stenosis ≥50%
4. Two or more anginal events in past 24 hours
5. Aspirin use in past 7 days
6. ST-segment changes
7. Positive cardiac markers
   TIMI Score = sum of applicable risk factors

Risk of Adverse Cardiac Event by TIMI Score

0–1: 4.7%

2: 8.3%   } Low Risk

3: 13.2%

4: 19.9%   } Intermediate Risk

5: 26.2%

6 to 7: 41%   } High Risk

MI, Myocardial infarction; TIMI, Thrombolysis in Myocardial Infarction.

TABLE 4-4 *TIMI Risk Score for ST-Segment Elevation MI*

Clinical Risk Factors	Points
History	
≥75 years old	3
65 to 74 years old	2
History of diabetes, hypertension, or angina	1
Physical examination	
Systolic blood pressure <100 mm Hg	3
Heart rate >100 beats/min	2
Killip class II to IV	2
Weight <67 kg	1
Presentation	
Anterior STEMI or left bundle branch block	1
Time to reperfusion therapy >4 hours	1
Total possible points	14

MI, Myocardial infarction; STEMI, ST-segment elevation myocardial infarction; TIMI, Thrombolysis in Myocardial Infarction.
Data from Morrow DA, Antman EM, Parsons L, et al. Application of the TIMI risk score for ST-elevation MI in the National Registry of Myocardial Infarction 3. *JAMA.* 2001;286:1356–1359.

- Patients with both ST-segment depression and elevated cardiac enzymes are at highest risk; those with one of the two factors are at intermediate risk; patients with neither of the two factors are at lower risk
- Calculate the Thrombolysis in Myocardial Infarction (TIMI) risk score for UA/NSTEMI (Box 4-2):
  - Scoring system uses seven factors to predict the risk of subsequent adverse cardiac events (defined as MI, persistent ischemia, or cardiac-related death)
    - A score of 0 to 2 is considered low risk, 3 to 4 is intermediate risk, 5 to 7 is high risk
  - Calculate GRACE (Global Registry of Acute Coronary Events) 2.0 risk score
    - Incorporates age, heart rate, systolic BP, Killip class, presence of cardiac arrest, ST-segment change, and troponins
    - Estimates 6-month mortality
  - **As a general rule, it is most appropriate to treat low-risk patients conservatively (i.e., noninvasive testing, medical management); more aggressive treatment (e.g., catheterization, PCI) is the best choice for intermediate-risk and high-risk patients**
- Risk stratification of STEMI
  - All patients who meet STEMI ECG criteria should be considered for rapid reperfusion with either PCI or thrombolytic therapy
  - Determine subsequent risk for adverse cardiac events:
    - Calculate TIMI risk score for STEMI: Assesses risk based on history, examination, and clinical presentation; there is an increased risk in 30-day

mortality rates, ranging from 1.1% to 30% for scores ranging from 0 to greater than 8, respectively (Table 4-4)
- Calculate GRACE 2.0 risk score:
  - Same risk calculator used for UA/NSTEMI
  - Estimates 6-month mortality
- **Always consider other diagnoses that can mimic ACS**
  - Chest pain and ECG changes can occur with other conditions, which require different management strategies, including the following:
    - Aortic dissection
      - Findings include abrupt, severe, "tearing" chest pain that radiates to the back or abdomen, unequal pulses and BP in the upper extremities, or a new murmur of aortic regurgitation
      - ECG can reveal ST-segment elevations if the dissection involves one or more of the coronary arteries (typically affects the right coronary artery first)
      - Thrombolytics and anticoagulants are contraindicated
    - Acute pericarditis
      - Findings include chest pain that may be pleuritic or is relieved by sitting up; pericardial friction rub may be present
      - ECG may reveal diffuse ST-segment elevation and PR interval depression
      - Thrombolytics and anticoagulants are contraindicated
    - Pulmonary embolism (PE)
      - Clinical clues include risk factors for PE (e.g., sedentary or immobile patient status, history of

deep venous thrombosis, leg trauma, or oral contraceptive use); symptoms include sudden-onset chest pain and dyspnea
  - ECG may show only sinus tachycardia, but classic findings include an S wave in lead I, Q wave in lead III, and T-wave inversion in lead III; can also present with new right bundle branch block or right axis deviation

TREATMENT OF ACUTE CORONARY SYNDROMES

- Management of UA and NSTEMI (Fig. 4-2)
  - Medical therapy
    - Antiplatelet therapy
      - **Aspirin: More than 50% relative reduction in risk of MI and death in patients with UA/NSTEMI; aspirin should be continued indefinitely**
      - Thienopyridines:
        - *Clopidogrel:* Reduces adverse cardiac events in patients with UA/NSTEMI when given in addition to aspirin; it should be continued for at least 12 months if PCI with drug-eluting stent is performed, 1 month if PCI with bare metal stent is performed, and for at least 9 months if no PCI is done
        - *Prasugrel:* When compared with clopidogrel, associated with lower rates of ischemic events but also with a higher risk of bleeding and should be avoided in patients who may be potential candidates for CABG
        - *Ticagrelor:* Similar to clopidogrel and prasugrel but does not require activation by CYP enzymes in the liver; compared with clopidogrel, it is a more effective and faster inhibitor of platelet activation, leading to lower rates of death and ischemic events with a slightly higher rate of bleeding
      - *Glycoprotein IIb/IIIa inhibitors:* Clear benefit demonstrated in both UA and NSTEMI; the greatest benefit is seen in patients who have positive troponins and are treated with PCI

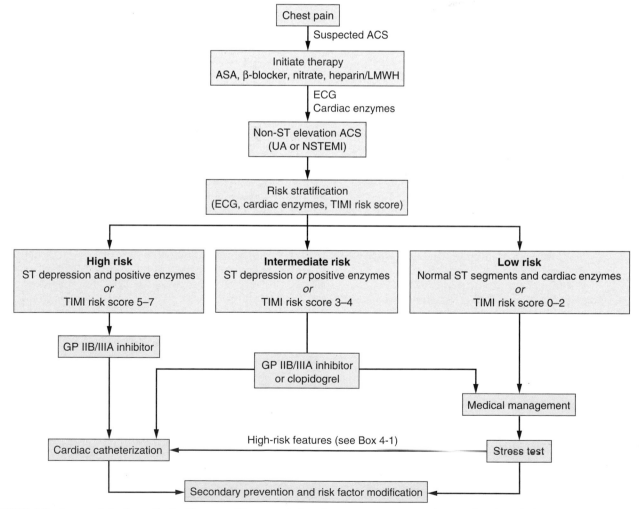

FIGURE 4-2 Approach to the patient with a non–ST-segment elevation acute coronary syndrome. The Thrombolysis in Myocardial Infarction (TIMI) risk score calculation appears in Box 4-2. *ACS,* Acute coronary syndrome; *ASA,* aspirin; *ECG,* electrocardiogram; *GP IIB/IIIA inhibitor,* glycoprotein IIb/IIIa inhibitor; *LMWH,* low-molecular-weight heparin; *NSTEMI,* non–ST-segment elevation myocardial infarction; *UA,* unstable angina. (Modified from Yang EH, Ardehali H, Achuff SC. Acute coronary syndromes: non-ST elevation. In: Cheng A, Zaas A, eds. *The Osler Medical Handbook.* St. Louis: Mosby; 2003: 95–110.)

- *Abciximab:* Fab fragment of a monoclonal antibody directed at the IIb/IIIa receptor; clear benefit for patients undergoing PCI; no benefit seen in patients with UA/NSTEMI who do not require PCI
  - *Eptifibatide:* A synthetic peptide; benefit demonstrated in UA/NSTEMI and PCI
  - *Tirofiban:* A nonpeptide molecule; benefit demonstrated in UA/NSTEMI
- Antithrombotic therapy
  - Associated with lower rates of myocardial infarction and death in patients with acute coronary syndromes
  - Unfractionated heparin (UFH)
  - Low-molecular-weight heparin (LMWH): Compared with UFH, has less nonspecific binding and causes less thrombocytopenia; can be dosed by body weight without need to follow activated partial thromboplastin time (aPTT)
    - *Enoxaparin:* Superior to UFH in reducing death, MI, and recurrent ischemic events in UA/NSTEMI patients who are treated conservatively; no difference compared with UFH in patients treated invasively, and also associated with higher rate of bleeding
    - *Fondaparinux:* Acts through antithrombin to neutralize factor Xa; can be used both with conservative strategy and as an invasive strategy in patients with UA/NSTEMI; preferable to UFH or enoxaparin in patients with increased risk of bleeding
  - Direct thrombin inhibitor
    - *Bivalirudin:* An option only in patients in whom an early invasive approach is planned; if high risk of bleeding exists, then bivalirudin monotherapy can be considered instead of heparin/glycoprotein IIb/IIIa inhibition combination
- β-Blockers:
  - In UA, β-blockers reduce ischemia and have been shown to reduce subsequent infarction
  - In NSTEMI, they decrease ischemia, reduce infarct size, help prevent reinfarction, and decrease mortality
  - Administer orally and only if there is no evidence of concomitant acute heart failure
- Nitrates: Decrease O_2 demand; quite effective in relieving anginal symptoms; have not been shown to improve survival
- Calcium channel blockers:
  - Not first-line treatment for UA or NSTEMI
  - The short-acting dihydropyridines have been associated with increased mortality in ACSs
  - Nondihydropyridine calcium channel blockers may be used to treat ischemia in patients refractory or intolerant to β-blockers and nitrates
  - Do not use diltiazem, verapamil, or nifedipine in patients with LVEF less than 40%
- Statins: In addition to lipid-lowering ability, these agents have been shown to have antiplatelet and antioxidant properties as well

- There is evidence to support their use during the acute presentation with UA/NSTEMI
- Should be administered even if lipid levels are low
- **Thrombolytics are not indicated in UA and NSTEMI**
- Cardiac catheterization in UA/NSTEMI
  - Emergent indications
    - Persistent ischemia despite medical therapy
    - Hemodynamic instability
    - Ventricular tachycardia, ventricular fibrillation, sudden death
  - Indications in patients stabilized with medication therapy
    - Stress test: positive–high-risk results
    - ECG: ST-segment depression suggesting ischemia in a large territory
    - ST-segment depression on ECG and elevated cardiac enzymes
    - Diabetes
    - Chronic kidney disease
    - Low EF
    - TIMI risk score: High or intermediate risk
    - **GRACE score: Patients with high GRACE risk scores (greater than 140) have less death, MI, and stroke events when treated with early PCI (less than 24 hours) compared with late intervention (more than 36 hours)**
- Management of STEMI (Fig. 4-3)
  - **Rapid recognition of a STEMI and immediate initiation of reperfusion therapy are crucial; the faster normal flow can be restored in the occluded artery, the better the prognosis**
  - Two major reperfusion strategies
    - Thrombolytic therapy
      - Approximately 60% successful
      - **Most effective when given in the first 6 hours, but can be given up to 12 hours after onset of chest pain**
      - **After 12 hours, the risk/benefit is unfavorable because the benefit decreases and the risk of myocardial rupture increases**
      - **Between 12 and 24 hours, only consider thrombolytics if there is no available PCI, and the patient has hemodynamic compromise or a large myocardial area at risk**
      - **Indications and contraindications:** see Table 4-5
      - Associated with hemorrhagic stroke: Increased risk in the elderly, women, hypertensives, and diabetics, as well as in patients with a previous stroke or treated with warfarin
      - Commonly used thrombolytics
        - Streptokinase: derived from group C streptococcus, inexpensive, can cause allergic reactions
        - Tissue plasminogen activator (tPA): faster and more clot-specific, more expensive, no allergic potential
        - Latest generation thrombolytics (e.g., reteplase [recombinant tPA], tenecteplase

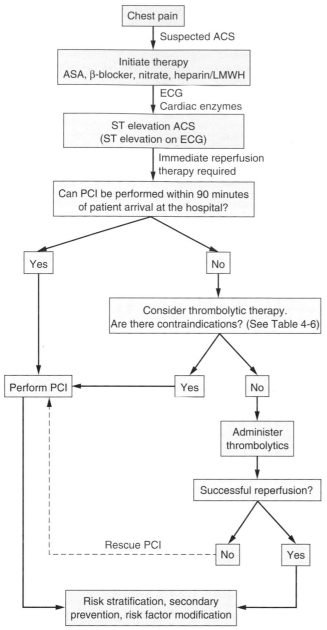

FIGURE 4-3 Approach to the patient with ST-segment elevation acute coronary syndrome. ACS, Acute coronary syndrome; ASA, aspirin; ECG, electrocardiogram; LMWH, low-molecular-weight heparin; PCI, percutaneous coronary intervention.

[TNK-tPA]): mutants of tPA; tend to be even more clot-specific but no differences in clinical outcomes between the latest generation thrombolytics and tPA

- PCI
  - Major advantages over thrombolytics:
    - Higher reperfusion rates (greater than 90% success rate of opening the occluded artery)
    - Decreased incidence of stroke
    - More effective than thrombolytics in patients with acute decompensated heart failure, cardiogenic shock, and prior bypass surgery
  - Major disadvantages:
    - Not available in all hospitals, and it may take too much time to get the patient to the appropriate facility
  - Terminology:
    - *Primary PCI:* Patient with STEMI is taken directly to the catheterization lab for PCI instead of receiving thrombolytics
    - *Rescue PCI:* urgent PCI after failure to reperfuse with thrombolytics
    - *Pharmacoinvasive PCI:* PCI after reperfusion with thrombolytics
  - Approximately 20% to 30% of patients receiving thrombolytics fail to reperfuse and have high mortality rates; they have better outcomes if they then undergo rescue PCI
- General management strategies
  - Perform reperfusion therapy emergently with either PCI or thrombolytics
    - **PCI is preferable if it can be performed in less than 90 minutes after patient arrival**
  - If PCI cannot be performed within 90 minutes of patient arrival, thrombolytics should be given if there are no contraindications
    - If the patient receives thrombolytics, he or she should be then considered for PCI (pharmaco-invasive PCI)
    - If a patient receives thrombolytics and fails to reperfuse, he or she should be referred for rescue PCI
  - **Of note, accelerated idioventricular rhythm suggests successful reperfusion after thrombolytic administration (or after PCI)**
- Other pharmacologic treatments
  - Medication recommendations are similar to UA/NSTEMI treatments

TABLE 4-5	*Thrombolytic Therapy in STEMI*	
Indication	**Absolute Contraindications**	**Relative Contraindications**
Duration of symptoms <12 hours	Any history of intracranial bleed Known cerebral vascular lesion (e.g., AVM) Known malignant intracranial neoplasm Ischemic stroke within 3 months Suspected aortic dissection Active bleeding or bleeding diathesis (excluding menses) Closed-head or facial trauma within 3 months	Systolic BP >180 mm Hg or diastolic BP >110 mm Hg at presentation History of ischemic stroke >3 months Prolonged CPR (>10 min) Major surgery within <3 weeks Recent internal bleeding (within 2–4 weeks) Pregnancy Active peptic ulcer disease For streptokinase/anistreplase: prior exposure >5 days ago or prior allergic reaction

AVM, Arteriovenous malformation; BP, blood pressure; CPR, cardiopulmonary resuscitation; ECG, electrocardiogram; STEMI, ST-segment elevation myocardial infarction.

- Aspirin, thienopyridines, antithrombotics, glycoprotein IIb/IIIa inhibitors, beta blockers, nitrates, calcium channel blockers, and statins all have similar benefits and risks when given to patients with STEMI as compared with UA/NSTEMI patients
- Additional recommendations:
  - ACE inhibitors: Proven benefit, particularly in patients with heart failure and LVEF less than 40%; can prevent adverse remodeling in patients with anterior wall MIs; angiotensin receptor blockers (ARBs) should be used if there is an ACE inhibitor intolerance
  - Heparin:
    - Indicated for all patients going for PCI (unless using LMWH or bivalrudin)
    - Administer concurrently with tPA and continue for at least 48 hours
    - Start 6 hours after treatment with a nonselective thrombolytic (e.g., streptokinase) once coagulation factors have normalized and continue for at least 48 hours
- Medications not recommended for STEMI treatment
  - Empirical antiarrhythmics: Prophylactic antiarrhythmic use can actually increase mortality in the peri-MI setting
  - Glycoprotein IIb/IIIa inhibitors: Only useful if undergoing PCI; not useful in conjunction with thrombolytics
- Monitor for complications of acute MI (see Table 4-6)

4

TABLE 4-6	*Complications of Myocardial Infarction*		
Complication	**Type of MI**	**Timing and Presentation**	**Treatment**
Bradyarrhythmias		Usually in first 24–48 hours for all types	
Mobitz type I block (Wenckebach)	Mobitz I: Usually seen with IMI; caused by ischemia or increased vagal tone; conduction block usually in AV node	Asymptomatic Hypotension	Mobitz I: Responds to atropine and usually resolves in 2 to 3 days
Mobitz type II block	Mobitz II: Usually AMI; block typically infranodal	Asymptomatic Hypotension	Mobitz II: Temporary pacer because high risk for progression to complete block; many will require permanent pacer
Third-degree block (complete heart block)	Third degree: AMI or IMI		Third degree: Permanent pacer usually required with AMI; often resolves spontaneously with IMI
Bundle branch block	Usually AMI	First 24 to 48 hours	Temporary pacer indicated for alternating left and right BBB; RBBB with alternating LAFB and LPFB; LBBB or RBBB with first degree AV block BBB associated with higher mortality
Premature ventricular contractions	Any MI	First 24–72 hours Usually asymptomatic	Treatment usually not required Avoid lidocaine (can ↑ mortality) Can use β-blockers
Ventricular tachycardia or fibrillation	Any territory, but commonly AMI	VT in first 24 hours: usually transient and benign Late VT: consider recurrent ischemia Most VF occurs in first 48 hours	Defibrillation for VF and hemodynamically significant VT For hemodynamically tolerated VT, medicines can be tried before cardioversion (e.g., amiodarone, lidocaine, procainamide) β-blockers decrease incidence of lethal VF
Papillary muscle rupture	Usually IMI	2–10 days after MI Sudden-onset CHF and hypotension caused by mitral regurgitation Large V waves on Swan-Ganz tracing	IABP to help stabilize Urgent surgery required

Continued on following page

TABLE 4-6	Complications of Myocardial Infarction (Continued)		
Complication	**Type of MI**	**Timing and Presentation**	**Treatment**
Ventricular septal rupture	Both AMI and IMI	1–20 days after MI Palpable thrill Pansystolic murmur Hypotension Increased pulmonary artery O_2 saturation by Swan-Ganz	IABP to help stabilize Urgent surgery required
Ventricular free wall rupture	Both AMI and IMI	2–14 days after STEMI Sudden PEA, tamponade, or death Elderly women at greatest risk	Emergency surgery Very high mortality
Right ventricular infarct	IMI	Classic triad: ↑ JVP, clear lungs, hypotension ECG: ST ↑ in V_4 with right-sided leads	Aggressive IV fluids to keep CVP 8–12 mm Hg Avoid agents that decrease preload (e.g., nitrates, morphine) May require inotrope support
Pericarditis	AMI or IMI	2–14 days after MI "Dressler syndrome" Pericardial rub ECG may show diffuse ST-segment elevation and P-R interval depression	Nonsteroidal antiinflammatory agents Avoid anticoagulation

AMI, Anterior myocardial infarction; AV, atrioventricular; BBB, bundle branch block; CHF, congestive heart failure; ECG, electrocardiogram; IABP, intraaortic balloon pump; IMI, inferior myocardial infarction; IV, intravenous; JVP, jugular venous pressure; LAFB, left anterior fascicular block; LBBB, left bundle branch block; LPFB, left posterior fascicular block; MI, myocardial infarction; PEA, pulseless electrical activity; RBBB, right bundle branch block; STEMI, ST-segment elevation myocardial infarction; VF, ventricular fibrillation; VT, ventricular tachycardia.

CARE FOLLOWING MYOCARDIAL INFARCTION AND SECONDARY PREVENTION

- Risk factor modification (e.g., diet and weight loss, BP control, control of blood glucose, lipid lowering, smoking cessation)
- Physical rehabilitation and exercise
  - Decreases hospitalizations, improves quality of life and functional capacity
  - Refer for 36 cardiac rehabilitation sessions (3 times/ week)
- Long-term medications
  - **Aspirin: Reduces rate of second MI and improves survival; should be taken indefinitely**
  - Thienopyridines: Use in combination with aspirin for at least 1 month, and ideally up to 12 months if patient is not at high risk for bleeding; should be used indefinitely in patients who have an intolerance or allergy to aspirin
    - In patients who undergo placement of a drug-eluting stent at the time of infarct, thienopyridine treatment should be used in combination with aspirin for at least a year
  - β-Blockers: Improve survival; should be used indefinitely in most patients following MI
  - ACE inhibitors (or ARBs): Decrease reinfarction rate and improve survival; should be used in all patients with LV dysfunction; help prevent remodeling in patients with anterior wall infarcts
  - Aldosterone blockers: Decrease morbidity and mortality; should be used long term for patients who do not have significant renal dysfunction or hyperkalemia, who are already on therapeutic doses of ACE inhibitor or ARB, have an LVEF less than 40%, and have either symptomatic HF or DM
  - Statins: Reduce reinfarction rates and improve survival in patients with both high and average cholesterol levels; should be used indefinitely
  - Warfarin: May benefit patients with severe LV dysfunction or apical thrombus; no survival benefit
- **Implantable defibrillators**
  - **Improve survival in patients with ischemic cardiomyopathy and low EF (even in the absence of ventricular arrhythmias)**
  - Measure EF at least 40 days after MI in patients who are being treated with goal-directed medical HF therapy
  - **ICD indicated if EF 30% or less with NYHA class I symptoms or if EF less than 35% with NYHA II or III symptoms**

Review Questions

For review questions, please go to ExpertConsult.com.

SUGGESTED READINGS

Antman EM, Cohen M, Bernink PJ, et al. The TIMI risk score for unstable angina/non-ST elevation MI: a method for prognostication and therapeutic decision making. *JAMA.* 2000;284:835-842.

Boden WE, O'Rourke RA, Teo KK, et al. Optimal medical therapy with or without PCI for stable coronary disease. *N Engl J Med.* 2007;356:1503-1516.

Fihn SD, Gardin JM, Abrams J, et al. 2012 ACCF/AHA/ACP/AATS/PCNA/SCAI/STS guideline for the diagnosis and management of patients with stable ischemic heart disease. *J Am Coll Cardiol.* 2012;60(24):e44-e164.

Jneid H, Anderson JL, Wright RS, et al. 2012 ACCF/AHA Focused Update of the Guideline for the Management of Patients with Unstable Angina/Non-ST Elevation Myocardial Infarction (Updating the 2007 Guideline and Replacing the 2011 Focused Update). *Circulation.* 2012;126:875-910.

Morrow DA, Antman EM, Parsons L, et al. Application of the TIMI risk score for ST-elevation MI in the National Registry of Myocardial Infarction 3. *JAMA.* 2001;286:1356-1359.

Morrow DA, Boden WE. Stable ischemic heart disease. In: *Braunwald's Heart Disease: A Textbook of Cardiovascular Medicine.* 9th ed. Philadelphia: Elsevier; 2011:1210-1270.

Moss AJ, Zareba W, Hall WJ, et al. Prophylactic implantation of a defibrillator in patients with myocardial infarction and reduced ejection fraction. *N Engl J Med.* 2002;346:877-883.

Mudd JO, Waters R, Keleman M. Acute coronary syndromes: ST elevation. In: Cheng A, Zaas A, eds. *The Osler Medical Handbook.* St. Louis: Mosby; 2003:111-122.

American College of Emergency Physicians; Society for Cardiovascular Angiography and Interventions, O'Gara PT, et al. 2013 ACCF/AHA guidelines for the management of ST-elevation myocardial: a report of the American College of Cardiology/American Heart Association Task Force on Practice Guidelines. *J Am Coll Cardiol.* 2013;61:e78-e140.

Velazquez EJ, Lee KL, Deja MA, et al. Coronary-artery bypass surgery in patients with left ventricular dysfunction. *N Engl J Med.* 2011;364:17.

Wright RS, Anderson JL, Adams CD, et al. 2011 AHA Focused Update of the Guidelines for the management of unstable angina/non ST elevation myocardial infarction. *Circulation.* 2011;123:2022.

Yang EH, Ardehali H, Achuff SC. Acute coronary syndromes: non-ST elevation. In: Cheng A, Zaas A, eds. *The Osler Medical Handbook.* St. Louis: Mosby; 2003:95-110.

4

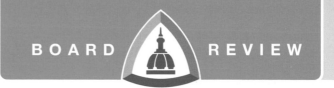
Arrhythmias

GRANT V. CHOW, MD; and JOSEPH E. MARINE, MD

Arrhythmias lead to significant morbidity and mortality and affect all age groups. They are classified as bradyarrhythmias or tachyarrhythmias based on heart rate. Bradyarrhythmias (heart rates <60 beats/min) can result from abnormalities at any point along the conduction path because of depressed automaticity, conduction delay, or block. Tachyarrhythmias (heart rates >100 beats/min) are typically classified as supraventricular or ventricular based on their site of origin. Treatment options for arrhythmias vary depending on the underlying cause and may encompass pharmacotherapy, electrical conversion, pacemaker or defibrillator insertion, or catheter or surgical ablation.

Bradyarrhythmias

BASIC INFORMATION

Bradyarrhythmias arise from abnormalities in one or more of three locations: sinoatrial node, atrioventricular node, or infranodal (Table 5-1).
- Sinoatrial (SA) node
  - Sinus node dysfunction (two forms)
    - Symptomatic sinus pauses (more than 2 seconds)
    - Chronotropic incompetence: inability to attain 80% of the maximum predicted heart rate in response to exercise associated with fatigue or other symptoms
    - Often coexists with atrial fibrillation (i.e., "tachy-brady" syndrome)
    - **Brief, asymptomatic sinus pauses are common; permanent pacemaker therapy is generally indicated only in the presence of symptoms**
- Atrioventricular (AV) node and His-Purkinje system
  - First-degree AV block
    - PR interval prolongation more than 200 ms
  - Second-degree AV block
    - Mobitz I (Wenckebach): progressive PR interval prolongation followed by single blocked P wave; most common site of block is in the AV node
    - Mobitz II: No progressive PR interval prolongation before blocked P wave; most common site of block is in the His-Purkinje system
  - Third-degree (complete) AV block
    - No association between P waves and QRS complexes
    - Narrow QRS (junctional) escape rhythm: usually blocked in AV node
    - Wide QRS (ventricular) escape rhythm: suggests block in His bundle or below

CLINICAL PRESENTATION

- Almost all patients with first-degree and most patients with Mobitz I second-degree AV block are asymptomatic
- Some patients with Mobitz II second-degree and third-degree AV block are asymptomatic; most present with fatigue, dyspnea on exertion, presyncope, or syncope
- Often better tolerated than tachyarrhythmias because they slowly progress, except for infranodal AV block, which may present with syncope or cardiac arrest

DIAGNOSIS AND EVALUATION

- Diagnostic clues are typically obtained from an electrocardiogram (ECG) (Table 5-2)
- Event recorders are useful in correlating symptoms with a suspected bradyarrhythmia

TREATMENT

- Acute management of bradyarrhythmias (see Table 5-1)
- Permanent pacemaker implantation for chronic management of bradyarrhythmias
  - **Indications:**
    - **Sinus node dysfunction and Mobitz I second-degree AV block in the presence of symptoms that correlate with the bradycardia**
    - **Mobitz II second-degree AV block and third-degree AV block, even when asymptomatic**
  - Device types:
    - Dual-chamber pacemaker (DDD, senses and paces right atrium and ventricle), unless permanent atrial fibrillation is present, in which case single-chamber ventricular (VVI) pacing is most appropriate
    - Biventricular pacemaker, which provides cardiac resynchronization therapy (CRT), increasingly used for patients with chronic systolic heart failure (ejection fraction [EF] 50% or less) who require frequent ventricular pacing

Supraventricular Tachyarrhythmias (SVTs)

AV NODAL REENTRANT TACHYCARDIA (AVNRT)

Basic Information (Table 5-3)

- Mechanism of arrhythmia: re-entrant pathway within the AV node complex (Fig. 5-1)

TABLE 5-1	*Bradyarrhythmias*			
Arrhythmia	**Location of Conduction Defect**	**Features**	**Acute Management**	
Sinus node dysfunction	Sinus node	Common with advanced age, coronary artery disease, and atrial fibrillation Very rare in young, healthy patients	Treat only if symptomatic Atropine Isoproterenol Rarely, temporary pacer (if symptomatic)	
First-degree AV block	Slowed conduction within AV node	PR interval ≥200 msec May limit medical therapy for other cardiac conditions	None required	
Second-degree AV block: Mobitz I (Wenckebach)	AV node dysfunction	Progressive prolongation of the PR interval until a P wave is blocked May occur with high vagal tone in healthy individuals at rest or during sleep Usually progresses slowly	Rarely, temporary pacer (if symptomatic)	
Second-degree AV block: Mobitz II	Lower conduction system (His-Purkinje) defect	Nonconducted P waves without progressive PR prolongation Often associated with LBBB or bifascicular block Often associated with prior MI cardiomyopathy, hypertension, or diabetes mellitus	Consider temporary pacemaker	
Third-degree (complete) AV block	Conduction system defect either within or below the AV node	Complete dissociation of P waves and QRS complexes	Level of urgency depends on symptoms, QRS width, and escape rate. If asymptomatic with narrow QRS: atropine or observation If symptomatic or with wide QRS: temporary pacemaker	

AV, Atrioventricular; LBBB, left bundle branch block; MI, myocardial infarction.

5

TABLE 5-2	*Electrocardiogram Examples of Common Bradyarrhythmias*
First-degree AV block	
Second-degree AV block Mobitz I	
Second-degree AV block Mobitz II	
Third-degree AV block	

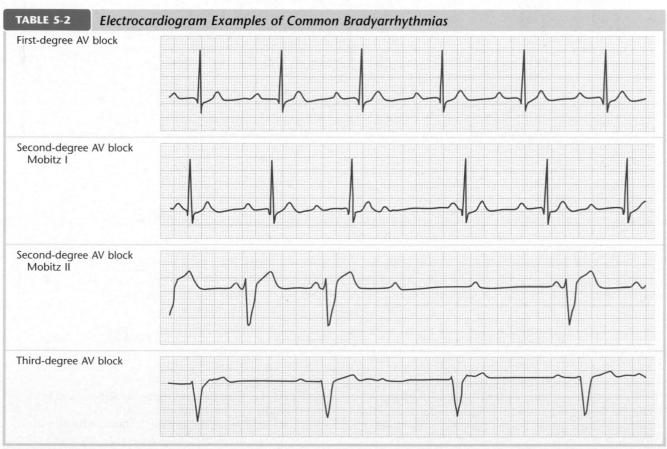

AV, Atrioventricular.

TABLE 5-3	*Narrow QRS Complex Tachycardias*			
Arrhythmia	**Atrial Rate (beats/min)**	**Ratio of Number of Atrial Waves (A) to QRS Complexes (V)**	**P-Wave Morphology**	**Response to Carotid Sinus Pressure**
Sinus tachycardia	100–180	1:1	Sinus	Slowing
AVNRT	150–230	1:1	Retrograde	Termination
ORT*	150–250	1:1	Eccentric	Termination
Atrial flutter	240–320	A > V	Sawtooth flutter waves	↑ AV block
Atrial fibrillation	350–500	A ≫ V	Fib (F) waves	↓ Ventricular rate
Atrial tachycardia	100–250	A ≥ V	Eccentric	↑ AV block
Junctional tachycardia	60–150	1:1	Retrograde	Slight slowing
MAT	100–180	A ≥ V	3 or more different types	Usually none

*Orthodromic AVRT with or without Wolff-Parkinson-White syndrome (tachyarrhythmia with pre-excitation on baseline electrocardiogram).
AV, Atrioventricular; AVNRT, atrioventricular nodal reentrant tachycardia; MAT, multifocal atrial tachycardia; ORT, orthodromic reciprocating tachycardia.

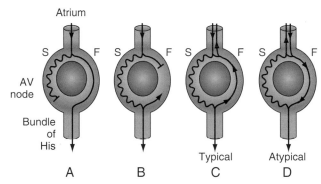

FIGURE 5-1 Reentrant pathways in atrioventricular (AV) nodal reentrant tachycardia (AVNRT). The AV node and perinodal tissue have dual physiology: a slow-conducting pathway with a short refractory period (S) and fast-conducting pathway with a long refractory period (F). **A,** A normal sinus beat conducts through the fast pathway, but conduction through the slow pathway is blocked when it hits a refractory period of the fast pathway. **B,** A premature atrial beat cannot traverse the fast pathway because it remains refractory after the previous (normal) beat. Rather, it conducts down the slow pathway. **C,** In the typical form of AVNRT, conduction occurs down the slow pathway, then retrograde up the fast pathway, with delivery of an echo beat (retrograde P wave immediately following or buried in the QRS complex on electrocardiogram) back up to the atrium. If the slow pathway has recovered, the impulse reenters the AV node, and reentrant tachycardia is established. **D,** In the atypical form of AVNRT, conduction occurs antegradely down the fast pathway and then retrogradely up the slow pathway. The echo atrial beat appears significantly later than the QRS complex because of slow retrograde conduction (RP > PR interval).

- Two functionally and anatomically distinct pathways within the AV node ("dual nodal physiology")
  - Slow-conducting path with short refractory period
  - Fast-conducting path with long refractory period
- **Typical form (90%) conducts antegrade down slow pathway; retrograde up the fast**
- **Atypical form conducts antegrade down fast pathway; retrograde up the slow**

- Although up to 10% of the general population may have dual nodal physiology, only a small proportion will experience AVNRT

Clinical Presentation

- **Notable for abrupt onset and termination of rapid, regular heart beat**
- Heart rate usually 150 to 220 beats/min
- Age of onset may range from childhood to old age
- Occasionally associated with syncope or near-syncope, but usually well tolerated

Diagnosis and Evaluation

- Event monitor may be useful in patients with intermittent palpitations
- Typical AVNRT findings on ECG (Table 5-4)
  - 1:1 relationship of P wave to QRS complex
  - RP interval less than PR interval ("short RP" tachycardia), if P wave can be seen
  - Retrograde P wave at end of QRS complex (pseudo-R′ in lead V₁; pseudo-S in lead II)
- Atypical AVNRT findings on ECG
  - RP interval more than PR interval ("long RP" tachycardia)

Treatment

- Acute management
  - **May respond to vagal maneuvers**
    - **Carotid sinus pressure**
    - **Valsalva maneuver**
  - IV adenosine (6 to 12 mg rapid push) is highly effective (90% conversion)
  - IV verapamil (2.5 to 10 mg) is also highly effective
- Chronic management
  - **Catheter ablation (AV node modification, with ablation of slow AV nodal pathway)**
    - **First-line treatment**
    - **Cures arrhythmia in more than 95% of patients**

TABLE 5-4	*Electrocardiogram Examples of Common Supraventricular Tachyarrhythmias*

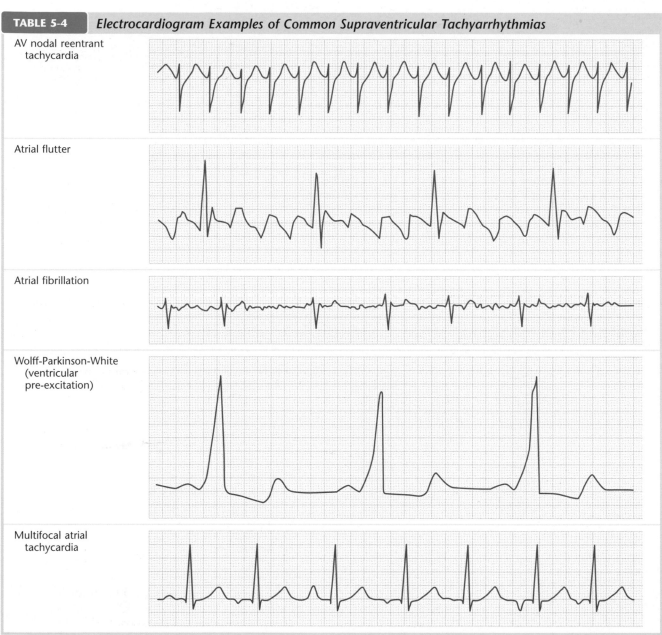

AV, Atrioventricular.

- Medications if not a candidate for ablation (Table 5-5)
  - Suppress AV node: verapamil, diltiazem, or β-blockers
  - Slow conduction within the re-entrant circuit: flecainide (sodium channel blocker)

WOLFF-PARKINSON-WHITE (WPW) SYNDROME

Basic Information (see Table 5-3)

- **Definition: Patients with both pre-excitation on ECG and an associated tachyarrhythmia**
  - Most common tachyarrhythmia is AV reciprocating tachycardia (AVRT)
  - Atrial fibrillation is the next most common arrhythmia, and may be life-threatening in this setting because of rapid conduction down the accessory pathway

- The accessory pathway is a congenital muscle fiber that connects the myocardium of the atrium to the ventricle outside of the AV node (Fig. 5-2)
- The accessory pathway may be:
  - Manifest: The accessory pathway conducts in the antegrade direction (atrium to ventricle) and usually the retrograde direction (ventricle to atrium) as well; ECG shows pre-excitation (short P-R interval and delta wave) and a slurred upstroke of the QRS complex (Table 5-4)
  - Concealed: The accessory pathway conducts only in the retrograde direction; baseline ECG appears normal
- Age of symptom onset is childhood through middle age

Clinical Presentation

- Some patients with accessory pathways may never develop symptomatic tachycardia (these patients technically do not have WPW *syndrome*, but rather have a WPW ECG)

TABLE 5-5	*Common Antiarrhythmic Drugs*		
Class	**Action**	**Examples**	**Notable Side Effects**
I	Block sodium channels; varying effects on maximal velocity of depolarization and duration of action potential	Class IA: quinidine, procainamide, disopyramide Class IB: lidocaine, mexiletine phenytoin Class IC: flecainide, propafenone	Class: nausea, vomiting Quinidine: hemolytic anemia, thrombocytopenia, tinnitus Procainamide: drug-induced lupus Lidocaine: dizziness, confusion, seizures, coma Mexiletine: tremor, ataxia, rash Flecainide: proarrhythmic toxicity, nausea, dizziness
II	β-Blockers; ↓ SA node automaticity and ↓ AV node conduction	Propranolol, metoprolol	CHF, bronchospasm, bradycardia, hypotension
III	Prolong action potential duration	Amiodarone, sotalol, dofetilide, dronedarone, ibutilide	Amiodarone: hepatitis, pulmonary toxicity, hypo- and hyperthyroidism, peripheral neuropathy Sotalol: bronchospasm, polymorphic VT Dofetilide: Polymorphic VT Ibutilide: 1%–2.5% risk of inducing polymorphic VT, requires telemetry during use and at least 4 hours afterward
IV	Calcium channel blockers; ↓ AV nodal conduction	Verapamil, diltiazem	AV block, hypotension, bradycardia, constipation

AV, Atrioventricular; CHF, congestive heart failure; SA, sinoatrial; VT, ventricular tachycardia.

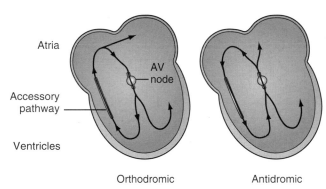

FIGURE 5-2 Reentrant tachycardia in Wolff-Parkinson-White syndrome. In orthodromic reentrant tachycardia (ORT), the impulse conducts down the atrioventricular (AV) node and then retrograde up the accessory pathway. Electrocardiography (ECG) during tachycardia shows a narrow QRS complex without the delta wave. In antidromic re-entrant tachycardia, the opposite circuit is established (conduction down the accessory pathway and up through the AV node). ECG shows a wide, bizarre QRS complex.

- Patients may present with tachycardia: AVRT (70%) or atrial fibrillation (30%)
- AVRT in WPW (see Fig. 5-2)
  - Classified into orthodromic or antidromic depending on the direction of conduction over the AV node
    - Orthodromic AV reciprocating tachycardia (ORT): Tachycardia conducts antegrade down the AV node and retrograde up the accessory pathway
      - Most common form of AVRT (95%)
      - May occur with manifest or concealed accessory pathways
      - ECG reveals a narrow-complex tachycardia
    - Antidromic AV reciprocating tachycardia (ART): Tachycardia conducts antegrade down the accessory pathway and retrograde up the AV node or a second accessory pathway

- Less common (5%)
- ECG reveals a **wide-complex tachycardia**; may be mistaken for ventricular tachycardia (VT)
- **Atrial fibrillation in WPW**
  - **Life-threatening**
  - **Accessory pathways often conduct rapidly with short refractory periods; may result in extremely rapid transmission of atrial fibrillation (AF) impulses to the ventricles**
  - **ECG shows a wide, irregular QRS complex morphology**
  - **May degenerate to ventricular fibrillation and cardiac arrest**

Diagnosis and Evaluation

- ECG findings with manifest accessory pathway (see Table 5-4)
  - **Short PR interval (<120 ms)**
  - **Delta wave with widened QRS complex**
    - Caused by dual ventricular activation through both the accessory pathway and the normal AV node/His-Purkinje conduction system, resulting in fused QRS complexes.

Treatment

- Asymptomatic patients
  - **Risk of sudden death is very low**
  - Equivocal benefits from electrophysiologic (EP) testing. Patients in high-risk occupations (e.g., pilot, competitive athletes) may need EP testing for medical clearance. Some studies support EP testing in younger asymptomatic individuals (younger than 35 years) as well. Older asymptomatic patients with a WPW ECG can be followed expectantly, unless symptoms occur.
- Symptomatic patients
  - **Acute management of AVRT: vagal maneuvers, IV AV nodal blockers (adenosine, β-blockers, verapamil)**

- **Acute management of atrial fibrillation with pre-excitation**
  - **First-line therapy: IV procainamide (slows accessory pathway and AV nodal conduction) or IV ibutilide (may convert acute-onset AF to sinus rhythm)**
  - **Avoid digoxin or calcium channel blockers, which cause even more rapid ventricular response via selective AV nodal blockade and shortening of atrial refractoriness**
  - **Urgent/emergent electrical cardioversion if patient hypotensive or otherwise unstable**
- Chronic management
  - Catheter ablation: first-line therapy in symptomatic patients
    - 2- to 4-hour procedure to localize and ablate (cauterize) the accessory pathway
    - 90% to 95% success rate depending on the site of the accessory pathway
    - Flecainide and β-blockers can be used to prevent further episodes of AVRT in patients awaiting catheter ablation, or if ablation is contraindicated or not accepted by the patient

ATRIAL FIBRILLATION AND ATRIAL FLUTTER

Basic Information (see Table 5-3)

- Atrial fibrillation (AF) and atrial flutter (AFL) are distinct arrhythmias that often occur in the same patient population
  - Atrial fibrillation
    - Most common sustained arrhythmia
    - Sustained by multiple reentrant wavelets within the atria; often triggered by atrial ectopy from the pulmonary veins
    - Incidence increases in older patients (older than 40 years of age) and in those with hypertension, diabetes, and structural heart disease
    - May be paroxysmal (episodes lasting less than 7 days) or persistent (more than 7 days)
      - Paroxysmal form initiated by premature atrial contractions (PACs) or by bursts of ectopic atrial activity (frequently originating in the pulmonary veins); often no structural heart disease present
      - Persistent form associated with one or more of the following:
        - Structural heart disease (mitral stenosis and other valvular diseases, atrial enlargement, hypertension, or congestive heart failure)
        - Hyperthyroidism (1% of AF cases)
  - Atrial flutter
    - Reentrant circuit usually confined to the right atrium, typically proceeds counterclockwise around the tricuspid valve annulus
    - Age of onset: Usually age 40 years or older, similar to AF

Clinical Presentation

- Atrial fibrillation: palpitations, fatigue, exertional dyspnea, dizziness

- Atrial flutter: palpitations, exertional dyspnea; may present with syncope or presyncope with 1:1 AV conduction

Diagnosis and Evaluation

- **ECG in AF (see Table 5-4)**
  - **Fibrillatory (F) waves instead of P waves; atrial rate 350 to 500 beats/min**
  - **Irregularly irregular QRS complexes often at a rapid rate**
- **ECG in typical atrial flutter (see Table 5-4)**
  - **"Sawtooth" P-wave pattern in inferior leads (II, III, aVF)**
  - **Atrial rate typically is at 300 beats/min with 2:1 AV conduction**
  - Carotid sinus massage or adenosine may slow AV conduction and reveal previously hidden flutter waves
    - 1:1 AV conduction can occur in younger patients when atrial flutter rate is relatively slow and excellent AV conduction is present, leading to significant discomfort

Treatment

- Acute management of AF and atrial flutter
  - Rate control with β-blocker, calcium channel blocker (verapamil, diltiazem)
  - Digoxin less useful but can be used if concomitant heart failure is present or if single-agent therapy is inadequate; digoxin is not effective for paroxysmal AF
  - Rate-controlling drugs generally do not terminate the arrhythmia or prevent recurrence
  - Attempt cardioversion if hemodynamically unstable (hypotension, congestive heart failure, angina, etc.)
- Chronic management options for AF
  - Rate control (β-blockers, calcium channel blockers, digoxin)
  - **If symptomatic despite rate-controlling agents, rhythm control with antiarrhythmic agents**
    - Class IC antiarrhythmic agents (flecainide, propafenone) are first-line in patients with structurally normal hearts
    - Amiodarone generally used in patients with systolic heart failure and in patients with severe left ventricular (LV) hypertrophy
    - Sotalol, dofetilide (class III agents) are acceptable alternatives in patients with coronary disease
    - Dronedarone is a newer class III agent similar to amiodarone
      - Appears to be somewhat safer, though less efficacious than amiodarone
      - Should not be used in patients with systolic heart failure or permanent AF
  - Can consider electrical cardioversion to achieve sinus rhythm in symptomatic patients
    - Before cardioversion, patients with AF or flutter for more than 36 to 48 hours should receive either:
      - Therapeutic anticoagulation treatment for at least 3 weeks before and 4 weeks after cardioversion

5

- Transesophageal echocardiography to exclude atrial thrombus, followed by 4 weeks of continuous anticoagulation after cardioversion
- **"Ablate and pace": In selected patients with refractory symptoms caused by rapid ventricular response, AV node ablation prevents conduction of rapid impulses to the ventricle and can decrease symptoms**
  - **Chronic anticoagulation remains necessary, because the atria still fibrillate**
  - **Requires permanent ventricular pacemaker placement because of resulting complete AV block**
  - Generally reserved for older patients with symptoms refractory to other therapies
- Consider pulmonary vein isolation (a catheter ablation procedure that does not involve AV node ablation) in symptomatic individuals with paroxysmal or short-duration persistent AF who are refractory to or intolerant of antiarrhythmic medications
- Chronic anticoagulation prevents stroke in both paroxysmal and persistent AF, and should be given depending primarily on the risk of stroke (CHA$_2$DS$_2$-VASc risk score; see Box 5-1)
  - Cardioembolic stroke risk assessment and indications for antithrombotic agents: Box 5-1
  - Patients on warfarin therapy should have international normalized ratios (INRs) checked weekly until a stable INR level between 2 to 3 is achieved
  - Novel, target-specific oral anticoagulants (NOACs: dabigatran, rivaroxaban, apixaban, edoxaban) are alternatives to warfarin for many patients with nonvalvular AF (Box 5-2).
    - NOACs do not require INR checks.
    - Require dose-adjustment depending on renal function and not recommended for use with end-stage renal disease
    - Should not be used in patients with rheumatic valve disease or mechanical prosthetic valves
- Chronic management of atrial flutter
  - Cardioversion (electrical or chemical)
  - Catheter ablation of re-entrant circuit: 90% to 95% permanent elimination
  - **Anticoagulation**
    - **Thromboembolic risk similar to AF; consider anticoagulant therapy based on CHA$_2$DS$_2$-VASc score and for all patients undergoing cardioversion (same guidelines as for AF; see Box 5-1)**

OTHER SUPRAVENTRICULAR TACHYCARDIAS

- Sinus tachycardia
  - Almost always caused by physiologic stimulus (e.g., fever, hypotension, infection, hemodynamic stress, endocrine disorder)
  - Features: see Table 5-3
  - Treatment
    - Identify and treat the underlying cause
    - **β-Blockade if caused by thyrotoxicosis, inappropriate sinus tachycardia, or if associated with cardiac ischemia**
- Focal atrial tachycardia
  - Arrhythmia usually caused by enhanced atrial automaticity or triggered activity (rare)
  - May be caused by digoxin toxicity
  - Features: see Table 5-3
  - Acute management: rate control or suppression with β-blocker or verapamil
  - Chronic management: rate control; suppression with flecainide, sotalol, or amiodarone; catheter ablation can eliminate arrhythmia in most patients

---

BOX 5-1	*Indications for Antithrombotic Agents in Atrial Fibrillation*

CHA$_2$DS$_2$-VASc risk score – 1 point for each of the following, except stroke:
  C = congestive heart failure (EF 40% or less)
  H = hypertension
  A = age > 65 years
  D = diabetes
  S = history of stroke (embolic or ischemic; not hemorrhagic, 2 points)
  V = peripheral vascular disease
  A = age > 75 years
  Sc = sex category (female gender)

Low risk (score = 0): No antithrombotic therapy
Moderate risk (score = 1): Either no antithrombotic therapy, aspirin alone, or anticoagulation with warfarin or new oral anticoagulant is reasonable.
High risk (score = 2+): Full anticoagulation with warfarin to INR 2-3 or newer oral anticoagulant
Additional indications for full anticoagulation:
  Mechanical heart valves
  Previous thromboembolism (stroke/TIA or systemic embolization)
  Rheumatic mitral stenosis
  Hypertrophic cardiomyopathy

EF, Ejection fraction; INR, International Normalized Ratio; TIA, transient ischemic attack.

BOX 5-2	*Novel, Target-Specific Oral Anticoagulants for Atrial Fibrillation*

Dabigatran: 150 mg twice daily if creatinine clearance (CrCl) >30 mL/min, 75 mg twice daily if CrCl 15 to 30 mL/min
Rivaroxaban: 20 mg once daily with the evening meal if CrCl >50 mL/min, 15 mg daily with the evening meal if CrCl 15 to 50 mL/min
Apixaban: 5 mg twice daily; 2.5 mg twice daily if any 2/3 conditions present: age ≥80 years, serum creatinine ≥1.5, body weight ≤60 kg
Edoxaban: 60 mg once daily if CrCl 51 to 95 mL/min; 30 mg once daily if CrCl 15 to 50 mL/min; do not use if CrCl > 95 mL/min

TABLE 5-6	*Ventricular Tachyarrhythmias*				
Arrhythmia	**Ventricular Rate (beats/min)**	**QRS Morphology**	**Substrate**	**Drug Therapy**	**Ablatable**
Sustained monomorphic VT	140–250	Any	Post-MI, cardiomyopathy	Amiodarone, Procainamide	Yes
Idiopathic RVOT VT	140–230	LBBB	Normal	β-Blockers, verapamil	Yes
Ventricular fibrillation	>300	Polymorphic	Ischemia, cardiomyopathy	Amiodarone, lidocaine	No
Torsades de pointes	200–300	Polymorphic	Long QTc interval	Magnesium, lidocaine	No

LBBB, Left bundle branch block; MI, myocardial infarction; RVOT, right ventricular outflow tract; VT, ventricular tachycardia.

- Multifocal atrial tachycardia
  - Arises from multiple automatic or triggered atrial foci
  - Occurs with elevated sympathetic tone, pulmonary disease (e.g., chronic obstructive pulmonary disease), hypoxemia, stimulant, or theophylline use
  - Features: see Table 5-3
  - **ECG: Three or more P-wave morphologies are present, usually with varying PR intervals (see Table 5-4)**
  - **Treatment: Treat underlying cause (e.g., hypoxemia); rate control with calcium channel or β-blockers**
    - Generally not amenable to catheter ablation
- Junctional tachycardia
  - Automatic rhythm arising from the AV node
  - Occurs in situations of enhanced automaticity (i.e., elevated sympathetic tone), after cardiac surgery, myocardial ischemia, or digoxin toxicity
  - Features: see Table 5-3
  - Acute management: Treat underlying cause
  - Chronic management: No therapy is usually required
    - Rare symptomatic cases require antiarrhythmic drug therapy; catheter ablation may lead to AV block

Ventricular Tachyarrhythmias

VENTRICULAR TACHYCARDIA

Basic Information

- Characterized by a wide QRS complex (Table 5-6)
- Majority (85%) of wide-complex tachycardias are ventricular; remainder are supraventricular with aberrant conduction
- Box 5-3 shows distinguishing characteristics of ventricular wide-complex tachycardias
- Several types of VTs (outlined in Table 5-6)
- VT may be nonsustained (3 beats to 30 sec) or sustained (>30 sec); monomorphic or polymorphic
- Prognosis and therapeutic approach are dependent on presence of underlying structural heart disease (Fig. 5-3)
- **Benign idiopathic VT may occur in otherwise healthy patients with structurally normal hearts;**

BOX 5-3	*Wide-Complex Tachycardia Characteristics Suggestive of Ventricular Origin (vs. Supraventricular Origin)*

History of structural or ischemic heart disease
Absence of an RS complex in all precordial leads (V_1-V_6)
Peak of R wave to nadir of S interval >100 ms in one precordial lead (V_1-V_6)
Presence of AV dissociation (P waves unrelated to QRS complexes)
Presence of fusion complexes (sinus QRS complex fuses with VT beats) or capture beats (sinus QRS complex appears between VT beats)
QRS duration >0.16 sec

AV, Atrioventricular; VT, ventricular tachycardia.

right ventricular outflow tract (RVOT) VT is the most common

Clinical Presentation

- Nonsustained VT: May be asymptomatic or cause occasional palpitations
- Sustained VT: More likely to cause palpitations, lightheadedness, near-syncope, syncope, or cardiac arrest

Diagnosis and Evaluation

- ECG findings (Table 5-7)
- Evaluation for structural heart disease: Should always include echocardiography; additional studies can include stress testing with imaging, computed tomography or conventional coronary angiography, and cardiac magnetic resonance imaging
- Monitoring: Depending on symptom frequency, may include 24- to 48-hour Holter monitor, 30-day event monitor, or long-term implantable loop recorder (ILR)
- Electrophysiologic study: Most useful in evaluation of monomorphic (rather than polymorphic) VT

Treatment

- If hemodynamically unstable, requires emergent cardioversion/defibrillation
- Chronic treatment of most VTs depends on the underlying presence of ischemic heart disease

5

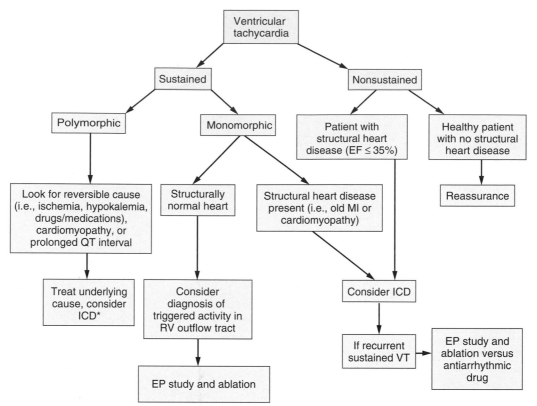

FIGURE 5-3 Approach to ventricular tachycardia. EF, Ejection fraction; EP, electrophysiology; ICD, implantable cardioverter-defibrillator; MI, myocardial infarction; RV, right ventricular; VT, ventricular tachycardia.*Polymorphic VT caused by congenital long QT syndrome or irreversible cardiomyopathy usually requires ICD implantation.

TABLE 5-7	*Electrocardiogram Examples of Common Ventricular Tachyarrhythmias*

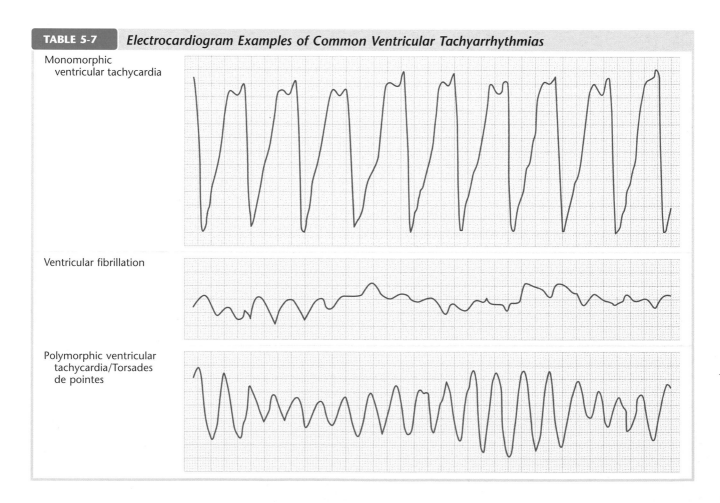

Monomorphic ventricular tachycardia

Ventricular fibrillation

Polymorphic ventricular tachycardia/Torsades de pointes

- Patients with monomorphic VT and no underlying structural heart disease (i.e., idiopathic VT) have a good prognosis and have 80% to 90% cure rates with catheter ablation
- Medications: see Table 5-6
  - Medical treatment: Depends on the etiology. Consider β-blockers, amiodarone, lidocaine, verapamil, sotalol, and others. Should be managed by a cardiologist.
- Patients with underlying heart disease and depressed LV function (EF ≤35%) are at increased risk of sudden death
  - Consider placing an implantable cardioverter-defibrillator (ICD), which has been shown to prolong survival in patients with:
    - Ischemic heart disease with previous myocardial infarction and LVEF 30% or less measured more than 3 months after revascularization and medical treatment
    - Ischemic or nonischemic cardiomyopathy (LVEF ≤35%), and New York Heart Association (NYHA) class II or III heart failure despite at least 3 months of guideline-directed medical therapy with β-blockers and afterload-reducing agents
  - EP study may be useful for risk stratification in some patients with milder forms of cardiomyopathy who have nonsustained VT or symptoms possibly related to VT (i.e., palpitations, syncope)
  - Catheter ablation is a useful adjunctive therapy for recurrent VT in patients with ICDs and can help prevent symptoms and recurrent ICD shocks

VENTRICULAR FIBRILLATION

Basic Information

- Characterized by irregular, chaotic, wide QRS complexes (see Table 5-6) with rates greater than 300 beats/min
- Causes:
  - Acute myocardial infarction
  - Myocardial ischemia
  - Cardiomyopathy
  - Metabolic disturbance (i.e., hypokalemia, acidosis)
  - Drugs (i.e., digoxin, tricyclic antidepressants, cocaine)

Clinical Presentation

- Cardiac arrest or sudden death

Diagnosis and Evaluation

- ECG findings: see Table 5-7

Treatment

- **Immediate electrical defibrillation**
- Medications: see Table 5-6
- Consider ICD placement for secondary prevention, unless ventricular fibrillation caused by a transient or reversible etiology (i.e., intoxication, acute myocardial infarction)

TORSADES DE POINTES

Basic Information

- **A form of polymorphic VT associated with prolonged ventricular repolarization, manifesting on ECG as a prolonged QT interval**
- Associated with both congenital and acquired long QT syndromes (LQTSs)
- Congenital LQTS usually results from mutations in cardiac ion channels affecting ventricular repolarization (most commonly potassium or sodium channels)
  - A genetic mutation can be identified in 60% to 70% of affected individuals/families
- Acquired LQTS is most commonly associated with administration of certain medications (see www.qtdrugs.org; Box 5-4) or electrolyte disturbances (i.e., hypokalemia, hypomagnesemia)
- Polymorphic VT is usually precipitated by a premature ventricular contraction occurring on the preceding T wave (R-on-T wave)

Clinical Presentation

- Sudden death, syncope, presyncope, or may be asymptomatic

Diagnosis and Evaluation

- ECG: polymorphic VT in patients with a prolonged QT interval at baseline (see Tables 5-6 and 5-7)

Treatment

- **Acute management**
  - **IV magnesium (2-g intravenous push, repeat as necessary)**
  - **Correct underlying metabolic abnormality or stop offending medication**
  - Consider Class IB antiarrhythmic (e.g., IV lidocaine (1 to 1.5 mg/kg over 2 min)
  - Increase heart rate to decrease QT duration:
    - IV isoproterenol
    - Place temporary pacer and overdrive pace to 90 to 100 beats/min

BOX 5-4	*Select Drugs Associated with Torsades de Pointes**

Class IA antiarrhythmics (quinidine, procainamide, disopyramide)
Class III antiarrhythmics (sotalol, dofetilide, ibutilide, amiodarone)
Methadone
Erythromycin
Ketoconazole
Haloperidol
Cisapride
Pentamidine

*See www.qtdrugs.org.

- Chronic management
  - Avoid QT-prolonging drugs
  - Avoid hypokalemia and hypomagnesemia
  - Use β-blockers in patients with congenital LQTS
  - **Consider ICD placement in patients with congenital LQTS and who have recurrent syncope or Torsades de Pointes on β-blockers, personal/family history of cardiac arrest, or other high-risk markers**

Syncope

BASIC INFORMATION

- Common (lifetime prevalence 20% to 25%)
- Etiologies categorized into cardiac, neurally mediated, and orthostatic diagnoses (Box 5-5)
  - Cause not identified in approximately 25% to 40% of cases

CLINICAL PRESENTATION

- **Transient, involuntary loss of consciousness and postural tone (lasting seconds to minutes) caused by cerebral hypoperfusion, followed by full spontaneous recovery**
  - Does *not* include loss of consciousness caused by seizure, hypoglycemia, cataplexy, etc.

DIAGNOSIS AND EVALUATION

- History and physical:
  - Ascertain history, symptoms, or signs of cardiac or neurologic disease
  - Determine precipitating factors, prodromal and recovery symptoms
  - Evaluate for possible offending medications
  - Obtain orthostatic vital signs

BOX 5-5 | *Causes of Syncope*

Cardiogenic Syncope
Anatomic: aortic stenosis, atrial myxoma, acute myocardial infarction, hypertrophic cardiomyopathy
Arrhythmic: bradycardia, tachycardia
Extracardiac obstructive: pericardial constriction or tamponade, pulmonary embolism, aortic dissection

Neurally Mediated (Reflex) Syncope
Vagally mediated/vasovagal
Carotid sinus syncope
Situational: cough, sneeze, micturition, post-exercise

Orthostatic Syncope
Volume depletion
Drug-induced: antihypertensives, alcohol, antidepressants
Primary autonomic failure: idiopathic dysautonomia, Lewy body dementia, multiple system atrophy, Parkinson disease with autonomic involvement
Secondary autonomic failure: diabetes, amyloidosis, spinal injury

Conditions with Altered Consciousness Commonly Miscategorized as Syncope
Metabolic: hyperventilation, hypoglycemia, hypoxemia
Neurologic: seizures, migraines

- A careful history and physical examination often provide important clues
- ECG is essential in all patients
- Echocardiogram often useful to assess for structural heart disease
- **In the presence of structural heart disease, arrhythmia is the most likely cause (often life threatening)**
  - Refer for EP evaluation
- **In the absence of structural heart disease, vasovagal syncope is the most likely cause**
  - Can consider tilt-table testing to evaluate autonomic system in patients with recurrent episodes

TREATMENT

- Treat the underlying condition; remove nonessential medications that may contribute to episodes
- Vasovagal syncope
  - Increase fluid and salt intake
  - Advise patients to stand slowly from a seated position
  - Eliminate offending medications
  - Consider midodrine or selective serotonin reuptake inhibitors (SSRIs) in refractory cases
  - Consider pacemaker placement in exceptional cases associated with documented prolonged asystole

Sudden Cardiac Death

BASIC INFORMATION

- *Sudden cardiac death* is defined as sudden unexpected death that occurs within 1 hour of symptoms because of a documented or presumed cardiac cause
- Ventricular fibrillation or pulseless VT is responsible for 30% to 60% of events, with a majority occurring in patients with structural heart disease
  - May represent the first manifestation of ischemic heart disease

DIAGNOSIS AND EVALUATION

- ECG for evidence of myocardial infarction or ischemia, accessory pathway (WPW syndrome), prolonged QT interval, Brugada syndrome
- Laboratory tests, including cardiac enzymes, electrolytes, drug levels, and urine toxicology screens
- Continuous telemetry to monitor for recurrent events until definitive treatment
- Echocardiogram to evaluate for structural heart disease
- Coronary angiography in most cases to exclude coronary artery disease or congenital coronary artery anomalies

TREATMENT

- Treat underlying causes
- Eliminate proarrhythmic medications
- Coronary artery revascularization in patients with ischemic heart disease
- IV amiodarone or lidocaine useful in acute management of repeated arrhythmia

| BOX 5-6 | *Indications for ICD Implantation* |

- Documented VT/VF cardiac arrest not caused by transient or reversible causes (i.e., MI, intoxication)
- Documented familial or inherited conditions with high risk of life-threatening arrhythmia, such as LQTS, HCM
- Documented previous MI (>40 days), LVEF <40%, inducible sustained VT or VF at EP study (MADIT-1 criteria)
- Documented previous MI, LVEF ≤30% either 40 days following medically managed MI or 3 months following revascularization (percutaneous coronary intervention or bypass surgery)
- Patients with ischemic or nonischemic dilated cardiomyopathy, measured LVEF ≤35%, and NYHA class II or III CHF despite at least three months of guideline-directed medical therapy
- Patients with NYHA class IV CHF who meet other requirements for cardiac resynchronization therapy

CABG, Coronary artery bypass grafting; CHF, congestive heart failure; EP, electrophysiology; HCM, hypertrophic cardiomyopathy; LQTS, long QT syndrome; LVEF, left ventricular ejection fraction; MADIT-1, Multicenter Automatic Defibrillator Implantation Trial 1; MI, myocardial infarction; NYHA, New York Heart Association; PTCA, percutaneous transluminal coronary angioplasty; VF, ventricular fibrillation; VT, ventricular tachycardia.

- ICD placement in most patients with VT or ventricular fibrillation causing cardiac arrest that is not caused by transient or reversible causes (Box 5-6)

Review Questions

For review questions, please go to ExpertConsult.com.

SUGGESTED READINGS

A comparison of antiarrhythmic-drug therapy with implantable defibrillators in patients resuscitated from near-fatal ventricular arrhythmias: The Antiarrhythmics Versus Implantable Defibrillators (AVID) investigators. *N Engl J Med.* 1997;337:1576-1583.

Bardy GH, Lee KL, Mark DB, et al. Amiodarone or an implantable cardioverter-defibrillator for congestive heart failure. *N Engl J Med.* 2005;352:225-237.

Bristow MR, Saxon LA, Boehmer J, et al. Cardiac-resynchronization therapy with or without an implantable defibrillator in advanced chronic heart failure. *N Engl J Med.* 2004;350:2140-2150.

Buxton AE, Lee KL, Fisher JD, et al. A randomized study of the prevention of sudden death in patients with coronary artery disease. Multicenter Unsustained Tachycardia Trial Investigators. *N Engl J Med.* 1999;341:1882-1890.

Calkins H, Yong P, Miller JM, et al. Catheter ablation of accessory pathways, atrioventricular nodal reentrant tachycardia, and the atrioventricular junction: final results of a prospective, multicenter clinical trial. The ATAKR multicenter investigators group. *Circulation.* 1999;99:195-197.

Epstein AE, DiMarco JP, Ellenbogen KA, et al. 2012 ACCF/AHA/HRS focused update incorporated into the ACCF/AHA/HRS 2008 Guidelines for Device-based Therapy of Cardiac Rhythm Abnormalities: a report of the American College of Cardiology Foundation/American Heart Association Task Force on Practice Guidelines and the Heart Rhythm Society. *J Am Coll Cardiol.* 2013;61:e6-e75.

Haissaguerre M, Jais P, Shah DC, et al. Spontaneous initiation of atrial fibrillation by ectopic beats originating in the pulmonary veins. *N Engl J Med.* 1998;339:659-666.

January CT, Wann LS, Alpert JS. 2014 AHA/ACC/HRS Guideline for the Management of Patients with Atrial Fibrillation: a report of the American College of Cardiology/American Heart Association Task Force on Practice Guidelines and the Heart Rhythm Society. *J Am Coll Cardiol.* 2014;64:e1-e76.

Moss AJ, Zareha W, Hall WJ, et al. Prophylactic implantation of a defibrillator in patients with myocardial infarction and reduced ejection fraction. *N Engl J Med.* 2002;346:877-883.

Moya A, Sutton R, Ammirati F, et al. Task Force for the Diagnosis and Management of Syncope; European Society of Cardiology (ESC); European Heart Rhythm Association (EHRA); Heart Failure Association (HFA); Heart Rhythm Society (HRS), Guidelines for the diagnosis and management of syncope (version 2009). *Eur Heart J.* 2009;30:2631-2671.

5

CHAPTER 6

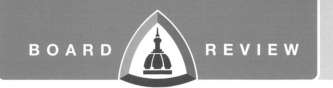

Heart Failure

ROSANNE ROUF, MD

Heart failure (HF) is common and leads to significant morbidity and mortality. In the United States, approximately 6 million people have HF, and up to 550,000 cases are newly diagnosed each year. Survival is poor, with only half of patients surviving longer than 5 years. HF exists when the heart can no longer meet the metabolic needs of the body. It can result from any disorder that impairs the ability of the ventricle to fill or pump blood. Identification of the cause, followed by aggressive treatment, is crucial.

BASIC INFORMATION

- **Definition: HF is a complex clinical syndrome that occurs when the heart or circulation is unable to meet the metabolic demands of peripheral tissue at normal cardiac filling pressures; it can occur in patients with normal or depressed systolic function**
- Commonly divided into systolic (HF with reduced ejection fraction, HFrEF) and nonsystolic HF (HF with preserved EF, HFpEF) (Table 6-1)
  - **Systolic (HFrEF): The left ventricle (LV) contracts poorly and empties inadequately, leading to depressed systolic function and reduced ejection fraction (EF)**
    - More common (60% of patients)
    - Often leads to right ventricular failure
    - Over time, the LV dilates, increasing wall stress and oxygen demand. Can result from pressure or volume overload causing abnormal hemodynamic stress and pathologic remodeling. Causes include:
      - Myocardial infarction, ischemia
      - Hypertension
      - Valvular heart disease (e.g., aortic stenosis, mitral regurgitation)
      - Intracardiac shunting (ventricular septal defect, atrial septal defect, patent ductus arteriosus)
    - Can also result from direct myocyte damage or abnormalities, including:
      - Toxins (alcohol, cocaine)
      - Drugs (chemotherapeutic agents)
      - Infection/inflammation (myocarditis)
      - Inherited/familial (dilated cardiomyopathy, muscular dystrophy, glycogen storage diseases)
  - **Nonsystolic (HFpEF): elevated diastolic filling pressures despite normal diastolic volumes and preserved (normal or near-normal) systolic function and EF**
    - Occurs in 40% of patients (and increasing in prevalence)
    - Poor LV filling can produce low cardiac output state and poor perfusion

- Can result from LV diastolic impairment because of impaired relaxation as a result of thickened or stiff ventricular walls due to:
  - Aging
  - Hypertension
  - Diabetes
  - Obesity
  - Ischemia
  - Constrictive pericarditis
  - Infiltrative disease (amyloid, sarcoid, hemochromatosis)
  - Inherited/familial (hypertrophic cardiomyopathy [HCM])
  - Fibrosis (scleroderma, radiation therapy/chemotherapy)
  - Idiopathic (restrictive cardiomyopathy)
- Can also result from high left atrial filling pressures with preserved LVEF from:
  - Valvular disease (mitral regurgitation or stenosis)
- Can also result from high output caused by increased metabolic demands or increased cardiac output such as:
  - Thyrotoxicosis, Paget disease, beriberi, liver disease
  - Sepsis
  - Severe anemia
  - Arteriovenous fistula
  - Persistent tachycardia (e.g., atrial arrhythmias)
- **Clinical signs and symptoms:**
  - Left heart failure: dyspnea, fatigue, pulmonary rales, inadequate organ perfusion, and arrhythmias
  - Right heart failure: peripheral edema, increased abdominal girth from ascites, enlarged liver, elevated JVP
- **Most common causes of HF**
  - **Coronary artery disease, myocardial ischemia and/or infarction**
  - **Hypertension**
- Causes of acute decompensated HF (ADHF)
  - Decompensation of preexisting chronic HF from a precipitating factor
    - Natural progression of underlying disease
    - Dietary indiscretion (excessive fluid or salt intake)
    - Medication nonadherence
    - Infection
    - New myocardial ischemia
    - Metabolic stress (e.g., anemia, hyperthyroidism)
    - Medication use (e.g., nonsteroidal antiinflammatory medications that lead to sodium retention)
  - Hypertensive crisis (e.g., hypertensive emergency)

- Myocardial infarction or ischemia, especially if: (1) a papillary muscle is involved, leading to severe mitral regurgitation; (2) a massive anterior myocardial infarction occurs; (3) a right ventricular infarct results in a low cardiac output state
- Acute tachyarrhythmia
- Acute endocarditis (leading to severe regurgitation)
- Acute dilated cardiomyopathy (e.g., myocarditis, cocaine, toxins)
- Cardiac tamponade
- High-output HF (e.g., Paget disease, thyrotoxicosis, beriberi, sepsis)
- **Cardiomyopathy: intrinsic heart muscle disease, possibly affecting myocytes, nonmyocytes, or myocardial interstitium, leading to impaired diastolic and/or systolic function. Classified into three broad types:**
  - **Dilated cardiomyopathy (Fig. 6-1): Ventricular dilation associated with decreased contractility (LVEF <45%); can result in HFrEF**

- **Most common type of cardiomyopathy**
- **Common causes: coronary artery disease (most common), idiopathic (second most common), inherited/familial (up to 1/3 of cases)**
- Comprehensive list shown in Box 6-1
- Usually presents as ADHF; can also see angina, systemic emboli (from LV wall thrombus), syncope, or death (from ventricular arrhythmias)
- Most worsen after an initial period of compensation, leading to eventual death or requiring advanced heart failure therapies such as cardiac transplant
- Prognosis depends on cause; some improve spontaneously (25% to 30%)
  - The more symptomatic, the worse the prognosis
  - New York Heart Association (NYHA) class IV (i.e., dyspnea at rest): 1-year mortality is 50%
  - For any given EF, an ischemic cause always has a worse prognosis
  - Predictors of poor prognosis: hyponatremia, high cardiac filling pressures, low cardiac index, poor kidney function

TABLE 6-1	*Comparison of Systolic Versus Nonsystolic Heart Failure*	
	Systolic Dysfunction (HFrEF)	**Nonsystolic Dysfunction (HFpEF)**
Incidence	60% of heart failure patients	40% of heart failure patients
Mechanism	Impaired ejection	Impaired filling
Physical findings	S_3 and/or S_4 Weak carotid upstroke Displaced apical impulse	S_4 more common Normal carotid upstroke Forceful apical impulse
Causes	Coronary artery disease Hypertension Valvular heart disease Myocarditis Drug-induced Toxin-induced Systemic disease Inherited/familial	Hypertension Diabetes mellitus Coronary artery disease (ischemia) Aging Obesity Pericardial disease Restrictive cardiomyopathy Hypertrophic cardiomyopathy Infiltrative disease (amyloidosis)

6

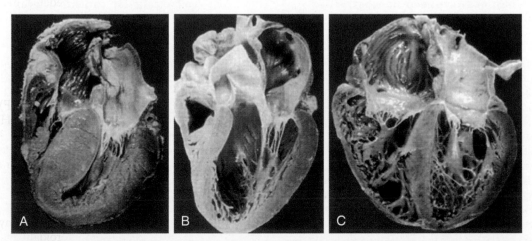

FIGURE 6-1 Gross pathology of hypertrophic and dilated cardiomyopathies. **A,** Hypertrophic cardiomyopathy showing marked hypertrophy, especially of the interventricular septum. **B,** Normal heart. **C,** Dilated cardiomyopathy with increased chamber size and spherical shape of the left ventricle. (From Seidman JG, Seidman C. The genetic basis for cardiomyopathy: from mutation identification to mechanistic paradigms. *Cell.* 2001;104:557.)

BOX 6-1	*Selected Causes of Dilated Cardiomyopathy*

Coronary artery disease
Hypertension
Idiopathic
Inherited/familial
Infections (viral, Chagas disease)
Myocarditis
Drugs (doxorubicin, cyclophosphamide, cocaine)
Alcohol
Peripartum
Glycogen storage disease
Thyroid disease
Vasculitis (lupus)
Pheochromocytoma
Neuromuscular diseases (Duchenne muscular dystrophy)
Uremia

- **Hypertrophic cardiomyopathy (HCM) (Fig. 6-1): Hypertrophy of left, right, or both ventricles with reduced or preserved contractility. Can result in HFpEF or rarely HFrEF.**
  - Hypertrophy may be generalized or regionally limited
  - Caused by gene mutations involved in contractile apparatus; β-myosin heavy chains (most common), troponin T, tropomyosin, and others
  - **Histologically characterized by myofibril disarray (also known as myocyte or myofibrillar disarray)**
  - Differential diagnosis: hypertrophy resulting from hypertension (called hypertensive HCM), renal failure, or Fabry disease
  - Hypertrophy almost always presents by age 30 years and symptoms by age 40 years
  - **All first-degree relatives should be undergo screening with echocardiography and electrocardiography (ECG)**
  - **Symptoms: most asymptomatic, others with dyspnea, palpitations, syncope, and sudden death**
  - **HCM types: obstructive or nonobstructive (more common)**
    - Obstructive HCM: Hypertrophic tissue obstructs the left ventricular outflow tract and can be worse when there is increased contractility and decreased preload
      - Diagnosed when there is a pressure difference more than 30 mm Hg in the areas before and after the obstruction
      - This can occur at rest or with inotropic stimulation (exercise, postventricular premature beat)
  - **Physical examination: Outflow murmur may be present because of turbulent blood flow in the obstructed left ventricular outflow tract region;** augmented with maneuvers that decrease preload (Valsalva, squat-to-stand) or medications that decrease afterload (amyl nitrite, vasodilators); carotid upstroke is rapid (versus delayed in aortic stenosis); parasternal heave may be present

- Prognosis: Variable
  - Most are asymptomatic
  - Sudden death can occur, and it is the leading cause of death in competing young athletes
  - Others develop HF; 5% will eventually develop dilated cardiomyopathy
- **Restrictive cardiomyopathy: Characterized by restrictive filling in the ventricles; typically presents as HFpEF, but depending on the etiology, can lead to reduced EF and HFrEF**
  - Least common form of cardiomyopathy
  - Characterized by significant diastolic dysfunction
  - Ventricular wall thickness is normal or increased but the ventricular cavity is not enlarged
  - Atria typically are enlarged
  - Usually clinically presents as right-sided HF
  - Etiologies:
    - Usually unknown (idiopathic or primary)
    - Infiltrative diseases
      - **Amyloid: Usually caused by primary (AL) form; echocardiogram often shows a refractile ground-glass myocardial appearance (starry-night appearance), and ECG is characterized by low voltages; associated with arrhythmias**
      - **Sarcoid: Typically subclinical; cardiac sarcoid can often lead to conduction disturbances**
      - Hemochromatosis: 15% have cardiac involvement; associated with arrhythmias; can rapidly lead to death if untreated
      - Danon and Fabry disease
    - Löffler syndrome/endocarditis, occurs in hypereosinophilic syndrome when eosinophils infiltrate the myocardium
    - Scleroderma
    - Radiation therapy/chemotherapy exposure
  - Prognosis depends on the cause
    - Idiopathic variety almost always associated with a slow, progressive decline
    - **Amyloid associated with high mortality in symptomatic HF patients (approximately 90% mortality at 6 months)**
- HF Pathophysiology
  - Neurohormonal mechanisms
    - Changes in norepinephrine, renin-angiotensin-aldosterone (RAA), vasopressin, endothelin, atrial natriuretic peptide, cytokines, nitric oxide, and other hormones (Fig. 6-2)
      - Alterations lead to vasoconstriction, increases systemic and pulmonic vascular resistance, and decreased renal blood flow
      - Neurohormonal activation is often initially compensatory but detrimental long term, leading to further ventricular dysfunction
      - Leads to ventricular hypertrophy, changes in interstitium, ischemia, and possibly programmed cell death (apoptosis)
      - Left ventricle further dilates (i.e., remodels) and becomes more spherical
    - RAA-vasopressin system

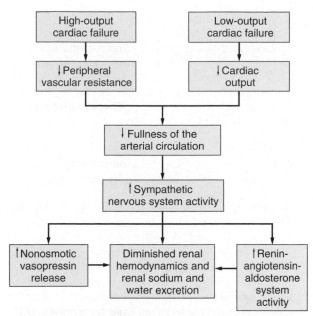

FIGURE 6-2 Pathophysiology of heart failure. Mechanism of high-output and low-output heart failure leading to activation of neurohormonal vasoconstrictor systems and renal sodium and water retention. (From Schrier RW, Abraham WT. Hormones and hemodynamics in heart failure. *N Engl J Med.* 1999;341:577.)

- Decreased renal blood flow activates the RAA system, increasing sodium and water retention
- Angiotensin II stimulates:
  - Aldosterone: Enhances sodium resorption and leads to myocardial collagen deposition and fibrosis
  - Vasopressin: Decreases renal excretion of free water, contributing to hyponatremia

CLINICAL PRESENTATION

- **HF symptoms and signs usually caused by fluid retention or poor cardiac output (or both) (Table 6-2)**
  - **NYHA classification: A measure of functional capacity (Table 6-3)**
  - **A to D staging system. An assessment of structural heart disease and symptoms (Table 6-4).**
- Key symptoms and physical examination findings are similar with most types of cardiomyopathy
- Physical examination findings: Left heart findings include bibasilar crackles, left ventricular heave with S_3 or S_4, cool extremities (if poor cardiac output). Right heart findings include elevated jugular venous pressure, enlarged liver, peripheral edema.
  - Findings associated with HCM:
    - S_4 more common (because of atrial contraction against a stiff ventricle)
    - Pulse may be bisferiens (two humps)
    - Outflow murmur is harsh, crescendo–decrescendo, located at lower sternal border, and (1) increased by standing, post-extrasystole, hypovolemia, Valsalva maneuver (during strain) (decreased preload increases the obstruction), and (2) decreased by squatting, isometric handgrip (increased afterload decreases the obstruction)

TABLE 6-2 — Symptoms and Signs of Congestive Heart Failure

Symptoms	Signs
Dyspnea	Increased jugular venous pressure
Cough (especially when recumbent)	Crackles (rales)
Orthopnea	Hepatojugular reflux
Paroxysmal nocturnal dyspnea	S_3 and/or S_4
Peripheral edema	Pedal edema and/or ascites
Poor appetite	Hepatomegaly
RUQ abdominal pain (hepatic congestion)	Tachycardia
	Decreased pulse pressure
Fatigue and poor exercise tolerance	Cachexia
	Hypotension
Anorexia and weight loss (end stage CHF)	Cool extremities

RUQ, Right upper quadrant.

TABLE 6-3 — New York Heart Association Classification

Class	Severity of Symptoms	Description
I	None to mild	No symptoms
II	Mild to moderate	Symptoms with moderate exertion
III	Moderate to severe	Symptoms with minimal exertion
IV	Severe	Symptoms at rest

TABLE 6-4 — Stages of Heart Failure

Class	Description
A	Risk factors only No structural heart disease No symptoms
B	Structural heart disease (MI, LVH, valvular heart disease) No symptoms
C	Structural heart disease Symptoms (previous or present)
D	Structural heart disease Symptoms (refractory, end-stage)

LVH, Left ventricular hypertrophy; MI, myocardial infarction.

- Findings associated with restrictive cardiomyopathy and pericardial disease (tamponade, constrictive pericarditis):
  - Present with predominately right-sided findings
  - Findings of infiltration often present in other organs in systemic disorders (e.g., amyloid also causes enlarged tongue and liver)

DIAGNOSIS AND EVALUATION

- **HF is a strictly clinical diagnosis and requires a careful history and physical examination**
- **Laboratory tests and other studies can assist in HF evaluation**

6

- ECG: Look for infarct and ischemia criteria, arrhythmias (e.g., tachyarrhythmias), and complex amplitude (suggesting either low voltage or hypertrophy)
- Echocardiogram: Most cost-effective way to evaluate systolic (HFrEF) versus nonsystolic (i.e., diastolic) dysfunction (HFpEF)
- Laboratory tests:
  - Electrolytes, liver profile, urinalysis to evaluate possible renal or hepatic disease contributing to fluid retention
  - **Brain natriuretic peptide (BNP) may be especially useful in distinguishing between cardiac and pulmonary causes of dyspnea**
  - **Most patients with ADHF have BNP values greater than 400 pg/mL, except for morbidly obese HF patients, who usually have normal BNP levels**
  - Thyroid function tests if patient is in atrial fibrillation, is greater than 60 years of age, or has thyroid disease symptoms
- Chest radiograph: Findings include cardiomegaly and pulmonary venous redistribution; patients with ADHF can also have enlarged hilar vessels and Kerley B lines (Fig. 6-3)
- Coronary artery disease evaluation: Consider stress testing to evaluate for subclinical ischemia *or* preferably coronary angiography, especially if the patient has angina, shows evidence of ischemia or infarction on ECG or stress test, or has multiple ASCVD risk factors

TREATMENT

- ADHF treatment
  - Reduce preload (preferably with loop diuretics)
  - Oxygen (if hypoxemia is present)
  - Reduce afterload (if systolic blood pressure >100 mm Hg); can use intravenous agents if hypertensive crisis is present (i.e., sodium nitroprusside)
  - Increase inotropy if there are signs of hypoperfusion (i.e., dobutamine, milrinone), but beware of increase in ventricular arrhythmias with inotropic agents
- **Chronic systolic HF (HFrEF) Treatment**
  - **Goal: (1) If asymptomatic, delay onset of symptoms, (2) if symptomatic, ameliorate symptoms, (3) prevent sudden death**

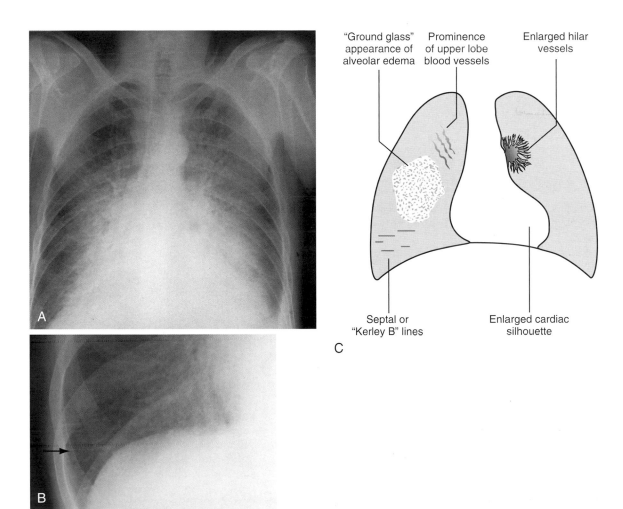

FIGURE 6-3 Radiologic features of heart failure. **A,** Chest radiograph of a patient with pulmonary edema. **B,** Enlargement of lung base showing Kerley B lines *(arrow).* **C,** Schematic highlighting the radiologic features of heart failure. (From Haslett C, Chilvers ER. *Davidson's Principles and Practice of Medicine,* 19th ed., Philadelphia: Churchill Livingstone; 2003: Figs. 12.22A, 12.22B, and 12.22C.)

- **First line therapy: angiotensin-converting enzyme inhibitors (ACEIs) and β-blockers increase survival and decrease morbidity**
- **ACEIs**
  - **All HFrEF patients should be considered for ACEI therapy**
  - Any ACEI therapy can be used; effects are the same for the entire class
  - Start with a low dose and titrate upward to the highest tolerated dose or doses used in clinical trials; need to monitor potassium and creatinine with each dose change
  - Do not stop increasing the dose unless creatinine increases by more than 30% or hyperkalemia is present; patients with hyponatremia, hypotension, and diabetes are most prone to problems
  - Side effects: cough, angioedema, renal dysfunction
  - Contraindications: bilateral renal artery stenosis, ACEI-associated angioedema; severe chronic kidney disease (relative contraindication)
  - Can consider angiotensin II receptor blocker (ARB) therapy, especially if patient develops cough with ACEI; clinical effects and side effects are similar
- **β-Blockers**
  - **All HFrEF patients should be considered for β-blocker therapy**
    - Only carvedilol, long-acting metoprolol (succinate), or bisoprolol have shown benefits in patients with HFrEF
    - Do not start when patient is in ADHF
    - Start at low dose and titrate up to highest tolerated dose or doses used in clinical trials
    - Side effects: fatigue, bradycardia, heart block
- Diuretics (if volume overload is present)
  - Loop diuretics most effective
  - Thiazides are synergistic, and can increase loop diuretic effectiveness (but can cause severe electrolyte disturbances and renal failure)
- **Aldosterone inhibitors (spironolactone or eplerenone) have a mortality benefit in patients with NYHA class II-IV HF, normal renal function, and normal potassium**
  - Should be considered in most patients with HFrEF
  - Carefully follow potassium levels because hyperkalemia is common
- **Hydralazine and isosorbide dinitrate therapy**
  - **Recommended for African American patients who continue to be symptomatic on ACEI and β-blocker therapy**
  - Should not be a substitute for ACEI or ARB therapy
  - Alternative if patient has a contraindication to ACEI and ARB therapy
- **Digoxin**
  - **Decreases morbidity (i.e., hospitalizations) but has no effect on mortality**
  - **Can use if symptomatic despite using ACEI, β-blocker, and loop diuretic therapy**
    - Use a low dose (0.125 mg/dL) and be careful in older adults, those with renal failure, and when

starting amiodarone (amiodarone decreases excretion)
  - Toxicity symptoms include visual disturbances (blurred or yellow vision), nausea, vomiting, and dizziness. Patients can also have heart block and atrial and ventricular tachycardias.
  - Toxicity exacerbated by hypokalemia
  - Toxicity treatments include digoxin immune antibody, atropine, potassium, and temporary pacing
- Other treatments: low-salt diet (2 g daily), fluid restriction (2 L daily), and flexibility in diuretic regimen in response to daily weight changes and HF symptoms
- Avoid: nonsteroidal antiinflammatory agents, calcium channel blockers (only vasoselective agents [e.g., amlodipine] are safe), antiarrhythmic drugs (only amiodarone and dofetilide do not affect mortality), alcohol, and tobacco
- Consider warfarin for treatment of atrial fibrillation, hypercoagulable state, or intracardiac thrombus
  - Also helpful in those with a previous embolic event
  - Controversial in dilated cardiomyopathy without a history of embolic events.
- **Cardiac resynchronization therapy (CRT or biventricular pacing): Decreases morbidity (and possibly mortality) if LVEF is less than 35%, and ECG shows sinus rhythm with an LBBB with QRS width greater than 150 ms, and if NYHA class is III or IV despite maximal medical therapy**
- **Implantable cardioverter-defibrillator (ICD): Prevents sudden cardiac death in patients with LVEF 35% or less and NYHA class II or III HF despite maximal medical therapy**
- Transplantation: Associated with 90% 1-year survival and 70% 5-year survival rates
  - Strict criteria for eligibility because of organ shortage
  - Major early problems are infection and rejection
  - Major late problem is transplant-associated coronary artery vasculopathy
- Mechanical circulatory support: Can be used for short-term support, "bridge" to transplantation, or "destination" (permanent) therapy for patients who are not candidates for transplantation
- **Chronic nonsystolic HF (HFpEF) treatment:**
- **No medication class (i.e., β-blockers, ACEI, ARBs, or aldosterone antagonists) has been shown to decrease morbidity or mortality**
- Recommendations:
  - Treat hypertension aggressively
  - Avoid atrial fibrillation because it shortens diastolic filling time, loses atrial kick
  - Treat myocardial ischemia
  - Use diuretics cautiously
  - Avoid digoxin and other inotropes
- Treatment considerations for specific causes of cardiomyopathy:
  - HCM: goal to ameliorate symptoms and prevent sudden death

6

- For symptomatic patients, use negative inotropic agents (β-blockers or verapamil) to slow heart rate and decrease inotropy; if symptoms persist, consider disopyramide
- Avoid volume depletion and drugs that reduce preload or afterload, which will worsen the LV outflow gradient
- Invasive septal reduction (preferably surgical myomectomy rather than catheter-based alcohol ablation) is rarely necessary; indicated with drug-refractory symptoms and a gradient greater than 50 mm Hg at rest or with provocation
- **ICD needed in patients with a history or family history of sudden death or unexplained syncope, sustained or nonsustained ventricular tachycardia (on telemetry monitoring), extreme hypertrophy (>30 mm) or an abnormal systolic BP response to exercise, or a high-risk genotype**
- **Perform screening ECGs and echocardiograms in family members**
- Treat HFrEF if patient eventually develops dilated cardiomyopathy
- Restrictive cardiomyopathy: goal to ameliorate symptoms
  - Judicious diuretic use (the noncompliant ventricle is preload dependent and will need higher filling pressures)
  - Decrease heart rate
- Avoid digoxin and verapamil, especially in patients with amyloid (high local cardiac digoxin levels lead to increased arrhythmias, and verapamil leads to an exaggerated decline in inotropy)
- Treat underlying cause
- **Make sure the patient does not have constrictive pericarditis, which is different and surgically correctable**

Review Questions

For review questions, please go to ExpertConsult.com.

SUGGESTED READINGS

Gersh BJ, Maron BJ, Bonow RO, et al. 2011 ACCF/AHA Guideline for the Diagnosis and Treatment of Hypertrophic Cardiomyopathy: executive summary: a report of the American College of Cardiology Foundation/American Heart Association Task Force on Practice Guidelines. *Circulation.* 2011;124:2761.

Jessup M, Brozena S. Heart failure. *N Engl J Med.* 2003;348:2007-2018.

Kushwaha SS, Fallon JT, Fuster V. Restrictive cardiomyopathy. *N Engl J Med.* 1997;336:267-276.

Nishimura RA, Holmes DR. Hypertrophic obstructive cardiomyopathy. *N Engl J Med.* 2004;350:1320-1327.

Yancy CW, Jessup M, Bozkurt B, et al. 2013 ACCF/AHA Guideline for the Management of Heart Failure: executive summary: a report of the American College of Cardiology Foundation/American Heart Association Task Force on Practice Guidelines. *Circulation.* 2013;128:1810.

CHAPTER 7

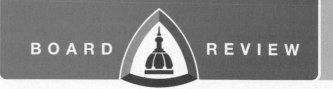
Valvular Heart Disease

THOMAS A. TRAILL, FRCP

Valvular heart disease is recognized by finding a heart murmur, thus highlighting the importance of physical findings in making a diagnosis and assessing severity. Often, physical examination findings trump the results of special testing, such as echocardiography. Murmurs can be first detected in an asymptomatic patient, perhaps a young athlete at a routine physical, or they can be the diagnostic clue in patients with heart failure, such as one with dyspnea and fluid retention. An experienced ear will be able to discern which murmurs require further investigation.

Aortic Stenosis

BASIC INFORMATION

- Causes and etiology
  - Congenital unicuspid valve
    - Usually severe
    - Symptoms present early in childhood
  - Congenital bicuspid valve
    - Murmur present from childhood
    - Common cause of aortic regurgitation (AR) and aortic stenosis (AS)
    - **Calcific AS commonly starts developing in patients in their 30s to 40s**
  - Degenerative calcific disease
    - Starts developing in patients aged 50 to 60 years old or more in a previously normal, trileaflet valve
    - 25% prevalence older than age 65 years
    - Earliest manifestation is **aortic sclerosis**, defined as thickening of the leaflets, presence of a heart murmur, and gradient less than 25 mm Hg
    - 20% of patients with aortic sclerosis develop stenosis within 10 years
      - Progression is biologically similar to atherosclerosis and is linked to the same risk factors
      - However, lipid-lowering agents and other risk factor treatments have not led to slower AS progression

CLINICAL PRESENTATION

- Physical signs
  - Slow-rising carotid upstroke (*parvus et tardus*)
  - May be difficult to detect in older patients with stiff vessels and wide pulse pressure; should be obvious in patients younger than 70 years of age
  - **Systolic ejection murmur**
    - **Synonyms: crescendo–decrescendo, diamond-shaped**

- **Intensity is no guide to severity**
- **Murmur of severe disease sounds "late-peaking"**
- May be conducted to the apex with a musical quality ("Gallavardin murmur")
- Reduced intensity of A_2 (aortic closure sound) with severe calcific disease (single S_2)
- Ejection sound (soon after S_1) signals bicuspid valve
- See Table 7-1 for effects of various maneuvers
- Natural history
  - Excellent prognosis in presymptomatic patients
  - **50% 3-year mortality in patients with symptoms**
    - Classic symptoms: angina, dyspnea, dizziness/syncope
    - Outflow tract velocity on Doppler echocardiography helps to anticipate onset of symptoms
    - If velocity greater than 4 m/sec (i.e., peak gradient >64 mm Hg), symptoms are likely within 3 years
  - Poor prognosis in patients with left ventricular (LV) dysfunction (in whom the outflow velocity and gradient may also be misleadingly low)

DIAGNOSIS AND EVALUATION

- Role of testing
  - Electrocardiogram (ECG):
    - Usually shows LV hypertrophy
    - Severe AS requiring operation is unusual in patients with a normal ECG
- Echocardiography:
  - Shows morphology of the valve
  - Allows Doppler measurement of outflow tract velocity
  - Can calculate gradient and valve area

TREATMENT

- No proven medical therapies
  - **Nitrates relatively contraindicated (may be dangerous to lower preload)**
- Surgery or percutaneous interventions are the only proven treatments
- Timing of interventions
  - Asymptomatic patients are followed, often for years
    - Intervention for a high gradient detected on echocardiography in the absence of symptoms is not routine
    - Intervention is indicated if LV ejection fraction (LVEF) is less than 50%
  - **Symptomatic patients, such as those with angina, dyspnea, fluid retention, syncope, or exertional dizziness, require prompt intervention**

TABLE 7-1	*Effects of Maneuvers on Valvular Murmurs*

	MANEUVERS: EFFECT ON MURMUR INTENSITY*			
Valve Abnormality	**Valsalva (during Continuous Strain)**	**Amyl Nitrite**	**Handgrip**	**Squatting**
Aortic stenosis	↓	↑	↓	↑
Hypertrophic cardiomyopathy (see Chapter 6)	↑	↑	↓	↓
Chronic aortic regurgitation	↓	↓	↑	↑
Chronic mitral regurgitation	↓	↓	↑	↑
Mitral valve prolapse	Moves click and murmur onset closer to S_1	Moves click and murmur onset closer to S_1	Moves click and murmur onset closer to S_2	Moves click and murmur onset closer to S_2
Mitral stenosis	↓	↑	↑	↑

*Valsalva maneuver: During continuous strain, increases intrathoracic pressure, thereby decreasing venous return and preload. After strain, arterial pressure drops and venous return subsequently increases.
Amyl nitrite inhalation: Systemic vasodilator causing a drop in blood pressure followed by a reflex increase in heart rate and myocardial contractility.
Handgrip (isometric exercise): Increases systemic pressure and increases afterload.
Squatting: Increases peripheral resistance, and thus increases venous return.

- Interventional options:
  - Mechanical or bioprosthetic valve replacement
  - Transcatheter aortic valve replacement procedures are increasingly performed, especially for older or frail patients
  - Pulmonary autograft surgery or percutaneous balloon valvotomy procedures are rarely useful

Aortic Regurgitation

BASIC INFORMATION

- Etiology and differential diagnosis
  - AR has a broad differential diagnosis, and it is critical to identify the underlying cause before determining management
  - Diseases of the valve
    - Bicuspid aortic valve
    - Previous endocarditis
    - Rheumatic valve disease
  - Diseases of the aorta
    - Connective tissue disorders
      - Marfan syndrome (Figure 7-1)
      - Familial aortic ectasia
      - Loeys-Dietz and other rare, inherited vascular disorders
    - Aortic dissection
    - Inflammatory disorders
      - Vasculitis (Takayasu disease)
      - Giant-cell arteritis
      - Syphilis
  - Diseases affecting aorta and valve
    - Spondyloarthropathies
      - Ankylosing spondylitis
      - Reactive arthritis
      - Psoriatic arthropathy

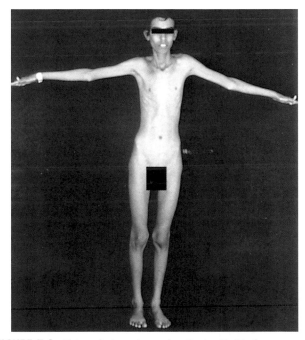

FIGURE 7-1 External phenotype of patient with Marfan syndrome, showing long extremities and digits, tall stature, and pectus carinatum. (From Zipes DP: *Braunwald's Heart Disease: A Textbook of Cardiovascular Medicine.* 7th ed. Philadelphia: Saunders; 2005: Fig. 70-7.)

CLINICAL PRESENTATION

- Acute AR:
  - Causes LV diastolic pressure to rise abruptly during diastole, so aortic diastolic pressure is not much reduced; pulse pressure is narrow, and patients present with cardiogenic shock, small-volume pulses, and an unimpressive or absent murmur

- Chronic AR:
  - Abnormal pulses, enlarged apical impulse, and a diastolic murmur
  - Pulses
    - **Bounding pulses reflect wide pulse pressure caused by runoff from the aorta**
    - In addition to AR, wider pulses can occur because of persistent ductus arteriosus (PDA), arteriovenous fistula, or hypertrophic cardiomyopathy
    - Various eponyms attached to AR pulses (Table 7-2)
  - Other peripheral findings (see Table 7-2)
  - Auscultatory findings
    - Early diastolic murmur starts at the instant of aortic closure, usually medium frequency
      - Longest and loudest when AR is chronic and the patient is doing well
      - When the LV diastolic pressure rises because of heart failure, a torrential leak, or in the acute setting, the murmur is less conspicuous
    - Austin Flint murmur: A second murmur, beginning in mid- or late diastole, caused by turbulent flow through the mitral orifice
      - It reflects high LV diastolic pressure, thus an adverse hemodynamic situation
      - Often indicates the need for surgical valve replacement
    - Effects of various maneuvers on murmur intensity: see Table 7-1

DIAGNOSIS AND EVALUATION

- Laboratory testing: as needed to investigate for underlying causes/conditions
- Echocardiography
  - Differentiates site leading to AR: valve or aortic wall
  - Determines valve morphology
  - Detects vegetations and perforations
  - Assesses associated disease of other valves
    - Mitral valve prolapse: connective tissue disorder
    - Mitral stenosis: rheumatic disease
    - Assesses LV cavity size and function

TREATMENT

- Treat associated medical issues
- No proven direct medical therapies for AR (afterload reduction is not beneficial)
- Surgery or percutaneous interventions are the only proven treatments (same treatments as for aortic stenosis, i.e., valve replacement)
- Timing of interventions
  - Acute AR is a medical emergency
    - **Surgery should not be delayed pending completion of antibiotic treatment for endocarditis**
  - In contrast to acute AR, chronic AR is often well tolerated for many years but will eventually lead to irreversible LV dilation (*cor bovinum*) and dysfunction
- Intervention (i.e., surgery) recommended for:
  - Symptomatic patients:
    - First hint of symptoms: dyspnea, fatigue, palpitations
    - Angina rare with AR; may reflect coronary ostial involvement by aortitis or unrelated coronary artery atherosclerosis
  - Asymptomatic patients:
    - Enlarging LV cavity: LV end-systolic dimension more than 5.5 cm or end-diastolic dimension more than 7 cm (implies combination of a large cavity and some reduction in function)
    - EF less than 50%
    - Aortic ectasia
    - Aortic root greater than 5 cm in Marfan or Loeys-Dietz syndromes, greater than 5.5 cm with other diagnoses

TABLE 7-2	*Peripheral Pulse Findings in Chronic Aortic Regurgitation*
Sign	**Description**
Quincke sign	Nail bed pulsation
Corrigan pulse	Visible carotid pulsation
de Musset sign	Head bobbing to pulse
Müller sign	Uvula bobbing to pulse
Duroziez sign	Diastolic bruit with compression of the femoral artery at the groin
Hill sign	Systolic pressure in the leg >10 mm Hg higher than the measurement at the brachial artery; reflects large stroke volume
Traube sign	Pistol-shot sounds best heard over the femoral artery
Water-hammer pulse	Slapping quality of pulse when the hand is held up and the arterial diastolic pressure is <25 mm Hg

Mitral Regurgitation

BASIC INFORMATION

- Differential diagnosis
  - Myxomatous (floppy) valve (i.e., mitral valve prolapse)
  - Ruptured chordae tendineae
  - Previous endocarditis
  - Papillary muscle dysfunction
  - Mitral annulus calcification
  - Rheumatic disease
  - "Functional" (i.e., from annulus or LV dilation)
  - Rarities (e.g., Libman-Sacks endocarditis caused by lupus)

CLINICAL PRESENTATION

- Acute mitral regurgitation (MR):
  - Causes a very abrupt tall V wave in the left atrium
  - **Hence, acute pulmonary edema, low cardiac output, and an unimpressive murmur that may sound like an ejection murmur**

7

- Chronic MR:
  - Hyperkinetic left ventricle (prominent apical impulse)
  - Pansystolic murmur
    - With acute severe MR, murmur may be shortened because of high left atrial pressure
    - **In general, loudness correlates with severity**
    - Effects of maneuvers on murmur: see Table 7-1
  - Signs of heart failure (e.g., presence of an S_3)

DIAGNOSIS AND EVALUATION

- Role of testing
  - Chest radiography: cardiomegaly, left atrial size, pulmonary congestion, pulmonary artery enlargement
  - ECG: May see atrial fibrillation
  - Echocardiogram
    - Distinguishes between functional and primary MR
    - Determines valve morphology; can detect vegetations and perforations
    - Assesses LV cavity size and function

TREATMENT

- Medical treatment with afterload-reducing medications can probably help, especially for "functional" MR
- Surgery is the only proven beneficial intervention for most types of MR
- Natural history and timing of surgery
  - Chronic MR is tolerated even better than AR; hence, there has been a tendency to operate too late, at a point when the LV is irremediably damaged
  - **It is important, therefore, to follow LV size carefully and be alert to even subtle changes in effort tolerance, stamina, and energy level**
    - **Palpitations could be caused by atrial fibrillation, which is an indication for surgery**
  - Asymptomatic patients need surgical evaluation when:
    - EF is less than 60% (EF should be higher than normal because the LV needs to pump blood adequate for systemic perfusion in addition to regurgitant volume)
    - End-systolic dimension greater than 4.5 cm (i.e., LV has enlarged)
    - Consider if pulmonary hypertension or atrial fibrillation
    - If other heart surgery needed
  - Surgical treatment: Mitral valve repair generally preferred over replacement
  - Interventional treatment: Remains investigational, in contrast to aortic valve interventions

Mitral Valve Prolapse

BASIC INFORMATION

- Etiology
  - Mitral valve prolapse (MVP) is the bulging of the mitral leaflets past the plane of the annulus into the left atrium (2% to 3% prevalence)
    - May be accompanied by MR, not necessarily severe
    - Is normally the result of myxomatous change (i.e., pathologic weakening), but can occur in a normal valve under certain conditions (e.g., hyperkinetic circulation with excessive sympathetic stimulation or an underfilled LV)

CLINICAL PRESENTATION

- **Physical signs (auscultation)**
  - **Midsystolic click**
  - **Late systolic murmur heard best at the apex**
- Natural history and complications
  - Generally benign
  - Infrequent complications
    - Slightly increased risk of endocarditis; antibiotic prophylaxis is not recommended
    - Progressive valve degeneration leading to severe regurgitation occurs in approximately 10% of patients
    - Atrial and ventricular arrhythmias
    - Sudden death: extremely rare; hence, virtually unpredictable
    - Stroke: very rare; thus, no routine antiplatelet or anticoagulant prophylaxis

Mitral Stenosis

BASIC INFORMATION

- Causes
  - **Acquired mitral stenosis (MS) is invariably from rheumatic fever; clinically significant 20 to 30 years after rheumatic fever**
  - Congenital MS is extremely rare

CLINICAL PRESENTATION

- Auscultatory findings
  - Loud S_1
  - Opening snap (follows S_2)
  - Low pitched middiastolic rumble (loudest apex)
    - Accentuates in late diastole caused by atrial contraction
  - Palpable P2
- Severe MS is associated with softening of S_1, dull or absent snap, and soft but long murmur
- Effect of various maneuvers (see Table 7-1)

DIAGNOSIS AND EVALUATION

- Chest radiography: Can show left atrial enlargement and pulmonary edema and right chamber enlargement
- Echocardiogram:
  - Assesses valve morphology
  - Assesses involvement of other valves
  - Transesophageal echocardiography (TEE) needed before percutaneous balloon valvotomy because left atrial thrombus rules precludes treatment

TREATMENT

- Asymptomatic patients: 80% survival rate at 10 years
  - No specific medical therapy
  - Percutaneous valvotomy if technically feasible in those with moderate or severe mitral stenosis
- Symptomatic patients (i.e., insidious progressive dyspnea, paroxysmal nocturnal dyspnea, hemoptysis,

palpitations caused by paroxysmal atrial fibrillation): 15% survival rate at 10 years
- No specific medical therapy
- Requires percutaneous valvotomy or mitral valve replacement/repair
- Percutaneous balloon valvotomy preferable as long as there is pure MS (without significant MR) with favorable valve characteristics and no left atrial thrombus by TEE
- Surgery preferable for calcified, immobile valve or subvalvular chordal disease
- If atrial fibrillation is present:
  - Associated with high rates of embolic stroke that need anticoagulation
- **Mitral stenosis and pregnancy**
  - **Common to have clinical decompensation caused by combined effects of increased blood volume and cardiac output**
  - Careful preconception assessment is indicated
  - In a pregnant woman with new-onset pulmonary edema, consider:
    - Mitral stenosis
    - Peripartum cardiomyopathy

Tricuspid Valve Disease

BASIC INFORMATION

- Causes and etiology
  - Primary disease
    - Rare
    - Mainly congenital
  - Acquired
    - Almost always manifests as tricuspid regurgitation (TR)
    - Etiologies
      - Left heart disease → leading to pulmonary hypertension and right ventricular (RV) dilatation
      - Primary pulmonary hypertension (cor pulmonale)
      - Endocarditis
      - Pacemaker lead injury
      - Carcinoid
      - Radiation
      - Trauma

CLINICAL PRESENTATION

- Physical signs
  - Signs of right heart failure (+S_3, RV heave, increased jugular venous distention, hepatic congestion, and edema)

TREATMENT

- Asymptomatic:
  - Usually associated with mild to moderate TR
  - No treatment
- Symptomatic (i.e., dyspnea, nausea/vomiting, edema)
  - Associated with severe TR

- Can medically treat with diuretics
- Can consider tricuspid valve repair or replacement

Pulmonary Valve Disease

BASIC INFORMATION

- Pulmonary valve stenosis is rare and associated with other congenital abnormalities (i.e., Noonan syndrome)
- Pulmonary regurgitation (PR)
  - Etiologies
    - Most often caused by previous pulmonary outflow tract surgery (i.e., tetralogy of Fallot repair)
    - Pulmonary hypertension
    - Previous endocarditis

TREATMENT

- Asymptomatic patients: associated with mild to moderate regurgitation
- Symptomatic patients (caused by right heart failure)
  - Consider surgery for:
    - Symptoms related to PR, including arrhythmias
    - Decreased RV systolic function (EF <40%)
    - Progressive RV dilation
    - Decline in functional aerobic capacity
    - Secondary severe TR related to progressive annular dilatation
    - Severe PR in a patient requiring another cardiac operation
    - Concern about risk of arrhythmia in patients with prolonged or increasing QRS duration (total QRS duration 180 ms or QRS duration increase of ≥3.5 ms/year)

Antibiotic Prophylaxis

- Goal is to prevent infective endocarditis
  - **Only four indications for prophylaxis:**
    - **Prosthetic heart valves (including bioprosthetics) or valve repair with additional prosthetic material**
    - **History of infective endocarditis**
    - **Cyanotic congenital heart disease (unrepaired or incompletely repaired or repaired using prosthetic material)**
    - **Any valve disease in a transplanted heart**
  - Not indicated for relatively low-risk valvular disorders, such as mitral valve prolapse, bicuspid aortic valve, acquired aortic and mitral valve disorders, or hypertrophic cardiomyopathy
- Procedures for prophylaxis include:
  - Dental procedures that involve manipulation of gingival tissue or periapical tooth region or mucosal perforation
  - Respiratory tract procedures that involve incision or biopsy
  - Procedures in patients with gastrointestinal or genitourinary tract infections
  - Procedures on infected skin or tissue

7

- Surgery to implant prosthetic valves or prosthetic intravascular or intracardiac materials

TREATMENT

- Standard regimen for most dental and respiratory procedures: amoxicillin 2 g given 30 to 60 minutes before procedure
- Alternatives for penicillin-allergic patients include cephalexin, azithromycin, clarithromycin, or clindamycin
- For other procedures, need to tailor antibiotic to likely organisms

Artificial Valves

- Valve repair preferred over replacement, but generally only possible for mitral valve disease
- Mechanical prosthetic valves require lifelong anticoagulation, but should obviate the need for future surgery
  - Especially consider if patient is in atrial fibrillation and needs to remain on anticoagulants
  - Of note, novel oral anticoagulants (i.e., apixiban) should not be used for anticoagulation at this time; use only warfarin and heparin compounds
- Biologic prosthetic valves last 15 to 20 years before degenerating
  - Biologic prostheses deteriorate more rapidly in young patients, those with kidney disease, or those on corticosteroids
  - Biologic prostheses do not need anticoagulant treatment
- Consider biologic valves rather than the more durable mechanical prostheses when:
  - There are plans for future pregnancy (and anticoagulants are undesirable)

- Anticoagulation is undesirable or risky
- Patients are older than 60 years of age (bioprosthesis should last long enough)
- In setting of high endocarditis risk because they are less likely to require removal in event of recurrent endocarditis
- Follow-up of prostheses
  - Prosthetic malfunction
    - Produces the same murmurs as in native valves (exception is paraprosthetic MR, which can be silent)
    - Consider in a patient with hemolysis
    - TEE often required for confirmation and assessing severity
- Interrupting anticoagulants
  - Relatively safe in patients with aortic prostheses
  - Should generally use heparin (or low-molecular-weight heparin) for bridging patients with mitral, tricuspid, or pulmonary prostheses. Also, heparin bridging is needed for older, more thrombogenic valves (e.g., ball-in-cage)

Review Questions

For review questions, please go to ExpertConsult.com.

SUGGESTED READINGS

Nishimura RA, Otto CM, Bonow RO, et al. 2014 ACC/AHA Guidelines for the management of patients with valvular heart disease. *J Am Coll Cardiol.* 2014;63:2438-2488.

Otto CM. Evaluation and management of chronic mitral regurgitation. *N Engl J Med.* 2001;345:740-746.

Otto CM. Valvular aortic stenosis: disease severity and timing of intervention. *J Am Coll Cardiol.* 2006;47:2141-2151.

CHAPTER 8

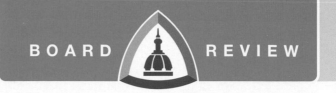

Pericardial Disease

MARY CORRETTI, MD

The pericardium suspends the heart in place, serves as a physical barrier to prevent spread of infection and malignancy from contiguous structures, and prevents acute cardiac dilation. It normally contains 15 to 50 mL of straw-colored serous pericardial fluid, a plasma ultrafiltrate, which acts as a lubricant to reduce interlayer friction during cardiac contraction. Pericardial disease can be caused by disturbances in the pericardial layers, which may also lead to increased pericardial fluid. This can be asymptomatic, or it can lead to tamponade, acute pericarditis, or chronic pericardial constriction. The etiologies are quite varied and can often be elucidated by a thorough history and physical examination.

Acute Pericarditis

- Signs and symptoms of pericardial inflammation that are less than 1 to 2 weeks in duration
- Relatively common: Accounts for approximately 5% of patients with nonischemic chest pain and 1% with ST-segment elevation on electrocardiogram (ECG)
- Major causes: idiopathic, infectious, neoplastic, autoimmune disorders, uremia, cardiac surgery, irradiation, traumatic events, and infarction (Table 8-1)
  - Most common: viral or idiopathic

CLINICAL PRESENTATION

- Antecedent history of fever and viral syndrome symptoms (common)
- Symptoms:
  - **Chest pain (can be severe)**
    - Sudden onset, sharp, and worse with inspiration, cough, and body movements
    - Pain is typically substernal or localized to left chest; left arm radiation is not typical
    - **Classically, pain is positional in nature—worse when patient is supine and relieved with sitting up and leaning forward**
    - May radiate to neck, back, left shoulder, or trapezius muscle ridge
    - May be persistent or wax and wane
  - Other symptoms include dyspnea (common), cough, dysphagia, and hiccups
- Examination findings:
  - Need to perform a complete physical examination for clues to etiology
  - 85% of patients have an audible friction rub

- High-pitched scratchy or squeaky sound best heard at the left sternal border at end-expiration with the patient leaning forward
- Can have up to three components, related to movement of the heart during the cardiac cycle: atrial systole, ventricular systole, and ventricular diastole
- Rub may be intermittent
- Special syndromes
  - Dressler syndrome
    - Results from an immunologic reaction weeks to months after a myocardial infarction (MI)
    - Findings include fever, malaise, serositis, pulmonary infiltrates, and pleural effusions in addition to a pericardial effusion
  - Postpericardiotomy syndrome
    - Etiology attributed to injured myocardial tissue hypersensitivity
    - Occurs weeks to months after cardiac surgery

DIAGNOSIS AND EVALUATION

- Consider the following tests:
  - Serial ECGs: Classically evolve through four stages (Fig. 8-1)
    - Stage I: Diffuse ST-segment elevation with concomitant PR interval depression in most leads (except aVR)
    - Stage II: Normalization of the ST segment and PR interval
    - Stage III: Widespread T-wave inversions
    - Stage IV: Normalization of the T waves
  - Chest radiography: Often normal in patients with uncomplicated acute idiopathic pericarditis
    - Occasional pleural effusions
    - Pulmonary vascular congestion (may indicate severe concomitant myocarditis and heart failure)
  - Echocardiography:
    - Typically normal in most patients with acute idiopathic pericarditis
    - May see effusions
      - May be loculated or diffuse
      - May contain blood, fibrinous, or inflammatory material
    - Can assess for tamponade or constrictive pericarditis physiology (see later discussion)
  - Laboratory studies:
    - Nonspecific markers of inflammation: usually only modestly increased
    - Cardiac enzymes: May be elevated in patients with concomitant adjacent myocardial inflammation

TABLE 8-1	*Causes of Acute Pericarditis*	
Process	**Examples**	
Infectious	Viral Bacterial Mycobacterial Fungal Protozoal HIV	
Neoplastic	Primary (mesothelioma, sarcomas, fibroma, lipoma) Secondary (breast, lung, melanoma, sarcoma, lymphoma, leukemia, ovarian)	
Immune/ inflammatory	Autoimmune and connective tissue disorders (e.g., SLE, RA, ankylosing spondylitis, scleroderma, sarcoidosis, dematomyositis, polyarteritis nodosa, Wegener granulomatosis, Sjögren syndrome) IBD Löffler syndrome Stevens-Johnson syndrome Myocardial infarction Dressler syndrome Postpericardiotomy syndrome Posttraumatic Pleural and pulmonary diseases	
Metabolic	Uremia Dialysis-associated Myxedema Gout	
Iatrogenic	Radiation injury Related to cardiac catheterization or placement of implantable cardioverter-defibrillators and pacemakers	
Traumatic	Blunt trauma Penetrating trauma Chylopericardium	
Drug-induced	Hydralazine, procainamide, minoxidil, isoniazid, anticoagulants	

HIV, Human immunodeficiency virus; IBD, inflammatory bowel disease; RA, rheumatoid arthritis; SLE, systemic lupus erythematosus.

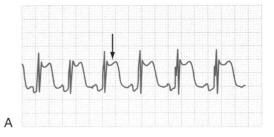

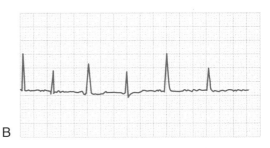

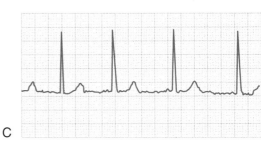

FIGURE 8-1 Electrocardiographic changes associated with pericarditis. **A**, Acute pericarditis. Note the raised ST segments, concave upward *(arrow)*. **B**, Chronic phase of pericarditis associated with a pericardial effusion. Note the T-wave flattening and inversions and alternation of the QRS amplitude (QRS alternans). **C**, The same patient after evacuation of the pericardial fluid. Note that the QRS voltage has increased and the T waves have returned to normal. (From Kumar P, Clark M. *Clinical Medicine.* 5th ed. Philadelphia: Saunders; 2005: Fig. 13.96.)

- Complete blood count
- Basic metabolic panel
- Antinuclear antibodies
- HIV testing, tuberculin skin test
- Other laboratory tests should be considered, depending on the suspected etiology
- Can consider pericardiocentesis for diagnostic purposes, but associated with risk and may not be definitive in those with small or moderate effusions

TREATMENT

- **Acute idiopathic or viral pericarditis is usually a benign, self-limited disease that typically resolves within 2 to 6 weeks**
- **Treatment is primarily supportive: nonsteroidal antiinflammatory drugs (NSAIDs), colchicine, and limitation of strenuous physical activity**
  - NSAIDS: such as aspirin (2 to 4 g/day), indomethacin (75 to 225 mg/day), ibuprofen (1600 to 3200 mg/day), or naproxen (1000 mg/day)

- Can begin tapering after 1 to 2 weeks of therapy if symptom free
- Colchicine: 0.6 to 1.2 mg twice daily for 3 months
  - Usually well tolerated, reduces symptoms, and decreases rate of recurrent pericarditis
- Limit strenuous physical activity for 2 to 6 months (not evidence-based)
- Other treatment recommendations
  - Avoid using corticosteroids because this leads to higher rates of recurrent pericarditis, especially during weaning
    - Can be necessary if there are refractory symptoms
    - If needed, administer high doses (60 to 80 mg/day of prednisone) and slowly taper off over a period of several months
  - Avoid NSAIDS or corticosteroids in patients with post-MI pericarditis
  - Avoid anticoagulants in the acute phase to decrease the risk of intrapericardial hemorrhage and tamponade

- Consider additional specific therapies if there is a treatable underlying cause
- Routine hospitalization is usually not necessary
- Hospitalization criteria:
  - Temperature greater than 38° C
  - Subacute onset (symptoms developing over several weeks)
  - Immunosuppression
  - Trauma-induced
  - Treatment with oral anticoagulants
  - Pericarditis with clinical or serologic evidence of myocardial involvement (i.e., myopericarditis)
  - Imaging suggesting a large pericardial effusion (>20 mm in width)
  - Signs of cardiac tamponade
  - Concomitant MI

Pericardial Effusion and Cardiac Tamponade

- Pericardial effusion
  - Fluid may be transudative or exudative
  - Occasionally occurs with acute pericarditis or fluid-retentive states (heart failure, renal failure, or cirrhosis)
  - Characteristics that can lead to clinical symptoms (caused by increased intrapericardial pressure and hemodynamic compromise) include:
    - Rapid fluid accumulation rate
    - Greater fluid volume
    - Pericardial compliance
    - **Gradual accumulations of up to 1 to 2 L are often well tolerated; whereas the rapid addition of even 80 to 200 mL will result in markedly increased intrapericardial pressures**
- Cardiac tamponade
  - Occurs in 15% of patients with acute pericarditis
  - Any cause of acute pericarditis and pericardial effusion can lead to tamponade, but the most common causes are neoplastic, uremic, or viral/idiopathic
  - Occurs when pericardial fluid accumulation increases intrapericardial pressure, exceeding intracardiac pressures, and resulting in cardiac chamber compression
  - Effects:
    - Limited diastolic filling
    - Decreased stroke volume and cardiac output
    - Elevated venous pressures
    - Decreased systemic blood pressure

CLINICAL PRESENTATION

- Symptoms
  - Can be asymptomatic or manifest with typical pericarditis symptoms
  - With large effusions, symptoms can include dull chest pain or pressure, or a nonspecific sense of discomfort
  - Other symptoms are related to mechanical compression of adjacent structures: dysphagia, cough, hoarseness (left recurrent laryngeal nerve

compression), hiccups (phrenic nerve compression), nausea, or abdominal fullness
  - If tamponade, symptoms include fatigue, lightheadedness, and dyspnea; patients may feel more comfortable sitting forward
- Signs
  - Small pericardial effusions: signs of pericarditis
  - Large pericardial effusions:
    - Heart sounds are often muffled
    - Ewart sign: Dullness to percussion and bronchial breath sounds beneath the left scapula caused by compressive atelectasis in the left lower lung field
  - Tamponade signs:
    - **Pulsus paradoxus: Greater than 10 mm Hg decrease in systolic blood pressure with inspiration**
    - **Classic presentation: Beck triad: (1) elevated jugular venous pressure, (2) arterial hypotension, and (3) quiet "muffled" heart sounds**
    - Tachypnea, diaphoresis, depressed sensorium, cool extremities, peripheral cyanosis
    - If gradual, blood pressure may be maintained and patients present with signs of right-heart failure (hepatomegaly, ascites, and lower extremity edema)

DIAGNOSIS AND EVALUATION

- Characteristic features of cardiac tamponade are shown in Table 8-2
- **Classic ECG findings: reduced QRS voltage, nonspecific T-wave flattening, and electrical alternans (change in QRS voltage from beat to beat)**
- Chest radiography: cardiac silhouette enlargement
- Echocardiogram (Fig. 8-2):
  - Highly useful for detecting pericardial effusions
  - Findings that support a diagnosis of tamponade:
    - Right atrial (RA) (late diastolic) and right ventricular (RV) (early diastolic) collapse
    - Exaggerated ventricular septal shift:
      - An increase in RV volume with inspiration shifts the septum toward the left ventricle in diastole
      - With expiration, a decrease in RV volume shifts the septum to the right
      - This pattern of motion, while normal, is exaggerated in patients with tamponade, and leads to pulsus paradoxus
    - Marked respiratory variation in Doppler echocardiography inflow velocities across mitral and tricuspid valves (flow velocity paradox); also seen in constrictive pericarditis
    - Enlargement of the inferior vena cava (correlates with increased jugular vein distention)
- Computed tomography (CT) or magnetic resonance imaging (MRI):
  - Can detect effusions but less useful than echocardiography
  - Pericardial thickness can be measured, which can help determine severity and chronicity of inflammation and elucidate pericardial disease etiologies.

8

TABLE 8-2	*Characteristic Features of Constrictive Pericarditis and Cardiac Tamponade*	
	Constrictive Pericarditis	**Cardiac Tamponade**
Equalization of end-diastolic pressures	Yes (within 5 mm Hg)	Yes (within 5 mm Hg)
Right atrial pressure waveform	Prominent X and Y descent (X = Y or Y > X)	Blunted or absent Y descent (X > Y)
Pericardium	Thickened (>3 to 4 mm)	Normal
Kussmaul sign	Present	Absent
Pulsus paradoxus	Absent	Present

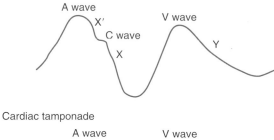

Right atrial pressure tracings—obtained from right heart catheterization (Swan-Ganz catheter)

Normal jugular venous pressure wave

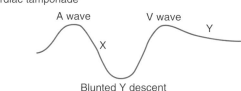

Cardiac tamponade

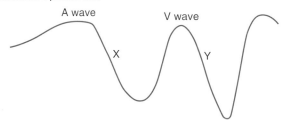

Blunted Y descent

Constrictive pericarditis

Left ventricular pressure tracing—obtained with catheter in the left ventricle

Constrictive pericarditis

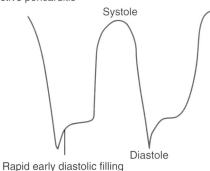

Rapid early diastolic filling followed by plateau phase— the square root sign

FIGURE 8-3 Typical catheterization findings in pericardial disease.

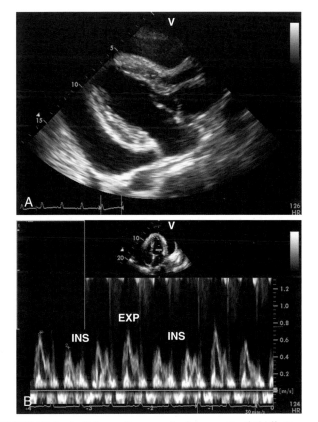

FIGURE 8-2 A, Echocardiogram of a large pericardial effusion with findings of tamponade physiology. Diastolic compression of the right ventricle on two-dimensional images. **B,** Marked variation of mitral inflow velocity by Doppler. EXP, Expiration; INS, inspiration.

- Right-heart catheterization (RHC)
  - RA pressure tracings normally composed of a series of waveforms (Fig. 8-3)
    - The A wave represents atrial contraction (and follows the P wave on ECG)
    - The X descent follows the A wave and represents atrial relaxation

- The V wave represents passive filling of the right atrium beginning after ventricular systole has closed the tricuspid valve
- The Y descent follows the V wave and represents the rapid flow of blood from the atrium into the ventricle in early diastole
- If tamponade is present:
  - RHC findings are diagnostic, although not typically performed
  - **Tamponade increases intrapericardial pressures, leading to equalization of RA, diastolic RV, and pulmonary capillary wedge pressures**

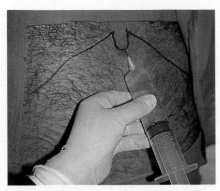

FIGURE 8-4 Aspiration of pericardial fluid. A wide-bore needle is inserted into the epigastrium below the xiphoid process and advanced in the direction of the medial third of the right clavicle. If the needle is connected to the V lead of an echocardiogram monitor, ST-segment elevation is usually seen if the needle touches the epicardium. This can be useful in distinguishing a bloody pericardial effusion from accidental puncture of the heart. Other complications of the procedure may include arrhythmias, vasovagal attack, and pneumothorax. (From Forbes C, Jackson W. *Color Atlas and Text of Clinical Medicine.* St. Louis: Mosby; 2003: Fig. 5.140.)

- The Y descent is blunted or absent (see Fig. 8-3) caused by a decrease in pressure gradients pushing blood from the right atrium to the ventricle in diastole
- The X descent, which corresponds to atrial relaxation, is preserved

TREATMENT

- Pericardial effusions:
    - Asymptomatic effusions, even large ones, may be followed indefinitely with serial echocardiograms and clinical assessments
    - **Pericardiocentesis (indications in Figure 8-4) only needed if fluid sampling is required to establish a diagnosis, especially if symptoms are suggestive of bacterial infection (i.e., purulent pericarditis)**
- Tamponade:
    - Medical emergency
    - **Pericardiocentesis or surgical evacuation of the fluid is the definitive treatment**
    - Temporizing measures before pericardial fluid evacuation include expansion of intravascular volume with fluids and administration of vasopressors
    - Recurrent episodes of pericardial effusion and tamponade treatment may require:
        - Repeated pericardiocenteses
        - Balloon pericardiotomy
        - Surgical creation of a pericardial window
        - Surgical pericardiectomy
        - Injection of a sclerosing agent into pericardial space to cause adherence of the visceral and parietal pericardium

Constrictive Pericarditis

- May occur following acute pericarditis as an inflammatory sequela resulting in a thickened (and often calcified) pericardium, which can then lead to constrictive pericarditis
- Any cause of acute pericarditis can lead to constrictive pericarditis
    - Most common are viral/idiopathic, uremic, post-surgery, tuberculosis, or postradiation therapy
    - Other causes include neoplasms, autoimmune, trauma, sarcoidosis, methysergide therapy, and implantable cardioverter-defibrillator patches
- Time course: months to years after the initial pericarditis episode
- Pathogenesis:
    - Pericardial effusion does not resorb, instead incorporating fibrin deposits
    - Pericardium then develops fibrous scarring and thickening
    - Calcium deposits into the pericardium, leading to further stiffening
    - Result is a rigid pericardium
    - Conceptually can be thought of as a normally contracting heart confined in a small box
        - Rigid pericardium impairs diastolic filling, resulting in increased and equal diastolic filling pressures in all cardiac chambers
        - Of note, the myocardium may be involved in the chronic inflammatory process, potentially leading to intrinsic contractile dysfunction
    - Result: increased systemic venous congestion and decreased cardiac output

CLINICAL PRESENTATION

- Symptoms:
    - Abdominal fullness (caused by hepatic congestion and ascites) and peripheral edema
    - Fatigue, weight loss, and muscle weakness
    - Less common to have orthopnea, dyspnea, or cough
- Physical examination:
    - Elevated jugular venous pressure
    - Signs of passive liver congestion (icterus, ascites)
    - Leg edema
    - **Kussmaul sign: increased jugular venous pressure with inspiration (normally decreases with inspiration)**
        - Occurs during inspiration because the rigid pericardium prevents the increased venous blood from fully filling the right cardiac chambers.
    - **Pericardial knock: Extra heart sound heard in early diastole (mimics an S$_3$), coinciding with abrupt cessation in ventricular filling because of the rigid pericardium**

DIAGNOSIS AND EVALUATION

- ECG: nonspecific findings such as T-wave flattening or inversions
- Chest radiography: may show a calcified pericardium (rare)
- Echocardiogram: Findings include abnormal diastolic ventricular septal motion caused by interventricular interdependence, marked respiratory variation in ventricular size/filling (>25%), plethoric inferior vena cava, and at times, a thickened pericardium (>4 mm)

8

- CT or MRI: most useful in identifying thickened (>4 mm) and calcified pericardium
- Right-heart catheterization
  - Important for diagnosing constrictive pericarditis
  - Reveals elevation and equalization of RA, RV diastolic, pulmonary capillary wedge, and left ventricular diastolic pressures
  - Prominent X and Y descents result in an M or W configuration of the RA pressure tracing (see Fig. 8-3)
  - **The early diastolic filling of the right and left ventricles shows a characteristic dip and plateau pattern, or square root sign, caused by early rapid diastolic filling of the ventricle and then its abrupt halt (see Fig. 8-3)**

TREATMENT

- Avoid calcium channel blockers and β-blockers because sinus tachycardia is a compensatory mechanism for impaired cardiac filling
- **Definitive treatment: total pericardiectomy (surgical removal of the pericardium)**
  - 90% of patients have symptomatic improvement; 50% with complete relief
  - Resolution of symptoms may take up to 6 months
  - Less effective when an underlying restrictive cardiomyopathy is also present, as seen after radiation therapy
  - Surgical mortality is 5% to 19%

Review Questions

For review questions, please go to ExpertConsult.com.

SUGGESTED READINGS

Ariyarajah V, Spodicak DH. Acute pericarditis: diagnostic cues and common electrocardiographic manifestations. *Cardiol Rev.* 2007;15:24-30.

Imazio M, Brucato A, Cemin R, et al. Colchicine for Recurrent Pericarditis (CORP): a randomized trial. *Ann Intern Med.* 2011;155:409-414.

Imazio M, Spodick MD, Brucato A, et al. Controversial issues in the management of pericardial diseases. *Circulation.* 2010;121:916-928.

Imazio M, Trinchero R, Brucato A, et al. Colchicine for the Prevention of the Post-Pericardiotomy Syndrome (COPPS): a multicentre, randomized, double-blind, placebo-controlled trial. *Eur Heart J.* 2010;31:2749-2754.

Khandaker MH, Espinosa RE, Nishimura RA, et al. Pericardial disease: diagnosis and management. *Mayo Clin Proc.* 2010;85:572-593.

Klein AL, Abbara S, Agler DA, et al. American Society of Echocardiography Clinical Recommendations for Multimodality Cardiovascular Imaging of Patients with Pericardial Disease. *J Am Soc Echocardiogr.* 2013;26:965-1012.

Lange RA, Hillis LD. Acute pericarditis. *N Engl J Med.* 2004;351:2195-2202.

Libby P, Bonow R, eds. *Braunwald's Heart Disease: A Textbook of Cardiovascular Medicine.* 8th ed. Philadelphia: Saunders; 2008.

Little WC, Freeman GL. Pericardial disease. *Circulation.* 2006;113:1622-1632.

Myers RB, Spodick DH. Constrictive pericarditis: clinical and pathophysiologic characteristics. *Am Heart J.* 1999;138:219-232.

Spodick DH. Acute cardiac tamponade. *N Engl J Med.* 2003;349:684-690.

Spodick DH. Acute pericarditis: current concepts and practice. *JAMA.* 2003;289:1150-1153.

CHAPTER 9

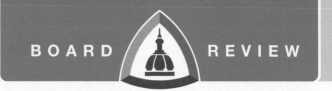
Electrocardiogram Review

BRENT G. PETTY, MD

The electrocardiogram (ECG) is important in diagnosing cardiac conditions. Interpretation requires a systematic approach and involves evaluating heart rate, rhythm, axis, intervals, and waveforms. In combination with the patient's clinical picture, ECG interpretation is critical in formulating a diagnosis and can lead to changes in treatment strategy.

Fundamental Features to Assess When Reading an Electrocardiogram

RATE (BEATS PER MINUTE)

- Normal is 60 to 100 beats/min
- Estimate rate by dividing 300 by the RR interval (as measured by number of large boxes (0.2 sec) from R to R)
  - For example, 300/2 large boxes = 150 beats/min
- Measure RR interval to nearest 0.01 sec and divide into 60 to calculate the rate more accurately
  - (e.g., 60/0.4 sec = 150 beats/min)
- For irregular rhythms, count the number of QRS complexes in 5, 6, 10, or 20 sec and multiply by the correct integer to get beats per minute.
  - For example, a standard ECG printout displays 10 sec of data, so if there is a total of 25 QRS complexes, multiply 25 × 6 = 150 beats/min

RHYTHM

(See Chapter 5 on arrhythmias for further details)
- Basic questions:
  - Too fast or too slow?
  - Regular or irregular?
  - Ventricular or supraventricular?

AXIS

- By convention, normal axis is between −30 and +90 degrees
- Determine axis quadrant by evaluating positive or negative deflection of the QRS complex in leads I and aVF (Table 9-1)
  - Suggested method:
    - Examine lead I (0 degrees) and lead aVF (90 degrees)
    - Axis is normal if both leads are in the net positive area (i.e., R-wave area > Q- + S-wave area)

- If QRS area is negative in lead aVF, examine lead II. If QRS area is positive in lead II (i.e., R wave area > Q + S wave area), axis remains normal (between 0 and 30 degrees). If QRS area is negative in lead II, then left-axis deviation is present (area between −30 and −90 degrees)
- If QRS area is negative in lead I, and positive in lead aVF, then right-axis deviation is present (area between +90 and 180 degrees)
- If QRS area is negative in leads I and aVF, then extreme axis deviation is present (−90 to 180 degrees or 180 to +270 degrees)

INTERVALS

Figure 9-1 illustrates intervals and waveforms of surface ECGs
- PR interval: Normal is 0.12 to 0.2 sec
- QRS duration: Normal is less than 0.12 sec
- QT interval varies with heart rate
  - Inversely proportional to heart rate
  - Roughly, prolonged QT is present when the QT interval is more than half the preceding RR interval (less reliable at faster heart rates)
  - Corrected QT ($QT_{corrected}$, or QT_c) adjusts for heart rate
    - Calculated as: QT divided by the square root of RR interval
- Normal QT_c is 0.36 to 0.41 sec

WAVEFORMS

- Pathologic Q waves (indicative of previous transmural ST-segment elevation myocardial infarction)
  - **To be considered pathologic, Q waves must be 1 small box wide and 1 small box deep (1 small box in width equals 0.04 sec at 25 mm/s)**
    - Septal: Any size Q waves are abnormal in leads V_1 to V_3
    - Anterior: pathologic Q waves in leads V_2 to V_4
    - Lateral: pathologic Q waves in leads I, aVL, V_5 to V_6
    - Apical: pathologic Q waves in leads V_5 to V_6
    - Inferior: pathologic Q waves in leads II, III, and aVF
    - Posterior: No Q waves are present with this type of myocardial infarction (MI); prominent R waves in leads V_1 and V_2
- ST segments (elevation or depression >1 mm)
- T-wave abnormalities (inversion or pseudonormalization)

TABLE 9-1	*Determination of Axis Quadrant on Electrocardiogram*			
	Lead I	**Lead AVF**	**Axis**	**Common Causes**
Normal			−30 to +90 degrees	Normal
Left-axis deviation			−30 to −90 degrees	LVH Left anterior fascicular block Inferior MI
Right-axis deviation			+90 to 180 degrees	Right ventricular hypertrophy Left posterior fascicular block Acute pulmonary disease (PE, pneumothorax)
Extreme axis deviation			−90 to 180 degrees (or 180 to +270 degrees)	Combination of left- and right-axis deviation causes

LVH, Left ventricular hypertrophy; MI, myocardial infarction; PE, pulmonary embolism.

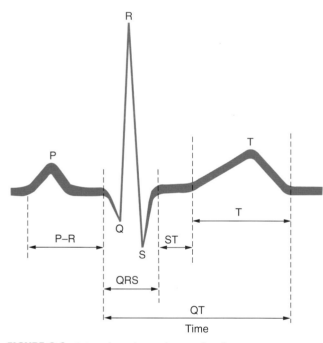

FIGURE 9-1 Intervals and waveforms of surface electrocardiogram.

Selected Electrocardiographic Abnormalities

ATRIOVENTRICULAR BLOCK

- First degree:
    - PR interval greater than 0.2 seconds
    - By itself, of no clinical consequence (can be exacerbated with atrioventricular (AV) nodal blocking agents, such as verapamil or digoxin)
- Second degree:
    - Mobitz type I (also called Wenckebach block)
        - Gradually increasing PR interval until a P wave is not followed by a QRS complex
        - Usually not clinically significant, but caution needed if administering AV nodal blocking agents

- **Mobitz type II:**
    - **Occasional dropped QRS complexes with no changes in PR interval for conducted beats; higher degree of block, where only a fraction of the P waves are followed by QRS complexes (e.g., 3:1)**
    - **Usually caused by disease of the His-Purkinje system rather than the AV node itself**
    - **Worrisome conduction pattern, often progressing to complete heart block (requiring pacemaker therapy)**
- Third degree:
    - Also known as complete heart block
    - **Characterized by AV dissociation, where the PP and RR intervals are different and the P waves are not responsible for subsequent QRS complexes**
        - QRS complexes are usually at a slow rate ("escape"), arising from intrinsic depolarization of the AV node (approximately 45 to 55 beats/min and with a narrow [<0.12-sec] QRS complex) or the ventricle (approximately 35 to 45 beats/min and with a wide [≥0.12-sec] QRS complex)
    - **Usually symptomatic (and requires pacemaker therapy)**

LOW VOLTAGE

- Definition:
    - No R or S wave in limb leads greater than 5 mm
    - No R or S wave in precordial leads greater than 10 mm
- Causes:
    - Obesity
    - Chronic obstructive pulmonary disease (increased thorax size)
    - Pericardial effusions or less commonly pleural effusions
    - Hypothyroidism
    - Addison disease
    - Infiltrative diseases (e.g., amyloidosis, hemochromatosis, sarcoidosis)
    - Diffuse myocardial infarctions

LEFT VENTRICULAR HYPERTROPHY

- ECG is not sensitive or specific for suggesting left ventricular hypertrophy (LVH) (echocardiogram is the gold standard)
- Many different ECG criteria exist for suggesting LVH
- Suggested method: increased QRS voltage plus evidence of "strain," left-axis deviation, or left atrial abnormality
  - Increased QRS voltage, as evidenced by one of the following:
    - R or S wave greater than 20 mm in any limb lead
    - S wave in leads V_1 to V_3 or R wave in leads V_4 to V_6 greater than 30 mm
    - R wave in lead V_5 + S wave in lead V_1 greater than 35 mm
    - R wave in lead aVL of 11 mm or more
    - R wave in aVL + S wave in lead V_3 of 28 mm or more (men) or 20 mm or more (women)
  - "Strain" pattern: ST-T changes (usually downward-sloping ST depression and T-wave inversion or biphasic T waves)
  - Left-axis deviation (see Table 9-1)
  - Left atrial abnormality: P wave greater than 0.12 sec (in lead II) *or* net negative P wave in lead V_1 (negative amplitude >0.1 mV)
- Causes
  - Hypertension
  - Aortic valve disease
  - Mitral insufficiency
  - Hypertrophic or dilated cardiomyopathy

WIDE QRS COMPLEX

- Definition: QRS complex 0.12 sec or more
- Potential causes:
  - Bundle branch block
  - Ventricular rhythm
  - Hyperkalemia
  - Wolff-Parkinson-White syndrome

BUNDLE BRANCH BLOCK

Figure 9-2 and Table 9-2 suggest criteria and methodology in diagnosing bundle branch blocks
- Causes:
  - Myocardial infarction
  - Infiltrative diseases (e.g., amyloidosis, hemochromatosis, sarcoidosis)
  - Conduction system degeneration

ST-SEGMENT ELEVATION ABNORMALITIES

- Consider myocardial infarction if:
  - Located regionally (i.e., anterior [leads V_2 to V_4], inferior [leads II, III, aVF], or lateral [leads V_4 to V_6])
  - ST-segment is convexed upward (sharp angle of takeoff from QRS complex) or horizontal
    - See Figure 9-3, which shows typical ECG changes associated with different stages of myocardial infarction
- Other causes include:
  - Early repolarization: typically diffuse concave upward ST-segment elevation

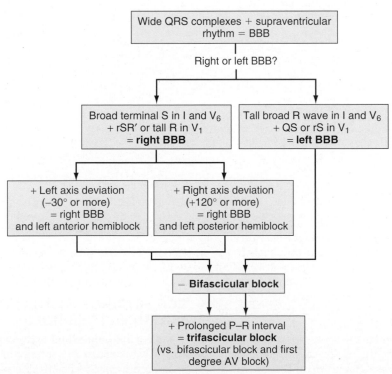

FIGURE 9-2 Bundle branch block (BBB) algorithm. AV, Atrioventricular.

TABLE 9-2	*Examples of Bundle Branch Block*	
Type of Bundle Branch Block	**Description**	**Example Electrocardiogram**
Right bundle branch block (RBBB)	Terminal S lead in I and lead V_6 + rSR' or tall R in lead V_1	
Left bundle branch block (LBBB)	Tall broad R in lead I and lead V_6 + QS or rS in lead V_1	
Bifascicular block	RBBB + left-axis deviation beyond −30 degrees (shown to right) *or* RBBB + right axis deviation at least +120 degrees *or* LBBB	
Trifascicular block	Bifascicular block (at right, LBBB) + prolonged PR interval	

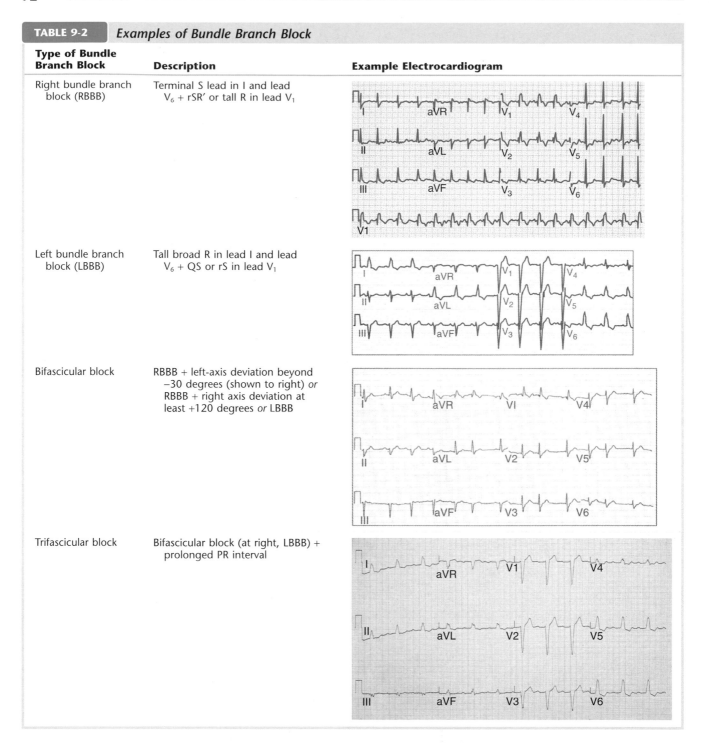

- Typically considered benign, but recent research suggests that it may be associated with slightly increased risk of early cardiac death, particularly if present in the inferior leads (II, III, and aVF)
- Ventricular aneurysm: acute, sharp-angled ST-segment elevation persisting after an ST-segment elevation myocardial infarction
- Pericarditis: diffuse ST-segment elevation and concave upward (smooth, curved takeoff from QRS complex) (also associated with PR segment depression)

OSBORN WAVES

- Positive deflection off declining shoulder of R wave
- Gives a "notched" appearance to the R wave
- Often seen with hypothermia (Figure 9-4)

ECG FINDINGS ASSOCIATED WITH PULMONARY EMBOLUS

- **Most common: sinus tachycardia**
- T-wave inversions in inferior and precordial leads
- Deep S wave in lead I (right-axis elevation) with a Q-wave and T-wave inversion in lead III ($S_1Q_3T_3$)

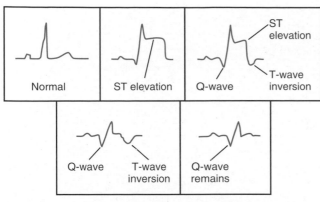

(in leads recording the area of MI)

FIGURE 9-3 Sequential electrocardiographic changes occurring in ST-segment elevation myocardial infarction (MI).

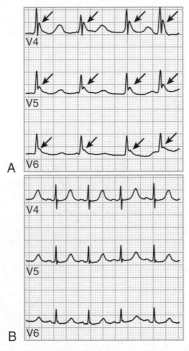

FIGURE 9-4 A, Initial echocardiogram (ECG) in a patient with hypothermia revealing atrial fibrillation and Osborn waves *(arrows).* **B,** Follow-up ECG after the patient was rewarmed, showing resolution of Osborn waves and reversion to sinus rhythm. (Courtesy Dr. Sammy Zakaria.)

ELECTRICAL ALTERNANS

- Alternating amplitude or direction of QRS complexes
- Associated with pericardial effusion caused by to-and-fro heart motion swinging in a fluid-filled pericardial sac

INVERTED T WAVES

- Nonspecific
- Potential causes
  - Intracranial hemorrhage or stroke: Classically associated with deep T-wave inversions and prolonged QT interval
  - Ischemia
  - Metabolic disorders
  - Stress cardiomyopathy ("broken heart syndrome"): Acute, temporary, often profound cardiomyopathy frequently following sudden fear or surprise

PROLONGED QT INTERVAL

- **Associated with Torsades de pointes and sudden death**
  - **Causes:**
    - **Genetic**
    - **Metabolic (hypokalemia, hypomagnesemia, hypocalcemia)**
    - **Medications (many cause QT prolongation)**
    - **Ischemia**

Review Questions

For review questions, please go to ExpertConsult.com.

SUGGESTED READINGS

Anguera I, Vallis V. Giant waves in hypothermia. *Circulation.* 2000;101:1627-1628.

Metkus T. *ECG Rounds.* New York: McGraw-Hill Education; 2014.

O'Keefe J, Hammill S, Freed M. *The Complete Guide to ECGs.* 4th ed. Jones & Bartlett Learning; planned for 2015.

Sakata K, Yoshino H, Houshaku H, et al. Myocardial damage and left ventricular dysfunction in patients with and without persistent negative T waves after Q-wave anterior myocardial infarction. *Am J Cardiol.* 2001;87:510-515.

Taylor GJ, Petty BG. Electrocardiogram. In: Taylor GJ, ed. *Primary Care and Management of Heart Disease.* St. Louis: Mosby; 2000:54-68.

Tikkanen JT, Anttonen O, Junttila MJ, et al. Long-term outcome associated with early repolarization on electrocardiography. *N Engl J Med.* 2009;361:2529-2537.

Wagner G, Strauss D. *Marriott's Practical Electrocardiography.* 12th ed. Philadelphia: Lippincott Williams & Wilkins; 2013.

Wittstein IS, Thiemann DR, Lima JAC, et al. Neurohumoral features of myocardial stunning due to sudden emotional stress. *N Engl J Med.* 2005;352:539-548.

9

SECTION TWO

BOARD REVIEW

Infectious Disease

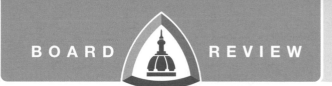
Respiratory Infections

PAUL G. AUWAERTER, MD

Infections of the respiratory tract result in more antibiotic prescriptions than any other group of medical disorders in the outpatient setting. **In many cases, respiratory tract infections do not require administration of antibiotics for cure.** The inappropriate prescription of antibiotics contributes to antibiotic resistance; this is particularly concerning in *Streptococcus pneumoniae* infections.

Bacterial Sinusitis

BASIC INFORMATION

- **Acute bacterial sinusitis (ABS) is often preceded by a viral upper respiratory tract infection (URTI), environmental allergen flare, trauma, or recent dental manipulation**
- Only 0.2% to 10% of all clinical sinusitis cases are bacterial in origin; on average, likely 2% of all cases
- Symptoms often mimicked by common cold or allergies
- Diagnosis is best made on clinical grounds, because history and physical findings are not specific
- Nasal passages are commonly involved (Fig. 10-1); some view this as rhinosinusitis
- **Chronic sinusitis is a poorly understood entity; it is diagnosed after at least 12 weeks of sinus symptoms and signs**
  - Results from chronic obstruction of sinus passages; the role of bacterial pathogens in this disorder is debated
- Microbiology of ABS shows that respiratory pathogens predominate (in order of decreasing frequency):
  - *S. pneumoniae*
  - *Haemophilus influenzae*
  - *Moraxella catarrhalis*
- Antibacterial resistance among these organisms is increasingly common
  - More than 40% of *H. influenzae* and 100% of *M. catarrhalis* are β-lactamase producers, meaning they are resistant to drugs that contain a β-lactam ring (such as amoxicillin)
  - High-level pneumococcal resistance to penicillin (PCN; defined as minimum inhibitory concentration [MIC] ≥8 mg/dL) for nonmeningeal isolates is uncommon, accounting for approximately 4% of isolates in the United States
  - The clinical importance of resistant bacteria in sinus conditions is debated
- Other pathogens, such as anaerobes, other streptococci, and *Staphylococcus aureus*, account for small percentages of isolates in ABS

- **In chronic sinusitis, *S. aureus*, *Staphylococcus epidermidis*, and anaerobes predominate. Whether or not antibiotic treatment helps this condition is unclear, but it is often used.**

CLINICAL PRESENTATION

- **ABS most commonly follows viral URTI**
- Change in color or character of nasal discharge is not specifically indicative of bacterial infection
- **ABS (as opposed to viral or allergic sinusitis) is unlikely if symptoms are less than 10 days in duration**
- History or physical findings suggestive of ABS include:
  - Persistent or worsening symptoms lasting at least 10 days

  or
  - Significant unilateral sinus pain or tenderness, fever higher than 39° C, purulent nasal discharge, maxillary, tooth, or facial pain (particularly unilateral) lasting at least 3 to 4 days in the beginning of the illness

  or
  - Worsening signs and symptoms of nasal discharge, headache, and fever after a URTI
    - Usually in this scenario the URTI symptoms lasted 5 to 6 days and were initially improving

DIAGNOSIS

- Gold standard is culture from sinus puncture (not commonly done)
- Best made on clinical grounds, usually only after symptoms have lasted for more than 10 days, although sensitivity and specificity of history and physical examination are poor
- **Imaging studies not recommended for uncomplicated cases of ABS because findings are no more sensitive or specific than clinical evaluation**

TREATMENT

- Many patients with signs and symptoms of sinusitis (even those with true ABS) will have resolution of their symptoms without antimicrobial therapy
  - The use of decongestants, analgesics, antipyretics is possibly helpful but not well studied
  - **Patients with moderate or severe symptoms should receive antibiotics (Fig. 10-2)**
  - Goals of ABS treatment: Avoid acute complications (e.g., brain abscess, meningitis, or osteomyelitis—all

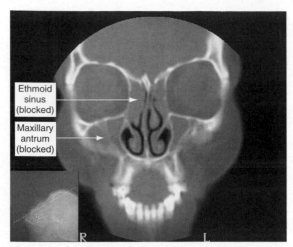

FIGURE 10-1 Coronal computed tomography scan showing ethmoid, labyrinth, and maxillary antral opacification in a patient with sinusitis. (From Swash M. *Hutchison's Clinical Methods.* 21st ed. Philadelphia: Saunders; 2002: Fig. 13.10.)

rare; Fig. 10-3) and chronic complications (e.g., chronic sinusitis)

- Antibiotic choice dictated by local sensitivities, cost, and drug allergy history
- Preferred drug: amoxicillin/clavulanate for 5 to 7 days; amoxicillin without clavulanate is no longer first-line because of high rates of resistance in sinus pathogens.
- Attempts to treat chronic sinusitis with antibiotics may result in little improvement; treatments should focus on relieving obstruction
- For chronic sinusitis, decrease mucosal swelling, exudates, and crusting by using nasal saline irrigation, topical nasal corticosteroids, antihistamines, decongestants, leukotriene antagonists
- **Sinus computed tomography (CT) scan can be helpful to evaluate for obstruction (e.g., polyps) in patients with suspected chronic sinusitis who are not responding to therapy; otolaryngology consultation is recommended**
- If a patient with chronic sinusitis has an acute flare, treatment with antibiotics against *S. pneumoniae* and *H. influenzae* should be given
- Recurrent ABS may indicate obstruction or immunodeficiency (e.g., HIV, hypogammaglobulinemia)

Otitis Media

BASIC INFORMATION

- Acute otitis media is an infection of the middle ear. It needs to be distinguished from otitis media with effusion (noninfectious)
    - Involves obstruction of the Eustachian tube, resulting in a pressure imbalance of the inner ear and subsequent bacterial infection
- Often initiated by either URTI or allergies
- **Uncommon in adults, less than 0.25% incidence**
- Intensively studied in children; less known about infection in adults

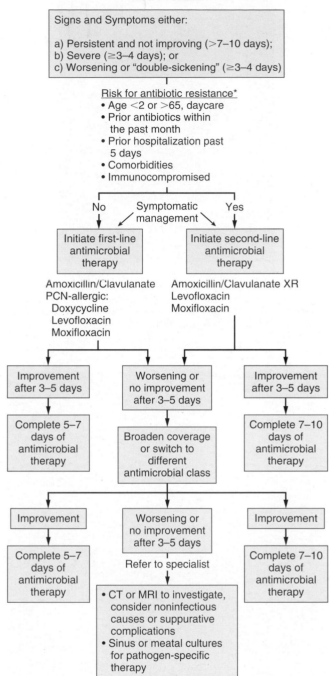

FIGURE 10-2 Management of acute bacterial sinusitis. *If patient is diabetic, immunocompromised, in an iron-overload state, and/or critically ill, consider rhinocerebral mucormycosis. ABS, Acute bacterial sinusitis; CT, computed tomography; MRI, magnetic resonance imaging; PCN, penicillin. (Modified from Chow AW, Benninger MS, Brook I, et al. IDSA clinical practice guideline for acute bacterial rhinosinusitis in children and adults. *Clin Infect Dis.* 2012;54:e72-e112.)

- *S. pneumoniae* and *H. influenzae* common isolates; unclear frequency of viral and allergic inflammation

CLINICAL PRESENTATION

- Commonly follows URTI or history of allergies
- **Otalgia and fever are most frequent symptoms**

10

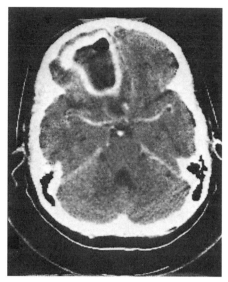

FIGURE 10-3 Cerebral abscess secondary to sinusitis. Right frontal abscess is demonstrated in a patient who had ethmoid sinusitis. An orbital abscess is also demonstrated. (From Forbes C, Jackson W. *Color Atlas and Text of Clinical Medicine.* 3rd ed. St. Louis: Mosby; 2003: Fig. 11.63.)

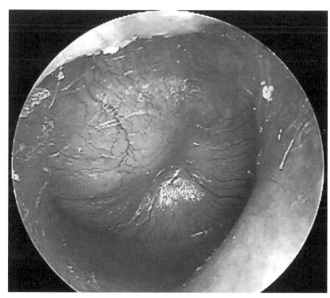

FIGURE 10-4 Acute left otitis media. (From Behrman RE. *Nelson Textbook of Pediatrics.* 16th ed. Philadelphia: Saunders; 2003: Fig. 630-3.)

- Severe cases may be complicated by meningitis, mastoiditis, or brain abscess (all rare)

DIAGNOSIS

- Physical examination in children imprecise, but accuracy increases with insufflation demonstrating decreased mobility of tympanic membrane
- **Examination findings in adults have not been studied, but typical presentation is bulging, red tympanic membrane (Fig. 10-4)**
- Perforation of tympanic membrane may occur and lead to drainage or crusting within ear canal

TREATMENT

- Antimicrobial therapy is not well defined: amoxicillin/clavulanate, cefuroxime axetil, and azithromycin possible options

Pharyngitis

BASIC INFORMATION

- Outpatient visits for pharyngitis account for 1% to 2% of all office visits
- **Viral etiology is most common cause in adults** (up to 80%)
  - Rhinovirus (20%) is most common
  - Coronavirus (5% to 10%), adenovirus (5%); herpes simplex (2% to 4%) is less common
  - Uncommon causes include parainfluenza (2%), influenza (1%), Epstein-Barr virus (EBV) (<1%), cytomegalovirus (<1%), acute HIV type 1 (<1%), coxsackievirus (<1%)
- ***Streptococcus pyogenes* most common bacterial cause in adults (5% to 10%)**
  - Other streptococci less common, usually group G or C
  - Rare bacterial causes include *Neisseria gonorrhoeae* (<1%), *Corynebacterium diphtheriae* (<1%), *Arcanobacterium haemolyticum* (often associated with rash, <1%), *Chlamydophila pneumoniae* (1%), or *Mycoplasma pneumoniae* (<1%)
- Bacterial infection is less common in adults than children; therefore, there is a much higher incidence of group A streptococci in children
- Some cases may be associated with evidence of more systemic infection (EBV, acute HIV infection); severe pharyngitis (*N. gonorrhoeae* or group A β-hemolytic streptococci [GABHS]); rheumatic fever (adult patients with a history of rheumatic fever should be managed differently, with lower threshold for prescription of antibiotics)
- In many cases the cause is unknown and presumed to be viral

CLINICAL PRESENTATION

- Typical presentations include sore throat and malaise, with possible fever or cervical lymphadenopathy
- Severe sore throat with inability to swallow secretions or associated dyspnea should be evaluated in an emergency department; may indicate epiglottitis
- Dehydration in severe cases may require IV hydration
- Red, beefy tonsils with exudates may have either bacterial or viral causes; the presence of exudate is not specific for bacterial cause (Fig. 10-5)
- **Primary infection with EBV (infectious mononucleosis) is easily confused with GABHS and may present with fever, sore throat, splenomegaly, and lymphadenopathy (either anterior and posterior cervical lymph nodes or generalized)**
  - In infectious mononucleosis, laboratory abnormalities may include predominance of lymphocytes or atypical lymphocytes

- In 90% of adult cases, the aspartate aminotransferase, alanine aminotransferase, or lactate dehydrogenase level is elevated to at least two to three times normal
- Prescription of amoxicillin for patients mistakenly believed to have GABHS or who have secondary concurrent GABHS predictably yields diffuse, pruritic, maculopapular rash in 95% to 100% of patients
    - **This rash does NOT mean patient is amoxicillin allergic (Fig. 10-6)**

DIAGNOSIS

- Because the signs and symptoms of GABHS and viral etiologies overlap, physicians are generally unable to include or exclude the diagnosis of streptococcal pharyngitis on epidemiologic and clinical grounds; therefore, laboratory testing should be done to determine whether group A streptococci are present in the pharynx (Fig. 10-7)

- Sensitivity and specificity of clinical presentation 50% to 75% for GABHS (Fig. 10-8)
- Throat culture is gold standard (90% sensitive); false positives may result from carrier state
- Rapid strep tests
    - Throat swab detects carbohydrate antigen
    - Sensitivity 80% to 90% in adults, but highly specific
    - **If positive test, treat as GABHS; no further culture required**
    - Because of a higher prevalence in children and adolescents, negative tests should be confirmed by standard culture. It is unclear whether this is necessary in adults

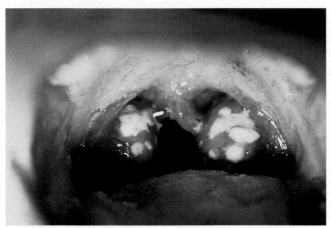

FIGURE 10-5 Acute streptococcal pharyngitis. Note purulent discharge in tonsillar crypts. A similar appearance may be seen with pharyngitis caused by infectious mononucleosis. (From Forbes C, Jackson W. *Color atlas and text of clinical medicine.* 3rd ed. St. Louis: Mosby; 2003, Fig. 1.82.)

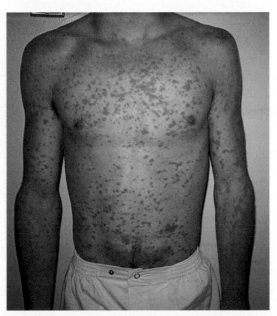

FIGURE 10-6 Generalized erythematous papular eruption of infectious mononucleosis precipitated by oral penicillin intake. (From Shah BR, Laude TA. *Atlas of pediatric clinical diagnosis.* Philadelphia: Saunders; 2000, Fig. 3-32.)

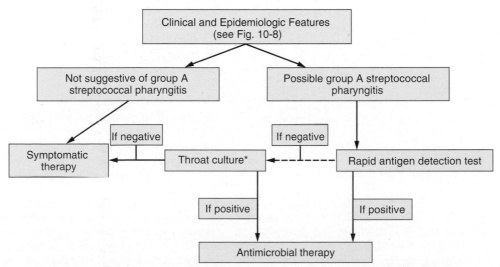

FIGURE 10-7 Diagnosis and management of pharyngitis. *Considered optional in adults.

10

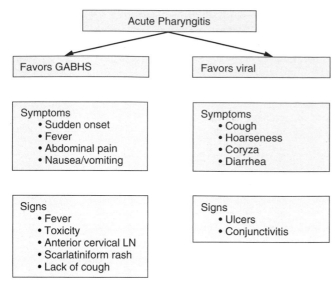

FIGURE 10-8 Differentiation of streptococcal (group A β-hemolytic streptococci [GABHS]) pharyngitis from viral causes. LN, Lymph nodes.

- Heterophile antibodies are used to diagnose infectious mononucleosis:
  - Occur in 90% of cases and are detected by blood testing with commercial kits (e.g., Monospot, Meridian Bioscience, Cincinnati, OH)
  - Are not directed against EBV; agglutinate either horse or sheep red blood cells (RBCs)
  - Detection of anti-EBV capsid immunoglobulin M (IgM) antibodies typically done if heterophilic antibodies are negative but EBV still suspected (approximately 10% of cases)
  - Anti-EBV immunoglobulin G (IgG) may be present at presentation in new infection or with preexisting infection and has less clinical utility in diagnosis of acute infection

TREATMENT

- Viral: Generally benign, self-limited illness remedied by rest, hydration, nonsteroidal drugs for pain or fever, and saltwater gargles
- GABHS: Historically, treatment is given to avoid complications of acute rheumatic fever; also may prevent suppurative complications such as tonsillar abscess
  - However, acute rheumatic fever is now rare in adults, and the main use of antibiotics is to shorten the duration of illness (16 to 24 hours); should be given within 72 hours of symptom onset
  - **All GABHS strains remain PCN sensitive**
  - PCN V is standard for adults
    - 250 mg four times daily or 500 mg twice daily orally OR long-acting intramuscular PCN given as one dose (1.2 million units benzathine ± procaine PCN G)
  - Options for PCN-allergic patients include clindamycin, azithromycin, or clarithromycin

Acute Bronchitis

BASIC INFORMATION

- **Most common cause of acute cough in the outpatient setting**
- Clinical challenge is to distinguish bronchitis from pneumonia
- **90% of cases are from nonbacterial causes in healthy nonsmokers**
- Purulent sputum may or may not indicate a bacterially induced process
- Viral causes predominate, especially coronaviruses, paramyxoviruses, rhinoviruses, and also, in season, influenza (A or B)
- **Pertussis is an uncommon cause of bronchitis, but is more likely if cough is severe or persists longer than 3 weeks**

CLINICAL PRESENTATION

- Acute respiratory infection with cough (with or without phlegm) for less than 3 weeks
- Wheezing may be present, including in those without asthma

DIAGNOSIS

- Diagnosis based on history and physical examination; sputum cultures are not recommended
- Pneumonia is uncommon if vital signs and chest examination are normal

TREATMENT

- Symptomatic support; antibiotics not recommended regardless of cough duration; prescription represents antibiotic abuse (Table 10-1; see notes on pertussis that follow)
- 50% will experience resolution of cough at 14 days; 90% will experience resolution at 21 days
- **Albuterol inhalation may decrease cough; most beneficial in those with documented reductions in peak airflow**
- Antitussives often prescribed, but few data to clarify role
- Consider antiviral therapy for influenza if early in course of illness (less than 48 hours) for ambulatory patients who are not significantly ill
- Pertussis should be suspected if cough persists beyond 3 weeks
  - Treatment initiation after 7 to 10 days of cough onset does not lead to reduction in cough duration (which can persist for 6 to 10 weeks regardless of therapy)
  - Historically, azithromycin or tetracycline was provided to limit the potential for transmission
    - Recently, routine use of macrolides in adults in outbreak situations has been discouraged because of lack of data to suggest staunching spread
  - **Because of risk of infant infection, routine treatment is now only suggested in pregnant women within 6 weeks of cough onset**
- Patient education essential: Patients not receiving an antibiotic are happier if told they have a chest cold rather than bronchitis

TABLE 10-1	*Treatment of Bronchitis*			
Basic Clinical State	**Symptoms/Risk Factors**	**Likely Pathogens**	**First-Line Treatment**	**Alternatives/ Treatment Failure**
Acute tracheobronchitis	Cough and sputum without previous pulmonary disease	Usually viral	None	Consider pertussis if >3 weeks of cough or if severe, especially in pregnant patient
Acute flare of chronic bronchitis without risk factors (group I)	Increased cough and sputum, sputum purulence, and increased dyspnea	*Haemophilus influenzae Haemophilus* spp. *Moraxella catarrhalis Streptococcus pneumoniae*	2nd-generation macrolide 2nd- or 3rd-generation cephalosporin Amoxicillin/clavulanate Doxycycline TMP-SMX Use an antibiotic from a different class if the patient has been treated with antibiotics in the last 3 months	Fluoroquinolone or β-lactam/β-lactamase inhibitor
Acute flare of chronic bronchitis with risk factors (group II)	Symptoms as in group I *plus* at least 1 of the following: FEV$_1$ <50% predicted Age > 65 years >3 exacerbations/year Cardiac disease Use of home oxygen Chronic oral steroid use Antibiotic use in past 3 months	Organisms as in group I, *plus Klebsiella* spp. Other gram-negative pathogens Increased probability of β-lactam resistance	Fluoroquinolone β-Lactam/β-lactamase inhibitor (e.g., amoxicillin/ clavulanate). Use an antibiotic from a different class if the patient has been treated with antibiotics in the last 3 months	May require parenteral therapy; consider referral to a specialist or hospital
Acute flare of chronic suppurative bronchitis (group III)	Symptoms as in group II, but with constant purulent sputum Some have bronchiectasis Multiple risk factors (e.g., frequent exacerbations and FEV$_1$ <50% predicted) Frequent administration of antibiotics (4 or more courses in last year) Recent hospitalization in the last 3 months	Organisms as in group II, *plus Pseudomonas aeruginosa* Multidrug-resistant Enterobacteriaceae	Ambulatory patients: Tailor treatment to airway pathogen (*P. aeruginosa* common; use ciprofloxacin and obtain sputum culture) Hospitalized patients: parenteral therapy usually required	

FEV$_1$, Forced expiratory volume in 1 second; TMP-SMX, trimethoprim-sulfamethoxazole.
Modified from Balter MS, LaForge J, Low DE, et al. Canadian guidelines for the management of acute exacerbations of chronic bronchitis. *Can Respir J*. 2003;10(Suppl B):3B–32B; and Sethi S, Murphy TF. Acute exacerbations of chronic bronchitis: new developments concerning microbiology and pathophysiology—impact on approaches to risk stratification and therapy. *Infect Dis Clin North Am*. 2004;18:861–882.

Chronic Bronchitis with Acute Exacerbation

BASIC INFORMATION

- Part of the clinical spectrum of chronic obstructive pulmonary disease (COPD)
- Cigarette smoking is major contributor to COPD, with less than 10% of patients with COPD having disease due to other reasons (such as α_1-antitrypsin deficiency, occupational or environmental exposure, and so on)
- Accounts for 5% of all deaths in United States
- Viral or bacterial infections may cause acute exacerbations of chronic bronchitis
  - Bacterial causes

- *H. influenzae* is the most common cause (approximately 22%), particularly in smokers
- *M. catarrhalis* (9% to 15%)
- *S. pneumoniae* (10% to 12%)
- *Pseudomonas aeruginosa* or other gram-negative bacteria (up to 15%)
  - Seen in those with recent previous antibiotic use or hospitalizations and in those with frequent flares
- Many cases without predominant bacterial species are presumed viral

CLINICAL PRESENTATION

- **Patients with COPD flare may have a combination of worsening dyspnea and increased sputum purulence and/or volume**

10

- Winnipeg criteria may be used to stratify severity of flares (Box 10-1)
  - Type 1 or type 2 flares require hospitalization and are associated with increased mortality (3% to 4%)
  - Mortality increases to 11% to 24% in-hospital if admission to intensive care unit is required
- Chest radiograph (CXR) abnormalities are common
- Consider deep venous thrombosis leading to pulmonary embolus as cause of exacerbation if no other clear etiology found

DIAGNOSIS

- Diagnosis made on clinical grounds
- **CXR, pulse oximetry, and arterial blood gas tests are beneficial to rule out pneumonia and gauge severity**
- May be difficult to differentiate from pneumonia if CXR has baseline abnormalities
- **Unlike in acute asthma exacerbations, acute spirometry considered unhelpful**
- Sputum culture not routinely recommended, but may be helpful in severe cases, patients with concurrent pneumonia, or cases with recent antibiotic use/hospitalization

TREATMENT

- Few good data to guide recommendations (see Table 10-1)
- **Bronchodilators and corticosteroids recommended**
- **Antibiotics recommended for moderate to severely ill patients (defined as patients with increased sputum purulence and either increased sputum volume or dyspnea *or* patients requiring ventilatory support)**
- **Antibiotics also recommended for patients with moderate to severe COPD exacerbation requiring hospitalization**
- Choice of antibiotic depends on patients' risk factors for pseudomonas and risk of complicated COPD
- Data using amoxicillin and tetracycline are more than 30 years old
  - Data are limited regarding optimal antibiotics for COPD exacerbations, but include macrolides and doxycyline for uncomplicated COPD exacerbations (patients older than 65 years of age with a forced expiratory volume during 1 sec greater than 50%, no cardiac disease, and greater than 3 exacerbations per year) and fluoroquinolones and amoxicillin/clavulanate for complicated COPD exacerbations
- Mucolytics and chest physiotherapy without clear benefit
- Oxygen helpful with hypoxemia, but may heighten risk of respiratory failure if patient has chronic hypoxemia.

Influenza

BASIC INFORMATION

- **Two major virus subtypes: influenza A and influenza B**
- Antigenic characteristics determined by surface-spike glycoproteins that have either hemagglutinin activity (HA) or neuraminidase activity (NA) (Fig. 10-9)
- Hemagglutinin attaches to erythrocytes and is responsible for initiation of infection
- Neuraminidase cleaves hemagglutinin protein, allowing viral release from infected cells
- Significant antigenic variation of HA or NA bypasses previous immune memory in the host infected with influenza in the past
- Antigenic drift: minor changes in HA or NA and minor changes in immunogenicity
- Antigenic shift: Major changes in HA or NA, resulting in completely new immunogenicity with risk of pandemic infection

BOX 10-1	*Winnipeg Criteria for Stratifying Severity of Acute Exacerbation of Chronic Bronchitis*

Symptoms

Increasing dyspnea
Increasing purulence of sputum
Increasing volume of sputum

Classification

Type 1: Severe, all three symptoms
Type 2: Moderate, two or three symptoms
Type 3: Mild, at least one symptom along with:
    Upper respiratory tract infection within last 5 days
    Fever without other apparent cause
    Increased wheezing
    Increased nonproductive cough
    Increased respirations or pulse >20% over baseline

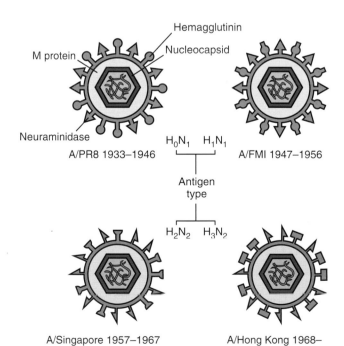

FIGURE 10-9 Schematic drawing of influenza A demonstrating hemagglutinin and neuraminidase. Hemagglutinin is responsible for attachment to cells; neuraminidase is responsible for viral release. Figure demonstrates antigenic shifts that have caused major influenza outbreaks. (From Roitt I, Brostoff J, Male D, eds. *Immunology.* 6th ed. St. Louis: Mosby; 2001: Fig. 14.9.)

- Avian influenza (H5N1) is a concern because of similarity to 1918 influenza severity; however, few cases to date in humans with limited human-to-human transmissibility
- The pandemic H1N1 strain in 2009 behaved similarly to seasonal influenza, with the exception that children and young adults were more often affected than the customary elderly populations; increased mortality was seen more often in those with co-morbidities

CLINICAL PRESENTATION

- Seasonal influenza outbreaks typically occur in an epidemic pattern, peaking at 2 to 3 weeks after introduction and completed after 5 to 6 weeks in any given community
- Seasonal peaks usually occur in winter, but may occur from early fall to late spring.
  - Influenza is uncommon in the summertime
- **Symptoms often begin abruptly with fever, rigors, malaise, headache, myalgia, and arthralgia**
- Fever, rigors, and myalgia peak at 3 days, after which respiratory symptoms (cough) and nasal congestion predominate
- **Major complication is postinfluenza pneumonia**
  - Viral pneumonia from influenza occurs early in course of disease and may be severe
  - **Postinfectious bacterial pneumonia often follows a period of recovery from influenza and is most often caused by *S. pneumoniae, S. aureus, S. pyogenes,* or *H. influenzae***
- Other complications may include rhabdomyolysis, myocarditis, encephalitis, or Guillain-Barré syndrome

DIAGNOSIS

- **Most commonly diagnosed based on clinical presentation during community outbreaks**
  - **If abrupt onset of cough and fever occurs in an adult living in a community with an outbreak, this is 70% specific for influenza**
- Seasonal strains of influenza may be detected from sputum, nasal or throat swab, or from nasopharyngeal aspirate by rapid antigen test
  - Sensitivity depends on testing kit; may be relatively insensitive (generally 40% to 70%). Specificity is usually 90% to 95%, but can range 85% to 100%
- Can also use molecular methods (90% to 100% specific), or culture (90% to 100% specific but slow)
- Only test if will change clinical care of the patient; treatment should not be delayed pending results if there is high suspicion

TREATMENT

- Optimal treatment is prevention, with influenza vaccine now universally recommended for all people older than the age of 6 months
- Can consider antiviral therapy for influenza if early in course of illness (less than 48 hours) for ambulatory patients who are not significantly ill
- Severely ill patients, hospitalized patients, and those at high risk for complications (pregnant, older than 65 years, immune suppressed, and other co-morbidities) should receive antiviral therapy even if initiated after 48 hours

- Clinical judgment should drive the decision to start antiviral therapy after 48 hours in high-risk outpatients
- Antiviral therapy should be initiated as early as possible for any patient with suspected influenza who is hospitalized, severely ill, or at high risk for complications. Do not wait for laboratory confirmation of the diagnosis to start antiviral therapy
- Amantadine and rimantadine block ion channel function only in influenza A virus and *should only be used if circulating strains are known to be susceptible;* these drugs have no role in treatment of influenza B
- Neuraminidase inhibitors (zanamivir, oseltamivir, and peramivir) prevent infection of cells by inhibiting influenza NA for both influenza A and influenza B
  - **Since 2009, neuraminidase inhibitors have been the preferred treatment for influenza because circulating strains have been resistant to amantadines.** Resistance profiles of circulating virus may change with every season, hence, check for up-to-date recommendations (ww.cdc.gov/flu/about/season/index.htm)
  - Oseltamivir is administered orally and may result in nausea
  - **Zanamivir is administered by inhalation and is well tolerated, but may result in bronchospasm and should be avoided in susceptible patients, such as those with asthma or COPD**
  - Peramivir is given by injection and is FDA (United States Food and Drug Administration) approved as a single dose for uncomplicated influenza; however, for patients who cannot take oral or inhaled drugs, it offers an unproven alternative treatment route for hospitalized patients

Pneumonia

BASIC INFORMATION

- Remains leading cause of infectious death in United States; seventh overall cause of death
- Mortality highest in older patients and in those with multiple co-morbidities
- ***S. pneumoniae* and *Legionella pneumophila* are the leading bacterial causes of pneumonia-related death**
- Microbiology is altered by host factors (e.g., age, immunosuppression, alcohol use) and geography
  - *S. pneumoniae* remains the most commonly diagnosed etiologic agent in studies of community-acquired pneumonia
    - High-level PCN resistance in *S. pneumoniae* is less frequent than previously thought (because of revised resistance breakpoints for non-meningeal isolates; approximately 4% in recent U.S. studies).
    - Clinical significance of antibiotic-resistant organisms in pneumonia is debated
- **Atypical agents account for 15% to 20% of community-acquired pneumonias, and include *L. pneumophila, M. pneumoniae,* and *C. pneumoniae***
- *H. influenzae, S. aureus,* and gram-negative bacilli each account for 3% to 10% of community-acquired pneumonias

10

- Viral pneumonia is uncommon in adults
  - Influenza A and B most common viral causes
  - Cytomegalovirus causes pneumonia only in immunosuppressed patients
  - Adenovirus, varicella-zoster virus, and EBV are rare causes of viral pneumonia in adults
  - Hantavirus, seen mostly in the southwestern United States, is a rare cause of viral pneumonia that quickly evolves to acute respiratory distress in previously health individuals and is associated with a high mortality rate
- Fungal infections
  - Rarely a cause of acute, community-acquired pneumonia
- More than 300 fungi capable of causing lung infection, mostly in immunocompromised patients
  - *Aspergillus* spp. and zygomycete organisms (*Rhizopus, Mucor* spp.) are the leading causes of serious clinical pulmonary infection in this population
- Endemic fungi (*Histoplasma capsulatum, Blastomyces dermatitidis, Coccidioides immitis,* and *Cryptococcus neoformans*) can infect normal hosts and cause lung disease, but greater than 60% of infections are asymptomatic and only a small percentage do not spontaneously resolve (Table 10-2)
- **Candida spp. are a very rare cause of pneumonia and should be considered as the causative agent**

TABLE 10-2	*Fungal Infections of the Lung*		
Organism	**Presentation**	**Diagnosis**	**Treatment**
Histoplasma capsulatum	Up to 60% asymptomatic; endemic to Ohio and Mississippi River valleys Acute infection: includes fever, infiltrates, pleurisy, hilar and mediastinal adenopathy ARDS, If inoculum sufficiently large, fulminant respiratory failure may result Progressive disseminated histoplasmosis: May result from primary infection or reactivation; more common in immunocompromised; diffuse lymphadenopathy, hepatosplenomegaly, and adrenal insufficiency may result Chronic pulmonary histoplasmosis: often in the setting of COPD; resembles tuberculosis with cavitation	Culture is gold standard, but takes 4–6 weeks *Histoplasma* antigen may be detected in serum and urine of patients with disseminated disease; may cross-react with blastomycosis and coccidioidomycosis Complement fixation of antibody to *H. capsulatum* may be used, including those with acute pulmonary infection (fourfold rise in titer consistent with acute infection)	Acute infection does not typically require treatment Chronic pulmonary infections may require treatment with itraconazole Disseminated infections treated with itraconazole or amphotericin High index of suspicion should be held for adrenal insufficiency in disseminated disease
Blastomyces dermatitidis	Endemic to region between Dakotas and Louisiana Disease may be self-limited or require treatment Pulmonary presentations include infiltrates, nodules, or cavitation Skin, bone, and genitourinary tract (prostate and epididymis) most common extrapulmonary sites of infection	Culture is gold standard Visualization of fungi in appropriate clinical setting used to initiate antimicrobial treatment Complement fixation is currently neither sensitive nor specific	Itraconazole in immune competent patients with mild to moderate disease Amphotericin in immune compromised or with CNS involvement
Coccidioides immitis	Endemic to dry regions of southwestern United States Acute pulmonary infection: Most common presentation, with fever, cough, and extensive alveolar infiltrates; may be accompanied by massive hilar and mediastinal adenopathy; cavitation may occur, with hemoptysis; erythema nodosum Dissemination may be widespread, with skin, muscle, bone, and CNS involvement	Stain and culture of infected fluid or tissues Elevated complement fixation titers to *C. immitis;* these may be followed as markers of disease, with rising titers a poor prognostic sign	Itraconazole or fluconazole Fluconazole used if CNS involvement or refractory disease
Aspergillus fumigatus	ABPA: A hypersensitivity reaction characterized by asthma and fleeting infiltrates accompanied by eosinophilia Aspergilloma (fungal ball or mycetoma): Most common noninvasive form, occurring in old scars, cavities, or blebs Invasive aspergillosis: Usually occurs in immunocompromised, with organ transplant and hematologic malignancies common predisposers; presents as acute pneumonia with cavitation, then invades locally along with hematogenous dissemination	Diagnosis of ABPA by positive sputum culture, elevated total IgE, elevated specific antibodies to *Aspergillus,* and cutaneous reaction to *Aspergillus* immunogen Aspergilloma diagnosed by clinical presentation Invasive aspergillosis diagnosed by clinical microbiologic and radiographic presentation and CT scan; biopsy with culture usually suggested to distinguish from colonization; serum galactomannan may be elevated	ABPA: Corticosteroids; role of antifungal treatment unclear Aspergilloma may require embolization or resection for control of hemoptysis; otherwise no antifungal treatment necessary Invasive aspergillosis: Voriconazole is treatment of choice

ABPA, Allergic bronchopulmonary aspergillosis; ARDS, acute respiratory distress syndrome; CNS, central nervous system; COPD, chronic obstructive pulmonary disease; CT, computed tomography; IgE, immunoglobulin E.

only in the profoundly immunosuppressed or neutropenic patient. Positive sputum cultures otherwise merely represent upper airway colonization.

CLINICAL PRESENTATION

- Cough, fever, and new pulmonary infiltrate constitute the classic triad
- Other common symptoms include pleurisy, dyspnea, malaise, headache, nausea, vomiting, abdominal pain, and diarrhea
- **Although no reliable clinical indicators have been established to differentiate typical pneumonia from atypical pneumonia, purulent sputum without identification of a pathogenic organism heightens suspicion for *Legionella, Mycoplasma,* and *Chlamydophilia* spp.**
- Certain presentations are associated with specific etiologic agents, noted in the following:
  - **_S. pneumoniae_ classically presents with sudden rigor, fever, and cough productive of rust-colored sputum (Fig. 10-10)**
  - ***Legionella* (which may occur sporadically or as part of an outbreak associated with aerosol spread of a contaminated water system) presents as a severe pneumonia with high-spiking fevers**
    - **Classically accompanied by diarrhea, and in some cases, relative bradycardia despite high fevers. Hyponatremia may be more common with *Legionella* than with other etiologic agents**
  - The hallmark of *Mycoplasma* infection is a paroxysmal, nonproductive cough, often with minimal findings on CXR; however, CXR may demonstrate diffuse pulmonary infiltrates and even effusions
    - Bullous myringitis, contrary to lore, is *not* a usual finding in *Mycoplasma* infection

- The production of cold agglutinins (IgM produced in *Mycoplasma* infection that reversibly agglutinates RBCs when blood is cooled) may lead to Raynaud phenomenon and even digital necrosis (particularly in patients with sickle cell anemia)
- *C. pneumoniae* results in a typically mild pneumonia that is slowly progressive and only rarely severe; it may follow URTI symptoms (pharyngitis, sinus infection) by 1 or 2 weeks
  - There is little clinically to differentiate *C. pneumoniae* from other causes of pneumonia
- Pneumonia is the most common initial acquired immune deficiency syndrome (AIDS)-defining illness, with *Pneumocystis jiroveci* (Fig. 10-11) and *S. pneumoniae* the leading etiologies
- Infiltrates with cavitation or subacute pneumonia, especially in an immunocompromised patient, warrant consideration of tuberculosis (1% to 2% of all cases of community-acquired pneumonia)

DIAGNOSIS

- Chest physical examination is unreliable to include or to exclude pneumonia diagnosis
- Abnormal vital signs heighten the likelihood of positive CXR
- CXR is critical to establish infiltrate and to decrease mistaken administration of antibiotics for acute bronchitis
- **Sputum with more than 25 polymorphonuclear neutrophils and less than 10 epithelial cells/high-powered field considered purulent specimen; may adequately reflect pathogen of pneumonia (Fig. 10-12)**
- Blood cultures are considered optional but should be obtained in certain patients (including those with

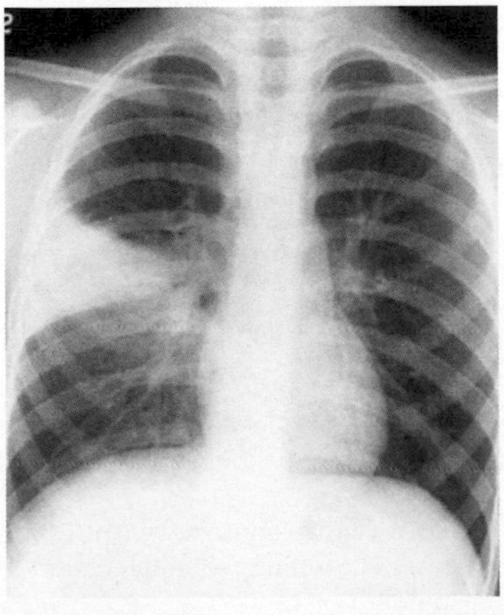

FIGURE 10-10 Right upper lobe pneumonia. On this posteroanterior chest radiograph, note that the right cardiac border is well seen. The alveolar infiltrate is seen in the right midlung. (From Mettler FA. *Essentials of Radiology.* 2nd ed. Philadelphia: Saunders; 2005: Fig. 3-44.)

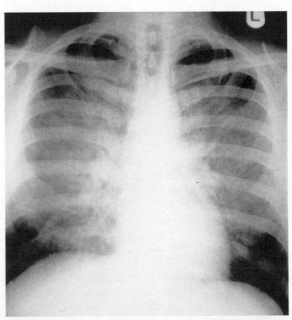

FIGURE 10-11 Chest radiograph of a patient with *Pneumocystis jiroveci* pneumonia. (From Haslett C, Chilvers ER, Boon NA, Colledge NR, eds. *Davidson's Principles and Practice of Medicine.* 19th ed. Edinburgh: Elsevier Science; 2002: Fig. 1.86.)

10

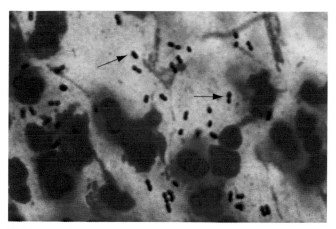

FIGURE 10-12 Purulent sputum in a patient with pneumococcal pneumonia. Gram stain shows gram-positive diplococci characteristic of *Streptococcus pneumoniae* (arrows). (From Haslett C, Chilvers ER, Boon NA, Colledge NR, eds. *Davidson's Principles and Practice of Medicine.* 19th ed. Edinburgh: Elsevier Science; 2002: Fig. 13.30.)

severe pneumonia, cavitary infiltrates, leukopenia, active alcohol abuse, chronic severe liver disease, asplenia, positive pneumococcal urinary antigen test, and pleural effusion)

- **If significant pleural effusion is seen at presentation, thoracentesis with analysis and culture should be performed**
- Cause of pneumonia is considered definitive only if bacteria are isolated from normally sterile space (blood, pleura)
- Cause is considered probable but not definitive if only cultured from sputum, unless sputum grows *Legionella,* tuberculosis, or some fungi
  - *Legionella* urinary antigen detects only serotype 1 *L. pneumophila*; sputum direct fluorescent antibody less reliable for *Legionella* spp.
- ***Chlamydophila* and *Mycoplasma* infections best diagnosed by polymerase chain reaction assay of respiratory specimen; serologic tests unreliable**

TREATMENT

Table 10-3 summarizes the initial therapy for suspected bacterial community-acquired pneumonia.
- First decision is whether to manage as outpatient or whether hospitalization is appropriate
  - Pneumonia severity index (PSI) or CURB-65 score may help guide hospitalization; PSI has higher sensitivity but lower specificity than CURB-65 (Tables 10-4 and 10-5)
  - **Hospitalization usually required for patients who have co-morbidities, highly abnormal vital signs, hypoxemia, laboratory abnormalities, or who are older adults**
- Initial antibiotic choice typically empiric and should cover S. *pneumoniae*

| TABLE 10-3 | *Recommended Empirical Antibiotics for Community-Acquired Pneumonia* |

Outpatient Treatment

1. Previously healthy and no use of antimicrobials within previous 3 months
   A macrolide (azithromycin, clarithromycin) (strong recommendation)
   Doxycycline (weak recommendation)
2. Presence of co-morbidities such as chronic heart, lung, liver, or renal disease; diabetes mellitus; alcoholism; malignancies; asplenia; immunosuppressing conditions or use of immunosuppressing drugs; or use of antimicrobials within the previous 3 months (in which case an alternative from a different class should be selected)
   A respiratory fluoroquinolone (moxifloxacin or levofloxacin) (strong recommendation)
   A β-lactam (amoxicillin/clavulanate, high-dose amoxicillin 1 g tid, cefpodoxime, or cefuroxime) plus a macrolide
3. In regions with a high rate (>25%) of infection with high-level (MIC ≥16 μg/mL) macrolide-resistant *Streptococcus pneumoniae,* consider use of alternative agents listed previously in (2) for patients without co-morbidities (moderate recommendation)

Inpatients, Non-ICU Treatment

A respiratory fluoroquinolone (strong recommendation)
A β-lactam (ceftriaxone, cefotaxime, ertapenem) plus a macrolide (strong recommendation)

Inpatients, ICU Treatment

A β-lactam (cefotaxime, ceftriaxone, or ampicillin/sulbactam) plus either azithromycin or a respiratory fluoroquinolone (strong recommendation) (for PCN-allergic patients, a respiratory fluoroquinolone and aztreonam are recommended)

Special Concerns

If there is high concern for *Pseudomonas* infection in sick patients: antipneumococcal, antipseudomonal β-lactam (piperacillin/tazobactam, cefepime, imipenem, or meropenem) plus either ciprofloxacin or levofloxacin (750 mg)
or
The above β-lactam plus an aminoglycoside and a respiratory fluoroquinolone (for PCN-allergic patients, substitute aztreonam for above β-lactam) (moderate recommendation)
If CA-MRSA is a consideration, add vancomycin or linezolid (moderate recommendation)

CA-MRSA, Community-acquired methicillin-resistant Staphylococcus aureus; ICU, intensive care unit; MIC, minimum inhibitory concentration.
Modified from Mandell LA, Wunderink RG, Anzueto A, et al. Infectious Diseases Society of America/American Thoracic Society consensus guidelines on the management of community-acquired pneumonia in adults. *Clin Infect Dis.* 2007;44:S27–S73.

  - Should also cover atypical agents and drug-resistant *Pneumococcus* if patient is severely ill (see Table 10-3)
- Timely antibiotic administration (within 6 hours of initial encounter) correlates with decreased mortality; considered standard of care
- Many guidelines exist with slight variations; consider individual patient factors when selecting empiric antibiotics

TABLE 10-4	*Pneumonia Severity Index**

Step 1. Is the patient at low risk (class I) based on the history and physical examination and not a resident of a nursing home?

Age ≤50 years

and

None of the co-existing conditions or physical examination findings listed in step 2

No: Go to step 2

Yes: Outpatient treatment is recommended

Step 2. Calculate risk score for classes II to V

Patient Characteristics	*Points Assigned*	*Patient's Points*
Demographic factors		
Age (years)		
Males	Age	____
Females	Age −10	____
Nursing home resident	+10	____
Co-existing conditions		
Neoplastic disease	+30	____
Liver disease	+20	____
Congestive heart failure	+10	____
Cerebrovascular disease	+10	____
Renal disease	+10	____
Initial physical examination findings		
Altered mental status	+20	____
Respiratory rate ≥30 breaths/min	+20	____
Systolic blood pressure <90 mm Hg	+20	____
Temperature <35°C (95°F) or ≥40°C (104°F)	+15	____
Pulse ≥125 beats/min	+10	____
Initial laboratory findings (score zero if not tested)		
pH <7.35	+30	____
Blood urea nitrogen >30 mg/dL (10.5 mmol/L)	+20	−
Sodium <130 mEq/L (130 mmol/L)	+20	____
Glucose ≥250 mg/dL (13.9 mmol/L)	+10	____
Hematocrit <30% (0.30)	+10	____
Arterial PO_2 <60 mm Hg or O_2 saturation <90%	+10	____
Pleural effusion	+10	____
Total score (sum of patient's points):		

30-Day Mortality Data by Risk Class

Total Score	Risk Class	Recommended Site of Treatment	Mortality Range Observed in Validation Cohorts (%)
None (see step 1)	I	Outpatient	0.1
≤70	II	Outpatient	0.5
71–90	III	Outpatient	0.9–2.8
91–130	IV	Inpatient	8.2–9.3
>130	V	Inpatient	27–29.2

*Step 1 identifies patients in risk class I on the basis of age of 50 years or younger and the absence of all co-morbid conditions and vital sign abnormalities listed in step 2. For all patients who are not classified as risk class I, the laboratory data listed in step 2 should be collected to calculate a pneumonia severity score. Risk class and recommended site of care based on the pneumonia severity score are listed in the final portion of the table. Thirty-day mortality data are based on two independent cohorts of 40,326 patients.

O_2, Oxygen; PO_2, partial pressure oxygen.

From Metlay JP, Fine MJ. Testing strategies in the initial management of patients with community-acquired pneumonia. *Ann Intern Med.* 2003;138:115.

10

TABLE 10-5	Clinical Feature Points (CURB-65) (score 1 point for each variable present)	
Confusion (defined as a mental test score ≤8, or disorientation in person, place, or time)	1	
Uremia: Blood urea ≥7 mmol/L (~19 mg/dL)	1	
Respiratory rate: ≥30 breaths/min	1	
Blood pressure: systolic ≤90 mm Hg or diastolic ≤60 mm Hg	1	
Age >65 years	1	
Total points		

Mortality Risks and Treatment Recommendations Based on CURB-65 Score

Score	Group
0 or 1	Mortality risk low (1.5%), consider home treatment
2	Mortality risk moderate (9.2%), consider hospital-supervised treatment
3	Mortality risk high (22%), manage in hospital
4 or 5	Consider admission to intensive care unit

From Lim WS, van der Eerden MM, Laing R, et al. Defining community acquired pneumonia severity on presentation to hospital: an international derivation and validation study. *Thorax.* 2003;58:377–382.

Review Questions

For review questions, please go to ExpertConsult.com.

SUGGESTED READINGS

Alcaide ML, Bisno AL. Pharyngitis and epiglottitis. *Infect Dis Clin North Am.* 2007;21:449-469.

Butorac-Petanjek B, Parnham MJ, Popovic-Grle S. Antibiotic therapy for exacerbations of chronic obstructive pulmonary disease (COPD). *J Chemother.* 2010;22:291-297.

Centers for Disease Control and Prevention [CDC]. Influenza, seasonal influenza, treatment-antiviral drugs. <www.cdc.gov/flu/antivirals/index.htm>.

Centers for Disease Control and Prevention [CDC]. Pertussis (whooping cough). <www.cdc.gov/pertussis/index.html>.

Chow AW, Benninger MS, Brook I, et al. IDSA clinical practice guideline for acute bacterial rhinosinusitis in children and adults. *Clin Infect Dis.* 2012;54:e72-e112.

Gonzales R, Bartlett JG, Besser RE, et al. Principles of appropriate antibiotic use for treatment of uncomplicated acute bronchitis: background. *Ann Intern Med.* 2001;134:521-529.

Liñares J, Ardanuy C, Pallares R, et al. Changes in antimicrobial resistance, serotypes and genotypes in *Streptococcus pneumoniae* over a 30-year period. *Clin Microbiol Infect.* 2010;16:402-410.

Mandell LA, Wunderink RG, Anzueto A, et al. Infectious Diseases Society of America/American Thoracic Society consensus guidelines on the management of community-acquired pneumonia in adults. *Clin Infect Dis.* 2007;44(suppl 2):S27-S72.

Pratter MR, Brightling CE, Boulet LP, et al. An empiric integrative approach to the management of cough: ACCP evidence-based guidelines. *Chest.* 2006;129(suppl 1):S222-S231.

Shulman ST, Bisno AL, Gerber MA, et al. Clinical practice guidelines for the diagnosis and management of Group A streptococcal pharyngitis: 2012 Update by the Infectious Diseases Society of America. *Clin Infect Dis.* 2012;55:1279-1282.

CHAPTER 11

Genitourinary Infections

KHALIL G. GHANEM, MD, PhD

Sexually transmitted diseases (STDs) may be classified according to syndromes. These include genital ulcer diseases, urethritis, cervicitis, pelvic inflammatory disease, epididymitis, vaginal discharge, genital warts, proctitis, and ectoparasite infestations. Urinary tract infections (UTIs) may involve the lower genitourinary tract or both the upper and lower tracts. Treatment differs based on the site involved.

Genital Ulcer Diseases

Table 11-1 provides a summary of the presentations and causes of urogenital ulcer diseases.

HERPES SIMPLEX VIRUS

Figure 11-3 shows an example of primary genital herpes

Basic Information

- Genital infections are caused by both herpes simplex virus (HSV)-2 and HSV-1; HSV-1 also causes orolabial herpes ("cold sores")
  - HSV-1 is now the predominant cause of genital herpes among young people
- Seroprevalence of HSV-2 and HSV-1 in adults in the United States is 17% and 60%, respectively
- **Up to 70% of cases of genital herpes are asymptomatic and unrecognized**
- Incubation period: 2 to 7 days
- Viral shedding occurs even in the absence of lesions; the amount of shedding declines over time
- Prior infection with HSV-1 does not protect against incident HSV-2 infection, although incident HSV-1 in persons infected with HSV-2 is rare

Clinical Presentation

- Primary genital herpes lesions are classically painful, multiple, and grouped on erythematous base, beginning as macules and papules, evolving to vesicles and ulcers
- Local symptoms may include pain, itching, dysuria, and tender inguinal adenopathy
- Primary lesions may be accompanied by fever, headache, malaise, and myalgias
- Recurrent disease is less severe than primary disease but may be severe in immunosuppressed individuals.
- Primary infections with HSV-1 and 2 are similar; recurrent infections with HSV-1 tend to be less severe and less frequent than recurrent infections with HSV-2
- Extragenital complications include central nervous system involvement (e.g. meningitis or encephalitis) and urinary retention

Diagnosis

- Clinical diagnosis can be confirmed by cell culture (gold standard but low sensitivity), detection of viral antigen (low sensitivity), polymerase chain reaction (PCR) (most sensitive), and serology (type-specific glycoprotein G1 and G2)
- Serology is the preferred method when no active lesions are present
- Tzanck preparation may show multinucleated giant cells (very low sensitivity)
- Serologic testing may be negative in primary infection; serologic false positives may occur, particularly if the pretest probability of having HSV is low
- Immunoglobulin M (IgM) serologies are neither sensitive nor specific for primary infections; there are no universal screening recommendations
- The presence of IgG antibodies to HSV-2 is diagnostic of genital infection; IgG antibodies to HSV-1 may reflect either orolabial infection or genital infection
- A combination of history, physical examination findings, and serologic test results are needed to assess whether a given patient's ulcer(s) are attributable to herpes

Treatment

- **Systemic antiviral drugs (e.g., acyclovir, famciclovir, or valacyclovir) can be used as episodic or suppressive therapy and they are all equally efficacious**
  - Episodic treatment does not eradicate the virus or reduce frequency of recurrences
  - **Daily suppressive therapy among patients with 6 or more recurrences per year can reduce the frequency by up to 80% and prevents recurrences in 25% to 30% of patients; frequency of episodes may diminish over time**
  - Suppressive therapy does not eliminate subclinical viral shedding
  - Once-daily valacyclovir in the infected partner, in addition to consistent condom use, may help decrease transmission to an uninfected partner by approximately 55%

SYPHILIS
Basic Information

- Systemic illness with protean manifestations caused by *Treponema pallidum*
- Major routes of transmission are via sexual intercourse and from mother to fetus

TABLE 11-1	*Urogenital Ulcer Disease*			
Ulcerative Disease	**Causative Agent**	**Clinical Presentation**	**Diagnosis**	**Treatment**
Genital herpes	HSV-2 > HSV-1	Cluster of vesicles on erythematous base **Painful** and pruritic Dysuria Lymphadenopathy	Tzanck preparation, multinucleated giant cells (low sensitivity) Viral culture (70% sensitivity) PCR Glycoprotein G-based serologies	Acyclovir or famciclovir or valacyclovir
Syphilitic chancre	*Treponema pallidum*	Single, **painless** ulcer at the site of inoculation Clean base and raised, firm border Painless lymphadenopathy	Darkfield examination Serology: Nontreponemal (RPR, VDRL) Treponemal (FTA-ABS, MHA-TP, TP-PA, EIAs)	Penicillin
Chancroid (Fig. 11-1)	*Haemophilus ducreyi*	**Painful** ulcer Tender inguinal adenopathy Occurs in outbreaks	Clinical diagnosis Culture available but not widely used	Azithromycin or ceftriaxone or ciprofloxacin
Donovanosis or granuloma inguinale	*Klebsiella granulomatis*	**Painless** papule or nodule erodes into beefy-red granulomatous ulcer with rolled edges. Endemic in Far East Asia and Southern Africa	Donovan bodies on biopsy	Doxycycline or trimethoprim-sulfamethoxazole Treat at least 3 weeks
Lymphogranuloma venereum (LGV; Fig. 11-2)	*Chlamydia trachomatis* serovar L1, L2, or L3	**Painless** genital ulcer; Painful inguinal lymphadenopathy (with groove sign) Proctitis	Clinical syndrome Serology Complement fixation titers of at least 1:64 Nucleic acid amplification tests	Doxycycline for 3 weeks

EIA, Enzyme immunoassay; FTA-ABS, fluorescent treponemal antibody, absorbed; HSV-1, herpes simplex virus type 1; HSV-2, herpes simplex virus type 2; MHA-TP, microhemagglutination-T. pallidum; PCR, polymerase chain reaction; RPR, rapid plasma regain; TP-PA, T. pallidum particle agglutination; VDRL, venereal disease research laboratory.

Clinical Presentation

- Primary syphilis (Fig. 11-4)
  - **Begins as a chancre (a single, painless papule) at the site of inoculation 2 to 3 weeks after exposure**
    - Quickly erodes and becomes indurated with a clean base and raised, firm borders
    - Atypical lesions occur in 60% of cases
    - Primary lesions may be accompanied by regional painless bilateral adenopathy
- Secondary or disseminated syphilis (Fig. 11-5)
  - Begins 2 to 8 weeks after appearance of chancre
  - **May be associated with flulike symptoms, generalized lymphadenopathy, and temporary patchy alopecia**
  - Characteristic rash may be macular, maculopapular, papular, or pustular, and may involve the whole body or palms and soles
  - **Condylomata lata appear as raised, painless, gray-white lesions; are highly infectious, and develop in intertriginous areas and on mucous membranes**
- Latent syphilis
  - Defined by a lack of clinical manifestations with positive serology
  - Latent syphilis acquired within the preceding year is early latent syphilis

- Late latent syphilis implies acquisition more than 1 year before diagnosis
- Tertiary syphilis
  - Implies late manifestations of syphilis
  - Gummatous syphilis results in skeletal, mucosal, ocular, and visceral lesions
  - Average time of onset is 4 to 12 years after infection
  - Cardiovascular syphilis causes endarteritis of the aortic vasovasorum
    - Average time of onset is 15 years
    - Presents as aortic aneurysm or aortic valve insufficiency
- Neurosyphilis
  - **Can occur at any syphilis stage (i.e., may be an early manifestation or a tertiary one)**
  - Early neurosyphilis (meningovascular syphilis) usually presents during the first year after infection as meningitis (often, a basilar meningitis involving cranial nerves) particularly among HIV-infected persons
  - Late neurosyphilis, occurring many years after primary infection, may be meningovascular (presenting as stroke), parenchymatous (manifesting as tabes dorsalis, electrical pains shooting down the legs), or general paresis (personality changes, hallucinations)
- Auditory manifestations may also occur during any stage of syphilis

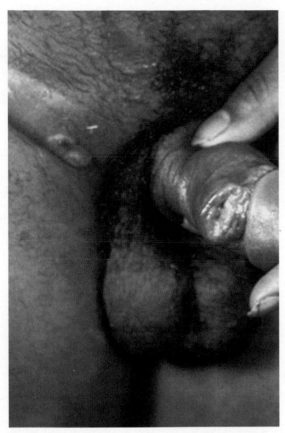

FIGURE 11-1 Chancroid presents as a painful ulcer and suppurative adenopathy. (From www.cdc.gov.)

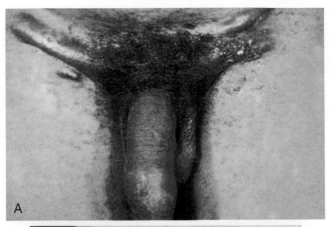

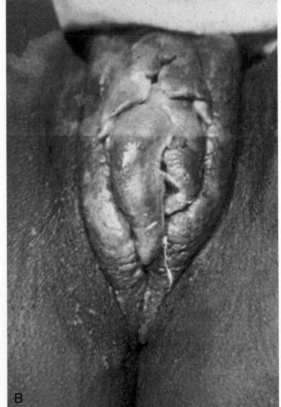

FIGURE 11-2 **A,** Early lymphogranuloma venereum (LGV) presents first as an ulcer and then as painful inguinal lymphadenopathy. **B,** Late complications of LGV include genital elephantiasis. (From www.cdc.gov.)

- Ophthalmic syphilis may occur at any stage and includes iritis, uveitis, neuroretinitis, and optic neuritis

Diagnosis

- Darkfield examination of genital lesions and direct fluorescent antibody tests of lesion exudates or tissue provide definitive evidence
- Two types of serologic tests are used for presumptive diagnosis:
  - Nontreponemal tests include rapid plasma reagin (RPR) and venereal disease research laboratory (VDRL) tests
    - Often used as screening tests
    - **Because of low specificity, must be confirmed by a treponemal test**
    - May revert to negative even in the absence of therapy
  - Treponemal tests include the fluorescent treponemal antibody, absorbed (FTA-ABS), *T. pallidum* particle agglutination tests (TP-PA), and newer automated tests (enzyme immunoassays [EIA] or chemoilluminescent assays [CIA])
    - **CIA or EIA now being used as screening tests instead of nontreponemal tests**
    - A positive test should reflex to a nontreponemal test; if the nontreponemal test is negative, a second different treponemal test (usually the TP-PA) should be done to confirm the first positive treponemal test

- Serologic tests may be negative in approximately 30% of primary syphilis cases but are approximately 100% sensitive in secondary syphilis
  - A negative RPR essentially rules out the diagnosis of secondary syphilis in the absence of a prozone reaction
- A confirmed positive treponemal test and a negative nontreponemal test may be seen with (1) old treated syphilis, (2) old untreated syphilis, (3) prozone reaction, and (4) early syphilis (where the treponemal tests became reactive before the nontreponemal ones)

11

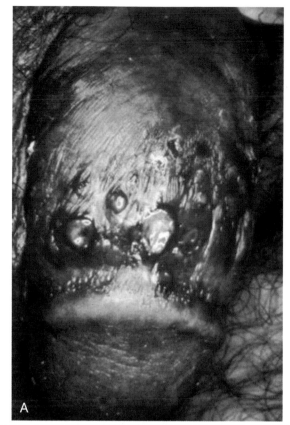

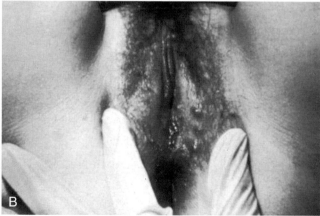

FIGURE 11-3 Primary genital herpes, **A**, along the shaft of the penis and **B**, in the vulvar area. (From www.cdc.gov.)

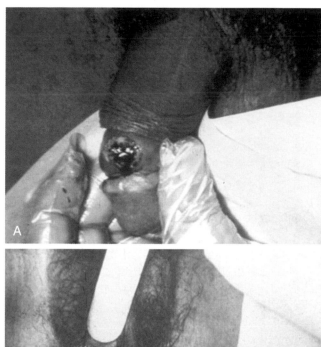

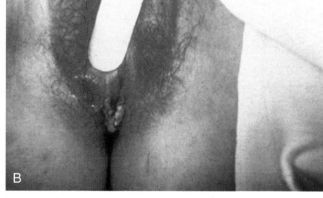

FIGURE 11-4 The chancre of primary syphilis shown in a man (**A**) and in a woman (**B**). (From www.cdc.gov.)

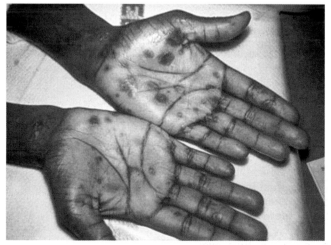

FIGURE 11-5 The characteristic rash of secondary syphilis, commonly involving the palms and soles (from www.cdc.gov).

- Diagnosis of neurosyphilis is based on a combination of serologic tests, cerebrospinal fluid (CSF) abnormalities (greater than 5 white blood cells [WBCs]/mm³ ± abnormal protein), or a reactive CSF VDRL
  - CSF VDRL is highly specific but insensitive (50%); negative study does not exclude the diagnosis
  - CSF FTA-ABS is less specific but very sensitive; negative study probably excludes neurosyphilis if the pretest probability is moderate to low
  - CSF examination is indicated in cases of neurologic or ophthalmologic abnormalities, evidence of active tertiary syphilis, or evidence of serologic treatment failure

- HIV infection with a CD4 count less than or equal to 350 cells/mm³, or an RPR greater than or equal to 1:32, is associated with increased risk of asymptomatic neurosyphilis; CSF examination may be considered

TABLE 11-2	*Recommended Treatment Regimens for Syphilis*
Clinical Stage	**Treatment**
Primary, secondary, and early latent syphilis	Benzathine penicillin G—2.4 million units IM in a single dose (if penicillin allergic—doxycycline 100 mg PO bid for 2 weeks, except pregnant patients, who should be desensitized and treated with penicillin)
Late latent syphilis, syphilis of unknown duration, or tertiary syphilis (gummatous and cardiovascular syphilis)	Benzathine penicillin G: 7.2 million units, administered as 3 doses of 2.4 million units IM each at 1-week intervals
Neurosyphilis	Aqueous crystalline penicillin G: 18 to 24 million units per day for 10 to 14 days

Bid, Twice daily; IM, intramuscularly; PO, orally.

Treatment

- **Parenteral penicillin G is the drug of choice (Table 11-2)**
  - Only accepted therapy with documented efficacy for neurosyphilis and syphilis during pregnancy is desensitization followed by penicillin therapy
- **The Jarisch-Herxheimer reaction**
  - Acute febrile reaction associated with headache and myalgias; thought to be activation of inflammatory cascade associated with lysis of spirochetes
  - **Can occur within the first 24 hours after therapy (particularly in early syphilis)**
  - Treatment is supportive
- Response to therapy is monitored by change in titer of a nontreponemal test (e.g., RPR) 12 (for primary, secondary, and early latent stages of syphilis) to 24 (for late syphilis) months after therapy
  - **A fourfold (or two-dilution) decrease in RPR or VDRL titer (e.g., from 1:64 to 1:16) indicates a cure**
  - No change or increase in titer indicates failure of therapy
  - Documentation of a titer response followed by a fourfold increase indicates reinfection
- **Treponemal test (e.g., FTA-ABS) titers do not correlate with disease activity or therapy and usually remain positive for life**
- In neurosyphilis, quantitative nontreponemal serologic tests should be repeated at 6, 12, and 24 months, and CSF examination should be repeated 6 months after therapy

Urethritis and Cervicitis

- Urethritis and cervicitis are characterized by discharge of mucopurulent or purulent material

- Principal etiologic agents are *Neisseria gonorrhoeae*, *Chlamydia trachomatis*, *Mycoplasma genitalium*, and *Trichomonas vaginalis*

GONORRHEA
Basic Information

- Can involve the genital tract, rectum, oropharynx, or be disseminated
- **Incubation period is 3 to 7 days; symptoms manifest within 10 to 14 days after exposure**
- Disseminated gonococcal infection (DGI) occurs in 1% to 3% of cases

Clinical Presentation

- In men, symptomatic disease occurs in approximately 50%, with purulent urethral discharge or dysuria; causes 30% of epididymitis cases in young men
- Women with cervicitis may have vaginal discharge or bleeding; 50% may be asymptomatic
  - Other syndromes in women include urethritis, Bartholin gland abscesses, or pelvic inflammatory disease (PID)
- **DGI may present as triad of (1) dermatitis with petechial or pustular acral skin lesions, (2) tenosynovitis, and (3) asymmetrical migratory polyarthralgias, or as purulent arthritis without skin lesions**
  - Perihepatitis, endocarditis, meningitis, and osteomyelitis occur less commonly

Diagnosis

- **Nucleic acid amplification (NAA) tests are the tests of choice for genital and extragenital sites; extragenital testing is not Food and Drug Administration cleared but is routinely performed**
- Sites for specimen collection for NAA tests include the vagina (preferred for women), cervix, urethra, urine (preferred for men), oropharynx, and rectum
- Gram stain may show gram-negative intracellular diplococci; low sensitivity in asymptomatic persons and women
- Culture using modified Thayer-Martin medium; sensitivity approximately 85% to 90%
- Screen high-risk men and women (e.g., men who have sex with men, new sex partner, recent sexually transmitted infection, HIV infection, high prevalence areas)
- **Retest all patients 3 months after completing therapy because reinfection rates are high**

Treatment

- **Ceftriaxone 250 mg intramuscular × 1 plus 1 g of oral azithromycin is first-line therapy;** intramuscular ceftriaxone has excellent activity; oral cephalosporins are approved alternate agents but they may have lower activity against pharyngeal gonorrhea
  - Patients with pharyngeal gonorrhea require a test-of-cure 2 weeks after therapy to verify response if treated with oral cephalosporins

- Monotherapy is not recommended because of increased prevalence of drug resistance
- **Azithromycin monotherapy (2 g) effective for both gonorrheal infections and chlamydial infections, but use is limited by gastrointestinal distress and emerging resistance**
- Sexual partners in the preceding 60 days or the last sexual partner should be referred for evaluation and treatment
- Patients with DGI should be hospitalized and treated parenterally with ceftriaxone and a single 2-g oral dose of azithromycin; may be discharged 24 hours after clinical response to complete a 7-day course of oral cephalosporin

CHLAMYDIA TRACHOMATIS

Basic Information

- *C. trachomatis* D through K serotypes are the most common bacterial STD in the United States (*C. trachomatis* L1–L3 serotypes cause lymphogranuloma venereum [LGV]; see Table 11-1)
- Single biggest risk factor for D through K serotypes is young age

Clinical Presentation

- **Infection in women may present as cervicitis or urethritis; may also have vaginal discharge, lower abdominal pain, or dysuria**
  - **Most cases are asymptomatic**
- Men may develop urethritis with dysuria and mucopurulent discharge; most are asymptomatic
  - Epididymitis manifests as unilateral testicular pain and tenderness, edema, and/or hydrocele

Diagnosis

- **Because asymptomatic infection is most common, annual screening of all sexually active women aged 25 years or younger and older at-risk women is recommended to prevent sequelae**
  - Untreated chlamydial infection in women is a major cause of PID, ectopic pregnancy, and infertility
- In men, untreated infection may result in prostatitis
- Diagnostic method of choice is NAA test

Treatment

- **Azithromycin or doxycycline are first-line agents; doxycycline is preferred for rectal infections**
  - Alternatives include fluoroquinolones and erythromycin
  - In pregnancy, doxycycline and fluoroquinolones are contraindicated
  - Test for cure is recommended after treatment with amoxicillin or erythromycin because these regimens may not be as efficacious, and side effects may discourage compliance
- Because reinfection following treatment is common and reinfection increases the risk for PID, repeat testing is warranted 3 months after therapy
- Sexual partners in the preceding 60 days or the last sexual partner should be referred for evaluation and treatment

MYCOPLASMA GENITALIUM

- Causes acute and chronic urethritis; moderate to strong association with cervicitis and PID
- **The most common cause of persistent urethritis in men**
- NAA tests are sensitive but none are FDA cleared
- Treatment: 1 g of azithromycin orally is effective but associated with emergence of resistance
  - Longer azithromycin courses are probably better; drug of choice if azithromycin resistance suspected is moxifloxacin 500 mg orally for 7 to 14 days

Pelvic Inflammatory Disease

Basic Information

- Encompasses endometritis, salpingitis, tubo-ovarian abscess, and pelvic peritonitis
- Most commonly implicated organisms include *N. gonorrhoeae* and *C. trachomatis*
  - Anaerobes, gram-negative bacilli, streptococci, and mycoplasma may also cause PID

Clinical Presentation

- Fever and lower abdominal pain (usually bilateral) are hallmarks of PID
- **Right upper quadrant tenderness from perihepatitis (Fitz-Hugh–Curtis syndrome) is seen in 10%**
- Pelvic examination may reveal cervical motion tenderness, adnexal tenderness, or purulent endocervical discharge
- A palpable adnexal mass suggests a tubo-ovarian abscess

Diagnosis

- **Clinical criteria for diagnosis:**
  - **One of the following: uterine tenderness, adnexal tenderness, or cervical motion tenderness**
  - Additional criteria include mucopurulent cervicitis, presence of WBCs in vaginal secretions, documented *N. gonorrhoeae* or *C. trachomatis*, oral temperature greater than 38.3° C, and elevated erythrocyte sedimentation rate or C-reactive protein
- Definitive criteria include histopathologic evidence of endometritis, radiologic evidence on transvaginal ultrasound, or laparoscopic evidence of PID

Treatment

- **Outpatient treatment: ceftriaxone *plus* doxycycline with or without metronidazole**
  - Empirical therapy is broad spectrum to cover *N. gonorrhoeae*, *C. trachomatis*, anaerobes, gram-negative bacteria, and streptococci
- Inpatient therapy is provided when surgical emergencies cannot be excluded, the patient is pregnant, there is lack of response to or inability to take oral antibiotics, or tubo-ovarian abscess is present

Epididymitis and Prostatitis

Basic Information

- *Epididymitis* is defined as inflammation of the epididymis caused by infection or trauma
  - In men younger than 35 years it is most often caused by *N. gonorrhoeae* (30%) or *C. trachomatis* (70%)
  - **In men older than 35 years nonsexually transmitted epididymitis is more commonly caused by gram-negative enteric organisms**
- Prostatitis, or inflammation of the prostate, may be acute or chronic
  - Acute infection is most often caused by *Escherichia coli* and occasionally by *N. gonorrhoeae*
  - Chronic prostatitis is most often caused by gram-negative bacilli (including *E. coli*) and enterococci

Clinical Presentation

- Epididymitis presents as unilateral testicular pain and tenderness, edema, and/or hydrocele
  - Must rule out testicular torsion, especially when onset of pain is sudden, and pain is severe
    - Pyuria is generally seen in epididymitis, but not torsion
    - **Doppler ultrasound will show decreased or absent blood flow to the affected testicle in torsion but normal or increased blood flow with epididymitis**
- Acute prostatitis presents with fever, chills, perineal pain, back pain, dysuria
  - The prostate gland is tender on examination
- Chronic prostatitis is often indolent

Diagnosis

- For urethritis, perform gram stain, culture, and/or NAA test of urethral exudates, intraurethral swabs, or urine
- Diagnosis of prostatitis is usually clinical
  - "Milking" the prostate by digital examination before voiding may induce pyuria

Treatment

- **For epididymitis most likely caused by gonococcal or chlamydial infection, treatment should cover both organisms**

- **For epididymitis in patients older than 35 years without risk of gonococcal or chlamydial infection, treatment should cover *E. coli***
- Treatment for acute prostatitis includes ceftriaxone, quinolones, or trimethoprim-sulfamethoxazole (TMP-SMX) for 14 days
- Treatment for chronic prostatitis includes 4 to 6 weeks of a quinolone or 6 to 12 weeks of TMP-SMX

Vaginitis

Table 11-3 provides a summary of the types of organisms causing vaginitis and their specific diagnoses.

Treatment

- Bacterial vaginosis is treated with a 7-day course of metronidazole (500 mg) twice daily
- Single dose (2-g) oral metronidazole is only recommended for the treatment of trichomoniasis
- Sex partners of women with trichomoniasis should be treated with 2 g of metronidazole
- Topical and oral antifungal agents may be used to treat vulvovaginal candidiasis

Proctitis

- Defined as inflammation of the lining of the rectum
- Major causes of sexually transmitted proctitis: *N. gonorrhoeae*; *Chlamydia trachomatis* serotypes D through K; *Chlamydia trachomatis* serotypes L1 through L3 (LGV); early syphilis; HSV-1 and 2
  - LGV has made a resurgence in the United States and Western Europe in the last few years (see Table 11-1); may cause strictures resembling Crohn disease
- All causes are indistinguishable based on symptoms; testing for all the previous pathogens should be considered.
  - NAA tests have the highest sensitivity to detect *N. gonorrhoeae* and *C. trachomatis* (even though not FDA cleared for extragenital sites)
  - Culture or PCR for HSV
  - Serology for syphilis

TABLE 11-3	*Vaginitis*			
Diagnosis	**Organism**	**Type of Organism**	**Discharge**	**Specific Diagnosis**
Bacterial vaginosis	Replacement of normal *Lactobacillus* spp. with anaerobes	Bacteria	White, noninflammatory coating discharge	Clue cells seen on microscopy Vaginal pH >4.5 + whiff test (fishy odor on addition of 10% KOH)
Trichomoniasis	*Trichomonas vaginalis*	Protozoan	Foul-smelling, frothy, yellow-green discharge	Organism seen on microscopy of secretions (<70% sensitive); culture; PCR now considered gold standard
Vulvovaginal candidiasis	Candida	Fungus (yeast)	White, "cottage cheese" discharge	Fungal elements seen on wet prep Vaginal pH 4 to 4.5

KOH, Potassium hydroxide; PCR, polymerase chain reaction.

11

- Empiric treatment with ceftriaxone and doxycycline may be considered until test results are available

Condylomata Acuminata (Anogenital Warts)

Basic Information

- **Caused by human papillomavirus (HPV) infection**
- The most common viral STD in the United States; most infections asymptomatic and self-limited
- **High-risk types 16, 18, 31, 33, and 35 have been strongly associated with cervical neoplasia**
  - The same types are also associated with dysplastic and neoplastic anal lesions
  - Low-risk HPV types 6 and 11 are rarely associated with neoplasia but cause approximately 90% of warts

Clinical Presentation

- Most infections are asymptomatic
- Exophytic verrucous white or pigmented lesions (Fig. 11-6)
- Symptoms vary according to site and size of the lesions

Diagnosis

- Diagnosis is based on visual inspection
  - Evaluation may include anoscopy, sigmoidoscopy, colposcopy, and/or vulvovaginal examination
  - Acetic acid 5% can be applied to facilitate identification
- **Biopsy serves to evaluate for dysplasia**
- HPV DNA used in conjunction with the Papanicolaou smear in women older than 30 years of age

Treatment

- Treatment of external genital warts depends on size, location, and patient and provider preference
- **Treatments include surgical removal, cryotherapy, or topical therapy with podophyllin, imiquimod, or trichloroacetic acid**
- Prevention (also see Chapter 73)
  - HPV virus-like–particle quadrivalent vaccine for types 6, 11, 16, and 18 and bivalent vaccine for types

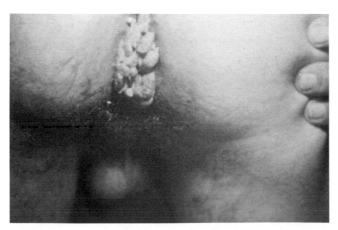

FIGURE 11-6 Anal condylomata acuminata appear as exophytic verrucous lesions. (From www.cdc.gov.)

16 and 18 are recommended for all females ages 9 to 26 years; quadrivalent vaccine may be given to males ages 9 to 26 years; also effective in HIV-infected persons with CD4 counts greater than 200 cells/mm³
- Vaccination does not eliminate the need for cervical cancer screening because not all cancer-causing HPV types are included in the vaccine

Urinary Tract Infections

Basic Information

- **Represent a broad spectrum of clinical illness, from uncomplicated cystitis to pyelonephritis with bacteremia**
- Pregnancy increases the risk of UTI because of dilation of the ureters, decreased ureteral peristalsis, and decreased bladder tone
  - Approximately 20% to 40% of patients with untreated bacteriuria early in gestation progress to pyelonephritis later in pregnancy
  - Pyelonephritis has been associated with premature delivery
  - Urine culture is therefore a routine part of prenatal screening

Clinical Presentation

- Uncomplicated acute bacterial cystitis
  - Characterized by dysuria, frequency, and urgency
  - Most often occurs in nonpregnant women with normal anatomy and no urologic instrumentation
  - Causative agent primarily *E. coli*
- Complicated UTI is defined by the presence of one of the following factors: pregnancy, male sex, immunosuppression, catheter or urologic instrumentation, stone or abnormal structure of the genitourinary tract, or functional abnormality of the genitourinary tract
- **Acute pyelonephritis manifests with fever, flank pain, and urinary symptoms**
- Development of perinephric abscess is suggested by an acute pyelonephritis-like illness with persistent fever and symptoms despite medical therapy
- Patients with bacteriuria (more than 10^5 colony-forming units [CFUs]/mL) but no symptoms are considered to have asymptomatic bacteriuria

Diagnosis

- Laboratory evaluation includes microscopic examination of the urine for pyuria and hematuria, or urine dipstick test for leukocyte esterase and nitrites
- **Urine culture is not necessary for uncomplicated UTI**
- **Microbiology of complicated UTI is less predictable and requires urine gram stain and culture**
- Diagnosis of pyelonephritis is supported by greater than 10^5 CFUs/mm³ of bacteriuria and pyuria of more than 10 WBCs/mm³
  - Leukocyte casts are seen in 20% to 50% of cases
  - Blood cultures are not required but are positive in 20% of cases

- Diagnosis of a perinephric abscess should be confirmed by ultrasound or computed tomography scan

Treatment

- Treatment of uncomplicated UTI is empirical and targeted to the most common etiologic bacteria
  - **Trimethoprim-sulfamethoxazole DS 1 tablet twice daily for 3 days is considered first-line in areas where resistance to the drug is less than 20%**
  - Other first-line agents include nitrofurantoin for 5 days or single-dose fosfomycin (avoid if any concern for pyelonephritis)
  - If cannot use the previous agents, can use fluoroquinolone but resistance and collateral damage a concern; can also consider β-lactams, but they have lower efficacy than other agents
    - **Amoxicillin or ampicillin should not be used for empiric treatment because of relatively poor efficacy**
- For complicated UTI, antibiotic selection is based on culture data
  - Duration of therapy is generally 7 to 14 days depending on chosen antimicrobial agent
- For pyelonephritis, treatment is based on severity of illness and is guided by urine and/or blood culture results
  - In mild cases, treatment includes oral quinolones for 7 days or TMP-SMX for a 14-day course
  - Moderate to severe illness may initially require intravenous therapy with quinolones, third-generation cephalosporins, or aminoglycosides
- Catheter-associated bacteriuria should only be treated in the setting of symptomatic infection, suspected sepsis, renal transplantation (controversial), or immunocompromise
  - In the catheterized patient, pyuria alone is not an indication for antibiotic therapy

- The presence, absence, or degree of pyuria should not be used to differentiate infection from asymptomatic bacteriuria
- **If possible, removal of catheter during treatment is advised**
- When long-term catheterization is required, intermittent catheterization rather than an indwelling catheter reduces the risk of infection
- For perinephric abscess, percutaneous drainage or surgery may be necessary
- Treat asymptomatic bacteriuria in pregnant women, before an invasive urologic procedure, in persons with renal transplant (controversial), or if neutropenia is present
  - Do NOT treat in diabetics and elderly persons.

Review Questions

For review questions, please go to ExpertConsult.com.

SUGGESTED READINGS

Centers for Disease Control and Prevention. Sexually transmitted diseases treatment guidelines 2010. *MMWR Recomm Rep.* 2010;59(RR-12):1-110.

Grigoryan L, Trautner BW, Gupta K. Diagnosis and management of urinary tract infections in the outpatient setting: a review. *JAMA.* 2014;312:1677-1684.

Hooton TM, Bradley SF, Cardenas DD, et al. Diagnosis, prevention, and treatment of catheter-associated urinary tract infection in adults: 2009 International Clinical Practice Guidelines from the Infectious Diseases Society of America. *Clin Infect Dis.* 2010;50:625-663.

Nicolle LE, Bradley S, Colgan R, et al. Infectious Diseases Society of America Guidelines for the Diagnosis and Treatment of Asymptomatic Bacteriuria in Adults. *Clin Infect Dis.* 2005;40:643-654.

CHAPTER 12

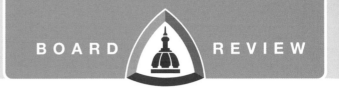
Human Immunodeficiency Virus Infection

GAIL BERKENBLIT, MD, PhD

There are more than 880,000 people infected with human immunodeficiency virus (HIV) living in the United States, and nearly 48,000 new cases per year. The continued development of more effective and tolerable antiretroviral therapy has led to an overall decline in mortality in the United States, as has the use of chemoprophylaxis for opportunistic infections. Although guidelines regarding HIV therapy are continuously changing and are usually the purview of HIV specialists, the presentation of acute HIV, common opportunistic infections, and complications of therapy should be recognized by all internists.

Basic Information

- Biology of retroviruses
  - HIV-1 and HIV-2 are RNA retroviruses that cause acquired immunodeficiency syndrome (AIDS)
  - HIV entry into T cells is mediated via binding of the CD4 receptor and associated co-factors
  - Reverse transcriptase converts the RNA genome into double-stranded DNA, which then integrates into the host genome and co-opts cellular machinery for replication
  - HIV infection selectively depletes CD4 cells, resulting in immunodeficiency
- Epidemiology
  - HIV-1 is the predominant subtype in the United States and worldwide
  - HIV-2 is found mainly in West Africa and has a slower clinical course
  - Both are spread via blood-borne exposure (e.g., needle sharing, transfusions), sexual intercourse, and maternal–fetal transmission

Clinical Presentation

- Acute retroviral syndrome
  - Typical onset of symptoms is 1 to 6 weeks after exposure to HIV (2 to 3 weeks most commonly)
  - Symptoms often mimic infectious mononucleosis
  - **Most common presentation: fever, lymphadenopathy, pharyngitis, rash (Fig. 12-1), myalgias, and arthralgias**
  - Also reported: thrombocytopenia, leukopenia, diarrhea, headache, elevated transaminases, hepatosplenomegaly, aseptic meningitis, encephalopathy

  - Symptoms resolve without treatment within 1 to 2 weeks
- Chronic HIV infection
  - May be clinically silent for years
  - Clinical manifestations depend on CD4 count (Table 12-1)

Diagnosis and Evaluation

- HIV screening
  - Voluntary routine screening recommended for all Americans ages 13 to 64 years
  - Need for repeat testing determined by risk assessment
- Diagnostic testing
  - Combination HIV antibody-HIV p24 antigen testing is able to diagnose infection within 12 to 16 days of infection
  - Older enzyme-linked immunosorbent assay (ELISA) antibody tests (followed by confirmatory Western blot) become positive 3 to 4 weeks after acute infection and remain the test of choice in screening for chronic infection
  - HIV RNA polymerase chain reaction (PCR)
    - Positive as early as 3 to 5 days after acute infection
    - **Test of choice in diagnosis of acute HIV infection (if exposure known to be less than 2 weeks previously)**
    - **Need to be wary of counts lower than 10,000 copies/mm³ because they may be false positives**
    - Correlates with rate of disease progression
    - Used to follow response to antiretroviral therapy (ART)
  - CD4 count
    - Measurement of immunodeficiency
    - Decline in CD4 cells confers susceptibility to opportunistic infections
    - **AIDS is defined as either a CD4 count lower than 200/mm³ or the presence of certain opportunistic illnesses**
  - HIV genotype
    - Detects mutations that confer resistance to ART
    - Should be obtained as part of initial panel of tests for an individual with HIV
    - In the United States, 10% to 20% of patients with new HIV infection have transmitted resistance to at least one class of antiretroviral medications

Antiretroviral Therapy

- There are six main classes of antiretroviral agents, each with different potential adverse effects (Table 12-2)
- Initiation of therapy
  - In the United States, ART is recommended for all HIV-infected individuals to reduce the risk of disease progression and prevent transmission
    - However, patients should understand the risks and benefits of ART and must be willing and able to commit to treatment
    - Patients may choose to postpone therapy, and providers on a case-by-case basis may elect to defer therapy based on clinical and/or psychosocial factors
    - **Indications favoring more urgent initiation of ART include pregnancy, AIDS-defining illness, low CD4 count, HIV-associated nephropathy (HIVAN), and hepatitis B co-infection**
  - **A combination of three antiretroviral agents from at least two different classes is recommended to prevent viral replication and inhibit the development of resistant HIV strains**
  - Selection of initial regimen should be individualized based on efficacy, baseline drug resistance profile, other co-morbid conditions, and potential adverse reactions
  - Initial recommended regimens for all patients include:
    - Efavirenz/tenofovir/emtricitabine
    - Ritonavir-boosted darunavir plus tenofovir/emtricitabine
    - Ritonavir-boosted atazanavir plus tenofovir/emtricitabine
    - Dolutegravir plus tenofovir/emtricitabine
    - Dolutegravir plus abacavir/lamivudine (only if HLA-B*5701 negative)
    - Elvitegravir/cobicistat plus tenofovir/emtricitabine (only if baseline creatinine clearance greater than 70 mL/min)
    - Raltegravir plus tenofovir/emtricitabine
  - Regimens that are also recommended but only for patients with pre-ART plasma HIV RNA greater than 100,000 copies/mL include:

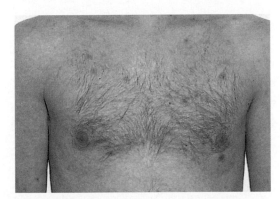

FIGURE 12-1 Typical morbilliform rash associated with acute retroviral syndrome. (From Forbes C, Jackson W. *Color Atlas and Text of Clinical Medicine.* 3rd ed. St. Louis: Mosby; 2003: Fig. 1-19.)

TABLE 12-1	*Complications and Recommended Chemoprophylaxis for Opportunistic Infections by CD4 Cell Count*	
CD4 Cell Count*	**Opportunistic Infections and Other HIV-Associated Conditions**	**Recommended Chemophylaxis Against Opportunistic Infections**
>500/mm³	Acute retroviral syndrome	None
200 to 500/mm³	Oral candidiasis Community-acquired pneumonia Pulmonary TB Kaposi sarcoma Herpes zoster CIN Lymphoma Anemia ITP HIV-associated nephropathy	None
<200/mm³	*Pneumocystis jiroveci* pneumonia (PCP) Disseminated histoplasmosis Extrapulmonary TB Wasting HIV dementia Progressive multifocal leukoencephalopathy	PCP prophylaxis with trimethoprim-sulfamethoxazole or dapsone or atovaquone or aerosolized pentamidine
<100/mm³	CNS toxoplasmosis Cryptococcosis CNS lymphoma	Toxoplasmosis prophylaxis (if patient is toxo IgG+) with trimethoprim-sulfamethoxazole *or* dapsone/pyrimethamine/folinic acid or atovaquone
<50/mm³	Disseminated MAI Disseminated CML	MAI prophylaxis with azithromycin or clarithromycin

*At each stage of decline in CD4 cell count, patients become at risk for further opportunistic infections and other conditions, and should receive appropriate chemoprophylaxis.
CIN, Cervical intraepithelial neoplasia; IgG, immunoglobulin G; ITP, idiopathic thrombocytopenia; MAI, Mycobacterium avium-intracellulare; TB, tuberculosis.

TABLE 12-2	*Antiretroviral Medications and Commonly Associated Adverse Effects*
Class of Antiretroviral Drug	**Adverse Effects**
Nucleoside Reverse Transcriptase Inhibitors	
Zidovudine (AZT)	Bone marrow suppression Lactic acidosis Presents with fatigue, nausea, myalgias Laboratory tests show anion gap acidosis and elevated lactic acid Can occur any time during therapy
Stavudine (d4T)	Peripheral neuropathy; lipodystrophy; lactic acidosis
Didanosine (ddI)	Peripheral neuropathy; pancreatitis; lactic acidosis
Lamivudine (3TC)	Can have severe hepatitis when discontinued in a patient co-infected with hepatitis B
Emtricitabine (FTC)	
Abacavir	Fatal hypersensitivity reaction Presents with fever, rash, flulike symptoms Usually in first 2 to 6 weeks after starting Can be fatal if drug not discontinued Screen for susceptibility to hypersensitivity with an HLA-B*5701 test before initiation
Tenofovir	Renal insufficiency Fanconi syndrome
Non-nucleoside Reverse Transcriptase Inhibitors	
Nevirapine	Rash Stevens-Johnson syndrome Hepatitis (especially at higher CD4 counts)
Efavirenz	Central nervous system side effects (confusion, nightmares); teratogenic
Etravirine	Hypersensitivity reactions characterized by rash, constitutional findings, organ dysfunction
Rilpivirine	Depression, nausea, headache
Protease Inhibitors	**General side effects include diarrhea, lipodystrophy, central obesity with peripheral wasting, hyperlipidemia, and insulin resistance**
Atazanavir	Indirect hyperbilirubinemia
Darunavir	Skin rash (has sulfonamide moiety)
Fosamprenavir	Skin rash (has sulfonamide moiety)
Indinavir	Nephrolithiasis
Lopinavir	
Nelfinavir	
Ritonavir	
Saquinavir	QT prolongation
Tipranivir	Intracranial hemorrhage
Membrane Fusion Inhibitors	
Enfuvirtide	Injection-site reactions
CCR5 Antagonist	
Maraviroc	Well tolerated, but only effective against CCR5 tropic virus
Integrase Inhibitor	
Raltegravir	Well tolerated, but twice daily
Dolutegravir	Hypersensitivity reactions characterized by rash, constitutional findings, organ dysfunction has been reported
Elvitegravir (co-formulated with cobicistat)	Renal impairment, do not use if creatinine clearance <70 mL/min

- Efavirenz plus abacavir/lamivudine (only if HLA-B*5701 negative)
- Rilpivirine/tenofovir/emtricitabine (only if CD4 greater than 200 cells/mm^3)
- Ritonavir-boosted atazanavir plus abacavir/lamivudine (only if HLA-B*5701 negative)
- Guidelines for monitoring and changing ART
  - Goal of therapy is viral suppression, meaning a viral load of less than 200 copies/mm^3.
  - CD4 count should be measured at initiation, at 3 months, and then at 3- to 6-month intervals for first 2 years of therapy; thereafter annually if viral load suppressed and CD4 consistently 300 to 500 cells/mm^3
  - When CD4 is consistently more than 500 cells/mm^3, and the patient has been on ART for 2 years or more (with a consistently suppressed viral load), CD4 count monitoring becomes optional
  - Viral load should be measured at ART initiation, 2 to 8 weeks after initiation of therapy, then every 4 to 8 weeks until viral load suppressed, then every 3 to 4 months once viral load suppressed. After 2 years or more of ART with consistent virologic suppression, time between viral load measurements can be extended to 6 months
  - **ART regimen should be changed if the patient has been adherent to therapy and fails to achieve virologic suppression in 24 to 48 weeks or has an increase in viral load (greater than 1000 copies/mm^3)**
    - If medications are changed for virologic failure, check viral loads as done for a treatment-naïve patient
  - **Obtain resistance testing if viral load is more than 500 copies/mm^3**
  - Generally, do not add a single drug to a failing regimen or switch single drugs in a regimen if there is ongoing viral replication
  - It is acceptable to switch single agents for side effect management if viral load is "undetectable"
    - If medications changed for toxicity or regimen simplification, check viral load 4 to 8 weeks after change to confirm continued virologic suppression
- Prevention of HIV transmission: ART for postexposure prophylaxis (PEP)
  - PEP should be given for both percutaneous and mucocutaneous exposures to blood, genital secretions, or other potentially infectious body fluids of a person known to be HIV-infected
  - PEP should be given without delay (first dose ideally within 1 to 2 hours)
  - The interval at which no benefit occurs is unknown, but likely to be less effective when started more than 72 hours after exposure
  - High-risk factors for percutaneous transmission include hollow needle, visible blood, needle in vessel, and high viral load
  - The recommended regimen is tenofovir/emtricitabine plus raltegravir
  - Exposed persons should be treated for 4 weeks
- Prevention of HIV transmission: ART for pre-exposure prophylaxis (PrEP)

- **PrEP with daily tenofovir/emtricitabine among high-risk HIV-negative men who have sex with men (MSM) has been shown reduce risk of acquiring HIV by 44%**
  - For patients whose tenofovir/emtricitabine blood levels suggested that at least four doses of the tablet were taken per week, the protective efficacy of PrEP increased to 96% or more per week
- The Centers for Disease Control and Prevention (CDC) recommends PrEP as one prevention option for sexually-active adult MSM at substantial risk of HIV acquisition, adult heterosexually active men and women at substantial risk of HIV acquisition, and injection drug users (IDUs) at substantial risk of HIV acquisition
- PrEP should also be discussed with heterosexually active women and men whose partners are known to have HIV infection as one of several options to protect the uninfected partner during conception and pregnancy
- Candidates for PrEP should be tested for HIV before initiation and at least every 3 months during use to avoid partial treatment of HIV infection
- Candidates for PrEP should be tested for hepatitis B, because tenofovir-emtricitabine is active against this infection, and patients may have a hepatitis flare were PrEP to be discontinued
- Other issues in the care of HIV-infected patients
  - Prophylaxis against certain opportunistic infections should be introduced once the CD4 count has declined to certain predetermined levels (see Table 12-1)
  - Immunizations are important, but most live attenuated virus vaccines should be avoided because of the risk of disseminated infection (Box 12-1)
  - **Screening purified protein derivative (PPD) or an interferon-gamma release assay should be done at diagnosis and then annually if patient is at risk; PPD greater than 5 mm is considered positive**
  - Screening and vaccination for viral hepatitis should be performed
  - Cancer screening is as per usual guidelines with the exception of cervical cancer (8- to 10-fold elevated risk in HIV patients)

BOX 12-1 | *Immunization in HIV Patients*

Indicated

Hepatitis A (if MSM, injection drug user, and/or chronic liver disease)
Hepatitis B
Human papillomavirus (through age 26 years)
Pneumococcus
Influenza
Tetanus-diphtheria/tetanus-diphtheria-acellular pertussis

Contraindicated (Live Virus)

Varicella
Measles-mumps-rubella
Bacille Calmette-Guérin
Smallpox

- Perform a Papanicolaou (Pap) smear at the time of diagnosis and again in 6 months; if normal, can screen annually

Opportunistic Infections and Other HIV-Associated Conditions

CANDIDIASIS

Clinical Presentation

- At higher risk when CD4 count is lower than 200/mm^3
- **Most commonly seen as oropharyngeal creamy white plaques (thrush) that are removable by scraping (Fig. 12-2)**
- Differential diagnosis includes oral hairy leukoplakia (Fig. 12-3), which are painless, white, nonremovable plaques associated with Epstein-Barr virus and typically located on the lateral and dorsal tongue

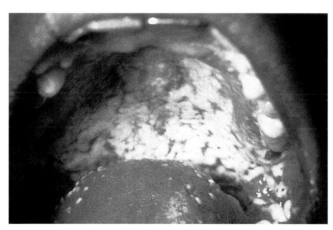

FIGURE 12-2 Oral candidiasis thrush. (From Mandell GL, Bennett JE, Dolin R, eds. *Principles and Practice of Infectious Diseases.* 6th ed. Philadelphia: Churchill Livingstone; 2005: Fig. 117-7.)

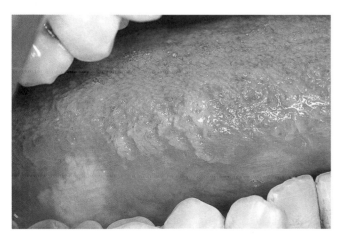

FIGURE 12-3 Oral hairy leukoplakia. Note the predilection for the lateral tongue surface and the vertical ridges. (From Cummings CW, Flint PW, Harker LA, et al, eds. *Cummings' Otolaryngology: Head and Neck Surgery.* 4th ed. Philadelphia: Mosby; 2005: Fig. 64-8.)

- Candida esophagitis is the most common cause of odynophagia in HIV-positive patients, followed by cytomegalovirus (CMV), herpes simplex virus (HSV), and aphthous ulcers

Diagnosis

- Oral candidiasis is usually diagnosed by appearance (see Fig. 12-2).
  - Swab or biopsy may be needed to differentiate from oral hairy leukoplakia
- Esophageal candidiasis is often diagnosed presumptively (odynophagia in HIV patient with low CD4 count)
  - Endoscopy is usually reserved for those who fail empiric therapy

Treatment

- Oral or vaginal candida infection may be treated with topical azole therapy
- Candida esophagitis is treated with a 2-week course of systemic fluconazole

PULMONARY INFECTIONS

See Table 12-3 and Figure 12-4 for common pulmonary conditions associated with HIV infection.

CENTRAL NERVOUS SYSTEM MANIFESTATIONS

See Table 12-4 and Figure 12-5 for common central nervous system (CNS) conditions associated with HIV infection.

DISSEMINATED *MYCOBACTERIUM AVIUM-INTRACELLULARE COMPLEX*

Clinical Presentation

- Typically presents when CD4 is less than 50/mm^3
- **Symptoms include fevers, malaise, wasting, abdominal pain, lymphadenopathy**
- Often associated with anemia and leukopenia
- **Elevated alkaline phosphatase is often a clue to this infection**

Diagnosis

- Most commonly diagnosed with mycobacterial blood cultures
  - Mycobacterium avium-intracellulare (MAI) is a slow growing mycobacterium; must hold cultures for weeks
- May suspect if acid-fast bacteria and granulomas are seen on biopsy of liver, lymph node, or bone marrow in a susceptible host (consider tuberculosis as well)

Treatment

- Treated with combination antimicrobial therapy (usually clarithromycin and ethambutol, with or without rifabutin)
- **Azithromycin chemoprophylaxis is recommended when CD4 is lower than 50/mm³**

CYTOMEGALOVIRUS

Clinical Presentation

- Typically presents when CD4 count is lower than 50/mm^3

TABLE 12-3	*Common Pulmonary Manifestations Associated with HIV Infection*				
	CD4 Count	**Clinical Presentation**	**Radiologic Appearance**	**Diagnostic Testing**	**Treatment**
Community-acquired pneumonia (CAP)	Any	Acute onset Fever Productive cough Pleuritic pain	Usually lobar infiltrate	Sputum gram stain and culture	Antibiotic coverage for *Streptococcus pneumoniae* and typical CAP pathogens; cover gram-negative rods if CD4 low
Pneumocystis jiroveci pneumonia (PCP)	Less than 200	Subacute onset Dry cough Hypoxia Fever Less likely if on prophylaxis	Usually "bat wing" perihilar infiltrate; 20% have normal chest radiograph	Immunofluorescence, silver stain, or culture of induced sputum or bronchoalveolar lavage	Trimethoprim-sulfamethoxazole first-line agent Alternatives: dapsone/trimethoprim; clindamycin/primaquine; atovaquone; or IV pentamidine Add corticosteroids if PaO$_2$ <70 or A-a gradient >35
Pulmonary histoplasmosis	<200	Subacute onset Dry cough Oral ulcers common Geographic risk	Diffuse interstitial infiltrates	*Histoplasma* urine antigen; bronchoalveolar lavage culture	Itraconazole or amphotericin B
Pulmonary tuberculosis	Any	Gradual onset Extrapulmonary manifestations common if CD4 <200	Diffuse interstitial infiltrates Noncavitary in advanced HIV	AFB stain/culture PPD >5 mm considered positive in HIV-infected patients	Four-drug TB regimen for 2 months, then two-drug maintenance for 6 month total therapy

A-a, Arterial-alveolar; AFB, acid-fast bacillus; PaO$_2$, arterial oxygen partial pressure; PPD, purified protein derivative; TB, tuberculosis.

- **Retinitis is most common end-organ complication of CMV (Fig. 12-6)**
  - Symptoms include floaters and decreased visual acuity
  - Less common sites of involvement include gastrointestinal (GI) tract (esophagitis and colitis), lung (pneumonitis), and CNS (encephalitis)

Diagnosis

- **Fundoscopy reveals characteristic "ketchup and cottage cheese" retinal lesions, representing perivascular hemorrhage and exudates (see Fig. 66-6)**
- Diagnosis at other sites is by CMV PCR, culture, or finding of characteristic viral inclusion bodies on histopathology

Treatment

- Systemic disease: treat with either systemic ganciclovir or foscarnet
- CMV retinitis: systemic ganciclovir, foscarnet, cidofovir, or oral valganciclovir (depending on the severity of disease)
  - Intravitreal injections of ganciclovir may be used
  - Ganciclovir implants no longer manufactured

KAPOSI SARCOMA

Clinical Presentation

- Can occur with any CD4 count, but more common when less than 200/mm^3
- **Presents with indurated or nodular violaceous growths on the skin, in the mouth, or in any visceral organ (Fig. 12-7)**
- Predominantly seen in men with same-sex contact as transmission risk

Diagnosis

- Biopsy shows proliferation of characteristic abnormal vascular structures on pathology
- Human herpesvirus 8 identified as causative agent, but not used diagnostically

Treatment

- Cytotoxic chemotherapy
- Intralesional chemotherapy (if cutaneous)
- May regress with effective ART

NON-HODGKIN LYMPHOMA

Clinical Presentation

- Usually seen at CD4 count less than 100/mm^3, but can occur with any CD4 count

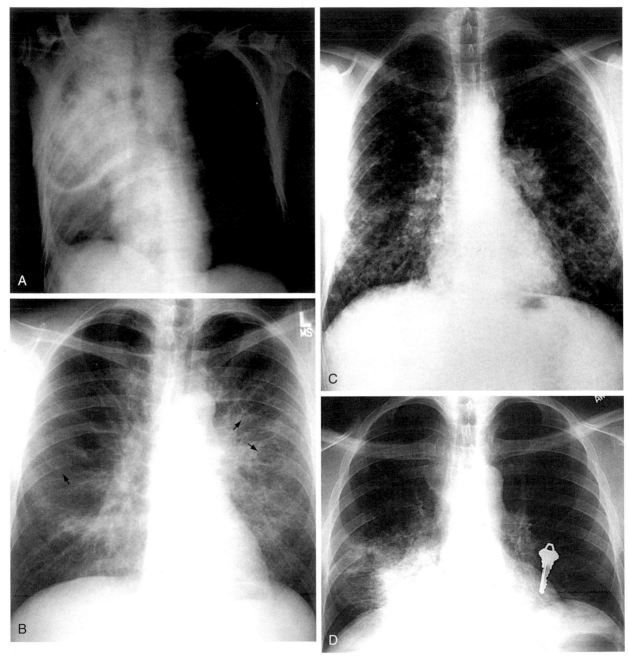

FIGURE 12-4 Chest radiographs of common pulmonary conditions associated with HIV infection. **A,** Streptococcal pneumonia, presenting with focal lobar infiltrate. **B,** *Pneumocystis* pneumonia, typical presentation with "bat wing" infiltrates *(arrows)*. **C,** Diffuse bilateral infiltrates in acute pulmonary histoplasmosis. **D,** Tuberculosis pneumonia, typically presents with noncavitary, lower lobe infiltrates in advanced disease (key is an overlying artifact). (**A, B,** and **D,** From Mason RJ. *Murray and Nadel's Textbook of Respiratory Medicine.* 4th ed. Philadelphia: Saunders; 2005: Figs. 75-1, 75-5, and 75-2; **C,** From Mandell GL, Bennett JE, Dolin R, eds. *Principles and Practice of Infectious Diseases.* 6th ed. Philadelphia: Churchill Livingstone; 2005: Fig. 262-5.)

| **TABLE 12-4** | *Common CNS Conditions Associated with HIV Infection* |

Disorder	CD4 Count	Clinical Scenario	Appearance on MRI	Diagnosis	Treatment
Toxoplasmosis	<100	Focal neurologic symptoms Seizures	Usually multiple ring-enhancing lesions Surrounding mass effect	Toxo IgG+ in 90% presumptive diagnosis Follow response to therapy Clinical improvement MRI in 2 weeks	Sulfadiazine + pyrimethamine Suppressive therapy until CD4 >200 for >3 months
CNS lymphoma	<100	Focal neurologic symptoms Seizures	Usually single solid or ring-enhancing lesions Surrounding mass effect	First step is usually trial of toxoplasmosis therapy If no response, brain biopsy to diagnose lymphoma	Radiation therapy Begin ART High-dose methotrexate
Cryptococcal meningitis	<100	Severe headache High intracranial pressure Extra-CNS manifestations: skin lesions, pneumonia	Normal in 90% of patients Mass lesion in 10%	Classically, India ink test Now, usually serum and CSF cryptococcal antigen CSF culture Low CSF WBC count is poor prognostic sign	Amphotericin B + fluconazole for suppressive therapy until CD4 >100–200 for >6 months Therapeutic lumbar punctures (to control elevated ICP)
Progressive multifocal leukoencephalopathy	Any	Rapidly progressive Focal neurologic symptoms Loss of speech, vision	Focal white matter changes No mass effect Definitive diagnosis requires brain biopsy	MRI appearance CSF for JC virus PCR	No specific therapy ART may be beneficial

ART, Antiretroviral therapy; CNS, central nervous system; CSF, cerebrospinal fluid; IgG, immunoglobulin G; MRI, magnetic resonance imaging; PCR, polymerase chain reaction; WBC, white blood cell.

- Heterogeneous group of malignancies
- 70% are B-cell derived
- Intermediate or high-grade B-cell lymphomas are considered AIDS-defining events
- **Extranodal presentation common (GI tract, visceral, bone marrow, etc.)**

Diagnosis

- For accessible lesions, diagnosis made by biopsy
- **Differential diagnosis includes toxoplasmosis**
  - Toxoplasmosis is more commonly multifocal, while lymphoma is more commonly unifocal
  - Biopsy warranted for CNS lesions that do not respond to empirical therapy for toxoplasmosis

Treatment

- Combination chemotherapy, brain radiation if CNS involvement, and ART

HIV-ASSOCIATED NEPHROPATHY

Clinical Presentation

- Can be seen at any CD4 level, but usually CD4 count is lower than 200/mm³

- Associated with high viral load
- **Presents with nephrotic syndrome**
- If untreated, leads to renal failure over 1 to 4 months

Diagnosis

- Large echogenic kidneys seen on ultrasound
- **Diagnosis made by biopsy that shows focal segmental glomerulosclerosis**

Treatment

- ART is the only effective treatment for HIVAN
- Steroid therapy may slow progression until viral suppression is achieved

IMMUNE RECONSTITUTION INFLAMMATORY SYNDROME

Clinical Presentation

- Occurs 2 to 12 weeks after initiating ART
- Paradoxical clinical worsening due to immune system's new ability to mount an inflammatory response against an underlying opportunistic infection or antigen (that was subclinical)
- Usually seen with low CD4 count (less than 100/mm³) and rapid decline in HIV viral load

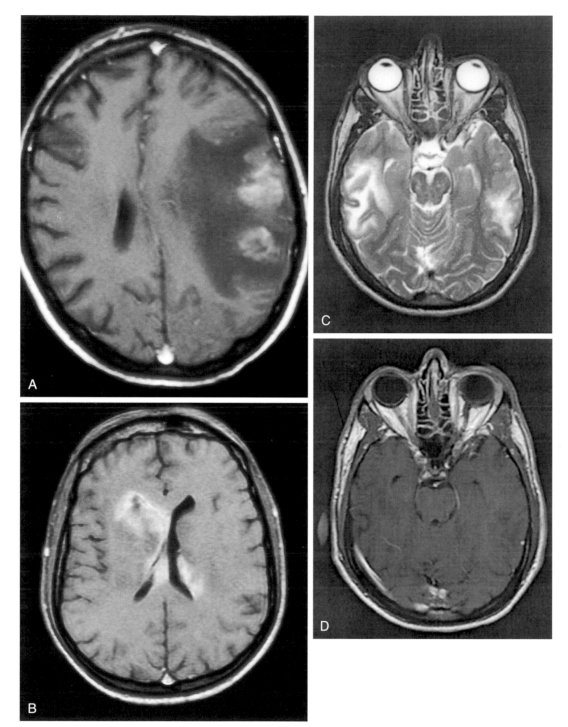

FIGURE 12-5 Imaging of common central nervous system (CNS) conditions associated with HIV. **A,** CNS toxoplasmosis presents as multiple ring-enhancing lesions. **B,** CNS lymphoma usually presents as a solitary ring-enhancing lesion. **C** and **D,** Progressive multifocal leukoencephalopathy lesions are seen as areas of high signal intensity in the subcortical white matter (**C**) and do not enhance with gadolinium (**D**). (**A** and **B,** From Haslett C, Chilvers ER, Boon NA, et al, eds. *Davidson's Principles and Practice of Medicine.* 19th ed. New York: Churchill Livingstone; 2002: Figs. 1.88 and 1.89; **C** and **D,** From Mandell GL, Bennett JE, Dolin R, eds. *Principles and Practice of Infectious Diseases.* 6th ed. Philadelphia: Churchill Livingstone; 2005: Fig. 120-4.)

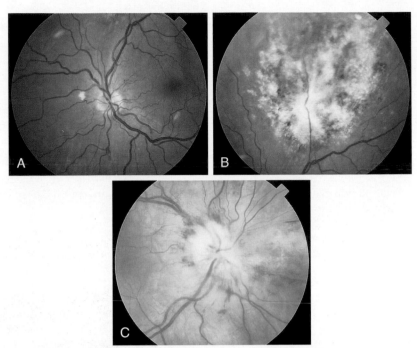

FIGURE 12-6 Cytomegalovirus (CMV) retinitis. **A,** Early disease with retinal involvement along blood vessels. **B,** Extensive retinal damage and retinal hemorrhages. **C,** CMV retinitis with papillitis. (From Mandell GL, Bennett JE, Dolin R, eds. *Principles and Practice of Infectious Diseases.* 6th ed. Philadelphia: Churchill Livingstone; 2005: Fig. 134-2.)

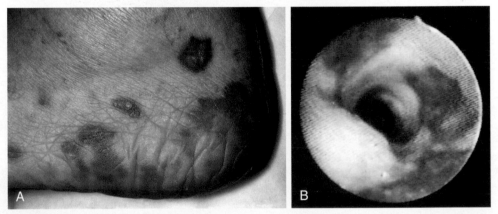

FIGURE 12-7 Kaposi sarcoma can present cutaneously (**A**), in the oral mucosa (**B**), and internally in the lungs or gastrointestinal tract (not shown). (**A,** From Mandell GL, Bennett JE, Dolin R, eds. *Principles and Practice of Infectious Diseases.* 6th ed. Philadelphia: Churchill Livingstone; 2005: Fig. 117-12; **B,** From Goldman L, Ausiello D. *Cecil Textbook of Medicine.* 23rd ed. Philadelphia: Saunders; 2008: Fig. 414-12.)

Diagnosis

- Presentations of opportunistic infections may be atypical because of brisk inflammation
- High index of suspicion needed

Treatment

- Diagnose and treat the underlying opportunistic infection
- Antiinflammatory treatment (corticosteroids or nonsteroidal antiinflammatory drugs) may be effective in specific conditions (tuberculosis, disseminated MAI, and so on), although no clinical trial data
- Continue ART

Review Questions

For review questions, please go to ExpertConsult.com.

SUGGESTED READINGS

Bartlett JG, Gallant JE, Pham PA. *Medical Management of HIV Infection.* 15th ed. Durham, NC: Knowledge Source Solutions; 2009–2010.

Kaplan JE, Benson C, Holmes KK, et al. Guidelines for prevention and treatment of opportunistic infections in HIV-infected adults and adolescents: recommendations from CDC, the National Institutes of Health, and the HIV Medicine Association of the Infectious Diseases Society of America. *MMWR Recomm Rep.* 2009;58:1-207.

Panel on Antiretroviral Guidelines for Adults and Adolescents. Guidelines for the use of antiretroviral agents in HIV-1-infected adults and adolescents. Department of Health and Human Services. <http://aidsinfo.nih.gov/ContentFiles/AdultandAdolescentGL.pdf>.

Sterling TR, Chaisson RE. General clinical manifestations of human immunodeficiency virus infection. In: Bennett JE, Dolin R, Blaser MJ, eds. *Principles and Practice of Infectious Diseases.* 8th ed. Philadelphia: Saunders; 2015.

CHAPTER 13

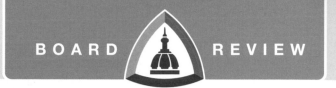
Mycobacterial Infections

KELLY E. DOOLEY, MD, PhD

Mycobacteria are aerobic bacteria that have the laboratory characteristic of retaining colorized stain when washed in an acid bath; hence they are "acid-fast" (Figure 13-1). *Mycobacterium tuberculosis*, *Mycobacterium leprae*, and *Mycobacterium avium* complex are clinically among the most important mycobacteria. However, with the rising prevalence of immunocompromised hosts, other mycobacterial species have become increasingly clinically relevant.

Tuberculosis

Basic Information

- Epidemiology
  - One-third of the world's population is infected with *M. tuberculosis*; most have latent (clinically silent) tuberculosis infection (LTBI)
  - There were 9582 tuberculosis (TB) cases reported in the United States in 2013. Foreign-born persons are disproportionately affected. Incidence is also higher in African Americans, Hispanics, and American Indian or Alaska Natives.
- Risk factors
  - Human immunodeficiency virus (HIV)
    - HIV increases risk of progression to active TB after *M. tuberculosis* infection
    - HIV increases risk of reactivation of LTBI
    - HIV increases mortality from TB
    - Highly active antiretroviral therapy decreases the risk of active TB in HIV-infected persons
  - Other risk factors
    - Systemic illness, including diabetes and chronic kidney disease
    - Nutritional status, including low body mass index and low vitamin D level
    - Other immunocompromising states, including use of tumor necrosis factor-alpha (TNF-α) blockers
- Multidrug-resistant TB (MDR TB)
  - **Defined as resistance to at least isoniazid and rifampin**
  - Clusters in geographic areas (Russia, India, China, Peru, South Africa are among the highest-burden countries)
  - Risk factors: previous TB treatment, poor adherence with TB treatment, adding one drug to a failing TB treatment regimen
  - Extensively drug-resistant TB (XDR TB) is defined as resistance to at least isoniazid, rifampin, at least one fluoroquinolone, and at least one of three injectable second-line drugs (amikacin, canamycin, capreomycin)

Clinical Features

- Transmission
  - Airborne transmission from patient with pulmonary TB disease
- **Primary infection: usually asymptomatic**
  - Most (greater than 90%) immunocompetent people control initial infection and develop clinically silent latent infection (Figure 13-2)
  - A minority of patients present with pleural effusion or pneumonia in mid- or lower lung fields with hilar or mediastinal lymphadenopathy
  - HIV-infected persons have high risk of progression to active TB after initial infection, even with a normal CD4 count. Can present with any chest radiographic pattern (including a normal radiograph)
- Reactivation TB disease
  - **Typically subacute illness over weeks or months with fever, sweats, weight loss, cough**
  - Although pulmonary disease is most common, nearly any organ system can be involved and clinical manifestations are protean, so a high index of suspicion is essential
  - In patients with HIV co-infection, increased prevalence of extrapulmonary and miliary TB
  - Miliary TB: Disease results from widespread hematogenous dissemination of bacilli. Classic chest radiographic appearance is innumerable tiny nodules (Figure 13-3)

Diagnosis and Evaluation

- Detection of *M. tuberculosis* infection (either LTBI or active disease)
  - Tuberculin skin test (TST)
    - Intradermal inoculation of mycobacterial purified protein derivative. Readout is induration 48 to 72 hours after inoculation
    - There are different cutoffs for positivity depending on patient characteristics (Table 13-1)
    - False-positive result can be caused by infection with nontuberculous mycobacteria (NTM) or previous bacille Calmette-Guérin (BCG) vaccination
    - False-negative test can result from immunosuppression
    - Positive TST with remote BCG vaccination (greater than 10 years) more difficult to interpret
    - If a patient is from an endemic country or is high risk for TB, the Centers for Disease Control and

Prevention recommendations are to interpret a positive TST as you would for someone who did not receive BCG

■ **Positive TST does not distinguish latent from active TB (See Figure 13-4 for diagnostic algorithm for distinguishing the two)**

■ Should not be relied upon as a test for active TB infection, because a negative result does not rule out active disease

■ Interferon-γ release assays (IGRAs)

■ Whole-blood tests that can be used to diagnose *M. tuberculosis* infection

■ Measures a person's immune reactivity to *M. tuberculosis*

■ Not a measurement of disease itself, and so does not directly correlate to disease activity or cure

■ May be used in most instances in place of the TST, though IGRA may be preferred in persons who have received BCG vaccine, and TST is preferred in young children

■ Like the TST, cannot distinguish LTBI from active TB

■ **Previous BCG vaccination will not cause a false-positive IGRA**

■ As with TST, should not be relied upon as a test for active TB infection, because a negative result does not rule out active disease

● Detection of TB disease (active TB)

■ Laboratory

■ Microscopic examination of sputum or other clinical specimen stained for acid-fast bacilli (AFB smear)

■ For diagnosis of pulmonary TB, obtain three morning sputum specimens (sent for AFB smear and mycobacterial culture)

13

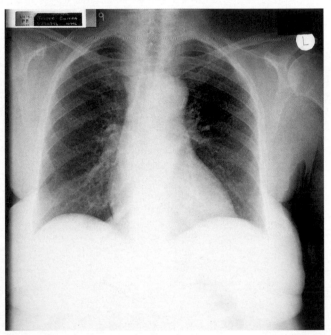

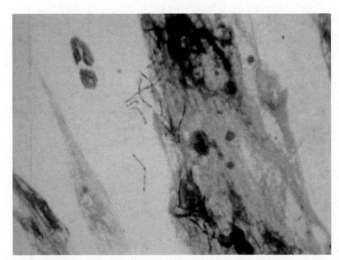

FIGURE 13-1 Ziehl-Neelsen staining of a sputum sample of a patient with pulmonary tuberculosis demonstrating acid-fast bacilli. (From Forbes C, Jackson W. *Color Atlas and Text of Clinical Medicine.* 3rd ed. St. Louis: Mosby; 2003: Fig. 4.14.)

FIGURE 13-3 Chest radiograph of a patient with miliary tuberculosis. (From Swash M. *Hutchinson's Clinical Methods.* 21st ed. Philadelphia: Saunders; 2002: Fig. 22.5.)

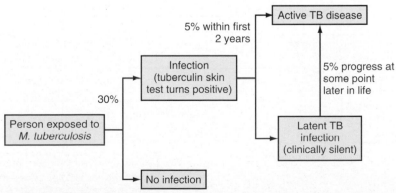

FIGURE 13-2 National history of tuberculosis (TB) in immune-competent individuals exposed to *Mycobacterium tuberculosis.* HIV infection (not shown in this figure) substantially increases the proportion of patients who develop active TB disease after initial exposure and the proportion of patients who progress from latent infection to active TB.

TABLE 13-1 *Criteria for a Positive Tuberculin Skin Test (TST), by Risk Group*

TST Induration Considered Positive	Risk Group
≥5 mm	HIV infection Recent contacts of patients with active tuberculosis (TB) Fibrotic changes on chest radiograph consistent with previous TB Immunosuppression, including organ transplant or prednisone ≥15 mg/day Use of antitumor necrosis factor-α drugs
≥10 mm	Recent immigrants (<5 years) from a high prevalence country Injection drug users Residents and employees of high-risk congregate settings (long-term care facilities, health care facilities, homeless shelters, prisons, or jails) Mycobacteriology laboratory workers Persons with medical conditions that put them at risk (silicosis, diabetes mellitus, chronic renal failure, some malignancies, gastrectomy or jejunoileal bypass, underweight) Children <4 years old Infants, children, or adolescents exposed to adults at high risk for TB
≥15 mm	Persons without any of above risk factors (TST not recommended in this group)

- AFB smear not sensitive and not specific for *M. tuberculosis* (but positive smear is highly predictive of TB in TB-endemic settings)
- Culture
  - Sensitive and specific (in combination with other tests done on cultured material) for *M. tuberculosis*
  - Slow: Takes 3 to 6 weeks for *M. tuberculosis* to grow in culture
  - Cannot check TB drug susceptibilities without a culture
- Nucleic acid amplification (NAA) tests
  - Used to evaluate respiratory specimens from untreated patients
  - Detects TB DNA, so highly specific for *M. tuberculosis*
  - Highly sensitive in AFB smear-positive patients; only 50% sensitive in AFB smear-negative patients
  - **If TB is suspected and NAA is negative, TB not excluded**
  - NAA test does not replace smear or culture
- Xpert MTB/RIF is a new, rapid test that can be used to diagnose TB and detect rifampin resistance from a sputum sample
  - Drug resistance detected with genetic test must be confirmed by culture with susceptibility testing
- Chest radiograph
  - Reactivation pulmonary disease typically involves upper lobe(s) or upper segments of lower lobe(s)

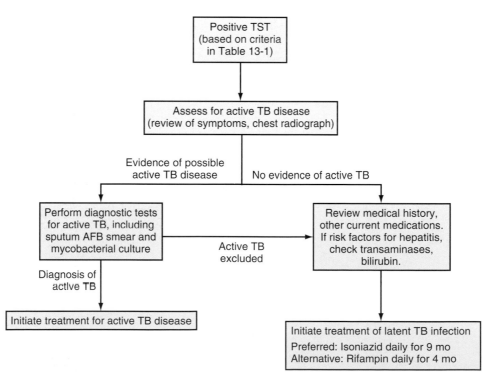

FIGURE 13-4 Clinical management of a positive tuberculin skin test (TST) or interferon-γ release assay. AFB, Acid-fast bacilli; TB, tuberculosis.

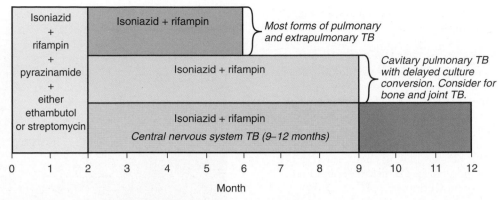

FIGURE 13-5 Recommended treatment for active tuberculosis (TB) disease, based on disease site.

TABLE 13-2	*Toxicities of First-Line Antituberculosis Medications*	
Drug	**Major Toxicities**	**Monitoring**
Isoniazid	Hepatotoxicity, peripheral neuropathy	Baseline liver chemistries Repeat if baseline is abnormal or if other hepatitis risk factors or symptoms of hepatotoxicity are present
Rifampin	Hepatotoxicity, fever, flulike syndrome, thrombocytopenia, drug–drug interactions	Baseline liver chemistries and CBC Repeat if baseline is abnormal or if other hepatitis risk factors or symptoms of adverse reaction are present
Pyrazinamide	Hepatotoxicity, arthralgia, rash	Baseline liver chemistries, uric acid Repeat if baseline is abnormal or if other hepatitis risk factors or symptoms of adverse reaction are present
Ethambutol	Optic neuritis	Baseline and monthly tests of visual acuity and color vision

CBC, Complete blood count.

- Cavitation is classic, but infiltrates may be lobar, nodular, or interstitial

Treatment
- Treatment of LTBI (TB prophylaxis) (Fig. 13-4)
  - Decision to treat is based on individual's risk of recent M. *tuberculosis* infection and risk of progression to active TB disease (Table 13-1)
  - **Must exclude active TB disease before starting treatment for latent TB**
  - Standard regimen: isoniazid daily for 9 months
  - Alternative regimens:
    - Rifampin daily for 4 months
    - Rifapentine plus isoniazid once-weekly for 3 months
      - Must use directly observed therapy
      - Cannot be used in HIV-infected patients on antiretroviral therapy, children under the age of 2, pregnant women, or women attempting to get pregnant
  - No age cutoff for treatment of LTBI
  - **If isoniazid used, pyridoxine (B6) supplementation should be provided to minimize risk of peripheral neuropathy caused by interference with pyridoxine metabolism**
- Treatment of drug-susceptible active TB disease
  - "Intensive phase" of treatment: isoniazid plus rifampin plus pyrazinamide plus ethambutol for 8 weeks

- "Continuation phase" of treatment: isoniazid plus rifampin for an additional 4 months (total treatment duration, 6 months; Fig. 13-5)
- Treatment extended to total of 9 months if delay (e.g., 2 to 3 months) in culture conversion
- Treatment extended to 9 to 12 months for central nervous system TB
- Pyrazinamide not generally recommended for use in pregnant women in the United States
- Pyridoxine (B6) supplementation should be given to pregnant women, persons with HIV infection, diabetes, renal failure, or alcoholism to prevent peripheral neuropathy
- Treatment of MDR-TB disease
  - Duration is 18 to 24 months, with complex multidrug regimen; toxicity is common
- Treatment of TB disease in HIV-infected persons
  - TB treatment duration not affected by HIV
  - Worsening of TB signs or symptoms can be seen in first several weeks after starting HIV and/or TB treatment (paradoxical worsening or immune reconstitution inflammatory syndrome)
  - Monitoring for drug toxicities important (Table 13-2)
  - Rifampin stimulates the cytochrome P450 system and enhances metabolism (thereby lowering blood levels and potentially decreasing effectiveness) of many drugs, including warfarin, oral contraceptives, methadone, and many HIV drugs (except nucleoside reverse transcriptase inhibitors). Adjustments to HIV

or TB regimen must generally be made to manage the drug interactions

Prevention of Tuberculosis Transmission

- Respiratory isolation should be initiated for all persons suspected of having pulmonary TB disease who are hospitalized or in otherwise congregate settings (e.g., prison, nursing home). Respiratory isolation can be discontinued once three sputum specimens collected more than 8 hours apart are smear negative.
- Care providers (for persons having or suspected of having infectious pulmonary TB disease) should use personal respiratory protection (e.g., N-95 mask)

Leprosy (Hansen Disease)

Basic Information

- Caused by M. *leprae*
- Prevalence highest in South America, Africa, Asia
- Rare indigenous leprosy in the United States in Louisiana, Texas, Hawaii

Clinical Presentation

- Predominantly affects skin, nerves, and upper airways
- Broad spectrum of disease, to include tuberculoid, borderline, and lepromatous forms:
  - Tuberculoid (paucibacillary): One or few asymmetrical anesthetic skin macules; nerve involvement (classically ulnar nerve at elbow) can be severe; biopsies of skin, nerves show few or no bacteria
  - Lepromatous (multibacillary): Symmetrical skin nodules and plaques on cool areas of body; affected tissues laden with mycobacteria; upper respiratory tract involvement common, manifest by nasal congestion, epistaxis, cartilage erosion/collapse (saddle-nose deformity; Fig. 13-6); peripheral neuropathy occurs late in the disease course

Diagnosis and Evaluation

- Diagnosis based on clinical presentation plus skin biopsy (demonstration of AFB and histology); M. *leprae* does not grow in culture

Treatment

- Tuberculoid (paucibacillary), skin smear negative, with five or fewer skin lesions: dapsone plus rifampin daily for 12 months
- Lepromatous (multibacillary), skin-smear positive, with more than five skin lesions: dapsone plus rifampin plus clofazimine daily for 24 months
- World Health Organization recommends shorter treatment durations (6 and 12 months, respectively) and less frequent dosing, largely because of resource limitations

Nontuberculous Mycobacteria

Basic Information

- Formerly known as mycobacteria other than tuberculosis (MOTT)

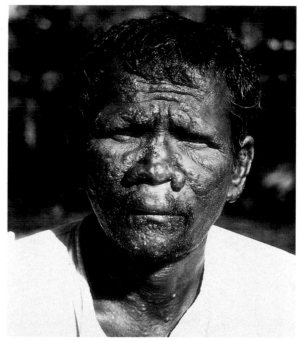

FIGURE 13-6 A patient with lepromatous leprosy demonstrating saddle-nose deformity. (From Haslett C, Chilvers ER, Boon NA, et al. *Davidson's Principles and Practice of Medicine.* 19th ed. New York: Churchill Livingstone; 2002: Fig. 1.69.)

- Rapid growers (visible growth within 7 days in culture): *Mycobacterium fortuitum, Mycobacterium chelonae, Mycobacterium abscessus*
- Slow growers (visible growth requires greater than 7 days in culture): *Mycobacterium kansasii, Mycobacterium avium intracellulare, Mycobacterium marinum*

Clinical Presentation

- Isolation of NTM from clinical specimen may result from contamination (e.g., from tap water), colonization in absence of NTM disease, or NTM disease
- Immunosuppression is a risk factor for NTM disease
- Common clinical syndromes listed in Table 13-3

Diagnosis and Evaluation

- Diagnosis is based on clinical presentation and positive culture of clinically relevant specimen (see Table 13-3)

Treatment

- Antimicrobial agents and treatment duration vary depending on organism and site of disease

Prevention

- In patients with HIV infection with CD4 count less than 50 cells/mm^3, azithromycin 1200 mg once weekly should be given to prevent M. *avium intracellulare* infection

TABLE 13-3	*Clinical Features of Infections Caused by Nontuberculous Mycobacteria*	
Species	**Reservoir**	**Common Clinical Manifestations**
Mycobacterium avium intracellulare complex	Birds, cattle, swine, water, soil	Disseminated disease in AIDS (fevers, sweats, diarrhea, mesenteric adenopathy) Pulmonary disease (cavity, infiltrate, or bronchiectasis) in persons with underlying lung disease (COPD, cystic fibrosis) or older women
Mycobacterium kansasii	Water	Pulmonary disease resembling TB, or disseminated disease, especially in HIV-infected persons
Mycobacterium marinum	Water, marine organisms	"Fish-tank granuloma" Infection follows trauma, usually to extremities, occurring in water Presents as enlarging nodule(s) that ulcerate, drain
Mycobacterium fortuitum *Mycobacterium abscessus* *Mycobacterium chelonae* (rapid growers)	Water	Cutaneous disease, catheter-related infections, surgical wound infections, keratitis *M. abscessus* can cause pulmonary disease in cystic fibrosis

COPD, Chronic obstructive pulmonary disease; TB, tuberculosis.

Review Questions

For review questions, please go to ExpertConsult.com.

SUGGESTED READINGS

American Thoracic Society. Centers for Disease Control and Prevention: treatment of tuberculosis. *Am J Respir Crit Care Med.* 2003;167:603-662.

Centers for Disease Control and Prevention. Latent tuberculosis infection: a guide for primary health care providers. 2013. <www.cdc.gov/tb/publications/ltbi/pdf/TargetedLTBI.pdf>.

Centers for Disease Control and Prevention. Tuberculosis. 2014. <www.cdc.gov/tb/>.

Griffith DE, Aksamit T, Brown-Elliott BA, et al. An official ATS/IDSA statement: diagnosis, treatment, and prevention of nontuberculous mycobacterial diseases. *Am J Respir Crit Care Med.* 2007;175:367-416.

Horsburgh CR Jr, Rubin EJ. Clinical practice: latent tuberculosis infection in the United States. *N Engl J Med.* 2011;364:1441-1448.

Rodrigues LC, Lockwood DNJ. Leprosy. *Lancet Inf Dis.* 2011;11:464-470.

Zumla A, Raviglione M, Hafner R, et al. Tuberculosis. *N Engl J Med.* 2013;368:745-755.

13

Infectious Diarrhea

CYNTHIA L. SEARS, MD

Infectious diarrhea is a leading cause of morbidity and mortality throughout the world, particularly among the extremes of age and in low-resource countries. In the United States, only a minority (approximately 10%) of those affected seek medical care. A systematic approach to the evaluation of the patient with diarrhea is useful in identifying the cause.

Approach to a Patient with Infectious Diarrhea

Clinical Presentation

- Acute diarrhea: three or more episodes of liquid stool in a 24-hour period; symptoms typically last less than 14 days
- Persistent diarrhea: duration of 14 days to 1 month
- Chronic diarrhea: duration exceeds 1 month
- Clinical classification of acute diarrhea (Table 14-1):
  - **Noninflammatory: large-volume watery stools without blood**
    - **Fecal inflammatory cells can be seen, but frank pus is absent**
  - **Inflammatory: Frequent, small-volume stools containing blood or pus. Fever and abdominal pain may be present.**
  - Clinical overlap does occur, such that common causes of inflammatory diarrhea appear to be noninflammatory diarrhea clinically

Diagnosis and Evaluation

- History should focus on duration of symptoms, features of stool (hematochezia, stool volume), associated symptoms (fever, abdominal pain, tenesmus), previous antibiotic use, immune status, travel history, exposure to children, and risk for food-borne illness
  - May be able to determine whether or not diarrhea is inflammatory by history alone
- Physical examination should include an evaluation of fever, hydration status, and abdominal tenderness
- Laboratory testing:
  - Laboratory assessment is typically unnecessary unless inflammatory diarrhea is suspected or the patient is unstable or immunocompromised
  - Fecal leukocytes: Can help differentiate inflammatory from noninflammatory, but sensitivity and specificity variable and imperfect
  - Stool culture: Indicated only if patient is clinically ill, immunocompromised, and/or history or presence of fecal leukocytes suggests an inflammatory process
  - Occult blood cards: Positive may indicate inflammatory diarrhea

- **Ova and parasites: Reserve for persistent diarrhea (>14 days) or high-risk individuals (e.g., travel history or immunocompromised)**
  - **Do not order routinely for acute diarrhea**
- Persistent and chronic diarrhea should be evaluated by both stool culture and ova and parasite examinations
  - Any etiology of acute diarrhea can cause persistent diarrheal illnesses

Treatment

- Hydration: Cornerstone of therapy for all patients; oral usually sufficient
- Diet: avoid caffeine, dairy products, and sorbitol
  - Transient lactase deficiency may occur
- Antidiarrheal medications
  - **Loperamide: Delays passage through the intestine; contraindicated in inflammatory diarrheas because of concern for decreased clearance of toxin or organism (particularly for Shiga toxin-producing *Escherichia coli* [STEC] and *Clostridium difficile*)**
  - Bismuth: Moderately effective but inconvenient, may darken tongue and stools.
    - Must consider potential toxicity caused by exposure to salicylate component
  - Diphenoxylate: Has central opiate effects and is linked to induction of toxic megacolon
- Antibiotics
  - Use is controversial; data are weak that antibiotics universally affect course of illness
  - Rarely indicated in noninflammatory diarrhea unless the patient is unstable or at high risk (e.g., immunocompromised, recent travel, older adult)
  - **Most guidelines recommend empirical use of fluoroquinolones in inflammatory diarrhea; azithromycin is second choice in clinically ill patients**
  - Organisms such as *Vibrio cholerae*, *Shigella*, and *Giardia* spp. should always be treated with antibiotics, but mild-to-moderate nontyphoidal *Salmonella* or *Campylobacter* typically do not require antibiotic therapy in stable, immunocompetent individuals. STEC does not require antibiotic therapy

Food-borne Illness

Basic Information (Table 14-2)

- Can be caused by bacteria, viruses, parasites, or bacterial toxins present in microbiologically contaminated foods

TABLE 14-1	Clinical Classification of Acute Diarrhea
Classification	**Organisms**
Noninflammatory	Noroviruses, rotavirus, enterotoxigenic *Escherichia coli*, *Clostridium perfringens*, *Vibrio cholera*, *Giardia lamblia*, *Cryptosporidium*
Inflammatory	*Salmonella*, *Shigella*, *Campylobacter*, Shiga toxin-producing *E. coli* (O157 and non-O157), enteroinvasive *E. coli*, *Clostridium difficile*, *Yersinia*, *Vibrio parahaemolyticus*, *Entamoeba histolytica*

TABLE 14-2	Potential Reportable Food-Borne Diseases
Category	**Illnesses or Organisms**
Bacteria	Botulism, brucellosis, cholera, enteric *Escherichia coli*, including *E. coli* O157 (Shiga toxin-producing *E. coli*) among others, campylobacteriosis, salmonellosis including typhoid fever, shigellosis, giardiasis, listeria, Yersinia
Viruses	Hepatitis A, norovirus
Parasites	Cryptosporidiosis, cyclosporiasis, trichinosis

- **It is important for physicians to report cases caused by certain organisms (e.g., *Salmonella*) to their local or state health departments.**

Clinical Presentation

- Typically presents with gastrointestinal symptoms (e.g., nausea, vomiting, diarrhea, abdominal pain)
- Neurologic symptoms may be present in certain conditions (e.g., botulism)

Diagnosis and Evaluation

- Patients should be asked about ingestion of raw or poorly cooked food (e.g., fish, eggs, meats, shellfish); unpasteurized milk; home-canned goods; or fresh produce
- Source of food (if known) can be important in identifying a particular causative organism
  - Shellfish: *Vibrio cholerae*, *Vibrio parahaemolyticus*
  - Poultry and eggs: *Campylobacter*, *Salmonella* spp.
  - Meat: *Clostridium perfringens*, *Salmonella*, STEC
  - Dairy: *Salmonella*, STEC, *Yersinia*
  - Prepared protein-rich foods: *Staphylococcus* (ingestion of preformed toxin; Table 14-3)
  - Deli foods: *Listeria monocytogenes* (causes bacteremia and meningitis)
- Etiologies can be narrowed by determining whether the diarrhea is inflammatory or noninflammatory (see Table 14-1)
- **Timing of illness (incubation period) may be helpful**
  - 1 to 6 hours: *Staphylococcus aureus*, *Bacillus cereus*
  - 8 to 16 hours: *C. perfringens*, *B. cereus*
  - 16 to 72 hours: *Campylobacter jejuni*, *Salmonella*, *Shigella*, *E. coli* (including STEC), *Yersinia*, *Vibrio*
    - Days to more than 1 month: *L. monocytogenes*

Common Pathogens

VIRAL PATHOGENS

- Account for at least 50% of all acute infectious diarrheal illnesses
- Usually the causative agent is never identified
- **Norovirus is the most commonly identified viral cause of endemic and epidemic diarrhea in adults**
  - Fecal–oral, food-borne, airborne, and fomite transmission common as a result of low inoculum required for disease
  - Incubation period is usually 24 to 48 hours
  - Noninflammatory diarrhea with or without vomiting
    - Approximately 80% have both vomiting and diarrhea
  - Low-grade fever in approximately 50%
  - Treatment is supportive because disease course is usually self-limited to a few days
- Rotavirus causes sporadic outbreaks in children; much less common in adults
  - Fecal–oral transmission usually seen
  - Vomiting, low-grade fever, transient lactase deficiency can be present
  - Episodes may last greater than 1 week
  - Treatment is supportive
- Hepatitis A (see Chapter 29)
  - Rare cause of food-borne disease
  - Long incubation period (15 to 50 days)
  - Transmitted by contaminated shellfish, raw produce, and foods contaminated after handling by infected people
  - Jaundice, abdominal pain, fever, elevated hepatic transaminases may be present
  - Diagnosis made by the presence of immunoglobulin M anti hepatitis A antibodies
  - Treatment is supportive
  - Contacts not previously vaccinated against hepatitis A may be given immunoglobulin

BACTERIAL PATHOGENS

See Table 14-3 for bacterial causes of diarrheal illness.

PARASITIC PATHOGENS

- *Giardia lamblia* (giardiasis)
  - Common cause of persistent or chronic diarrhea
  - Diarrhea usually watery, but steatorrhea/malabsorption can arise
  - Bloating and mild nausea are common
  - **Major source is drinking water (often well water); person-to-person spread occurs**
  - Usually responds to treatment with metronidazole
  - *Giardia* stool enzyme immunoassay (EIA) available for diagnosis
- *Cryptosporidium parvum* (cryptosporidiosis)
  - Regionally variable, but can be similar in incidence to *Giardia*

TABLE 14-3	Bacterial Causes of Diarrheal Illness*		
Organism	**Usual Incubation Period**	**Associated Foods**	**Comments**
Bacillus cereus (preformed bacterial enterotoxin)	1–6 hr	Fried rice, other starchy foods	Usually presents as sudden nausea and vomiting Diarrhea may be present
Bacillus cereus (diarrhea toxin)	6–24 hr	Meats, vegetables	Diarrhea is the major manifestation
Campylobacter jejuni	1–3 days	Poultry, milk, water	Common bacterial pathogen Rarely, patients can develop Guillain-Barré syndrome or reactive arthritis after infection
Clostridium botulinum	3–30 days	Home-canned foods	Presents with vomiting, diarrhea, blurred vision, diplopia, and descending muscle weakness
Clostridium perfringens (diarrhea toxin)	6–24 hr	Meat, poultry, or gravy	Diarrhea is the major manifestation
Escherichia coli O157:H7/ other STEC	1–3 days	Beef, apple cider, water, unpasteurized milk, sprouts, vegetables	5% to 10% of infections lead to hemolytic uremic syndrome (HUS) Antibiotics usually not recommended because they may increase risk of HUS If infection suspected, enzyme immunoassay for Shiga-like toxin and stool culture for specific organism must be requested
Salmonella (nontyphoidal)	1–3 days	Poultry, eggs, milk, juice, fruits, vegetables (many foods possible)	Nontyphoidal *Salmonella* (many serotypes) are common causes of bacterial diarrhea In typhoid fever (*S. typhi*), diarrhea is uncommon; fever, fatigue, myalgias predominate
Shigella	1–3 days	Primarily person-to-person spread; 20% of cases are food-borne	Variable presentation depending on infecting species Always treat with antibiotics for public health reasons
Staphylococcus aureus (preformed bacterial enterotoxin)	1–6 hr	Cream pastries, salads, poultry	Sudden onset of nausea and vomiting, followed later by diarrhea in some
Vibrio cholerae	1–3 days	Shellfish, contaminated water	Massive, noninflammatory diarrhea Antibiotics reduce length of illness
Vibrio parahaemolyticus	1–3 days	Raw fish, shellfish	Inflammatory diarrhea
Yersinia	1–3 days	Pork, milk	Inflammatory diarrhea Can cause right lower quadrant pain (pseudoappendicitis)

*Most causes of diarrhea can lead to postdiarrheal reactive arthritis and irritable bowel syndrome.
STEC, Shiga toxin-producing E. coli.

- **Source is often water, but can be transmitted through person-to-person, fecal–oral routes**
- Usually self-limited in normal host but can cause persistent or chronic diarrhea
  - In human immunodeficiency virus (HIV)-infected host with CD4 counts less than 150 cells/mm³, often a chronic illness
- Symptoms are variable, but can cause large-volume losses or malabsorption; may be relapsing
  - Abdominal pain, fever, and vomiting can occur
- Stool oocysts can be detected by modified acid fast stain (Fig. 14-1A)
- On histopathology, life-cycle forms can be detected in the brush border of the intestinal mucosa
- *Cryptosporidium* stool EIA available for diagnosis
- Most immunocompetent persons recover spontaneously

- Primary treatment for HIV-infected persons is highly active antiretroviral therapy
- Nitazoxanide available for treatment of persistent and/or severe disease
- *Cyclospora cayetanensis*
  - More commonly seen in HIV but can infect immunocompetent hosts (e.g., outbreaks associated with imported raspberries, salad greens, cilantro)
  - Symptoms similar to *Cryptosporidium*
  - Responds to trimethoprim-sulfamethoxazole (TMP-SMX)
  - Stool oocysts are also acid-fast but twice the size of *Crytosporidium* (see Fig. 14-1B)
- **Entamoeba histolytica**
  - **Presents as an inflammatory process, often chronic, with bloody diarrhea and lower abdominal pain (similar to Shigella); can**

14

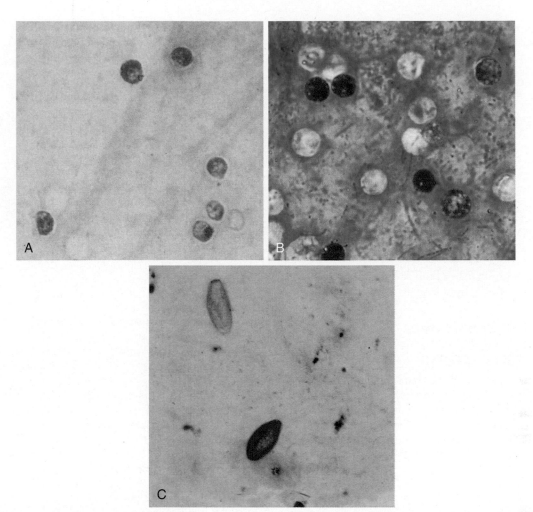

FIGURE 14-1   Acid-fast stain of intestinal pathogens. **A,** *Cryptosporidium* spp., 4 to 6 mm in diameter. **B,** *Cyclospora* spp., 8 to 10 mm in diameter. **C,** Elliptical-shaped *Isospora belli*. (From Cohen J, Powderly W. *Infectious Diseases*. 2nd ed. St. Louis: Mosby; 2004: Fig. 243-3.)

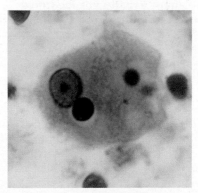

FIGURE 14-2   Trophozoite of *Entamoeba histolytica*. Note the ingested red blood cells. (From Cohen J, Powderly W. *Infectious Diseases*. 2nd ed. St. Louis: Mosby; 2004: Fig. 242-1.)

cause extraintestinal disease, especially liver abscess
- Diagnose by examining stool for cysts or trophozoites (Fig. 14-2), but morphologically indistinguishable from nonpathogenic *Entamoeba dispar* or *Entamoeba moshkovskii* strains
- Antigen detection methods for serum and stool to distinguish *E. histolytica* and *E. dispar* are available

- Metronidazole is effective; attention to elimination of tissue and fecal cyst forms is important
- *Trichinella spiralis*
  - Causes diarrhea, vomiting, abdominal pain, myalgias, fever, periorbital edema
  - Occurs days to weeks after ingestion of raw or undercooked meat (e.g., pork, bear, moose)
  - Cardiac involvement is not common, but can lead to myocarditis with life-threatening arrhythmias
  - Eosinophilia usually present
  - Treatment is supportive for mild cases. Mebendazole or albendazole is used in more severe cases. Prednisone is added if inflammation is severe.

TOXIN-PRODUCING ORGANISMS

- *Staphylococcus aureus*, *Bacillus cereus*, and *Clostridium perfringens* are the most common toxin-mediated causes of food-borne disease
  - Consider botulism if neurologic symptoms are present
- Ciguatera fish poisoning
  - Illness caused by toxins concentrated in the fish
  - **Causes diarrhea, nausea, and abdominal cramps followed by neurologic symptoms and signs**

such as tooth pain and paresthesias of the lips, tongue, and oropharynx
- Can lead to respiratory paralysis and bradycardia
- Incubation is 1 to 6 hours
- In the United States, primarily seen in Florida, primarily seen in Florida and Hawaii because it is found in tropical fish (e.g., barracuda, moray eel, some mackerel, grouper, red snapper)
- Duration of illness can be days to months
- Scombroid fish poisoning
  - Ingestion of histamine present in fish results in abdominal cramps, nausea, and diarrhea, and rarely, bronchospasm
  - Predominantly associated with eating dark-meat fish (tuna, mackerel, skip-jack, bonito)
  - Incubation is less than an hour; duration is a few hours
  - Treat with antihistamines in severe cases
  - Often mistaken as an allergy to fish

Special Circumstances

HIV-INFECTED PATIENTS
- An absolute CD4 count less than 200 cells/mm^3 is a major risk factor for persistent/chronic infectious diarrhea. In addition to directed antimicrobial therapy, antiretroviral therapy is required to resolve persistent or chronic diarrhea caused by opportunistic infections
- Patients with HIV can develop diarrhea secondary to antiretroviral therapy
- Common infections:
  - *C. difficile* is the leading bacterial cause of diarrhea in HIV/AIDS; risk increases with lower CD4 cell counts
  - ***Cryptosporidium* (see preceding discussion): Most common protozoal cause of diarrhea in patients with AIDS**
  - *Cytomegalovirus* (CMV)
    - Most common cause of viral colonic disease in HIV patients
    - Typically seen with CD4 counts below 50/mm^3
    - Presentation is variable and can range from mild diarrhea to an acute abdomen
    - Biopsy is required for diagnosis
      - Characteristic "owl's-eye" nucleus with basophilic intranuclear inclusion surrounded by clear halo (Fig. 14-3)
  - *Mycobacterium avium* complex (MAC)
    - Most infections seen when CD4 counts are less than 50/mm^3
    - Can involve small or large bowel; mucosa can appear normal on colonoscopy
    - May present with abdominal pain, lymphadenopathy, and prominent liver/spleen
    - Diagnose by mycobacterial blood culture or tissue biopsy; stool culture alone is not diagnostic and may represent colonization
      - Positive stool culture is predictive of risk of disease over time
    - Combination therapy is important; treat with clarithromycin and ethambutol, with or without rifabutin

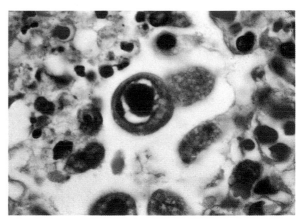

FIGURE 14-3 Cytomegalovirus colitis. Biopsy specimen reveals the typical "owl's-eye" cell. (From Kumar P, Clark M. *Clinical Medicine.* 6th ed. Philadelphia: Saunders; 2005: Fig. 2.16.)

  - *Microsporidium*
    - Obligate intracellular pathogen
    - Seen almost exclusively in AIDS with CD4 count less than 100/mm^3; causes chronic diarrhea
    - Can visualize the organisms on small-bowel biopsies or on fecal examination using special stains, such as fluorescence with calcofluor white
  - *Isospora belli*
    - Endemic to tropical areas; rare in the United States
    - Diagnose by ova and parasite examination or biopsy (see Fig. 14-1C)
    - Can treat with TMP-SMX
  - Herpes simplex virus
    - Usually causes proctitis with anorectal pain and tenesmus

TRAVELER'S DIARRHEA
- **Causative agent usually not identified**
  - **Enterotoxigenic *E. coli* most common identified cause**
- Up to 80% of cases are bacterial in origin
- Antibiotics shorten illness to approximately 24 to 48 hours; without treatment lasts 4 to 7 days
- Patients should be advised to avoid tap water, ice, unpeeled or raw fruits and vegetables, and undercooked meats in low-resource countries
- **Fluoroquinolones are the empiric antibiotics of choice**
  - Azithromycin is alternative therapy because of increasing bacterial resistance, particularly in Southeast Asia where fluoroquinolone-resistant C. jejuni is a common cause of traveler's diarrhea
- Prophylaxis (with TMP-SMX or fluoroquinolones) considered only for high-risk patients

Antibiotic-Associated Diarrhea

- **Noninfectious diarrhea can occur in up to 20% of patients receiving certain antibiotics (e.g., ampicillin, amoxicillin/clavulanate, cefixime, clindamycin)**

- Most cases of mild diarrhea caused by antibiotic use is because of noninfectious causes

Clostridium difficile

- Only 10% to 20% of cases of antibiotic-associated diarrhea are caused by C. difficile infection
  - C. difficile does, however, account for most cases of colitis caused by antibiotics
  - Rates of C. difficile disease presenting from the community have increased
    - Most have health care or antibiotic exposure
    - Specific risk groups of concern include peripartum women with young infants, children between ages 1 and 5 years, and patients with inflammatory bowel disease
    - Patients 65 years of age and older are at increased risk for severe disease

Clinical Presentation

- **Severe disease is defined by fever, low albumin, renal insufficiency, white blood cell (WBC) count more than 15,0000/mm³, and/or colon wall thickening on abdominal computed tomography**
- Fever occurs in only 10% to 15% of C. difficile patients but, if present, is a sign of severe disease
- C. difficile disease symptoms can range from mild, loose, or watery bowel movements to acute severe colitis with leukocytosis and abdominal pain
- Symptoms of C. difficile can be delayed up to 4 to 8 weeks after antibiotic exposure

Diagnosis and Evaluation

- Need to rule out C. difficile infection in most cases of diarrhea that are not mild and self-limited after antibiotic exposure
- Diagnosis is dependent on detection of C. difficile toxins in stool
  - Polymerase chain reaction (PCR)-based tests offer high sensitivity and specificity and are tests of choice
    - One negative PCR is often enough to exclude diagnosis
    - EIAs for C. difficile toxins have a false-negative rate of 10% to 30% and are suboptimal for diagnosis
- Most cases of C. difficile involve toxins A *and* B, and less frequently, toxin B alone

Treatment

- Antibiotic-associated diarrhea not caused by C. difficile is self-limited after discontinuation of the antibiotic
- Avoid antiperistaltic agents until C. difficile-associated disease excluded

- C. difficile infection should be treated and the inciting antibiotics discontinued if clinically feasible
  - Current guidelines are for 10 to 14 days of treatment, with drug selection based on severity of disease
    - Initial episode, mild: Oral metronidazole, 500 mg every 8 hours, although some experts recommend oral vancomycin for all initial episodes
    - Severe disease: Start with oral vancomycin, 125 mg every 6 hours
    - Initial episode, severe and complicated: oral vancomycin, 500 mg every 6 hours, plus IV metronidazole 500 mg every 8 hours
      - If complete ileus, consider adding rectal instillation of vancomycin and surgical consult
- **There is a high relapse rate (20% to 25%) after initial treatment for C. difficile**
  - Initial relapses of mild disease can be treated with metronidazole if WBC is less than 15,000/mm³ and serum creatinine not rising
  - Otherwise, treat initial relapses with oral vancomycin
  - Method of treatment of patients with more than one relapse is controversial
    - Prolonged, tapered treatment with vancomycin is most often used
    - Do not use metronidazole for fear of cumulative neurotoxicity
    - Sequential therapy with vancomycin followed by rifaximin or fidaxomicin may be useful for recurrences
  - Fidaxomicin may be useful in patients with relapsing C. difficile and in patients who cannot tolerate or do not respond to vancomycin
    - For severe disease (any): IV metronidazole, vancomycin by nasogastric tube or enema, and surgical consult; consider IV immunoglobulin (investigational)
    - Fecal transplantation may be an option for recurrent, severe disease

Review Questions

For review questions, please go to ExpertConsult.com.

SUGGESTED READINGS

Cohen SH, Gerding DN, Johnson S, et al. Clinical practice guidelines for Clostridium difficile infections in adults: 2010 update by the Society for Healthcare Epidemiology of America (SHEA) and the Infectious Diseases Society of America (IDSA). *Infect Control Hosp Epidemiol.* 2014;31:431-455.

Dupont HL. Acute infectious diarrhea in immunocompetent adults. *N Engl J Med.* 2014;370:1532-1540.

Johnson S, Louie TJ, Gerding DN, et al. Vancomycin, metronidazole or tolevamer for Clostridium difficile infection: results from two multinational, randomized, controlled trials. *Clin Infect Dis.* 2014;59:345-354.

Surawicz CM, Brandt LJ, Binion DG, et al. Guidelines for diagnosis, treatment and prevention of Clostridium difficile infections. *Am J Gastroenterol.* 2013;108:478-498.

14

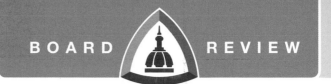
Selected Topics in Infectious Disease I

JULIE B. TRIVEDI, MD

Internists in both the inpatient and outpatient settings often care for patients with infections; they are therefore responsible for managing a variety of infectious processes. This chapter provides an overview of the infections with which internists are most commonly confronted, including meningitis, encephalitis, skin and soft tissue infections, infectious arthritis, and osteomyelitis. In addition, an approach to the patient with fever of unknown origin (FUO) is reviewed.

Meningitis

Basic Information

- Defined as inflammation of the leptomeninges, which are the tissues surrounding the brain and spinal cord
- May be caused by bacteria, viruses, fungi, or noninfectious processes
- Specific pathogens of acute bacterial meningitis: see Table 15-1
- Aseptic meningitis is defined as meningeal inflammation with an absence of bacteria on cerebrospinal fluid (CSF) examination and culture
  - Lymphocytic or monocytic pleocytosis and a normal glucose level are often seen
  - Can result from a number of different causes (Table 15-2)
  - Most commonly caused by viral pathogens, particularly enteroviruses
- Some pathogens may cause chronic meningitis, in which symptoms are present for 4 or more weeks
  - Cryptococcal meningitis is more commonly seen in immunocompromised hosts, especially in advanced AIDS (see Chapter 12); however, it can also rarely occur in seemingly healthy individuals
  - Tuberculous meningitis typically follows a protracted course. The CSF profile usually reveals a lymphocytic pleocytosis, elevated protein level, and lowered glucose concentration

Clinical Presentation

- Fever, headache, and nuchal rigidity (neck stiffness) are seen in most cases
- Unlike in encephalitis, brain function can be normal; however, mental status changes and seizures can occur

- A diffuse maculopapular rash that becomes petechial can be seen with meningococcemia (Fig. 15-1)
- Physical examination may reveal signs of meningeal irritation, but these findings occur in less than 5% of patients
  - Kernig sign: Pain in the back is elicited with passive extension of the knee while the hip is flexed
  - Brudzinski sign: Passive flexion of the neck results in spontaneous flexion of the hips and knees

Diagnosis

- Blood cultures should be obtained immediately
- Diagnosis relies on examination of the CSF (Table 15-3)
- **Neuroimaging with computed tomography (CT) or magnetic resonance imaging (MRI) is only needed in select situations before performing a lumbar puncture (Table 15-4)**
- **If neuroimaging is needed, empiric antibiotic therapy (and dexamethasone if indicated) should be started before scanning**

Treatment

- Bacterial meningitis
  - Empiric therapy
    - Age younger than 1 month: ampicillin plus cefotaxime or ampicillin plus aminoglycoside
    - Age 1 month to 50 years: vancomycin plus a third-generation cephalosporin (ceftriaxone or cefotaxime)
    - Older than 50 years: ampicillin (to cover *Listeria* spp.) plus vancomycin plus a third-generation cephalosporin
    - Penetrating head trauma, post-neurosurgery, or CSF shunt: vancomycin plus cefepime, ceftazidime, or meropenem
  - Role of adjunctive dexamethasone
    - **Recommended in adults with suspected or proven pneumococcal meningitis**
    - First dose ideally given 10 to 20 minutes before the first dose of antibiotics
    - If not given before the first dose of antibiotics, then give concomitantly with the first dose
    - Dosing: 0.15 mg/kg IV every 6 hours for 2 to 4 days
  - Organism-specific therapy (see Table 15-1)

TABLE 15-1	*Common Etiologic Agents Causing Acute Bacterial Meningitis in Adults*	
Pathogen	**Description**	**Recommended Treatment**
Streptococcus pneumoniae	Most common etiologic agent in United States Mortality 19% to 26% Sometimes associated with other foci of infection (e.g., pneumonia, endocarditis)	Vancomycin + third-generation cephalosporin until antimicrobial susceptibility is known (some experts add rifampin if dexamethasone is given)
Neisseria meningitides	Affects mostly children and young adults Patients with terminal complement deficiency are at increased risk Maculopapular rash progresses to petechiae on the trunk, extremities, and mucous membranes	Third-generation cephalosporin Switch to penicillin G or ampicillin once confirmed to be highly sensitive Chemoprophylaxis: rifampin (or ciprofloxacin or ceftriaxone) recommended for household contacts, day care center members, those directly exposed to oral secretions
Haemophilus influenzae	Mostly occurs in children Disease in adults usually associated with sinusitis, otitis media, pneumonia, sickle cell disease, splenectomy, diabetes, immune deficiency, head trauma with cerebrospinal fluid (CSF) leak, or alcoholism	Third-generation cephalosporin
Listeria monocytogenes	Disease of neonates, older adults, and immunocompromised (including poorly controlled diabetics and pregnant women) Outbreaks associated with contaminated produce, coleslaw, milk, cheese Associated with hematologic malignancy, steroid use, iron overload	Ampicillin (or penicillin G) ± aminoglycoside
Staphylococcus aureus	Usually seen after head trauma, in postoperative settings, or when hardware is present	Nafcillin or oxacillin (if methicillin-susceptible) Vancomycin ± rifampin (if methicillin-resistant)

15

TABLE 15-2	*Causes of Aseptic Meningitis*
Category	**Examples**
Viral	Enteroviruses, mumps, echovirus, poliovirus, coxsackievirus, HSV, CMV, VZV, arboviruses, acute HIV, influenza
Bacterial	Tuberculosis, rickettsiae, syphilis, *Borrelia burgdorferi*
Fungal	Cryptococcus, coccidioides, histoplasma, candida, molds (aspergillus, exserohilum)
Miscellaneous infections	Toxoplasma, malaria, Whipple disease, leptospira
Noninfectious diseases	Brain tumors, sarcoidosis, lupus, meningeal carcinomatosis
Drugs	Trimethoprim-sulfamethoxazole, ibuprofen, carbamazepine

CMV, Cytomegalovirus; HSV, herpes simplex virus; VZV, varicella zoster virus.

- Aseptic meningitis
  - Treatment is generally supportive

Encephalitis

Basic Information

- Inflammation of the brain parenchyma with neurologic dysfunction

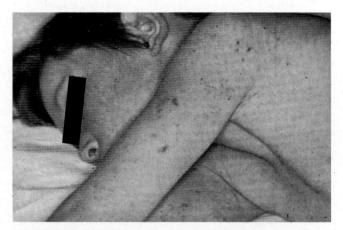

FIGURE 15-1 Typical rash of meningococcal sepsis. Fine erythematous macules and petechiae are present in some areas. (From Cohen J, Powderly W: *Infectious Diseases*. 2nd ed. St. Louis: Mosby: 2004: Fig. 227.9.)

- Frequently concurrent with meningitis (meningoencephalitis) or inflammation of the spinal cord (encephalomyelitis)
- Can be caused by a number of different pathogens (Table 15-5)
- In patients who had a recent viral illness or vaccination and who present with encephalitis, consider a diagnosis of acute disseminated encephalomyelitis (ADEM)

Clinical Presentation

- Headache, fever, nuchal rigidity in meningoencephalitis (as in meningitis)

TABLE 15-3	*Typical Cerebrospinal Fluid Abnormalities in Acute Bacterial and Aseptic Meningitis*	
	Bacterial	**Aseptic**
Opening pressure	>20 cm H_2O	<25 cm H_2O
White blood cells	10 to 10,000/mm³	10 to 1000/mm³
Differential	Neutrophils predominate	Mononuclear cells predominate*
Glucose	<40 mg/dL	>45 mg/dL
Protein	>100 mg/dL	<200 mg/dL
Gram stain	Positive in 60% to 90% of cases	Negative
Culture	Positive in 70% to 85% of cases who have not received previous antimicrobials	Negative
PCR of CMV, EBV, viral nucleic acid	Negative	Positive in some cases (i.e., HSV, CMV, EBV, VZV, enteroviruses)

*Neutrophils may predominate in very early viral meningitis.
CMV, Cytomegalovirus; EBV, Epstein-Barr virus; HSV, herpes simplex virus; PCR, polymerase chain reaction; VZV, varicella zoster virus.

TABLE 15-4	*Indications for Head CT before Lumbar Puncture When Acute Bacterial Meningitis Is Suspected*	
Category	**Specific Indication**	
Immunocompromised host	HIV/AIDS, transplant patient, patient on immunosuppressive medications	
History of CNS disease	Mass lesion, stroke, focal infection	
Papilledema	Especially if no venous pulsations	
New-onset seizure	Onset within 1 week of presentation	
Focal neurologic deficit	Dilated nonreactive pupil, ocular motility abnormalities, abnormal visual fields, gaze palsy, arm or leg drift	
Abnormal level of consciousness	Inability to follow 2 consecutive commands or answer 2 consecutive questions	

AIDS, Acquired immunodeficiency syndrome; CNS, central nervous system; CT, computed tomography; HIV, human immunodeficiency virus.

- Alterations in consciousness may help distinguish from meningitis
  - Bizarre behavior, hallucinations, expressive aphasia can be seen with temporal lobe involvement with herpes simplex virus (HSV) infection (Fig. 15-2)
  - Focal neurologic signs and seizures can also develop
  - West Nile virus may be associated with flaccid weakness and reduced or absent reflexes

Diagnosis

- CSF: lymphocytic pleocytosis, normal glucose level, and elevated protein level
- CSF polymerase chain reactions (PCRs) are useful for the detection of HSV, cytomegalovirus, Epstein-Barr virus, varicella-zoster virus, JC virus, West Nile virus, and enteroviruses
- CSF serologic testing is useful for the detection of arboviruses

- Serum and/or CSF serologic testing and PCRs can help diagnose tick-borne and spirochetal disease
- Brain biopsy only needed in patients who continue to deteriorate on acyclovir and who have a negative diagnostic workup
- CSF culture is useful for fungal, mycobacterial, and bacterial causes of encephalitis
- Perform respiratory viral panel testing if there is a suspicion of respiratory viral disease
- MRI of the brain should be performed in all cases; if not possible, then CT scanning should be done

Treatment

- Treatment is generally supportive (see Table 15-5)
- HSV encephalitis should be treated with intravenous (IV) acyclovir to lower morbidity and mortality
- Postexposure prophylaxis with antiserum should be given for rabies exposure
- Initiate empiric doxycycline when there is a high suspicion of rickettsial or ehrlichial disease
- Tailor treatment to etiologic agent, if found

Skin and Soft Tissue Infections

See Figure 15-3 and Table 15-6 for examples and summary of skin and soft tissue infections.

Basic Information

- Range from minor superficial infections to life-threatening conditions, such as necrotizing fasciitis
- Generally categorized into purulent versus nonpurulent infections
- Purulence usually denotes staphylococcal disease
- Increasing incidence of infections caused by community-acquired methicillin-resistant *Staphylococcus aureus* (MRSA)

Clinical Presentation

- Most present with isolated skin or soft tissue findings; some develop necrotizing pneumonia, necrotizing fasciitis, endocarditis, osteomyelitis, or sepsis

TABLE 15-5	*Selected Pathogens Causing Encephalitis*			
Virus	**Transmission**	**Diagnosis**	**Treatment**	**Comments**
Arboviruses California encephalitis (LaCrosse)	Mosquito	Serologic testing	Supportive	Mortality is low
St. Louis encephalitis	Mosquito	Serologic testing	Supportive	Mortality seen in up to 20% of patients
West Nile	Mosquito	PCR and IgM in CSF or serum Convalescent titers in serum	Supportive	Most infected patients present with febrile illness Advanced age is greatest risk factor for severe disease
Enteroviruses	Fecal–oral	CSF PCR	Supportive	Usually occurs in summer Rash, conjunctivitis, pleurodynia may occur
Herpes simplex virus	Contact with mucosal surfaces	CSF PCR	Acyclovir	HSV-1 usually causes encephalitis, HSV-2 usually causes meningitis MRI may reveal abnormalities in the temporal lobe with encephalitis
Rabies virus	Bite from a rabid animal (dog, cat, bat)	Viral antigen from a nape-of-neck biopsy	Supportive treatment Postexposure prophylaxis with antiserum and active immunization is important	Brainstem dysfunction causes diplopia, neuritis, excessive salivation, respiratory paralysis Consider diagnosis in spelunkers

CSF, Cerebrospinal fluid; HSV, herpes simplex virus; IgM, immunoglobulin M; MRI, magnetic resonance imaging; PCR, polymerase chain reaction.

15

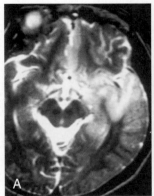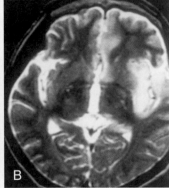

FIGURE 15-2   A and **B**, Herpes simplex encephalitis. T2-weighted magnetic resonance imaging views showing increased signal in left medial temporal lobe, inferior frontal lobe, and insular cortex. (From Bradley WG, Daroff RB, Fenichel GM, et al. *Neurology in Clinical Practice.* 4th ed. Burlington, MA: Butterworth-Heinemann; 2004: Fig. 59B.1.)

- Erythema without pain, fever, warmth, or leukocytosis should lead to consideration of alternative diagnoses

Treatment

- Treatment options for MRSA
  - Incision and drainage is the primary treatment for cutaneous abscesses
  - Vancomycin is the drug of choice for hospitalized patients; linezolid is an alternative

- Many community-acquired MRSA strains may be sensitive to trimethoprim-sulfamethoxazole; other options for outpatients include clindamycin (although resistance can be inducible) and doxycycline
  - Other newer agents such as daptomycin, telavancin, and ceftaroline can be considered
  - Consider empirical treatment for patients with purulent disease pending culture results
- Nonpurulent infections
  - Most are caused by β-hemolytic Streptococci, making β-lactam therapy (e.g., amoxicillin) the treatment of choice

Acute Bacterial Arthritis

Basic Information

- Usually involves one joint (*monoarticular*)
- Route of infection is usually hematogenous, but direct inoculation of bacteria from penetrating trauma can occur
- Significant morbidity/mortality when treatment is delayed
- *S. aureus* most common etiologic agent
- *Neisseria gonorrhoeae* should be considered in healthy young adults (Fig. 15-4)
- Groups A, B, C, and G streptococci, *Streptococcus pneumoniae*, and gram-negative bacilli account for most other infections

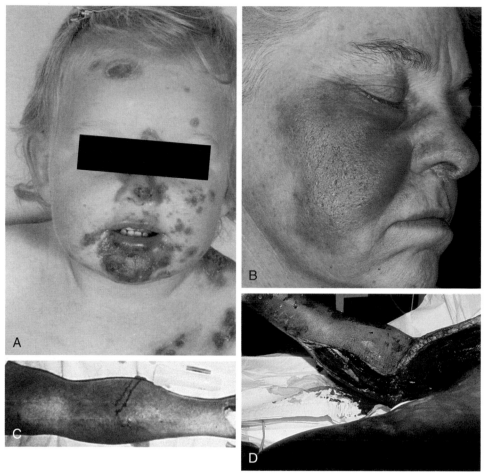

FIGURE 15-3 **A,** Impetigo. **B,** Erysipelas. **C,** Necrotizing fasciitis. **D,** Extensive gas gangrene of the arm. (**A, C,** and **D,** From Cohen J, Powderly W. *Infectious Diseases.* 2nd ed. St. Louis: Mosby; 2004: Figs. 225.18, 225.20, and 10.19. **B,** From Habif TP. *Clinical Dermatology.* 4th ed. St. Louis: Mosby; 2004: Fig. 9-12.)

TABLE 15-6	*Skin and Soft Tissue Infections*			
	Description	**Pathogens**	**Treatment**	**Comments**
Impetigo or ethyma (see Fig. 15-3A)	Superficial infection Vesicular with golden crusts	Group A streptococci *Staphylococcus aureus* (MSSA or MRSA)	Topical antibiotics (mupirocin or retapamulin) or oral antibiotics if impetigo and single lesion; oral antibiotics if ecthyma or impetigo with multiple lesions	Consider culture/gram stain of pus/exudate to identify if staphylococcal or streptococcal Can form bullae
Furuncle (boil) or abscesses	Furuncle is a deep infection of hair follicle Usually on buttocks, face, neck Painful and tender	*S. aureus*	Moist heat Incision and drainage alone often sufficient Oral antibiotics may be needed if systemic symptoms or surrounding cellulitis	Consider gram stain/culture of purulence Carbuncles are infections of contiguous follicles that extend into subcutaneous fat For recurrent disease consider 5-day decolonization with intranasal mupirocin and chlorhexidine washes
Erysipelas (see Fig. 15-3B)	Superficial infection Involves cutaneous lymphatics More superficial than cellulitis Usually involves face or extremities Raised, violaceous, painful, spreading lesions with distinct border	Group A streptococci	Oral or IV penicillin (PCN)	Bullae can develop Systemic toxicity can occur Cultures not routinely recommended in non–immune-compromised hosts/simple disease

TABLE 15-6 | *Skin and Soft Tissue Infections (Continued)*

	Description	Pathogens	Treatment	Comments
Cellulitis	Spreading infection of deeper dermis and subcutaneous fat Localized pain, swelling, and warmth No distinct border	Most common: group A streptococci Purulent: *S. aureus* Diabetics: mixed gram-positive and gram-negative aerobic/anaerobic bacteria Lymphedema: groups A, B, C, G streptococci Penetrating trauma, Injection drug use: MRSA	Mild: oral PCN, dicloxacillin, cephalexin, or clindamycin Severe: vancomycin + piperacillin-tazobactam or vancomycin + imipenem or meropenem Diabetic: broad coverage Lymphedema: IV PCN; Can use oral PCN to prevent recurrences Penetrating trauma, IDU: vancomycin or other agent with MRSA activity	Cultures not routinely recommended in non–immune-compromised hosts/simple disease Elevation of affected area important Tinea pedis may be a portal of entry in some patients Bullae may be present In patients with liver disease and saltwater exposure, consider *Vibrio vulnificus*
Necrotizing fasciitis (see Fig. 15-3C)	Severe infection of the subcutaneous soft tissues along superficial fascia Erythema and swelling progress rapidly to bullae and cutaneous gangrene Predilection for lower extremities, abdominal wall, and perineum (Fournier gangrene)	Polymicrobial: (anaerobes + streptococci + Enterobacteriaceae) Monomicrobial: group A streptococci *S. aureus* (MRSA or MSSA) *V. vulificus* Aeromonas hydrophila Anaerobic streptococci	Early surgical exploration critical Broad-spectrum antibiotics Vancomycin or linezolid + piperacillin-tazobactam or + carbapenem or + ceftriaxone and flagyl PCN + clindamycin if documented group A strep	Risk factors include diabetes, peripheral vascular disease, surgery, trauma, including injection drug use or insect bites Systemic toxicity develops rapidly High mortality rate if surgical exploration not immediate Imaging should not delay surgical exploration
Pyomyositis	Pus within individual muscle groups Usually in an extremity Localized pain with a firm "woody" feel	*S. aureus* (90%) Group A streptococci *S. pneumoniae* Gram-negative enterics	Early drainage important Vancomycin with antibiotics tailored to organism Immune compromised: vancomycin + piperacillin-tazobactam orampicillin-sulbactam or carbapenem If MSSA: cefazolin or oxacillin or nafcillin	Usually in tropics Temperate climate: HIV and DM CK may be elevated, but often normal if single muscle group Blood and abscess material cultures should be obtained MRI is recommended imaging modality; CT if not available
Gas gangrene (anaerobic cellulitis; see Fig. 15-3D)	Begins as a localized infection in a superficial wound Rapidly spreads across fascial planes, causing severe pain and swelling Crepitance may be palpable	*Clostridium perfringens* or other species Other anaerobes	Surgical exploration Penicillin + clindamycin if clostridial Vancomycin + piperacillin/tazobactam or a carbapenem if unclear etiology	Progresses from cellulitis to myositis to myonecrosis rapidly High mortality rate
Staphylococcal toxic shock syndrome	Fever, sunburn rash, hypotension progressing to multiorgan failure Desquamation occurs late	Associated with colonization of wound/vagina with toxin-producing *S. aureus* without invasive disease	IV fluid resuscitation Removal/drainage of the colonizing source Antibiotics: PCN or first-generation cephalosporins	Most commonly seen in the setting of menstruation Bacteremia or overt infection with *S. aureus* not usually seen
Streptococcal toxic shock syndrome	Fever and hypotension progressing to multiorgan failure Rash and desquamation usually not present	Usually associated with skin/soft tissue infection with toxin-producing group A streptococci	IV fluids PCN + clindamycin	Most patients are bacteremic

CK, Creatine kinase; CT, computerized tomography; DM, diabetes mellitus; HIV, human immunodeficiency virus; IDU, injection drug users; IV, intravenous; MRI, magnetic resonance imaging; MRSA, methicillin-resistant *S. aureus*; MSSA, methicillin-susceptible *S. aureus*; PCN, penicillin.

15

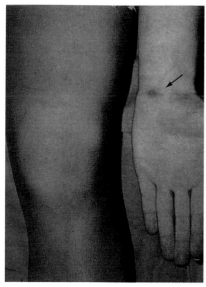

FIGURE 15-4 Gonococcal septic arthritis with an associated papular skin lesion *(arrow)*. (From Forbes C, Jackson W. *Color Atlas and Text of Clinical Medicine.* 3rd ed. St. Louis: Mosby; 2003: Fig. 3.8.)

TABLE 15-7	**Organisms Causing Acute Bacterial Arthritis**
Organism	**Predisposing Factors and Conditions**
Neisseria gonorrhoeae	Age <30 years
Staphylococcus aureus	Glucocorticoid therapy Rheumatoid arthritis Diabetes Postsurgical Injection drug use
Streptococcus pneumoniae	HIV Alcoholism Sickle cell anemia Less than half have another focus of *S. pneumoniae* infection
Mycoplasma spp.	Primary immunoglobulin deficiency
Salmonella spp.	HIV Sickle cell disease
Pasteurella multocida	Cat bites or scratches
Other gram-negative bacilli	Injection drug use Immunodeficiency Neonates Elderly Nursing home residents

- Specific organisms should be suspected based on the underlying host (Table 15-7)

Clinical Presentation

- Pain, decreased range of motion, effusion, and erythema are typically seen
- Fever not always present
- Knee or hip most commonly affected

Diagnosis

- Aspiration of synovial fluid is essential for diagnosis
  - Ultrasonography, CT scan, or MRI may be helpful for detection and aspiration with involvement of certain joints (e.g., hip, sacroiliac joint)
  - **White blood cell (WBC) counts in the synovial fluid are usually greater than 50,000/mm³ with greater than 75% neutrophils**
  - **Glucose is usually less than 40 mg/dL**
  - The presence of crystals does not rule out infection, because crystal-induced arthritis and septic arthritis can occur together
  - Gram stain is positive in one third of cases
  - **Joint fluid cultures are positive in up to 90% of nongonococcal bacterial arthritis, but in less than 50% of gonococcal (GC) arthritis**
  - Often need genital or pharyngeal culture and/or nucleic acid amplification (NAA) to confirm GC, or NAA on joint fluid or urine
- Blood cultures should be obtained
  - Blood cultures are positive in up to 60% of cases of *S. aureus*, but are less sensitive in diagnosing other pathogens

Treatment

- Empirical antimicrobial therapy after blood cultures and joint aspiration largely depends on gram stain
  - If GC arthritis is suspected, ceftriaxone should be started
  - If *S. aureus* is suspected, vancomycin should be started. This can be narrowed to a penicillinase-resistant penicillin (e.g., oxacillin or nafcillin) if methicillin-susceptible *S. aureus* (MSSA) is present
  - If Streptococcal disease is suspected, penicillin or ampicillin should be started
  - If gram-negative infection is suspected, ceftazidime or cefepime are appropriate empiric choices
- Repeated aspirations may be necessary if effusions reaccumulate
- Indications for surgical drainage
  - Hip joint involvement (except in cases of GC)
  - Delay of therapy (>1 week after onset of symptoms)
  - Loculated infection or exudate too thick to aspirate
  - Poor response to therapy (e.g., failure to decrease synovial WBC)
  - Prosthetic joint infection (Box 15-1)

Chronic Monoarticular Arthritis

Basic Information

- Frequently caused by bacteria (and mycobacteria), fungi, and rarely, parasites (Table 15-8)
- If joint culture is negative, synovial biopsy is necessary
- Treatment guided toward specific organism

Viral Arthritis

Basic Information

- Caused by direct invasion of the synovium or by an immune reaction involving certain joints

- Usually a migratory polyarthritis
- Many viruses implicated
  - Rubella
    - Can occur following infection or immunization
    - Usually seen in women
    - Disease typically self-limited but can rarely persist for years
  - Mumps
    - More common in men
    - Develops within 2 weeks of parotitis
  - Parvovirus B19
    - Small joints of the hands most frequently involved
    - Infection in adults can occur without fever or rash
    - Self-limited: usually resolves within 8 to 10 weeks
  - Hepatitis B
    - Can manifest as arthralgias or symmetrical arthritis

- Symptoms (arthralgias or arthritis) occur before jaundice and resolve when jaundice develops
- Most are self-limited: No specific treatment for the arthritis is available

Osteomyelitis

Basic Information

- Defined as an infection of bone
- Two basic types based on the route of infection
  - Hematogenous source
    - Caused by seeding of the bone during bacteremia
    - Primarily occurs in children and older adults
    - Injection drug users
      - May have involvement of the vertebrae, sternoclavicular, or sacroiliac joints, or the symphysis pubis
      - *S. aureus*, *Pseudomonas*, *Serratia*, and *Eikenella* are common pathogens for this group
    - *S. aureus* is the organism most frequently isolated
    - Patients with sickle cell disease may be infected with *S. aureus* or *Salmonella*
    - Vertebral involvement can be caused by *S. aureus*, gram-negative bacilli, tuberculosis (TB; Pott disease), or *Candida*
  - Contiguous source
    - Accounts for most cases of osteomyelitis in adults
    - Includes infections extending from adjacent soft tissue, injury, or surgery
    - Presentation is more indolent than with hematogenous spread
    - Diabetic foot ulcers and decubitus ulcers are common sources
    - **Most infections are polymicrobial, although *S. aureus* is still frequently found**

BOX 15-1	*Prosthetic Joint Infection*

Early infection: Within 1 to 3 months, acquired at surgery, acute symptoms (cellulitis, erythema, pain, drainage); usually caused by *Staphylococcus aureus*, gram-negative bacilli, anaerobes, or polymicrobial

Delayed infection: 3 to 12 months, acquired at surgery, indolent symptoms of joint pain and/or loosening of prosthesis; usually low-virulence pathogens (e.g., *Propionibacterium acnes*, coagulase-negative staphylococci, enterococci)

Late infection: After 12 months, commonly via hematogenous seeding; usual pathogens are *S. aureus*, β-hemolytic streptococci, or gram-negative bacilli

Definitive diagnosis made by arthrocentesis or surgical débridement

Most successful therapy is removal of entire prosthesis with 6 weeks of antibiotic therapy

---

TABLE 15-8	*Selected Pathogens Causing Chronic Monoarticular Arthritis*
Borrelia burgdorferi (Lyme disease)	Up to 50% of untreated patients develop monoarthritis or oligoarthritis of large joint(s) Serology is universally positive See Chapter 16 for further information
Mycobacterium tuberculosis	Usually involves large joints (hips, knees, or ankles) Swelling and pain worsen over months to years; systemic signs and symptoms are frequently absent; synovial fluid examination reveals approximately 50% neutrophils; acid-fast stain is positive in less than half of cases; culture is frequently positive; synovial biopsy culture has higher yield Treat for 6 to 9 months with multiple agents (see Chapter 13)
Atypical mycobacteria	Usually involves smaller joints (wrists, hands) Infection occurs from inoculation from water or soil, so may see as a result of gardening or water-related activities Synovial biopsy often necessary to make the diagnosis
Brucella spp.	Can cause acute or chronic monoarthritis or asymmetrical polyarthritis Febrile illness frequently coexists Transmission is through ingestion of unpasteurized milk or cheese, ingestion of raw meat, or inhalation during contact with animals (e.g., slaughterhouse workers) Treat with doxycycline + aminoglycoside
Sporothrix schenckii	Seen in gardeners or those who work with soil
Candida spp.	Results from surgical procedures or articular injections Injection drug users may have involvement of spine or sacroiliac joint Treat with drainage and antifungal therapy

15

- ■ ***Pseudomonas aeruginosa* should be considered in the setting of a puncture wound of the foot**

Clinical Presentation

- ■ Fever
- ■ Bone pain over the affected site

Diagnosis

- ■ Blood studies
  - ■ Sedimentation rate and C-reactive protein (CRP) elevated in most cases
  - ■ Blood cultures more likely to be positive in cases of hematogenous spread
- ■ Radiologic and imaging studies
  - ■ Plain radiographs
    - ■ May show periosteal elevation, soft tissue swelling, or lytic changes (Fig. 15-5)
    - ■ Findings may not be present during early or acute infection, but if seen are adequate for diagnosis
  - ■ MRI
    - ■ **Best identifies early changes consistent with acute osteomyelitis, such as bone marrow edema**
    - ■ **Test of choice for vertebral osteomyelitis because it better defines the surrounding soft tissue**
  - ■ CT
    - ■ Can be helpful if hardware present
  - ■ Technetium bone scan:
    - ■ Can detect early lesions with high sensitivity
    - ■ Can be falsely negative in acute and chronic infection
    - ■ Best when bone was previously normal (false positives common with previously abnormal bone)
    - ■ Cannot distinguish infection from tumor, fracture, or infarction

- ■ Consider if MRI and CT not available or contraindicated
- ■ **Bone biopsy for culture is recommended to make a definitive diagnosis if blood cultures are negative**
- ■ Swab cultures of sinus tract or ulcer base are unreliable for making a microbiologic diagnosis; however, they can be useful if treatment is to be empiric to determine if therapy needs to include coverage against virulent pathogens such as *S. aureus* or *P. aeruginosa*

Treatment

- ■ Early diagnosis and treatment are important to prevent bone necrosis
- ■ Therapy for acute osteomyelitis usually consists of 6 weeks of intravenous (IV) antibiotics directed by the culture results
  - ■ Depending on organism and antimicrobial susceptibilities, oral therapy after an initial 2 weeks of IV antibiotics may be considered in select cases if the antibiotic to be used has adequate bioavailability and bone penetration
- ■ Chronic osteomyelitis often requires surgical débridement to remove devitalized bone or restore vascular supply in conjunction with antimicrobial therapy. Antimicrobial therapy in the absence of débridement is suppressive, not curative.
- ■ Monitoring of erythrocyte sedimentation rate (ESR) and CRP over time is helpful

Fever of Unknown Origin

Basic Information

- ■ Classified by a patient's condition and setting in which the fever manifests (Table 15-9)

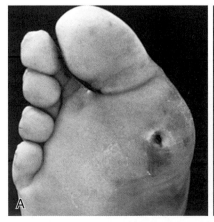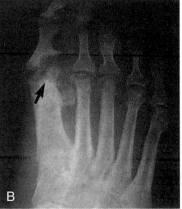

FIGURE 15-5   Diabetic abscess. **A**, Note discoloration proximal to abscess beneath first metatarsal head. **B**, Results of osteomyelitis of the first metatarsal with bony erosion *(arrow)* seen on radiograph. (**A**, From Canale ST. *Campbell's Operative Orthopaedics.* 10th ed. St. Louis: Mosby; 2003: Fig. 82-11A. **B**, From Forbes C, Jackson W. *Color Atlas and Text of Clinical Medicine.* 3rd ed. St. Louis: Mosby; 2003: Fig. 3.152.)

TABLE 15-9	**Classification of Fever of Unknown Origin**	
Category	**Definition**	**Common Underlying Causes**
Classic FUO	Fever 38.3° C for ≥3 weeks Blood cultures negative Lack of diagnosis with 3 outpatient visits or 3 inpatient days	Infection Malignancy Collagen vascular diseases Granulomatous disease
Nosocomial FUO	Hospitalized patient with no fever on admission 3 days of investigation 2 days of negative incubating cultures	*Clostridium difficile* Phlebitis or venous thromboembolism Sinusitis Drug fever
Neutropenic FUO	Absolute neutrophil count <500/μL 3 days of investigation 2 days of negative incubating cultures	Perianal infection *Aspergillus* spp. *Candida* spp.
HIV-associated FUO	HIV-positive patient Fever ≥3 weeks in outpatients or >3 days for inpatients 3 days of investigation 2 days of negative incubating cultures	Mycobacteria, including TB Lymphoma Drug fever Cytomegalovirus *Pneumocystis jiroveci* (previously *P. carinii*) pneumonia

FUO, Fever of unknown origin; TB, tuberculosis.

TABLE 15-10	**Etiologic Considerations for Classic Fever of Unknown Origin**
History	**Disease**
Foreign-born individuals	Extrapulmonary tuberculosis
Age >50 years	Malignancy Giant cell arteritis Polymyalgia rheumatica
High fevers with arthralgias/arthritis and rash	Adult Still disease
Medical background with undocumented fevers	Factitious fever
Returning traveler	From endemic countries: *Plasmodium* spp., Dengue, *Salmonella* spp., tick-borne diseases
Recurrent episodic fevers	Hereditary periodic fevers

- Traditionally defined as fever for greater than 3 weeks with negative workup while hospitalized for more than 1 week
- Most accept a definition of fever for more than 3 weeks without a diagnosis after two outpatient visits or 3 days of hospitalization
- Most cases are caused by infections, noninfectious inflammatory diseases, or neoplasms
- Specific etiologies of classic FUO may be suggested by the patient's history (Table 15-10)

Diagnosis

- A thorough history, including travel, hobbies, history of TB exposure, human immunodeficiency virus (HIV) risk factors, and medications, should be obtained to guide the evaluation
- Repeated physical examinations may be necessary to detect slowly progressing diseases
- Basic testing should include the following:
  - Complete blood count (CBC)
  - Comprehensive metabolic panel
  - Urinalysis
  - ESR and CRP
  - Blood cultures (greater than 3 sets)
  - Chest radiograph
  - Antinuclear antibodies (ANA)
  - HIV
- Purified protein derivative or interferon-γ release assay (IGRA) testing should be considered
- CT scan of the chest, abdomen, and pelvis should be considered in the absence of other localizing signs
- Further evaluation should be based on findings from the history, physical examination, and basic laboratory tests
- Administration of naproxen may help distinguish between neoplasia and infection because the fever from neoplasms is thought to be more responsive to the medication
- Try to avoid empirical antibiotics because they may suppress an occult infection without curing it, and may interfere with the ability to make a diagnosis
- Drug-induced fever should be considered a diagnosis of exclusion; it is confirmed by stopping the potentially offending agent
  - Usually patients do not appear as toxic as with other causes of FUO
  - **Rash and eosinophilia are sometimes present, but their absence does not rule out drug fever**
  - Common causes include sulfonamides, β-lactam antibiotics, phenytoin, amiodarone, and nitrofurantoin
- Figure 15-6 shows an algorithm for diagnostic approach to FUO
- The cause of the FUO may not be found in approximately 30% of adults, but most of those without a diagnosis have a good prognosis

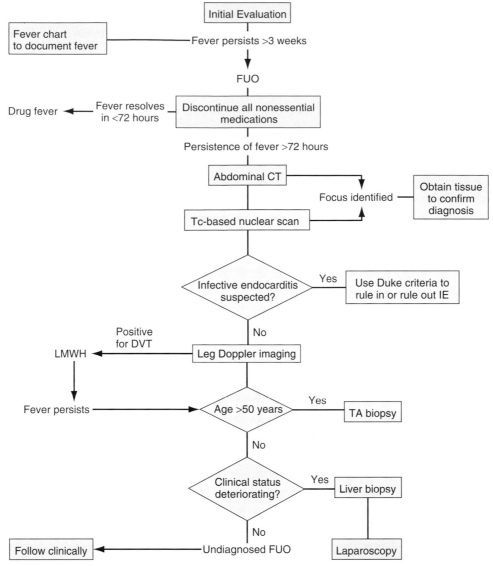

FIGURE 15-6 Diagnostic approach to fever of unknown origin (FUO). CT, Computed tomography; DVT, deep vein thrombosis; IE, infective endocarditis; LMWH, low-molecular-weight heparin; TA, temporal artery. (From Mourad O, Palda V, Detsky AS. A comprehensive evidence-based approach to fever of unknown origin. *Arch Intern Med.* 2003; 163:549: Fig. 2.)

Acknowledgment

The author would like to thank Aruna K. Subramanian, MD, for her work on previous editions of this chapter.

Review Questions

For review questions, please go to ExpertConsult.com.

SUGGESTED READINGS

Cunha BA. Fever of unknown origin. *Infect Dis Clin North Am.* 2007;21:867-915.

Durack DT, Street AC. Fever of unknown origin reexamined and redefined. *Curr Clin Top Infect Dis.* 1991;11:35-51.

Hussein QA, Anaya DA. Necrotizing soft tissue infections. *Crit Care Clin.* 2013;29:795-806.

Smith JW, Chalupa P, Shabaz Hasan M. Infectious arthritis: clinical features, laboratory findings and treatment. *Clin Microbiol Infect.* 2006;12:309-314.

Stevens DL, Bisno AL, Chambers HF, et al. Practice guidelines for the diagnosis and management of skin and soft tissue infections: 2014 update by the Infectious Disease Society of America. *Clin Infect Dis.* 2014;9:e10-e52.

Tunkel AR, Hartman BJ, Kaplan SL, et al. Practice guidelines for the management of bacterial meningitis. *Clin Infect Dis.* 2004;39:1267-1284.

Venkatesan A, Tunkel AR, Bloch KC, et al. Case definitions, diagnostic algorithms, and priorities in encephalitis: consensus statement of the International Encephalitis Consortium. *Clin Infect Dis.* 2013;57:1114-1128.

Zimmerli W. Vertebral osteomyelitis. *N Engl J Med.* 2010;362:1022-1029.

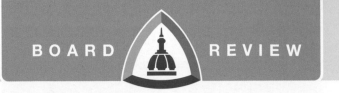
Selected Topics in Infectious Disease II

JOHN N. AUCOTT, MD; and MICHAEL A. CHATTERGOON, MD, PhD

This chapter is divided into three sections on selected topics in infectious disease encountered by the internist: (1) endocarditis, (2) tick-borne illnesses, and (3) infections from bite and scratch wounds.

Infective Endocarditis

Basic Information

- **Infective endocarditis refers to infection of the endocardium and most commonly refers to infection of one of the heart valves**
  - Infective endocarditis may present acutely with devastating consequences or be slowly progressive and have subtle clinical findings
  - Bacterial and fungal organisms may cause infective endocarditis
  - Noninfective endocarditis may be caused by inflammatory conditions of the endocardium and valves (e.g., Libman-Sacks endocarditis associated with systemic lupus erythematosus)
- Types of infective endocarditis
  - Native valve endocarditis, acute and subacute
  - Prosthetic valve endocarditis, early and late
  - Intravenous drug use-related endocarditis
- The classic clinical presentation and course of infective endocarditis have been historically characterized as either acute or subacute
  - Acute native valve endocarditis is usually aggressive and is typically caused by virulent organisms, e.g., *Staphylococcus aureus* and group B *streptococci*. (Fig. 16-1)
  - Subacute native valve endocarditis typically affects abnormal valves. It is often an indolent infection and is more commonly caused by organisms such as the viridans group *streptococci*
    - In subacute bacterial endocarditis, left-sided valvular infection is more common than right-sided valvular infection. Tricuspid valve involvement is much less common. Infection of the pulmonic valve is rare
  - The increasing prevalence of prosthetic heart valves, along with the evolving infectious etiologies of endocarditis, have made the acute versus subacute distinction less clinically useful
    - **Because the etiologic agent is what determines treatment, infective endocarditis is now**
      classified by organism, rather than the time course of the infection
- Predisposing factors
  - Age older than 60 years
  - Male sex
  - Abnormal cardiac anatomy
    - Having an abnormal native heart valve is the most common predisposing factor
    - Mitral valve prolapse is among the most common associated abnormalities (20% to 30% of cases); the presence of a murmur or thickened valve associated with highest risk
    - Rheumatic heart disease becoming less common in developed nations
    - Bicuspid aortic valves can be seen as a predisposing factor
    - Congenital heart disease, including atrial and ventricular septal defects and patent ductus arteriosus
    - Presence of prosthetic valves
  - Injection drug use
  - Poor dentition
  - Presence of an intravascular device, such as a catheter
  - Previous endocarditis
  - Hemodialysis
  - HIV infection

Clinical Presentation

- Signs and symptoms
  - Symptoms are often nonspecific and include fever, malaise, chest pain, night sweats
  - **Cardiac findings that may be seen include new murmurs, vegetations on echocardiography (absence of a visible vegetation does not exclude diagnosis), conduction abnormalities (especially with endocarditis of aortic valve), and congestive heart failure**
  - Cough, pleurisy, and cavitating pulmonary infiltrates can be seen in right-sided endocarditis
  - Signs of systemic inflammation, such as fever, fatigue or failure to thrive, and arthralgias can be seen
  - Systemic emboli are seen in up to 45% of patients; may involve any organ; can lead to renal infarcts, splenic infarcts, pulmonary embolism, myocardial infarction if central nervous system is involved;

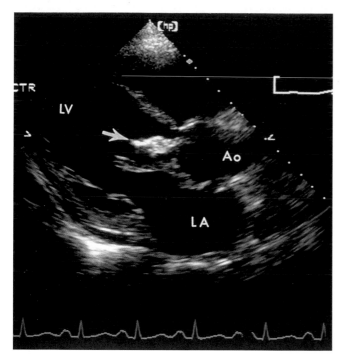

FIGURE 16-1 Infective endocarditis. Parasternal long-axis view echocardiogram of a patient with a large aortic valve vegetation *(arrow)*. Ao, Aorta; CTR, cardiothoracic; LA, left atrium; LV, left ventricle. (From Zipes DP. *Braunwald's Heart Disease: A Textbook of Cardiovascular Medicine.* 7th ed. Philadelphia: Saunders; 2005: Fig. 11-81.)

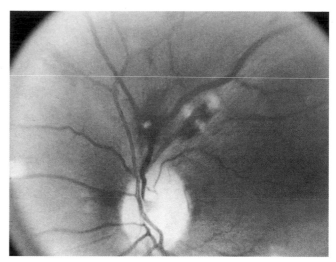

FIGURE 16-2 Roth spots in a patient with infective endocarditis. (From Zipes DP. *Braunwald's Heart Disease: A Textbook of Cardiovascular Medicine.* 7th ed. Philadelphia: Saunders; 2005: Fig. 58-5.)

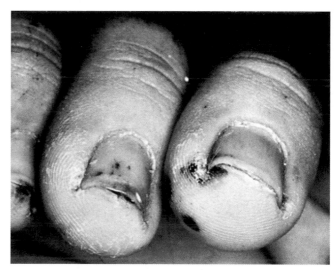

FIGURE 16-3 Splinter hemorrhages and petechiae in a patient with infective endocarditis. (From Zipes DP: *Braunwald's Heart Disease: A Textbook of Cardiovascular Medicine.* 7th ed. Philadelphia: Saunders; 2005: Fig. 58-4.)

middle cerebral artery territory is most commonly affected. Large emboli are more common in fungal endocarditis.
- Mycotic aneurysms are aneurysms associated with infective endocarditis; they usually arise in the cerebral arteries and aorta, but may also involve other major arteries
- Metastatic infection from bacteremia or fungemia can occur (e.g., vertebral osteomyelitis)
- Immune complex disease more often occurs in patients with subacute bacterial endocarditis; findings include glomerulonephritis, Roth spots (retinal hemorrhages; Fig. 16-2), and Osler nodes (tender nodules on finger or toe pads)
- Other: Splinter hemorrhages (especially in proximal nail beds; Fig. 16-3), Janeway lesions (nodular hemorrhages on palms of hands and soles of feet, caused by microabscesses), petechiae, splenomegaly, digital clubbing
- Etiologic agents (Table 16-1)
  - *Streptococci* spp. and *staphylococci* spp. account for the majority of infective endocarditis, but a variety of bacteria and fungi may be implicated
    - **Staphylococci spp. account for the majority of cases of health care-associated infective endocarditis**
    - **Staphylococci spp. and streptococci spp. occur in roughly equal proportions in with community-acquired infective endocarditis**
  - Viridans group *streptococci* are the most common *streptococci* spp.

- Pyogenic strep: groups A, C rarely cause endocarditis
- *Streptococcus gallolyticus* subspecies *gallolyticus* (*Streptococcus bovis* biotype I): Associated with gastrointestinal (GI) neoplasms; should prompt evaluation of the colon for malignancy
- *Streptococcus mutans*: An oral pathogen; may cause endocarditis in the susceptible host with poor dentition
- S. *aureus* is the most commonly implicated *Staphylococci* spp.
  - S. *aureus* infective endocarditis may involve normal heart valves and result in rapid progression with valve destruction. It is the most common cause of acute endocarditis
- **Enterococcus spp. are an increasingly prevalent cause of endocarditis and can be seen in older**

TABLE 16-1	*Causes of Bacterial Endocarditis*	
Endocarditis Subtype	**Most Common Organism**	**Other Common Organisms**
"Typical"	*Staphylococcus aureus*	Viridans group *streptococci* *Enterococcus* spp. Coagulase-negative *staphylococcus* spp. *Streptococcus bovis* biotype I Other *Streptococcus* spp.
"HACEK" group		*Haemophilus aphrophilus* *Haemophilus parainfluenzae* *Actinobacillus actinomycetemcomitans* *Cardiobacterium hominis* *Eikenella corrodens* *Kingella kingii*
Injection drug use	*S. aureus*	Viridans group *streptococci* *Enterococcus* spp. *Pseudomonas aeruginosa* *Candida* spp. *S. epidermidis* Polymicrobial
Unusual causes	No dominant organism	*Candida* spp. *Aspergillus* spp. *Coxiella burnetii* *Bartonella* spp. *Chlamydia* spp. *Legionella* spp. *Brucella* spp. *Mycoplasma*
Early prosthetic valve	*S. aureus* and coagulase negative- *Staphylococcus* spp. (*S. epidermidis*)	Gram-negative bacilli *Enterococcus* spp. Diphtheroids Fungi
Late prosthetic valve	Viridans group *streptococci*, *S. aureus*	Coagulase negative *Staphylococcus* spp. Gram-negative bacilli *Enterococcus* spp.

16

men following genitourinary (GU) instrumentation and in women following obstetric procedures
- *Pseudomonas spp.*: Very uncommon; typically occurs in those with history of intravenous (IV) drug use; usually right-sided
- Culture-negative infective endocarditis: May present with endocardial vegetation or embolic events
  - HACEK (*Haemophilus aphrophilus*, *Actinobacillus actinomycetemcomitans*, *Cardiobacterium hominis*, *Eikenella corrodens*, and *Kingella kingae*) organisms are now readily cultured with contemporary blood culture systems; this group accounts for 3% to 5% of native valve infections (see Table 16-1)
  - May need to hold blood cultures for 3 weeks if organisms such as *Bartonella* and *Brucella* are suspected
- Unusual infective endocarditis organisms
  - *Coxiella burnetii* (Q fever): Diagnosed by serology; culture often negative
  - Fungi: *Candida* spp. most common, followed by *Aspergillus* spp.; susceptible hosts include those with history of injection drug use, prosthetic heart valve recipients, and immunocompromised hosts
  - *Bartonella*, *Chlamydia*, *Legionella*, *Brucella*, *Mycoplasma* spp. are rare causes of infective endocarditis

- Prosthetic valves
  - Early prosthetic valve endocarditis occurs within 2 months of valve insertion
  - Late prosthetic valve endocarditis occurs 12 months after valve insertion
  - **The risk of prosthetic valve endocarditis is highest in the first 6 months following valve placement; infections less than 2 months after surgery are often nosocomial, although those that occur more than 2 months after surgery are more likely to be community-acquired**
  - *S. aureus* and *coagulase negative staphylococci* spp. are the most common causes of prosthetic valve endocarditis
  - Viridans group *streptococci* are a rare cause of early prosthetic valve endocarditis, but are a relatively common cause of late prosthetic valve endocarditis

Diagnosis and Evaluation

- Diagnosing endocarditis requires a high index of suspicion
- Definite bacterial endocarditis is a pathologic diagnosis made by culture cardiac tissue
  - Clinical criteria are often used to diagnose endocarditis (Table 16-2); typically requires a demonstration of persistent bacteremia by blood

TABLE 16-2	*Diagnostic Criteria for Endocarditis**	
Major Criteria	**Minor Criteria**	
Positive Blood Cultures Two separate positive blood cultures for a typical organism. Persistent bacteremia with any organism; defined as blood cultures drawn more than 12 hours apart, *or* 3 of 3 or 4 positive sets of blood cultures drawn over the course of at least 1 hour *or* the majority of more than 4 cultures positive from any period of time Positive *Coxiella burnetti* culture or serology **Evidence of Echocardiographic Involvement** Vegetation Abscess New dehiscence of prosthetic valve **Physical Examination** New regurgitant murmur; change in preexisting murmur not sufficient	**Fever ≥38°C** Predisposing heart condition: Previous endocarditis, injection drug use, prosthetic valve, ventricular septal defect, calcified valve, patent ductus, mitral valve regurgitation, or other valvular disease **Vascular or Embolic Events** Arterial or pulmonary emboli, conjunctival or retinal splinter or intracranial hemorrhage, mycotic aneurysm, Janeway lesions **Immunologic Phenomenon** Osler nodes, glomerulonephritis, rheumatoid factor, Roth spots Positive blood cultures that do not meet major microbiologic criteria or serologic evidence of acute infection with an organism known to cause endocarditis	

*Definite endocarditis is diagnosed with two major criteria or *one major plus three minor criteria* or *five minor criteria.*
Modified from AHA Scientific Statement on Infective Endocarditis. *Circulation.* 2005;111:e394-434.

culture with an organism likely to cause endocarditis, along with echocardiographic and/or clinical findings
- Blood cultures: Three separate sets of cultures drawn should be drawn, ideally from three different sites. They should also be separated in time, ideally 6 hours apart.
- Transthoracic echocardiography (TTE): First step in patients with native valves, no congenital heart disease, and no previous endocarditis; sensitivity is up to 62%. If intermediate-to-high probability of having endocarditis, proceed to transesophageal echocardiography (TEE).
- TEE: Can consider as a first step in patients with prosthetic valves, congenital heart disease, and previous endocarditis/valve abnormalities; sometimes a first step in patients with limited transthoracic windows, clear stigmata of endocarditis, and new murmurs
  - Sensitivity ranges from 90% to 100% in native valve endocarditis, and is lower in prosthetic valve endocarditis; a negative TEE does not necessarily rule out infective endocarditis
- Possible endocarditis, in which diagnostic criteria are not met, should be treated as endocarditis until an alternate diagnosis is confirmed

Treatment
- Treatment principles in endocarditis
  - Parenteral antibiotics preferred to ensure consistent and therapeutic antibiotic levels

- Extended therapy indicated—usually 4 to 6 weeks, depending on the etiologic agent (shorter courses associated with risk of relapse)
- Bactericidal antibiotics are preferred to bacteriostatic antibiotics
  - **Antibiotic choice should be guided by culture and sensitivity results (Table 16-3)**
- When to consider surgery:
  - Failure of medical therapy (i.e., persistent bacteremia or fungemia)
  - Infection with difficult to treat organisms (e.g., fungal organisms, *Pseudomonas* spp. or *Brucella* spp. endocarditis)
  - Major embolic events
  - New congestive heart failure; particularly with moderate to severe aortic or mitral regurgitation
  - Significant valve dysfunction, especially in prosthetic valves
  - Paravalvular extension; may be manifested by prolonged fever, aortic valve ring abscess, atrioventricular conduction abnormalities, and/or fistulas and mycotic aneurysms
  - Prosthetic valve and organisms such as *S. aureus*, *Pseudomonas* spp., fungi, and resistant enterococci

Prevention of Endocarditis
- Endocarditis prophylaxis
  - Endocarditis prophylaxis recommendations were revised in 2007 because the risk of endocarditis from dental procedures is less than previously estimated
  - Prophylaxis should be offered to patients with high-risk cardiac conditions who are undergoing procedures that are likely to cause bacteremia
  - Procedures likely to cause bacteremia include:
    - Dental procedures that involve manipulation of the gingiva or periapical region of the teeth, or perforation of the oral mucosa (not routine dental cleaning)
    - Procedures of the respiratory tract that will lead to an incision or biopsy of the respiratory mucosa
    - GI or GU procedures, only in patients with active GI/GU infections
    - Procedures involving infected skin or musculoskeletal tissue
    - Cardiac surgery involving placement of prosthetic material
  - High-risk cardiac conditions include:
    - Prosthetic cardiac valves, bioprosthetic and homograft
    - Presence of prosthetic material used for valve repair
    - Previous infective endocarditis
    - Unrepaired cyanotic congenital heart disease, including palliative shunts and conduits
    - Completely repaired congenital heart defect with prosthetic material or device during the first 6 months after the procedure
    - Repaired congenital heart disease with residual defects at the site or next to the prosthesis
    - Cardiac transplant recipients who develop cardiac valvulopathy

TABLE 16-3	*Synopsis of Treatment of Bacterial Endocarditis*	
Organism	**Standard Treatment**	**Comments**
Viridans group *streptococci* or *Streptococcus bovis* biotype I, with PCN MIC <0.12 μg/mL	4 weeks PCN G; if non-severe penicillin allergy use ceftriaxone	2 weeks PCN or ceftriaxone, combined with gentamicin reasonable alternative for select patients with select infections (including prosthetic valve infection). Severe PCN allergy: use vancomycin
Viridans group *streptococci*, with PCN MIC >0.12 and <0.5 μg/mL	4 weeks PCN G or ceftriaxone, combined with gentamicin for first 2 weeks	Severe PCN allergy: use vancomycin If prosthetic valve infection, use combination therapy for 6 weeks
Methicillin-susceptible *Staphylococcus aureus*, native valve, left-sided	4 weeks of nafcillin or oxacillin for uncomplicated disease; for complicated disease (e.g., perivalvular abscess, metastatic disease, uncontrolled diabetes), 6 weeks	
Methicillin-susceptible *S. aureus*, native valve, right-sided	2 weeks nafcillin or oxacillin only if criteria for 2 weeks of therapy met	Several patient and clinical criteria make patients inappropriate candidates for 2-week treatment. Treatment decisions need to be individualized and should be made in consultation with an infectious disease physician
Methicillin-resistant *S. aureus*, native valve	4 to 6 weeks vancomycin targeting a trough of 15 to 20 μg/mL	Complicated infections require at least 6-week course and discussion with infectious diseases and cardiac surgery consultants
S. aureus, prosthetic valve	6 weeks therapy with nafcillin or oxacillin, or vancomycin (depending on pathogen and sensitivities) in combination with aminoglycoside for initial 2 weeks and rifampin for 6 weeks after blood cultures have cleared (for *S. aureus*)	Early surgical consultation advised.
Enterococcus spp.	4 to 6 weeks ampicillin combined with gentamicin or streptomycin if susceptible	Must ensure isolate susceptible to both ampicillin and gentamicin If PCN allergic, consider desensitization, but if anaphylaxis consider vancomycin If aminoglycoside resistance demonstrated, pursue combination therapy with ampicillin + ceftriaxone; other antimicrobial resistance common and should prompt infectious diseases consultation
Fungal	Early surgery usually required	

MIC, Minimum infective concentration; PCN, penicillin.

16

- Antibiotic recommendations
  - Single-dose oral amoxicillin (2 g) 30 to 60 min before procedure (clindamycin, clarithromycin, or azithromycin if penicillin allergic)
  - Parenteral alternative: ampicillin 2 g IV or intramuscularly (cefazolin or ceftriaxone 1 g IM or IV are also acceptable)
  - If patient has a severe penicillin allergy and is unable to take oral medications, a single dose of clindamycin (600 mg), azithromycin (500 mg), or vancomycin 15 mg/kg can be used
  - If biopsy through active infection, consider vancomycin if methicillin-resistant *S. aureus* (MRSA) is a concern
- Low-risk patients for whom antibiotic prophylaxis is not recommended
  - Mitral valve prolapse
  - Bicuspid aortic valve
  - Acquired aortic or mitral valve disease

- Pacemakers
- Defibrillators
- Low-risk procedures for which endocarditis prophylaxis is not recommended:
  - GI endoscopy (except sclerosis or dilatation/ endoscopic retrograde cholangiopancreatography)
  - Restorative dentistry
  - Gynecologic procedures: vaginal hysterectomy, vaginal delivery, cesarean section
  - Cardiac procedures: cardiac catheterization, balloon angioplasty

Tick-Borne Illnesses

Basic Information

- Tick-borne illnesses are best understood by recognizing not only their clinical manifestations but also their vectors, reservoirs, geographic distribution, and seasonal variations (Table 16-4)

TABLE 16-4	*Comparison of Tick-Borne Illnesses*			
Illness	**Etiologic Agent**	**Vector**	**Reservoir**	**Geographic Distribution**
Rocky Mountain spotted fever	*Rickettsia rickettsii*	Eastern United States: Dog tick (*Dermacentor variabilis*) Western United States: Rocky Mountain wood tick (*Dermacentor andersoni*)	Vector tick is also reservoir	South-central and mid-Atlantic states (uncommon in western United States and Rocky Mountains)
Human monocytic ehrlichiosis	*Ehrlichia chaffeensis*	Lone-star tick (*Amblyomma americanum*)	Deer	Midwest; south-central and southeastern United States
Human granulocytic anaplasmosis	*Anaplasma phagocytophilum*	Deer tick (*Ixodes scapularis*)	Unknown	Scattered east and west coast states; northern states; Florida
Babesiosis	United States: *Babesia microti* Europe: *Babesia divergens, Babesia bovis*	Ticks (*I. scapularis*)	Rodents (especially white-footed mouse); cattle	Northeast coastal states
Lyme disease	*Borrelia burgdorferi*	Deer tick (*I. scapularis*)	Mouse	Northeast; mid-Atlantic; Wisconsin and Minnesota

- Most people with tick-borne infections do not remember a recent tick bite, and most tick bites do not result in a tick-borne infection
- Transmission of infection usually requires attachment for multiple hours; time depends on pathogen
- **In most cases, early manifestations of tick-borne disease are nonspecific flulike symptoms of fever, fatigue, and generalized achiness with or without a rash**
- Lyme disease may present with later symptoms of arthritis, neurologic manifestations of cranial nerve VII palsy, aseptic meningitis, or neuroradiculitis

Clinical Presentation

Table 16-5 compares the clinical features of tick-borne illnesses
- Rocky Mountain spotted fever (RMSF)
  - After an average incubation period of 4 days (range of 2 to 14 days), flulike symptoms of fever, headache, myalgias, and GI upset develop
  - Characteristic rash develops 3 to 5 days after onset of fever (Fig. 16-4)
  - **Disease may be fatal, especially if not diagnosed and treated early in illness (case fatality rate approaches 20%)**
- Ehrlichiosis and anaplasmosis (human monocytic ehrlichiosis [HME] and human granulocytic anaplasmosis [HGA])
  - After an incubation period of 7 days, flulike symptoms of fever (often higher than 39.44°C [103°F]), headache, myalgias, and malaise develop; often accompanied by thrombocytopenia and mild elevation of aspartate aminotransferase (AST) and alanine aminotransferase (ALT)

- **Presenting symptoms may be mild; rash is uncommon, and its absence helps distinguish these disorders from RMSF and Lyme disease**
- HGA may occur as co-infection with Lyme disease
- Although most patients have mild illness, severe illness, including renal failure and respiratory insufficiency, can occur
- Babesiosis
  - Infect erythrocytes, much like malaria
  - **Mild symptoms are the rule in North America, except in patients with asplenia, immune compromise, and older adults. These patients may experience overwhelming infection with hypotension and acute respiratory distress syndrome**
  - After an incubation period of 1 to 3 weeks, flulike symptoms of fever, headache, myalgias, and arthralgias occur, often accompanied by dark urine (resulting from hemolysis). Cough may also be present and can be misleading
  - Coinfection with *Borrelia burgdorferi* (Lyme disease) is not uncommon and should be considered in all patients with babesiosis; co-infection with HGA can also occur
  - Has been associated with transfusions caused by asymptomatic carriers
- Lyme disease
  - Can occur as an acute localized cutaneous rash and/or with disseminated early and late manifestations; always consider co-infection with babesiosis or HGA when diagnosing Lyme disease
    - **Localized erythema migrans is the most common acute presentation** (spreading erythematous rash; minority of rashes have central clearing or classic "bull's-eye" appearance; Figs. 16-5 and 16-6)
      - The rash is noted in at least 80% of cases

- Malaise, headache, migratory myalgias, and arthralgias are common and may occur with or without rash
  - Disseminated infection may occur within days to weeks of infection (Fig. 16-7)
    - Cutaneous dissemination with multiple areas of distant skin involvement with pleomorphic-appearing rash

- Neurologic symptoms may include cranial neuritis (most commonly cranial nerve VII), meningitis, radicular pain syndromes
- Cardiac symptoms may include atrioventricular block and myocarditis
- Late infection results from persistent infection at systemic sites seeded during primary infection

TABLE 16-5	Comparison of Clinical Features of Tick-Borne Illnesses		
	Rash	**Laboratory**	**Diagnostic Test of Choice**
Rocky Mountain spotted fever	Begins distally (palms or soles) Spreads to involve arms, legs, then trunk Begins as maculopapular eruption, evolving to petechial or purpuric appearance Seen in 90%	Laboratory findings nonspecific WBC typically normal Renal insufficiency and acute tubular necrosis common CSF may show elevated protein if neurologic involvement	Early clinical diagnosis required to prevent death; occasionally rickettsiae may be demonstrated in biopsy of rash; diagnosis may be confirmed by acute and convalescent serology
Human monocytic ehrlichiosis (HME)	Rash seen in one third Maculopapular eruption; rarely petechial	Leukopenia and thrombocytopenia common Transaminitis and renal insufficiency common	Clinical diagnosis but fourfold increase in antibody titer to *Ehrlichia chaffeensis;* monocytic inclusions may be seen
Hemolytic granulocytic anaplasmosis (HGA)	Rare; if present, should prompt consideration of co-infection with *B. burgdorferi*	Same as HME	Clinical diagnosis, but fourfold increase in antibody titer to *Anaplasma phacocytophilum* granulocytic inclusions may be seen. PCR available for acute diagnosis.
Babesiosis	Rash from babesiosis unusual, but coinfection with Lyme disease is common and should be investigated in all patients with babesiosis	Hemolytic anemia (can be pronounced) Mild transaminitis	Thick or thin blood smear demonstrates intraerythrocytic parasites PCR of blood
Lyme disease	Erythema migrans rash 80% Rarely bull's-eye rash; uniform erythematous eruption most common	WBC typically normal Mild transaminitis rare	ELISA; negative in 70% to 80% in weeks 1 to 2; positive when repeated weeks 4 to 6

CSF, Cerebrospinal fluid; ELISA, enzyme-linked immunosorbent assay; PCR, polymerase chain reaction; WBC, white blood cell.

16

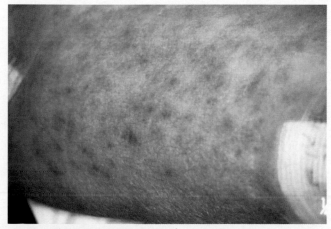

FIGURE 16-4   Florid petechial rash on the arm of a patient with Rocky Mountain spotted fever. (From Mandell GL, Bennett JE, Dolin R, eds. *Principles and Practice of Infectious Diseases.* 6th ed. Philadelphia: Churchill Livingstone; 2005: Fig. 184-4.)

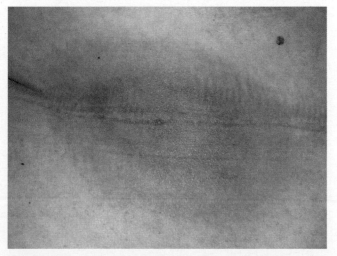

FIGURE 16-5   Erythema migrans rash of Lyme disease with classic bull's-eye appearance.

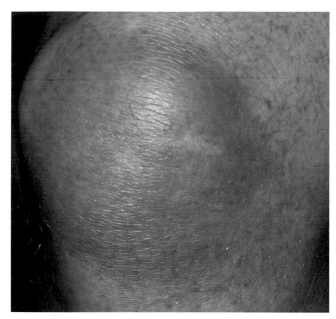

FIGURE 16-6 Erythema migrans rash of Lyme disease with uniform erythema.

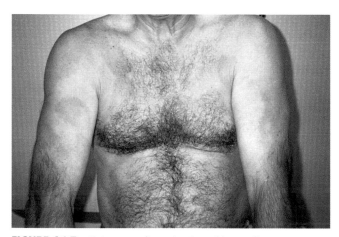

FIGURE 16-7 Cutaneous dissemination of Lyme disease presenting with pleomorphic rash.

- Late manifestations occur months after infection, manifested primarily with musculoskeletal disease
- **Classic manifestation is monoarthritis of the knee, with effusion occurring months after infection**
- Radiculopathy or symmetrical sensory neuropathy can occur

Diagnosis

Figure 16-8 provides an algorithm of the history of untreated Lyme disease (see also Table 16-5)

- Early features of most tick-borne illnesses are similar; high index of suspicion coupled with geographic distribution and season contribute to diagnosis
- Clinical presentation of many of these disorders should prompt initiation of treatment before definitive test results available

- Rash may assist in diagnosis of patients, particularly with RMSF and Lyme disease (see Table 16-5)
- **Some laboratory features may support diagnosis, such as thrombocytopenia (which suggests anaplasmosis), but many findings (such as mild elevation of AST and ALT) are shared across disorders**
- HME, HGA, and babesiosis may all be diagnosed via PCR on whole blood
- HME, HGA, and babesiosis may also be diagnosed via serology titers; criteria are different for each organism
- Babesiosis can be diagnosed via thin/thick blood smears with Giemsa or Wright-Giemsa stains; may see intraerythrocytic ring forms

Treatment

- **RMSF, ehrlichiosis, anaplasmosis, and Lyme disease all respond to doxycycline**
  - RMSF: doxycycline 100 mg twice daily for 1 week
  - Anaplasmosis and ehrlichiosis: doxycycline 100 mg twice daily for 10 days
  - Lyme disease: doxycycline 100 mg twice daily for 10–21 days; 10 days sufficient to treat acute infection
    - Amoxicillin used for children, because doxycycline is contraindicated
  - Lyme arthritis: 28 days oral doxycycline or amoxicillin; retreatment for recurrent arthritis: 28 days of oral therapy or 14 to 28 days of IV ceftriaxone
  - Neuroborreliosis (i.e., meningitis or radiculopathy because of Lyme disease) or cardiac involvement: ceftriaxone IV for 14 to 28 days
  - Lyme disease prophylaxis
    - A 200-mg single dose of doxycycline may be effective as postexposure prophylaxis; the Infectious Disease Society of America recommends its use only when all of the following criteria are met:
      - Attached tick identified as an adult or nymphal *Ixodes scapularis* tick (deer tick)
      - Tick is estimated to have been attached for 36 hours or more (by degree of engorgement or time of exposure)
      - Prophylaxis can begin within 72 hours of tick removal
      - Local rate of infection of ticks with *B. burgdorferi* is 20% or more (these rates of infection have been shown to occur in parts of New England, parts of the mid-Atlantic states, and parts of Minnesota and Wisconsin)
    - Vaccine for Lyme disease discontinued; long-term protection unclear, especially without availability of boosters
- Babesiosis may be asymptomatic and may not require treatment
  - Symptomatic patients and those with asplenia or immune compromise should be treated with atovaquone and azithromycin
  - Exchange transfusion may be necessary in cases with high-grade parasitemia greater than 10%
  - Relapses of symptomatic disease have been observed in patients with asplenia or underlying malignancy

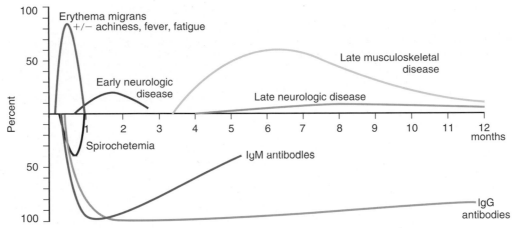

FIGURE 16-8 Natural history of untreated Lyme disease showing both acute and chronic phases of illness. IgG, Immunoglobulin G; IgM, immunoglobulin M.

Infection from Bite and Scratch Wounds

Basic Information

- Humans, dogs, and cats harbor bacterial pathogens in the oral cavity that can cause significant infection in humans who experience bites
- Antibiotic prophylaxis is indicated for high-risk wounds, which include:
  - Deep puncture wounds
  - Severe injury
  - Crush injuries
  - Bone or joint penetration
  - Wounds on the hand, face, or genitalia
  - Wounds in immune compromised patients
- Immunization for tetanus should be current (or updated, if not), and consideration should be given to the possibility of rabies

Clinical Presentation

- Most bite wounds occur on the upper extremities but are also commonly seen on the face and lower extremities
- **Superficial abrasions should be cleaned and otherwise need no treatment**
  - Deep bite wounds and wounds inflicted on a closed fist may need extensive debridement and surgical evaluation
- Human bites may introduce infection with viridans group *streptococci*, *S. epidermidis*, *S. aureus*, *Eikenella* spp., and other organisms
- Dog bites may introduce infection with *Pasteurella multocida*, *S. aureus*, and, less commonly, *Bacteroides*, *Fusobacterium*, and *Capnocytophagia*
- **Cat bites may introduce infection with *P. multocida* or *S. aureus*; deep bites risk the development of osteomyelitis**
- The major risk from cat scratches (almost always from kittens) is infection with *Bartonella henselae* (i.e., cat-scratch disease)
  - Regional adenopathy developing 2 weeks after a cat scratch (by which time the injury is likely to have

healed) is the most common presentation and may be accompanied by malaise and fever
  - Adenopathy may progress to lymphadenitis and rarely to suppuration
  - More serious manifestations include seizures and coma and are more common in children

Diagnosis

- Bite wounds present with an obvious history and present little in the way of clinical dilemmas
  - Cat-scratch disease may be missed in a patient presenting with adenopathy unless an inciting injury is specifically queried
  - Antibody titers for *B. henselae* are available, but unlikely to be of use in the acute setting; often an empiric diagnosis, especially because the organism is difficult to culture and takes weeks to grow
- *Pasteurella* infection typically becomes symptomatic in 24 hours and can lead to a necrotizing infection
- If the patient with a history of cat bite presents late (i.e., days or weeks after injury), consideration should be given to osteomyelitis if the clinical history and findings are appropriate

Treatment

- Treatment for bite wounds is empirical and not based on culture results
- **Optimal empiric therapy for both human and animal bites includes amoxicillin/clavulanate, or for more severe infections, ampicillin/sulbactam or a carbapenem**
- The major consideration for pathogens in animal bites, particularly in cat bites, is treatment to cover infection with *P. multocida*
  - *P. multocida* is resistant to typical agents used to cover cellulitis (i.e., dicloxacillin, cephalexin, erythromycin)
  - **Treatment is typically with amoxicillin/ clavulanate or clindamycin plus a fluoroquinolone (in penicillin-allergic patients); doxycycline also has excellent coverage**
- Dog bites may introduce *P. multocida* and rarely cause infection with *Capnocytophagia*, which in asplenic

16

patients or patients with liver disease patients may result in sepsis

- *Capnocytophagia* infection responds to β-lactam/β-lactamase inhibitors, such as ampicillin/sulbactam (for severe infections) or amoxicillin/clavulanate; for penicillin-allergic patients, can also consider clindamycin
- If rabies is a consideration, treatment should include the administration of rabies immune globulin and rabies vaccine
- Human bites are more commonly associated with cellulitis from *Staphylococcus* or *Streptococcus* spp. and should be treated with amoxicillin/clavulanate or clindamycin
  - *Eikenella* spp. may be resistant to both and often require a fluoroquinolone for treatment
- Cat-scratch disease is treated with macrolides (clarithromycin, azithromycin) or fluoroquinolones

Review Questions

For review questions, please go to ExpertConsult.com.

SUGGESTED READINGS

Durack DT, Lukes AS, Bright DK. New criteria for diagnosis of infective endocarditis: utilization of specific echocardiographic findings. Duke Endocarditis Service. *Am J Med.* 1994;96:200-209.

Ellis R, Ellis C. Dog and cat bites. *Am Fam Physician.* 2014;90:239-243.

Shapiro ED. Clinical practice. Lyme disease. *N Engl J Med.* 2014;370:1724-1731.

Wilson W, Taubert KA, Gewitz M, et al. Prevention of infective endocarditis: guidelines from the American Heart Association. A Guideline from the American Heart Association Rheumatic Fever, Endocarditis, and Kawasaki Disease Committee, Council on Cardiovascular Disease in the Young, and the Council on Clinical Cardiology, Council on Cardiovascular Surgery and Anesthesia, and the Quality of Care and Outcomes Research Interdisciplinary Working Group. *Circulation.* 2007;116:1736-1754.

Wilson WR, Karchmer AW, Dajani AS, et al. Antibiotic treatment of adults with infective endocarditis caused by streptococci, enterococci, staphylococci, and HACEK microorganisms. American Heart Association. *JAMA.* 1995;274:1706-1713.

Wormser GP, Dattwyler RJ, Shapiro ED, et al. The clinical assessment, treatment, and prevention of Lyme disease, human granulocytic anaplasmosis, and babesiosis: clinical practice guidelines by the Infectious Diseases Society of America. *Clin Infect Dis.* 2006;43:1089-1134.

SECTION THREE

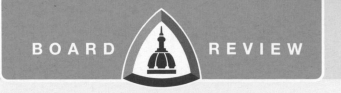

BOARD REVIEW

Pulmonary and Critical Care Medicine

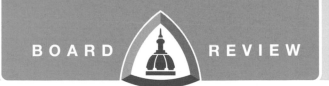
Obstructive Lung Disease

ROBERT A. WISE, MD; and M. BRADLEY DRUMMOND, MD, MHS

Obstructive lung disease encompasses a wide range of processes all involving obstruction to airflow. Approximately 50% of patients die within 10 years of initial diagnosis of smoking-related chronic obstructive pulmonary disease (COPD). The most common chronic obstructive lung diseases include those that are smoking-related (chronic bronchitis and emphysema) and those that are not smoking-related (asthma, bronchiectasis, cystic fibrosis [CF], and bronchiolitis obliterans).

Asthma

Basic Information

- **Asthma is a chronic inflammatory disease of the airways that is characterized by episodes of cough, wheezing, and dyspnea**
- **Asthma is also characterized by increased sensitivity of the airways to constrict in response to nonspecific stimulation (i.e., bronchial hyperreactivity)**
- **Approximately 80% of patients with asthma have an allergic tendency (atopy) characterized by positive immediate hypersensitivity skin tests (Fig. 17-1)**

Clinical Presentation

- Asthma may manifest with different syndromes, often overlapping
- Extrinsic asthma
  - **Usual onset in childhood**
  - **Attacks triggered by exposure to inhaled allergen**
    - Dust mites
    - Cockroaches
    - Cat antigen
    - Molds, particularly *Alternaria*
    - Pollens (e.g., ragweed, trees, grasses)
- Intrinsic asthma
  - Usual onset in **early adulthood**
  - **Attacks triggered by viral infections, nonspecific irritants**
  - May lead to chronic asthmatic bronchitis
  - Obesity is a risk factor, particularly for women
- Exercise-induced asthma
  - **Characterized by bronchospasm 10 to 20 minutes after exhausting exercise (Fig. 17-2)**
  - Occurs in majority of asthmatics, but may occur as sole manifestation of asthma
  - **Triggered by drying or cooling (or both) of airways with hyperventilation, particularly cold, dry air**

- **Can be prevented with inhaled bronchodilators (e.g., albuterol), or leukotriene antagonists (e.g., montelukast)**
- Triad asthma (Samter syndrome)
  - **Asthma, often requiring systemic corticosteroids for control**
  - **Nasal polyps (Fig. 17-3)**
  - **Aspirin (or other nonsteroidal antiinflammatory drug) sensitivity**
  - May require leukotriene antagonist for control of symptoms
- Cough-variant asthma
  - **May manifest as cough in the absence of wheezing**
  - Responds to treatment for asthma
  - Airways hyperreactivity present
  - **One of the three most common causes of chronic cough (along with gastroesophageal reflux disease and chronic sinusitis/postnasal drip syndrome)**
- Occupational asthma
  - **Presents as "Monday morning" symptoms that abate during weekends**
  - Symptoms usually worse in the evening, better in the morning
  - Prolonged exposures may lead to irreversible airflow obstruction
  - Common causes
    - Pigeons, chickens
    - Epoxy resins
    - Laboratory animals
    - Metals (nickel, chromium)
    - Plastics and rubber
- Refractory asthma
  - **Chronic unremitting wheezing requiring long-term systemic corticosteroids**
  - Often leads to chronic airway remodeling with chronic airflow obstruction
  - Possible causes for refractory asthma (Box 17-1)
- **Disorders that may mimic asthma**
  - Congestive heart failure
  - Mitral stenosis
  - Upper airway obstructions (e.g., laryngeal tumors, subglottic stenosis, Wegener granulomatosis)
  - Paradoxical vocal cord dysfunction (more common in women and health care workers)

Evaluation and Diagnosis

- **Consider diagnosis of asthma in patients with history of wheezing or variable dyspnea with specific triggers**

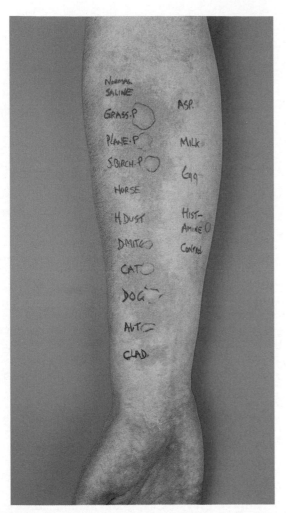

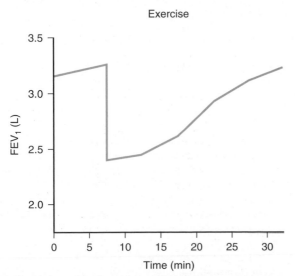

FIGURE 17-1 Multiple positive skin test results in a patient with extrinsic asthma. (From Forbes CD, Jackson WF: *Color Atlas and Text of Clinical Medicine*. 3rd ed. St. Louis: Mosby; 2003: Fig. 4.18.)

Exercise

FIGURE 17-2 Forced expiratory volume in 1 sec (FEV_1) in a patient with exercise-induced asthma. Note the sudden fall of FEV_1, followed by gradual recovery. (From Haslett C, Chilvers ER, Boon NA, et al. *Davidson's Principles and Practice of Medicine*. 19th ed. New York: Churchill Livingstone; 2003: Fig. 13.25.)

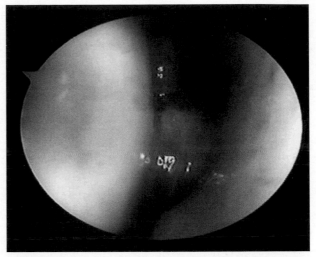

FIGURE 17-3 Endoscopic view of nasal polyps protruding from middle meatus. (From Adkinson NF Jr, Yunginger J, Busse W, et al. *Middleton's Allergy: Principles and Practice*. 6th ed. St. Louis: Mosby; 2003: Fig. 78-1.)

BOX 17-1	*Causes of Refractory Asthma*

Chronic exposure to an allergen (e.g., molds), irritant (e.g., air pollution), or sensitizing agent (e.g., toluene di-isocyanate)
Use of β-blockers (e.g., timolol eye drops for glaucoma)
Use of aspirin-containing drugs
Mucocutaneous fungal infections
Allergic bronchopulmonary aspergillosis
Churg-Strauss vasculitis

- **Diagnosis confirmed by presence of obstructive lung disease on pulmonary function tests at the time of symptoms that normalize when asymptomatic**
- Diffusing capacity of the lungs for carbon monoxide (DL_{CO}) normal between episodes
- Home monitoring with peak flow meter may be helpful for diagnosing or monitoring disease
- **Negative methacholine challenge test makes active asthma unlikely**

Treatment

Figure 17-4 shows a stepwise approach to asthma treatment.
- **The goal of asthma treatment is to avoid symptoms, minimize use of short-acting bronchodilators for relief of symptoms, prevent nocturnal awakening from asthma, and minimize systemic side effects of treatment**
- Four components of asthma treatment
  - **Monitor symptoms and pulmonary function**
  - **Control environmental exposures**
  - **Educate patients regarding proper treatment and avoidance of triggers**
  - **Drug treatment (Box 17-2)**
- Stepwise drug treatment of chronic asthma (see Fig. 17-4)

17

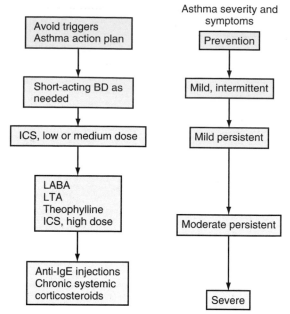

FIGURE 17-4 Stepwise approach to asthma treatment. Severity of asthma is defined by the abnormality of lung function, frequency of symptomatic use of bronchodilators, and frequency of nocturnal awakenings. For patients who use their short-acting bronchodilator more than twice weekly, drugs are prescribed to control or prevent symptoms. Usually treatment is initiated with inhaled corticosteroids, and then additional controller drugs are added. Patients with recalcitrant asthma may require long-term corticosteroids or anti-immunoglobulin E (anti-IgE) therapy. BD, Bronchodilator; ICS, inhaled corticosteroids; IgE, immunoglobulin E; LABA, long-acting β-agonist; LTA, leukotriene antagonist.

BOX 17-2	*Drug Therapy for Asthma*

β2-Agonists
   Short-acting (albuterol)
   Long-acting (salmeterol, formoterol, arformoterol) (used
     in combination with inhaled corticosteroids)
Antimuscarinics
   Tiotropium
   Theophylline, aminophylline
Corticosteroids
   Systemic
   Inhaled
Antileukotrienes
   Leukotriene receptor antagonist
   Lipoxygenase inhibitors

- **For intermittent symptoms (up to two episodes per week), occasional inhaled short-acting bronchodilators**
- **For persistent symptoms (e.g., use of short-acting bronchodilator more than twice per week), controller therapy with inhaled corticosteroids or leukotriene antagonists, supplemented by bronchodilators as needed**
- **For persistent symptoms that do not respond to moderate doses of inhaled corticosteroids, leukotriene antagonists, theophylline, or long-acting β-agonists (e.g., salmeterol, formoterol) may be added to inhaled corticosteroids.**

- **Long-acting antimuscarinics (e.g., tiotropium) are also effective for asthma if other agents are not tolerated.**
- **For persistently low lung function, frequent exacerbations, or severe attack, systemic corticosteroids may be needed to gain control of disease**
- Review treatment at 1- to 6-month intervals. Consider step-down of therapy if asthma has been well controlled for at least 3 months
- Treatment of an acute asthmatic attack
  - **Inhaled short-acting bronchodilators (e.g., albuterol) every 20 minutes for 3 doses**
  - **Inhaled ipratropium for individuals with severe airflow obstruction failing to improve after repeated short-acting β-agonist treatment**
  - **Supplemental oxygen if hypoxemia is present**
  - Intravenous magnesium sulfate (2 g infused over 20 minutes) can be helpful in individuals with severe attacks
  - **If no relief, systemic corticosteroids (e.g., prednisone 60 to 120 mg orally or intravenously and repeat every 6 hours as needed)**
  - Systemic bronchodilators (e.g., subcutaneous terbutaline or intravenous aminophylline) may be used in selected cases
- Indications for hospitalization
  - **Peak flow less than 40% of baseline after 4 to 6 hours of treatment**
  - **Persistent hypoxemia**
  - **Hypercapnia: Blood gas pH may normalize if severe attack and patient is becoming fatigued**
  - **Altered sensorium**
  - **History of previous near-fatal asthma attacks**

Smoking-Related Chronic Obstructive Pulmonary Disease

Basic Information

- Chronic bronchitis (chronic mucus hypersecretion syndrome)
  - **Occurs in approximately one of three smokers**
  - Can occur with occupational exposures to dust
  - **Often remits when exposure to dust or tobacco ceases**
  - Definition
    - **Daily production of sputum for 3 or more months per year for 2 consecutive years**
    - With obstructive ventilatory defect, may be called chronic obstructive bronchitis
  - Morbid anatomy
    - **Hyperplasia of the airway mucous glands and goblet cells**
    - Mucus plugging, thickening, tortuosity, and fibrosis of the peripheral airways (Fig. 17-5)
  - Pathophysiology
    - Not always associated with obstructive ventilatory defect
    - Airway resistance may be increased
  - Chest radiograph

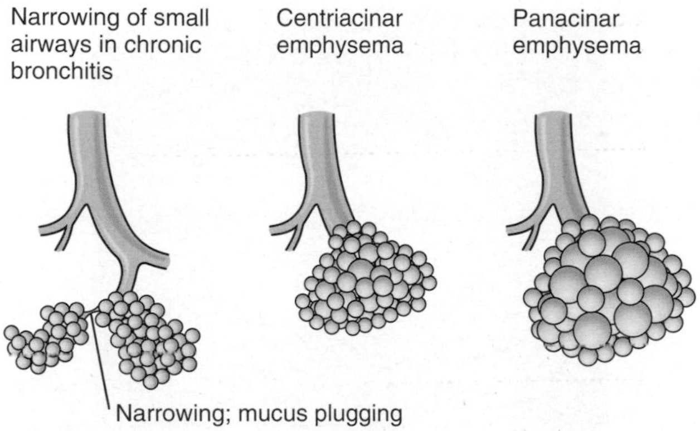

Narrowing of small airways in chronic bronchitis   Centriacinar emphysema   Panacinar emphysema

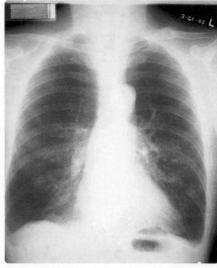

Narrowing; mucus plugging

FIGURE 17-5 Pathologic features of chronic bronchitis and emphysema. (From Kumar P, Clark M. *Clinical Medicine.* 5th ed. Philadelphia: Saunders; 2005: Fig. 14.23.)

- **Hyperinflation**
- **Increased peribronchial markings at lung bases**
- Thickening of airway walls
- Emphysema
  - **Progressive destruction of alveolar septa and capillaries**
  - Airspace enlargement and the development of macroscopic bullae
  - Smoking-related disease usually involves respiratory bronchiole in the center of the pulmonary lobule (centrilobular or centriacinar emphysema; see Fig. 17-5)
  - α_1-Antitrypsin deficiency usually involves the entire pulmonary lobule (panlobular or panacinar) emphysema (see later discussion)
  - **Centrilobular emphysema mostly affects the upper lung zones**
  - **Panacinar emphysema mostly affects the lower lung zones**
  - Pathophysiology
    - Reduced elastic recoil of the lung (increased compliance)
    - Slowing of maximum expiratory airflow (decreased forced expiratory volume in 1 sec/forced vital capacity [FEV_1/FVC] ratio)
    - Hyperinflation (increased static lung volumes)
    - Decreased alveolar surface area for gas exchange (reduction in DL_{CO}); ventilation-perfusion mismatch (hypoxemia)
  - Chest radiograph
    - **Flattening of the diaphragm (**Fig. 17-6**)**
    - Attenuation of vascular markings
    - Enlargement of the central pulmonary arteries
    - Hyperinflation
    - Enlargement of the anterior airspace
    - Increase of the sternophrenic angle
  - Computed tomography (CT) of chest
    - **Bullae (avascular regions)**
    - Regions of decreased lung density (less than −910/−950 Hounsfield units)
- Natural history of COPD (Fig. 17-7)
  - One in seven patients who smoke develops COPD
  - COPD develops over many years of smoking

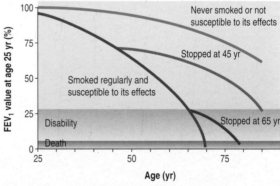

FIGURE 17-6 Chest radiograph of patient with severe chronic obstructive pulmonary disease, showing arterial deficiency pattern of emphysema. Lungs are hyperinflated, diaphragms are low and flat, and there is paucity of vascular markings. (From Weinberger SE. *Principles of Pulmonary Medicine.* 4th ed. Philadelphia: Saunders; 2004: Fig. 6-8.)

FIGURE 17-7 Natural history of chronic obstructive pulmonary disease (COPD). Nonsmokers and smokers who are not susceptible to develop COPD lose approximately 25% of the early adulthood forced expiratory volume in 1 sec (FEV_1) as a consequence of aging. Susceptible smokers lose lung function at a rate two to three times faster. By middle age, they develop symptomatic obstructive lung disease. If they continue to smoke, the disease progresses and eventually leads to disability and death. At any degree of impairment of lung function, smoking cessation leads to slowing of disease progression and extends the period of relative health.

- **Those who develop COPD have increased rate of FEV_1 decline**
- **Smoking cessation stops accelerated loss of lung function and prolongs survival**
- **Patients are usually asymptomatic until FEV_1 is 30% to 50% predicted**
- Risk factors for development of COPD in smokers (Box 17-3)
- Survival is lower in patients with higher BODE index based on
  - Low **B**ody mass index
  - Severe **O**bstructive ventilatory defect
  - Severe **D**yspnea
  - Poor **E**xercise tolerance on 6-minute walk test

| BOX 17-3 | Risk Factors for Development of Chronic Obstructive Pulmonary Disease in Smokers |

Airways reactivity
Family history of COPD
Childhood lung disease
Occupational dust exposures (e.g., silica, cotton dust, grain dust)

COPD, Chronic obstructive pulmonary disease.

TABLE 17-1	Clinical Spectrum of Chronic Obstructive Pulmonary Disease	
Characteristic	**Type A**	**Type B**
Underlying lung disease	Emphysema	Chronic bronchitis
Lung volumes	Hyperinflated	May be normal
Physique	Slender	Obese
Dyspnea	Very dyspneic	Not dyspneic
PaCO$_2$	Low until end stage	Elevated
Oxygenation with exercise	Worsens	May improve
Oxygenation at rest	Satisfactory	Low

PaCO$_2$, Arterial partial pressure of carbon dioxide.

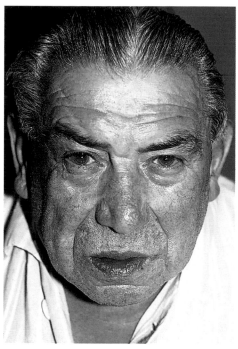

FIGURE 17-8 Respiratory failure. The patient is breathless at rest and exhibits central cyanosis with blueness of the lips and face. The lips are pursed during expiration, a characteristic feature of chronic obstructive pulmonary disease. This facial appearance is often accompanied by heart failure with peripheral edema (cor pulmonale). The term *blue bloater* derives from this combination of cyanosis and edema. (From Swash M, Glynn M. *Hutchison's Clinical Methods.* 22nd ed. Philadelphia: Saunders; 2007: Fig. 6.1.)

Clinical Presentation

- Spectrum of COPD (Table 17-1)
  - COPD includes patients with chronic obstructive bronchitis, emphysema, or both
- Physical findings in COPD (Figs. 17-8 and 17-9; Box 17-4)
  - **Physical examination not helpful in detecting mild COPD**
  - **Physical examination not helpful in ruling out COPD**
  - An abnormal physical examination is approximately 90% specific for a diagnosis of COPD

Diagnosis

- Spirometry in COPD
  - **Most sensitive measure of disease presence and progression**
  - Earliest abnormalities are decreased maximal flow at low lung volumes (seen on flow-volume loops)
  - FEV$_1$/FVC less than 70% is a reasonable threshold for diagnosing obstructive lung disease, but this may be within the normal range in older adult patients and may underdiagnose younger patients
  - **FEV$_1$ determines the severity (<30% predicted is very severe)**

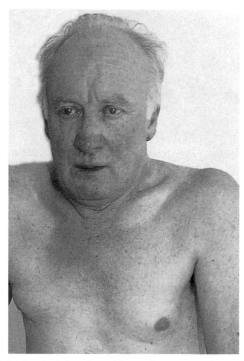

FIGURE 17-9 A pink puffer with emphysema. PaO$_2$ is maintained, but breathlessness is common, combined in the term *pink puffer*. (From Forbes CD, Jackson WF. *Color Atlas and Text of Clinical Medicine.* 3rd ed. St. Louis: Mosby; 2003: Fig. 4.91.)

Treatment

- Treatment of stable COPD (Fig. 17-10)
  - **Smoking cessation**
    - Strong personalized message
    - Nicotine replacement (e.g., gum, patch, inhaler, lozenge, nasal spray)
  - Bupropion
  - Varenicline
  - Set quit date
  - Group support
  - Follow-up
  - See Chapter 71 regarding discontinuation of addictive substances
- Bronchodilators for maintenance bronchodilation
  - Anticholinergic (e.g., ipratropium, tiotropium)
  - β-Agonists (e.g., salmeterol, formoterol, arformoterol, indacaterol)
  - Short-acting for symptom relief (e.g., albuterol)
  - Oral theophylline or phosphodiesterase type 4 inhibitors (roflumilast)

BOX 17-4	*Physical Findings in Moderate Chronic Pulmonary Disorder*

Diaphragm moves <2 cm
Hyperresonant percussion
Decreased cardiac dullness
Decreased breath sounds
Forced expiration time >10 sec
Abdominal point of maximum cardiac impulse

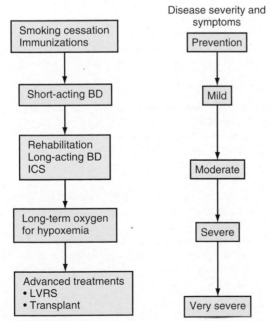

FIGURE 17-10 The stepwise approach to treatment of chronic obstructive pulmonary disease. The severity of disease is judged by the impairment of forced expiratory volume in 1 sec (FEV_1) as a percent predicted: greater than 80%, mild; 50% to 80%, moderate; 30% to 50%, severe; and less than 30%, very severe. BD, Bronchodilator, either β-agonist or anticholinergic or combined; ICS, inhaled corticosteroids; LVRS, lung volume reduction surgery.

- Inhaled corticosteroids to reduce exacerbation frequency
  - Not useful to prevent disease progression
  - Reduce frequency of exacerbations
  - Associated with an increased risk of pneumonia
- Exercise training/rehabilitation to improve exercise tolerance
  - Improves efficiency of exercise
  - No effect on lung function
- Long-term low-flow oxygen therapy (e.g., 2 L/min by nasal cannula)
  - **Improves survival in patients with hypoxemia**
  - Indications
    - Partial pressure of oxygen (PaO_2) less than 55 mm Hg (O_2 saturation less than 89%) in usual health
    - PaO_2 less than 60 mm Hg (O_2 saturation less than 90%) with evidence of cor pulmonale or neurocognitive impairment
- Lung transplantation candidates
  - **FEV_1 less than 20% predicted**
  - **Age younger than 60 to 65 years**
  - Sufficient social support
  - **Lung volume reduction surgery (LVRS)**
    - Procedure removes 20% to 30% of lung volume
    - Best results in patients with upper lung zone emphysema and poor exercise capacity after rehabilitation
  - **Bullectomy**
    - For single bulla occupying one third of a hemithorax
    - Best results with normal compressed lung and normal DL_{CO}
- Treatment of COPD exacerbation
  - **Approximately 50% are associated with lower airway bacterial infection**
    - **Antibiotics if change in sputum volume, color, associated dyspnea**
  - Bronchodilators by metered-dose inhaler as effective as by nebulizer in compliant patients
  - Systemic corticosteroids shorten duration of exacerbation
    - **No benefit of more than 2 weeks of corticosteroids**

Other Forms of Obstructive Lung Disease

$α_1$-ANTITRYPSIN DEFICIENCY

Basic Information

- Autosomal recessive trait
  - Also referred to as $α_1$-antiprotease deficiency
- Alleles of antiprotease activity (3 most common of more than 75 identified)
  - M: Normal
  - S: Intermediate
  - Z: Marked decrease
  - Null: Absent (rare)
- Phenotypes
  - **M, MS, MZ: No increased risk**
  - **SZ: Mild increased risk**

17

- **ZZ: Increased risk for emphysema; 10% also develop chronic liver disease**
- **Panacinar emphysema is the typical manifestation of ZZ disease**
  - Affects entire respiratory lobule uniformly
  - Predominates at lung bases

Clinical Presentation

- **Found in approximately 1% of patients with emphysema**
- Premature lung disease (age 30 to 40 years in smokers, age 50 to 60 years in nonsmokers)
- Absence of the antiprotease enzyme allows proteases from inflammatory cells to damage alveolar septae
- **Bronchiectasis and chronic bronchitis may occur along with mucous gland hyperplasia**
- **Approximately 10% of patients have concomitant liver disease**
- Many patients have COPD that is not distinguishable from other smoking-related presentations

Diagnosis

- Low α_1 fraction on serum protein electrophoresis
- Plasma levels of α_1-antitrypsin reduced
- Direct genotyping

Treatment

- Smoking cessation
- Genetic counseling
- **Augmentation therapy with human α_1-protease inhibitor is most useful in those with moderate disease severity**

BRONCHIOLITIS OBLITERANS

Basic Information

- Causes of bronchiolitis obliterans (BO)
  - **Inhalation of toxic fumes**
    - Methane
    - Hydrochloric acid
    - Chlorine
    - Ammonia
    - Sulfuric acid
    - Nitric acid (silo filler's disease)
  - Viral infections (e.g., respiratory syncytial virus, adenovirus, and influenza)
  - Connective tissue diseases—rheumatoid arthritis
  - **Organ transplantation: lung, heart, and bone marrow**
  - Neuroendocrine cell hyperplasia
  - Idiopathic

Clinical Presentation

- Cough
- Dyspnea
- Airflow obstruction
- Air trapping
- Physical findings
  - **Inspiratory squeaks and diffuse crackles**
  - Chest may be quiet

Diagnosis

- Chest CT
  - May appear normal
  - Diffuse centriacinar nodules
  - Diffuse ground-glass infiltrates
  - Mosaic pattern with segmental hyperinflation on expiratory views
- Histology
  - Often requires lung biopsy for diagnosis
  - Inflammation, thickening, occlusion, and disappearance of bronchioles

Treatment

- Immunosuppressive drugs, but often there is little response
- Macrolide antibiotics useful in some cases, particularly after lung transplantation
- **Bronchiolitis obliterans (BO) should not be confused with bronchiolitis obliterans with organizing pneumonia (BOOP; also called cryptogenic organizing pneumonia, or COP),** which is a different entity involving plugging of airways with granulation tissue and postobstructive chronic pneumonia. BOOP is often responsive to corticosteroids, whereas BO is not (see Chapter 20).

ALLERGIC BRONCHOPULMONARY ASPERGILLOSIS

Basic Information

- **Hypersensitivity reaction to *Aspergillus* manifesting as worsening asthma**
- Patients with CF are also susceptible to allergic bronchopulmonary aspergillosis (ABPA), and this may be an important factor in rapid clinical deterioration

Clinical Presentation

- **Chronic steroid-dependent asthma or rapidly progressive CF**
- **Recurrent pulmonary infiltrates**
- **Brown, black, or green sputum plugs and airway casts expectorated (Fig. 17-11)**
- Culture of *Aspergillus* species from sputum
- Perihilar evanescent oval shadows on chest radiograph from mucoid impactions
- **Marked eosinophilia**
- **Elevated serum immunoglobulin E (IgE)**
- Positive *Aspergillus* skin test and serum precipitins
- Dilation of central airways, "gloved finger" bronchiectasis

Pathophysiology

- Immune arthus-type reaction to *Aspergillus* colonizing airways

Diagnosis

- Major criteria
  - **Asthma**
  - **Blood eosinophilia**

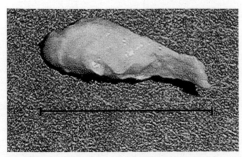

FIGURE 17-11 Typical sputum plug of allergic bronchopulmonary aspergillosis. (From Forbes CD, Jackson WF. *Color Atlas and Text of Clinical Medicine.* 3rd ed. St. Louis: Mosby; 2003: Fig. 4.12.)

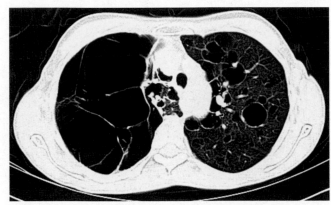

FIGURE 17-12 Characteristic computerized tomography scan from patient with lymphangioleiomyomatosis. The bullae within the left lung appear as typical punched-out "Swiss cheese" lesions. The interlobular septae are thickened, giving the remaining lung parenchyma a more opaque appearance.

- Immediate skin reactivity (IgE-dependent reaction) to *Aspergillus* antigens
- Immunoglobulin G (IgG) antibodies (type III reaction) to *Aspergillus* antigens
- **Transient or fixed pulmonary infiltrates**
- Central bronchiectasis
- **High serum IgE titer (normal level in symptomatic patient excludes ABPA)**
- Minor criteria
  - Presence of *Aspergillus* in sputum
  - Expectoration of brown mucous plugs
  - Late-phase skin test reactivity to *Aspergillus* antigen

Treatment

- **Corticosteroids with dose adjusted by IgE levels**
- Oral antifungal agents may help in some cases
- Check for CF genotype in affected patients

LYMPHANGIOLEIOMYOMATOSIS

See Figure 17-12 for a characteristic computerized tomography (CT) scan showing lymphangioleiomyomatosis.

Basic Information

- This is a rare disorder; etiology is unknown
- **Affects only fertile women**
- Excess proliferation of lymphatic smooth muscle
- Cystic lung disease with increased interstitial markings
- Associated in some cases with polymorphisms of tuberous sclerosis gene complex

Clinical Presentation

- Presents with progressive dyspnea
- Repeated hemoptysis may occur
- Interstitial infiltrates and airflow obstruction
- May present with pneumothorax or chylothorax

Diagnosis

- Obstructive pattern on pulmonary function tests; low DL_{CO}
- **Characteristic "Swiss cheese" appearance on chest CT from multiple cystic spaces**
- **Diffuse proliferation of smooth muscle within the airway walls, interstitium, and lymphatics**

Treatment

- **Sirolimus (rapamycin) prevents disease progression**
- **Lung transplantation for severe disease**

CYSTIC FIBROSIS

Basic Information

- **Most common lethal autosomal recessive disease in whites in the United States**
- Obstruction of exocrine glands by viscous secretion
- Forty percent may not be diagnosed until adolescence
- ABPA and asthma are seen more frequently in patients with CF

Clinical Presentation

- COPD
- Bronchiectasis
- **Nasal polyps**
- **Pancreatic insufficiency**
- **Hemoptysis**
- Chronic mucoid *Pseudomonas* infection

Diagnosis

- Abnormal sweat chloride test (elevated chloride)
- Genotyping

Treatment

- Management of obstructive lung disease
- Chest physiotherapy with manual percussion, flutter valves, pneumatic vest
- Long-term antibiotics, including inhaled antibiotics
- Nutritional support and replacement of pancreatic enzymes
- Newer drugs that target the defective CFTR channel have shown promise

UNUSUAL CAUSES OF OBSTRUCTIVE LUNG DISEASE

- Immunoglobulin deficiency with bronchiectasis
  - Immunoglobulin A (IgA), IgG subclasses 2 and 4

17

- Immotile cilia syndromes
  - Kartagener syndrome with situs inversus
  - Absence of dynein arms of cilia on electron microscopy
- Yellow nails syndrome with bronchiectasis
  - Pleural effusions, lymphedema, yellow nails
- Sarcoidosis with upper or lower airway involvement (see Chapter 20)
- Eosinophilic granuloma
- Sjögren syndrome
- HIV with premature emphysema

Review Questions

For review questions, please go to ExpertConsult.com.

SUGGESTED READINGS

Celli BR, MacNee W. ATS/ERS Task Force. Standards for the diagnosis and treatment of patients with COPD: a summary of the ATS/ERS position paper. *Eur Respir J.* 2004;23:932-946.

Global Initiative for Asthma (GINA). Global strategy for asthma management and prevention (updated 2010). <www.ginasthma.com>.

Global Initiative for Chronic Obstructive Lung Disease (GOLD). Global strategy for the diagnosis, management, and prevention of chronic obstructive pulmonary disease (updated 2010). <www.goldcopd.org>.

National Asthma Education and Prevention Program Expert Panel Report III. Guidelines for the diagnosis and management of asthma: update of selected topics, 2008. <www.nhlbi.nih.gov/guidelines/asthma/>.

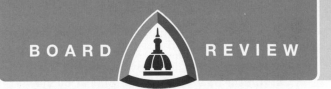
Pulmonary Function Testing

ROBERT A. WISE, MD; and MEREDITH C. McCORMACK, MD, MHS

Pulmonary function tests (PFTs) are used in the evaluation of lung diseases. The quality of the tests may vary depending on the patient's effort. The most commonly used tests are spirometry, flow-volume loops, bronchoprovocation testing, carbon monoxide diffusing capacity, lung volume measurements, and measures of respiratory muscle strength. The 6-minute walk test, a simple measure of functional exercise capacity, is also performed in many pulmonary laboratories.

Pulmonary Function Tests

Spirometry

- Widely available and the most useful pulmonary function test
  - Can be performed in office or clinic, as well as laboratory setting
  - Measured using flow sensors (pneumotachometers) or volume sensors (spirometers)
- **Helpful in evaluation of obstructive lung disease (e.g., chronic obstructive pulmonary disease [COPD]/asthma)**
- Performed as a forced expiration following maximum inspiration
- Recorded as volume of air expired per unit of time
- **Forced expiratory volume is the volume expired in 1 sec (FEV_1) (Fig. 18-1)**
  - Correlated with maximum ventilation and with exercise
  - **Reduced in both obstructive and restrictive disorders**
  - Predictive of mortality in the general population, lung cancer risk, disability
- Forced vital capacity (FVC) is the maximum volume expired from the lung (see Fig. 18-1)
  - **May be reduced because of low total lung capacity (TLC) in restrictive ventilatory defect or caused by elevated residual volume (RV) from air trapping in obstructive disease**
- **FEV_1/FVC is an index of the rate of emptying of the lung**
  - **A reduced FEV_1/FVC *usually* indicates an obstructive ventilatory defect (Box 18-1)**
- **To define a low FEV_1/FVC:**
  - **FEV_1/FVC below the lower limit of normal (LLN)**
    - **LLN is defined by the 5th percentile of expected normal values accounting for a patient's sex, age, and height**

- **FEV_1/FVC less than 0.70 is a rule of thumb that usually indicates obstruction but is more subject to misclassification (does not account for expected changes caused by age, height, or sex)**
- Maximum midexpiratory flow rate (MMFR) or forced expiratory flow (FEF) 25% to 75% (forced expiratory flow at 25% to 75% of vital capacity) measures the mean flow during the middle 50% of expiration
  - Often considered a measure of small airways function; the test is variable and nonspecific

Flow-Volume Loops

Figure 18-2 illustrates flow-volume loops
- Displays forced expiratory and inspiratory maneuvers as flow (i.e., slope of spirogram) versus volume
- **Useful for diagnosis of upper airway obstruction**
  - Abnormality in both inspiration and expiration (fixed)
  - Abnormality in inspiration only (variable extrathoracic obstruction)
  - Abnormality in expiration only (variable intrathoracic obstruction)
- Fixed upper airway obstructions
  - Cause greater reduction in peak expiratory flow rates, but inspiratory flow rate also decreased
  - Common causes
    - **Bilateral vocal cord paralysis**
    - **Tracheal stenosis** (e.g., following prolonged endotracheal intubation or in relapsing polychondritis)
    - **Laryngeal or tracheal tumors**
    - **Granulomatous diseases** (e.g., sarcoidosis, Wegener granulomatosis)
- Variable extrathoracic obstruction
  - Flow during inspiration is normally greater than expiratory flow
  - In variable extrathoracic obstruction, **inspiratory flow is less than expiratory flow at middle lung volumes**
  - **Common with vocal cord dysfunction or unilateral vocal cord paralysis**
  - Found in obese individuals and those with **sleep apnea** syndrome
- Variable intrathoracic obstruction
  - Expiratory flow is decreased but inspiratory flow is not altered
  - **Tracheal tumors, subglottic stenosis** may present this way

- Chronic obstructive pulmonary disease
  - **Curvilinear flow volume loop caused by slowly emptying lung units**
  - Peak flow is relatively preserved, making it a poor measure of COPD severity
  - Flow rates at low lung volumes are more impaired
  - Asthma produces similar curve shape but with reduced flow rates at all lung volumes, including peak flow

---

BOX 18-1 *Potential Indications for Spirometry*

Diagnosis of obstructive lung disease
Evaluation of severity of lung disease
Screen high-risk individuals (e.g., smokers)
Preoperative assessment (see Chapter 72)
Evaluation of disability/impairment
Monitoring of treatment
Assess toxic effects of exposure or drug toxicity

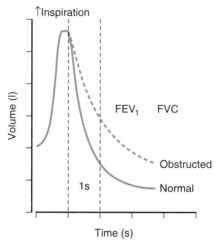

FIGURE 18-1 A spirometer tracing. The patient breathes out as fast as possible after maximum inhalation. Volume expelled is related to lung capacity. The forced expiratory volume in 1 sec (FEV_1) is compared with the forced vital capacity (FVC). In the normal person, this ratio is greater than 80%; a reduced FEV_1/FVC indicates an obstructive defect. (From Davies A, Blakeley A, Kidd C. *Human Physiology*. New York: Churchill Livingstone; 2001: Fig. 7.1.9.)

- Vocal cord dysfunction (VCD)
  - **VCD presents as asthma but without hyperinflation on chest radiograph, and is unresponsive to steroids**
  - More common in women than men
  - Definitive diagnosis is made by visualizing vocal cord abnormalities with laryngoscopy during an attack
  - Diagnosis may be suggested by abnormal inspiratory flow patterns on flow-volume loops (presents as variable extrathoracic obstruction)

Bronchoprovocation Testing

See Figure 18-3 for a methacholine challenge test.
- Performed by inhaling increasing concentrations of methacholine, followed by spirometry after each concentration
- **A positive test is defined by achieving a 20% or greater fall in FEV_1 with a dose of 16 to 25 mg/mL methacholine or less**
- The concentration required to achieve a 20% fall in FEV_1 is called the PC_{20}
- Half of COPD patients have positive methacholine challenge testing
- **A positive test is nonspecific; negative methacholine challenge makes active asthma unlikely**
- **Useful in the case of chronic cough to rule out cough-variant asthma**

Carbon Monoxide Diffusing Capacity

- Tests the integrity of the alveolar-capillary surface area for gas exchange
  - **Carbon monoxide diffusing capacity (DL_{CO}) less than 80% predicted is abnormal**
  - DL_{CO} less than 50% predicted predicts oxygen desaturation with exercise
- **DL_{CO} is decreased in disorders that decrease pulmonary capillary blood volume**
  - **Interstitial lung diseases**
  - **Emphysema**
  - **Pulmonary vascular disease**
- **Normal DL_{CO} makes clinically important interstitial disease unlikely**
- DL_{CO} changes in disease states (Table 18-1)
- Uses:
  - **Distinguishing emphysema from asthma (low in emphysema, normal or high in asthma)**

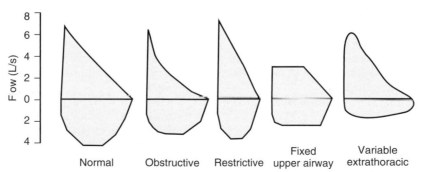

FIGURE 18-2 Flow-volume loops. Curve begins at left axis, and with forced expiration, follows a clockwise pattern. The normal pattern appears as a triangle over a half circle. With development of chronic obstructive pulmonary disease, the expiratory limb becomes curvilinear. In restrictive lung diseases, the flows are relatively preserved, and the width of the curve is narrowed. With a fixed upper airway obstruction, the inspiratory and expiratory limbs are flattened.

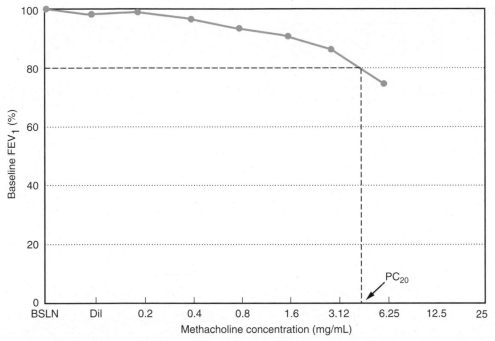

FIGURE 18-3 Methacholine challenge test. Progressively greater concentrations of inhaled methacholine are given with a nebulizer. After each concentration, spirometry is performed. In patients with airways reactivity, the forced expiratory volume in 1 sec (FEV$_1$) will decline by more than 20% before the maximum concentration is reached (usually 25 mg/mL). The provocative concentration (PC$_{20}$) is determined by interpolation between concentrations. Patients with active asthma will usually show a drop in FEV$_1$ at less than 10 mg/mL. A positive test for airways reactivity is not diagnostic, however, because many normal individuals and patients with chronic obstructive pulmonary disease have a positive test.

TABLE 18-1	*DL$_{CO}$ Changes in Disease States*
DL$_{CO}$ Normal or Increased	**DL$_{CO}$ Decreased**
Asthma	Emphysema
Polycythemia	Anemia
Obesity	Interstitial lung disease
Left-to-right shunt	Pneumonectomy
Supine position	Pulmonary hypertension
Postexercise	Pulmonary embolism
Pulmonary hemorrhage	

DL$_{CO}$, Diffusing capacity of the lungs for carbon monoxide.

- Evaluation of dyspnea
- Monitoring occupational/toxic exposures (e.g., bleomycin, amiodarone)

Lung Volume Measurements

- Useful for distinguishing restrictive lung diseases from obstructive lung diseases (Figs. 18-4 and 18-5)
    - **Restrictive ventilatory defects have a reduction in all subdivisions of lung volume, including TLC, vital capacity (VC), and RV**
    - **Obstructive ventilatory defects typically cause elevation of TLC (hyperinflation) and RV (gas trapping) with reduction in VC**
- Obesity typically causes a disproportionate reduction in end-expiratory lung volume (functional residual capacity) with small reductions in TLC and VC

Respiratory Muscle Strength

- Maximum inspiratory pressure (MIP) is useful for screening for respiratory muscle weakness (i.e., diaphragmatic weakness/paralysis)
    - **Normal values between −100 and −140 cm H$_2$O**
- Maximum sniff nasal pressure (SNIP) is also useful for diagnosing and following the course of patients with neuromuscular disease
- Bilateral diaphragm paralysis usually causes hypercapnia at moderate levels of restriction
- **Clues to diaphragm paralysis include orthopnea and paradoxical abdominal motion with inspiration**

Six-Minute Walk Test

- Simple assessment of functional exercise capacity
- Used to assess functional status (e.g., lung transplantation evaluation) and response to treatment (e.g., pulmonary hypertension; heart failure)
- Predicts morbidity and mortality (e.g., in COPD, pulmonary hypertension, and heart failure)
- Test is performed under standard conditions
    - Patient walks as far as possible in 6 minutes
    - Patient can stop and rest during the 6 minutes as needed (clock continues)
    - Patients can use oxygen and necessary walking aids, such as canes
    - Scripted language at each minute interval without coaching
    - Dyspnea and leg pain are recorded pre- and post-test
- Results reported as absolute and percent predicted

18

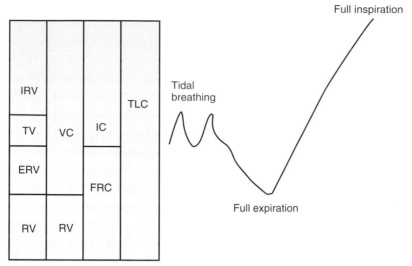

FIGURE 18-4 Lung volume subdivisions. Lung volumes are determined by measurement of functional residual capacity (FRC) using a resident gas method (nitrogen washout or helium dilution) or the Boyle law method (body plethysmography). The remaining lung volumes are calculated from a period of tidal breathing followed by a slow vital capacity maneuver as shown in the right panel. ERV, Expiratory reserve volume; IC, inspiratory capacity; IRV, inspiratory reserve volume; RV, residual volume; TLC, total lung capacity; TV, tidal volume; VC, vital capacity.

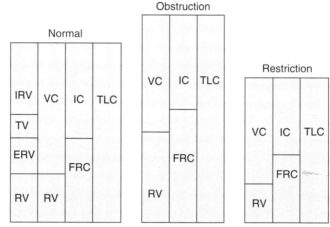

FIGURE 18-5 Abnormalities of lung volumes. Obstructive lung diseases cause elevation of total lung capacity (TLC) (hyperinflation) and residual volume (RV) (air trapping) with a net increase in the ratio of RV/TLC and a reduction in vital capacity (VC). Restrictive lung diseases cause proportionate reduction in all of the lung volumes. In obesity, however, a mild reduction in TLC is accompanied by a more marked reduction in functional residual capacity (FRC). ERV, Expiratory reserve volume; IC, inspiratory capacity; IRV, inspiratory reserve volume; RV, residual volume; TLC, total lung capacity; TV, tidal volume; VC, vital capacity.

Review Questions

For review questions, please go to ExpertConsult.com.

SUGGESTED READINGS

American Thoracic Society. ATS Statement: guidelines for the six-minute walk test. *Am J Respir Crit Care Med.* 2002;166:111-117.

Macintyre N, Crapo RO, Viegi G, et al. Standardisation of the single-breath determination of carbon monoxide uptake in the lung. *Eur Respir J.* 2005;26:720-735.

Miller MR, Hankinson J, Brusasco V, et al. Standardisation of spirometry. *Eur Respir J.* 2005;26:319-338.

Pellegrino R, Viegi G, Brusasco RO, et al. Interpretative strategies for lung function tests. *Eur Respir J.* 2005;26:948-968.

Wanger J, Clausen JL, Coates A, et al. Standardisation of the measurement of lung volumes. *Eur Respir J.* 2005;26:511-522.

West JB. *Respiratory Physiology: The Essentials.* Philadelphia: Lippincott, Williams & Wilkins; 2004.

CHAPTER 19

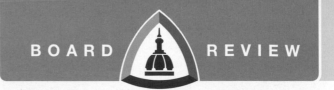
Chest Radiograph Review

CHRISTIAN A. MERLO, MD, MPH; and PETER B. TERRY, MD, MA

Pattern recognition is used by most radiologists to narrow the differential diagnosis when interpreting chest radiographs. This entails evaluation of both the character (e.g., nodule, mass, or infiltrate) and distribution (e.g., upper vs lower lung field; unilateral vs bilateral) of pulmonary abnormalities.

Nodules and Masses

Basic Information

- **A nodule (Fig. 19-1) is defined as a lesion that measures less than 4 cm in diameter. A mass (Figs. 19-2 to 19-5) is one that is greater than 4 cm in diameter. Lesions greater than 3 cm in diameter have a greater than 75% probability of being malignant.**

Clinical Presentation

- **Smaller lesions are usually benign** because to be visible on a chest radiograph, they must be of high density, a property usually associated with calcification. Certain patterns of calcification suggest that the nodule is benign. **Eccentric calcification, although usually benign, may be associated with a malignant cause.** More benign patterns of calcification include:
  - Diffuse complete calcification
  - Laminated calcification
  - Eggshell calcification
  - Central/"bull's-eye" calcification
  - Popcorn calcification
  - Onion skin calcification

(See Chapter 22 for a more in-depth review of the solitary pulmonary nodule and calcification patterns.)

Diagnosis and Evaluation

- **The differential diagnosis of nodules includes:**
  - Infections
    - Bacterial (including abscesses)
    - Mycobacterial
    - Fungal
    - Parasitic (e.g., human infection with *Dirofilaria immitis* [dog heartworm])
  - Granulomata
  - Rheumatoid nodules
  - Granulomatosis with polyangiitis (formerly Wegener granulomatosis)
  - Vascular malformations
  - Bronchogenic cysts

- Hamartoma
- Primary or secondary lung neoplasms
- **The differential diagnosis of masses includes the previously listed possibilities and is expanded to include sarcomas, fibromas, and progressive massive fibrosis (PMF)**
- **The differential diagnosis for anterior mediastinal masses ("terrible Ts") deserves particular attention and includes:**
  - **T**eratoma
  - **T**hymoma
  - **T**hymolipoma
  - **T**hymic carcinoma/carcinoid
  - **T**hymic cyst
  - **T**horacic thyroid
  - **T**errible lymphoma

Infiltrates

Basic Information

- The radiographic pattern of infiltrates provides clues to the etiology

Clinical Presentation

- **Alveolar infiltrates (Figs. 19-6 and 19-7) are marked by their homogeneity, their irregular and often fluffy appearance, and the presence of air bronchograms (Fig. 19-8).** They may consist of:
  - Water
    - Cardiogenic pulmonary edema
    - Noncardiogenic pulmonary edema
  - Blood
    - Goodpasture syndrome
    - Idiopathic pulmonary hemosiderosis
    - Systemic lupus erythematosus (SLE)
    - Alveolar hemorrhage of any cause
  - Cells
    - Malignant
      - Bronchoalveolar cell carcinoma
    - Benign
      - Eosinophilic pneumonia
      - Desquamative interstitial pneumonitis
  - Pus
    - Bacterial pneumonia
  - Protein
    - Alveolar proteinosis
    - *Pneumocystis jiroveci* pneumonia–associated protein in alveoli

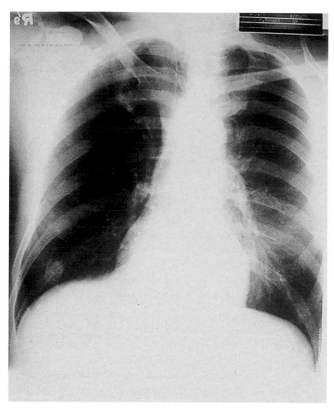

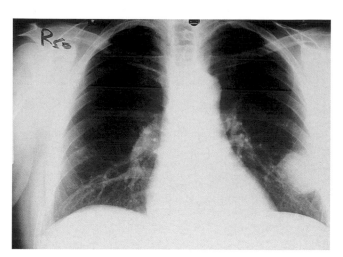

FIGURE 19-2   Mass in the lower left thorax. The acute angle between the mass and the chest wall suggests an intraparenchymal mass rather than a pleural-based mass.

FIGURE 19-1   Well-circumscribed nodule in the right lower lobe with central calcification suggestive of an old granuloma.

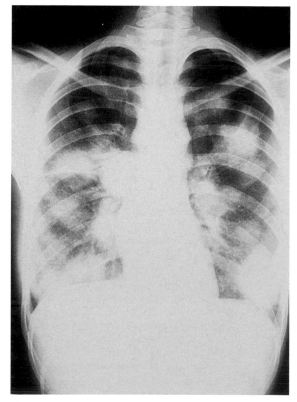

FIGURE 19-3   Multiple bilateral masses of sarcoidosis. A mass that "respects the fissure" as seen in the right upper lobe as it abuts the minor fissure is usually benign.

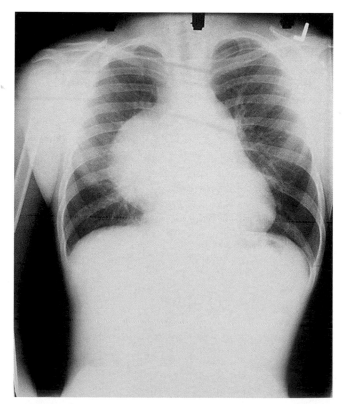

FIGURE 19-4   A mediastinal mass in a patient with thymoma.

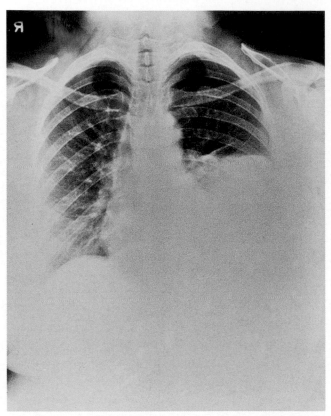

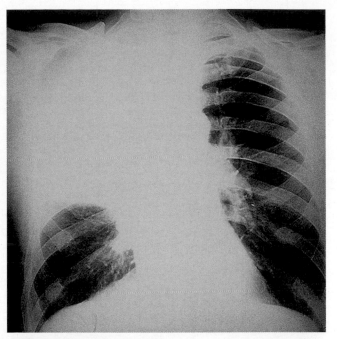

FIGURE 19-6 An alveolar infiltrate, as seen in this patient with pneumonia, can sometimes mimic a mass.

FIGURE 19-5 Partial whiteout of the left hemithorax. This is either from atelectasis, effusion, or a mass. This is a case of sarcoma.

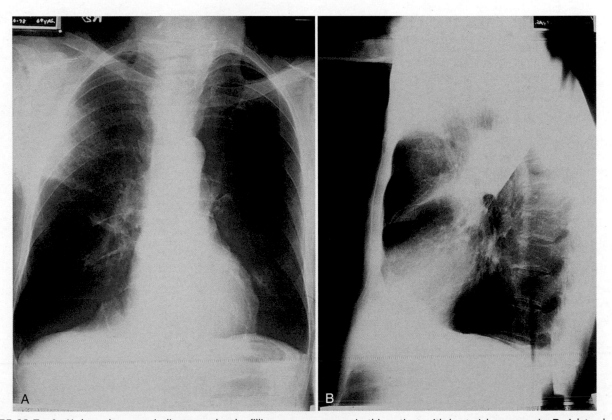

FIGURE 19-7 **A,** Air bronchograms indicate an alveolar filling process as seen in this patient with bacterial pneumonia. **B,** A lateral view shows that the infiltrate is in the posterior segment of the right upper lobe.

19

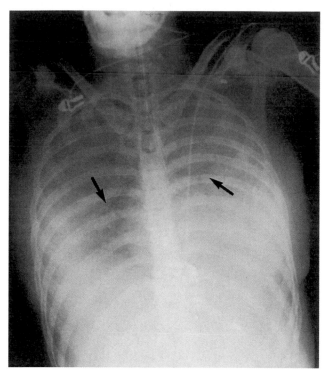

FIGURE 19-8   Air bronchograms *(arrows)* in a patient with alveolar infiltrates caused by *Pneumocystis jiroveci* pneumonia. (From Souhami R. *Textbook of Medicine.* New York: Churchill Livingstone; 2002: Fig. 13.12.)

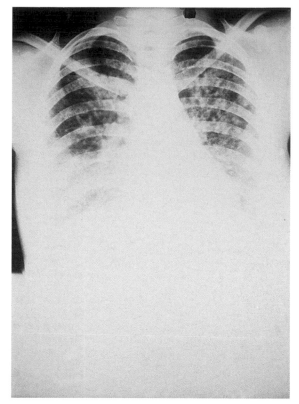

FIGURE 19-9   Interstitial infiltrate in a critically ill patient with varicella pneumonia. Notice the nodular appearance and lack of air bronchograms.

- Calcium
  - Alveolar microlithiasis (very rare)
- **Interstitial infiltrates (Figs. 19-9 and 19-10) have a broad differential diagnosis, although the pattern helps to narrow the diagnostic possibilities:**
  - Reticular
  - Nodular
  - Combined: a very common pattern with a broad differential diagnosis
  - Linear
  - **Honeycomb: Implies scarring and end-stage disease and is usually seen with idiopathic pulmonary fibrosis (IPF)**
  - Ground glass
    - Bronchiolitis obliterans with organizing pneumonia
    - Sarcoidosis
    - Viral pneumonitis

Diagnosis and Evaluation

- **The pattern of distribution of interstitial infiltrates may provide clues to the specific diagnosis**
- **The differential diagnosis of upper lobe infiltrates is generally small** and depends on the clinical history and whether the abnormality is unilateral or bilateral
  - Diffuse bilateral upper lobe infiltrates (Figs. 19-11 and 19-12)
    - Sarcoidosis
    - Eosinophilic granuloma
    - Ankylosing spondylitis
    - Cystic fibrosis

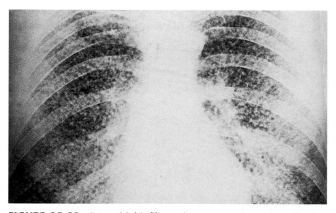

FIGURE 19-10   Interstitial infiltrate in an asymptomatic patient with sarcoidosis. Sarcoidosis is one of the few diseases in which a patient may have minimal symptoms yet have dramatic findings on a chest radiograph.

  - Hypersensitivity pneumonitis
  - Old tuberculosis or histoplasmosis
  - Pneumoconiosis (e.g., silicosis)
  - Unilateral upper lobe infiltrates (Figs. 19-13 to 19-15)
    - Infections
      - Tuberculosis
      - Histoplasmosis
      - Coccidioidomycosis
      - *Klebsiella* pneumonia
    - Primary lung neoplasms

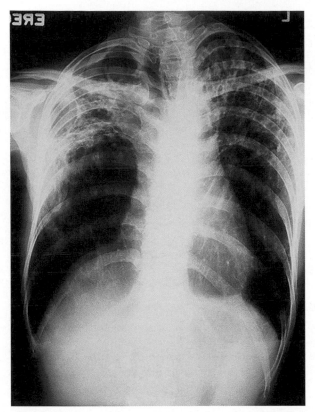

FIGURE 19-11 Fibrocystic sarcoidosis involving the upper lobes.

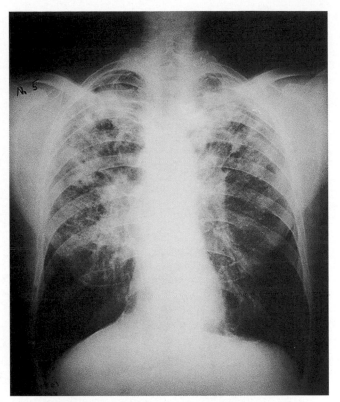

FIGURE 19-12 Cystic fibrosis involving the upper lobes.

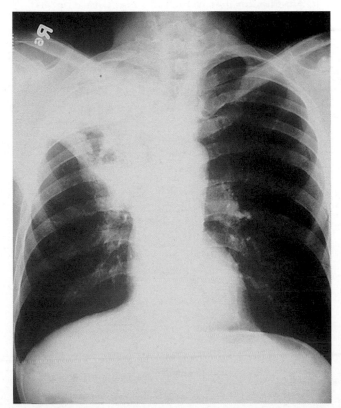

FIGURE 19-13 Unilateral infiltrate with partial collapse of the right upper lobe in an alcoholic with *Klebsiella* pneumonia.

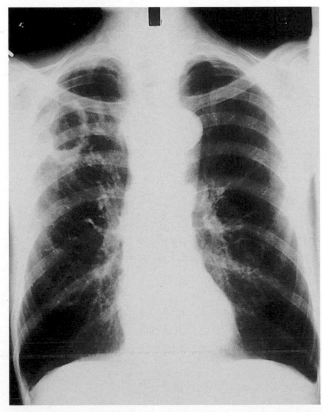

FIGURE 19-14 Unilateral upper lobe infiltrate with cavitation in a patient with squamous cell carcinoma.

19

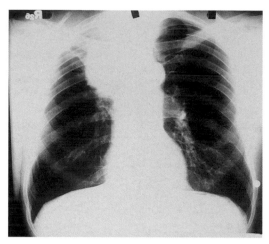

FIGURE 19-15 Unilateral upper lobe infiltrate with the "reverse S sign" highly suggestive of malignancy. The reverse S is comprised of a mass (oftentimes in the hilum) and the resulting collapsed right upper lobe.

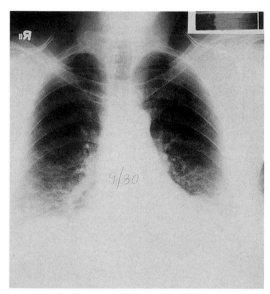

FIGURE 19-16 Bilateral lower lobe interstitial infiltrates in a patient with idiopathic pulmonary fibrosis.

- **The differential diagnosis of lower lobe infiltrates (Fig. 19-16) is generally much broader, but 80% of the time the differential is found within the following:**
  - Bronchiectasis (look for "tram tracks")
  - Aspiration (usually found in the superior or posterior basilar segments)
  - Dermatomyositis/polymyositis
  - Asbestosis (always associated with crackles on examination)
  - Scleroderma, SLE, Sjögren syndrome
  - Sarcoidosis (pleural thickening and effusions are seldom seen)
  - Early Hamman-Rich syndrome/IPF (pleural disease is uncommon)
  - Rheumatoid arthritis

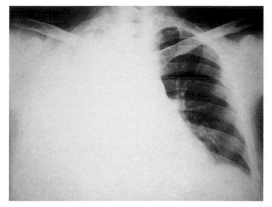

FIGURE 19-17 A large right-sided pleural effusion in a patient with hepatic hydrothorax.

Pleural Effusions

Basic Information

- **Both the size and side of a pleural effusion provide clues to its etiology**
  - **A pleural effusion filling more than half (Fig. 19-17) of the hemithorax is likely caused by:**
    - Trauma
    - Tumor
    - Tuberculosis
    - Hepatic hydrothorax (in patients with cirrhosis and ascites)
    - Chylothorax (caused by thoracic duct obstruction or disruption)
  - **An effusion that is bilateral and with a normal heart is generally caused by:**
    - Tumor
    - Connective tissue disease
    - Viral infection
    - Congestive heart failure (less often)
  - **An effusion that is bilateral and with an enlarged heart is generally caused by congestive heart failure**
  - Right-sided effusions suggest:
    - Congestive heart failure
    - Hepatic hydrothorax
    - Meigs syndrome (in patients with benign ovarian tumors or fibroids)
  - Left-sided effusions suggest:
    - Aortic aneurysm dissection
    - Boerhaave syndrome (esophageal rupture)
    - Pancreatitis
    - Splenic rupture or infarction

Review Questions

For review questions, please go to ExpertConsult.com.

SUGGESTED READINGS

Fraser RG, Pare JAP, Pare PD, et al. *Diagnosis of Diseases of the Chest.* Philadelphia: WB Saunders; 1991.

Sherman CB. Inflammatory disease of the lung. In: Barondess JA, Carpenter CJ, eds. *Differential Diagnosis.* Philadelphia: Lea & Febiger; 1994.

Teeter JG, Terry PB. Pulmonary nodules, masses and mediastinal disease. In: Barondess JA, Carpenter CJ, eds. *Differential Diagnosis.* Philadelphia: Lea & Febiger; 1994.

Interstitial Lung Disease

MAUREEN R. HORTON, MD; and CHRISTINE L. VIGELAND, MD

The term interstitial lung disease (ILD) describes a number of distinct disorders that cause inflammation in the pulmonary interstitium and may lead to pulmonary fibrosis. Some are primary pulmonary diseases; others are seen in association with systemic disorders. The pace of symptom onset, the presence or absence of extrapulmonary signs and symptoms, and the radiographic pattern of the process often provide clues to the etiology.

Idiopathic Interstitial Pneumonia

Basic Information

- Collection of ILDs with no known etiology (Table 20-1).
- Diagnosis based on clinical presentation, high-resolution computed tomography (HRCT), and lung histology

Idiopathic Pulmonary Fibrosis

Basic Information

- **Most common idiopathic interstitial pneumonia; more than 60% of cases (see Table 20-1).**
- No known cause or cure, although two new drugs have been shown to possibly slow disease progression

Clinical Presentation

- **Two thirds of patients have disease onset when older than 60 years of age**
  - Majority of patients have a history of smoking; environmental exposures may play a role
  - Rare familial forms (<5%)
  - Slight male predominance
- Insidious onset over years; symptoms usually present 3 to 5 years before diagnosis
- Acute exacerbations portend a worse prognosis
- **Exertional dyspnea; nonproductive cough; rare constitutional symptoms**
- Physical examination
  - Dry, Velcro-like crackles
  - Clubbing
  - Signs of elevated right-sided pressure on cardiac examination late in disease (e.g., elevated jugular venous pressure, edema, and right ventricular heave)

Diagnosis, Evaluation, and Treatment

- Imaging: HRCT
  - **Subpleural, reticular infiltrates with basilar predominance and areas of honeycombing (Figs. 20-1 and 20-2)**
  - Minimal ground glass infiltrates
  - May be asymmetric
- Laboratory results are nonspecific
- Pulmonary function tests (PFTs)
  - **Restrictive disease with decreased forced vital capacity (FVC), total lung capacity (TLC), and diffusing capacity for carbon monoxide (DLCO)**
- Diagnosis
  - Made from the constellation of clinical history, classic HRCT findings, and the absence of other identifiable causes for fibrosis (e.g., environmental exposures, connective tissue disease, drug toxicity)
  - Surgical lung biopsy is only needed if there is a disconnect between the clinical picture and HRCT findings. Biopsy pathology shows a usual interstitial pneumonitis (UIP) pattern, although other diseases may also cause UIP.
  - Table 20-1 lists diagnostic categories of alternative idiopathic interstitial pneumonias
- Therapy/natural history
  - Chronic, slowly progressive dyspnea on exertion and exertional hypoxemia
  - No cure or treatment to reverse fibrosis
  - Pirfenidone (a tumor growth factor β-antagonist) and nintedanib (a tyrosine kinase inhibitor) have been shown to slow loss of lung function and were recently approved by the Food and Drug Administration for use in the United States
  - Although often used in acute exacerbations, steroids have not proven effective, with historic response rates less than 5% to 10%
  - Cytotoxic agents (e.g., azathioprine, cyclophosphamide, and so on) are ineffective, have no role in treatment, and may actually cause harm
  - Lung transplantation remains the only effective therapy for patients with progressive or end-stage disease

Acute Interstitial Pneumonia

Basic Information

- Commonly referred to as the Hamman-Rich syndrome
- Presents with acute onset of cough and shortness of breath rapidly progressing to hypoxic respiratory failure
- Most patients require mechanical ventilation

Imaging

- Diffuse bilateral ground-glass infiltrates on chest x-ray and HRCT

TABLE 20-1	Idiopathic Interstitial Pneumonias			
	IPF	**DIP**	**AIP**	**NSIP**
Onset	Insidious	Insidious	Acute	Subacute
Steroid response	Poor	Good	Poor	Good
Complete recovery possible?	No	Yes	Yes	Yes

AIP, Acute interstitial pneumonitis; DIP, desquamative interstitial pneumonitis; IPF, idiopathic pulmonary fibrosis; NSIP, nonspecific interstitial pneumonitis.

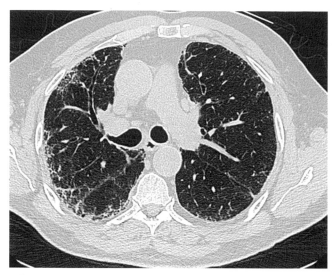

FIGURE 20-1 Reticular infiltrates in a patient with idiopathic pulmonary fibrosis. Note subpleural, peripheral distribution of infiltrates.

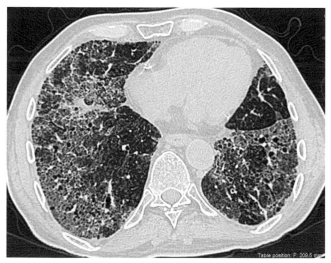

FIGURE 20-2 Lungs of a patient with end-stage idiopathic pulmonary fibrosis.

Diagnosis

- Based on clinical presentation, imaging, and ruling out alternative diagnoses
- Histology shows diffuse alveolar damage

Treatment

- Supportive treatment with mechanical ventilation if necessary

- Steroids have been used, but have not been clearly shown to be beneficial
- Recrudescence reported during recovery, possibly caused by steroid tapering

Connective Tissue Disease Related Interstitial Lung Disease

Basic Information

- **Many connective tissue diseases are associated with ILD**
- **Treatment is most often directed toward the underlying connective tissue disease**

SYSTEMIC LUPUS ERYTHEMATOSUS

Basic Information

- Systemic lupus erythematosus (SLE) is a systemic, autoimmune disease that may involve the lung or pleura
- Rarely causes chronic ILD
- More than one manifestation may be present in a single patient

Clinical Presentation

Table 20-2 summarizes the main pulmonary presentations of SLE.
- Additional lung manifestations:
  - **Alveolar hemorrhage**
    - Acute fever, dyspnea, cough, with or without hemoptysis
    - **Falling hematocrit with new infiltrates suggests alveolar hemorrhage**
    - Diagnosed by bronchoscopy showing progressively bloody bronchial washings
    - May be seen in the presence or absence of the antiphospholipid antibody syndrome
  - **Shrinking lung syndrome**
    - Restrictive lung disease in the absence of parenchymal disease
    - Etiology is debated, but possibilities include diaphragmatic weakness, phrenic nerve involvement, or pleural inflammation.

RHEUMATOID ARTHRITIS

Basic Information

- **Although rheumatoid arthritis (RA) is more common in females, RA lung disease is more common in males (3:1)**

TABLE 20-2	*Pulmonary Manifestations of Connective Tissue Diseases*			
	SLE	**RA**	**Scleroderma**	**PM**
Acute pneumonitis	May be initial manifestation of SLE Acute onset fever, pneumonic symptoms Diffuse or patchy infiltrates Pleuritis, pericarditis are common	None	Aspiration pneumonia is common consequence of esophageal dysmotility	None
Interstitial disease	Progression from acute pneumonitis gradual; dyspnea ± pleuritis ± productive cough Lower lobe infiltrates, with increasing restriction of PFTs	Similar to IPF Dyspnea and cough are common Clubbing is common Lower lobe infiltrates, with or without honeycombing Variable response to corticosteroids	Can be seen in patients with CREST or diffuse disease Usually after skin disease Infiltrates are predominantly lower lobe Clubbing is rare Recurrent aspiration may present as interstitial disease	Progressive DOE ± Muscle symptoms Lower lobe infiltrates
Pleural disease	Pain, dyspnea, fever, and effusion are common Pleural fluid is exudative, with normal glucose and normal PH Pleural fluid ANA may be increased LE cells diagnostic	Symptoms related to pleural disease are present in 20% of patients Pleural fluid: low pH, glucose <30 mg/dL in 70% to 80% of patients Pleural fluid RF may be increased and greater than serum RF	Thickening or effusions in 10% to 25%, but rarely symptomatic	None
Pulmonary hypertension	Rare without parenchymal disease May be primary arteriolar disease or secondary to interstitial lung disease	Secondary to hypoxia with severe ILD Idiopathic or secondary to RA	Seen in 10% of patients with CREST Primary vascular disease occurs independent of parenchymal disease	Usually secondary to parenchymal disease

ANA, Antinuclear antibody; CREST, calcinosis, Raynaud syndrome, esophageal dysmotility, sclerodactyly, telangiectasia; DOE, dyspnea on exertion; ILD, interstitial lung disease; IPF, idiopathic pulmonary fibrosis; LE, lupus erythematosus; PFTs, pulmonary function tests; PM, polymyositis; RA, rheumatoid arthritis; RF, rheumatoid factor; SLE, systemic lupus erythematosus.

- **Symptoms from RA lung involvement precede joint disease in 20% of cases**
- Multiple pulmonary manifestations of RA

Clinical Presentation

See Table 20-2 for a summary of the main pulmonary manifestations of RA.
- Additional lung manifestations:
  - **Rheumatoid (necrobiotic) nodules**
    - **May be single or multiple; may cavitate**
    - Pathology of nodules reveals histiocytic palisades specific for RA
    - Caplan syndrome: rheumatoid nodules in coal miners
  - **Constrictive bronchiolitis (or bronchiolitis obliterans)**
    - **Dyspnea, dry cough; chest radiograph clear or hyperinflated**
    - Obstruction on PFTs that does not respond to bronchodilators

- Pathology reveals narrowing and eventual replacement of respiratory bronchioles by peribronchiolar and submucosal fibrosis
- Poor response to therapy
- **Cricoarytenoid arthritis**
  - **Pain, hoarseness, dyspnea, stridor, obstruction**
  - Symptoms in 25% of patients with RA

SCLERODERMA

Basic Information

- **60% to 100% of patients with scleroderma have ILD at autopsy**
- Pulmonary hypertension occurs in 5% to 37% of patients and is more common with CREST (calcinosis, Raynaud phenomenon, esophageal dysmotility, sclerodactyly, and telangiectasia) syndrome. It can be secondary to ILD or to primary vascular involvement.
- **Cyclophosphamide has been shown to decrease the progression of ILD**

20

Clinical Presentation

See Table 20-2

POLYMYOSITIS/DERMATOMYOSITIS

Basic Information

- More common in females
- 10% present with ILD before myositis
- Associated with anti-Jo, anti-PL-12, or other antisynthetase antibodies
  - Biopsy can show UIP or nonspecific interstitial pneumonitis pattern
- The antisynthetase syndrome is often characterized by subclinical myositis, ILD, Raynaud, mechanic's hands, and symmetric polyarthritis of small joints
- Often steroid-responsive

Clinical Presentation

- Dyspnea on exertion (DOE), proximal muscle weakness, skin rash, "heliotrope" rash around eyes, "mechanic's hands." Although often present, elevated creatine kinase and aldolase are not needed for the diagnosis.

Antineutrophil Cytoplasmic Antibody-Associated Vasculitides

GRANULOMATOSIS WITH POLYANGIITIS (FORMERLY WEGENER GRANULOMATOSIS)

Basic Information

- 90% of cases have antineutrophil cytoplasmic antibody (ANCA) antibodies
- Two forms described
  - **Classic disease: involving the upper and lower respiratory tracts and kidney**
  - **Limited disease: isolated respiratory tract involvement; up to 40% may be negative for ANCA antibodies**
- Characteristic pathology reveals necrotizing granulomatous inflammation and small-vessel vasculitis of the upper and lower respiratory tracts and necrotizing glomerulonephritis in the kidney
- Majority of cases demonstrate positive PR3-ANCA

Clinical Presentation

See Table 20-3

MICROSCOPIC POLYANGIITIS

Basic Information

- Most common ANCA-associated small vessel vasculitis
- Similar to granulomatosis with polyangiitis, only without the presence of granulomas on
- biopsy
- Upper respiratory tract involvement is much less common
- Majority of cases demonstrate positive microscopic polyangiitis (MPO)-ANCA
- Less likely to relapse than granulomatosis with polyangiitis

EOSINOPHILIC GRANULOMATOSIS WITH POLYANGIITIS (CHURG-STRAUSS SYNDROME)

Basic Information

- 50% are ANCA positive; MPO-ANCA is most common
- Discussed later in Eosinophilic Lung Diseases section

GOODPASTURE SYNDROME

Basic Information

- **Disease affecting the lung and kidney associated with circulating antiglomerular basement membrane antibodies that may be the cause of the process (Fig. 20-3)**
- MPO-ANCA can be positive in 10% to 40% of cases
- **The lung and kidney are both involved in 60% to 80% of cases; in the remainder, the kidney alone is involved**

Clinical Presentation

See Table 20-3

Eosinophilic Lung Diseases

Basic Information

- Comprise a diverse group of diseases, all of which exhibit blood or tissue eosinophilia

Clinical Presentation and Treatment

- **Acute eosinophilic pneumonia**
  - Acute presentation with infiltrates and hypoxemia with or without peripheral eosinophilia
  - **Diagnosis requires eosinophilia in bronchoalveolar lavage (BAL) fluid or lung tissue**
  - **Steroid-responsive**
- **Chronic eosinophilic pneumonia**
  - **Subacute presentation with constitutional symptoms, cough, dyspnea, and peripheral eosinophilia**
  - **Chest radiograph with peripheral infiltrates (reverse pulmonary edema) (Fig. 20-4)**
  - Diagnosis requires BAL eosinophilia (>40% diagnostic) or lung tissue eosinophilia
  - Steroid-responsive
  - May develop severe asthma and require chronic steroid use
- **Hypereosinophilic syndrome**
  - Defined as more than 1500 eosinophils/mm^3 in peripheral blood for 6 months
  - Primary targets include the heart, central nervous system, peripheral nervous system, and skin. The lung is less commonly involved.
  - Treat with corticosteroids or cytotoxic agents (or both)
- **Allergic bronchopulmonary aspergillosis (ABPA)**
  - **Clinical constellation of asthma, elevated IgE levels, eosinophilia, infiltrates, and mucous plugs**
  - Central bronchiectasis (Fig. 20-5)

TABLE 20-3	Comparison of Pulmonary–Renal Disorders		
	Granulomatosis with Polyangiitis	**Microscopic Polyangiitis**	**Goodpasture Syndrome**
Presentation	Ears, nose, and throat are involved in 85% of patients Kidney is ultimately involved in 85% of cases Cough and dyspnea Pleural effusion, subglottic/bronchial stenoses or endobronchial lesions seen Can involve skin, joints, eyes, and neurologic system	Upper respiratory tract is involved in only 35% Kidneys are most common organ affected (90%) Cough and dyspnea Pleural effusion, subglottic/bronchial stenoses or endobronchial lesions Can involve skin, joints, eyes, and neurologic system	Hemoptysis, dyspnea, cough, and fatigue are the primary symptoms Fever, chills, and weight loss occur in <25% of patients
Radiographic findings	Infiltrates, nodules, or cavitation may be seen Infiltrates or nodules may be unilateral or bilateral	Similar to granulomatosis with polyangiitis	Bilateral infiltrates are the most common chest radiographic finding
Diagnostic studies	ESR commonly increased Abnormal urinalysis 80% PR3-ANCA most strongly correlated, but sensitivity and specificity variable MPO-ANCA can be positive in up to 20% of cases Lung or kidney biopsy demonstrates granulomatous inflammation	Elevated ESR Abnormal urinalysis MPO-ANCA is most strongly correlated with MPA, but PR3-ANCA can also be positive No granulomas on biopsy; most common lung findings are pulmonary capillaritis	Anemia is common Hematuria and proteinuria are seen in 90% of patients Anti-GBM antibodies are seen in 90% of patients Suspect when patient has the constellation of alveolar infiltrates, anemia, and renal disease Linear IgG in biopsy, or anti-GBM antibodies are diagnostic
Treatment	Limited disease: methotrexate plus prednisone Life- or organ-threatening disease: oral daily cytoxan plus prednisone If patient is severely ill, give solumedrol 1 g/d for 3 days followed by oral prednisone Cyclophosphamide for 3 to 6 months; taper steroids over 6 months 75% to 90% complete remission Plasmapharesis is only indicated for severe pulmonary hemorrhage or cases with positive anti-GBM	Treatment is the same as for granulomatosis with polyangiitis MPA is less likely to relapse	Corticosteroids, cyclophosphamide, plasmapheresis

ANCA, Antineutrophil cytoplasmic antibody; ESR, erythrocyte sedimentation rate; GBM, glomerular basement membrane; IgG, immunoglobulin; MPA, microscopic polyangiitis; MPO, microscopic polyangiitis.

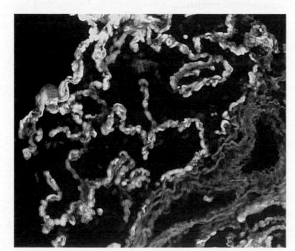

FIGURE 20-3 Immunofluorescence study demonstrating linear staining (immunoglobulin G) of alveolar walls in a patient with Goodpasture syndrome. (Original magnification ×10.) (From Mason RJ. *Murray and Nadel's Textbook of Respiratory Medicine.* 4th ed. London: Elsevier; 2005: Fig. 56.8.)

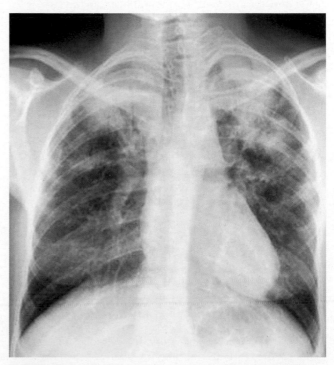

FIGURE 20-4 Chest radiograph of a patient with idiopathic chronic eosinophilic pneumonia showing bilateral alveolar opacities predominating in the upper lobes (reverse pulmonary edema). (From Mason RJ. *Murray and Nadel's Textbook of Respiratory Medicine.* 4th ed. London: Elsevier; 2005: Fig. 57-3.)

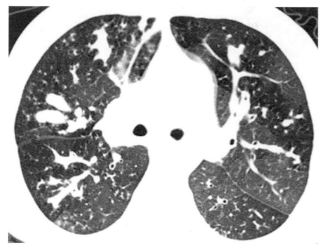

FIGURE 20-5 Axial computed tomographic scan of a patient with allergic bronchopulmonary aspergillosis showing central bronchiectasis with mucoid impaction. Diffuse bilateral inhomogeneous lung opacity is present, with areas of low attenuation throughout the pulmonary parenchyma, representing mosaic perfusion resulting from a combination of large and small airway inflammation. (From Mason RJ. *Murray and Nadel's Textbook of Respiratory Medicine.* 4th ed. London: Elsevier; 2005: Fig. 57-7.)

- Diagnosis is made by demonstrating eosinophilia, a positive skin test or antibodies to *Aspergillus*, an increased total and specific IgE, and recurrent infiltrates on chest film
- **Responsive to corticosteroids and itraconazole**
  - See Chapter 17 for more information
- **Eosinophilic granulomatosis with polyangiitis (Churg-Strauss syndrome)**
  - **Clinical constellation of asthma, eosinophilia, and systemic vasculitis**
  - Lung biopsy reveals eosinophilia and extravascular granulomas
  - Asthma is present in more than 80% of patients and radiographic infiltrates are present in more than 90% of patients; 30% have pleural effusions
  - Disease may be unmasked after tapering systemic steroids in an asthmatic
  - **This is a systemic illness, with skin (75% of patients) and peripheral nervous system (mononeuritis multiplex in 60% of cases) involvement**
    - Mononeuritis multiplex is the most common peripheral nervous system feature
    - The heart and gastrointestinal tract may also be involved
    - The kidneys are rarely involved
  - Usually responsive to corticosteroids
- **Eosinophilic granuloma (pulmonary Langerhans cell histiocytosis, pulmonary histiocytosis X)**
  - Variant of histiocytosis X seen almost exclusively in smoking adults (Box 20-1)
  - Progressive dyspnea; 10% to 20% develop spontaneous pneumothorax
  - HRCT ranges from small peribronchiolar nodular opacities early to multiple irregularly-shaped cysts, usually in a mid- to upper-zone distribution
  - Histology reveals proliferation of Langerhans cells in the bronchiolar and bronchial epithelium. Resulting

BOX 20-1 | *Eosinophilic Granuloma*

Pulmonary Langerhans cell histiocytosis
Cough and dyspnea in two thirds of patients
Smoking history in 90% of patients
Radiographic manifestations: progression from diffuse nodules to reticulonodular pattern to diffuse cystic changes in severe disease
Spares costophrenic angles
Pneumothorax common
May have associated central diabetes insipidus and bone cysts
Biopsies reveal CD1a(+), s100+ Langerhans cells on light microscopy with Birbeck granules on electron microscopy
Prognosis usually good with smoking cessation

granulomas cause traction on the central bronchiole and can lead to cyst formation. Electron microscopy may reveal characteristic Birbeck granules.
- Treatment includes smoking cessation with lung transplant in severe cases. Steroids are generally ineffective.

Bronchiolitis Obliterans Organizing Pneumonia/Cryptogenic Organizing Pneumonia

Basic Information

- Pathologic diagnosis of fibroblast and inflammatory cell plugs filling bronchioles, alveolar ducts, and alveoli
- **Nonspecific histologic reaction that can be seen in response to infections, connective tissue diseases, drugs or idiopathic**
- Often coexists with other ILDs
- **This is a different entity from bronchiolitis obliterans (or obliterative bronchiolitis) (Box 20-2)**

Clinical Presentation

- Idiopathic bronchiolitis obliterans organizing pneumonia (BOOP) commonly presents as a subacute illness with infectious-like symptoms
  - Cough, dyspnea, and fever are the most common symptoms; may be diagnosed as recurrent pneumonias unresponsive to antibiotics
  - **Crackles or squeaks are present on lung examination in 75% of patients**

Evaluation and Diagnosis

- **Patchy, migratory infiltrates on HRCT**
- Pulmonary function tests reveal restriction and a decreased diffusing capacity, in contrast to obliterative bronchiolitis, which is predominantly characterized by obstruction and air-trapping
- Obstruction is seen in only 20% of patients with BOOP and is most often associated with smoking

Treatment

- **Idiopathic BOOP is steroid-responsive, with typical doses 0.75 to 1.5 mg/kg prednisone/day**

BOX 20-2 | *Obliterative Bronchiolitis*

Basic Information

A variety of associations, including postinfection (primarily viral); posttransplant (lung or bone marrow); toxin/inhalational exposure; drugs (e.g., penicillamine, gold); and connective tissue diseases.

There is also an idiopathic form.

Clinical Presentation

The primary clinical manifestation is dyspnea.

Evaluation and Diagnosis

Pulmonary function tests reveal obstruction or air-trapping with high residual volumes.

Chest radiographs may reveal hyperinflation or may be normal.

High-resolution computed tomography shows air-trapping and mosaic perfusion accentuated on expiratory images.

Lung biopsies demonstrate replacement of small airways by peribronchiolar and submucosal fibrosis (i.e., constrictive bronchiolitis), but not organizing pneumonia.

Treatment

The response to corticosteroid therapy is generally poor.

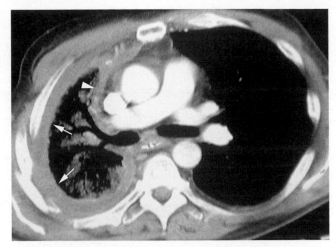

FIGURE 20-6 Mesothelioma. Axial thoracic computed tomographic scan shows diffuse right pleural thickening *(arrows)* associated with marked volume loss in the right thorax. Note the presence of mediastinal pleural involvement *(arrowhead)*. (From Mason RJ: *Murray and Nadel's Textbook of Respiratory Medicine.* 4th ed. London: Elsevier; 2005: Fig. 70.2.)

- Relapse is common if the duration of therapy is less than 6 months
- The response to therapy in drug- and connective tissue disease-associated BOOP is much less predictable

Asbestos-Related Lung Disease

Basic Information

- Disease results from chronic exposure over prolonged periods, usually years
- Sources of exposure include the auto industry (brakes), construction, demolition, shipbuilding and renovation, the cement industry, and mining

Clinical Presentation

- **Asbestosis**
  - Manifests as progressive dyspnea, usually 10 years or longer after exposure
  - Intensity of asbestos exposure affects expression and latency
  - Interstitial fibrosis, primarily in the lower lobes, similar to IPF
- **Pleural disease**
  - Benign pleural disease is typically the first manifestation, includes pleural plaques, thickening, and benign effusions
    - Mesothelioma is a malignant tumor of the pleura, presenting with chest pain (often pleuritic), dyspnea, weight loss, and cough, after a latency of 20 to 40 years (Fig. 20-6)
    - **Mesothelioma risk does not appear to be affected by smoking**
    - There is no effective therapy
- **Lung cancer and asbestos**
  - The risk of lung cancer in an asbestos-exposed individual is **increased fourfold to fivefold in nonsmokers and fiftyfold in smokers**, compared with nonsmokers who have not been exposed to asbestos

Sarcoidosis

Basic Information

- Sarcoidosis is a systemic disease of unknown origin
- **Pathologic hallmark is noncaseating granulomas**
- Presentation
  - Most instances (70% to 80%) occur between the ages of 20 and 50 years
  - More common in African Americans and females in the United States
  - 30% to 60% of cases are asymptomatic

Clinical Presentation

- Constitutional symptoms may include weight loss, fatigue, fever, and malaise
- Respiratory tract
  - Lung is involved in more than 90% of cases
  - Cough, dyspnea, sputum production, and hemoptysis can be seen
  - Endobronchial disease may produce obstructive symptoms
  - Upper respiratory tract can be involved, producing nasal and upper airway obstruction or hoarseness
  - Mycetomas can be seen in patients with fibrocystic sarcoid
- Eye
  - Uveitis, keratoconjunctivitis
  - Sicca syndrome (dry eyes and mouth)
  - Uveoparotid fever in sarcoidosis (Heerfordt-Waldenström syndrome) is the constellation of bilateral lacrimal and parotid gland enlargement, fever, and anterior uveitis

- Heart
  - Myocardial granulomatous inflammation can produce conduction abnormalities, tachyarrhythmias, cardiomyopathy, and sudden death
- Neurologic
  - Up to 5% of patients with sarcoidosis have neurologic manifestations
  - Cranial nerves (II, VII, VIII, IX, X), meninges, and pituitary gland are most often involved
- Skin
  - Erythema nodosum most common skin finding (Fig. 20-7)
    - **Löfgren syndrome: erythema nodosum with hilar adenopathy, arthralgias, and fever; spontaneous resolution common**
  - Lupus pernio: purplish nodules or plaques on cheeks, nose, and ears
  - Treatment of skin disease may be with chloroquine or pentoxifylline, rather than corticosteroids

- Liver
  - Hepatic granulomas in 75% of patients
  - Only 35% have elevated liver function test results; alkaline phosphatase is the best clinical predictor

Evaluation and Diagnosis

- Chest radiographs in patients with sarcoidosis have been typed (or staged) based on the pattern of abnormalities (Table 20-4 and Fig. 20-8)
- Disease progression is not necessarily from one stage to the next
- **Tissue biopsy revealing noncaseating granulomas is required for the diagnosis**
- Serum angiotensin-converting enzyme level may be elevated in patients with sarcoidosis and may track with disease activity. However, it is nonspecific and nondiagnostic, so its role in management is undefined

Treatment

- Treatment should be limited to symptomatic or progressive pulmonary disease or any involvement of heart, eye, or nervous system

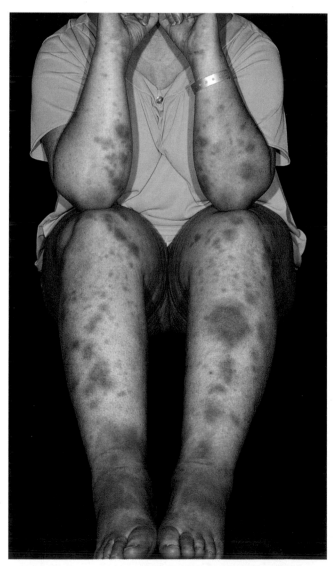

FIGURE 20-7 Erythema nodosum. (From Habif TP. *Clinical Dermatology: A Color Guide to Diagnostic Therapy.* 4th ed. St. Louis: Mosby; 2004: Fig. 18-9.)

TABLE 20-4	*Chest Radiographic Staging in Sarcoidosis*	
Type	**Distribution**	**Frequency (%)**
0	Normal	5 to 10
I	Hilar nodes	45 to 65
II	Hilar nodes + reticular opacities	25 to 30
III	Reticular opacities alone	15
IV	Pulmonary fibrosis and fibrocystic disease	5 to 10

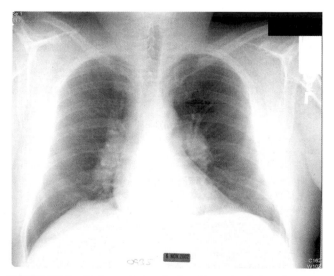

FIGURE 20-8 Posteroanterior chest radiograph of stage I sarcoidosis. Important features include prominent hilar lymphadenopathy and normal lung fields. (From Mason RJ. *Murray and Nadel's Textbook of Respiratory Medicine.* 4th ed. London: Elsevier; 2005: Fig. 55-1.)

- Corticosteroids (usually low to moderate doses) are the mainstay of therapy; alternative regimens including methotrexate or azathioprine may be used in refractory cases or as steroid-sparing agents

Review Questions

For review questions, please go to ExpertConsult.com.

SUGGESTED READINGS

Browne K. Asbestos-related disorders. In: Parkes WR, ed. *Occupational Lung Disorders*. Boston: Butterworth Heinemann; 1994.

Delaney P. Neurologic manifestations of sarcoidosis. *Ann Intern Med.* 1997;87:336-345.

Epler GR, ed. *Diseases of the Bronchioles*. New York: Raven Press; 1994.

Johns CJ, Scott PP, Schonfeld SA. Sarcoidosis. *Annu Rev Med.* 1989;40:353-371.

Katzenstein A-L. *Katzenstein and Askin's Surgical Pathology of Non-neoplastic Lung Disease*. Philadelphia: WB Saunders; 1997.

Katzenstein A-L, Myers JL. Idiopathic pulmonary fibrosis. *Am J Respir Crit Care Med.* 1998;157:1301-1315.

Ragu GA, Collard HR, Egan JJ, et al. An Official ATS/ERS/JRS/ALAT Statement: idiopathic pulmonary fibrosis: evidence-based guidelines for diagnosis and management. *Am J Respir Crit Care Med.* 2011;181:788-824.

Schwarz MI, King TE, Cherniak RM. Principles of and approach to the patient with interstitial lung disease. In: Murray JF, Nadel JA, eds. *Textbook of Respiratory Medicine*. 3rd ed. Philadelphia: Saunders; 2000.

Venous Thromboembolic Disease

DAVID B. PEARSE, MD

Venous thromboembolism (VTE), which includes deep venous thrombosis (DVT) and pulmonary thromboembolism (PE), has an annual incidence of 0.1% to 0.3% and a cumulative lifetime population incidence of 5% in the United States. **More than 80% of clinically significant pulmonary emboli occur from DVTs in the lower extremities;** the remaining emboli originate from pelvic and upper extremity veins. The estimated short-term mortality rate from untreated PE (30%) is markedly reduced (to less than 5%) by successful diagnosis and appropriate therapy. Unfortunately, the diagnoses of DVT and PE are frequently missed, and effective prophylactic treatment is underused.

Deep Venous Thrombosis

Basic Information

- Virchow triad
  - **Venous stasis**
    - Immobility
    - Elevated venous pressure
    - Elevated blood viscosity
  - **Vessel wall damage**
  - **Increased blood coagulability**
    - Activation of clotting
    - Inhibition of fibrinolytic system
    - Deficiencies of coagulation factors
- Mechanisms
  - **Most important clinical risk is venous stasis from immobility**

Clinical Risk Factors

- Lower extremity DVT
  - Recent surgery
  - **Major trauma (more than 50% develop DVT if prophylaxis not implemented)**
  - Previous DVT **(25% recurrence over 5 years after first DVT)**
  - Increasing age (exponential increase after age 50 years)
  - Pregnancy/puerperium (PE is second leading cause of death; 75% occur postpartum)
  - Oral contraception
  - Medical conditions with immobility/hypercoagulability
    - Common: cancer, heart failure, myocardial infarction, obesity, myeloproliferative disorder, nephrotic syndrome

- Uncommon: systemic lupus erythematosus, antiphospholipid antibody, sickle cell anemia, homocystinuria, Behçet syndrome
- Upper extremity DVT
  - Central venous catheter
  - Cancer
  - Anatomic abnormality of costoclavicular junction

Familial Thrombophilic Disorders

- Common
  - Activated protein C resistance (factor V Leiden)
    - Autosomal dominant defect of factor V (incomplete penetrance): prevents inactivation by protein C
    - Five percent normal white population is heterozygous; rare in those of African or Asian descent
    - Twenty percent unselected DVT patients; 60% idiopathic, recurrent DVT are heterozygous
    - **DVT recurrence risk significant in homozygotes; insignificant in heterozygotes**
  - Prothrombin 20210A
    - Gene defect causing increased prothrombin and thrombin
    - Two percent normal white population; rare in those of African or Asian descent
    - Five percent unselected DVT, problematic when coexisting with other defects
- Rare
  - Deficiencies of antithrombin III, protein C, protein S
    - Autosomal dominant
    - **Protein C or S deficiency associated with warfarin-induced skin necrosis**

Clinical Presentation

- Symptoms and signs neither sensitive nor specific
  - Only 20% of symptomatic patients have leg DVT
  - Leg pain or swelling may be present
  - Homans sign (pain and tenderness with dorsiflexion of ankle) present in less than 40%
- Starts in calf (except leg trauma, orthopedic surgery); most are self-limited
- Twenty-five percent of calf DVT extend to thigh
- **Thigh DVT strongly associated with PE**
  - Untreated symptomatic proximal DVT: 20% mortality from acute PE
  - Forty percent to 50% of patients with symptomatic thigh DVT have silent PE

- DVT can be a recurrent disease (after anticoagulation stopped)
  - Overall recurs in 25% by 5 years; 50% of recurrences are in contralateral leg
  - Recurrence risk after unprovoked (no major risk factors) DVT nearly double

Diagnosis and Evaluation

- Noninvasive
  - B-mode compression ultrasonography (US)
    - Visualizes noncompressable clot in proximal veins
    - 99% sensitive and specific for symptomatic proximal leg DVT
    - Thirty percent to 60% sensitive, 99% specific for asymptomatic proximal leg DVT
    - **Initial test of choice for upper extremity DVT evaluation,** but sensitivity and specificity 80%
    - Addition of Doppler flow or color adds little to sensitivity
  - Computed tomography (CT) venography
    - Performed with CT angiography; able to visualize clot in thigh, pelvic veins, inferior vena cava (IVC)
    - **Sensitivity and specificity comparable to compression US, so not routinely recommended; useful if injured or casted leg because US cannot be performed in this scenario**
  - Magnetic resonance imaging (MRI)
    - Able to visualize clot in calf, thigh, pelvic veins, IVC, upper extremities
    - Performed with injured or casted leg because US cannot be performed in this scenario
    - Requires administration of high-dose gadolinium
      - Can cause nephrogenic systemic fibrosis, especially in the context of renal insufficiency
    - **Sensitivity and specificity greater than 90%**
- D-Dimer
  - Degradation product of cross-linked fibrin
  - Elevated in DVT/PE (95% sensitivity), but specificity low (40%) because of nonspecific elevations in patients with:
    - Surgery, trauma, malignancy, disseminated intravascular coagulopathy, pregnancy, and infection and in normal elderly persons
  - Assay
    - Enzyme-linked immunosorbent assay (ELISA) more sensitive than latex agglutination
    - **Positive D-dimer not helpful; negative (i.e., normal) D-dimer more clinically useful** as follows:
      - Normal D-dimer with low or intermediate pretest probability for DVT or PE excludes thromboembolism
      - Normal highly sensitive D-dimer with nondiagnostic *ventilation/perfusion* ($\dot{V}/\dot{Q}$) scan excludes PE
  - Usefulness limited in inpatients and older adults because of nonspecific elevated levels
  - **DVT diagnosis in the symptomatic lower extremity**
    - Determine pretest clinical risk using the Wells prediction rule (Table 21-1)
    - Low or moderate clinical suspicion and normal D-dimer

TABLE 21-1	*Wells Assessment of Pretest Probability of Deep Vein Thrombosis (DVT)*	
Variables		**Points**
Active cancer		1
Paralysis, paresis, or recent plaster immobilization of lower extremities		1
Bedridden >3 days or major surgery within 12 weeks		1
Localized tenderness along deep veins		1
Swelling of entire leg		1
Calf swelling >3 cm larger than other side		1
Pitting edema of symptomatic leg		1
Collateral superficial veins		1
Alternative diagnosis at least as likely as DVT		–2

Clinical pretest probability for PE: low, <1; intermediate, 1 to 2; high, >2.
Data from Wells PS, Hirsh J, Anderson DR, et al. Accuracy of clinical assessment of deep-vein thrombosis. *Lancet.* 1995;345:1326–1330.

  - Further testing unnecessary, low incidence of DVT/PE if no therapy given
  - Low or moderate clinical suspicion and negative US (if D-dimer not available)
    - Further testing unnecessary, low incidence of DVT/PE if no therapy given
  - High clinical suspicion: US necessary (regardless of D-dimer result)
  - **Negative bilateral whole leg US excludes DVT**
  - **Negative initial thigh US (without calf testing):** 15% of these patients have calf DVT, 20% to 30% of which will extend to thigh
    - US should be repeated at 1 week
  - Negative serial US: Acceptable 1% to 2% risk of thromboembolism if untreated
  - **Positive compression US prompts treatment regardless of pretest risk or symptoms**

Deep Vein Thrombosis Treatment/Prophylaxis

- Treatment of DVT: see PE treatment
- Prophylaxis choice depends on the risk of thrombosis for an individual (Tables 21-2 and 21-3)

Pulmonary Embolism

Basic Information

- Effects of pulmonary emboli on gas exchange
  - **Dead space (i.e., ventilated, but not perfused) increased but arterial partial pressure of carbon dioxide ($PaCO_2$) normal or low (from increased ventilation in perfused lung)**
  - **Hypoxemia variable because it is an epiphenomenon of thrombus (e.g., atelectasis, edema, interatrial shunting, low-mixed venous oxygen tension)**

21

- Effects of pulmonary emboli on pulmonary and systemic hemodynamics
  - In previously healthy patients
    - Peripheral vascular resistance (PVR) increases proportionally to obstruction

- Pulmonary artery pressure (Ppa) increases after 30% to 50% bed occluded
- Normal right ventricle (RV): maximal mean Ppa of 40 mm Hg
- In patients with preexisting heart/lung disease
  - No correlation of clot burden with PVR or Ppa
- Shock
  - Increased right atrial pressure decreases venous return
  - RV distension leads to shift of interventricular septum, causing impaired left ventricular function

TABLE 21-2	Padua Risk Assessment for Deep Vein Thrombosis (DVT) in Noncritically Ill Medical Patients

Variables	Points
Active cancer	3
Previous VTE (excluding superficial vein thrombosis)	3
Bed rest for ≥3 days (with or without bathroom privileges)	3
Known thrombophilic disorder	3
Recent (≤1 month) trauma or surgery	2
Age ≥70 years	1
Heart or respiratory failure	1
Acute MI or ischemic stroke	1
Acute infection or rheumatologic disorder	1
Obesity (BMI ≥30 kg/m^2)	1
Ongoing hormonal therapy	1

Risk for DVT: lower, <4; higher, ≥4.
BMI, Body mass index; MI, myocardial infarction; VTE, venous thromboembolism.
Data from Kahn SR, Lim W, Dunn AS, et al. Prevention of VTE in nonsurgical patients. Antithrombotic therapy and prevention of thrombosis. 9th ed. American College of Chest Physicians Evidenced-Based Clinical Practice Guidelines. *Chest.* 2012;141(2) (suppl):e195S–e226S.

Clinical Presentation

- **PE presents as:**
  - **Infarction-like syndrome: chest pain, cough, hemoptysis (44%)**
  - **Uncomplicated dyspnea (36%)**
  - **Tachypnea or tachycardia plus evidence suggesting DVT (12%)**
  - **Circulatory collapse (8%)**
- **Major symptoms: dyspnea, chest pain, cough**
- **Major signs: tachypnea, crackles, tachycardia**
  - **Dyspnea, tachypnea, pleuritic chest pain, or signs of DVT present in 97% of PE**

Diagnosis and Evaluation

See Figures 21-1 and 21-2
- Chest radiograph and electrocardiogram (ECG)
  - Abnormal 70% to 90%, but nonspecific
    - Atelectasis, consolidation, diaphragm elevation on chest film
    - Nonspecific ST changes on ECG
- Arterial blood gases
  - **Increased alveolar-to-arterial O$_2$ gradient**
  - **Respiratory alkalosis**
  - Hypoxemia with the following caveats:

TABLE 21-3	DVT Prophylaxis		
	Clinical Risks	**Prophylaxis**	
Low risk (<2% DVT*)	Minor surgery in mobile patients	Early ambulation	
	Medical patients (Padua score <4)	None	
Moderate risk (6% to 30% DVT)	Most general, open gynecologic or urogenital surgery	LMWH (e.g., enoxaparin 40 mg SQ daily)	
	Non-ICU medical patients (Padua score ≥4); ICU medical patients	LDUH (5000 U SQ bid or tid), fondaparinux Mechanical thromboprophylaxis†	
High risk (40% to 80% DVT)	Hip or knee arthroplasty Hip fracture surgery Extensive trauma Stroke, spinal cord injury Major cancer surgery or major surgery in elderly or with history of DVT	LMWH (preferred), fondaparinux, dabigatran, apixaban, rivaroxaban adjusted-dose warfarin (continue LMWH after hospital discharge for 35 days after orthopedic or cancer surgery) LMWH, LDUFH or fondaparinux for stroke or trauma patients Mechanical thromboprophylaxis†	

*Rates based on objective diagnostic screening for DVT in patients not receiving thromboprophylaxis.
†Mechanical thromboprophylaxis includes intermittent pneumatic compression (preferred) and/or graduated compression stockings for patients with substantial bleeding risk. In high-risk patients, intermittent pneumatic compression suggested *in addition* to pharmacologic prophylaxis.
bid, Twice daily; DVT, deep vein thromboembolism; ICU, intensive care unit; LDUH, low-dose unfractionated heparin; LMWH, low-molecular-weight heparin; SQ, subcutaneously; tid, three times daily.
From Kahn SR, Lim W, Dunn AS, et al. Prevention of VTE in nonsurgical patients. Antithrombotic therapy and prevention of thrombosis. 9th ed. American College of Chest Physicians Evidenced-Based Clinical Practice Guidelines. *Chest.* 2012;141(2)(suppl):e195S–e226S; Gould MK, Garcia DA, Wren SM, et al. Prevention of VTE in nonorthopedic surgical patients. Antithrombotic therapy and prevention of thrombosis. 9th ed. American College of Chest Physicians Evidenced-Based Clinical Practice Guidelines. *Chest.* 2012;141(2)(suppl):e227S–e277S; and Falck-Ytter Y, Francis CW, Johanson NA, et al. Prevention of VTE in orthopedic surgical patients. Antithrombotic therapy and prevention of thrombosis. 9th ed. American College of Chest Physicians Evidenced-Based Clinical Practice Guidelines. *Chest.* 2012;141(2)(suppl):e278S–e325S.

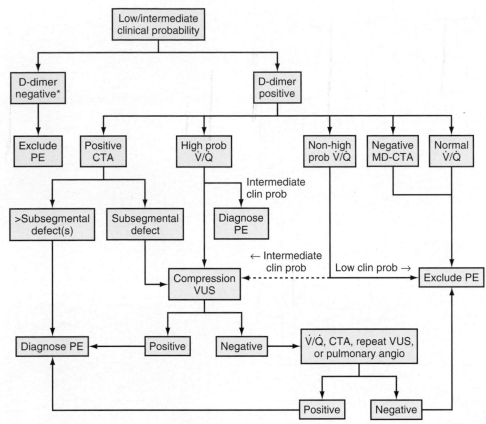

FIGURE 21-1 Proposed diagnostic algorithm for pulmonary embolism (PE) in patients with low or intermediate pretest probability using either V̇/Q̇ scan or computed tomographic angiography (CTA) as initial test. *Dashed line* indicates optional choice. *Using a highly sensitive assay. MD-CTA, Multidetector CTA; V̇/Q̇, ventilation perfusion scan; VUS, venous ultrasound. (Modified from Torbicki A, Perrier A, Konstantinides S, et al. Guidelines on the diagnosis and management of acute pulmonary embolism. *Eur Heart J.* 2008;29:2276–2315.)

- Twelve percent to 25% of patients have an arterial oxygen partial pressure (PaO$_2$) greater than 80 mm Hg
  - **20% have normal age-defined alveolar-to-arterial O$_2$ gradient**
- PE diagnosis in the symptomatic patient
  - Determine pretest clinical risk using the Well prediction rule (Table 21-4)
  - Low or intermediate clinical risk and normal D-dimer
    - Further testing unnecessary, low incidence of DVT/PE if no therapy given
  - Low/intermediate clinical risk and elevated D-dimer or high clinical risk
    - Lung imaging with V̇/Q̇ scan (Fig. 21-3 and Table 21-5) or CT angiography (CTA)
  - **Normal V̇/Q̇ scan rules out PE regardless of clinical suspicion or ventilation scan findings**
  - High probability V̇/Q̇ and moderate/high clinical probability: 88% to 96% positive predictive value
  - High probability V̇/Q̇ and low clinical probability: 50% positive predictive value
  - All other abnormal V̇/Q̇ scan/clinical probability combinations: PE risk unpredictable but substantial (20% to 40%)
  - Specificity of high probability V̇/Q̇ not altered by underlying lung disease such as chronic obstructive pulmonary disease

- Proximal filling defects on CTA diagnostic (Fig. 21-4); single distal filling defects can be false positive, so further testing may be justified
- Negative multidetector CTA adequate stopping point only if low or intermediate pretest risk
- If additional testing needed, can perform V̇/Q̇, CTA, pulmonary angiography, or lower extremity US as secondary test depending on initial test choice
- Role for serial leg studies following V̇/Q̇ testing
  - Low/intermediate clinical probability, indeterminate probability V̇/Q̇, negative leg US, and good cardiopulmonary reserve (no shock, syncope, RV dysfunction, or respiratory failure)
    - Two additional leg studies at 7 and 14 days after anticoagulant withdrawn; if negative, no treatment
    - If cardiopulmonary reserve poor, proceed with lung imaging with CTA or conventional angiography
  - This strategy results in
    - Less than 10% overall need for pulmonary angiography in PE work-up
    - Less than 3% subsequent thromboembolism at 3 months if anticoagulant withheld

Treatment

- Acceptable forms of therapy
  - Low-molecular-weight heparin (LMWH), most commonly enoxaparin 1 mg/kg every 12 hours or

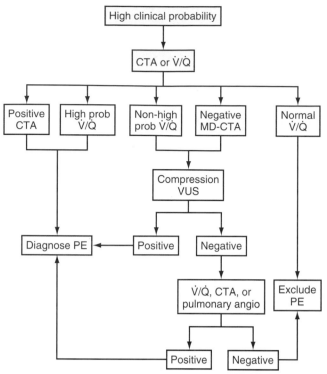

FIGURE 21-2 Proposed diagnostic algorithm for pulmonary embolism (PE) in patients with high pretest probability using either V̇/Q̇ scan or computed tomographic angiography (CTA) as initial test. MD-CTA, Multidetector CTA; V̇/Q̇, ventilation perfusion scan; VUS, venous ultrasound. (Modified from Torbicki A, Perrier A, Konstantinides S, et al. Guidelines on the diagnosis and management of acute pulmonary embolism. *Eur Heart J.* 2008;29:2276–2315.)

TABLE 21-4	Assessment of Pretest Probability of Pulmonary Embolism	
Variables		**Points**
Clinical signs and symptoms of DVT		3.0
Alternative diagnosis less likely than PE		3.0
Heart rate >100 beats/min		1.5
Immobilization or surgery in preceding 4 weeks		1.5
Previous DVT or PE		1.5
Hemoptysis		1.0
Cancer		1.0

Clinical pretest probability for PE: low, <2; intermediate, 2 to 6; high, >6. DVT, Deep vein thromboembolism; PE, pulmonary thromboembolism. From Wells PS, Ginsberg JS, Anderson DR, et al. Use of a clinical model for safe management of patients with suspected pulmonary embolism. *Ann Intern Med.* 1998;129:997–1005.

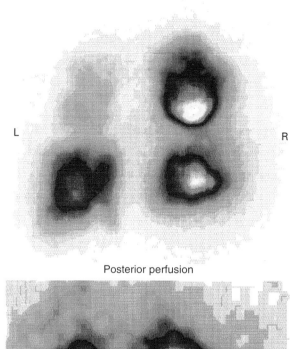

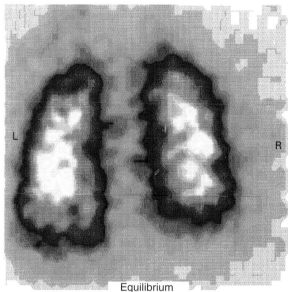

FIGURE 21-3 Lung ventilation and perfusion scintigraphy. **A,** Multiple perfusion defects in left upper lobe and right midzone on perfusion scan. **B,** Normal ventilation scan. This combination is consistent with high probability of pulmonary embolism. (From Haslett C, Chilvers ER, Boon NA, et al. *Davidson's Principles and Practice of Medicine.* 19th ed. New York: Churchill Livingstone; 2002: Fig. 13.6.)

1.5 mg/kg once per day (minimum 5 days, no monitoring, contraindicated in renal failure)
or
- Unfractionated heparin (UH) 80 U/kg IV bolus, 18 U/kg/hour, activated partial thromboplastin time 1.5 to 2.5 continuous (minimum 5 days)
or
- Fondaparinux (50 to 100 kg: 7.5 mg subcutaneously once a day) for minimum 5 days (no monitoring, contraindicated if renal failure)

then
- Warfarin 5 or 10 mg/day started day 1, target international normalized ratio (INR) 2 to 3
  - Protein C and S decline when warfarin is started during an active thrombotic state. This decline causes an increase in thrombogenic potential. Heparin can counteract this temporary procoagulant effect
- Rivaroxaban 15 mg orally twice daily for 3 weeks, then 20 mg orally once a day
- LMWH treatment of choice for VTE during pregnancy
- UH treatment of choice for submassive PE (nonhypotensive but RV dysfunction) because may need to escalate therapy to thrombolysis or surgical embolectomy

TABLE 21-5	*Ventilation/Perfusion Lung Scanning: The PIOPED Study Criteria*	
Scan Pattern (Prevalence)	**Original Definition**	**Revised Definition**
High probability (13%)	Segmental mismatches ≥2 large 1 large + 2 moderate ≥4 moderate	≥2 moderate/large segmental mismatch
Intermediate (39%)	Not high or low	1 moderate/large segmental mismatch or match Not high or low
Low (34%)	1 moderate/large segmental mismatch ≤4 moderate/large segmental match	>3 small subsegmental defects Nonsegmental perfusion defects
Very low/normal (14%)	Normal perfusion ≤3 small subsegmental perfusion defects	Normal perfusion ≤3 small subsegmental perfusion defects

PIOPED, Prospective investigation of pulmonary embolism diagnosis.

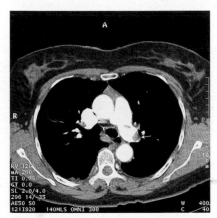

FIGURE 21-4 Computed tomographic scan demonstrating filling defect in proximal left pulmonary artery *(arrow)* from thrombus. Distal branches of artery are occluded. (From Souhami R. *Textbook of Medicine.* New York: Churchill Livingstone; 2002: Fig. 13.6.2A.)

- PE/DVT: Duration of therapy
  - **Three months after reversible major risk factors: provoked VTE**
  - **Three months to indefinite: first unprovoked VTE**
    - Indefinite if low bleeding risk and patient agrees
    - Three months if significant bleeding risk or patient refuses indefinite treatment
  - **Indefinite for**
    - First DVT/PE with active cancer
    - *or*
    - Second unprovoked DVT/PE
- Thrombolytic therapy (TT)
  - TT indicated for
    - **PE with severe hemodynamic/oxygenation compromise**
      - In PE, TT accelerates resolution of physiologic abnormalities and scan defects
      - However, no difference at 7 days compared with heparin
    - **Extensive iliofemoral DVT**
      - Prevents ischemic injury
      - Decreases postphlebitic syndrome
    - Use of TT in submassive PE controversial
    - Submassive PE (30% of all PEs) associated with small in-hospital mortality increase on heparin therapy

- TT in this subgroup decreased escalation of therapy, increased serious hemorrhage, and did not decrease mortality
  - **Increased monitoring but not routine TT in submassive PE**
  - Risk of TT
    - Serious bleeding 6% to 45% (threefold greater than heparin)
    - Fatal bleeding 2% (tenfold greater than heparin)
  - Approved drugs
    - Recombinant tissue-type plasminogen activator (rt-PA) infusion over 2 hours
    - Streptokinase infusion over 24 hours
    - Urokinase infusion over 12 to 24 hours
  - Contraindications of TT
    - Absolute
      - **Intracranial or intraspinal disorders, surgery, trauma in preceding 2 months**
      - **Active bleeding**
    - Relative
      - Surgery, organ biopsy, large vessel puncture, cardiopulmonary resuscitation, within 10 days postpartum
- Surgical or catheter embolectomy
  - Alternative to TT when TT contraindications present
  - Effective in small case series; morbidity and mortality poorly defined
- Optional (retrievable) inferior vena caval filters
  - Indications
    - Contraindication to anticoagulation
    - Recurrence of DVT/PE on therapeutic anticoagulation
  - Effects
    - Decrease early recurrent PE after anticoagulation without mortality effect
    - Increase incidence of later DVT
  - **Remove after resolution of indication**

Review Questions

For review questions, please go to ExpertConsult.com.

SUGGESTED READINGS

Bounameaux H, Perrier A, Righini M. Diagnosis of venous thromboembolism: an update. *Vasc Med.* 2010;15:399-406.

21

Carrier M, Righini M, Djurabi RK. VIDAS D-dimer in combination with clinical pre-test probability to rule out pulmonary embolism. *Thromb Haemost.* 2009;101:886-892.

Decousus H, Leizorovicz A, Parent F, et al. A clinical trial of vena caval filters in the prevention of pulmonary embolism in patients with proximal deep-vein thrombosis. *N Engl J Med.* 1998;338:409-415.

Elliott CG, Lovelace TD, Brown LM, et al. Diagnosis: imaging techniques. *Clin Chest Med.* 2010;31:641-657.

Falck-Ytter Y, Francis CW, Johanson NA, et al. Prevention of VTE in orthopedic surgical patients. Antithrombotic therapy and prevention of thrombosis, 9th ed: American College of Chest Physicians Evidenced-Based Clinical Practice Guidelines. *Chest.* 2012;141(suppl 2):e278S-e325S.

Goldhaber SZ, Bounameaux H. Pulmonary embolism and deep vein thrombosis. *Lancet.* 2012;379:1835-1846.

Gould MK, Garcia DA, Wren SM, et al. Prevention of VTE in nonorthopedic surgical patients. Antithrombotic therapy and prevention of thrombosis, 9th ed: American College of Chest Physicians Evidenced-Based Clinical Practice Guidelines. *Chest.* 2012;141(suppl 2):e227S-e277S.

Grant JD, Stevens SM, Woller SC, et al. Diagnosis and management of upper extremity deep-vein thrombosis in adults. *Thromb Haemost.* 2012;108:1097-1108.

Kahn SR, Lim W, Dunn AS, et al. Prevention of VTE in nonsurgical patients. Antithrombotic therapy and prevention of thrombosis, 9th ed: American College of Chest Physicians Evidenced-Based Clinical Practice Guidelines. *Chest.* 2012;141(suppl 2):e195S-e226S.

Kearon C, Aki EA. Duraton of anticoagulant therapy for deep vein thrombosis and pulmonary embolism. *Blood.* 2014;123:1794-1801.

Qaseem A, Snow V, Barry P, et al. Current diagnosis of venous thromboembolism in primary care: a clinical practice guideline from AAFP and ACP. *Ann Fam Med.* 2007;5:57-62.

Stein PD, Beemath A, Matta F, et al. Clinical characteristics of patients with acute pulmonary embolism: data from PIOPED II. *Am J Med.* 2007;120:871-879.

Stein PD, Fowler SE, Goodman LR, et al. For PIOPED II. Multidetector computed tomography for acute pulmonary embolism. *N Engl J Med.* 2006;354:2317-2327.

Todd JL, Tapson VF. Thrombolytic therapy for acute pulmonary embolism. *Chest.* 2009;135:1321-1329.

Wells P, Anderson D. The diagnosis and treatment of venous thromboembolism. *Hematol Am Soc Hematol Educ Program.* 2013;2013:457-463.

Wells PS, Forgie MA, Rodger MA. Treatment of venous thromboembolism. *JAMA.* 2014;311:717-728.

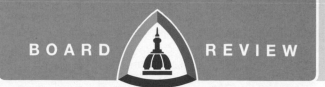
Selected Topics in Pulmonary Medicine

ALBERT J. POLITO, MD

Pulmonary medicine encompasses a variety of disorders that fall outside the traditionally broad topics of chronic obstructive pulmonary disease (COPD), asthma, interstitial lung disease, and thromboembolic disease. This chapter addresses four important smaller topics: (1) sleep disorders, (2) the solitary pulmonary nodule, (3) hemoptysis, and (4) pulmonary hypertension.

Sleep Disorders and Obstructive Sleep Apnea

Basic Information

- Apnea: Cessation of airflow for more than 10 sec
- **Obstructive apnea: Patient continues to make respiratory efforts against an obstruction (typically a narrowing or closure in the upper airway)**
  - Occurs in 3% to 4% of women and 6% to 9% of men (Box 22-1 lists risk factors)
  - Recurrent decrements in airflow (i.e., apneas or hypopneas) most commonly occur during sleep (obstructive sleep apnea [OSA])
  - Events usually more prominent during rapid eye movement sleep, caused by associated hypotonia of upper airway musculature
- **Central apnea: Patient makes no respiratory effort during the apnea** (Box 22-2 lists diseases associated with central apnea)
  - Occurs most commonly during sleep (central sleep apnea [CSA])
  - During sleep, transient abnormalities of central drive to the respiratory muscles occur in affected individuals
  - Much less common than OSA
- Mixed apnea: apnea with features of both OSA and CSA
- Hypopnea: A 50% or greater decrease in airflow or a less than 50% decrease in airflow associated with at least a 4% drop in oxygen saturation or an arousal
- Apnea-hypopnea index (AHI) is the total number of apneas and hypopneas per hour of sleep; normal is five or fewer events per hour
- Respiratory disturbance index (RDI) is frequently larger than the AHI because it includes not only apneas and hypopneas, but other respiratory disturbances that can disrupt sleep (e.g., respiratory effort–related arousals [RERAs])
- Upper airway resistance syndrome (UARS)
  - Repeated arousals secondary to increased upper airway resistance ("crescendo snoring")
  - AHI is normal; RDI is elevated
  - No significant oxygen desaturation episodes
- Obesity-hypoventilation syndrome (Pickwickian syndrome)
  - Syndrome of morbid obesity and chronic hypoventilation with daytime hypercapnia (arterial partial pressure of carbon dioxide [$PaCO_2$] greater than 45 mm Hg)
  - OSA present in majority of patients
- Cheyne-Stokes respirations
  - Cyclic rise and fall in respiratory pattern with recurrent periods of apnea
  - Apneas are typically central
  - Most commonly seen with congestive heart failure, central neurologic disease, or administration of sedative agents, but may occur in patients without these conditions or not taking these medications

Clinical Presentation

- OSA
  - History obtained from the patient alone may be unreliable
    - Input of bed partner or housemate often helpful
    - Symptoms of OSA include loud, disruptive snoring (patient "wakes the dead"); daytime sleepiness; and witnessed apneas (most sensitive medical history question: "Have you ever been told that you stop breathing while you are sleeping?")
    - Patients also describe sleep as nonrefreshing, complain of morning headaches, and experience irritability/personality change/depression, cognitive impairment, and decreased libido
    - Nocturia/enuresis may also be seen
  - **Physical examination findings in OSA include obesity, increased neck circumference, large tonsils and adenoids, large uvula, low soft palate, systemic hypertension, and lower extremity edema**
    - Retrognathia, micrognathia, and other craniofacial abnormalities also described
    - Medical consequences of OSA are listed in Table 22-1

BOX 22-1 | *Risk Factors for Obstructive Sleep Apnea*

Gender
  Male:female ratio, 2:1
  Risk increases for postmenopausal women
Age
  Predominantly 40 to 70 years old
Body habitus
  Obese (body mass index >30 kg/m^2)
Alcohol use
Medications
  Sedatives
  Hypnotics
Endocrine disease
  Acromegaly
  Hypothyroidism

BOX 22-2 | *Clinical Conditions and Diseases Associated with Central Sleep Apnea*

Stroke
Stable methadone maintenance treatment
Multiple system atrophy (Shy-Drager syndrome)
Autonomic dysfunction
Myasthenia gravis
Neuromuscular disease
Bulbar poliomyelitis
Encephalitis

TABLE 22-1 | *Medical Consequences of Obstructive Sleep Apnea*

Cardiovascular Effects	Noncardiovascular Effects
Systemic hypertension	Cognitive impairment
Pulmonary hypertension	Motor vehicle accidents
Congestive heart failure	Work-related accidents
Coronary artery disease	Sexual dysfunction
Nocturnal arrhythmias	Impaired quality of life
Stroke	

- CSA
  - History findings include daytime sleepiness and witnessed apneas
    - Snoring not a prominent finding
  - Physical examination findings in CSA:
    - Patients may have any body habitus
    - Underlying neurologic disease, if present, determines many of the physical findings

Diagnosis and Evaluation

- Diagnosis of an apnea syndrome is made by an overnight polysomnogram (PSG) sleep study (Fig. 22-1)
- Physiologic parameters measured include airflow, chest/abdominal wall effort, oxygen saturation, electroencephalogram (EEG), electrocardiogram (ECG), electrooculogram (EOG), and body position
- Recording time should be 6 to 8 hours

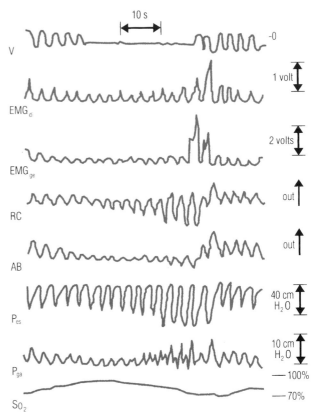

FIGURE 22-1 Polysomnogram in obstructive sleep apnea. The study shows a period when ventilation is obstructed and there is no airflow (V). At this time, the diaphragm continues to contract (EMG$_{di}$), esophageal (P$_{es}$) and gastric (P$_{ga}$) pressure swings occur, and there is ribcage and abdominal movement (RC and AB). As obstruction continues, arterial oxygen saturation (SO$_2$) falls. Eventually the activity of the upper airway muscles, including the genioglossus muscle (EMG$_{ge}$), increases, the upper airway becomes patent, and airflow is restored. Patients can have hundreds of similar episodes during the night. (From Onal E, Lopata M, O'Connor T. Pathogenesis of apneas in hypersomnia-sleep syndrome. *Am Rev Respir Dis.* 1982;125:167; and Souhami R. *Textbook of Medicine.* New York: Churchill Livingstone; 2002: Fig. 13.42.)

- **If AHI is more than five events per hour, sleep study is positive for sleep apnea**
  - **OSA versus CSA is determined by presence versus absence of chest/abdominal wall efforts, respectively**
    - Mild: 6 to 15 events per hour
    - Moderate: 16 to 30 events per hour
    - Severe: more than 30 events per hour

Treatment

- OSA
  - Three components to treatment: behavioral, medical, and surgical (Table 22-2)
  - **Behavioral treatment is commonly the only intervention recommended for patients with mild OSA**
  - Compliance is a major problem with nasal continuous positive airway pressure (CPAP) (Fig. 22-2); discomfort of apparatus, claustrophobia,

aerophagia, and difficulty with exhalation are common side effects
- CSA
  - Nasal CPAP usually not effective
  - Treatment of choice: nocturnal nasal noninvasive ventilation with a backup respiratory rate and bilevel (inspiratory and expiratory) positive airway pressure (BiPAP) settings
  - Ventilatory stimulants (e.g., acetazolamide) have not proven useful

Solitary Pulmonary Nodule

Basic Information

- Pulmonary nodule: A single, well-defined lesion, usually rounded or slightly ovoid, surrounded by normal lung tissue
  - **Diameter must be 3 cm or less**
    - **If diameter greater than 3 cm, process is called a mass, of which 90% are malignant**

- Solitary pulmonary nodules are found in 1 of every 500 chest radiographs
  - Nodular mimics: nipple shadows, skin moles, prominent costochondral junction
- Etiologies (Table 22-3)
  - **Sixty percent benign (most common: healed granulomas secondary to tuberculosis or fungal infection)**
  - **Forty percent malignant (most common: bronchogenic carcinoma)**

Clinical Presentation

- The solitary pulmonary nodule is usually an unexpected finding on routine chest film
  - Most patients are asymptomatic; some have cough

Diagnosis and Evaluation

- Key features of the history include
  - Age (malignancy uncommon in patients younger than 35 years old)
  - Smoking (increases likelihood of malignancy)
  - Occupational exposure (e.g., asbestos, silica)

TABLE 22-2	*Treatment of Obstructive Sleep Apnea*	
Modality	**Options**	**Comments**
Behavioral	Weight loss Avoidance of alcohol, sedatives, and hypnotics Position therapy	Small amounts of weight loss can significantly improve symptoms Lateral decubitus sleeping position helps alleviate symptoms in many
Medical	Nasal continuous positive airway pressure (CPAP) Oral appliances Protriptyline Medroxyprogesterone acetate Oxygen	Nasal CPAP is treatment of choice for moderate to severe obstructive sleep apnea (OSA); apnea, snoring, daytime somnolence, and hypertension all may improve Oral appliances most useful in retrognathia and micrognathia; not effective in severe OSA No medication has been shown to be successful in treating OSA Medroxyprogesterone increases respiratory drive and improves daytime arterial blood gases but has no effect on OSA
Surgical	Nasal surgery (e.g., septoplasty, sinus surgery) Tonsillectomy/adenoidectomy Uvulopalatopharyngoplasty (UPPP) Laser-assisted uvuloplasty Maxillofacial surgery Tracheostomy	Nasal surgery rarely effective in directly treating OSA Tonsillectomy/adenoidectomy most effective in children UPPP most common surgical procedure for OSA but at least 50% will not improve Tracheostomy 100% effective but should be reserved for patients with severe/incapacitating disease that has failed standard aggressive therapy

Untreated OSA

Obstructive sleep apnea treated with CPAP

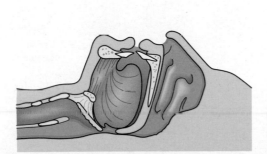 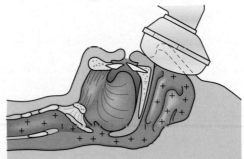

FIGURE 22-2 Effect of continuous positive airway pressure (CPAP) on obstructive sleep apnea (OSA). The chief mechanism of CPAP in the treatment of OSA is airway splinting and dilation of obstructed pharyngeal segments. (From Albert RK, Spiro SG, Jett JR. *Clinical Respiratory Medicine.* 2nd ed. St. Louis: Mosby; 2004: Fig. 71-9.)

| TABLE 22-3 | Causes of the Solitary Pulmonary Nodule |

Benign Causes	Malignant Causes
Infectious granuloma (tuberculosis, histoplasmosis, coccidioidomycosis)	Bronchogenic carcinoma
Hamartoma	Bronchial carcinoid
"Round" pneumonia	Pulmonary lymphoma
Bronchogenic cyst	Pulmonary sarcoma
Pulmonary infarction	Solitary metastasis from extrapulmonary site
Arteriovenous malformation	
Rheumatoid nodule	
Wegener granulomatosis	
Amyloidosis	
Parasitic infection (e.g., *Ascaris, Echinococcus*)	

- History of cancer
- Travel or history of living in endemic area
  - **Mississippi and Ohio River valleys: suggests histoplasmosis (most common); blastomycosis**
  - **Southwestern United States: suggests coccidioidomycosis**
- Physical examination
  - Most patients have a normal lung examination
  - Occasionally, with a proximally located nodule, a localized wheeze (from airway impingement) may be present
  - Clubbing may be present with a malignant pulmonary nodule
- Further imaging (Fig. 22-3)
  - The initial step is always to locate older chest imaging to evaluate stability or change in size of the nodule; allows approximate calculation of doubling time
  - **Doubling time of 25 to 450 days suggests a malignant process**
  - **Doubling time of less than 25 days or more than 450 days suggests a benign process**
  - Doubling time refers to the volume of the nodule (i.e., an increase of 28% in nodule diameter indicates doubling)
- Chest computed tomography (CT): Important for defining the characteristics of the nodule (Table 22-4)
- The pattern of calcification, if present, may be useful in diagnosis (Figs. 22-4 and 22-5)
  - Hamartomas have a "popcorn" calcification pattern or areas of low-attenuation fat deposits (or both) (Fig. 22-6)
  - Pulmonary arteriovenous malformations (AVMs) fill with contrast material
- Positron emission tomography (PET): Used to define metabolic activity of pulmonary nodule
  - In general, malignant lesions have an increased rate of label uptake compared with benign lesions or normal tissue; however, active infections, granulomatous diseases, and other inflammatory conditions also can have increased uptake (false positives)
  - False negatives can occur with small tumors (<1 cm), tumors with low metabolic activity (e.g., bronchial carcinoid), and hyperglycemia

| TABLE 22-4 | Characteristics Suggestive of Benign and Malignant Pulmonary Nodules |

Characteristic	Benign	Malignant
Size	<2 cm	>2 cm
Edge	Smooth, sharp	Spiculated, ragged
Cavitation	No	Yes
Satellite lesions	Yes	No
Doubling time	<25 days or >450 days	25 to 450 days

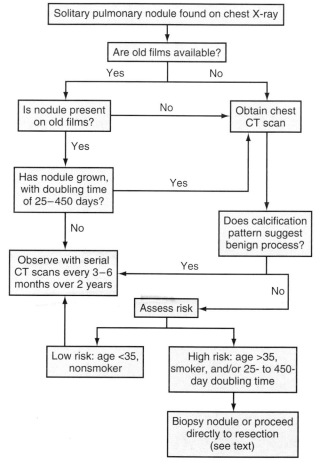

FIGURE 22-3 Management of the solitary pulmonary nodule. CT, Computed tomography.

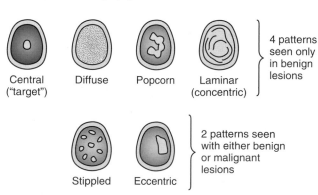

FIGURE 22-4 Calcification patterns in solitary pulmonary nodules. (Modified from Lillington GA. Management of solitary pulmonary nodules. *Dis Mon.* 1991;37:271.)

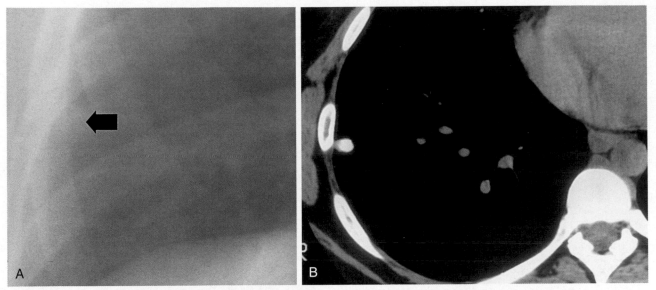

FIGURE 22-5 The use of computed tomography (CT) to characterize a solitary pulmonary nodule. **A,** Chest radiograph shows a peripheral nodule *(arrow)* that does not appear to be calcified. **B,** CT scan through the nodule demonstrates dense, diffuse calcification, consistent with a benign lesion. The other gray densities on the scan are pulmonary vessels rather than nodules. (From Mason RJ. *Murray and Nadel's Textbook of Respiratory Medicine.* 4th ed. Philadelphia: Saunders; 2005: Fig. 20-36.)

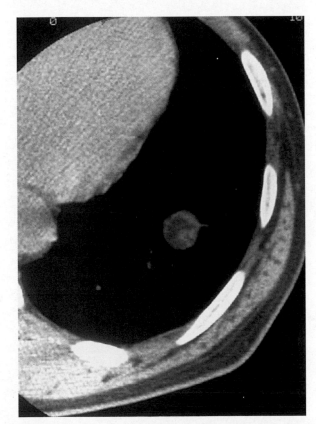

FIGURE 22-6 Hamartoma. Computed tomography scan shows low attenuation within the solitary pulmonary nodule, consistent with fat. (From Mason RJ. *Murray and Nadel's Textbook of Respiratory Medicine.* 4th ed. Philadelphia: Saunders; 2005: Fig. 20-37.)

- For diagnosis of malignant solitary pulmonary nodules, sensitivity is 97%, and specificity is 82%
- Role in evaluating solitary pulmonary nodules is still being determined; most useful in borderline cases, with biopsy recommended if PET scan positive

Treatment

- General principles
  - The Fleischner Society recommendations provide widely used guidance for the follow-up of the solitary pulmonary nodule (Table 22-5)
  - If a nodule has grown with a doubling time of 25 to 450 days and the patient's cardiopulmonary status permits surgery, thoracotomy with resection is indicated
  - **Solid pulmonary nodules less than 1 cm in size** that are stable for 2 years are most likely benign and do not require further follow-up
  - If no previous films are available, the patient's risk of cancer must be assessed to determine whether the approach should be observation or biopsy (see Fig. 22-3)
- Biopsy techniques
  - Fiberoptic bronchoscopy: Limited usefulness in evaluation of the solitary pulmonary nodule
    - Most useful if the nodule is greater than 2 cm in diameter, is located proximally, or has a bronchus leading into it on chest CT
    - Diagnostic yield: 10% to 20% if less than 2 cm, 55% if greater than 2 cm
  - Percutaneous transthoracic needle aspiration: Usually performed with CT guidance
    - Most useful for peripheral lesions in the outer one third of the lung
    - **Higher diagnostic yield than bronchoscopic biopsy: 80% to 95% (even in lesions less than 2 cm)**

22

TABLE 22-5	*Fleischner Society Guidelines for Nodule Follow-up*	
Nodule Size (mm)	**Low-Risk* Patient**	**High-Risk† Patient**
<4	No follow-up needed	Follow-up computed tomography (CT) at 12 months; if unchanged, no further follow-up
>4–6	Follow-up CT at 12 months; if unchanged, no further follow-up	Initial follow-up CT at 6 to 12 months, then at 18 to 24 months if no change
>6–8	Initial follow-up CT at 6 to 12 months, then at 18 to 24 months if no change	Initial follow-up CT at 3 to 6 months, then at 9 to 12 months if no change
>8	Follow-up at around 3, 9, and 24 months, dynamic contrast-enhanced CT, positron emission tomography, biopsy	Same as for low-risk patients

*Low risk: Minimal or no smoking history and no other risk factors (e.g., family history of lung cancer in a first degree relative, exposure to asbestos, radon, or uranium).
†High risk: Smoking history or other risk factors.
From Padley SPG, Lazoura O. Pulmonary neoplasms. In Adam A, Dixon AK, et al, eds. *Grainger & Allison's Diagnostic Radiology.* 6th ed. Philadelphia: Churchill Livingstone; 2015: Table 15.1; Modified from MacMahon H, Austin JH, Gamsu G, et al. Guidelines for management of small pulmonary nodules detected on CT scans: a statement from the Fleischner Society. *Radiology.* 2005;237:395–400.

- Major limitation: 10% to 30% rate of pneumothorax
- Once diagnosis is confirmed, treatment can be directed appropriately

Hemoptysis

Basic Information

- Hemoptysis: expectoration of blood from the airways
- Pathophysiology: **In the majority of cases, hemoptysis originates from bronchial arterial circulation**
  - Bronchial arteries increase in size and number in the setting of chronic inflammation (e.g., bronchiectasis) or malignancy and are susceptible to rupture
  - Bleeding may be profuse because of the high pressure of the systemic circulation
  - **Clinically significant bleeding from pulmonary arterial circulation is rare because it is a low-pressure system, and hypoxic pulmonary vasoconstriction diverts blood flow away from diseased portions of the lung**
- Causes are listed in Box 22-3
  - Bronchitis and bronchogenic carcinoma, the two most common causes, account for 40% and 25% of cases, respectively

Clinical Presentation

- Amount of blood may be small or large; massive hemoptysis is defined most commonly as a loss of more than 600 mL of blood in 24 hours
- Hemoptysis may be accompanied by mucopurulent sputum and fever (bacterial pneumonia), hematuria (pulmonary–renal syndromes, including Goodpasture syndrome), or prominent sinusitis (i.e., granulomatosis with polyangiitis), the presence of which may offer clues to etiology

Diagnosis and Evaluation

- Key features of the history start with a careful questioning of the patient's symptoms to help determine source of blood; many patients confuse hemoptysis with hematemesis or epistaxis

BOX 22-3	*Causes of Hemoptysis*

Infectious
Bronchitis
Bronchiectasis
Pneumonia
Tuberculosis

Neoplastic
Bronchogenic carcinoma
Bronchial carcinoid
Pulmonary metastasis from other site

Cardiovascular
Congestive heart failure
Mitral stenosis
Pulmonary embolism/infarction
Pulmonary arteriovenous malformation

Miscellaneous
Idiopathic (as much as 20% to 30% of cases)
Lung contusion
Goodpasture syndrome
Granulomatosis with polyangiitis
Smoking freebase cocaine ("crack")
Pseudohemoptysis (from *Serratia marcescens* pneumonia)

- Other features include estimation of the quantity of blood and the duration of bleeding
- Physical examination
  - Crackles or rhonchi may be present in the area of the bleeding and can help localize site of bleeding
- Radiographic studies
  - Chest radiograph should be obtained in every patient and may suggest the diagnosis
    - Nodule or mass suggests neoplasm
    - Lobar atelectasis suggests obstructing endobronchial lesion
    - **Mass within a cavity ("air crescent sign") suggests aspergilloma (fungus ball)** (Fig. 22-7)
  - Thickened bronchial walls ("tram tracking") suggest bronchiectasis
  - Thirty percent of patients have normal or nonlocalizing chest films

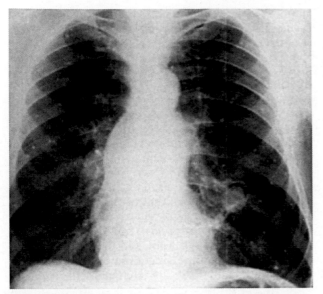

FIGURE 22-7 Chest radiograph showing an aspergilloma in the left lower lung zone of an asymptomatic patient. A dark rim of air is readily seen around the upper edge of the fungus ball ("air crescent sign"). (From Mason RJ. *Murray and Nadel's Textbook of Respiratory Medicine.* 4th ed. Philadelphia: Saunders; 2005: Fig. 34-15.)

- Chest CT is generally not an important tool for evaluation of hemoptysis, except in those patients with normal or nonlocalizing chest radiographs
- Fiberoptic bronchoscopy: the invasive procedure of choice for nonmassive hemoptysis
  - Helpful for localizing the bleeding side or the specific site of bleeding
  - Not useful for massive hemoptysis (field of vision through bronchoscope is obscured by large amounts of blood)

Treatment

- Therapy should be directed at the underlying cause of the hemoptysis (e.g., antibiotics for bronchitis or pneumonia; diuresis for congestive heart failure; resection and chemotherapy/radiotherapy for bronchogenic carcinoma)
- Massive hemoptysis requires special attention
  - **Airway protection: Position patient with the bleeding lung in the dependent position (prevents spillage of blood into the nonbleeding lung)**
    - Intubation may be needed to isolate the lungs from each other, using a double-lumen endotracheal tube
  - Fluid resuscitation to support volume
    - Initial management: crystalloid intravenous fluids
    - Blood products in patients who are anemic, coagulopathic, and/or bleeding rapidly
  - Gentle cough suppression to prevent the airway trauma of vigorous coughing
    - Avoid excessive cough suppression because airway compromise can result
  - Correction of coagulopathy, if present
  - Bronchial artery embolization is effective at immediately halting bleeding in 80% to 95% of patients
    - Thirty percent will re-bleed within 3 months

BOX 22-4 *Causes of Secondary Pulmonary Hypertension*

Cardiac Disease
Congenital
Eisenmenger syndrome
Left-sided heart failure

Parenchymal Lung Disease
Chronic obstructive pulmonary disease
Interstitial lung disease

Vascular Impairment
Chronic thromboembolic disease
Pulmonary veno-occlusive disease
Sickle cell disease

Infections
HIV
Schistosomiasis

Drugs/Toxins
Anorexigens

Miscellaneous
Obstructive sleep apnea
Collagen vascular diseases (through either direct vascular effect or interstitial changes in the parenchyma)

- Surgery: Indicated for massive, unilateral hemoptysis unresponsive to other measures, provided that the patient has adequate pulmonary reserve
  - High mortality rate (35%) for patients actively bleeding at time of surgery

Pulmonary Hypertension

Basic Information

- Normal pulmonary artery (PA) pressures are 18 to 30 mm Hg systolic and 4 to 12 mm Hg diastolic
- **Pulmonary hypertension is defined as mean PA pressure greater than 25 mm Hg at rest**
  - Severe pulmonary hypertension is defined as mean PA pressure 40 mm Hg or greater at rest
- **Traditionally classified as either primary or secondary (Box 22-4 lists causes of secondary pulmonary hypertension)**

Clinical Presentation

- Demographics
  - **Primary pulmonary hypertension, now usually called idiopathic pulmonary arterial hypertension (IPAH), is three times more common in women than in men and generally occurs in younger patients (typical age of onset is 20 to 40 years)**
- Symptoms
  - Similar for both primary and secondary etiologies, though for the latter, other symptoms of the underlying disorder may be present (e.g., snoring and hypersomnolence in OSA, skin changes in scleroderma)
  - Patients with mild pulmonary hypertension are usually asymptomatic

- Exertional dyspnea is most common presenting complaint
- May also have chest pain or dizziness; syncope portends a poor prognosis

Diagnosis and Evaluation

- Physical examination
  - **Prominent pulmonic component (P$_2$) of the S$_2$ is a reliable indicator of elevated PA pressure**
  - May also see elevated jugular venous pressure with large A wave, left parasternal heave (from right ventricular hypertrophy), right-sided S$_3$, or tricuspid regurgitation murmur
  - Pedal edema common
- Chest radiography
  - Shows enlarged pulmonary arteries with rapid tapering of vessels toward the periphery of the lungs (a "pruned tree" appearance) (Fig. 22-8)
  - May also see right-heart enlargement
  - For secondary pulmonary hypertension caused by parenchymal lung disease, look for hyperinflation and bullous disease (suggestive of COPD) or increased interstitial markings (suggestive of interstitial lung disease)
- Other studies
  - Echocardiography:
    - Permits evaluation for signs of right ventricular pressure overload, including paradoxical bulging of the septum into the left ventricle during systole and hypertrophy of the right ventricular free wall
    - Doppler estimates of PA pressure based on velocity of tricuspid regurgitation can suggest the presence of pulmonary hypertension but do not correlate well with directly measured PA pressure

- Pulmonary function tests: Typically show decreased diffusing capacity
- Ventilation-perfusion scan: Helps identify patients with secondary pulmonary hypertension caused by chronic thromboembolic disease, but IPAH can also produce abnormal scans
- Right-heart catheterization: Permits direct measurement of PA pressure, and with angiography, a definitive diagnosis of chronic thromboembolic disease

Treatment

- IPAH
  - Right-heart catheterization should be performed in all patients to determine if there is a positive response to acute administration of a vasodilator (typically nitric oxide)
    - **Five percent to 10% of patients are "responders" (PA pressure declines by at least 10 mm Hg to a value less than 40 mm Hg) and should be treated with oral calcium channel blockers**
    - **"Nonresponders" have an increased risk of death with calcium channel blockers and should receive other therapy (prostacyclin, endothelin receptor antagonist, or phosphodiesterase-5 inhibitor)**
  - Continuous infusion of epoprostenol (prostacyclin), a direct pulmonary vasodilator, is indicated in patients with New York Heart Association class III or IV symptoms
    - Adverse effects of epoprostenol include flushing and diarrhea
    - Prostacyclin analogues: treprostinil, iloprost

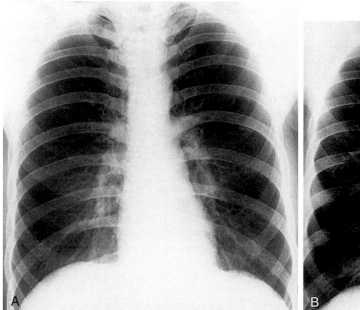 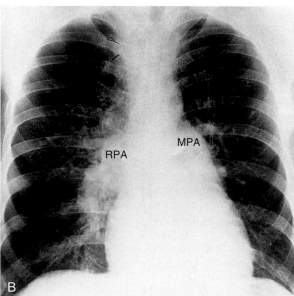

FIGURE 22-8 Progressive pulmonary arterial hypertension. **A,** The patient initially had a normal chest radiograph. **B,** Several years later, however, increasing heart size and marked dilation of the main pulmonary artery (MPA) and right pulmonary artery (RPA) are noted. Pulmonary artery enlargement can be recognized by a bulging along the left cardiac border just below the aortic arch. (From Mettler FA. *Essentials of Radiology.* 2nd ed. Philadelphia: Saunders; 2005: Fig. 5-12.)

- Other treatment options
  - Endothelin receptor antagonists (e.g., bosentan, ambrisentan) directly oppose the vasoconstricting effects of endothelin-1
  - Phosphodiesterase-5 inhibitors (e.g., sildenafil, tadalafil) enhance nitric oxide-mediated vasodilation
  - Clinical studies are evaluating combination therapy with more than one of the various classes of drugs
  - **Long-term anticoagulation is indicated in all patients to prevent intravascular thrombosis in the pulmonary circulation as well as deep venous thrombosis**
  - Many patients require long-term diuretic therapy
  - Supplemental oxygen
- Secondary pulmonary hypertension
  - Treat underlying disease
  - Epoprostenol and bosentan are used frequently for secondary pulmonary hypertension caused by scleroderma
  - Sildenafil is used increasingly in a variety of secondary settings
  - Long-term anticoagulation should be instituted for all patients with severe pulmonary hypertension, provided there is no contraindication
  - Supplemental oxygen helps reduce hypoxic pulmonary vasoconstriction
  - For severe chronic thromboembolic pulmonary hypertension, consider pulmonary thromboendarterectomy

Review Questions

For review questions, please go to ExpertConsult.com.

SUGGESTED READINGS

Badesch DB, Champion HC, Sanchez MA, et al. Diagnosis and assessment of pulmonary arterial hypertension. *J Am Coll Cardiol.* 2009;54:S55-S66.

Corder R. Hemoptysis. *Emerg Med Clin North Am.* 2003;21:421-435.

Epstein LJ, Kristo D, Strollo PJ Jr, et al. Clinical guideline for the evaluation, management and long-term care of obstructive sleep apnea in adults. *J Clin Sleep Med.* 2009;5:263-276.

Flemons WW. Clinical practice: obstructive sleep apnea. *N Engl J Med.* 2002;347:498-504.

Galiè N, Corris PA, Frost A, et al. Updated treatment algorithm of pulmonary arterial hypertension. *J Am Coll Cardiol.* 2013;62:D60-D72.

Jean-Baptiste E. Clinical assessment and management of massive hemoptysis. *Crit Care Med.* 2000;28:1642-1647.

Lillington GA. Management of solitary pulmonary nodules. *Dis Mon.* 1991;37:271-318.

Malhotra A, White DP. Obstructive sleep apnoea. *Lancet.* 2002;360:237-245.

Ost D, Fein AM, Feinsilver SH. Clinical practice: the solitary pulmonary nodule. *N Engl J Med.* 2003;348:2535-2542.

Runo JR, Loyd JE. Primary pulmonary hypertension. *Lancet.* 2003;361:1533-1544.

Wahidi MM, Govert JA, Goudar RK, et al. Evidence for the treatment of patients with pulmonary nodules: when is it lung cancer? ACCP evidence-based clinical practice guidelines (ed 2). *Chest.* 2007;132:94S-107S.

Critical Care Medicine

DAVID N. HAGER, MD, PhD

Critical care medicine focuses on the management of life-threatening illnesses often caused by acute organ failure. This chapter addresses common presenting syndromes and diagnoses encountered in the Medical Intensive Care Unit (MICU). These include acute respiratory failure (acute respiratory distress syndrome [ARDS], chronic obstructive pulmonary disease [COPD], pneumonia), sepsis and septic shock, and toxin exposures. Recent emphasis on minimizing and preventing the complications of critical care therapies is also highlighted here, with special mention of delirium assessment and management. Although patients who experience failure of other organ systems (e.g., heart, liver, kidney, central nervous system) are frequently managed in the MICU, the critical care required to manage those systems is captured in other chapters of this book.

Acute Respiratory Failure

Basic Information

- Two pathophysiologic causes of acute respiratory failure:
  - **Failure of oxygenation**
    - **Defined as an inadequate arterial partial pressure of O_2 (PaO_2 less than 60 mm Hg) despite high levels of supplemental inspired O_2**
    - Five major etiologic classes of hypoxemia
      - Right-to-left shunt via pathologic vascular communications (e.g., pulmonary arteriovenous malformations [AVMs], intracardiac right-to-left shunts) or space-filling pulmonary parenchymal lesions (e.g., atelectasis or pneumonia)
      - Supplemental O_2 should be administered, but frequently has very modest effect on PaO_2; alveolar-arterial (A–a) gradient remains high
      - Ventilation-perfusion ($\dot{V}/\dot{Q}$) mismatch: Regional imbalances between ventilation and blood flow (e.g., COPD, asthma, other lung parenchymal disease, and pulmonary embolism)
        - Corrects partially or completely, with the addition of supplemental O_2; A–a gradient improves
      - Reduced diffusion capacity (e.g., interstitial lung disease, emphysema). Little to no hypoxemia at rest
        - More pronounced with exercise
        - Supplemental O_2 improves oxygenation; A–a gradient improves
      - Alveolar hypoventilation (e.g., from central nervous system [CNS] depression, neuromuscular disease, chest wall abnormality, acute increase in dead space as with pulmonary embolism)
        - Normal (A–a) gradient
        - Easily managed with ventilatory support and/or supplemental O_2
      - Low partial pressure of inspired O_2 (e.g., high altitude). Normal A–a gradient at rest, which may increase with exertion. Easily managed with supplemental O_2
  - **Failure of ventilation**
    - Defined as elevated arterial partial pressure of carbon dioxide (PaCO_2 greater than 45 mm Hg) with decreased pH
    - Caused by either
      - Increased CO_2 production (e.g., sepsis, overfeeding, thyrotoxicosis, burns)
      - Decreased CO_2 elimination
    - Ultimately because of decreased alveolar ventilation
      - Airways disease (e.g., COPD, asthma)
      - Acute increase in dead space (e.g., pneumonia or large pulmonary embolus) in the absence of maintained alveolar ventilation
    - Decreased minute ventilation (e.g., CNS depression, obesity hypoventilation, Guillain-Barré, myasthenia gravis, amyotrophic lateral sclerosis)

Clinical Presentation

- Depends on underlying cause
- Agitation or altered mental status commonly seen in hypoxia and hypercarbia
- **Cyanosis occurs only after deoxyhemoglobin level is greater than 5 g/dL, which corresponds to an arterial O_2 saturation (SaO_2) at approximately 67%**

Diagnosis and Evaluation

- **Pulse oximeter may be unreliable in the following situations:**
  - On the steep portion of the oxyhemoglobin dissociation curve (i.e., at saturation levels less than 90%; Fig. 23-1)
  - Patients with carboxyhemoglobin or methemoglobin (may overestimate oxyhemoglobin)
  - Patients with decreased peripheral perfusion (e.g., shock)
  - Patients with pigmented skin or nail polish
- Arterial blood gas measurement is the gold standard
  - Most O_2 is delivered to tissues bound to hemoglobin, which is reflected in measured saturation obtained

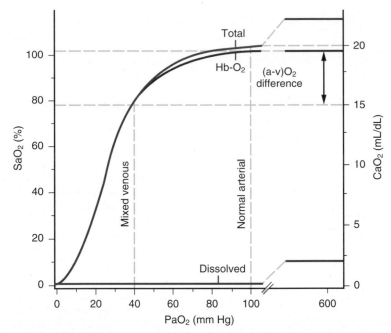

FIGURE 23-1 Oxyhemoglobin dissociation curve. (a-v)O_2 difference, Arteriovenous O_2 difference; CaO_2, arterial O_2 content; Hb-O_2, O_2 bound to hemoglobin; SaO_2, arterial O_2 saturation; PaO_2, arterial partial pressure of O_2. (From Goldman L, Bennett JC, Ausiello D. *Cecil Textbook of Medicine*. 22nd ed. Philadelphia; Saunders: 2004: Fig. 100.5.)

TABLE 23-1	*Criteria for Use of Noninvasive Ventilation*	
Disease	**Patient Characteristics**	**Contraindications**
COPD exacerbation	Hypercapnic respiratory failure (pH 7.25 to 7.35, RR 20 to 25) Able to manage secretions	Shock Not able to tolerate mask GCS score <8
Respiratory failure in immunosuppressed patients with bilateral infiltrates	Immunosuppression (e.g., bone marrow transplantation, HIV, or postchemotherapy neutropenia)	Shock Not able to tolerate mask GCS score <8

COPD, Chronic obstructive pulmonary disease; GCS, Glasgow Coma Scale; HIV, human immunodeficiency virus; RR, respiratory rate.

with arterial blood gas (SaO_2) rather than dissolved in the plasma (i.e., measured by PaO_2)

- **Consider positive pressure ventilation, in conjunction with a tight-fitting mask (noninvasive) or endotracheal intubation when PaO_2 is less than 60 to 70 mm Hg with FiO_2 greater than 80% or PaCO_2 45 mm Hg or more with pH less than 7.30**
- **Work of breathing (high respiratory rate with use of accessory muscles) and ability to protect airway are additional important considerations**

Treatment

- **Supplemental O_2 to maintain O_2 saturation greater than 88% or PaO_2 greater than 55 mm Hg**
- Do not deliver inadequate amounts of O_2 because of concern over suppressing central respiratory drive; this is a rare complication. A target O_2 saturation of 88% to 92% should limit likelihood of suppressing a hypercapnic patient's hypoxic drive to breathe
- Consider whether patient is a noninvasive ventilation candidate (Table 23-1)

- A trial of noninvasive ventilation in patients not requiring immediate intubation is reasonable in some patients, but a low threshold to convert to invasive ventilation should be maintained if the patient does not stabilize quickly
- Noninvasive ventilation decreases complications such as ventilator-associated pneumonia, decreases length of ICU stay, and improves mortality rates for selected patients with hypercarbic respiratory failure in the setting of COPD, cardiogenic pulmonary edema, and immunosuppressed patients with bilateral infiltrates and hypoxemic respiratory failure
- Mechanical ventilation (Box 23-1)
  - Treat underlying cause of respiratory failure (e.g., antibiotics for pneumonia, bronchodilators and corticosteroids for status asthmaticus)
  - Protocol-driven interruptions of sedation combined with daily spontaneous breathing trials decreases ventilator days, ICU length of stay, and 1-year mortality
  - Benzodiazepines should be limited when possible because they contribute to agitated delirium and increase time spent on the ventilator, especially when used as a continuous infusion

BOX 23-1 | *Mechanical Ventilation*

Types

Volume cycled: Ventilator delivers a set volume, using whatever pressure is required to overcome airway resistance and lung compliance. Examples include assist volume control and synchronized intermittent mandatory ventilation.

Assist volume control: Patient receives a set tidal volume for every initiated breath. A preset number of breaths/min prevents hypoventilation.

Synchronized intermittent mandatory ventilation (SIMV): Patient receives a set tidal volume for only a designated number of breaths/min. Additional nonmandatory breaths have either no support or limited pressure support. Size of nonmandatory breaths dependent on patient effort and magnitude of pressure support provided.

Pressure cycled: Ventilator maintains a set pressure; tidal volume delivered depends on lung mechanics. Examples include assist pressure control and pressure support ventilation.

Assist pressure control: Patient receives set inspiratory pressure and mandatory minimum respiratory rate. The magnitude of all breaths (programmed or patient-initiated) are dependent on respiratory system compliance and patient effort.

Pressure support: Ventilator provides a constant preset pressure for each patient-initiated breath. Size of nonmandatory breaths dependent on patient effort and magnitude of pressure support provided. Often used as a weaning mode. Should not be used in patients without intact respiratory drive.

Complications

Auto–positive end-expiratory pressure (PEEP) (dynamic hyperinflation): Caused by air trapping because of inadequate emptying during expiration in patient with airflow obstruction (e.g., asthma or chronic obstructive pulmonary disease)

The increased intrathoracic pressure causes increased work of breathing and may decrease venous return to the heart, producing hypotension

Treatment includes disconnecting the patient from the ventilator as a temporary measure if decompensating; changing the ventilator parameters to allow increased expiratory time by increasing inspiratory flow rate; decreasing tidal volume and respiratory rate; and increasing sedation

Volutrauma or barotrauma: Can cause pneumothorax, pneumomediastinum, and diffuse alveolar damage

Increased infection rate: Ventilator-associated pneumonia

Endotracheal tube complications: Subglottal stenosis, vocal cord dysfunction, tracheoesophageal fistula, sinusitis

Noninvasive Ventilation

Definition: Mechanical ventilation without endotracheal intubation

Does not protect airway; avoid using in patients with depressed level of consciousness

Continuous positive airway pressure (CPAP): Constant pressure provided throughout respiratory cycle

Bilevel positive airway pressure (BiPAP): Different pressures provided upon inspiration and expiration

- Consider antipsychotics (e.g.; haloperidol, quetiapine) for management of agitated delirium rather than persistent use of benzodiazepines and narcotics (check daily electrocardiogram for QT prolongation)

Acute Respiratory Distress Syndrome

Definition

The Berlin definition of ARDS requires the following:

- **Respiratory symptom onset within 7 days following known insult *or* progressively worsening symptoms over the past 7 days**
- **Diffuse bilateral infiltrates consistent with pulmonary edema on chest x-ray or chest computed tomographic scan (Fig. 23-2);** infiltrates cannot be explained by pleural effusions, atelectasis, or nodules
- **Respiratory failure cannot be caused by cardiac failure or volume overload.** In the absence of risk factors for ARDS, an echocardiogram to exclude cardiogenic source of infiltrates is needed
- **Severity is based on PaO_2/FiO_2 ratio while on CPAP 5 cm H_2O or greater or end-expiratory pressure of 5 cm H_2O or greater**
  - Mild: PaO_2/FiO_2 less than 300 mm Hg and more than 200 mm Hg
  - Moderate: PaO_2/FiO_2 200 mm Hg or less and more than 100 mm Hg
  - Severe: PaO_2/FiO_2 100 mm Hg or less

Basic Information

- Divided into pulmonary and nonpulmonary causes (although no clear difference in outcomes)
  - **Sepsis and pneumonia are the most common causes**

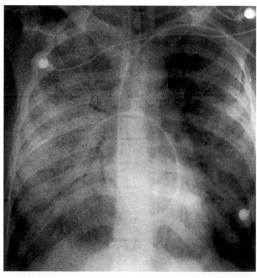

FIGURE 23-2 Chest radiograph of a patient with acute respiratory distress syndrome. Note diffuse bilateral infiltrates. (From Mason RJ. *Murray and Nadel's Textbook of Respiratory Medicine.* 4th ed. Philadelphia: Saunders; 2005: Fig. 51.2.)

- Other common causes: aspiration, irritant gases and smoke inhalation, medications, blood transfusions, burns, pancreatitis, and trauma
  - Rare causes: amniotic fluid embolus, fat emboli, air emboli
- Incidence increases with increasing age
  - At-risk patients who develop ARDS generally do so within 48 to 72 hours of acquiring a risk factor, although some may take as long as a week to meet criteria
- **Overall mortality related to number of organ system failures**
  - Single-organ system failure mortality rate 25% to 40%
  - Three-organ system failure has up to 90% mortality rate
  - Mortality rates increase with age
- **Sepsis and multiorgan system failure most common causes of death**
  - Rare for patients to die solely from intractable hypoxemia
- Survivors of ARDS may have long-term sequelae
  - Two thirds of survivors have minimal to moderate respiratory impairment 1 year after event
  - Recent studies have reported muscle wasting, weakness, and posttraumatic stress disorder as late as 1 year after illness in survivors of ARDS. Only half of the survivors return to work 1 year after discharge. Some neuromuscular and psychiatric sequelae persist 5 years after hospital discharge.

Prevention

- **Early antibiotics and resuscitation for severe sepsis, use of lower tidal volumes in at-risk patients, and conservative use of blood and blood products may reduce the incidence of ARDS**
- The early administration of continuous positive airway pressure (CPAP) ventilation in hematologic malignancy patients with signs of respiratory failure decreases incidence of ARDS

Treatment

- **Use lung-protective ventilatory strategy**
  - **Small tidal volumes (6 mL/kg) coupled with low plateau pressures (less than 30 cm H_2O) help to minimize ventilator-induced lung injury**
  - This approach decreases mortality from ARDS, reduces incidence of multiorgan system failure, and decreases measures of local and systemic inflammation
  - Higher levels of positive end-expiratory pressure (PEEP) coupled with small tidal volume ventilation do not change mortality rates in patients with ARDS
- Use of a conservative fluid management strategy (limiting fluid balance after initial resuscitation has been accomplished) improves lung function and decreases the need for mechanical ventilation without increasing rates of cardiovascular or renal failure
- Prone positioning for at least 16 hours/day for patients with severe ARDS (PaO$_2$/FiO$_2$ of less than 150 mm Hg while on FiO$_2$ of 0.6 and PEEP 5 cm H_2O or greater) in

conjunction with low tidal volumes may reduce mortality from ARDS
- Cis-atracurium infusion in the first 48 hours of mechanical ventilation in patients with severe ARDS (PaO$_2$/FiO$_2$ of less than 150 mm Hg while on PEEP 5 cm H_2O or greater) may also decrease mortality. Increased rates of prolonged neuromuscular weakness were not observed
- Supportive care
  - Mechanical ventilation, treatment of underlying cause, hemodynamic and renal support, and nutritional support if necessary
  - The timing and formulation of enteral nutrition remain controversial
- Attempts to modulate proinflammatory mediators have not led to improved outcomes
- **Corticosteroids to treat late-phase ARDS may be of benefit in carefully selected patients**
- Inhaled nitric oxide improves oxygenation in many patients but has no proven effect on length of ventilation or survival
- Alternate modes of mechanical ventilation, such as high-frequency oscillatory ventilation (HFOV) and airway pressure release ventilation (APRV), may be considered in patients who fail conventional therapy but there is no evidence that they are beneficial. It is reasonable to consider transfer of patients failing standard therapy to high-volume centers with expertise in rescue modes of ventilation, including extracorporeal membrane oxygenation.

Shock

Basic Information

- **Shock is defined as inadequate end-organ perfusion (not synonymous with hypotension)**
- Four types of shock are described (Table 23-2) and result from
  - Failed vascular performance (vasodilatory/distributive shock)
  - Hypovolemia (hemorrhage or other volume loss)
  - Cardiac failure (cardiomyopathy, arrhythmia, valvular lesions)
  - Obstruction to cardiac output (pulmonary embolus, tension pneumothorax, pericardial effusion)

Clinical Presentation

- Decreased urine output
- Decreased peripheral perfusion (e.g., cool extremities, cyanosis)
- Altered mental status
- Tissue hypoxia (elevated lactic acid)

Diagnosis

See Fig. 23-3 for a diagnostic and management algorithm for treating shock.
- The pulmonary artery catheter (PAC) may be useful to distinguish between different types of shock and is the gold standard for measuring cardiac output and cardiac filling pressures. However:
  - Interpretation skills vary

TABLE 23-2	Differentiation of the Four Different Types of Shock*		
Type of Shock	**Cardiac Output**	**Filling Pressure**	**SVR**
Distributive	↑	↓ or normal	↓
Septic Anaphylactic Neurogenic			
Hypovolemic	↓	↓	↑
Volume depletion Hemorrhagic			
Cardiogenic (pump failure)	↓	↑	↑
Extracardiac obstructive	↓	↓ or ↑	↑
Pericardial tamponade Acute PE Air embolism			

*Can be made based on pulmonary artery catheter parameters.
PE, Pulmonary embolism; SVR, systemic vascular resistance.

- Cardiac filling pressures (including wedge pressure) are not always a good surrogate for left ventricular end-diastolic volume
- Routine placement of a PAC does not improve clinical outcomes

Sepsis

Basic Information

- Etiology
  - Bacterial products (e.g., endotoxin, peptidoglycans, teichoic acid) stimulate host defense cells
  - Host defense cells produce proinflammatory mediators (e.g., tumor necrosis factor-α [TNF-α], interleukin-1 [IL-1], IL-6, arachidonic acid metabolites, platelet-activating factor, complement components, and nitric oxide), which recruit PMNs and macrophages
  - Excessive local proinflammatory mediators are released into the systemic circulation and trigger widespread cellular injury
  - **Systemic vasodilatation, hypotension, and vascular permeability follow**
  - Inflammatory mediators promote leukocyte-endothelial adhesion and subsequent endothelial injury, with tissue factor-mediated dysregulation of the coagulation cascade
  - At the tissue level, microthrombi impair O_2 and nutrient delivery, leading to end-organ damage/injury
- Epidemiology
  - Incidence: 80 cases per 100,000 population
    - More common at the extremes of age (i.e., very young or very old)
    - More common in men and in African Americans
  - May occur in the setting of a wide number of infections (i.e., gram-positive, gram-negative, viral, or fungal organisms)
  - The lungs, central venous catheters, and bladder catheters are the most common sites of nosocomial infections in ICU patients
- **Gram-positive organisms now most common cause of sepsis, followed closely by gram-negative organisms**
- Mortality related to severity of sepsis (may also be affected by underlying disease)
  - Sepsis: 10% to 20%
  - Severe sepsis: 20% to 50%
  - Septic shock: 40% to 80%
- Mortality increases with each additional organ system that fails

Clinical Presentation and Diagnosis

- **Bacteremia is defined as the presence of bacteria in the bloodstream**
- **Sepsis syndrome** is defined as the presence of infection (high probability or documented) and at least two of the following signs of systemic inflammation:
  - Temperature (higher than 38°C or lower than 36°C)
  - Pulse (more than 90 beats/min)
  - Respiration rate more than 20 breaths/min (or $PaCO_2$ less than 32)
  - White blood cell count (greater than 12,000/mm³ or less than 4000/mm³) or more than 10% band forms
- Note: Positive blood, urine, or sputum cultures, positive gram stain, or presence of pus not required because patients are sometimes on antibiotics when sepsis develops
- Note: Definition of syndrome is not specific because there are many causes of elevated pulse, temperature, respiration rate in hospitalized patients
- **Severe sepsis defined as sepsis plus organ failure (e.g., renal, hematologic, respiratory, cardiovascular, neurologic)**
- **Septic shock is defined as sepsis with hypotension unresponsive to fluid resuscitation and the presence of end-organ damage**

Treatment

- Timely antibiotics, fluids, and hemodynamic support; renal support if necessary

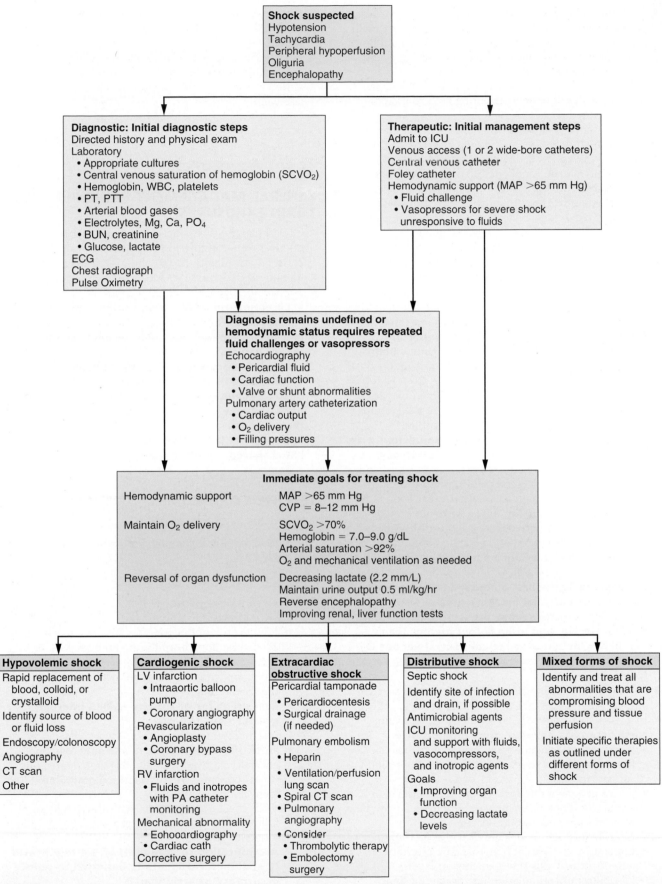

FIGURE 23-3 Diagnosis of shock. BUN, Blood urea nitrogen; Ca, calcium; CT, computed tomography; CVP, central venous pressure; ECG, electrocardiogram; ICU, intensive care unit; LV, left ventricular; MAP, mean arterial pressure; Mg, magnesium; MRI, magnetic resonance imaging; PA, pulmonary artery; PCWP, pulmonary capillary wedge pressure; PO4, phosphate; PT, prothrombin time; PTT, partial thromboplastin time; RV, right ventricular; SCVO2, central venous O2 saturation; WBC, white blood cells. (Modified from Goldman L, Bennett JC, Ausiello D. *Cecil Textbook of Medicine.* 22nd ed. Philadelphia; Saunders: 2004: Fig. 102.3.)

- Volume challenge with 30 mL/kg crystalloids to treat sepsis-related tissue hypoperfusion. Many patients will benefit from more volume, provided they remain fluid responsive based on improvements in pulse pressure, stroke volume, arterial pressure, and heart rate
  - No proven benefit to use of colloids (e.g., albumin) in critically ill patients requiring fluid resuscitation in randomized trials
  - Some forms of volume-expanding starches may worsen clinical outcomes
- Vasopressor support to maintain organ perfusion
  - Norepinephrine is preferred to dopamine as first-line vasopressor in septic shock because of a nonsignificant trend towards increased mortality among patients managed with dopamine. Dopamine is more likely to cause tachyarrhythmias
  - Norepinephrine is a more potent vasopressor
- Vasopressin reduces norepinephrine requirements compared with using norepinephrine alone
  - There may be a mortality benefit to adding vasopressin to patients with less severe shock
- **Antibiotics directed at likely pathogens (site of infection and location of infection important determinants) should be infused within 1 hour** in patients with hypotension caused by sepsis (door-to-infusion time less than 1 hour)
  - Selection of antibiotics should be driven by patient characteristics and the location where the patient developed infection (i.e., home vs hospital)
- **Early antibiotic administration in conjunction with early goal-directed therapy improves outcome** (e.g., protocol-based strategy using fluids, vasopressors, and, if necessary, packed red blood cell transfusions, and endotracheal intubation/mechanical ventilation)
  - In patients with critical illness without coronary artery disease or active bleeding, a transfusion threshold hemoglobin of 7 g/dL is as effective as, and possibly superior to, using a transfusion threshold hemoglobin of 10 g/dL
- **Appropriate early (first 6 hours) treatment goals include mean arterial pressure greater than 65 mm Hg, central venous pressure greater than 8 to 12 mm Hg, and urine output greater than 0.5 mL/kg/h; may also include central venous O₂ saturation greater than 70% and decreasing lactate levels**
- Similar goal-directed therapy late in management (i.e., after 24 hours) does not improve outcomes
- In patients without adrenal suppression at baseline, **corticosteroids have no effect on mortality**
  - Corticosteroids may reduce the incidence of hypotension and shorten duration of vasopressor support in sepsis
  - There may be a role for steroids in patients with sepsis who remain hypotensive despite adequate fluid resuscitation and vasopressor use
  - No role for high-dose (pulsed) corticosteroids
  - Laboratory analyses of hypothalamic-pituitary-adrenocortical axis (random cortisol levels, corticotrophin stimulation testing) are of limited value in selecting whether to use stress-dose steroids in septic shock

- Patients with adrenal suppression at baseline (i.e., on corticosteroids chronically) should receive stress dose steroids
- No benefit seen with attempts to modulate proinflammatory cytokines (e.g., anti-TNF monoclonal antibody, soluble TNF receptor, IL-1 receptor antagonist)
- Supplemental O₂ should be used to increase O₂ delivery

Toxin Exposures

GENERAL MANAGEMENT PRINCIPLES FOR TOXIN EXPOSURES

- Obtain history: time since ingestion, number and type of pills taken, formulation (e.g., extended release), concomitant ingestions (alcohol, illicit drugs)
- Obtain intravenous (IV) access, nasogastric intubation
- Activated charcoal blocks absorption of most drugs
  - **Exceptions include alkali, lithium, iron, and insecticides**
- **Ipecac is no longer routinely recommended to induce emesis**
  - May be used in the alert, awake patient or via nasogastric tube in a patient with poor mental status
- **Gastric lavage is of unproven efficacy, but is often used and may be useful if recent ingestion (less than 1 hour)**
- **Endotracheal intubation should be considered in patients who are obtunded or have a poor gag reflex**

SPECIFIC TOXIDROMES

Analgesics and Sedatives

See Table 23-3 for a summary of analgesic and sedative toxin exposures

Cardioactive Medications

- Tricyclic antidepressants
  - Basic information
    - Possess anticholinergic, α-adrenergic blocking, and adrenergic uptake-inhibiting properties
    - Ingestion of 10 to 20 mg/kg may cause moderate to severe toxicity, and 30 to 40 mg/kg may be life-threatening
    - **Best predictor of toxicity is QRS interval greater than 100 ms**
  - Clinical presentation
    - Arrhythmias, hypotension, and anticholinergic effects (e.g., hyperthermia, flushing, dilated pupils, intestinal ileus, urinary retention, and sinus tachycardia) (Fig. 23-4)
    - CNS effects are common, with initial agitation followed by seizures and depressed consciousness
  - Treatment
    - **Alkalinization to serum pH of 7.4 to 7.5 with IV sodium bicarbonate is indicated to reduce occurrence of arrhythmias**
    - If patient is on a ventilator, may also hyperventilate

TABLE 23-3	*Toxin Exposures: Analgesics and Sedatives*			
Toxin Exposure	**Basic Information**	**Clinical Picture**	**Diagnosis**	**Treatment**
Acetaminophen	Toxicity caused by reactive metabolite Metabolite detoxified by glutathione	Hepatotoxicity: If ingestion >7.5 g, less in alcoholics	Acetaminophen level Nomogram helpful in determining potential for toxicity over time	*N*-Acetylcysteine Best results within 8 hours of exposure May be beneficial up to 24 hours
Salicylate	Uncouples oxidative phosphorylation	Acute toxicity: Respiratory alkalosis Anion gap acidosis Hyperthermia, Coagulopathy Pulmonary edema Hyper- or hypoglycemia Seizures	Salicylate level: >40 mg/dL in acute ingestion >30 mg/dL in chronic ingestion Potential toxicity by dose: <150 mg/kg low risk >300 mg/kg severe toxicity >500 mg/kg may be lethal	Hydration alkalinization of urine Gastric lavage, activated charcoal hemodialysis (for seizures, refractory acidosis, or levels >90 to 100 mg/dL)
Opiates	Bind opiate receptors	Hypotension Respiratory depression CNS depression	Urine testing for opiate metabolites	Naloxone Opiate antagonist Short-acting
Benzodiazepines	Bind the GABA receptor	Hypotension Respiratory depression CNS depression Synergistic effect with opiates	Urine testing for metabolites	Flumazenil Benzodiazepine receptor antagonist Short acting. Use with caution. May precipitate seizures in patients with long-term benzodiazepine use or concomitant TCA overdose

CNS, Central nervous system; GABA, γ-aminobutyric acid; TCA, tricyclic antidepressant.

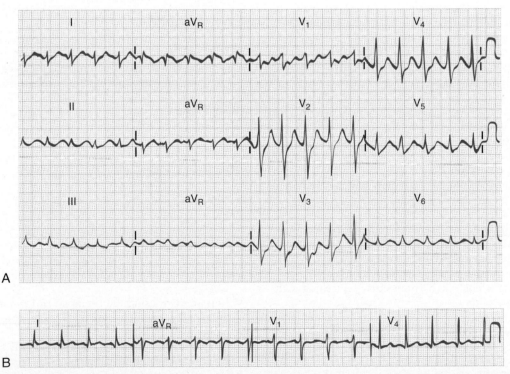

FIGURE 23-4 Electrocardiogram (ECG) in tricyclic antidepressant overdose. **A,** Sinus tachycardia, QRS widening, and QT prolongation in a patient with tricyclic antidepressant overdose. **B,** Normal ECG in the same individual 4 days later. (From Goldberger AL. *Clinical Electrocardiography: A Simplified Approach.* 6th ed. St. Louis; Mosby: 1999: Fig. 10-4.)

- Carefully monitor pH during therapy (pH greater than 7.55 increases risk of seizures)
- β-Blockers
  - Basic information
    - Negative inotropic and chronotropic effects
    - Non–β_1-selective agents may have respiratory effects, and lipophilic agents (e.g., propranolol) can cross blood-brain barrier, causing CNS depression
  - Clinical presentation
    - Hypotension, bradycardia, and varying degrees of heart block
  - Treatment
    - Glucagon
    - IV fluids if hypotensive
    - If needed, pacing and vasopressor or inotrope with β_1 activity
- Calcium channel blockers
  - Basic information
    - Negative inotropic and chronotropic effects
  - Clinical presentation
    - Hypotension, bradycardia, and low cardiac output
  - Treatment
    - 10% calcium chloride
    - If needed, pacing and vasopressor with β and α activity
- Digitalis
  - Basic information
    - Therapeutic inotropic agent/antiarrhythmic with a narrow therapeutic window
  - Clinical presentation
    - Nausea, malaise, weakness, bradycardia, heart block, hyperkalemia, visual complaints of seeing yellow halos around lights
  - Treatment
    - **Digoxin-specific antibody is indicated for hemodynamically compromising conduction disturbances or for hyperkalemia**
    - Calcium is relatively contraindicated because hypercalcemia may potentiate digitalis toxicity
    - Cardiac monitor for at least 6 hours after ingestion
- Theophylline
  - Basic information
    - Methylxanthine bronchodilator with a narrow therapeutic window
  - Clinical presentation
    - Nausea and vomiting, agitation, seizures and arrhythmias, especially supraventricular
  - Treatment
    - **Hemodialysis or charcoal hemoperfusion may be initiated for markedly elevated levels (more than 60 to 100 mg/mL), seizures, or persistently unstable hemodynamics**
    - Supraventricular arrhythmias may be treated with β-blockers

Toxins That Alter Hemoglobin/O_2-Binding Properties

- Carbon monoxide poisoning
  - Basic information
    - Colorless, odorless gas emitted by faulty heaters
    - Seen primarily in winter months
  - Clinical presentation
    - Dizziness, headache, weakness, confusion, dyspnea, chest pain
    - In severe cases: loss of consciousness, focal CNS symptoms, cardiac ischemia
    - Lips and skin may appear cherry red, but this is an insensitive sign
    - Diagnosis is made by measurement of carboxyhemoglobin
  - Treatment
    - Remove patient from the source
    - **Deliver 100% FiO_2 by nonrebreathing mask**
    - **Hyperbaric O_2** appears to prevent delayed neurologic sequelae in high-risk patients (loss of consciousness, confusion, lactic acidosis)
- Methemoglobinemia
  - Basic information
    - Occurs when the ferrous ions (Fe^{2+}) of heme are oxidized to the ferric (Fe^{3+}) state that has a lower affinity for O_2
    - Methemoglobin formation may be caused by exogenous agents, including sulfonamides, nitrates, topical anesthetics, antimalarials, and occupational exposures
    - Higher levels of methemoglobin occur in individuals with deficiency of the cytochrome b_5 reductase enzyme, which reduces Fe^{3+} to the Fe^{2+} state
  - Clinical presentation
    - Hypoxia, cyanosis, and chocolate color of arterial blood
    - **Suggested in a patient with a low pulse oximetry reading, but a normal arterial blood gas PaO_2**
  - Diagnosis
    - Measurement of methemoglobin level by co-oximetry
  - Treatment
    - Discontinuation of the offending agent
    - **Administration of methylene blue to reduce the methemoglobin to hemoglobin**

Alcohols
See Table 23-4 for a summary of alcohol-induced toxicity

Preventing Complications

- Most life-sustaining therapies used in the ICU have potential mechanical or infectious complications (e.g., ventilator-induced lung injury, ventilator-associated pneumonia, central line-associated bloodstream infections, catheter-associated urinary tract infections, medication-induced delirium, critical illness weakness)
- Important to use these therapies only when necessary and to discontinue when risk/benefit ratio no longer favors use
- Use ventilator protocols, especially daily spontaneous breathing trials, to wean patients off ventilators
- Use sterile technique to place catheters; full-body as opposed to local sterile field preferred, chlorhexidine should be used, povidone-iodine solution no longer considered adequate

TABLE 23-4	*Alcohol-induced Toxicity*				
Alcohol	**Example**	**Clinical Presentation**	**Anion Gap***	**Osmolar Gap†**	**Treatment**
Methanol	Antifreeze Bootleg whiskey	Abdominal pain Nausea/vomiting Loss of vision	+	+	Fomepizole (alcohol dehydrogenase inhibitor)
Ethylene glycol	Antifreeze Windshield deicer	Ataxia Seizures, Abdominal pain Nausea/vomiting	+	+	Fomepizole
Isopropanol	Rubbing alcohol	Abdominal pain Nausea/vomiting Headache Ataxia Coma	−	+	Fomepizole

*Anion gap = $[Na^+] - ([Cl-] + [HCO_3-])$.
†Osmolar gap = measured osmolality − $\{2[Na^+] + (BUN/2.8) + ([glucose]/18)\}$.

- Subclavian or internal jugular site less likely to have mechanical or infectious complications than femoral site
- Central venous catheters should be placed under bedside ultrasound guidance when available
- Remove catheters when no longer essential
- Use deep venous thromboembolism prophylaxis for all ICU patients without a strong contraindication
- Stress ulcer prophylaxis for at-risk patients (mechanical ventilation longer than 48 hours or coagulopathy)
- Tight glucose control is no longer indicated given the risks of hypoglycemia, though hyperglycemia should be avoided as well; glucose values should be maintained between 100 and 150 mg/dL
- Sedation protocols to minimize dose of sedatives
  - Daily interruption or nurse-driven protocols are both acceptable
  - Both decrease length of intubation, ICU stay, and days in ICU without delirium
- **Assess for and manage delirium in all patients**
  - ICU delirium is associated with longer hospitalizations and higher long-term mortality
  - Assess for delirium using a validated tool (e.g., Confusion Assessment Method-ICU)
  - Correct/treat physiologic triggers (e.g., electrolyte abnormalities; hypoxia/hypercarbia; uremia; infections)
  - Avoid deliriogenic medications when possible (e.g., narcotics; benzodiazepines; diphenhydramine; metoclopramide; anticholinergics)
  - Avoid/minimize restraints/lines/catheters, redirect/reorient patient frequently, return glasses, hearing aids, and facilitate improved day/night cycles
  - Antipsychotics (e.g., haloperidol/quetiapine) for agitated delirium and as sleep aids rather than benzodiazepines
- Elevation of head of bed 30 to 45 degrees to reduce risk of ventilator-associated pneumonia in intubated patients
- The use of checklists (e.g., when placing a central line; performing a thoracentesis; daily rounding checklists) decreases complications, nosocomial infections, and lengths of stay in critically ill patients in the ICU
- Early mobility, ideally through a nurse-directed protocol to identify eligible patients, should be used in most ICU patients, including many who are still orally intubated

Review Questions

For review questions, please go to ExpertConsult.com.

SUGGESTED READINGS

The Acute Respiratory Distress Syndrome Network. Ventilation with lower tidal volumes as compared with traditional tidal volumes for acute lung injury and the acute respiratory distress syndrome. *N Engl J Med.* 2000;342:1301-1308.

Angus DC, van der Poll T. Severe sepsis and septic shock. *N Engl J Med.* 2013;369:840.

Dellinger RP, Levy MM, Rhodes A, et al. Surviving sepsis campaign: international guidelines for management of severe sepsis and septic shock. *Crit Care Med.* 2012;41:580-637.

Finfer S, Bellamo R, Boyce N, et al. A comparison of albumin and saline for fluid resuscitation in the intensive care unit. *N Engl J Med.* 2004;350:2247-2256.

Girard TD, Kress JP, Fuchs BD, et al. Efficacy and safety of a paired sedation and ventilator weaning protocol for mechanically ventilated patients in intensive care (Awakening and Breathing Controlled trial): a randomized controlled trial. *Lancet.* 2008;371:126-134.

Harvey S, Harrison DA, Singer M, et al. Assessment of the clinical effectiveness of pulmonary artery catheters in management of patients in intensive care (PAC-Man): a randomized controlled trial. *Lancet.* 2005;366:472-477.

Hebert PC, Wells G, Blajchman MA, et al. A multicenter, randomized, controlled clinical trial of transfusion requirements in critical care. Transfusion Requirements in Critical Care Investigators, Canadian Critical Care Trials Group. *N Engl J Med.* 1999;340:409-417.

Herridge MS, Tansey CM, Matté A, et al. Canadian Critical Care Trials Group. Functional disability 5 years after acute respiratory distress syndrome. *N Engl J Med.* 2011;364:1293-1304.

Knaus WA, Zimmerman JE, Wagner DP, et al. APACHE—Acute Physiology and Chronic Health Evaluation: physiologically based classification system. *Crit Care Med.* 1981;9:591-597.

National Heart, Lung, and Blood Institute. Acute Respiratory Distress Syndrome (ARDS) Clinical Trials Network: comparison of two fluid-management strategies in acute lung injury. *N Engl J Med.* 2006;354:2564-2575.

Rubenfeld GD, Caldwell E, Peabody E, et al. Incidence and outcomes of acute lung injury. *N Engl J Med.* 2005;353:1685-1693.

Slutsky AS, Ranieeri VM. Ventilator-induced lung injury. *N Engl J Med.* 2013;369:2126.

Tobin MJ. Advances in mechanical ventilation. *N Engl J Med.* 2001;344:1986-1996.

Vincent JL, De Backer D. Circulatory shock. *N Engl J Med.* 2013;369:1726.

Pleural Disease

ALBERT J. POLITO, MD

Pleural diseases are among the most frequently encountered problems in chest medicine. Two of the most common entities are pleural effusion and pneumothorax. The former reflects an excessive accumulation of fluid in the pleural space; the latter occurs when air enters the pleural space.

Pleural Effusions

Basic Information

- **The most common causes of pleural effusion in the United States are congestive heart failure, pneumonia, malignancy, and pulmonary embolism**
- Pathophysiology of pleural effusions
  - Pleural fluid originates from capillaries in parietal pleura and is drained by lymphatics in parietal pleura
  - Pleural effusion forms when more fluid is formed than can be reabsorbed
  - Effusion can also originate from the interstitial spaces in the lung, intrathoracic lymphatics, or peritoneal cavity
    - Mechanisms of pleural fluid accumulation are shown in Table 24-1
  - Subpulmonic effusions develop when fluid becomes loculated between the lower aspect of the lung and the diaphragm
  - Parapneumonic effusions and empyema are pleural effusions associated with bacterial pneumonia or lung abscess; they are associated with a higher mortality rate than pneumonia and abscess without effusions

Clinical Presentation

- Symptoms of pleural effusion differ markedly according to cause and rapidity of onset
  - Pleural effusions are often asymptomatic, but small to moderate effusions may be symptomatic if they develop rapidly
  - Dyspnea, pleuritic chest pain (although pain may be dull and aching), and a dry nonproductive cough are typical symptoms of pleural effusion
    - Patients with infectious causes (e.g., pneumonia, tuberculosis) present with acute febrile illness and chest pain
    - **Patients with malignant pleural effusions typically present with dyspnea**
      - **Malignancy is the most common cause of massive pleural effusions that cause complete opacification of one hemithorax**
    - Patients with a pulmonary embolus may present with pleuritic chest pain and dyspnea

- Effusions (seen in 30% to 50% of cases) are usually small to moderate in size and unilateral
- Rheumatoid pleurisy may be asymptomatic and occur in the absence of joint disease activity
  - Classic presentation is an older man with subcutaneous rheumatoid nodules and a unilateral pleural effusion
  - **Frequently mimics a complicated parapneumonic effusion, with high lactate dehydrogenase (>1000 U/L), low glucose (<40 mg/dL), and low pH (<7.2)**
- Lupus pleuritis is typically painful and occurs in 15% to 40% of patients with lupus at some point in the disease
  - Small, bilateral effusions commonly seen
  - It is the presenting feature of lupus in 5% of cases
  - **Lupus pleuritis may be seen in drug-induced lupus secondary to procainamide, hydralazine, or isoniazid, among others**
- Chylothorax manifests with (typically) unilateral pleural effusion (Fig. 24-1)
  - Thoracic duct course (Fig. 24-2): Originates in abdomen as cisterna chyli, enters the thorax with the aorta, runs along the right anterolateral surface of the vertebrae, crosses the midline at the fourth thoracic vertebra, continues up along the left anterolateral vertebral surface, and empties into the junction of the left internal jugular and subclavian veins
  - **Site of interruption of thoracic duct determines side of pleural effusion (right-sided if below the fourth thoracic vertebra; left-sided if above it)**
  - **Lymphoma is cause in 75% of cases**
  - Thoracic duct trauma from injury or surgery makes up the majority of the remainder of cases
  - Occasionally idiopathic; rarely seen with tuberculosis or sarcoid
- Patients with asbestos exposure may present with benign asbestos pleural effusion 5 to 15 years after exposure to asbestos
  - Effusions are typically unilateral, persist for a mean of 4 months, and resolve spontaneously
  - Patients may go on to develop pleural plaques (20 years after exposure) or mesothelioma (20 to 30 years after exposure)
- **Physical examination findings over the site of the effusion include dullness to percussion, with**

decreased or absent breath sounds and absence of tactile fremitus
- Pleural rub (creaky, leathery sound) not common; suggests pleural inflammation alone or with small effusion
- Other physical findings vary depending on cause of effusion

Diagnosis and Evaluation

- Evaluation of pleural effusions is done by imaging of the effusion and sampling of the effusion by thoracentesis
- Imaging
  - As pleural effusion develops, small amounts of fluid obscure posterior costophrenic angle on lateral imaging, followed by blunting of lateral costophrenic angle on posteroanterior imaging (Fig. 24-3)
    - Sensitivity of posteroanterior and lateral films is 200 mL

- Lateral decubitus film extremely helpful in detecting effusion; can detect as little as 15 mL of fluid
- **If lateral decubitus film shows fluid is free-flowing and depth of pleural fluid is greater than 10 mm, diagnostic thoracentesis can be performed at the bedside**

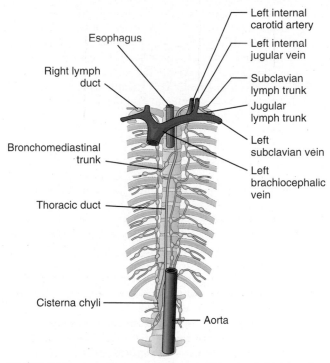

FIGURE 24-2 Lymphatics of the thorax. (From Jacob S. *Atlas of Human Anatomy*. New York: Churchill Livingstone; 2002: Fig. 3.4h.)

TABLE 24-1	Mechanisms of Pleural Fluid Accumulation	
Mechanism	**Representative Disease State**
Increased hydrostatic pressure of vasculature	Congestive heart failure
Decreased oncotic pressure of vasculature	Nephrotic syndrome
Decreased pleural pressure	Atelectasis
Obstruction of lymphatic drainage	Malignancy
Increased capillary permeability	Parapneumonic effusion
Rupture of thoracic duct	Chylothorax
Increased fluid in peritoneal cavity	Hepatic hydrothorax
Iatrogenic	Placement of central line into pleural space

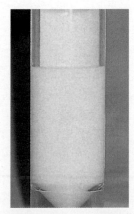

FIGURE 24-1 Chylothorax. The classic milky-appearing pleural fluid of a chylothorax. (From Forbes CD, Jackson WF. *Color Atlas and Text of Clinical Medicine*. 3rd ed. St. Louis: Mosby; 2003: Fig. 4.53.)

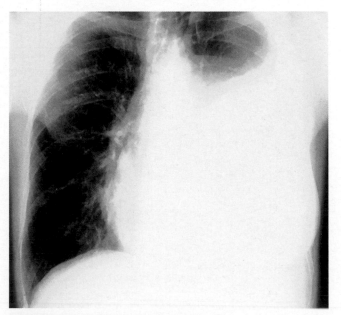

FIGURE 24-3 Large left pleural effusion. This patient had a previous mastectomy on the right, and the pleural effusion is malignant. The mediastinal shift to the right results from the space-occupying effects of the fluid. (From Albert RK, Spiro SG, Jett JR. *Clinical Respiratory Medicine*. 2nd ed. St. Louis: Mosby; 2004: Fig. 1.83.)

- Use of ultrasound guidance decreases complication rate, permits sampling of small and/or loculated effusions, and is rapidly becoming the standard of care for thoracentesis
- Consider subpulmonic effusion if one hemidiaphragm appears elevated and apex of diaphragm is laterally displaced
  - On left side, consider if the top of the hemidiaphragm is separated from gastric air bubble
- Ultrasound is useful for identifying loculated areas of pleural fluid, localizing placement of thoracentesis needle, and distinguishing pleural fluid from pleural thickening
- Computed tomography (CT) scanning helps distinguish between pleural and parenchymal disease and can differentiate between empyema and lung abscess
- Thoracentesis
  - Thoracentesis is indicated for undiagnosed pleural effusions
  - Differential diagnosis of pleural effusion is narrowed by determining whether pleural fluid is transudate or exudate (Fig. 24-4)
    - Note that pulmonary embolus usually (80%) results in an exudative effusion, but may be transudative in 20% of cases
  - If any one of the three criteria shown in Figure 24-4 (known as light criteria) is met, the effusion is classified as an exudate
    - Application of light criteria occasionally leads to misclassification of a transudate as an exudate, but does not lead to misclassifying exudates

- Cytopathology: important for diagnosing malignant effusions
  - Most common causes of malignant pleural effusions include lung cancer (33%, usually adenocarcinoma), breast cancer (25%), and lymphoma/leukemia (15%)
  - Sensitivity of a single thoracentesis sample for diagnosing malignancy is 60%; three sequential thoracenteses increase sensitivity to 80%
  - Cytology more likely to be positive with pleural metastases or with mediastinal lymph node involvement
- Culture
  - Most common organisms in empyemas are *Staphylococcus aureus*, anaerobes such as *Bacteroides* and *Peptostreptococcus*, *Streptococcus pneumoniae*, and gram-negative organisms such as *Escherichia coli* and *Klebsiella*
  - Yield for mycobacterial cultures is only 35%; pleural biopsy typically performed if tuberculosis suspected
    - With pleural biopsy, granulomas seen in 80% of cases, acid-fast bacteria (AFB) stain positive in 25% of cases, and AFB culture positive in 55% of cases
    - Tuberculin skin test (purified protein derivative) positive in only two thirds of patients with a tuberculous pleural effusion
- Other tests used in evaluation of pleural fluid are shown in Table 24-2
- In patients with pneumonia, characteristics used to distinguish parapneumonic effusion from empyema are shown in Table 24-3

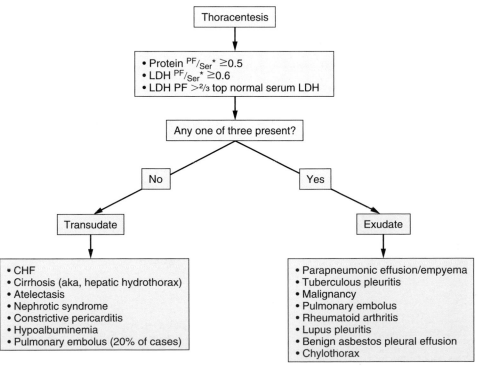

FIGURE 24-4 Transudates and exudates. CHF, Congestive heart failure; LDH, lactate dehydrogenase. *Pleural fluid value (PF) divided by serum value (Ser).

TABLE 24-2	*Tests Used in the Evaluation of Pleural Fluid*
Test	**Result**

Cell counts	RBC count >100,000/μL suggests:
	  Trauma
	  Malignancy
	  Pulmonary embolism with infarction
	WBC count
	  <1000/μL suggests transudate
	  >1000/μL suggests exudate
	WBC differential
	  >10,000 neutrophils/μL suggests parapneumonic effusion or empyema; occasionally seen with pulmonary embolus, pancreatitis, or early tuberculosis
	  >50% lymphocytes suggests tuberculosis or malignancy; also seen after coronary artery bypass graft surgery
	  Eosinophilia nonspecific, but may suggest parasitic infection, drug reaction, malignant effusion, or Churg-Strauss syndrome

pH	pH <7.2 suggests:
	  Complicated parapneumonic effusion
	  Empyema
	  Esophageal rupture
	  Rheumatoid pleurisy
	  Malignant effusion
	pH >7.8 suggests *Proteus* infection

Glucose	Glucose <60 mg/dL suggests:
	  Parapneumonic effusion
	  Empyema
	  Rheumatoid pleurisy
	  Malignant effusion
	  Tuberculous pleuritis

Amylase	If elevated, suggests:
	  Pancreatic disease
	  Esophageal rupture (salivary isoenzymes elevated); typically results in left-sided effusion
	  Malignant effusion (salivary isoenzymes not elevated)

Triglycerides (TG)	TG >110 mg/dL indicates chylothorax If TG 50 to 110 mg/dL, send fluid for chylomicrons Presence of chylomicrons indicates chylothorax TG <50 mg/dL indicates no chylothorax

Cholesterol	Causes a "pseudochylothorax" (milky fluid but not a true chylothorax)
	Usually seen in long-standing effusions
	  Old tuberculous effusion
	  Rheumatoid pleurisy
	  Nephrotic syndrome

Antinuclear antibody (ANA)	Pleural fluid ANA titer commonly elevated to >1:160 in lupus, but is not specific for the disease
Adenosine deaminase	Typically >50 units/L in tuberculous pleurisy
Interferon-γ	Elevated in tuberculous pleurisy but cutoff value not well established Note that interferon-γ release assays, such as commercially available QuantiFERON-TB Gold and T-SPOT.TB, are not useful for diagnosing tuberculous pleuritis

RBC, Red blood cell; WBC, white blood cell.

Treatment

- Treatment of pleural effusions determined by size of effusion, presence of symptoms, and cause of effusion
- Treatment of underlying etiology of effusion is most important, but definitive mechanical removal of fluid may also be needed
  - Options include therapeutic thoracentesis, chest tube drainage, indwelling pleural catheter placement, thoracotomy with decortication, and pleurodesis (fusion of visceral and parietal pleura to prevent recurrence of symptomatic effusion; particularly useful with empyemas and malignant effusions)
- Chemical pleurodesis: Sclerosing agent is introduced through chest tube after fluid is drained and the lung has reexpanded
  - **Talc, administered in a slurry, is the most effective agent but does carry a small risk of respiratory failure**
  - Doxycycline also is commonly used—slightly less effective than talc but not associated with respiratory failure
- Surgical pleurodesis via thoracotomy using one of two techniques:
  - Mechanical abrasion of pleura
  - Insufflation of talc (equally effective as talc slurry, and with same risk of respiratory failure)

TABLE 24-3	Parapneumonic Effusions and Empyema	
Effusion Type	**Definition**	**Treatment***
Simple parapneumonic effusion	pH >7.2 Glucose >40 mg/dL LDH <3 times top normal serum LDH	Antibiotics alone often sufficient
Complicated parapneumonic effusion	Gross appearance does not resemble pus pH <7.0 Glucose <40 mg/dL "Borderline" complicated pH 7.0 to 7.2, with glucose >40 mg/dL and/or LDH <3 times normal	Antibiotics Chest tube Serial thoracentesis acceptable in borderline cases
Empyema	Appearance of frank pus pH <7.0 Glucose <40 mg/dL WBC count typically >15,000/μL Bacterial culture commonly positive	Antibiotics Chest tube Decortication may be required Fibrinolytics or thoracoscopy occasionally used if loculations present

*Treatment of each disorder will be determined in part by volume of fluid and presence of loculations.
LDH, Lactate dehydrogenase; WBC, white blood cell.

- Specific treatment
  - Parapneumonic effusion (see Table 24-3)
  - **Chylothorax: Treatment includes chest tube, bed rest, enteral feeding with medium-chain triglycerides (absorbed to circulation via portal vein, avoiding thoracic duct)**
    - Occasionally thoracic duct ligation or placement of pleuroperitoneal shunt needed
    - Lack of treatment results in loss of protein, fat, and lymphocytes, risking malnutrition and infection

Pneumothorax

Basic Information

- Pneumothorax results from the introduction of air into the pleural space
  - May occur spontaneously or result from trauma or iatrogenic causes (e.g., surgery, central venous access placement, thoracentesis)
- Primary spontaneous pneumothorax occurs when no clinically apparent lung disease is present
  - **Male predominance (6:1)**
  - **Typical patient is a tall, thin male smoker younger than age 40 years.** Most patients have radiographically inapparent subpleural bullae.
- Secondary spontaneous pneumothorax occurs as a result of underlying lung disease
  - Obstructive lung diseases associated with secondary spontaneous pneumothorax include asthma, chronic obstructive pulmonary disease, and cystic fibrosis
  - Associated interstitial lung diseases include idiopathic pulmonary fibrosis, eosinophilic granuloma, and lymphangioleiomyomatosis
  - *Pneumocystis jiroveci* (formerly *carinii*) pneumonia and Marfan syndrome are also associated with secondary spontaneous pneumothorax

Clinical Presentation

- Typical symptoms include ipsilateral pleuritic chest pain and dyspnea

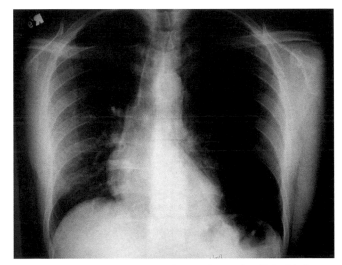

FIGURE 24-5 Anteroposterior chest radiograph of left-sided pneumothorax. Note absence of lung markings on the affected side and deviation of the trachea contralaterally. (From Roberts JR. *Clinical Procedures in Emergency Medicine.* 4th ed. Philadelphia: Saunders; 2004: Fig. 10-1.)

- Physical findings normal with small pneumothorax (<15% of hemithorax)
  - **Tachycardia is the most common finding in pneumothorax**
  - **Hyperresonance to percussion, decreased chest wall movement, decreased fremitus, and decreased or absent breath sounds common with large pneumothorax**
  - Hypotension, cyanosis, and shift of the trachea to the contralateral side seen with tension pneumothorax

Diagnosis and Evaluation

- Radiographic imaging used to confirm diagnosis
  - Visceral pleural edge separated from chest wall on chest radiograph (Fig. 24-5)
  - May be difficult to diagnose with underlying lung disease (e.g., bullous emphysema)
  - Chest computed tomography (CT) may be needed if suggested but not apparent on chest film

Treatment

- Treatment is similar for primary and secondary spontaneous pneumothorax, although the threshold for placing a chest tube is lower (i.e., done sooner) for secondary spontaneous pneumothorax
  - **Administer 100% oxygen and observe patient if pneumothorax is small (<15% of hemithorax)**
    - **Increases rate of reabsorption of air from pleural space fourfold**
  - Larger (>15% of hemithorax) pneumothoraces require removal of air, either with catheter (works best with young patients) or with chest tube (required for most patients)
- Recurrence rate
  - Similar for primary and secondary forms
  - **Thirty percent after first episode; more than 50% after second episode**
  - Usually occurs within 2 years after initial pneumothorax
  - Advise patients to avoid scuba diving
  - **After second pneumothorax, recommend intervention to prevent recurrence**
    - Chemical pleurodesis through chest tube
    - If present, blebs/bullae should be surgically resected, with concomitant surgical pleurodesis

- Pleurodesis agents and techniques are the same as those used for persistent pleural effusions (see Pleural Effusion section)

Review Questions

For review questions, please go to ExpertConsult.com.

SUGGESTED READINGS

Haynes D, Baumann MH. Management of pneumothorax. *Semin Respir Crit Care Med.* 2010;31:769-780.

Heffner JE, Klein JS. Recent advances in the diagnosis and management of malignant pleural effusions. *Mayo Clin Proc.* 2008;83:235-250.

Light RW. *Pleural Diseases.* 5th ed. Philadelphia: Lippincott, Williams & Wilkins; 2007.

Light RW. Update on tuberculous pleural effusion. *Respirology.* 2010;15:451-458.

Sahn SA. Getting the most from pleural fluid analysis. *Respirology.* 2012;17:270-277.

Schiza S, Siafakas SM. Clinical presentation and management of empyema, lung abscess, and pleural effusion. *Curr Opin Pulm Med.* 2006;12:205-211.

Wrightson JM, Davies RJ. The approach to the patient with a parapneumonic effusion. *Semin Respir Crit Care Med.* 2010;31:706-715.

SECTION FOUR

BOARD REVIEW

Gastroenterology

Peptic Ulcer Disease and Gastrointestinal Bleeding

EDUARDO J. GONZALEZ-VELEZ, MD; and JOHN O. CLARKE, MD

Causes of gastrointestinal (GI) blood loss have been traditionally divided into two basic categories based on the anatomic location of the bleeding source in relation to the ligament of Treitz. *Upper GI bleeding* refers to blood loss originating above this area, whereas *lower GI bleeding* stems from sources below this area. The advent of new technology such as the wireless capsule and deep enteroscopy has improved our ability to evaluate the region from the ampulla of Vater to the terminal ileum. The ability to evaluate this region is of particular importance because 10% to 20% of patients presenting with GI bleeding have an etiology that remains unclear despite upper endoscopy and colonoscopy. This chapter focuses on the approach to patients with suspected upper or lower GI bleeding and describes the most common specific causes within each category. The approach to the diagnosis of obscure overt GI bleeding will also be reviewed.

Background

Stomach Anatomy

Figure 25-1 illustrates the anatomy of the stomach
- Antrum
  - Pyloric glands
    - G cells: Secrete gastrin, which stimulates acid production
    - D cells: Secrete somatostatin, which inhibits gastrin secretion
    - Goblet cells: Secrete mucus to coat and protect the stomach from corrosive injury
- Fundus/body
  - Oxyntic glands
    - Parietal cells: Secrete acid (HCl)
    - Chief cells: Secrete pepsinogen, which is converted to pepsin by HCl. Pepsin can damage the gastric epithelium.

Gastric Acid Secretion

- Three pathways by which acid production/secretion occurs
  - Vagus innervation leads to release of acetylcholine, which leads to stimulation of H^+/K^+-adenosine triphosphatase (ATPase) and acid production/secretion
  - Gastrin release leads to direct stimulation of H^+/K^+-ATPase, which leads to acid production/secretion

- Histamine release leads to stimulation of adenylate cyclase, which leads to cyclic adenosine monophosphate (cAMP), which leads to stimulation of H^+/K^+-ATPase and leads to acid production/ secretion
- Regulation of acid secretion
  - Basal acid secretion: Mediated by vagal tone, highest levels at nighttime
  - Food-stimulated secretion
    - Cephalic phase: Sight, smell, and taste stimulate the vagus nerve
    - Gastric phase: Triggered by gastric distention and protein digestion caused by food entering the stomach; gastrin is then released
    - Intestinal phase: Triggered by protein in the small bowel

Peptic Ulcer Disease

Causes

- Direct mucosal injury (e.g., toxins, ethanol, nonsteroidal anti-inflammatory drugs [NSAIDs], *Helicobacter pylori*, bile)
- Inhibition of prostaglandin synthesis (NSAIDs)
- Disruption of the protective mucus layer (NSAIDs, *H. pylori*)
- Increased gastric acid secretion (*H. pylori*, gastrinoma, hypercalcemia, sepsis, central nervous system, burns)
- Mucosal ischemia (anastomotic ulcers)

Epidemiology

- **Most patients have normal acid secretion**
- Gastric ulcers may represent an underlying malignancy (approximately 3%)
- Duodenal ulcers rarely represent an underlying malignancy
- Lifetime prevalence of peptic ulcer disease (PUD) is 5% to 10%

Clinical Presentation

- Epigastric abdominal pain is the most common symptom
- Nausea and vomiting may occur
- GI bleeding (see later discussion): 20% of patients will bleed and can present with hematemesis, coffee-grounds emesis, hematochezia, or melena

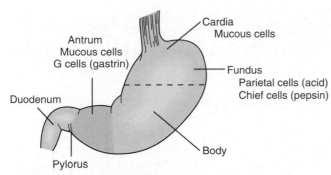

FIGURE 25-1 Anatomy of the stomach. (From Kumar V, Fausto N, Abbas A. *Robbins & Cotran's Pathologic Basis of Disease.* 7th ed. Philadelphia: Saunders; 2004: Fig. 17-12A.)

- Perforation
  - Seen in 5% of patients
  - Abdominal examination reveals rigid abdomen with rebound tenderness
  - Duodenal ulcers may penetrate posterior to the pancreas, resulting in elevations in amylase and lipase
- Gastric outlet obstruction
  - Usually caused by peripyloric scar formation
  - Presents with abdominal bloating, nausea, vomiting, weight loss

Diagnosis

- Endoscopy has been shown to be far superior to barium studies for the detection of gastric and duodenal ulcers

Therapy

- Antacids
  - Neutralize acid
  - **Magnesium and aluminum compounds can be toxic in patients with renal failure**
  - Calcium carbonate antacids can cause milk-alkali syndrome (hypercalcemia, hyperphosphatemia) with prolonged use
- Histamine$_2$ (H$_2$) blockers (e.g., cimetidine, ranitidine, famotidine, nizatidine)
  - Block H$_2$ receptor on parietal cells
  - **Work relatively quickly (approximately 30 minutes)**
  - Effective for both duodenal and gastric ulcers
  - Associated with tachyphylaxis and may not provide long-term benefit (but effective in acute treatment or intermittent use)
  - Inhibit cytochrome P-450 drug metabolism (more common with cimetidine); need to monitor levels of some drugs (e.g., warfarin, phenytoin, theophylline)
- Proton pump (H$^+$/K$^+$-ATPase) inhibitors (PPIs) (e.g., omeprazole, lansoprazole, rabeprazole, pantoprazole, esomeprazole, dexlansoprazole)
  - **Irreversibly block H$^+$/K$^+$-ATPase; take 3 days to block 90% of pumps**
  - Increase gastrin levels
  - Most effective when given before meals (typically before breakfast if once daily and before breakfast and before dinner if twice daily)
  - Effective for both duodenal and gastric ulcers

- Can interfere with the absorption of other drugs (e.g., ketoconazole, ampicillin, iron, digoxin)
- Emerging data document potential side effects associated with the use of PPIs, including decreased bone mineral density, increased community-acquired infection, *Clostridium difficile* infection, and hypomagnesemia
- PPI use with clopidogrel
  - Compared with other PPIs, omeprazole and esomeprazole have a greater effect on CYP2C19-mediated conversion of clopidogrel to its active metabolite, thus diminishing its effect on platelets
  - **New labeling from the Food and Drug Administration suggests that PPI use among patients taking clopidogrel be limited to pantoprazole, rabeprazole, lansoprazole, or dexlansoprazole**
- PPIs have not been shown to increase the risk of gastric cancers
- Can be associated with rebound acid hypersecretion upon cessation
- Sucralfate
  - Stimulates endogenous prostaglandins and enhances mucosal defenses and repair
  - Effective for duodenal ulcer
  - Avoid in patients with renal insufficiency because of the potential for aluminum toxicity

Duration of Therapy

- Duodenal ulcers: 4 to 6 weeks
- Gastric ulcers: 6 to 8 weeks; repeat endoscopy with biopsies to rule out gastric cancer in 8 weeks

NSAID-Associated GI Toxicity

Epidemiology

- Dyspepsia occurs in 10% to 20% of patients taking NSAIDs
- 1.3% of those taking NSAIDs for arthritis have a serious GI complication
- Mortality rate for those hospitalized with NSAID-related bleeding is 5% to 10%
- **An increased risk of GI bleeding is associated with even low-dose aspirin use (<75 mg/day)**
- Enteric-coated aspirin has a rate of complications similar to non–enteric-coated preparations

Risk Factors

- History of ulcer
- Concomitant use of corticosteroids
- Concomitant use of other anticoagulants
- High doses of NSAIDs
- Advanced age (older than 70 years)
- *H. pylori*: controversial

Mechanisms

- Topical: NSAIDs are acidic and can migrate through the protective layer of mucus to the gastric epithelium, where they dissociate into the ionized form. The disruption in the layer of mucus also permits further injury by gastric acid and pepsin.

25

- Inhibition of prostaglandin synthesis: most important cause of gastroduodenal NSAID injury

Therapy

- Stop NSAIDs
- Treat *H. pylori* (see later discussion) if ulcer is present
- PPI

Prophylaxis

- Not indicated in the absence of prior PUD or symptoms
- Misoprostol
  - Prostaglandin E derivative shown to decrease the incidence of NSAID-induced ulceration
  - Diarrhea is a common side effect
  - Contraindicated in pregnancy (or in women considering pregnancy because it acts as an abortifacient)
- PPI is also effective
- H_2 blockers found to be inferior to PPIs and misoprostol
- **Eradicate *H. pylori* before initiating NSAID therapy if patient is *H. pylori* positive and has a history of PUD**

Alternative to Prophylaxis

- Cyclooxygenase-2 (COX-2)–selective inhibitors
- Based on the fact that cyclooxygenase-1 (COX-1) is constitutively expressed and maintains GI mucosal integrity and COX-2 expression is induced by inflammation
- **Studies show that COX-2–selective inhibitors are less likely to cause PUD than nonselective NSAIDs**
- Lack cardiovascular protective effects (COX-1 participates in platelet aggregation)
- There are increasing data that all drugs in this class appear to have potential cardiovascular risk that may be dose-dependent. Should be used with caution in patients with cardiac risk factors.
- Protective effect of COX-2–selective inhibitor is lost if the patient uses regular or baby acetylsalicylic acid concomitantly

Helicobacter pylori Infection

Features

- Gram-negative, spiral-shaped, flagellated rod
- **Accounts for most cases of PUD in the United States**
- Found in mucus layer; produces a urease that splits urea into ammonia and bicarbonate
- Humans are the principal reservoir
- Mode of transmission thought to be fecal–oral and/or oral–oral routes
- Infection thought to occur in childhood
- In the United States, 40% to 50% of those older than 60 years are infected
- More prevalent in developing countries
- Risk factors for infection include low socioeconomic status, domestic crowding, exposure to unclean food or water

- Over half the world is infected with *H. pylori*; however, only approximately 15% of people with *H. pylori* report GI symptoms

Diagnosis

- Noninvasive tests
  - Serum immunoglobulin G (IgG)
    - Approximately 90% sensitivity
    - Serum qualitative antibody test
    - Whole-blood qualitative antibody test
    - Quantitative antibody test: A 30% decrease in titer can be used to document post-treatment eradication (rarely done). A qualitative test is not useful to document post-treatment eradication because IgG remains positive after treatment.
  - Urea breath test (95% sensitivity; greater than 95% specificity)
    - Urea labeled with C-13 or C-14 cleaved by urease into ammonia and carbon dioxide.
    - Stop PPI 1 week and antibiotics 4 weeks before test; should also stop bismuth and high doses of H_2-receptor antagonists
  - Stool *H. pylori* antigen test
    - Sensitivity 93%, specificity 93%
    - Useful for initial diagnosis and also documentation of post-therapy eradication
    - More widely available than breath test
- Invasive tests
  - Rapid urease test (approximately 90% sensitivity; greater than 95% specificity)
    - Biopsy is placed on a card that is spotted with urea; when urease is present, it cleaves the urea, inducing a pH and color change on the card
  - Histology
    - Presence of active chronic gastritis suggests the presence of *H. pylori* even in the absence of visible organisms
    - Organisms can be detected by Giemsa, hematoxylin and eosin, and silver stains
  - Culture
    - Useful only for detecting antibiotic resistance and not often obtained in clinical practice
- Use of *H. pylori* testing
  - Antibody tests are useful in those who have not been previously treated
  - **Stool antigen test or urea breath test is useful to detect active infections or to monitor response to therapy**
  - Endoscopy is useful to detect *H. pylori*-associated ulcers or cancers; of note, although endoscopy with histology is specific for *H. pylori*, sensitivity is less than either the stool antigen test or urea breath test

Therapy

- Overview
  - **Triple-drug therapy superior to dual-drug therapy**
  - Reinfection is rare
  - Clarithromycin resistance is increasing because of population exposure to macrolides, resulting in

recent fall in the success rates of *H. pylori* eradication treatment

- If failure after first-line triple drug therapy with amoxicillin, clarithromycin, and a PPI is documented, then second-line therapy generally consists of bismuth-based quadruple therapy (bismuth subcitrate potassium, metronidazole, tetracycline, and a PPI). Sequential strategy has also been proposed
- In patients with a penicillin allergy, a first-line treatment with bismuth-containing quadruple therapy (PPI–bismuth–tetracycline–metronidazole) seems to be a better option than the triple regimen (PPI–clarithromycin–metronidazole)
- Rescue regimens include levofloxacin or rifabutin
- Cultures for *H. pylori* sensitivity can be considered after failure with rescue therapy regimens
- Treatment regimens
  - Triple therapy for 7 to 14 days (7-day therapy is approved with rabeprazole; 10-day therapy is approved with lansoprazole, omeprazole, pantoprazole, and esomeprazole).
    - PPI twice a day
    - Amoxicillin 1 g oral twice a day
    - Clarithromycin 500 mg twice a day
  - Quadruple therapy for 10 to 14 days
    - PPI twice a day
    - Bismuth 120 mg four times a day
    - Tetracycline 500 mg four times a day
    - Metronidazole 250 mg four times a day
  - Sequential therapy
    - Days 1 to 5
      - PPI twice a day
      - Amoxicillin, 1 g twice a day
    - Days 6 to 10
      - PPI twice a day
      - Clarithromycin 500 mg twice a day
      - Tinidazole 500 mg twice a day

Diseases Associated with *H. pylori*

- PUD
  - **_H. pylori_ is present in 70% of patients with gastric ulcers and in nearly 100% of patients with duodenal ulcers**
- Active chronic gastritis
- Gastric adenocarcinoma
- **Gastric mucosa-associated lymphoid tissue (MALT) lymphoma: Treatment of infection results in tumor regression in most patients with this disease**

Zollinger-Ellison Syndrome

Basic Information

- Hypersecretion of gastrin from tumors arising from the pancreas or wall of the duodenum (*gastrinoma*)
- Presents with peptic ulceration, which may be refractory to treatment
- Ulceration may be single or multiple and involve the stomach, duodenum, or jejunum (classic location is postbulbar duodenum)
- Diarrhea results from the high volumes of gastric acid produced. Steatorrhea may result from inactivation of

pancreatic enzymes as a result of the high volume of gastric acid in the duodenum.

- Two thirds of gastrinomas are malignant and may metastasize to the lymph nodes or liver
- About one third of gastrinomas are associated with multiple endocrine neoplasia type 1 (MEN 1), so adenomas of the parathyroid (causing hypercalcemia) and pituitary may also be seen

Diagnosis

- Elevated basal acid output levels (not sensitive)
- **Increased serum gastrin levels (value greater than 1000 pg/mL) with a gastric pH l less than 2 mEq/mL is virtually diagnostic**
- Patients with gastrin levels less than 1000 pg/mL and with a pH less than 2 mEq/mL need provocative testing
- Secretin test: IV infusion of secretin results in a paradoxic rise in serum gastrin in patients with Zollinger-Ellison syndrome but not in other conditions. A secretin stimulation test has a sensitivity of approximately 85%.
- Calcium infusion test has a much lower sensitivity and specificity and should be used only if the secretin test does not confirm the diagnosis and suspicion is high
- Tumor localization
  - Radiologic imaging: Abdominal computed tomography (CT)—90% of gastrinomas are located within the gastrinoma triangle, bordered by the head of the pancreas, the second portion of the duodenum, and the cystic and common bile ducts
  - Octreotide scintigraphy scan: ^{111}In-DTPA-D-Phe1 octreotide binds to the somatostatin type 2 receptors on gastrinomas. Using whole-body scintigraphy, gastrinomas can be localized with a sensitivity of 71% to 75% and a specificity of 86% to 100%.

Dyspepsia

- Definition: chronic or recurrent epigastric pain in the absence of reflux symptoms, acute severe pain, abdominal wall pain, or dysphagia
- Differential diagnosis of dyspepsia
  - Functional dyspepsia: 60% of cases
  - Disordered motility
    - Visceral hypersensitivity
    - Altered intestinogastric reflexes
    - Psychological stress
  - PUD: 15% to 25% of cases
  - Gastroesophageal reflux disease: 5% to 15% of cases
  - Malignancy: less than 2% of cases
- Clinical evaluation and therapy
  - 2005 American Gastroenterology Association Guidelines
    - If age younger than 55 years and no warning symptoms (e.g., weight loss, dysphagia, anemia), check for *H. pylori* (breath test or stool antigen test preferred), and treat if positive; trial of antisecretory therapy if serology negative; if no response, then endoscopy
    - If age older than 55 years or warning symptoms are present, proceed directly to endoscopy

Gastrointestinal Bleeding

Approach to the Patient with Gastrointestinal Bleeding

- Evaluation
  - Determine heart rate, blood pressure, presence of orthostatic hypotension
  - Check hematocrit; may initially be misleadingly normal in patients with severe bleeding
  - Volume resuscitation with IV fluids or blood
  - Differentiate between upper GI bleeding (UGIB) and lower GI bleeding (LGIB)
    - Hematemesis: Indicates an upper source (above the ligament of Treitz)
    - Melena: Indicates that blood has been present in the GI tract for a number of hours; can be seen in upper GI as well as proximal lower (i.e., right colon) GI bleeding
    - Hematochezia: Usually suggests a lower GI source, but can be from a massive upper GI bleed
    - **Nasogastric aspirate: Has very limited utility in assessment and management**
- Diagnosis (Fig. 25-2)
  - Suspected UGIB: Proceed with upper endoscopy
  - Suspected LGIB: controversial
    - Many sources recommend performing sigmoidoscopy or colonoscopy because the most common cause of lower GI bleeding is diverticula, and colonoscopy could offer a means for hemostasis by clip placement or thermocoagulation; however, risk may be higher in the context of a poorly prepped colon and diverticulosis
    - **If the patient is presenting with massive bleeding with significant blood transfusion**

requirements and hemodynamic instability, then angiography can lead to both diagnosis and treatment
  - Because of issues of preparation and timing and with significant bleeding, the role of colonoscopy versus angiography could be altered
  - Technetium-99m (^{99m}Tc)-labeled red cell scan can also be used on occasion for localization
- Hematochezia with hemodynamic instability: Initially perform upper endoscopy to rule out an upper GI source
- Occult GI bleed: Refers to hemoccult-positive stool without a clear source; workup usually consists of upper and lower endoscopy (yield, approximately 50%); if negative, the small bowel should be evaluated (push enteroscopy, video capsule endoscopy, single/double balloon enteroscopy, or small bowel series; yield of additional studies approximately 70%) (see Chronic Bleeding section for more details)
- Treatment: Based on the cause of the bleed:
  - H_2 blockers and PPIs do not reduce the risk of rebleeding in the absence of endoscopic stigmata of recent bleeding
  - **If UGIB is suspected, may wish to start intravenous (IV) PPI empirically because multiple studies have now shown that IV PPIs reduce the rate of rebleeding and need for surgery in patients with bleeding ulcers**

Etiology

See Table 25-1 for a summary of the causes of GI bleeding
- Upper GI source
  - Consider in a patient who presents with melena, hematemesis, or brisk hematochezia associated with orthostatic hypotension

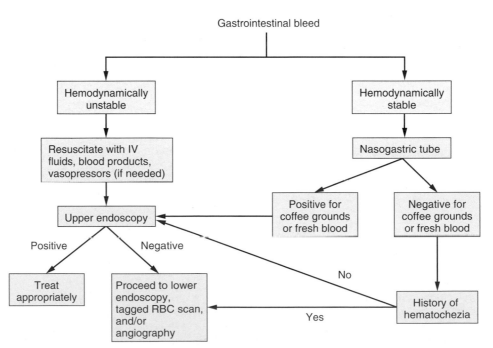

FIGURE 25-2 Evaluation of patient with gastrointestinal bleeding. IV, Intravenous; RBC, red blood cell.

TABLE 25-1	*Causes of Gastrointestinal Bleeding*		
	Upper GI		**Lower GI**
Acute GI bleeding	Peptic ulcer disease Gastric erosions Esophagitis Mallory-Weiss tear (5%–15%) Portal hypertension-related Dieulafoy lesion		Diverticulosis Vascular ectasia Colitis Neoplasms
Chronic GI bleeding	Esophagitis Gastric ulcer Gastritis Duodenal ulcer Vascular ectasia		Adenomas >1 cm Carcinoma Colitis Vascular ectasia

GI, Gastrointestinal.

25

- Lower GI source
  - Accounts for only 20% of all episodes of acute GI bleeding
  - Consider in a patient who presents with hematochezia, occasionally with melena
  - **In more than half the cases of acute LGIB, diverticular bleed is the cause**

Specific Etiologies

- Gastric/duodenal ulcers
  - Bleeding ulcers tend to be located on the lesser curve or in the posterior duodenal bulb, where erosion into large vessels may occur
  - *H. pylori* does not appear to be a risk factor for ulcer bleeding, unlike age and NSAID use
  - **Endoscopic therapy is warranted in patients with a visible vessel observed in an ulcer crater, even if there is no active bleeding; chance of rebleeding is 50% to 70% without therapy, 20% with therapy**
  - IV omeprazole administered after endoscopic therapy decreased the rate of recurrent bleeding from 22.5% to 6.7%
  - Refer patients for surgery if endoscopic therapy is unsuccessful
  - Consider long-term prophylactic therapy in those who have bled; 33% PUD recurrence rate in 3 years without prophylaxis
- Mallory-Weiss tear
  - Laceration of the mucosa at the gastroesophageal junction
  - Often associated with a history of vomiting or dry heaves before the bleeding episode
  - May also be associated with heavy alcohol use
  - Bleeding usually stops spontaneously, although rebleeding may occur in 5% of patients
  - Angiography with embolization can be performed; surgery is rarely required
  - Distinguished from Boerhaave syndrome, which is esophageal perforation caused by retching
- Vascular malformations
  - Angiodysplasia
    - Flat, red lesions; can be found anywhere in the small intestine and colon
    - Diagnosed by endoscopy
    - Associated with chronic renal failure, valvular heart disease

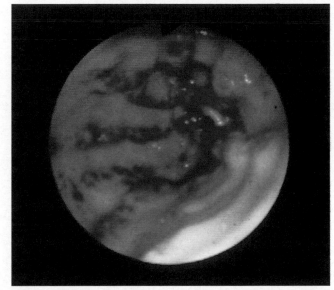

FIGURE 25-3 Endoscopic view of watermelon stomach. (From Feldman M. *Sleisenger and Fordtran's Gastrointestinal and Liver Disease.* 7th ed. Philadelphia: Saunders; 2002: Fig. 120-9.)

    - Treat with iron supplements or with estrogens
    - Brisk bleeds can be evaluated by bleeding scan or arteriography and treated by embolization, surgical resection
- Watermelon stomach (Fig. 25-3)
  - Vascular ectasia of the gastric antrum
  - Seen predominantly in elderly women
  - **Association with chronic liver disease and scleroderma**
  - Usually manifests as iron-deficiency anemia
  - Treat with iron supplementation
  - Sometimes cautery, or rarely, surgery is necessary
- Dieulafoy lesion
  - Ectatic artery that erodes into the stomach, causing brisk bleeding
  - Endoscopy may fail to identify the lesion if the bleeding has ceased
  - Treat endoscopically with cautery or hemoclip; embolization or surgery may be necessary
  - Uncommon (1% of upper GI bleeds) but can be catastrophic

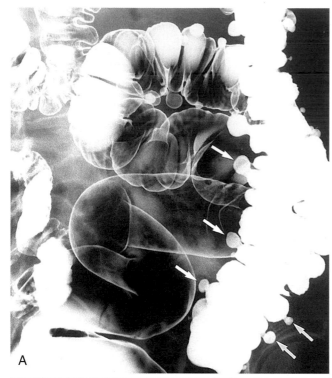

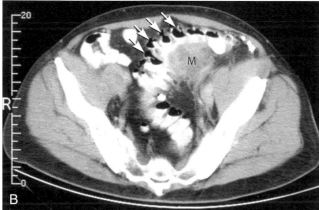

FIGURE 25-4 Diverticulosis of the colon. **A,** Double-contrast barium enema showing outpouchings *(arrows)* that represent diverticula. **B,** Computed tomographic scan showing outpouchings *(arrows)* and a focal mass (M), a developing abscess. (From Mettler FA. *Essentials of Radiology.* 2nd ed. Philadelphia: Saunders; 2005: Fig. 6-73.)

- Diverticulosis: "outpouchings" of colonic mucosa and submucosa (Fig. 25-4)
  - Most common cause of acute LGIB
  - Usually affects the left colon, but bleeding is often from the right colon
  - Low recurrence rate of bleeding
  - In only 20% of cases will the bleeding diverticulum be identified
  - **Most patients do well, and bleeding stops spontaneously**
  - Resection in those with refractory bleeding or recurrent bleeding
  - Diverticulitis
    - Inflammation around the diverticular sac
    - Usually occurs in the left colon

- Typically presents with abdominal pain, fever, and leukocytosis
- Microscopic bleeding can occur commonly, but gross bleeding is rare
- **CT scan can aid in the diagnosis. Barium enema and colonoscopy should be avoided with acute infection.**
- Complications include perforation, peritonitis, abscess, and fistula formation
- Treatment
  - **Mild cases may not require antibiotics**
  - More severe cases should be treated with broad-spectrum antibiotics (e.g., oral ciprofloxacin plus metronidazole or IV pipercillin/tazobactam) to cover gram-negative aerobes and anaerobes
  - Surgery may be necessary in patients with complications or those not improving with antibiotic therapy
  - Role of prophylactic hemicolectomy to prevent recurrences of diverticulitis is controversial and should be individualized
- Bleeding associated with portal hypertension
  - Bleeding can occur if portal pressure is greater than 12 mm Hg
  - Prevent bleeding with nonselective β-blockers, which also reduce mortality associated with bleeding
  - Esophageal/gastric varices
    - Likelihood of varices in cirrhotic patients is 35% to 80%, with 30% experiencing bleeding
    - Mortality rate for each bleeding episode is 35% to 50%
    - **Poor prognostic indicator: Only one third of patients with a history of variceal bleeding are alive at 1 year**
    - Acute therapy
      - Volume replacement/blood products
    - Sengstaken-Blakemore tube is only a temporizing measure for another therapy
    - Octreotide (minimal impact on systemic hemodynamics, in contrast to vasopressin)
    - Prophylactic antibiotics in patients with cirrhosis and GI hemorrhage with or without ascites has been shown not only to decrease bacterial infection but also to increase survival. IV ceftriaxone or norfloxacin administered orally at a dose of 400 mg twice daily for 7 days is standard
    - Endoscopic sclerotherapy or band ligation
    - Transjugular intrahepatic portosystemic shunt (TIPS)
      - No mortality advantage over endoscopic therapy
      - High incidence of hepatic encephalopathy
      - Useful as a bridge to transplantation
    - Surgical shunting
    - Orthotopic liver transplantation
  - Portal hypertensive gastropathy
    - Vascular congestion of the gastric mucosa; imparts a mosaic appearance endoscopically
    - Treat with somatostatin to lower splanchnic blood flow
    - Consider TIPS

- Secondary prevention of recurrent bleeding associated with portal hypertension
  - Nonselective β-adrenergic blocker drugs (e.g., propranolol)
  - Variceal banding: Useful for esophageal varices only, not gastropathy or gastric varices
  - TIPS
- Colitis
  - Infectious (see Chapter 14)
  - Inflammatory: Crohn disease, ulcerative colitis (see Chapter 28)
  - Ischemic
    - Patients usually older than age 60 years
    - Arises from low flow rate, not occlusion
    - **Watershed areas more often affected (e.g., splenic flexure, rectum)**
    - Symptoms include mild abdominal pain, cramping, bloody diarrhea
    - Diagnose by clinical presentation, colonoscopy
    - Can be associated with estrogen use, hypercoagulable states, vasculitis
- Chronic GI bleeding
  - Definitions
    - Obscure bleeding is defined as bleeding from the GI tract that persists or recurs without identifiable source after upper endoscopy, colonoscopy, and radiologic evaluation
    - Occult bleeding is defined as a positive fecal occult blood test (FOBT) result and/or iron-deficiency anemia without the patient or physician seeing visible blood
    - Obscure GI bleeding can be either occult or overt
  - Methods for evaluating the small bowel include wireless capsule endoscopy, single or double balloon enteroscopy, and radiological imaging (CT and magnetic resonance imaging [MRI] enterography, enteroclysis)
  - Algorithms for obscure overt and occult GI bleeding also give the option for repeat upper and lower endoscopy because video capsule endoscopy and deep enteroscopy studies have documented that 20% to 30% of the obscure GI bleeding lesions were subsequently found to be within the reach of adult upper and lower endoscopes
  - In patients who present with obscure overt GI bleeding, video capsule endoscopy has been recommended as the next step
  - If patient presents with massive bleeding, angiography can offer diagnostic and therapeutic intent
    - The amount of hemorrhage needed for positive angiography is a rate of blood loss of 1 mL/min of bleeding in the setting of hemodynamic instability (Fig. 25-5)
  - Common missed lesions in the upper GI tract are as follows: Cameron erosions in a large hiatal hernia, fundic varices, PUD, angioectasia, Dieulafoy lesion, and gastric antral vascular ectasia

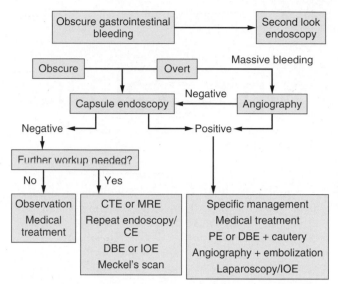

FIGURE 25-5 Clinical algorithm for the management of patients with obscure gastrointestinal hemorrhage. CE, Capsule endoscopy; CTE, computed tomography enterography; DBE, double balloon enteroscopy; IOE, intraoperative endoscopy; MRE, magnetic resonance enterography, PE, push enteroscopy. (Modified from Gerson LB. Editorial: is there a role for angiography in patients with obscure overt bleeding? *Am J Gastroenterol.* 2012;107:1377–1379, with permission from Macmillan Publishers Ltd.)

- Common missed lesion in the colonoscopy: angioectasia and neoplasms
- Most common etiologies of the small bowel is dependent on age
  - Younger than 40 years old: small bowel tumor, Meckel diverticulum, Dieulafoy lesion and Crohn disease
  - Older than 40 years old: vascular lesion and NSAID-induced enteropathy

Review Questions

For review questions, please go to ExpertConsult.com.

SUGGESTED READINGS

Barkun AN, Bardou M, Kuipers EJ, et al. International consensus recommendations on the management of patients with nonvariceal upper gastrointestinal bleeding. *Ann Intern Med.* 2010;152:101-113.

Gerson LB. Is there a role for angiography in patients with obscure overt bleeding? *Am J Gastroenterol.* 2012;107:1377-1379.

Lanza FL, Chan FK, Quigley EM. Guidelines for prevention of NSAID related ulcer complications. *Am J Gastroenterol.* 2009;104:728-738.

Overland MK. Dyspepsia. *Med Clin North Am.* 2014;98:549-564.

Prasad Kerlin M, Tokar JL. Acute gastrointestinal bleeding. *Ann Intern Med.* 2013;159:ITC2-ITC1.

Raju GS, Gerson L, Das A, et al. American Gastroenterological Association Institute medical position statement on obscure gastrointestinal bleeding. *Gastroenterology.* 2007;133:1694-1696.

Wong Kee Song LM, Baron TH. Endoscopic management of acute lower gastrointestinal bleeding. *Am J Gastroenterol.* 2008;103: 1881-1887.

Esophageal Disease

KRISTLE L. LYNCH, MD; and JOHN O. CLARKE, MD

Diseases of the esophagus include a number of conditions caused by abnormalities in anatomic structure or function. This chapter reviews many of those conditions, including gastroesophageal reflux disease (GERD), esophagitis, esophageal cancer, and dysmotility syndromes. Before describing specific disease processes, basic esophageal anatomy is reviewed.

Normal Esophageal Structure and Function

Figure 26-1 shows the anatomy of the esophagus.
- Upper esophageal sphincter
  - Striated muscle
  - Relaxes in response to a swallow
  - Functions to prevent aspiration
- Esophageal body
  - Upper one third striated muscle, lower two thirds smooth muscle
  - Innervated by the vagus nerve
  - Swallowing initiates contractions in the upper esophagus, and the enteric nervous system perpetuates them through the body
- Lower esophageal sphincter (LES)
  - High-pressure zone in distal esophagus
  - Relaxes in response to a swallow (vagally mediated)
  - Prevents GERD
  - Relaxation regulated by a variety of neuropeptides and hormones

Gastroesophageal Reflux Disease

Basic Information
- Protective mechanisms against reflux include the LES, peristalsis, saliva, and gravity
- Caused by increased frequency of transient relaxations of the LES and decreased LES tone
- An acid pocket forms as newly secreted acid layers on top of less acidic chyme in the stomach
- There are numerous potential complications of GERD (Box 26-1)

Clinical Presentation
- Heartburn, indigestion
- Acid regurgitation
- Water brash: vagal-mediated saliva production that occurs in response to esophagitis; distinguished from regurgitation

- Dyspnea: vagal-mediated bronchoconstriction, microaspiration
- Dysphagia: triggered by esophageal spasm
- Chronic cough
- Hoarseness
- Chest pain

Diagnosis and Evaluation
- **Testing not necessary in patients who present typically (heartburn and/or acid regurgitation); a therapeutic trial (see later) may be sufficient**
- Testing is indicated for atypical presentations, refractory symptoms, or presence of alarm findings (e.g., weight loss and dysphagia)
- Endoscopy with biopsies
  - Often the first-line diagnostic study
  - Very specific for reflux (greater than 95%) if esophagitis or Barrett esophagus is identified
  - Relatively insensitive (approximately 20% in most studies)
- A 24-hour catheter-based pH probe has been the traditional gold standard when symptoms are persistent, and endoscopy is unrevealing
- Newer diagnostic modalities
  - Wireless pH capsule that can be attached temporarily to the esophageal wall and records the pH telemetrically
    - Allows pH testing without the need for a nasal tube; increased patient comfort
    - Permits longer duration of testing (up to 96 hours)
  - Combined 24-hour pH/impedance, which combines standard pH monitoring with impedance flow, thereby allowing detection of flow (allowing detection of nonacid reflux)
    - Improves sensitivity because nonacid reflux can be detected
- Barium swallow: Used primarily to evaluate dysphagia; insensitive for nonerosive reflux
- Bernstein test (acid infusion): A provocative test to evaluate atypical chest pain. Symptoms are reproduced with the infusion of 0.1 N HCl but not with the infusion of saline; not used clinically in most centers and of limited diagnostic use.

Treatment
- Greater amount of acid suppression is needed to control GERD than to control peptic ulcer disease
- Lifestyle changes
  - Smoking cessation
  - Avoidance of alcohol

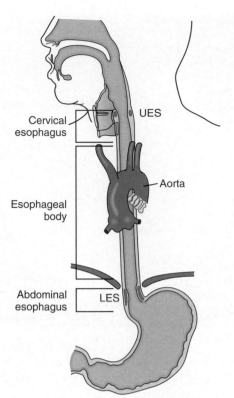

FIGURE 26-1 Anatomy of the esophagus showing the upper esophageal sphincter (UES), lower esophageal sphincter (LES), and esophageal body.

BOX 26-1	*Potential Complications of Gastroesophageal Reflux Disease*

Esophagitis
Esophageal ulceration
Esophageal stricture
Pulmonary aspiration
Barrett esophagus
    Occurs in up to 14% of patients with reflux symptoms
        undergoing endoscopy
    Replacement of the squamous epithelium with columnar
        epithelium
    Increased cancer risk associated only with specialized
        columnar epithelium (i.e., goblet cells present)
    Increased rate of adenocarcinoma estimated to be 10%
    Surveillance endoscopy every 3 years with biopsies from
        multiple levels is recommended, but has not yet been
        shown to reduce mortality
    Treatment is antireflux therapy, although this may not
        cause regression of Barrett esophagus or reduce the
        risk of progression to high-grade dysplasia or cancer
    Presence of high-grade dysplasia is an indication for
        endoscopic ablative therapy, particularly for those
        patients who are not good surgical candidates,
        or potentially esophagectomy

- Low-fat diet (fat can delay gastric emptying)
- Elevate the head of the bed (6 inches)
- Eat several hours before going to bed
- Avoid medications that lower LES tone (e.g., anticholinergics, sedatives, nitrates, calcium channel blockers, theophylline)

- Avoid foods known to lower LES tone (e.g., tomatoes, citrus, garlic, onions, peppermint, chocolate)
- Medical therapy
  - Antacids: treat symptoms, not esophagitis
  - Histamine₂ (H₂) blockers (cimetidine, ranitidine, famotidine, nizatidine) are useful for cases of moderate severity
  - Proton pump inhibitors (PPIs) (omeprazole, pantoprazole, rabeprazole, lansoprazole, dexlansoprazole, esomeprazole)
    - Superior to H₂ blockers in controlling symptoms and healing esophagitis
    - Duration of therapy should be at least 2 weeks
    - Prolonged use is necessary for severe cases
    - **No increased risk of tumors (carcinoid or gastrinoma) with long-term use**
    - Emerging data to suggest long-term use may be associated with decreased bone mineral density and increase in community-acquired infections
    - May interfere with the antiplatelet activity of clopidogrel
  - Prokinetic agents (e.g., metoclopramide) increase LES pressure and/or gastric emptying
  - γ-Aminobutyric acid (GABA) agonists (e.g., baclofen) decrease the frequency of transient LES relaxation and subsequently the number of reflux episodes; limited use because of dose-related side effects
- Endoscopic antireflux devices
  - Operate on the assumption that either plication of the gastroesophageal junction provides an increased mechanical barrier to reflux (EsopHyx) or that energy deposition at the gastroesophageal junction modifies distensibility and neural response (Stretta)
  - Long-term data are still emerging, and these are not considered first-line therapies
- Surgical antireflux options:
  - Antireflux surgery (fundoplication) is indicated in patients with refractory symptoms. Laparoscopic Nissen fundoplication is a proven effective alternative to PPI use and may be effective in up to 90% of cases.
  - The LINX reflux management system was approved by the Food and Drug Administration in 2013 for patients with mild to moderate GERD, but only if there is no hiatal hernia or a hernia smaller than 3 cm. Short-term results are positive but long-term results are still pending.
- **In cases of refractory GERD, consider alternative diagnoses, such as gastroparesis, gastrinoma (rare), gallbladder dysfunction, eosinophilic esophagitis, or cardiac etiology**

Esophagitis

Causes

- GERD (see earlier)
- Pill-induced
  - Common offenders include KCl, nonsteroidal antiinflammatory drugs (NSAIDs), tetracycline, alendronate, quinidine, FeSO₄, and ascorbic acid
  - Occurs more often in elderly patients

26

- Caustic ingestion
  - **Ingestion of alkali is worse than acid**
  - Induction of vomiting is not recommended for lye ingestion
  - Increased risk of squamous cell carcinoma with lye strictures
  - Stricture formation is common
  - Can also cause perforation, bleeding, and death
- Eosinophilic esophagitis
  - Deposition of eosinophils in esophagus leads to a ringed or furrowed esophagus
  - Results in solid-food dysphagia
  - Can also result in various types of esophageal dysmotility and decreased esophageal distensibility
  - Believed to be related to either food or airborne allergies but mechanism uncertain
  - Clusters with asthma and atopic disorders
  - Classically associated with white men with mean age of diagnosis 38 years
  - Diagnosed with endoscopic biopsy
  - Increasing markedly in incidence and prevalence
    - **Most common cause of dysphagia in patients younger than 40 years old**
    - **Accounts for at least half of food-impaction cases presenting to the emergency room (ER)**
  - Treated in most cases with dietary modification or topical steroids
- Infectious
  - Presence or absence of oral lesions does not correlate with esophagitis
  - Diagnosis best made by endoscopy
  - Viral esophagitis
    - Cytomegalovirus
      - Typically seen in immunocompromised patients
      - Endoscopy shows serpiginous ulcers within normal mucosa
      - Histology shows intranuclear and intracytoplasmic inclusions
      - Treat with ganciclovir or foscarnet (if resistance occurs)
    - Herpes simplex virus (HSV)
      - Type 1 rarely causes esophagitis in immunocompetent patients
      - Type 1 or 2 can cause esophagitis in immunosuppressed patients
      - Endoscopy shows vesicles and small ulcers
      - Histology can show eosinophilic intranuclear inclusions and giant cell formation
      - Treat with acyclovir or foscarnet (if acyclovir resistance occurs)
    - Varicella-zoster virus
      - Can cause esophagitis in immunocompetent and immunosuppressed patients
      - Similar presentation to HSV
      - Acyclovir can reduce symptom duration
    - Human immunodeficiency virus (HIV) (see Chapter 12)
      - Self-limited ulceration can accompany seroconversion

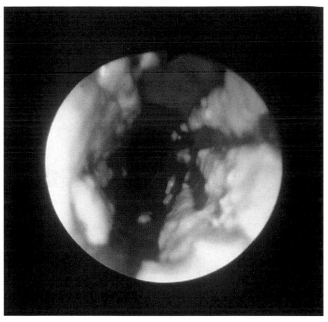

FIGURE 26-2 Endoscopic appearance of candidal esophagitis. (From Cohen J, Powderly W. *Infectious Diseases.* 2nd ed. St. Louis: Mosby; 2004: Fig. 237-2.)

- Persistent ulceration can exist in patients with more advanced disease; glucocorticoids or thalidomide may be used to treat
- Candidal esophagitis
  - Endoscopy shows whitish-yellow plaques (Fig. 26-2)
  - Diagnose by demonstrating yeast or hyphal forms on potassium hydroxide (KOH) preparation
  - Fluconazole is the preferred treatment
  - Ketoconazole and amphotericin are acceptable alternatives
- Bacterial esophagitis (rare): In immunocompromised hosts, *Lactobacillus* and β-hemolytic streptococci can be the cause

Structural Disorders

- Zenker diverticulum
  - Outpouching of the wall above the upper esophageal sphincter
  - Symptoms include halitosis and regurgitation of saliva, pills, and food
  - Commonly associated with underlying dysmotility
  - Treatment with surgery (cricopharyngeal myotomy/diverticulectomy) if needed
- Esophageal webs and rings
  - Schatzki ring
    - Causes intermittent dysphagia to solids ("steakhouse syndrome")
    - Congenital ring at distal esophagus just above or at the LES
    - Endoscopic dilation usually effective in treating

- Plummer-Vinson syndrome
  - Web(s) in cervical esophagus
  - Presents as intermittent dysphagia
  - Associated with iron-deficiency anemia
  - Associated with squamous cell esophageal cancer
- Hiatal hernia: movement of part of the stomach into the thoracic cavity
  - Sliding type
    - Very common with increasing age
    - Gastroesophageal junction (GEJ) and fundus slide upward
    - Can contribute to reflux esophagitis
  - Paraesophageal type
    - GEJ remains fixed
    - Pouch of stomach herniates through the esophageal hiatus next to the GEJ
    - Can cause bleeding and strangulation
    - **Surgery is often necessary for symptomatic or large hernias of this type**

Esophageal Dysmotility Syndromes

- Oropharyngeal dysmotility
  - Diminished ability to move food to esophagus
  - Characterized by dysphagia, nasal regurgitation, coughing, and aspiration
  - Most often caused by neurologic disorders (e.g., myasthenia gravis, multiple sclerosis, amyotrophic lateral sclerosis, cerebrovascular events)
  - Collagen vascular diseases that affect striated muscle (polymyositis, dermatomyositis) can also cause oropharyngeal dysmotility
- Achalasia
  - Most cases in the United States are idiopathic
  - Presentation: dysphagia, regurgitation, chest pain, weight loss
  - Diagnosis: Barium swallow can be highly suggestive, but manometry is the most sensitive study
    - Radiologic studies
      - Barium swallow: dilated esophagus that tapers to a "bird's beak" and air-fluid level in the esophagus (Fig. 26-3)
      - Chest radiograph: absent gastric bubble
    - Esophageal manometry: absence of peristalsis and failure of the LES to relax in response to a swallow
    - Esophagogastroduodenoscopy is necessary to rule out pseudoachalasia/secondary cause; sometimes an endoscopic ultrasound (EUS) is also performed if suspicion for a secondary process is high
  - Therapy
    - Endoscopic dilation of LES (success rates of 60% to 90%)
    - Myotomy: open, laparoscopic (Heller), or endoscopic (per-oral endoscopic myotomy); reflux esophagitis and stricture may be a complication of surgery, but this is viewed as the most successful option with reported success rates of up to 90%

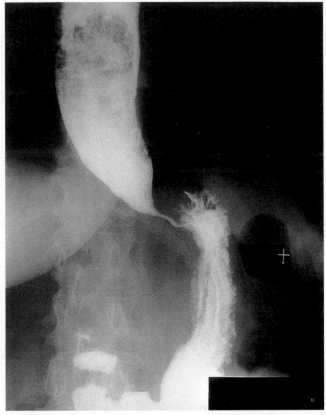

FIGURE 26-3 Barium swallow showing an air-fluid level in the esophagus and a "bird's beak" deformity consistent with achalasia.

  - Botulinum toxin produces short-term results only, but can be diagnostically helpful in atypical presentations
  - Medications (smooth muscle relaxants): rarely effective
- Secondary causes
  - Gastric cancer involving the GEJ (pseudoachalasia)
  - Neurologic disorders (e.g., myasthenia gravis, amyotrophic lateral sclerosis)
  - Chagas disease (American trypanosomiasis)
    - Transmission: Through reduviid bugs carrying the parasite *Trypanosoma cruzi*; transmission also occurs through blood transfusions
    - Epidemiology: Found mainly in Central and South America, although cases have been reported in the southern United States
    - Presentation
      - Acute disease (usually self-limited): Skin induration (chagoma), fever, lymphadenopathy; myocarditis and heart failure can occur
      - Chronic disease (years or decades after primary infection): cardiomyopathy, arrhythmias, megaesophagus, megacolon, aspiration pneumonia
      - Diagnosis: Examination of blood smear for parasites in acute disease; serologic tests for antibodies to *T. cruzi* for chronic disease

■ Treatment: Nifurtimox or benznidazole recommended; referral for cardiac transplantation may be needed for severe cardiomyopathy
- Scleroderma (see Chapter 45)
  - Presentation: Severe GERD, dysphagia
  - More than 90% have esophageal involvement
  - More than 90% have Raynaud phenomenon
  - Peptic stricture in distal esophagus may occur
  - Diagnosis
    - **Esophageal manometry shows absent peristalsis and low LES tone**
    - Barium swallow shows dilation and loss of peristaltic contractions; of note these patterns are consistent with a scleroderma diagnosis but can be seen in other conditions and are not pathognomonically specific
  - Therapy
    - PPIs
    - Esophageal dilation for peptic stricture
- Diffuse esophageal spasm
  - Presentation: dysphagia, chest pain that can be aggravated by stress
  - Commonly associated with GERD (70%)
  - Diagnosis
    - Esophageal manometry test may be normal if patient is asymptomatic at the time
    - Barium swallow can show "corkscrew" esophagus, uncoordinated contractions along the esophageal wall (Fig. 26-4)
  - Treatment
    - Treat GERD
    - Smooth muscle relaxants (isosorbide dinitrate, dicyclomine, calcium channel blockers) if GERD is not present
    - Antidepressants (selective serotonin reuptake inhibitors, trazodone)
    - Benzodiazepines

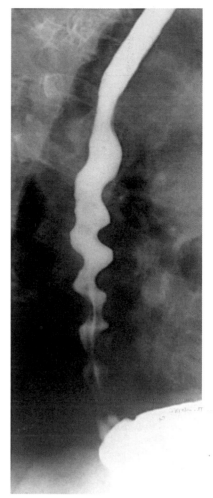

FIGURE 26-4 Diffuse esophageal spasm leading to "corkscrew" esophagus. (From Feldman M. *Sleisenger and Fordtran's Gastrointestinal and Liver Disease.* 7th ed. Philadelphia: Saunders; 2002: Fig. 32-14.)

Esophageal Cancer

- Can present with solid-food dysphagia, odynophagia, weight loss, and/or pneumonia from tracheoesophageal fistulas
- Squamous cell carcinoma
  - Incidence decreasing
  - More common in men and African Americans
  - Usually occurs in mid- to lower esophagus
  - Risk factors include alcohol, smoking, achalasia, nitrate consumption, lye ingestion, Plummer-Vinson syndrome
- Adenocarcinoma
  - Incidence increasing
  - More common in men and in whites
  - Usually occurs in the distal esophagus
  - Major risk factor is GERD and Barrett esophagus (see Box 26-1)
  - Diagnosis: endoscopic biopsy and tumor brushings; computed tomographic scan and endoscopic ultrasound to assess regional spread
  - Therapy
    - Prognosis is generally poor (5-year survival is 5%)

- Surgical resection appropriate for less than half of patients; 5-year survival rate after esophagectomy is approximately 20%
- Palliative measures include radiation, chemotherapy, photodynamic therapy, stenting, and endoscopic fulguration with lasers

Approach to the Patient with Dysphagia/Odynophagia

- Age, gender, immunosuppression, duration of symptoms, and associated symptoms (e.g., weight loss, chest pain) may suggest a particular cause
- Barium swallow has traditionally been the first test to obtain; however, if suspicion for eosinophilic esophagitis or infectious etiology is high, endoscopy is a reasonable alternative for initial evaluation
  - **With the emergence of eosinophilic esophagitis, many authorities now start with endoscopy as the initial test**
- Symptom-based evaluation is often helpful (Fig. 26-5)

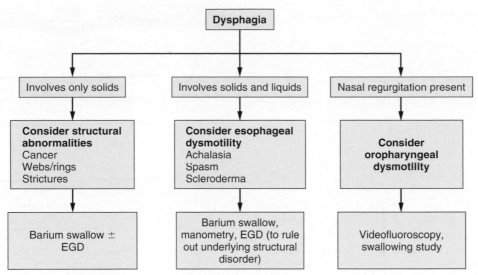

FIGURE 26-5 Evaluation of dysphagia. EGD, Esophagogastroduodenoscopy.

26

Review Questions

For review questions, please go to ExpertConsult.com.

SUGGESTED READINGS

ASGE Standards of Practice Committee. The role of endoscopy in the evaluation and management of dysphagia. *Gastrointest Endosc.* 2014;79:191-201.

Boeckxstaens GE, Zaninotto G, Richter JE. Achalasia. *Lancet.* 2014;383:83-93.

Boeckxstaens G, El-Serag HB, Smout AJ, Kahrilas PJ. Symptomatic reflux disease: the present, the past and the future. *Gut.* 2014;63:1185-1193.

Dellon ES, Gonsalves N, Hirano I, et al. ACG clinical guideline: evidenced based approach to the diagnosis and management of esophageal eosinophilia and eosinophilic esophagitis (EoE). *Am J Gastroenterol.* 2013;108:679-692.

Spechler SJ, Souza RF. Barrett's esophagus. *N Engl J Med.* 2014;371: 836-845.

Pancreatic and Biliary Disease

EUN JI SHIN, MD, PhD

The pancreas is a lobular structure responsible for secretion of digestive enzymes, bicarbonate, and certain hormones. The gallbladder and biliary tree serve to excrete cholesterol, assist in the absorption of fats, and influence water and electrolyte transport. Diseases of the pancreas and biliary system include a number of acute and chronic conditions responsible for frequent visits to both internists and gastroenterologists.

Pancreatic Disease

OVERVIEW OF PANCREATIC STRUCTURE AND FUNCTION

- Anatomy and physiology (Fig. 27-1A)
  - Pancreas: soft, elongated gland that lies in the retroperitoneum
  - Anatomic parts of the pancreas are the head with the uncinate process, the neck, the body, and the tail
  - Main pancreatic duct (duct of Wirsung) opens in the major duodenal papilla
  - The accessory pancreatic duct (duct of Santorini) drains via the minor duodenal papilla
  - The pancreas has a lobular structure and consists of an exocrine portion, which secretes digestive enzymes and bicarbonate, and an endocrine portion, which secretes hormones into the blood
  - The exocrine portion is composed of ductal, acinar, and centroacinar cells
  - **More than 95% of pancreatic cancer arise from the exocrine portion**
  - The endocrine pancreas consists of islet cells (1% to 2%) that produce insulin, glucagon, somatostatin, and pancreatic polypeptide
  - Exocrine pancreatic secretion occurs via acinar cell secretion into pancreatic ductules; islet cells secrete hormones directly into the blood
- Developmental abnormalities
  - Pancreas divisum (see Fig. 27-1B)
    - Incomplete fusion of the ducts results in the duct of Wirsung draining only the ventral pancreas and the duct of Santorini draining the entire dorsal pancreas
    - Present in 5% to 10% of the general population
    - Can be associated with pancreatitis, but most are asymptomatic
  - A long common channel between the bile duct and pancreatic duct may facilitate reflux of bile into the pancreatic duct. This can increase the risk of acute pancreatitis.

- Annular pancreas
  - Congenital anomaly in which a concentric band of pancreatic tissue forms around the duodenum
  - Typically presents in infancy as duodenal obstruction, but can also present in adulthood
  - Can be seen with other congenital abnormalities, such as intestinal malrotation, Meckel diverticulum, Down syndrome, tracheoesophageal fistulas, imperforate anus, and cardiac abnormalities

ACUTE PANCREATITIS

Basic Information

- Epidemiology
  - Acute pancreatitis is a common disorder that results in thousands of hospitalizations
  - The incidence of acute pancreatitis ranges from 5 to 35 per 100,000 per year
- Etiology (Table 27-1)
  - **Gallstones and ethanol are the two most common causes of acute pancreatitis in the United States**
  - Drug-induced pancreatitis usually occurs within the first month of drug administration
  - The incidence of postendoscopic retrograde cholangiopancreatography (ERCP) pancreatitis is 1% to 10%, and may be as high as 30% following sphincter of Oddi manometry
  - Autoimmune pancreatitis causes recurrent episodes of acute pancreatitis and chronic pancreatitis
    - Characterized by pancreatic and biliary strictures
    - Computed tomography (CT) shows diffuse enlargement of the pancreas or a focal inflammatory mass
    - Serum immunoglobulin G, subclass 4 (IgG4), can be elevated
    - Responds to corticosteroids
  - Biliary sludge, or microlithiasis, can cause recurrent acute pancreatitis
  - Approximately 10% to 30% of acute pancreatitis is idiopathic
- Pathophysiology
  - Poorly understood, but the triggering event is thought to vary according to the cause
  - The initiating event includes intraacinar activation of pancreatic enzymes. Trypsinogen is converted to trypsin with damage to the microcirculation and autodigestion of the pancreas
  - Activation and release of phospholipase, elastase, kallikrein, complement, and coagulation factors

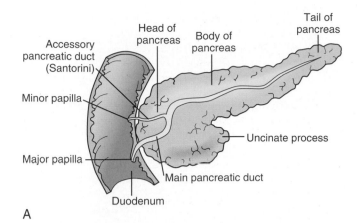

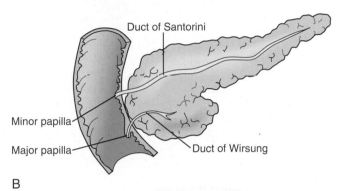

FIGURE 27-1 **A,** Normal anatomy of the pancreatic ductal system. **B,** Pancreas divisum.

further damage the pancreas. Release of cytokines can lead to systemic inflammatory response syndrome in severe cases of pancreatitis.

Clinical Presentation

- Symptoms
  - Epigastric abdominal pain radiating to the back
  - Nausea, vomiting, abdominal distention
- Physical examination
  - Fever, tachycardia, hypotension
  - Abdominal tenderness
  - Diminished bowel sounds
  - **Ecchymoses around umbilicus (Cullen sign) or flanks (Grey-Turner sign) suggests hemoperitoneum and hemorrhagic pancreatitis**
- Clinical course and complications
  - Most patients with acute pancreatitis have mild, self-limited disease
  - In those with recurrent attacks, the first attack is usually the most severe and has the highest associated risk of death
  - Early complications are those that develop less than 14 days from admission (Box 27-1)
  - Late complications are those that develop after 14 days
    - Pseudocyst formation with or without infection (Fig. 27-2)
      - Most pseudocysts resolve spontaneously within 6 weeks
      - Those that persist, enlarge, become infected, or become symptomatic need endoscopic, percutaneous, or surgical drainage
    - Infected pancreatic necrosis leading to phlegmon

27

TABLE 27-1	*Etiologic Association of Acute Pancreatitis*
Category	**Examples**
Obstruction	Choledocholithiasis, biliary microlithiasis, ampullary or pancreatic tumor, pancreas divisum, mucinous ductal ectasia or intraductal papillary mucinous neoplasm, choledochocele, parasites, periampullary duodenal diverticula, hypertensive sphincter of Oddi, duodenal loop obstruction
Toxins	Ethanol, methanol, scorpion venom, organophosphorus insecticides, cigarette smoking
Drugs	Azathioprine, 6-mercaptopurine, valproic acid, estrogens, tetracycline, metronidazole, pentamidine, furosemide, sulfonamides, methyldopa, cimetidine, ranitidine, sulindac, dideoxyinosine, nitrofurantoin
Metabolic	Hypertriglyceridemia (types I, IV, V), hypercalcemia
Trauma	Blunt trauma to abdomen, postoperative, post-ERCP/endoscopic sphincterotomy/sphincter of Oddi manometry
Infections	Parasites (ascariasis, chlonorchiasis), viral (mumps; rubella; hepatitis: A, B, non-A, non-B; coxsackievirus; echovirus; adenovirus; cytomegalovirus; varicella; Epstein-Barr virus; HIV)
Vascular	Ischemia (after cardiac surgery), atherosclerotic emboli, malignant hypertension, vasculitis (SLE, PAN)
Miscellaneous	Penetrating peptic ulcer, Crohn disease of the duodenum, autoimmune pancreatitis, pregnancy-associated, Reye syndrome, idiopathic
Hereditary	Mutations of *PRSS1, SPINK1,* and *CFTR;* can develop into chronic pancreatitis
Idiopathic	

ERCP, Endoscopic retrograde cholangiopancreatography; HIV, human immunodeficiency virus; PAN, polyarteritis nodosa; SLE, systemic lupus erythematosus.

- Pancreatic sepsis is the most common cause of death in patients with severe acute pancreatitis

Diagnosis and Evaluation

- Blood tests
  - Serum amylase and lipase: Most often used to diagnose acute pancreatitis
    - Amylase is the most commonly used test, but it is less sensitive and specific than serum lipase
    - Pancreatitis is more likely when amylase and lipase are elevated to at least three times the upper limit of normal
    - **If amylase is elevated but lipase is not, consider a nonpancreatic process**
  - Both amylase and lipase can be elevated in other intra-abdominal processes (e.g., bowel infarction, perforation, or obstruction) that may also present with an acute abdomen
  - **The levels of pancreatic enzymes do not correlate with the severity of disease**

BOX 27-1   *Early Complications of Pancreatitis*

Vascular instability and SIRS
Pulmonary complications: ARDS, effusions, atelectasis
Renal: acute renal failure, acute tubular necrosis
Endocrine and metabolic derangements: hyperglycemia,
    acidosis, hypocalcemia
Infected pancreatic necrosis
Pancreatic or retroperitoneal hemorrhage
Hemosuccus pancreaticus: massive GI bleeding caused by
    pseudoaneurysm of the splenic artery
Disseminated intravascular coagulation
Splenic vein thrombosis

ARDS, Acute respiratory distress syndrome; GI, gastrointestinal;
  SIRS, systemic inflammatory response syndrome.

- Renal failure alone and diabetic ketoacidosis (without pancreatitis) may be associated with elevated amylase and lipase
- Serum liver function tests
  - Serum alanine aminotransferase (ALT) is a useful predictor of biliary origin of pancreatitis. An ALT more than three times the upper limit of normal is suggestive of gallstone pancreatitis. However, a normal ALT does not rule out gallstone pancreatitis because sensitivity is low
  - Elevations of serum bilirubin and alkaline phosphatase are not specific for the diagnosis of gallstone pancreatitis
- Radiologic tests
  - Plain radiographs
    - Useful for detecting free air, which suggests bowel perforation
    - Abnormal gas signs in pancreatitis include local "sentinel loop" and general small bowel ileus
    - Chest radiograph may show pleural effusions (left greater than right), atelectasis, or acute respiratory distress syndrome-like pattern
  - Transabdominal ultrasonography
    - Useful for diagnosis of gallstone disease and bile duct dilation in gallstone pancreatitis
    - Not usually helpful in visualizing the pancreas itself because of overlying bowel gas
  - **Abdominal CT is often the most informative radiologic test**
    - Mild pancreatitis may be associated with a normal CT scan
    - Severe pancreatitis can result in pancreatic enlargement, peripancreatic fluid or debris, abdominal fluid collections, hemorrhage, and necrosis. Intravenous (IV) contrast can help identify pancreatic necrosis (Fig. 27-3).

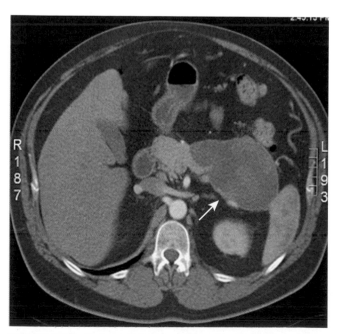

FIGURE 27-2 Computed tomographic scan: pancreatic pseudocyst in the tail of the pancreas *(arrow)*.

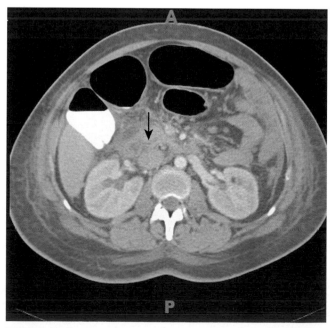

FIGURE 27-3 Computed tomographic scan: acute pancreatitis *(arrow)*.

- Serial CT scans can be helpful in detecting pancreatic abscesses; gas in fluid collections may suggest a pancreatic abscess caused by gas-forming organisms
- Magnetic resonance cholangiopancreatography (MRCP) can be used to identify the cause of acute pancreatitis and stage severity
  - Provides a better view of pancreatic and bile ducts than CT
  - Can detect choledocholithiasis, fluid collections, necrosis, and pseudocysts
- ERCP helps to diagnose the cause of acute recurrent pancreatitis, such as choledocholithiasis (gallstone pancreatitis), papillary stenosis, complete or incomplete pancreas divisum, tumor, stones, and sphincter of Oddi dysfunction
- Endoscopic ultrasonography (EUS) may be helpful for diagnosing tumors not evident by CT scan that may present with acute pancreatitis
- Clinical measurements of severity
  - Ranson criteria (Table 27-2)
    - Traditionally used for predicting mortality
    - Fulfillment of three or more criteria indicates severe disease and poor prognosis. Those with three or four risk factors have a 15% mortality rate; those with seven or more risk factors have a 100% mortality rate
    - More recent studies have suggested that the Ranson score is not an adequate predictor of severity
  - Acute Physiology and Chronic Health Evaluation II score
    - Also used to assess illness severity. Uses vital signs, selected laboratory studies (white blood cell count, hematocrit, arterial pH, creatinine), age, and comorbid illnesses to predict mortality
  - CT scan: The presence of pancreatic necrosis, abscess, or pseudocyst usually predicts severe disease

Treatment

- Supportive care: bowel rest, IV fluids, analgesic and antiemetic medications
- Enteral nutrition: Jejunal feeding in acute pancreatitis reduces the incidence of infection and shortens length of hospital stay
- Parenteral nutrition: May be required for moderate and severe pancreatitis
- Antibiotics
  - Use of antibiotics in pancreatitis is a source of controversy, with studies showing conflicting results
  - Empiric antibiotic therapy is not recommended for most cases
  - Patients with severe necrotizing pancreatitis are most likely to benefit from antibiotics
    - Imipenem and meropenem achieve high pancreatic tissue levels and may be effective for reducing the incidence of pancreatic sepsis in patients with severe necrotizing pancreatitis
  - **Empiric antibiotic therapy is currently recommended for this group**
- A CT scan can be obtained if there is no clinical improvement within 72 hours. If necrosis is found and infection is suspected, endoscopic or CT-guided fine-needle aspiration and drainage can be considered.
- Surgery is only indicated for drainage of pancreatic abscess and débridement of infected pancreatic phlegmon, not amenable to less invasive interventions
- ERCP
  - Urgent ERCP is indicated for gallstone pancreatitis, especially with coexisting cholangitis, jaundice, dilated common bile duct, or in patients with clinical deterioration (Fig. 27-4)
  - ERCP with sphincterotomy and stenting of the minor papilla is also useful for treatment of acute recurrent pancreatitis in patients with pancreas divisum
- Cholecystectomy is recommended for patients with gallstone pancreatitis after recovery
- Nasogastric tube suction, histamine₂ (H₂) receptor antagonists, fresh-frozen plasma, and peritoneal lavage

TABLE 27-2	*Ranson Criteria for Acute Pancreatitis*	
On Admission	**Within 48 Hours**
Age >55 years	Hematocrit decrease = 10%
WBC >16,000/mm³	BUN increase = 5 mg/dL
Glucose >200 mg/dL	Calcium <8 mg/dL
Lactate dehydrogenase >350 U/L	PO_2 <60 mm Hg
Aspartate aminotransferase >250 U/L	Base deficit >4 mEq/L
	Fluid deficit >6 L

BUN, Blood urea nitrogen; PO_2, partial pressure of oxygen; WBC, white blood cell count.

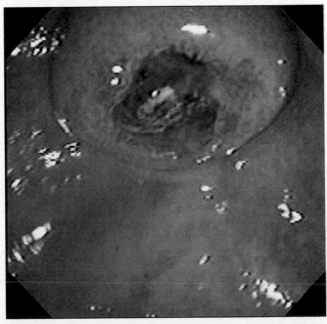

FIGURE 27-4 Endoscopic retrograde cholangiopancreatography: gallstone pancreatitis caused by stone impacted in major duodenal papilla.

27

have no proven efficacy for treatment of acute pancreatitis. Pancreatic duct stents have been shown to reduce the risk of post-ERCP pancreatitis

CHRONIC PANCREATITIS

Basic Information

- Definition and cause
  - Chronic pancreatitis is manifested by abdominal pain and abnormal secretory function of the exocrine pancreas associated with histologic findings of atrophy and fibrosis of exocrine parenchyma
  - If alcohol use is excluded, most patients in the United States with chronic pancreatitis have no identifiable cause
  - Idiopathic chronic pancreatitis can present at any age
  - Hereditary pancreatitis: Several mutations lead to hereditary pancreatitis
    - *PRSS1*: Autosomal dominant mutation in the serine protease 1 gene. Can present as acute or chronic pancreatitis with prominent pancreatolithiasis.
    - *SPINK1*: Acute or chronic pancreatitis caused by mutations in the serine protease inhibitor Kazal type 1 gene. Inheritance pattern is complex.
    - *CFTR*: Autosomal recessive mutation of the cystic fibrosis transmembrane conductance regulator gene
  - Autoimmune pancreatitis can also cause chronic pancreatitis
  - Cigarette smoking increases the risk of chronic pancreatitis

- Pathophysiology
  - Pancreatic duct obstruction occurs from hypersecretion of pancreatic fluid, rich in protein and calcium carbonate, which can precipitate in branches of the pancreatic duct
  - Patchy mononuclear cell parenchymal infiltration, atrophy, and fibrosis of the exocrine tissue may be seen on pathology

Clinical Presentation

- Signs and symptoms
  - May be asymptomatic
  - Abdominal pain: recurrent episodes or continuous pain
  - Pancreatic insufficiency: diarrhea (steatorrhea) and weight loss caused by malabsorption
  - Diabetes: Occurs in advanced chronic pancreatitis
  - Occasionally, patients may have no pain but may have malabsorption with or without diabetes
- **Painful attacks tend to diminish over time (5 to 10 years) as the exocrine and endocrine insufficiency progresses**
- Cessation of alcohol intake may decrease the frequency of painful attacks, but pancreatic insufficiency may still develop despite abstinence
- Complications include pseudocysts, ascites, and biliary obstruction (Fig. 27-5)

Diagnosis and Evaluation

- Blood tests
  - Amylase and lipase levels can be normal

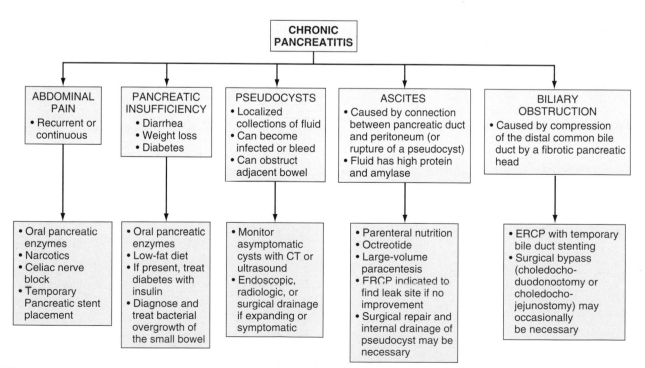

FIGURE 27-5 Sequelae and treatment of chronic pancreatitis. *CT,* Computed tomography; *ERCP,* endoscopic retrograde cholangiopancreatography.

- Pancreatic function tests
  - Bentiromide test
    - Bentiromide is N-benzoyl-L-tyrosyl-*para*-aminobenzoic acid (NBT-PABA), which is cleaved by pancreatic chymotrypsin in the duodenum
    - PABA is absorbed by the small intestine, conjugated by the liver, and excreted in the urine if pancreatic exocrine function is normal
    - Assuming small-bowel function is normal, decreased urinary excretion or serum levels suggest pancreatic exocrine insufficiency
    - Mainly of historical interest, not commonly used clinically
  - Direct pancreatic function tests: Bicarbonate and enzyme concentrations measured from direct samples obtained from an endoscopy after administration of secretin
- Stool tests
  - 72-hour fecal fat collection
    - **The most definitive test for diagnosing steatorrhea, which may be pancreatic or nonpancreatic**
    - Greater than 7 g/24 hours of fecal fat while consuming a high-fat diet is considered abnormal
    - Pancreatic steatorrhea does not occur until the pancreatic lipase output decreases to less than 5% to 10% of normal
  - Fecal chymotrypsin and fecal elastase are simpler tests of pancreatic exocrine function
    - Low fecal levels of chymotrypsin or fecal elastase suggest pancreatic dysfunction, but may not be sensitive for mild cases of chronic pancreatitis
- Radiology and imaging studies
  - Plain radiographs: Useful for detecting pancreatic calcifications, which are suggestive of chronic pancreatitis
  - Transabdominal ultrasound: Can occasionally see portions of the pancreas, but often the tail and body are obscured by bowel gas. Not the test of choice.
  - CT scan: Can detect atrophy, pancreatic calcifications, pseudocysts, tumors, focal fibrotic masses, and associated bile duct and/or pancreatic duct dilation
  - MRCP: Best for visualizing the pancreatic duct and cysts and in diagnosing pancreas divisum. Can detect calcifications, pseudocysts, tumors.
  - ERCP: Useful for evaluating pancreatic ductal changes, but can be normal in mild cases. Because of the risk of post-ERCP pancreatitis, ERCP is performed infrequently for diagnosis alone.
  - EUS: High-resolution images of the pancreas identify irregularities in the pancreatic ducts, cysts, parenchymal atrophy and lobularity, calcifications, and masses. Can help in diagnosing early chronic pancreatitis, even when ERCP and/or other imaging is normal.

Treatment

See Figure 27-5 for treatment options.

PANCREATIC CANCER

Basic Information

- Epidemiology
  - Pancreatic cancer is the second most common gastrointestinal (GI) malignancy (after colorectal cancer) in the United States
  - Types of pancreatic cancer
    - Adenocarcinoma is the most common type of malignancy in the pancreas and has the worst prognosis
    - Cystadenocarcinoma, papillary cystic carcinoma, ampullary carcinoma, neuroendocrine tumors, and lymphoma are less likely
  - Intraductal papillary mucinous neoplasms (IPMNs) are cystic lesions of the pancreas
    - Can be associated with acute and chronic pancreatitis
    - Risk of pancreatic adenocarcinoma depends on IPMN type, size, and features
    - Many are detected incidentally on imaging studies (e.g., CT, magnetic resonance imaging of the abdomen) in patients with no history of pancreatitis
    - Evaluation with CT, MRCP, and EUS-guided FNA can be used
    - Large cysts, cysts with a solid component, dilation of the pancreatic duct, and symptomatic cysts have a higher risk of malignancy and should be considered for surgical resection
- Etiology
  - Risk factors for pancreatic cancer include cigarette smoking, obesity, age, male sex, African American race, chronic pancreatitis
  - Most cases of pancreatic cancer are sporadic
  - Cases of familial pancreatic cancer suggest a genetic linkage
  - Gene mutations in hereditary chronic pancreatitis, Peutz-Jeghers syndrome, and hereditary breast cancer (*BRCA2*) are associated with pancreatic cancer

Clinical Presentation

- Most common presenting symptoms are abdominal pain (frequently radiating to the back), weight loss, and jaundice
- Jaundice caused by biliary obstruction commonly found in patients with tumors of the pancreatic head
- On examination, a palpable gallbladder (Courvoisier sign) may be present but is not sensitive or specific
- Glucose intolerance, venous thrombosis (Trousseau syndrome), and GI variceal bleeding (from compression of the portal system) may occur
- **Most patients present with advanced disease**

Diagnosis and Evaluation

- CT scan (Fig. 27-6)
  - A specific diagnosis of a pancreatic mass can be made with up to 95% accuracy
  - Pancreatic protocol (high-resolution CT with IV contrast and water contrast in the stomach) improves sensitivity

27

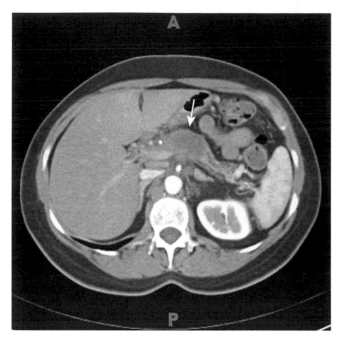

FIGURE 27-6 Computed tomographic scan: mass in the body of the pancreas.

- Necessary for staging and to rule out metastatic disease
- Serum cancer antigen (CA) 19-9
  - Has a sensitivity of 80% to 90% and specificity of 85% to 95% in patients with signs and symptoms of pancreatic cancer
  - In patients with pancreatic masses on CT scan, high levels may be suggestive of malignancy
  - Can also be elevated in colon, gastric, and bile duct cancers
  - **Not considered an appropriate screening test at this time**
- EUS: Can diagnose small tumors (<1 to 2 cm) not seen by CT scan and/or magnetic resonance imaging
  - Provides staging information as well as histology (via EUS-guided FNA) during the same procedure
  - EUS is also useful in diagnosing and localizing pancreatic endocrine tumors, including gastrinomas (associated with Zollinger-Ellison syndrome) and insulinomas (associated with hypoglycemia)
- ERCP
  - Compression of the main pancreatic duct and common bile duct, the "double duct" sign, is suggestive of pancreatic cancer
  - Cytologic sampling and/or biopsy at the time of ERCP is possible, but the yield can be lower than with EUS-guided FNA
  - ERCP is most useful in the setting of biliary obstruction because endoscopic sphincterotomy and biliary stent placement for decompression can be done during the same procedure

Treatment

- Surgery: In curative resections, 5-year survival results vary from 0% to 35%, with better outcome in ampullary carcinomas (up to 50% survival)

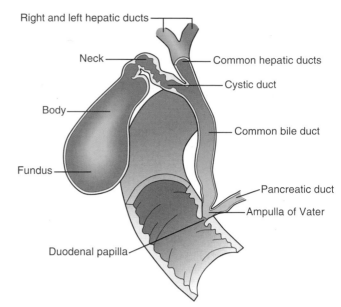

FIGURE 27-7 Gallbladder and biliary tree.

- Patients who have the best chance for curative resection are those who present with painless obstructive jaundice
- **Patients with tumors in the body or tail are rarely eligible for resection for cure (because of late presentation)**
- Chemotherapy and chemoradiotherapy: 5-fluorouracil (5-FU) and gemcitabine are the most commonly used chemotherapy agents. Often used as adjuvant therapy after surgery.
- Palliation
  - Endoscopic or percutaneous stenting or biliary bypass at the time of surgery may relieve obstruction and jaundice
  - Pain can be palliated with celiac axis nerve block during surgery or under CT or EUS guidance
  - Chemotherapy with gemcitabine and 5-FU–based chemoradiotherapy are also used for palliative treatment

Biliary Diseases

Overview of Anatomy and Physiology

- Gallbladder (Fig. 27-7)
  - The anatomic parts of the gallbladder are the fundus, body, infundibulum, and neck
  - Accumulates and concentrates bile and stores concentrated bile between meals
  - Filling and emptying of the gallbladder are controlled by neural and hormonal factors, including cholecystokinin (CCK), cholinergic vagal stimulation, motilin, and pancreatic polypeptide
  - In response to hormonal stimulation after meals, the gallbladder releases concentrated bile into the duodenum for activation of digestive enzymes and digestion of dietary lipids

- Extrahepatic biliary tree
  - Main right and left hepatic ducts join to form the common hepatic duct, which joins with the cystic duct to form the common bile duct (CBD); in most patients, the CBD joins with the pancreatic duct to open into the major duodenal papilla
  - Bile flow from liver to duodenum is controlled by gallbladder contraction and sphincter of Oddi activity

GALLSTONE DISEASE

Basic Information

- Definition and epidemiology
  - Cholelithiasis refers to the presence of microscopic crystals or large stones in the gallbladder
  - Choledocholithiasis refers to the presence of gallstones in extrahepatic bile ducts
  - **Women are diagnosed with gallstones two to three times more often than men of the same age**
  - Most gallstones are cholesterol stones (contain greater than 50% cholesterol) that have centers with calcium, pigment, and glycoprotein
  - A minority of gallstones are pigment stones (have <20% cholesterol content) that contain calcium salts of carbonate, phosphate, and bilirubin distributed evenly throughout the stone; these usually form in the setting of hemolysis (e.g., sickle cell anemia), cirrhosis, or chronic biliary infection
- Pathogenesis and risk factors
  - The healthy gallbladder prevents gallstone formation by acidifying bile, absorbing cholesterol, concentrating bile (which in turn promotes micelle formation), and expelling crystals and sludge
  - Risk factors for development of cholelithiasis (Box 27-2)

Clinical Presentation

- Biliary colic
  - Transient episodes of pain caused by intermittent obstruction of the cystic duct or CBD by a passing stone or sludge
  - The pain typically occurs in the right upper quadrant or epigastrium and can radiate to the shoulder or back. May be associated with nausea and vomiting.

BOX 27-2	*Risk Factors for the Development of Cholelithiasis*

Genetic predisposition (Pima Indians, other Native Americans, Mexican Americans, Scandinavians)
Older age (>50 years)
Obesity
Pregnancy
Medications (e.g., oral contraceptives, octreotide, ceftriaxone)
Prolonged total parenteral nutrition
Rapid weight loss
Diseases of the terminal ileum causing decreased reabsorption of bile acids

- **The pain can be sharp and intense, often related to meals (particularly fatty food)**
- Acute cholecystitis
  - Results from lasting obstruction of the cystic duct by a gallstone
  - Abdominal pain is more intense and prolonged than that of biliary colic
  - Fevers, chills, nausea, and vomiting commonly accompany the pain
  - Obstructive jaundice may occur when migration of the gallstone into the extrahepatic bile duct with obstruction of the duct occurs; it may also occur when a cystic duct stone erodes into or compresses the adjacent common bile duct (Mirizzi syndrome)
- Acalculous cholecystitis
  - May be seen in up to 10% of patients with cholecystitis symptoms
  - Often associated with other underlying illness (e.g., patients in the intensive care unit, those with diabetes)
  - Has a higher morbidity and mortality rate than calculous cholecystitis
- Chronic cholecystitis: chronic inflammation and fibrosis of the gallbladder
  - Typically associated with cholelithiasis
  - Can by seen with dyskinesia of the gallbladder
  - Symptoms include biliary colic
- Complications of cholecystitis
  - Gangrenous cholecystitis: From ischemia of the gallbladder wall; advanced age and diabetes are commonly present
  - Emphysematous cholecystitis may occur with gangrene and infection of the gallbladder with gas-forming bacteria
  - Perforation: Can occur with gangrenous or emphysematous cholecystitis with abscess and sepsis
  - Gallstone ileus: bowel obstruction caused by large stones that erode into the duodenum from an inflamed gallbladder (Bouveret syndrome) or pass into the small bowel from the bile duct
- Cholangitis: Patients present with spiking fever, right upper quadrant abdominal pain, jaundice, tachycardia, nausea and vomiting
  - Caused by obstruction of the CBD
  - IV antibiotics and IV fluids are essential for management
  - Urgent ERCP with sphincterotomy ± biliary stent placement is helpful for removing obstructing stones and sludge and decompressing the biliary tree
- Gallstone pancreatitis
  - Caused by acute impaction of gallstones in the CBD or at the major papilla
  - Urgent ERCP with sphincterotomy is necessary to remove the impacted stone and to restore adequate drainage from biliary and pancreatic ducts

Diagnosis and Evaluation

- Physical examination
  - Acute cholecystitis
    - Right upper quadrant tenderness with or without peritoneal signs

27

- Murphy sign: inspiratory arrest with right upper quadrant palpation
- The gallbladder is palpable in less than half of cases
  - Acute cholangitis
    - Charcot triad: fever, right upper quadrant pain, jaundice
    - Reynold pentad: hypotension, confusion, and Charcot triad
    - Most patient with cholangitis do not have all the previous symptoms
- Leukocytosis and elevated liver function tests commonly noted in cases of acute cholecystitis or cholangitis
- Most common organisms cultured are *Escherichia coli*, *Klebsiella* spp., group D *Streptococcus*, *Staphylococcus* spp., and *Clostridium* spp.
- Lipase and amylase will be elevated in gallstone pancreatitis. Bilirubin and liver function tests may also be elevated
- Radiologic tests can be helpful (Fig. 27-8)

Treatment

See Figure 27-8 for treatment options.

POSTCHOLECYSTECTOMY SYNDROME

Basic Information

- Postcholecystectomy syndrome: Abdominal discomfort, pain, and nausea persisting or presenting after cholecystectomy. Can be associated with abnormal liver function tests, and occasionally with an abnormal amylase and lipase.

- Most common causes of the postcholecystectomy syndrome
  - Papillary stenosis: Fixed narrowing of the distal CBD and/or pancreatic duct as a result of fibrosis
  - Retained bile duct stone
  - Consequences of the intraoperative bile duct injury (strictures, bile leak)
  - Biliary dyskinesia (also called *sphincter of Oddi dysfunction* [SOD]): Primary motility disorder of the sphincter of Oddi, leading to elevated intraductal pressure

Clinical Presentation

- Persistent or recurrent pain in the right upper quadrant and/or epigastric area that can be accompanied by nausea and vomiting and that resembles symptoms that occurred before cholecystectomy
- Patients with postoperative bile duct strictures can present with pruritus, jaundice, or cholangitis

Diagnosis and Evaluation

- A biliary cause for postcholecystectomy pain should be suspected in the presence of bile duct dilation and abnormalities in liver function tests during painful attacks
- If ductal dilation and laboratory abnormalities are absent, patients may require ERCP with sphincter of Oddi manometry to document an elevated intraductal pressure. There is a high risk of post-ERCP pancreatitis after sphincter of Oddi manometry.
- The less-invasive CCK–hepatobiliary iminodiacetic acid (HIDA) scan with SOD score can discriminate patients with SOD

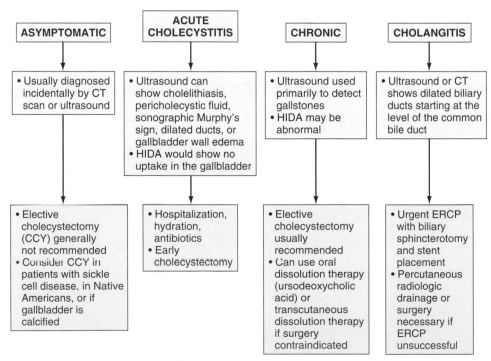

FIGURE 27-8 Diagnosis and treatment of gallstone disease. CT, Computed tomography; ERCP, endoscopic retrograde cholangiopancreatography; HIDA, hepatobiliary iminodiacetic acid.

- Patients with unexplained pain after cholecystectomy, with normal imaging and laboratory results, should have a careful evaluation for other causes of pain before proceeding with ERCP with sphincter of Oddi manometry

Treatment

- Most causes of postcholecystectomy syndrome, particularly those with imaging and laboratory abnormalities, can be corrected endoscopically during ERCP

CHOLANGIOCARCINOMA
Basic Information

- Rare tumor of the biliary tree that is challenging to diagnose, accounting for 3% of all GI cancers
- Defined as a primary malignant tumor originating from cells resembling biliary epithelium and distinguished from gallbladder cancer. These tumors may arise from:
  - Small peripheral intrahepatic bile ducts
  - Larger intrahepatic bile ducts at or near the hilar confluence of the right and left hepatic ducts (Klatskin tumor)
  - Extrahepatic bile ducts (distal bile duct carcinoma)
- Associated risk factors include the following:
  - Primary sclerosing cholangitis (PSC) (lifetime risk of 15%); between 50% and 90% of PSC patients have ulcerative colitis
  - Chronic parasitic infection of the biliary tree with *Clonorchis sinensis*, *Opisthorchis* spp., *Ascaris*, and other parasites
  - Exposure to thorium dioxide (Thorotrast, a radiocontrast medium used in the 1930s and 1940s)
  - Choledochal cysts (Box 27-3)
  - Oriental cholangiohepatitis: Brown pigment intrahepatic biliary stones develop as a result of chronic inflammation from chronic bacterial infection
  - Multiple biliary papillomatosis
  - Hereditary nonpolyposis colorectal cancer (Lynch syndrome)
  - Increasing age, male gender

BOX 27-3 | *Choledochal Cysts*

- Cystic dilations of any segment of the biliary system (intrahepatic and/or extrahepatic)
- Can present with abdominal pain, jaundice, and right upper quadrant mass
- Bile duct obstruction and pancreatitis can occur
- Surgical excision can be indicated to prevent malignant transformation
- Types of choledochal cysts:
  Type I: cystic dilation of the common bile duct (most common)
  Type III: choledochocele. Intraduodenal choledochal cyst
  Type V: Caroli syndrome
- Autosomal-recessive condition
- Patients have widespread saccular dilations of the bile ducts
- Bile collections may become infected
- Associated with polycystic kidney disease

Clinical Presentation

- **Patients typically present with jaundice, weight loss, abdominal pain, and pruritus; may also have dark urine and acholic stools**
- Physical examination
  - Courvoisier sign: palpable gallbladder
  - Hepatomegaly may be present
  - Jaundice
- Bilirubin, alkaline phosphatase, γ-glutamyltransferase (GGT) may be elevated. Aspartate aminotransferase and ALT are often normal early in disease.

Diagnosis and Evaluation

- Transabdominal ultrasonography, CT scan, or MRCP may show biliary dilation, a level of obstruction, and possibly a ductal mass
- Cholangiography (percutaneous or endoscopic via ERCP) will show irregular, tight strictures with proximal dilation and allow for histologic sampling; however, brushings and biopsies may be falsely negative
- EUS can be used to identify small tumors and lymph nodes. Histologic sampling can be performed by FNA.
- CA 19-9 may be elevated but is nonspecific for cholangiocarcinoma and can be falsely negative

Treatment

- The overall prognosis is poor, with a 5-year survival rate of 5%
- **The diagnosis is often made late and many patients are unresectable at diagnosis**
- Surgical resection may be possible in up to 20% of patients
- Chemotherapy and radiation therapy can also be used, but long-term survival is poor

GALLBLADDER CANCER
Basic Information

- Rare GI cancer that presents late in life and is usually unresectable when symptomatic
- It is potentially curable when incidentally found or removed by cholecystectomy (seen in up to 2% of gallbladders removed for symptomatic gallstones or cholecystitis)
- Predisposing risk factors include
  - Cholelithiasis: Present in up to 90% of patients with gallbladder cancer. However, the incidence is rare in patients with gallstones (0.5% to 3%).
  - Older age
  - Female gender
  - Obesity
  - Gallbladder adenomas/polyps (particularly those >1 cm in diameter)
  - Chronic cholecystitis (e.g., large gallstones)
  - Chronic *Salmonella typhi* infection
  - Calcified or (porcelain) gallbladder
  - Some carcinogenic occupational chemical exposures

Clinical Presentation

- Weight loss, abdominal pain, biliary obstruction, nausea, or right upper quadrant mass

27

Diagnosis and Evaluation

- Ultrasound may show a mass, thickening of the gallbladder wall, or extraluminal extension of the tumor
- CT and MRCP can also be used to identify gallbladder masses and polyps
- Laboratory studies are less helpful; alkaline phosphatase and bilirubin can be elevated if biliary obstruction is present

Treatment

- **The prognosis is very poor because these cancers are very aggressive and patients usually present with an advanced form of disease**
- Surgery for very limited disease may be curative. Overall survival rates for more advanced disease are poor.
- Treatment options are limited for tumors that extend beyond the gallbladder and include aggressive surgery, chemotherapy, and radiation

Acknowledgment

The author is grateful to Dr. Kerry B. Dunbar for her work on previous drafts of this chapter for previous editions of this textbook.

Review Questions

For review questions, please go to ExpertConsult.com.

SUGGESTED READINGS

Braganza JM, Lee SH, McCloy RF, et al. Chronic pancreatitis. *Lancet.* 2011;377:1184-1197.

Forsmark CE. Management of chronic pancreatitis. *Gastroenterology.* 2013;144:1282-1291.

Johnson CD, Besselink MG, Carter R. Acute pancreatitis. *BMJ.* 2014;349:g4859.

Rizvi S, Gores GJ. Pathogenesis, diagnosis, and management of cholangiocarcinoma. *Gastroenterology.* 2013;145:1215-1229.

Soares KC, Arnaoutakis DJ, Kamel I, et al. Choledochal cysts: presentation, clinical differentiation, and management. *J Am Coll Surg.* 2014;219:1167-1180.

Disorders of the Small and Large Intestine

ELLEN STEIN, MD

The small and large bowels are responsible for absorption of nutrients and fluid and for excretion of waste. Diseases that affect the intestinal system are likely to interfere with at least one of these two functions and lead to problems with motility or malabsorption. Diseases that disrupt the mucosal integrity can also cause bleeding, as discussed in Chapter 25.

Diarrhea: General Principles

Basic Information

- Defined as an increase in the fluidity, frequency, or volume of stool output; usually results in increased daily stool weight (more than 200 g/day in the United States)
- Diarrhea can be described by many features, one classic comparison is **osmotic** (reduced oral intake eliminates/ decreases diarrhea) versus **secretory** (reduced oral intake does not alter diarrhea). Other comparisons may include bloody versus nonbloody, inflammatory versus noninflammatory, steatorrhea (fatty stools) versus normal fat content, infectious versus noninfectious.
- Mechanisms of diarrhea (Table 28-1)
  - Osmotic diarrhea
    - Osmotically active solutes are not absorbed well from the gut lumen and cause increased stool frequency
    - Higher osmolality in the lumen causes passive water loss across the mucosa of the duodenum and jejunum, overwhelming the absorptive capacities of the ileum and colon
    - **Diarrhea stops when oral intake stops**
    - Volume is usually less than 1 L/day
  - Secretory diarrhea
    - Increased fluid secretion and impaired electrolyte absorption across the intestinal mucosa
    - **Diarrhea continues even when oral intake stops**
    - Volume usually large (more than 1 L/day), watery, without pus or blood
  - Altered motility
    - Increased motility
      - Causes decreased contact time between the gut and digesting food (*chyme*)
      - Leads to less absorption and large amounts of fluid delivered to the colon

- Decreased motility
  - Causes bacterial overgrowth
  - Leads to impaired bile salt malabsorption
- Altered mucosa and exudative diarrhea
  - Inflamed or ulcerated mucosa permits mucus, blood, and pus to leak into lumen
  - Diarrhea can result directly from the increased osmotic load, increased motility (stimulation of the enteric nervous system), or secretion of the products of inflammation
  - Stool volume can be large or small, depending on the part of the bowel affected
  - Bloody diarrhea can be related to *campylobacter, shigella, salmonella, E. coli,* amebiasis, inflammatory bowel disease (IBD), malignancy, adenocarcinoma, colitis (infectious or ischemic)
- Anorectal dysfunction or injury
  - Leads to the inability to retain feces
  - Characterized by fecal incontinence and small-volume stools
- Most diarrheal illnesses have more than one mechanism of stool generation (e.g., diseases of malabsorption)

Clinical Presentation

- Acute diarrhea
  - Usually self-limited (shorter than 4 weeks' duration)
  - Most cases infectious (see Chapter 14)
  - Consider medications (e.g., laxatives, magnesium-containing antacids, proton pump inhibitors, colchicine, furosemide)
  - **If abdominal pain and bloody diarrhea occur together in a patient older than 50 years or with known vascular disease, consider ischemic colitis**
- Chronic diarrhea
  - Lasts longer than 4 weeks
  - Stools can be watery, bloody, contain grease, and be foul-smelling
  - Steatorrhea is defined as more than 7 g of fat/day over 72-hour fecal fat collection while on a high-fat diet (100 g fat/day)
  - Abdominal pain or cramping is often present
  - Associated signs and symptoms that suggest an organic rather than a functional (e.g., irritable bowel syndrome [IBS]) cause are:
    - Fever
    - Weight loss

TABLE 28-1	Mechanisms of Diarrheal Disease	
Category	**Example Conditions**	**Comments**
Osmotic	Maldigestion of carbohydrates (e.g., lactose, fructose) Ingestion of nonabsorbed solutes (e.g., mannitol, sorbitol) Ingestion of poorly absorbed salts (magnesium hydroxide)	Small stool volume Osmolar gap present Stops with fasting Stool pH <6
Secretory	Bacterial toxins (e.g., cholera, *Escherichia coli*) Hormonal secretagogues (e.g., vasoactive intestinal peptides, serotonin) Gastric hypersecretion (e.g., Zollinger-Ellison syndrome) Laxatives (e.g., senna, phenolphthalein) Bile salt malabsorption	Large volume of stool No osmolar gap Persistent diarrhea with fasting
Abnormal motility	Increased motility: hyperthyroid, carcinoid, post-gastrectomy, dumping syndrome Decreased motility: diabetes, hypothyroidism, scleroderma, amyloidosis, postvagotomy syndromes	Bacterial overgrowth motility usually secondary to decreased motility
Abnormal mucosa/ Exudative	Inflammatory bowel disease Bacterial pathogens (e.g., *Salmonella, Shigella*) Vasculitis Radiation enteritis Severe diverticulitis Ischemic injury	Volume can be small or large
Anorectal dysfunction	Neurologic disease Postsurgical complication Inflammatory bowel disease	Small volume of stools

- Arthritis
- Anemia
- Signs of malabsorption (Table 28-2)
- Chronic diarrhea can result from a number of different etiologies (Table 28-3)

Diagnosis and Evaluation

- **Acute diarrhea in an immune-competent patient does not require evaluation unless signs of dehydration, bloody stools, fever, or severe abdominal pain are present (see Chapter 14)**
- History and physical examination
  - Ask about stool character (bloody, watery, floating/hard to flush, frequency, urgency, night symptoms, accidents/leakage), associated symptoms (pain, fever, joint problems, eye redness), and predisposing conditions (e.g., travel history, human immunodeficiency virus [HIV] status, pets, camping, family history of IBD, recent antibiotic use)
- Diagnostic tests for chronic diarrhea
  - General blood studies: complete blood count (CBC) with differential, chemistry panel that includes renal and liver function
- Use of further testing needs to be guided by history, physical findings, and results of general blood studies
  - Stool studies
    - Fecal occult blood
    - Fecal leukocytes: Suggest inflammatory or infectious process if present

TABLE 28-2	Nutrient Malabsorption	
Location of Normal Absorption	**Nutrient**	**Consequences of Malabsorption**
Proximal small bowel	Iron	Glossitis Pallor Anemia, Pica
	Calcium	Bone pain Tetany Osteoporosis
	Folate	Glossitis Pallor Anemia Depression
Distal small bowel	Vitamin A	Night blindness Hyperkeratosis Corneal ulcers
	Vitamin D	Bone pain Muscle weakness Osteomalacia
	Vitamin E	Peripheral neuropathy Retinopathy
	Vitamin K	Bleeding Easy bruising
	Vitamin B_{12}	Peripheral neuropathy Subacute combined degeneration of the spinal cord Dementia Neuropsychiatric effects Anemia

TABLE 28-3	*Selected Causes of Chronic Diarrhea*
Category	**Examples**
Infections	Amebiasis Giardiasis *Clostridium difficile* HIV enteropathy *Yersinia* *Campylobacter* *Cryptosporidium* *Cyclospora* Intestinal schistosomiasis
Inflammatory	Ulcerative colitis Crohn disease Microscopic colitis Eosinophilic gastroenteritis
Hormonal abnormalities/ tumors	Diabetes Hyperthyroidism Adrenal insufficiency Vasoactive intestinal peptide tumors (VIPomas) Carcinoid syndrome Medullary thyroid cancer Gastrinoma Mastocytosis
Nonendocrine neoplasms	Villous adenoma secreting bicarbonate Obstructive colon cancer causing impaction and overflow diarrhea of liquid feces
Steatorrheal causes— maldigestion	Pancreatic exocrine insufficiency Bacterial overgrowth Liver disease
Steatorrheal causes— mucosal malabsorption	Celiac sprue Tropical sprue Whipple disease Ischemia
Structural	Bile salt diarrhea after ileal resection Vagotomy Short-gut syndrome
Osmotic	Laxatives (magnesium) Carbohydrate enzyme deficiencies (e.g., lactase) Sorbitol, lactulose ingestion
Functional	Irritable bowel syndrome
Anorectal dysfunction	Neurologic disease

- Fecal calprotecin: Suggests inflammatory process (IBD) if present
- Bacterial culture: most useful for acute diarrhea
- Ova and parasites
- *Clostridium difficile* toxin assay or *C. difficile* gene assay: Particularly useful if recent exposure to antibiotics reported
- Seventy-two-hour quantitative stool collection; how much is released
- Spot fecal fat or 72-hour qualitative and quantitative stool collection for volume (needs to be on 100 g fat/day diet); how fatty is the stool
- Stool electrolytes can be collected (stool sodium [Na], potassium [K]) and then used to calculate osmolar gap

- Measure stool Na^+ and K^+ concentrations
- **Osmolar gap = 290 − ([Na^+] + [K^+]) × 2**
  - **If osmolar gap is greater than 40, osmotic diarrhea likely**
  - **If osmolar gap is less than 40, secretory diarrhea likely**
- If laxative abuse is suspected, a stool phenolphthalein or laxative screen can be performed (rarely needed)
- Tests for malabsorption
  - D-Xylose test
    - Measures the absorptive capacity of the proximal small bowel
    - Urine and blood are collected after 25 g oral xylose is administered
    - Abnormal test suggests small bowel mucosal disease or bacterial overgrowth
    - Normal test in pancreatic enzyme deficiency
  - Hydrogen breath test for lactose intolerance
    - Tests for lactose digestion
    - After ingestion of lactose, the amount of hydrogen in expired air is measured
    - If substantial levels are recorded, lactose intolerance is suggested
    - **Alternative test is dietary restriction followed by a milk challenge. If dietary rechallenge produces typical symptoms, lactose maldigestion is likely.**
  - Hydrogen breath test for bacterial overgrowth
    - Tests for lactulose digestion
    - After ingestion of lactulose, the amount of hydrogen and methane in expired air is measured
    - If substantial levels are recorded, bacterial overgrowth is suggested
- Endoscopy
  - Upper endoscopy not routinely indicated, but small bowel biopsy may be helpful in some suspected cases of celiac disease, small-bowel overgrowth, or enteropathy
  - Colonoscopy and sigmoidoscopy are useful in cases where bloody diarrhea is present, or where inflammatory markers suggest mucosal injury
    - Colonic biopsies are needed to diagnose microscopic colitis or IBD
- Radiologic studies may also be useful in certain cases
- Capsule endoscopy may be helpful to evaluate the cause of suspected small intestinal diarrhea if radiology and endoscopy are nondiagnostic
- Specific blood and urine studies assist in searching for particular etiologies

Treatment

- Directed at the specific cause when identified
- Treat dehydration
- Avoid caffeine and other secretagogues
- Antimotility agents (e.g., loperamide) can be useful if infection has been ruled out

28

Diarrheal Diseases

CELIAC SPRUE (GLUTEN-SENSITIVE ENTEROPATHY)

Basic Information

- Predominantly seen in white population
- Causes flattened villi of the proximal small bowel (Fig. 28-1)
- Most patients have a genetic predisposition to sprue and will express human leukocyte antigen (HLA) DQ2 or DQ8. (Note: genetic testing should not be routinely performed for diagnosis.)
- **Serology studies (tissue transglutaminase IGA) suggest celiac disease has a prevalence of approximately 1 in 200 individuals in the United States**
- Type 1 diabetes mellitus and celiac disease share common alleles, suggesting that they share biologic mechanisms

Clinical Presentation

- Diarrhea is common but might not be present
- Iron-deficiency anemia seen in 50% of adults with celiac disease

- Osteomalacia and osteoporosis can develop from vitamin D and calcium malabsorption
- Most adult patients do not present with classic features of malabsorption (e.g., steatorrhea)
- Forty-two percent of patients with celiac disease have elevation of aminotransferases (liver function will return to normal when placed on gluten-free diet)
- **Diagnosis is often delayed for many years after the onset of symptoms**
- **Patients often have been given a diagnosis of IBS**
- Associated with a number of diseases:
  - Dermatitis herpetiformis (papulovesicular rash usually on the elbows, knees, buttocks, or scalp; Fig. 28-2)
  - Type 1 diabetes mellitus and other autoimmune disorders
  - Autoimmune hepatitis
  - Autoimmune thyroid disease
  - It is also more common in people with Down, Turner, or Williams syndrome
  - Increased incidence of small-bowel lymphoma

DIAGNOSIS AND EVALUATION

- Initial screening is usually performed with antibody testing: Check total serum immunoglobulin A (IgA) level and tissue transglutaminase (tTG) IgA as first-line screening
  - Antiendomysial antibody is an IgA antibody that is 85% to 98% sensitive and 97% to 100% specific
  - Tissue transglutaminase IgA antibody is 90% to 98% sensitive and 95% to 97% specific
  - Antigliadin antibody (immunoglobulin G [IgG] and IgA) has lower sensitivity and specificity
- **If there is high suspicion, but tTG IgA is negative, further tests can be useful, such as IgG assays (tTG IgG), or upper endoscopy with biopsy**
- In some cases, the diagnosis of celiac disease requires a small-bowel biopsy, which demonstrates flattened or blunted villi and increased lymphocytes (see Fig. 28-1A)

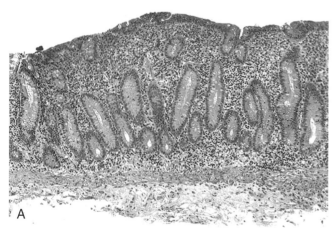

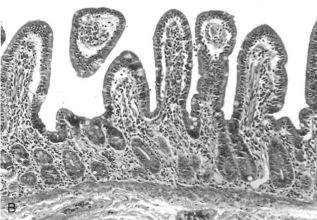

FIGURE 28-1 Celiac disease (gluten-sensitive enteropathy). **A,** A jejunal biopsy specimen of diseased mucosa shows diffuse severe atrophy and blunting of villi, with a chronic inflammatory infiltrate of the lamina propria. **B,** A normal mucosal biopsy. (From Kumar V, Fausto N, Abbas A. *Robbins and Cotran: Pathologic Basis of Disease.* 7th ed. Philadelphia; Saunders: 2005: Fig. 17-38.)

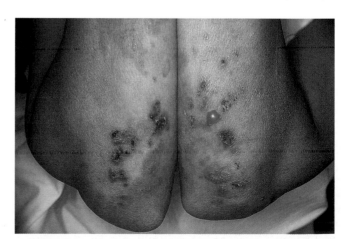

FIGURE 28-2 Dermatitis herpetiformis of the elbows. (From Callen JP. *Color Atlas of Dermatology.* 2nd ed. Philadelphia; Saunders: 2000.)

- The gold standard for the confirmation of diagnosis of celiac disease includes a repeat endoscopy with biopsies after initiating a strict gluten-free diet. After dietary challenge, biopsies should show healing and resolution of the histologic changes (restoration of villi). In absence of symptoms after initiating gluten-free diet, follow-up endoscopy is less commonly performed to confirm a diagnosis, but is very useful in patients who do not seem to be improving.

Treatment

- Lifelong completely gluten-free diet is highly effective in resolving symptoms and reversing pathologic abnormalities
- Most relapses are caused by dietary noncompliance or hidden sources of gluten
- Refractory cases may require steroids or other immunosuppressives
- The possibility of early-onset small-bowel lymphoma should be considered in refractory cases
- Response to treatment should be monitored with antibody testing, either IgA tTG antibody or IgA antigliadin antibody. If dietary adherence is present, the antibodies should return to normal within 3 to 12 months after initiation of gluten-free diet
- Nutritional deficiencies (iron, calcium, phosphorus, folate, vitamin B_{12}, fat-soluble vitamins) should be identified and treated
- Patients should be screened for osteoporosis

TROPICAL SPRUE (RARE OUTSIDE OF TROPICAL AREAS)

- Suspect in patients with chronic diarrhea and malabsorption after traveling to or living in a tropical area
- **Most patients have evidence of folate deficiency**
- Infectious agents (e.g., *Klebsiella*) have been implicated
- Pathology findings from a small-bowel biopsy can be similar to celiac sprue, but the patient is unresponsive to a gluten-free diet
- Treatment is with tetracycline and folate

WHIPPLE DISEASE

- Usually seen in middle-aged men
- **Caused by gram-positive bacillus (*Tropheryma whippelii*)**
- Presents with diarrhea, steatorrhea, abdominal pain, weight loss, migratory arthritis, and fever
- Neurologic (dementia, ocular disturbances, meningoencephalitis, cerebellar symptoms), cardiac (congestive heart failure, pericarditis, valvular heart disease), and ophthalmologic features may be present
- The diagnosis is made by showing periodic acid–Schiff (PAS)-positive macrophages containing the small bacillus in any affected tissue (usually small bowel). Antibodies to the protein and polymerase chain reaction (PCR) to the DNA of *Tropheryma whippelii* can also help to establish the diagnosis
- Treatment is with trimethoprim-sulfamethoxazole for 1 year

BACTERIAL OVERGROWTH SYNDROME

Basic Information

- Caused by
  - Small-bowel stasis
    - Anatomic abnormalities (postsurgical anatomy, diverticulae)
    - Abnormal small-bowel motility (scleroderma, diabetes mellitus)
  - Abnormal communication (Crohn fistula, resection of the ileocecal valve) between the small bowel and colon
  - Multifactorial (chronic pancreatitis, cirrhosis, achlorhydria, immunodeficiency)

Clinical Presentation

- Bloating, flatulence, abdominal pain
- Diarrhea
- Steatorrhea is caused by impaired micelle formation because of bacterial deconjugation of bile acids in the proximal small bowel
- Weight loss
- Dermatitis, arthritis
- Vitamin deficiencies:
  - Vitamin B_{12} deficiency is common
  - Vitamin A deficiency with night blindness
  - Hypocalcemia secondary to vitamin D deficiency
  - Folate may be elevated because it is produced by enteric bacteria

Diagnosis and Evaluation

- The gold standard is small-bowel aspirate demonstrating bacterial overgrowth (greater than 10^5 colony-forming units/mL), but aspirate is difficult to perform well, costly, and not widely available. Therefore, it is not required in most cases.
- Breath testing can be performed more readily at less cost, but the validity of the results is controversial. Testing has a high false-positive rate and issues with sensitivity and specificity tests include:
  - Glucose breath testing
    - Glucose is administered, hydrogen is measured in breath
  - Lactulose: hydrogen breath test
    - Lactulose is normally broken down in the colon. In bacterial overgrowth, an early hydrogen peak is seen.
  - ^{14}C-glycocholate breath test: infrequently available or performed
  - ^{14}C-D-xylose breath test:
    - Detect the release of radiolabeled carbon dioxide resulting from bacterial deconjugation of bile acid and metabolism of xylose
- Normalization of the Schilling test after antibiotics is highly suggestive of bacterial overgrowth (see Chapter 46)

Treatment

- Destroy the overgrowth
  - Broad-spectrum antibiotics can be used for several weeks; sometimes cycling of antibiotics or recurrent courses are needed.

28

- Nonabsorbable options: rifaximin, neomycin
- Absorbable options: ciprofloxacin, tetracycline, metronidazole
- Eliminate the underlying cause, when feasible
  - Some patients require surgery (e.g., small-bowel diverticulosis)
- Improve gut motility
  - If slow transit is noted, improving rate of transit can help
- Eliminate nutritional deficiencies with supplementation

BILE ACID MALABSORPTION

- Bile acids are absorbed in the ileum. Diseases that affect the ileum (i.e., Crohn disease [CD]) or where the ileum has been resected can contribute to bile acid diarrhea.
- Two basic forms of the disease:
  - Bile acid diarrhea
    - Associated with limited ileal abnormality or resection
    - Impaired bile acid absorption in the ileum leads to chloride and water secretion in the colon
    - Steatorrhea does not develop because the liver is able to compensate for the loss of bile acids in the stool
    - Responds to cholestyramine
  - Fatty acid diarrhea
    - Associated with extensive ileal abnormality/resection
    - Liver is unable to compensate for the loss of bile acids in the stool, so steatorrhea develops
    - Does not respond to cholestyramine
    - May respond to low-fat diet

MICROSCOPIC COLITIS

Basic Information

- Usually occurs in patients in their 50s and 60s
- **Accounts for up to 10% of cases of chronic diarrhea**
- There are two types of microscopic colitis based on histology: collagenous colitis and lymphocytic colitis
  - Lymphocytic colitis is more common
  - Collagenous colitis occurs more frequently in women
- Microscopic colitis is associated with certain drugs, especially nonsteroidal antiinflammatory drugs (NSAIDs). Other drugs implicated include ticlodipine, olmesartan, ranitidine, lansoprazole, and several others.
- Associated with other diseases, especially celiac disease
- Consider in the differential diagnosis of patient with celiac disease adhering to a strict diet but who continues to have symptoms

Clinical Presentation

- Microcytic anemia
- Diarrhea
- Weight loss
- Abdominal discomfort
- Fatigue

Diagnosis and Evaluation

- Colonoscopy with biopsy of right and left colon
  - May be grossly normal endoscopically, but biopsies from both the right and left colon may show injury

- **Diagnosis is made by histologic examination**
  - Histologic criteria for diagnosing microscopic colitis are:
    - Increased chronic inflammatory infiltrate in the lamina propria
    - Increased number of intraepithelial lymphocytes (more than 15 to 20 lymphocytes per 1000 epithelial cells)
    - Damage of the surface epithelium with flattening of the epithelial cells
  - The presence of subepithelial collagenous band is pathognomonic of collagenous colitis, and differentiates it from lymphocytic colitis, which lacks such a band

Treatment

- Microscopic colitis can resolve spontaneously if there is an inciting factor that is identified and removed
  - Stop NSAIDs or associated drugs
- **Most patient require medical therapy**
  - **First-line treatment is budesonide**
  - **Other choices: 5-aminosalicylic acid (5-ASA) like mesalamine or sulfasalazine, bismuth, prednisone, and rarely, strong immune-suppressive agents or biologics**
- Symptoms of diarrhea may respond to cholestyramine

OTHER DISEASES

See Table 28-4 for selected diseases that cause chronic diarrhea.

Constipation

Basic Information

- Subjectively defined as difficult-to-pass or hard feces, or bowel movements occurring less frequently than usual
- Objective definition is less than three bowel movements per week
- Increases with age
- Women have a greater incidence than men
- Can result from a number of different conditions (Table 28-5)

Clinical Presentation

- Can be acute or chronic
- New-onset, persistent constipation can be a symptom of underlying organic disease
- Abdominal discomfort may also be present but is less prominent than in patients with constipation-predominant IBS

Diagnosis and Evaluation

- History and physical examination should look for secondary causes of constipation. History may point to low fiber intake or new medications. Rectal examination may point to anorectal dysfunction
- Blood work should include CBC, electrolytes, calcium, thyroid-stimulating hormone
- In problematic cases, consider abdominal radiograph, colonic transit studies, colonoscopy (for those with a change in bowel habits, those who are elderly, or those

TABLE 28-4 *Selected Diseases Causing Chronic Diarrhea*

Category/Disease	Extradiarrheal Manifestations	Diagnosis	Treatment	Comments
Infections				
Giardia lamblia	Bloating Nausea	Stool examination for ova and parasites of *Giardia* antigen	Metronidazole	Suspect in those with exposure to surface water (e.g., campers)
Secretory				
Vasoactive intestinal peptide tumors (VIPomas)	Hypokalemia Achlorhydria Nonanion gap metabolic acidosis	Elevated plasma VIP	Somatostatin analogues Surgery	Causes massive diarrhea WDHA syndrome (watery diarrhea, hypokalemia, achlorhydria)
Carcinoid syndrome	Flushing Abdominal pain Wheezing Right-sided valvular disease	Elevated urinary 5-hydroxyindoleacetic acid and/or elevated serum chromogranin	Somatostatin analogues	Syndrome generally present when hepatic metastases present
Mastocytosis	Pruritus Flushing Abdominal pain Headache Urticaria pigmentosa: macular lesions that urticate when stroked (Darier sign)	Elevated 24-hour urine for histamine and metabolites Elevated serum tryptase levels Skin biopsy	Histamine receptor blockers Glucocorticoids	Symptoms can be episodic
Osmotic				
Lactase deficiency	Abdominal cramps Flatulence	Empirical trial of lactose-free diet Hydrogen breath test	Lactose-free diet	Common disorder Symptoms typically occur after ingestion of dairy products
Inflammatory				
Microscopic/collagenous colitis	None	Colonoscopy shows grossly normal colon Increased collagen or in basement membrane or lymphocytic infiltrate microscopically	Corticosteroids 5-Aminosalicylic acid	More commonly seen in women older than age 50 years

28

who have not received their screening examinations); anorectal motility testing can be considered after initial therapy is tried

- Constipation is often caused by slow transit. Occasionally it is because of pelvic floor dysfunction. With pelvic floor dysfunction, straining is a dominant symptom and soft stool and even enemas may be difficult to pass.

Treatment

- Functional constipation
  - Hydration
  - Exercise
  - Dietary fiber (15 to 25 g/day)
  - Consider osmotic laxatives (e.g., polyethylene glycol, lactulose, sorbitol)
  - Reserve stimulant laxatives (e.g., bisacodyl, senna) for acute constipation
  - Psychological counseling
- Pelvic floor dysfunction requires enemas, physical therapy, and biofeedback

- Secondary causes
  - Remove offending drugs
  - Treat specific condition

Irritable Bowel Syndrome

Basic Information

- Characterized by chronic recurrent abdominal pain and altered bowel habits in absence of structural disorder
- Patients may have predominant diarrhea (almost never nocturnal), constipation, or intermittent episodes of the two. Pain is often relieved with defecation.
- Affects 20% of Western adults
- Women more often affected than men
- Second leading cause of work absenteeism (next to the common cold)
- Patient characteristics
  - Diet may be unhealthy: fast foods, low-fiber diet
  - Emotional or psychological factors: Stress is associated with increase in symptoms; sexual abuse is

TABLE 28-5   *Causes of Constipation*

Functional (most common)	Psychogenic Irritable bowel syndrome Mental illness (e.g., depression, eating disorders) Inactivity Low dietary fiber
Drugs	Side effects from anticholinergics, calcium channel blockers, diuretics, calcium/aluminum antacids, opiates Laxative abuse leading to diminished neurologic function of the colon Metal toxicity (e.g., arsenic, lead, mercury, phosphates)
Endocrine/ metabolic	Hypothyroidism Diabetes Hypokalemia Hypercalcemia Uremia Amyloid neuropathy Porphyria
Neurogenic	Colonic pseudo-obstruction. Occurs postoperatively, with infections, narcotic use, or electrolyte disorders; risk of perforation when cecum >13 cm Peripheral nerve injury: cauda equina syndrome Hirschsprung disease. Can present in adults as chronic constipation Rectal biopsy shows aganglionosis Autonomic neuropathy CNS disorders (e.g., MS, Parkinson disease, stroke)
Diseases of the large bowel and rectum	Tumors Volvulus, hernia Colitis, proctitis Infection Scleroderma
Anorectal diseases	Fissure Rectal prolapse, rectocele, pelvic floor injury

CNS, Central nervous system; MS, multiple sclerosis.

more common in these patients; an increase in anxiety and depression, but possibly only in those who seek medical attention
- Innate sensitivity or susceptibility: Positive family history of irritable bowel, increased occurrence of other disorders with somatization features (e.g., fibromyalgia)
- Motility disturbance (slower myoelectric rhythm in colon) and abnormal sensitivity to rectal distention have been demonstrated
- Postinfectious: Infectious gastroenteritis predisposes to the development of IBS
- Small-bowel bacterial overgrowth may cause IBS symptoms and is found in a minority of patients diagnosed with IBS
- Celiac disease may contribute to IBS symptoms

BOX 28-1   *Diagnostic Criteria for Irritable Bowel Syndrome (Rome III)*

Symptoms of recurrent abdominal pain or discomfort and a marked change in bowel habit for at least 6 months, with symptoms experienced on at least 3 days of at least 3 months. Two or more of the following must apply:
- Pain is relieved by a bowel movement
- Onset of pain is related to a change in frequency of stool
- Onset of pain is related to a change in the appearance of stool

Clinical Presentation

- Pain most commonly in left iliac fossa or hypogastrium
- Knotting, burning, cramping sensation
- Distention, bloating, fullness, especially postprandially
- Small-volume stools whether diarrhea or constipation
- **Constipation stools often scybalous (pebble-like); diarrhea often in morning, following normal bowel movements; mucus is common**
- **Relief of pain often with passage of bowel movement**
- Dyspepsia, heartburn, nausea, headaches, urinary frequency, dysmenorrhea can also be seen
- Warning symptoms are not present. No history of weight loss, awakening from sleep, rectal bleeding, fever, or rigidity on examination (if present, think of other disorders).
- No specific findings on examination, except for mild abdominal tenderness, more often over sigmoid colon

Diagnosis and Evaluation

- Diagnostic criteria (Rome III criteria) are based on history alone (Box 28-1). Extensive investigation is usually not necessary, especially because many patients with classic IBS are otherwise healthy young women. Patients with new-onset symptoms or who are older than 50 years should be properly investigated.
- CBC, erythrocyte sedimentation rate, stool studies, occult blood examination are normal
- With diarrhea-predominant IBS, need to rule out lactose intolerance, celiac disease, IBD
- In more severe or unresponsive cases, stool volume (should be normal) can be examined and sigmoidoscopy performed
- If constipation is severe, rule out hypothyroidism, hyperparathyroidism, diverticulosis, anorectal dysfunction, and malignancy
- Occasionally, pelvic pain and altered bowel habit with gynecologic conditions, such as endometriosis, can mimic IBS; be wary of patients with risk factors for ovarian cancer (such as *BRCA* mutation or family history of ovarian cancer). A thorough age-appropriate gynecologic evaluation should be considered as required before making a diagnosis of IBS

Treatment

- Educate patient about condition: it is benign
- Adding soluble fiber in the diet or via supplementation can help those with IBS

- Reducing or remove offending foods (e.g., high-fat, high-carbohydrate). Some reported benefits when reducing foods containing FODMAP (Fermentable Oligo-Disaccharides, Monosaccharides And Polyols)
- Antispasmodics (e.g., dicyclomine, hyoscyamine) and low-dose tricyclics are helpful for abdominal pain by reducing spasm and hypersensitivity, respectively
- Antimotility agents (e.g., loperamide) may be helpful for diarrhea
- Probiotics have been used in small trials, particularly for postinfectious IBS
- Gas symptoms may respond to diet changes, simethicone, or bismuth
- Treat depression and anxiety (avoid narcotics and benzodiazepines)
- Drugs
  - Linzess is a guanylate cyclase C agonist indicated for constipation-predominant or pain-predominant IBS-C
  - Amitiza is a chloride-channel agonist indicated for constipation-predominant or IBS-C
  - Prucalopride is approved in Europe for treatment of IBS, but this drug is not yet available in the US
  - Removed from market in the United States: Tegaserod, a 5-hydroxytryptamine receptor 4 partial agonist, which was useful for women with constipation-predominant symptoms. Cardiovascular events prompted removal from the US market.
  - Alosetron, a 5-hydroxytryptamine receptor 3 agonist, modulates visceral afferent activity from the gastrointestinal (GI) tract and was found to be helpful in IBS in women with diarrhea-predominant symptoms. This drug can be prescribed through a special postmarketing program to dedicated registered prescribers, but is not in general use because of reported episodes of ischemic colitis.

Inflammatory Bowel Disease

Basic Information

- Defined as an idiopathic chronic inflammation of the GI tract: primarily CD and ulcerative colitis (UC)
- **Bimodal peak age distribution: initial 15 to 25 years, second peak 50 to 80 years**
- Significantly greater incidence in Western developed countries
- Smoking as a risk factor
  - Increased risk in CD
  - Decreased risk of current smokers and increased risk of ex-smokers in UC
- Genetics
  - Ten percent to 20% of patients with IBD have additional relatives with IBD
  - First-degree relatives of patients with IBD are 3 to 20 times more likely to develop the disease than the general population
  - Increased risk of IBD in patients with other autoimmune diseases
  - NOD2/CARD15 mutation is a risk factor for CD but not UC (mutation carriers often do not have disease)

- CD can affect any part of the bowel from the mouth to the anus. It can have "skip lesions" with a normal section of bowel between diseased sections
  - Eighty percent of patients have small-bowel involvement, usually in the distal ileum
  - Fifty percent have involvement of both the ileum and the colon
  - A small number of patients have involvement of the upper GI tract (esophagus, stomach, proximal small bowel)
  - Thirty percent have perianal disease
- UC affects the large bowel and is continuous from the rectum to the proximal extent of the disease
  - Proctitis: ulcerative colitis limited to the rectum
  - Distal colitis: affects the rectum and sigmoid colon
  - Left-sided colitis: affects area from the rectum to the splenic flexure
  - Extensive colitis: extends from the rectum past the splenic flexure but does not involve the cecum
  - Pancolitis: extends from the rectum to the cecum

Clinical Presentation

- Typically characterized by recurrence of a number of symptoms
  - Diarrhea, often with urgency, sometimes with night symptoms
  - Abdominal pain
  - Weight loss
  - Rectal bleeding
  - Fever
- Causes of exacerbations
  - Usually not identifiable
  - NSAID use, tobacco use (in CD), infections, and medication noncompliance may predispose to attacks
- Extraintestinal manifestations may present without symptoms of abdominal disease (Box 28-2)
- Cancer
  - Colorectal cancer
    - The risk is related to the duration and extent of the disease
    - **Overall risk in UC and extensive colitis from CD is 2% to 5%**
    - **Screen for dysplasia and cancer beginning 8 to 10 years after diagnosis of IBD is made, then every 1 to 2 years**
  - Small-bowel cancer risk increased in CD

Diagnosis and Evaluation

- Laboratory tests
  - Increased C-reactive protein and sedimentation rate; leukocytosis, anemia, and thrombocytosis are commonly seen. Fecal calprotectin elevated.
  - Stool studies for ova and parasites, culture, and C. difficile should be obtained to rule out infection
  - Peripheral antineutrophil cytoplasmic antibody (p-ANCA) is elevated in 60% of patients with CD or UC. Anti–Saccharomyces cerevisiae antibody is elevated in 80% of CD patients. Neither is adequate for diagnosis, but in some cases of indeterminate colitis, antibodies can help guide diagnosis.

28

Extra-Intestinal Manifestations and Complications of Inflammatory Bowel Disease

Arthritis
  Peripheral arthritis involving large joints
  Spondyloarthropathy/ankylosing spondylitis
Uveitis/iritis
Skin manifestations
Pyoderma gangrenosum
Erythema nodosum
Hepatobiliary manifestations
Primary sclerosing cholangitis (PSC)
  70% of PSC patients have inflammatory bowel disease (IBD)
  All PSC patients should be screened for IBD with colonoscopy
Cholelithiasis
Fistulas (Crohn disease [CD])
  Often involves perianal area, but any area of bowel may be involved, can lead to abscess formation
  Usually extend to skin, bowel, or vagina
Hemorrhage
Bowel obstruction/perforation
  Stricturing can lead to obstruction
  Spontaneous perforation more common in CD
  Toxic megacolon (abdominal distention, diarrhea, colonic dilation on radiograph)
  More commonly seen in ulcerative colitis
  Fever, tachycardia, leukocytosis, anemia
  50% of patients will require surgery
  15% mortality rate
Nutritional manifestations/malabsorption
Malnutrition
Dehydration
Anemia (iron deficiency, vitamin B_{12} deficiency)
Osteoporosis
  Can occur even without corticosteroid use
  Bone density scans should be checked routinely
Thromboembolism
Spontaneous abortion/premature delivery
Protein-losing enteropathy
Nephrolithiasis (calcium oxalate and uric acid stones)
Amyloid
Colorectal carcinoma

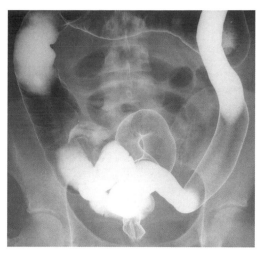

FIGURE 28-3 Air-contrast barium enema demonstrating luminal narrowing and loss of haustral markings in the sigmoid and descending colon in a patient with ulcerative colitis. (From Goldman L, Bennett JC, Ausiello D. *Cecil Textbook of Medicine.* 22nd ed. Philadelphia; Saunders: 2004: Fig. 142-1.)

TABLE 28-6 *Differentiating Ulcerative Colitis from Crohn Disease**

	UC	CD
Perianal disease	−	+
Fistula formation	−	+
Small bowel involvement	−	+
Granuloma formation on biopsy	−	+
Transmural inflammation	−	+
Inflammation limited to mucosa	+	−
Continuous colonic inflammation	+	−

*In 10% of patients, ulcerative colitis (UC) and Crohn disease (CD) will be indistinguishable.

- Radiographic features
  - Barium enema can show mucosal granularity or ulceration (in UC; Fig. 28-3).
  - Small-bowel series may show ulcerations in between normal mucosa, fistulas ("cobblestoning"), or strictures (in CD)
  - Magnetic resonance imaging (MRI) with enterography is also helpful in evaluating CD, particularly of the small intestine. MRI of the pelvis is helpful in evaluating rectal or perirectal disease and fistula.
  - CT scan of abdomen and pelvis or CT enterography can also be useful in some cases
- Sigmoidoscopy or colonoscopy is most often used to make the diagnosis and to distinguish between UC and colonic CD (Table 28-6)
- Capsule endoscopy is useful for staging or identifying small-bowel CD

- Complications of IBD and therapies, such as malnutrition, osteoporosis, and gallstones, should be sought and treated (e.g., nutritional supplementation, bone densitometry; see Box 28-2)
- Assessment of severity of a disease flare
  - Mild to moderate: able to tolerate oral diet; no dehydration, toxicity, abdominal tenderness, mass or obstruction; for UC, less than 4 stools per day
  - Moderate to severe: Failed treatment for mild to moderate disease or symptoms of fever, weight loss, abdominal pain and tenderness, intermittent nausea, vomiting, or anemia; moderate UC (greater than 4 stools per day); severe UC (greater than 6 stools per day with signs of toxicity).
  - Severe: Fulminant. Persisting symptoms despite treatment with steroids or high temperature, persistent vomiting, intestinal obstruction, rebound tenderness, cachexia, or abscess. Fulminant UC: greater than 10 bloody stools per day, with signs of toxicity; tenderness, distension, dilated colon, fever, tachycardia.

Treatment

- Medical management(Table 28-7)
  - 5-ASA medications (sulfasalazine, mesalamine, olsalazine)
    - Mainstay of therapy for mild to moderate cases of UC and CD
    - Inhibit lipoxygenase pathway, prostaglandin cytokine synthesis, free radical scavengers
  - Corticosteroids
    - **Initial therapy for most moderate cases and all severe cases**
    - Can be used intravenously, orally, or as an enema (for isolated rectal involvement or proctitis)
    - Oral budesonide undergoes extensive first-pass metabolism and has fewer side effects
  - Antibiotics (metronidazole, ciprofloxacin)
    - No clear role in treatment of UC
    - Most effective in fistulizing and perianal disease of CD

TABLE 28-7	Medications Used for the Treatment of Inflammatory Bowel Disease
Medication	**Side Effects**
Sulfasalazine	Gastrointestinal (GI) distress Allergy (fever and rash, similar to other sulfa drugs) Folic acid deficiency Hemolysis Neutropenia Male infertility
Other aminosalicylates (mesalamine, olsalazine, balsalazide)	Fewer than sulfasalazine; no hemolysis or infertility; rarely nephritis
Corticosteroids (including budesonide)	Hyperglycemia Cataracts Mood disorders Avascular necrosis Osteoporosis
Metronidazole	Metallic taste Peripheral neuropathy
Ciprofloxacin	GI distress Photosensitivity Elevated transaminases
Azathioprine/6-mercaptopurine	Pancreatitis Leukopenia Elevated transaminases Skin malignancies Lymphoma
Cyclosporine	Hypertension Renal failure Tremors Paresthesias Seizures Serious infections
Methotrexate	Leukopenia Hepatic fibrosis Pneumonitis
Infliximab (and other biologic agents)	Infusion reaction Tuberculosis reactivation Infections related to immunosuppression Lupus-like syndrome

- Some role suggested in postoperative care to prevent recurrence
- Immunosuppressants
  - Used to spare steroid use in patients who have moderate to severe disease
  - Most commonly indicated in steroid-resistant or steroid-dependent patients
  - Nonbiologic agents
    - Azathioprine (aza)/6-mercaptopurine (6-mp): Most frequently used. These agents are used both to induce and to maintain remission.
    - Cyclosporine: Used in some cases for UC, not CD; given over 2 to 4 months to induce remission
    - Methotrexate: Mainly used for CD
  - Biologic agents (used alone or in combination with 6-mp/aza to induce and maintain remission)
    - Anti–tumor necrosis factor (TNF) therapies
      - Infliximab: Chimeric mouse/human monoclonal antibody against TNF-α; given as intravenous (IV) infusion for both CD and UC to induce and maintain remission; also used to treat fistulizing CD
      - Adalimumab: Recombinant human immunoglobulin G 1 (IgG1) monoclonal antibody against TNF-α; subcutaneous administration every 2 weeks; can be used in patients who have lost response to infliximab
      - Certolizumab: Humanized monoclonal antibody Fab fragment linked to polyethylene glycol, which neutralizes TNF; subcutaneous administration every 4 weeks
    - Newer integrin therapies
      - Natalizumab: α4 integrin antibody. Was initially not recommended for routine use after cases of progressive multifocal leukencephalopathy (PML) were reported in patients using this drug. Presence of John Cunningham (JC) virus should be checked before administration. In some cases, this medication can still be used clinically if patient is JC virus negative.
      - Vedolizumab: a4b7 integrin antibody that blocks leukocytes from binding and traveling to the gut. Approved for UC and CD in adults with moderate to severe disease.
      - Other agents are under study, including ustekinumab
    - Patients need to be screened for tuberculosis (TB) before initiating biologic agents because any anti-TNF therapy dramatically increases risk of TB reactivation and other serious infections
    - If patient has appropriate risk factors, testing for hepatitis B virus (HBV) is also to be considered
    - Lymphoma risk is also slightly increased, as is risk for demyelinating disease, hematologic disease, and liver toxicity
- Surgical
  - UC
    - Because UC is limited to the colon, total proctocolectomy cures UC. An ileal pouch can be

28

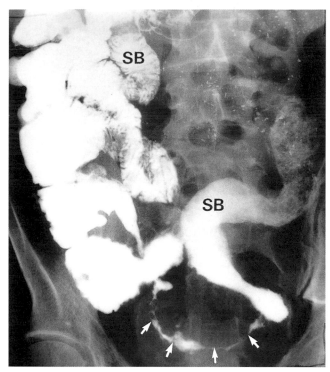

FIGURE 28-4 Small bowel (SB) of a patient with Crohn disease. Note the stricture in the terminal ileum *(arrows)*. (From Burkitt GH, Quick CRG. *Essential Surgery.* 3rd ed. New York; Churchill Livingstone: 2002: Fig. 21.8.)

formed, replacing the rectum. This can be affected by pouchitis.

- Indications for surgery:
  - Fulminant disease (toxic megacolon)
  - Colitis refractory to medical therapy
  - Dysplasia or concern for colorectal cancer
  - Stricture
  - Massive bleeding
- CD (Fig. 28-4)
  - Indications for surgery include obstructive symptoms, refractory severe inflammation, and repair of fistulas

- More than 40% of patients require surgery within first 10 years of diagnosis
- Up to 80% of patients will have evidence of recurrence endoscopically, and 10% to 15% will have clinical recurrence
- There is an increased risk of recurrence in patients who smoke or have perforating disease
- The aim of surgery is to preserve as much small bowel as possible
- A stricturoplasty can be performed to treat strictures, avoiding removing large sections of bowel
- Bile salt diarrhea and fat malabsorption may occur following ileal resection
- Nutritional (enteral therapy)
  - Effective therapy in patients with active CD for treating flare and decreasing fistula output
  - Useful in children, but adults can find enteral therapy unpalatable
  - Not effective as lone therapy in UC

Review Questions

For review questions, please go to ExpertConsult.com.

SUGGESTED READINGS

Dassopoulos T, Sultan TS, Falck-Ytter YT, et al. American Gastroenterological Association Institute technical review on the use of thiopurines, methotrexate, and anti-TNF-alpha biologic drugs for the induction and maintenance of remission in inflammatory Crohn's disease. *Gastroenterology.* 2013;145:1464-1478.

Ford AC, Moayyedi P, Lacy BE, et al. American College of Gastroenterology monograph on the management of irritable bowel syndrome and chronic idiopathic constipation. *Am J Gastroenterol.* 2014;109:S2-S26.

Pardi DS. Microscopic colitis. *Clin Geriatr Med.* 2014;30:55-65.

Rubio-Tapio A, Hill ID, Kelly CP, et al. ACG Clinical guidelines: diagnosis and management of celiac disease. *Am J Gastroenterol.* 2013;108:656-676.

Sandborn WJ. Crohn's disease clinical evaluation and treatment: clinical decision tool. *Gastroenterology.* 2014;147:702-705.

CHAPTER 29

Acute and Chronic Liver Disease

PO-HUNG CHEN, MD; and JAMES P. HAMILTON, MD

The widespread use of serum liver chemistries has led to an increase in the identification of diseases of the liver. Diseases such as hepatitis C, hemochromatosis, and nonalcoholic fatty liver disease have been found to be quite prevalent in the general population. A systematic approach designed to assess liver function and disease severity via laboratory testing and imaging can direct the need for more invasive evaluation and defined treatment.

Evaluation of Elevated Liver Tests

Basic Information

- Biochemical liver tests lack sensitivity and specificity, but both the pattern and degree of elevation may sometimes give clues to disease processes
- **Persistently or markedly (more than 10 times normal for aminotransferases or more than 4 times normal for alkaline phosphatase [AP]) elevated liver tests should always be fully evaluated**

Clinical Presentation

- Elevated aminotransferases (aspartate aminotransferase [AST] and alanine aminotransferase [ALT]) are usually indicative of hepatic inflammation and hepatocyte injury
  - Alcoholic hepatitis, viral hepatitis, drug-induced injury, autoimmune hepatitis, toxic injury, and nonalcoholic fatty liver disease are common causes
  - **The pattern of enzyme elevation (i.e., hepatocellular versus cholestatic) is a critical first step in the interpretation of liver chemistries**
  - **An AST/ALT ratio of greater than 2 is suggestive of alcoholic liver disease in the appropriate clinical scenario**
  - AST and ALT values greater than 1000 IU/mL are usually indicative of acute viral, toxic, or ischemic hepatitis. Alcoholic hepatitis almost never raises aminotransferases above 400 IU/mL.
- AP is elevated in diseases associated with impaired flow of bile, such as cholestatic diseases, infiltrative diseases, biliary tract obstruction, and drug-induced toxic injury
- γ-Glutamyl transpeptidase (GGT) and 5′-nucleotidase are tests that can confirm whether an elevation in AP

originates from the hepatobiliary system or another source (e.g., bone)
- Liver function tests (bilirubin, prothrombin time [PT], and albumin) reflect synthetic capacity of the liver
  - Bilirubin is elevated in a variety of hepatocellular and biliary diseases in addition to some nonhepatic causes (e.g., hemolysis)
  - PT is prolonged when coagulation factors of the extrinsic pathway (i.e., factors I, II, V, VII, and X) are insufficiently synthesized by the liver. This can occur because of vitamin K malabsorption in cholestatic liver disease or impaired production in cirrhosis.
  - Albumin is produced by the liver, has a half-life of 3 weeks, and decreases as synthetic function of the liver fails
  - Contrary to the popular term "LFTs," aminotransferases and AP are not true liver function tests

Diagnosis: Investigating Elevated Liver Enzymes

- The pattern of elevation dictates the evaluation process and diseases to be considered (Table 29-1)
- A careful history and a review of patient's medications, both prescribed and over-the-counter, are critical
- Elevated aminotransferases should first be evaluated by serologic and biochemical tests (Fig. 29-1)
- Elevated bilirubin or AP should be evaluated by an ultrasound of the biliary tree and an antimitochondrial antibody (see Fig. 29-1)
- If ascites is present, Doppler studies of hepatic veins should be performed to rule out outflow obstruction of the liver (e.g., hepatic vein thrombosis [Budd-Chiari syndrome])
- **Liver biopsy should be considered when diagnostic confirmation is required or if serologic and biochemical tests have not revealed the cause of liver enzyme abnormality**
- Endoscopic retrograde cholangiopancreatography (ERCP) or magnetic resonance cholangiopancreatography (MRCP) can be used to evaluate biliary tract disease
- Computed tomography (CT) and magnetic resonance imaging (MRI) scans can be used in place of or to complement ultrasound studies

TABLE 29-1	Summary of Common Liver Disorders		
Disease	**Liver Test Abnormalities**	**Diagnostic Testing**	**Treatment**
Autoimmune hepatitis	AST, ALT	ANA, antismooth muscle Ab, immunoglobulins	Prednisone plus azathioprine, transplant
Primary biliary cirrhosis	AP	Antimitochondrial Ab	UDCA, transplant
Primary sclerosing cholangitis	AP	ERCP, MRCP, pANCA	Stenting of strictures, transplant
Alcoholic liver disease	AST/ALT ratio >2	History suggestive; improvement with abstention from alcohol	Pentoxifylline, corticosteroids, transplant
Hemochromatosis	AST, ALT	Iron saturation, ferritin, genetic analysis	Phlebotomy, transplant
Wilson disease	AST, ALT	AP low, ceruloplasmin low, high 24-h urine copper, hepatic copper high	Chelation, transplant
Hepatitis A	AST, ALT	Anti-HAV IgM	Supportive
Hepatitis B	AST, ALT	HBsAg, HBc-IgM, HBeAg, HBV DNA	Nucleoside and nucleotide analogues, interferon-α, transplant
Hepatitis C	AST, ALT	Anti-HCV, HCV RNA	Oral direct-acting antiviral medications

Ab, Antibody; ALT, alanine aminotransferase; ANA, antinuclear antibodies; AP, alkaline phosphatase; AST, aspartate aminotransferase; DNA, deoxyribonucleic acid; ERCP, endoscopic retrograde cholangiopancreatography; MRCP, magnetic resonance cholangiopancreatography; HAV, hepatitis A virus; HBc, hepatitis B core; HBsAg, hepatitis B surface antigen; HBV, hepatitis B virus; HCV, hepatitis C virus; HBeAg, hepatitis B e antigen; IgM, immunoglobulin M; pANCA, perinuclear antineutrophil cytoplasmic antibody; RNA, ribonucleic acid; UDCA, ursodeoxycholic acid.

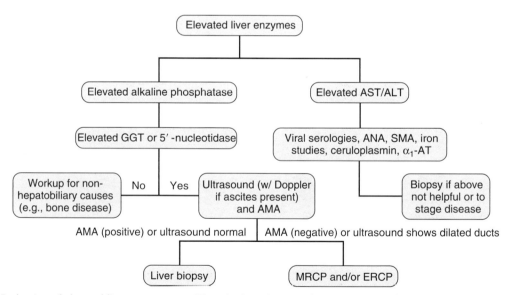

FIGURE 29-1 Evaluation of elevated liver enzymes. α$_1$-AT, α$_1$-Antitrypsin; ALT, alanine aminotransferase; AMA, antimitochondrial antibody; ANA, antinuclear antibody; AST, aspartate aminotransferase; AT, antitrypsin; ERCP, endoscopic retrograde cholangiopancreatography; GGT, γ-glutamyl transpeptidase; MRCP, magnetic resonance cholangiopancreatography; SMA, smooth muscle antibody.

Acute Liver Failure

Basic Information

- Acute liver failure (ALF) is defined as an onset of coagulopathy (i.e., international normalized ratio [INR] >1.5) and encephalopathy within 26 weeks of disease presentation, and without a history of liver disease. Jaundice is often present as well.

- Most commonly caused by medications, toxins (e.g., Amanita mushrooms), or viruses (e.g., hepatitis B, herpes simplex)
- **Acetaminophen toxicity is the most common cause of ALF in the United States (35% to 40% of reported cases).** Worldwide, viral hepatitis is the most common cause.
- Other causes of ALF are Wilson disease, Budd-Chiari syndrome, acute fatty liver of pregnancy, autoimmune

hepatitis, Reye syndrome, and other idiosyncratic drug reactions (e.g., isoniazid, phenytoin, sulfonamides, propylthiouracil, azoles)
- No specific cause of ALF is identified in approximately 20% of cases

Clinical Presentation

- Patients may present with encephalopathy, the severity of which is related to the presence of cerebral edema. Cerebral edema can result in brainstem herniation, which is the leading cause of death in ALF.
- Some patients present with abdominal pain, nausea, fever, lethargy, and massive elevations of serum aminotransferases (>1000 IU/mL)
- Patients who present with jaundice and then develop encephalopathy after several days have worse prognosis
- Presentation is often complicated by sepsis, multisystem organ failure (including renal failure and pancreatitis), gastrointestinal bleeding, and coagulopathy
- With progressive coagulopathy, spontaneous hemorrhage is commonly seen
- Widespread hepatocyte necrosis leads to loss of glycogen stores and impaired gluconeogenesis, causing hypoglycemia

Diagnosis

- Careful history from family and friends, history of toxin exposure, drug use, medications
- Toxicology screen, including acetaminophen level, should be obtained immediately
- Viral serologies, Doppler study of hepatic vasculature, CT imaging, ceruloplasmin, and 24-hour urinary copper excretion may be helpful in establishing the underlying diagnosis
- Prognosis can be made using King's College criteria (Box 29-1) or the Clichy criteria

Treatment

- Monitor PT, pH, glucose level, liver enzymes, cultures, fluid and electrolyte balance, central venous pressure
- Enteral feeding, dextrose infusion, thiamine
- Prophylactic antibiotics, antifungals
- Proton-pump inhibitor or H_2 receptor antagonist
- **N-Acetylcysteine for all causes, especially acetaminophen toxicity**
- Mechanical ventilation to protect airway in patients with delirium
- Elevate head of bed, hyperventilate initially, induce hypothermia, and administer mannitol if serum osmolality is less than 320 mOsm to keep intracranial pressure (ICP) low; avoid procedures that may elevate ICP.
- ICP monitor, when available, should be used to monitor perfusion pressures and ICP
- Continuous venovenous hemofiltration for renal failure
- **Transfuse clotting factors (including recombinant factor VII) only for active bleeding or before invasive procedures**
- Disease-specific treatments such as penicillin G and silibinin for Amanita poisoning or acyclovir for herpes hepatitis. There is some evidence to support empiric use of acyclovir in idiopathic cases.

BOX 29-1	*Indicators of Poor Prognosis in Acute Liver Failure (King's College Criteria)*

Acetaminophen Toxicity

Arterial pH <7.3 after adequate fluid resuscitation
Or all of the following within a 24-hour period:
  PT >100 sec (INR >6.5)
  Serum Cr >3.4 mg/dL
  Grade 3 to 4 HE

Non-Acetaminophen Causes of ALF

PT >100 sec (INR >6.5) and HE (irrespective of grade)
Or any *three* of the following:
  Wilson disease, idiosyncratic drug reaction, seronegative, or indeterminate hepatitis
  Jaundice >7 days before HE
  Age <10 or >40 years
  PT >50 sec (INR >3.5)
  Bilirubin ≥17 mg/dL

ALF, Acute liver failure; Cr, creatinine; HE, hepatic encephalopathy; INR, international normalized ratio; PT, prothrombin time.

- Early transfer to liver transplantation center results in improved survival

Drug-Induced Liver Injury

Basic Information

- *Drug-induced liver injury* (DILI) is the most common cause of ALF (>50% of cases) in the United States
- 6% of all adverse drug reactions involve the liver
- DILI is the most common reason for postmarketing withdrawal of medications
- Reactions can be dose-dependent or idiosyncratic

Clinical Presentation

- Symptoms range from asymptomatic to nonspecific complaints, such as fatigue, nausea, vomiting, and/or mild right upper quadrant discomfort
- Can follow several patterns of injury: hepatitis, cholestasis, mixed cholestatic hepatitis, and progressive bile duct injury known as *vanishing bile duct syndrome*
- Injury pattern can give clue to offending agent (Table 29-2)
- Some cases can be immune-mediated, and hypereosinophilia is present (both in serum and on liver biopsy)
- Most biochemical parameters return to normal after eliminating the offending drug
- Several medications require regular monitoring (Table 29-3)

Diagnosis

- Diagnosis of exclusion: first exclude other more common causes of liver disease
- Thorough history is critical to diagnosis
- Temporal relationship to medication/herbal exposure may assist in the diagnosis
- Rechallenging with the suspected drug is *not* recommended: If the liver injury is immune-mediated, second exposure may be more severe than the initial episode

29

Treatment

- Discontinue medication and do not rechallenge
- Biopsy liver if enzymes do not improve within several weeks of discontinuation or if diagnosis is in question
- Transfer to transplant ation center if liver failure ensues (coagulopathy and encephalopathy)

Herbal Remedies and Natural Products

Basic Information

- Increased use of herbal remedies has led to recognition of potential hepatotoxicity

TABLE 29-2	Hepatic Injury Caused by Various Medications
Injury Pattern	**Drug**
Nonspecific or viral-like hepatitis	Aspirin, amiodarone, diclofenac, isoniazid, methyldopa, nitrofurantoin, phenytoin, propylthiouracil, sulfonamides
Cholestasis	Carbamazepine, chlorpromazine, cotrimoxazole, haloperidol, tricyclics, estrogens, 17-α substituted steroids
Steatosis	Alcohol, prednisone, tetracycline, valproic acid, amiodarone, zidovudine
Granulomatous hepatitis	Allopurinol, quinidine, sulfonamides, sulfonylurea agents
Veno-occlusive disease	Antineoplastics, azathioprine, pyrrolizidine alkaloids
Adenomas and hepatocellular carcinoma	Estrogens and anabolic steroids

- Herbals are implicated in 10% of all DILI in the United States
- Few over-the-counter agents have been put through any rigorous scientific testing
- **Most reactions are idiosyncratic, although some are dose-dependent**

Clinical Presentation

- Wide-ranging presentations, including elevated aminotransferases, steatosis, fibrosis, portal hypertension, venoocclusive disease, and hepatic necrosis
  - Eosinophilia and rash can also be seen
- Cirrhosis or liver failure can occur with ongoing use of offending agent
- Some herbals can exacerbate pre-existing liver disease (e.g., *ma-huang* and autoimmune hepatitis)
- Table 29-4 lists herbs and associated hepatic injuries

Diagnosis

- Thorough history (patients often do not consider herbal supplements as medicines)
- Exclude other forms of liver disease. Liver biopsy findings often nonspecific.

Treatment

- Discontinue herbal medication and do not rechallenge
- Monitor liver enzymes and biopsy liver if enzymes do not normalize within several weeks of discontinuation
- Transfer to transplantation center if liver failure ensues (coagulopathy and encephalopathy)

Autoimmune Hepatitis

Basic Information

- Autoimmune hepatitis (AIH) is an idiopathic, chronic hepatitis characterized by lymphoplasmacytic, periportal infiltrates on liver biopsy, positive serum autoantbodies, and hypergammaglobulinemia

TABLE 29-3	Liver Monitoring Schedule for Hepatotoxic Medications		
Medication	**Every Month**	**Every Month for 3 Months, Then Every 3 Months**	**Every 3 Months**
Amiodarone			✓
Antiepileptics			✓
Azathioprine	✓		
Diclofenac			✓
HMG-CoA reductase inhibitors			✓
Herbal remedies			✓
All azoles (e.g., fluconazole)	✓		
Nicotinic acid		✓	
NSAIDs (other)			✓ (3 to 6 months)
Tacrine		✓	
Protease inhibitors	✓		

HMG-CoA, 3-Hydroxy-3-methylglutaryl-coenzyme A; NSAIDs, nonsteroidal antiinflammatory drugs.

TABLE 29-4	Herbs and Associated Hepatic Injuries	
Remedy	**Toxic Component**	**Injury**
Chinese herbal tea	Many	Hepatitis, veno-occlusive disease
Chaparral leaf	*Larrea tridentata*	Necrosis, chronic hepatitis
Dai-saiko-to and Sho-saiko-to	Scutellaria, others	Hepatitis, steatosis, fibrosis
Germander	*Teucrium chamaedrys L.*	Hepatitis, fibrosis, necrosis
Gordolobo yerba tea, comfrey	Pyrrolizidine alkaloids	Veno-occlusive disease
Jin Bu Huan	*Lycopodium serratum*	Hepatitis, steatosis, fibrosis
Kava	Kavalactones	Cholestatic hepatitis
Ma-huang	Ephedrine	Hepatitis, exacerbates autoimmune hepatitis
Mistletoe, skullcap, valerian	Unknown	Hepatitis
"Natural laxatives"	Senna, podophyllin	Hepatitis, cholestatic hepatitis
Red yeast rice	HMG-CoA reductase inhibitors	Hepatitis

HMG-CoA, 3-Hydroxy-3-methylglutaryl-coenzyme A.

TABLE 29-5	Serologic Features of Autoimmune Hepatitis Variants	
Serologic Features	**Type 1 (Classic)**	**Type 2**
Antismooth muscle Ab	+/−	−
Antinuclear Ab	+/−	−
Antiliver kidney microsomal type 1 Ab	−	+
Anti-F actin Ab	+/−	−
Antiliver cytosol-1	−	+/−
Antisoluble liver antigen/liver pancreas antigen	+/−	−

Ab, Antibody.

- Concomitant autoimmune diseases (e.g., thyroiditis, type 1 diabetes, systemic lupus erythematosus, Sjögren syndrome) are common
- Liver enzyme elevations tend to wax and wane

Diagnosis

- Elevated liver enzymes with negative viral hepatitis serologies, elevated gamma globulin (especially immunoglobulin G [IgG])
- Supported by histologic pattern of interface hepatitis, plasma cell infiltrate, and portal tract inflammation
- Autoantibodies usually but not invariably present (see Table 29-5)

Treatment

- Treatment indicated in patients with aminotransferases greater than 10 times normal; aminotransferases greater than 5 times normal plus gamma globulin greater than 2 times normal; or significant inflammation and/or necrosis on liver biopsy. Many clinicians treat AIH before the aminotransferases reach this degree of elevation.
- **Prednisone with or without azathioprine for at least 18 to 36 months (majority of patients require lifelong therapy)**
- Patients not responsive to the standard regimen may require more potent immunosuppressives (e.g., mycophenolate mofetil, cyclosporine, or tacrolimus)
- Treatment progress is followed by monitoring aminotransferases, gamma globulin levels, and liver biopsies
- After cessation of therapy, 80% of patients in remission eventually relapse, 50% within 6 months
- Consider liver transplantation for decompensated cirrhosis
- 30% recurrence rate after transplantation, with an average time to recurrence of 5 years

Primary Biliary Cirrhosis

Basic Information

- Immune-mediated destruction of small bile ducts
- Genetic predisposition plus triggering event such as viral infection or medication underlie many cases

29

- **Should be considered when aminotransferases are elevated, the patient has negative viral serologies, and no drug injury is implicated**
- Cause of AIH is not known, but pathogenesis likely involves genetic susceptibility with an etiologic trigger, such as viral infection or medication
- Variant, overlapping, or mixed forms of AIH exist that share features with other autoimmune liver diseases, such as primary biliary cirrhosis and primary sclerosing cholangitis

Clinical Presentation

- Two established forms of AIH with different autoantibodies (Table 29-5)
  - Both are more common in women
  - Distinction between subtypes not particularly useful with respect to management
- Type 1 AIH (80%) has a peak incidence between ages 16 and 30 years, but more than 20% of patients are older than 60 years
- Type 2 AIH (20%) typically presents acutely in childhood
- Range of presentation varies from mild enzyme elevations to liver failure
- Symptoms include nonspecific fatigue, lethargy, abdominal pain, rash, and arthralgias

- Highest incidence and prevalence in northern Europe
- First-degree relatives have a 50- to 100-fold higher relative risk compared to general population

Clinical Presentation

- Median age at diagnosis is 50 years, with a broad range from 20 to 90 years
- **90% of patients are women**
- Intermittent pruritus, fatigue, and abdominal pain; jaundice late in disease
- Long-term survival excellent in those responding to treatment in the first year of treatment (70% survival after 20 years). Response measured by fall in AP to within 1.67 times upper limit of normal.
- Impaired fat-soluble vitamin (A, D, E, K) absorption leading to osteoporosis, night blindness, etc.
- Elevated total cholesterol with unclear effect on cardiovascular risk (mostly high-density lipoprotein; classic dogma is no increased risk, but this has recently been challenged)
- May lead to cirrhosis, portal hypertension, and hepatocellular carcinoma

Diagnosis

- AP almost always elevated
- Aminotransferases typically mildly elevated
- Antimitochondrial antibody (AMA) is present in 95% of cases (and less than 1% of healthy population)
- Antinuclear antibody (ANA) is also positive in most cases
- Liver biopsy reveals portal tract infiltrates with injury/destruction of intrahepatic bile ducts (Fig. 29-2)

Treatment

- Ursodeoxycholic acid (UDCA, 13 to 15 mg/kg/day) improves transplant-free survival, improves liver chemistries, and slows histological progression
  - Exact mechanism is uncertain, but possibly increases canalicular excretion of toxic bile acids, inhibits intestinal bile acid reabsorption, and scavenges reactive oxygen species
  - Should be continued indefinitely

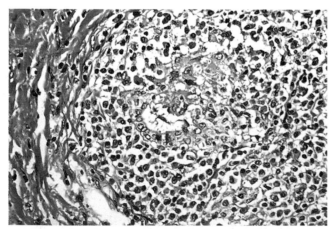

FIGURE 29-2 Primary biliary cirrhosis. Note the portal tract inflammation and injury to the bile duct. (From Kumar V, Fausto N, Abbas A: *Robbins and Cotran's Pathologic Basis of Disease.* 7th ed. Philadelphia: Saunders; 2005: Fig. 18-31.)

- Corticosteroids, colchicine, and other immunosuppressants may improve liver chemistries, but they do not alter disease progression and are not recommended
- Bile acid sequestrants (cholestyramine/colestipol) for pruritus; second-line agents are rifampin, opioid antagonists, or selective serotonin reuptake inhibitors.
- Liver transplantation should be considered once cirrhosis and jaundice develop. The 5-year post-transplantation survival rate is greater than 80% (among the highest for all liver diseases).
- Primary biliary cirrhosis recurs in 20% to 25% of patients by 10 years posttransplantation

Primary Sclerosing Cholangitis

Basic Information

- Idiopathic, progressive, inflammatory disease leading to stricturing and scarring of the medium and large bile ducts
  - Median age at diagnosis is 40 years
- 60% to 70% of patients are men
- **Most (80%) cases are associated with inflammatory bowel diseases, particularly ulcerative colitis (UC)**
  - 2.5% to 7.5% of patients with UC have primary sclerosing cholangitis (PSC)
  - Increased risk of colon cancer in patients with UC and PSC (more than UC alone)
  - 10% to 15% of patients with PSC have Crohn colitis
- Prevalence is 8.5 to 13.5 per 100,000 in the northern hemisphere
- Increased risk of cholangiocarcinoma: 10-year cumulative incidence of 7% to 9%

Clinical Presentation

- May present with abdominal pain, jaundice, cholangitis, and pruritus, or asymptomatic elevation of AP
- Osteopenia/osteoporosis can occur in advanced PSC
- Median survival of 9.5 to 12 years from diagnosis to death or liver transplantation
- Small duct PSC has better prognosis than large duct PSC

Diagnosis

- AP is elevated, with mild elevation of aminotransferases
- Bilirubin can be normal, except when common hepatic duct or common bile duct is involved and in late stages of disease
- Autoantibodies have no role in the routine diagnosis of PSC
  - No specific autoantibodies have been recognized for PSC
  - Perinuclear antineutrophil cytoplasmic antibody (pANCA) detectable in 50% to 80% of cases, but is not specific to PSC
- Diagnosis made by ERCP or MRCP, which demonstrates strictures or beading of the intrahepatic or extrahepatic bile ducts (Fig. 29-3)
  - ERCP is considered the gold standard, but is invasive
  - MRCP is 80% or more sensitive and 87% or more specific for the diagnosis of PSC

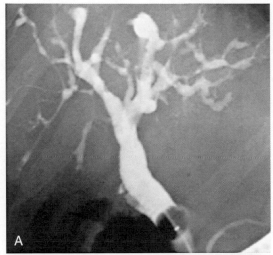
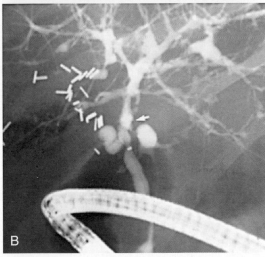

FIGURE 29-3 **A,** Primary sclerosing cholangitis. **B,** Endoscopic retrograde cholangiopancreatography showing beading and strictures of the intrahepatic ducts *(arrow).* (From Feldman M. *Sleisenger and Fordtran's Gastrointestinal and Liver Disease.* 8th ed. Philadelphia: Saunders; 2006: Fig. 65-1.)

- Liver biopsy classically shows periductal concentric fibrosis ("onion skin") but is often nondiagnostic, especially in early disease
    - Not essential for the diagnosis of PSC
    - Can be helpful in assessing possible overlap syndromes and liver fibrosis

Treatment

- Low-dose (13 to 15 mg/kg/day) UDCA may improve biochemical tests but does not alter symptoms, progression to cirrhosis, or survival. Some experts advocate for the use of low-dose UDCA if there is a reduction in AP after 6 to 12 months of use. High-dose (28 to 30 mg/kg/day) UDCA may be associated with increased serious adverse events and is not recommended.
- Periodic dilation of strictures via ERCP or percutaneous approach may be necessary
- Annual screening for colon cancer in patients with concomitant colitis

- Annual screening for gallbladder mass lesions and cholangiocarcinoma with serum cancer antigen 19-9 and MRI/MRC
- Liver transplantation should be offered to those with advanced liver disease or repeated bouts of cholangitis
- PSC recurs in 20% to 25% of patients 5 to 10 years after transplantation

Alcoholic Liver Disease

Basic Information

- Alcoholic liver disease (ALD) spans a spectrum of presentations, from simple steatosis to acute hepatitis to cirrhosis. Acute chronic liver disease is not uncommon
- 10% to 35% of heavy drinkers (>60 g/day of alcohol) develop acute alcoholic hepatitis
- Cirrhosis occurs in 8% to 20% of heavy drinkers
- Variables contributing to higher likelihood of ALD include increased quantity of ingested alcohol, malnutrition, female gender, and concomitant hepatitis C
- Pathophysiology related to increased reactive oxygen species and inflammatory cytokines (e.g., tumor necrosis factor [TNF]-α): this is the rationale for antiinflammatory therapy (see later discussion)
- Alcoholic cirrhosis has worse prognosis than other forms of cirrhosis. Hepatorenal syndrome is a frequent cause of death in severe acute alcoholic liver disease.

Clinical Presentation

- Physical examination in acute alcoholic hepatitis can reveal fever, malnutrition, jaundice, encephalopathy, tremor, parotid gland enlargement, hepatomegaly, right upper quadrant pain, ascites, spider nevi, and leukocytosis
- Tender hepatomegaly can occur secondary to fatty infiltration
- Can develop portal hypertension and ascites
- May have coexisting cardiomyopathy, pancreatic insufficiency, and/or neurotoxicity

Diagnosis

- History of excessive alcohol use (>60 to 80 g/day for men and >20 g/day for women for 10 years or longer) associated with chronic alcoholic liver disease
- **Modestly elevated aminotransferases (usually AST <400 IU and ALT <200 IU), often with AST:ALT ratio greater than 2:1**
- Bilirubin and PT may be elevated
- GGT and red blood cell mean corpuscular volume are often increased
- Serum immunoglobulin A may be elevated
- Low-grade fever and leukocytosis may be present in acute alcoholic hepatitis
- Liver biopsy can be used to stage fibrosis and exclude other forms of liver disease
- Histopathology varies depending on the nature of injury, and may include macrovesicular steatosis, lobular inflammation, ballooning degeneration (in alcoholic

29

hepatitis), parenchymal necrosis (in alcoholic hepatitis), periportal fibrosis, or cirrhosis
- Mallory bodies are a classic finding on biopsy, but are not specific for ALD

Treatment

- Abstinence is the most critical component of therapy
  - Baclofen given orally 5 mg 3 times a day for 3 days followed by 10 mg 3 times a day can reduce alcohol craving and consumption
- Reversal of portal hypertension and remarkable clinical improvement can be seen after prolonged abstinence
- Adequate nutrition is important. Nutritional intervention may be at least as efficacious as corticosteroid therapy in the treatment of acute alcoholic hepatitis.
- Prednisolone 40 mg/day for 4 weeks ± taper over 2 to 4 weeks may offer modest benefit in improving short-term survival in acute alcoholic hepatitis
  - The discriminant function (DF) = 4.6 × [PT − control (in seconds)] + serum bilirubin (in milligrams per deciliter) determines the severity of disease
  - **DF scores of 32 or greater predict 30% to 50% mortality at 1 month.** This signals the need to consider medical therapy
  - Long-term survival benefits of corticosteroids in acute alcoholic hepatitis have not been shown
- Pentoxifylline 400 mg 3 times daily for 4 weeks may improve short-term survival in acute alcoholic hepatitis by decreasing the risk of hepatorenal syndrome
  - Consider pentoxifylline when DF score 32 or greater if corticosteroids are contraindicated (e.g., active infection)
  - Pentoxifylline is a phosphodiesterase inhibitor that also reduces the production of inflammatory cytokines such as TNF-α, interleukin (IL)-5, IL-10, and IL-12
- Nephrotoxins should be carefully avoided (including contrast dye)
- Liver transplantation may be considered if a patient has abstained from alcohol use for the period of time required by the local transplantation program (usually at least 6 months)

Nonalcoholic Fatty Liver Disease

Basic Information

- Nonalcoholic fatty liver disease (NAFLD) comprises nonalcoholic fatty liver (NAFL) and nonalcoholic steatohepatitis (NASH)
- **Most common liver disorder causing elevated liver enzymes in the United States**
- Prevalence as high as 40% depending on definition used and population studied
  - Accounts for one-third of cases of chronic liver disease in the primary care setting
  - In the United States, Hispanics have the highest prevalence and African Americans have the lowest
- Histologically similar to alcoholic liver disease
- **Leading cause of death is cardiovascular disease**
- Spectrum of disease ranges from hepatic steatosis to steatohepatitis and can progress to fibrosis and cirrhosis

BOX 29-2	*Risk Factors for Nonalcoholic Fatty Liver Disease*

Obesity
Diabetes mellitus
Hyperlipidemia
Polycystic ovary syndrome
Jejunoileal bypass and rapid weight loss
Severe malnutrition
Prolonged total parenteral nutrition
Celiac disease
Small-bowel bacterial overgrowth
Advanced HIV/AIDS with lipodystrophy
Medications
   Amiodarone
   Corticosteroids
   Anabolic steroids
   Tamoxifen
   Perihexiline maleate
   Tetracycline
   Calcium channel blockers
   Methotrexate
Wilson disease

HIV/AIDS, Human immunodeficiency virus/acquired immunodeficiency syndrome.

- 15% to 20% of patients with NASH eventually progress to cirrhosis

Clinical Presentation

- The main risk factor is coexisting features of metabolic syndrome, most notably obesity and diabetes mellitus. Insulin resistance is a hallmark of the disease.
- Other risk factors of NAFLD are listed in Box 29-2
- Elevated aminotransferases usually AST:ALT less than 1, unless advanced fibrosis or cirrhosis; then AST:ALT greater than 1
- Hepatomegaly caused by steatosis. Can present with signs of portal hypertension in more advanced disease.

Diagnosis

- Heavy alcohol use (more than 21 drinks/week in men and more than 14 drinks/week in women) should be ruled out by history
- Imaging with ultrasound, CT, or MR scanning often reveals hepatomegaly and suggests fatty infiltration. Ultrasound is limited by body habitus, but is less expensive.
- Liver chemistry elevation pattern not typically helpful in diagnosis
- Histology is the gold standard for diagnosis, revealing either steatosis or steatonecrosis with or without fibrosis (Fig. 29-4)
- In advanced stages, histology loses characteristic fatty infiltration and may be called "cryptogenic" cirrhosis

Treatment

- Weight loss, strict glucose control, treatment of hypertension, and lipid management are recommended
- Vitamin E (800 IU/day) improves liver histology in biopsy-proven NASH. Its effects are unknown in patients with diabetes or cirrhosis

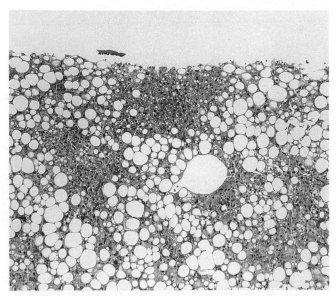

FIGURE 29-4 Nonalcoholic fatty liver disease. Liver biopsy specimen showing diffuse steatosis and focal inflammation and necrosis. (From Feldman M: *Sleisenger and Fordtran's Gastrointestinal and Liver Disease.* 8th ed. Philadelphia: Saunders; 2006: Fig. 82-3.)

- Insulin sensitizers and lipid-lowering agents have not conclusively shown benefit
- Potentially offending medications should be discontinued
- Avoid heavy consumption of alcohol
- One-year survival after liver transplantation is worse in patients aged 60 or older, body mass index 30 kg/m² or greater, and diabetes. Recurrence of NAFLD and NASH after transplantation is well-described.

Hereditary Hemochromatosis

Basic Information

- Most common genetic liver disease of Caucasians, particularly those of northern European origin (10% heterozygous carriers)
- Most cases of hereditary hemochromatosis (HH) are *HFE*-related
- Mutant *HFE* gene identified on chromosome 6, autosomal recessive inheritance
- Disease may present in C282Y homozygotes, H63D homozygotes, or C282Y/H63D compound heterozygotes
  - 85% to 90% of patients with HH in the United States are C282Y homozygotes
  - Numerous other *HFE* mutations (e.g., S65C, G93R) have been described
  - All mutations have incomplete biochemical and clinical disease penetrance
- Pathogenesis involves increased intestinal iron absorption, possibly caused by decreased production of the hepatic hormone hepcidin, resulting in hepatic accumulation of iron
- Non-*HFE*–related HH include mutations of hemojuvelin (*HJV*) gene, hepcidin (*HAMP*) gene, and

transferrin receptor 2 (*TfR2*) gene. African iron overload (Bantu siderosis) is a non-*HFE*–related HH that is worsened by dietary iron loading

Clinical Presentation

- Symptomatic HH is 10 times more common in men than women
- Peak presentation in men between 40 and 60 years, and in postmenopausal women
- Nonspecific elevation of liver enzymes
- **In addition to the liver, the joints (caused by calcium pyrophosphate deposition), pituitary gland, testes, pancreas, and heart can be affected**
- Nonspecific symptoms include weakness, lethargy, weight loss, loss of libido
- Hepatomegaly may be present, especially early in disease
- As disease advances, patients can develop skin pigmentation, diabetes, cardiomyopathy, arrhythmias, or arthalgias
- Significant hepatocellular carcinoma risk (5% per year) once cirrhosis develops

Diagnosis

- Screening for high-risk groups, including those with suggestive organ involvement and first-degree relatives of known HH
- **Transferrin saturation greater than 45% or elevated ferritin in high-risk groups should prompt *HFE* mutation analysis to detect C282Y or H63D mutations**
- If compound heterozygote (C282Y/H63D), C282Y heterozygote, or non-C282Y, need to rule out concomitant liver (e.g., hepatitis C virus [HCV], hepatitis B virus [HBV], ALD, NAFLD) or hematologic (e.g., thalassemia major, frequent blood transfusions, chronic hemodialysis) conditions that may lead to secondary iron overload
- Liver biopsy when ferritin >1000 µg/L or elevated liver enzymes to stage the degree of liver fibrosis or cirrhosis, or when not C282Y homozygote to rule out other liver diseases
- Screen first-degree family members either via serum transferrin saturation and ferritin, or by genetic testing

Treatment

- Phlebotomy of 1 unit of blood weekly or biweekly (as tolerated) until goal serum ferritin of 50 to 100 µg/L, followed by maintenance phlebotomy at intervals
  - Can improve cardiac function, diabetes, skin hyperpigmentation
  - No reversal of arthropathy, established cirrhosis, testicular atrophy, or cardiomyopathy
- Iron chelation (e.g., deferoxamine) is a reasonable alternative when phlebotomy is restricted by anemia. It is also the first-line therapy for iron overload because of ineffective erythropoiesis.
- Avoid vitamin C supplements
- Consider liver transplantation once cirrhosis has developed

29

α₁-*Antitrypsin Deficiency*

Basic Information

- α₁-Antitrypsin (AAT) is a protease inhibitor produced by hepatocytes that prevents proteolytic enzymes such as elastase from degrading normal host tissue
- Mutated AAT proteins become abnormally folded and cannot exit hepatocytes
  - Normal alleles (M) are associated with normal AAT activity
  - Deficient alleles (many, most commonly Z) are associated with decreased AAT levels
  - Null alleles are associated with undetectable AAT levels
- **Absolute AAT deficiency leads to lung disease alone, although relative deficiency leads to liver and/or lung disease**
  - Lung disease results from an imbalance between destructive neutrophil elastase and protective AAT in the lung
  - Liver injury is a consequence of intrahepatocytic AAT accumulation within the rough endoplasmic reticulum
- Highest incidence of homozygous ZZ is among people of Scandinavian and northern European ancestries. Occurs in up to 1 in 600 live births.
- Incidence from 1 in 2000 to 1 in 3000 among North American Caucasian populations
- The most common genetic cause of pediatric liver disease
- The most common genetic cause of chronic obstructive pulmonary disease

Clinical Presentation

- Persistent jaundice, elevated aminotransferases, and hepatomegaly may manifest as early as 4 to 8 weeks of age
- Portal hypertension (e.g., ascites, hematemesis) may develop in late childhood or early adolescence
- May progress to chronic hepatitis or cirrhosis by adulthood
- High risk for the development of hepatocellular carcinoma in adulthood
- Chronic obstructive pulmonary disease, particularly panacinar emphysema, may manifest alone or in addition to cirrhosis depending on degree of AAT deficiency
- May rarely be associated with necrotizing panniculitis and Wegener granulomatosis

Diagnosis

- Consider screening in adults with chronic idiopathic hepatitis or cryptogenic cirrhosis
- Screen for disease using serum AAT levels
- Obtain phenotype analysis if AAT level is below normal
  - ZZ phenotype associated with advanced liver disease
- Histopathology features periodic acid-Schiff (PAS)-positive, diastase-resistant globules in hepatocytic endoplasmic reticulum

Treatment

- Avoid cigarette smoking to prevent the acceleration of destructive lung disease
- Intravenous infusions of AAT derived from pooled plasma or obtained by recombinant deoxyribonucleic acid (DNA) methods are under investigation for treatment of pulmonary disease but have not been successfully used for liver disease
- **Liver transplantation is the only viable therapy for the liver disease component and is curative**
  - 5-year posttransplant survival of 80% to 85% in adults

Wilson Disease

Basic Information

- Also known as hepatolenticular degeneration
- Autosomal recessive disorder of copper metabolism
- Mutation in *ATP7B* gene leads to decreased biliary excretion of hepatocellular copper, resulting in accumulation in the liver, brain, cornea, and kidneys with subsequent injury thought to caused by oxidative stress
- *ATP7B* mutation also prevents integration of copper into ceruloplasmin (i.e., apoceruloplamin), which shortens ceruloplasmin's half-life, causing lower blood concentrations
- Affects around 30 individuals per million population worldwide

Clinical Presentation

- Most patients present at younger than 40 years old
- Manifests as liver disease, neurologic abnormalities, psychiatric illness, or any combination of these
- Spectrum of liver disease ranges from asymptomatic aminotransferase abnormalities to acute liver failure
- Acute liver failure can present with Coombs-negative hemolytic anemia and acute renal failure
  - AP can be inappropriately subnormal
  - In one study, AP:bilirubin ratio less than 4 *plus* AST:ALT ratio greater than 2.2 had 100% sensitivity and specificity for identifying acute liver failure because of Wilson disease
- Possible neurologic presentations include movement disorders, dysarthria, dysautonomia, seizures, and insomnia
- Psychiatric symptoms may involve depression, psychosis, or personality changes
- Can also affect kidneys (nephrolithiasis), heart (cardiomyopathy), pancreas (pancreatitis), endocrine system (hypoparathyroidism, infertility), or skeletal system (osteoporosis)

Diagnosis

- Consider in any individual between ages 3 and 55 with acute hepatitis or jaundice of unclear causes
- **Kayser-Fleischer rings are present in 95% of patients with neurologic presentation (Fig. 29-5)**
  - Only present in 40% to 60% of patients with mainly hepatic manifestations

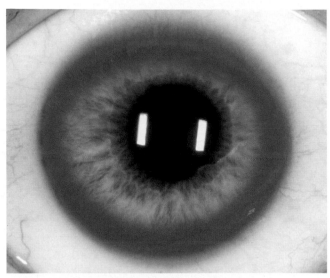

FIGURE 29-5 Kayser-Fleischer ring in a patient with Wilson disease. Note the brown-green pigment around the cornea. (From Goldman, L, Bennett JC, Aussiello D: *Cecil Textbook of Medicine.* 22nd ed. Philadelphia: Saunders; 2004: Fig. 224-1.)

- Rings represent copper deposition in the cornea
- Not specific for Wilson disease; can manifest in chronic cholestatic diseases
- Requires slit-lamp evaluation by an experienced ophthalmologist
- Serum ceruloplasmin is usually markedly low, but may be normal or even mildly elevated in the setting of acute inflammation
- 24-hour urine copper excretion is typically greater than 100 μg, but even levels greater than 40 μg warrant further work-up
  - Not specific; levels greater than 100 μg can be seen in autoimmune hepatitis and other chronic liver diseases
  - Penicillamine challenge during 24-hour urine collection has only been standardized in children
- Liver biopsy for copper quantification and histology should be obtained when biochemical testing is indeterminate
  - Copper greater than 250 μg/g of dry liver weight confirms diagnosis, less than 50 μg/g in untreated patients excludes diagnosis
  - Early histology shows micro-/macrovesicular steatosis, glycogenated hepatocytic nuclei, and focal necrosis
- Consider molecular genetic testing if liver biopsy is inconclusive

Treatment

- Primary therapy is chelation with oral D-penicillamine or trientine. Trientine is better tolerated and more commonly used in the United States
  - Neurologic exacerbation after starting treatment is more common with D-penicillamine
  - Monitor treatment using 24-hour urinary copper excretion
- Oral zinc induces enterocyte metallothionein, which binds dietary copper and prevents its gastrointestinal absorption. Use in presymptomatic patients or those on maintenance therapy.
- Avoid foods and water (e.g., shellfish, mushrooms, chocolate, organ meats) with high copper concentrations
- Lifelong pharmacologic treatment unless liver transplantation takes place
- Liver transplantation corrects the fundamental defect in hepatic copper excretion and should be offered to patients with advanced or acute fulminant disease

Pregnancy-Specific Liver Diseases

Basic Information

- Abnormal liver tests occur in 3% to 5% of all pregnancies
- Several different disease processes but no clearly defined causes
- **Abnormal intramitochondrial fatty acid oxidation has been linked to acute fatty liver of pregnancy (AFLP).** This is less established in HELLP (hemolysis, elevated liver enzymes, low platelets) syndrome.
  - Several possible mutations, particularly of long-chain 3-hydroxyachyl-CoA dehydrogenase (LCHAD)
  - Babies of mothers with AFLP should undergo genetic screening for LCHAD mutations
- All pregnancy-specific liver diseases tend to be recurrent in subsequent pregnancies, except for AFLP
  - Notable exception is women who carry LCHAD mutation → recurrence in 20% to 70% of subsequent pregnancies

Clinical Presentation

See Table 29-6 for a summary of liver diseases in pregnancy.

Diagnosis

See Table 29-6.

Treatment

See Table 29-6.

Viral Hepatitis

Overview

- Several human hepatatropic viruses exist, the most significant being hepatitis A, B, and C
- Hepatitis A is commonly found in developing countries, with occasional outbreaks in the United States
- Hepatitis B is the most common chronic viral hepatitis worldwide
- Hepatitis C is the most common chronic viral hepatitis in the United States

HEPATITIS A

Basic Information

- 37% of the U.S. adult population is positive for anti-hepatitis A virus (HAV)
- Incubation period of 2 to 6 weeks
- Fecal–oral transmission

29

TABLE 29-6 *Liver Diseases of Pregnancy*

Disease	Symptoms/Signs	Lab(s)	Treatment	Mortality Risk: Mother/Fetus
Hyperemesis gravidarum	Intractable N/V, dehydration in 1st trimester	Bilirubin up to 5× normal AST/ALT rarely 20× normal	Antiemetics, intravenous hydration	–/– (Resolves spontaneously)
Intrahepatic cholestasis of pregnancy	Pruritus, jaundice, steatorrhea in 2nd or 3rd trimester	Bilirubin up to 5× normal AST/ALT up to 20× normal Bile acid up to 100× normal	UDCA, dexamethasone; deliver if fetal distress	–/Low
Preeclampsia/eclampsia	HTN, edema, proteinuria, seizures/coma in late 2nd or 3rd trimester	Bilirubin <5 mg/dL AST/ALT up to 10 to 20× normal	Treat HTN and edema; magnesium sulfate; deliver in severe cases	+/Low
HELLP syndrome (subset of severe preeclampsia)	RUQ pain, N/V, HTN, edema, proteinuria in late 2nd/3rd trimester or postpartum period	AST/ALT up to 10 to 20× normal Low haptoglobin LDH >600 U/L Platelets <100 K	Delivery	+/+
Acute fatty liver of pregnancy	RUQ pain, N/V, fatigue, jaundice, ascites, encephalopathy, renal failure in 3rd trimester	Bilirubin commonly <5 mg/dL, but is higher in severe disease AST/ALT up to 1000 Hyperammonemia Azotemia Hypoglycemia Disseminated intravascular coagulation can develop	Delivery	+/+
Hepatic rupture	Severe abdominal pain, shock in 3rd trimester	Variable	Immediate surgery	+/+

ALT, Alanine aminotransferase; AST, aspartate aminotransferase; HELLP, hemolysis, elevated liver enzymes, low platelet count; HTN, hypertension; LDH, lactate dehydrogenase; N/V, nausea/vomiting; RUQ, right upper quadrant; UDCA, ursodeoxycholic acid.

Clinical Presentation

- Usually mild or even subclinical in children younger than 5 years of age; more marked and prolonged in older children and adults
  - Low mortality in previously healthy individuals, including pregnant women
- Prodromal symptoms of fatigue, anorexia, nausea, vomiting, abdominal pain, diarrhea
- Several clinical patterns: self-limited hepatitis ± jaundice (typical), prolonged cholestasis (uncommon), protracted relapsing course (uncommon), and fulminant liver failure (rare)
- 2% to 15% of cases develop a prolonged and relapsing course with associated arthritis, vasculitis, or cryoglobulinemia
  - Relapses resemble the original episode, including serum anti-HAV IgM positivity
- Complete clinical recovery in most cases by 6 months
- The elderly and those with concomitant chronic liver disease have increased risk for fulminant liver failure
- **Never results in chronic infection**

Diagnosis

- Acute disease is diagnosed by serum anti-HAV IgM
- Immunity conferred by presence of anti-HAV IgG or HAV total AB

Treatment

- Supportive care
- Attention to sanitation

- **Vaccinate high-risk individuals, including travelers to endemic areas, military workers, intravenous drug users, those with chronic liver disease, and family members of infected patients**
- Immune globulin prophylaxis is 80% to 90% effective if given within 2 weeks following exposure
- In the prolonged cholestatic variant, prednisolone 30 mg daily tapered over 21 days may shorten the duration of jaundice and pruritus

HEPATITIS B

Basic Information

- 350 million individuals chronically infected worldwide, but carrier rates vary greatly depending on geographic region
  - Low prevalence (0.1% to 2%): United States, Australia, Western Europe
  - Intermediate prevalence (3% to 7%): Japan, Mediterranean basin, Latin America, Middle East
  - High prevalence (8% to 20%): China, Southeast Asia, sub-Saharan Africa
- 15% to 40% of chronic HBV carriers eventually develop serious complications
- Transmitted parenterally, by sexual contact, and via vertical transmission
- Elevated vertical transmission risk (85% to 90%) in mothers with high serum HBV DNA levels and presence of hepatitis B e antigen (HBeAg)

- High-risk adults include health care workers, intravenous drug users, hemodialysis patients, men who have sex with men, sexually promiscuous individuals, institutionalized patients, immigrants from HBV-endemic regions, and household members of chronic carriers
- **Majority of those infected as adults will clear virus spontaneously**; less than 5% progress to chronic hepatitis and 0.1 to 0.5% develop fulminant liver failure
    - This is in contrast to approximately 90% who become chronic HBV for infections at birth, or 25% to 50% for infections occurring between ages 1 and 5 years
    - Mortality from fulminant course approaches 80% without liver transplantation
- Persistent presence of HBeAg and elevated serum HBV DNA are associated with an increased risk of hepatocellular carcinoma (HCC), even without cirrhosis

Clinical Presentation

- Incubation period of acute infection is 1 to 4 months
- Symptomatic acute hepatitis (e.g., abdominal pain, low-grade fever, nausea, jaundice) occurs in 30% of adults, but in only 10% of children younger than 4 years of age
    - Clinical symptoms usually normalize after 1 to 3 months
- Many are chronic inactive carriers with normal liver chemistries, presence of anti-HBe, and minimal serum HBV DNA. Inactive carriers remain at risk for HCC. This phase of the disease is also known as *immune tolerance.*
- Reactivation of HBV replication (presence of anti-HBe, high serum HBV DNA, intermittently elevated ALT) can occur in the setting of immunosuppression (i.e., chemotherapy)
- **Extrahepatic manifestations (in 10% to 20% of chronic HBV) include polyarteritis nodosa, membranous or membranoproliferative glomerulonephritis, and mixed cryoglobulinemia**

Diagnosis

- Based on serologic patterns (Table 29-7) and positive HBV DNA PCR.
- **Hepatitis B surface antigen (HBsAg) is the first positive marker of acute infection (Fig. 29-6)**
    - **Persistence for longer than 6 months is considered chronic HBV infection**
- Presence of hepatitis B core-IgM (HBc-IgM) indicates acute infection; whereas HBc-IgG marks a history of infection
- HBeAg positivity indicates active replication and infectivity. Seroconversion to anti-HBe is usually associated with a marked decline in serum HBV DNA.
    - Precore or core promoter variants can show high HBV DNA levels despite positive anti-HBe
- Serum HBV DNA signifies active viremia and infectivity
- **Presence of anti-HBs indicates immunity to HBV**

Treatment

- **Indications for treatment**
    - **HBeAg-positive: HBV DNA greater than 20,000 IU/mL, plus ALT greater than 2 times normal or moderate inflammation/significant fibrosis on liver biopsy**
    - **HBeAg-negative: HBV DNA greater than 2000 IU/mL, plus ALT greater than 2 times normal or moderate inflammation/significant fibrosis on liver biopsy**
    - **Presence of cirrhosis, plus HBV DNA greater than 2000 IU/mL or persistent ALT elevation**
- Standard-interferon-α, pegylated-interferon-α, and nucleos(t)ide analogues including lamivudine, adefovir, entecavir, tenofovir, and telbivudine are all U.S. Food and Drug Administration-approved for the treatment of chronic HBV
- Interferon-α is administered for a predefined duration and has the highest rate of HbeAg seroconversion (up to 50%), but is associated with significant side effects (e.g., flulike symptoms, bone marrow suppression, hair loss, and mood changes)

29

TABLE 29-7	*Serologic Diagnosis of Hepatitis B*						
HBsAg	**Anti-HBs**	**HBc–IgM**	**HBc–IgG**	**HBeAg**	**Anti-HBe**	**HBV DNA**	**Disease Pattern**
+	−	+	−	+	−	++	Acute infection, early period
−	−	+	+	−	+	+	Acute infection, window period
−	+	−	+	−	+	+/−	Acute infection, recovery period
+	−	−	+	+/−	+/−	Variable	Chronic infection
+	−	+/−	+	+/−	+/+	++	Reactivation/exacerbation
−	+	−	+	−	+	−	Resolved previous infection
−	+	−	−	−	−	−	HBV immunization

DNA, Deoxyribonucleic acid; HBc, Hepatitis B core protein; HBeAg, hepatitis B e antigen; HBsAg, hepatitis B surface antigen; HBV, hepatitis B virus; IgM/IgG, immunoglobulin M/G.

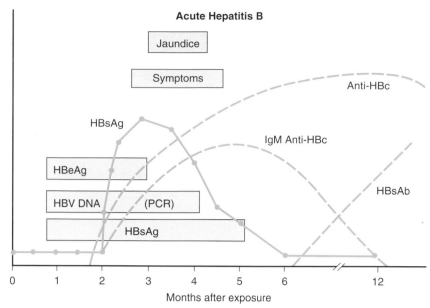

FIGURE 29-6 Serologic response to acute hepatitis B infection. DNA, Deoxyribonucleic acid; HBc, hepatitis B core protein; HBsAg, hepatitis B surface antigen; HBsAb, hepatitis B surface antibody; HBV, hepatitis B virus; IgM, immunoglobulin M; PCR, polymerase chain reaction.

- Predictors of HBeAg seroconversion include elevated pretreatment ALT, high histologic activity index, low serum HBV DNA, and HBV genotypes A and B
  - Contraindicated in decompensated liver disease
- Entecavir and tenofovir are associated with the most impressive reductions in HBV DNA and the lowest resistance rates among the nucleos(t)ide analogues. Variable durations of therapy depend on pretreatment HBeAg status and viral response.
  - HBeAg-positive: Continue treatment for at least 6 months after HBeAg seroconversion and undetectable serum HBV DNA
  - HBeAg-negative: Continue treatment indefinitely until HBsAg clearance
  - Decompensated cirrhosis: Life-long treatment
  - These medicines are generally very well tolerated
- **Antiviral therapy is generally not needed in acute HBV because of a greater than 95% spontaneous recovery among immunocompetent adults**
  - Exceptions are fulminant liver disease and protracted severe course
  - May use lamivudine or telbivudine when anticipating short treatment duration
  - Less preferable: adefovir (weak antiviral activity, nephrotoxic potential) and tenofovir (nephrotoxic potential)
  - Interferon-α is contraindicated
- Mainstays of prevention are "universal precaution" and vaccination
  - HBV vaccine is part of universal immunization program for newborns in the United States
  - Consider vaccination in high-risk adults (see previously)
  - Hepatitis B immune globulin (HBIG) can also prevent infection if given within hours of exposure (e.g., newborns of HBsAg-positive mothers). Always initiate HBV vaccination in conjunction with HBIG.

- Verification of vaccine response is unnecessary except in health care workers, chronic hemodialysis or immunocompromised patients, sexual partners of chronic carriers, and infants of HBsAg-positive mothers
  - Check anti-HBs titer 1 to 2 months after the completion of vaccine series, or at 9 to 15 months of age in infants. Levels 10 mIU/mL or higher are considered protective
  - Annual follow-up testing for patients on chronic hemodialysis
  - Consider booster dose(s) if anti-HBs concentration less than 10 mIU/mL
- **Routine HCC surveillance in high-risk HBV carriers including Asian men older than 40 years of age, Asian women older than 50 years of age, Africans older than 20 years of age, and cirrhotic patients**
  - Consider liver transplantation in fulminant or advanced liver disease

HEPATITIS C

Basic Information

- HCV is a heterogeneous ribonucleic acid (RNA) virus with at least 6 major genotypes
- Genotypes vary in geographic distribution. Genotype 1 is most common in North/South Americas, Australia, and Europe; genotype 4, the Middle East and Egypt; genotype 5, South Africa; and genotype 6, Southeast Asia.
- Overall global prevalence of 2% to 3%, highest in Africa (e.g., Egypt), eastern Mediterranean region, and Southeast Asia
  - Can reach prevalence of 50% among intravenous drug users
- Most common hepatotropic viral infection in the United States. Four million people are estimated to be anti-HCV positive.

- Currently the leading indication for liver transplantation in North America and Europe
- Transmitted parenterally (most common), via vertical transmission (4% to 6%, higher with human immunodeficiency virus [HIV]/HCV co-infection), and through sexual contact (rare)
- Highest risk for chronic infection among hepatotropic viral infections; chronicity develops in 60% to 85% of adult infections, and 55% to 70% of pediatric cases
- Heavy alcohol use, older age at initial HCV infection, obesity, or co-infection with HIV may accelerate the progression of fibrosis
- **Risk factors for HCV infection include birthdate from 1945 to 1965, history of intravenous drug use, transfusions or organ transplants before 1992, history of long-term hemodialysis, HIV infection, Vietnam War era veterans, and known exposures to HCV (including being born to HCV-positive mothers)**

Clinical Presentation

- Incubation period ranges from 2 to 12 weeks, but acute infections are often clinically mild or asymptomatic. Jaundice occurs infrequently (<20%), but may be associated with increased spontaneous viral clearance.
  - Acute fulminant hepatitis is rare
- Common symptoms of chronic HCV include fatigue, anorexia, myalgias, and arthralgias
- Approximately 20% of patients progress to cirrhosis after 20 years of chronic HCV
  - Once cirrhotic, 4% annual risk of clinical decompensation (e.g., ascites), 3% annual risk of HCC
- Extrahepatic manifestations include mixed cryoglobulinemia, leukocytoclastic vasculitis, membranous glomerulonephritis, porphyria cutanea tarda, insulin resistance, and non-Hodgkin lymphoma

Diagnosis

- Screen all patients for risk factors of HCV infection (see previously). HCV testing should be offered to at-risk individuals.
  - Since 2012, the U.S. Centers for Disease Control and Prevention (CDC) has recommended one-time testing for HCV in adults born during 1945 to 1965
- **Anti-HCV is the first-line screening test. It indicates past or chronic HCV infection, but does not imply immunity.**
  - Anti-HCV becomes detectable within 2 to 3 months postinfection, so it may miss acute cases
- Check serum HCV RNA if (1) anti-HCV is positive, (2) considering HCV antiviral therapy, or (3) suspicion for infection remains despite negative anti-HCV
  - Presence of HCV RNA suggests active viral replication
  - HCV RNA is detectable in serum within 2 weeks of infection
  - Persistence for more than 6 months defines chronic HCV infection
  - RNA titer does not correlate with disease activity or progression
- Obtain HCV genotyping to guide appropriate antiviral therapy

- Single-nucleotide polymorphism at the *IL28B* gene on chromosome 19 predicts spontaneous viral clearance and response to antiviral therapy
  - CC genotype is associated with the most favorable spontaneous and treatment-induced clearance rates. TT is least favorable.
  - Frequency of C allele is highest in East Asia, intermediate in Europe, and lowest in Africa
  - May be less clinically relevant with the advent of more efficacious newer generation direct-acting antivirals (DAAs, see following)
- For prognosis, it is useful to ascertain liver fibrotic stage and degree of inflammatory activity. Liver biopsy is gold standard but invasive; noninvasive options include serum biomarker panels and imaging (MR or ultrasound) with elastography.
- Aminotransferases do not help differentiate the presence or absence of disease because 25% to 50% of chronic HCV patients may have persistently normal levels

Treatment

- Historical therapies for chronic HCV are pegylated-interferon and ribavirin ± an NS3/4A protease inhibitor (i.e., telaprevir or boceprevir) for up to 12 months. These regimens were 30% to 70% effective, and fraught with side effects.
- **In 2013, two new DAAs were approved for treatment of chronic HCV: simeprevir (an NS3/4A protease inhibitor) and sofosbuvir (an NS5B polymerase inhibitor). Recommended regimens vary depending on HCV genotype and history of HCV therapy. A host of new, very effective, and well-tolerated oral medications are in advanced clinical trials.**
  - Sofosbuvir and ledipisvir are combined in the first-ever interferon-free regimen for chronic HCV
  - Treatment success rates after 12 to 24 weeks of therapy are greater than 90%. Sustained viral clearance 6 months after treatment is considered a cure.
  - Much better tolerated than previous regimens. Main barrier to treatment is cost.
  - Use of interferon and ribavirin requires monitoring of routine laboratory tests and thyroid-stimulating hormone.
  - Testing of HCV RNA titer after 4 weeks on antivirals, at the conclusion of therapy, and 24 weeks after completion of therapy is typically performed
- Treatment is generally recommended for acute HCV infection that does not spontaneously clear within 12 weeks
  - Viral response to conventional, non-DAA therapy is significantly better in acute HCV
  - Pegylated-interferon monotherapy for at least 12 weeks results in viral clearance in 80% to over 90% of acute HCV
  - At the time of writing, there are no recommendations yet regarding DAAs in the treatment of acute HCV
- Liver transplantation is indicated for advanced liver disease (hepatitis C is the most common cause of HCC

29

and indication for liver transplant in United States and Europe)

HEPATITIS D

Basic Information

- Hepatitis D virus (HDV) is a partial/defective RNA virus that requires the presence of HBV surface antigen for infection and replication
- Similar routes of transmission as HBV, though vertical transmission is rare
- Can co-infect with HBV or superinfect a chronic HBsAg carrier
- High prevalence in Mediterranean countries, East Africa, and Central and Northern Asia

Clinical Presentation

- Co-infection
  - Biphasic aminotransferase elevations separated by a few weeks because of distinct acute effects of HBV and HDV
  - Chronic HDV infection occurs in only 2% of cases
- Superinfection: Hepatitis is more severe with higher rates of fulminant liver disease (more common in HDV than other types of viral hepatitis)
  - Progression to chronic infection in more than 90% of cases

Diagnosis

- **HBsAg must be present to diagnose HDV infection**
- Co-infection
  - Positive anti-HDV-IgM is preceded by the appearance of anti-HBc-IgM 1 to 2 weeks earlier
  - Anti-HDV-IgM disappears after 1.5 to 3 months, and is followed by anti-HDV-IgG positivity
  - Hepatitis D antigen (HDAg) appears early in serum but is short-lived (because of sequestration in antibody complexes), thus often escapes detection
- Superinfection
  - Rising titers of both anti-HDV-IgM *and* anti-HDV-IgG
  - Early and short-lived presence of serum HDAg
  - Negative anti-HBc-IgM, positive anti-HBc-IgG

Treatment

- No effective antiviral therapies exist for acute HDV
- One-year course of standard interferon-α or pegylated-interferon offers modest efficacy for viral suppression in chronic HDV; pegylated-interferon tends to be better tolerated
  - Contraindicated in decompensated liver disease
- Nucleoside or nucleotide analogues used against HBV have no effect on HDV replication
- Consider liver transplantation in fulminant or advanced liver disease

HEPATITIS E

Basic Information

- **Hepatitis E (HEV) is an RNA virus typically distributed via fecal–oral route, through contaminated food or water supply**
  - Transmission by blood products and organ transplantation has also been reported
- Endemic in India and parts of Asia
  - Anti-HEV has seroprevalence of approximately 25% in the United States
- Two- to 8-week incubation period

Clinical Presentation

- Generally mild acute disease and often subclinical
  - Malaise, fever, anorexia, nausea, abdominal pain, jaundice
- **Rarely fatal except during pregnancy, when case fatality can reach 25%**
- Usually self-limited, with rare cases of chronicity in postliver transplant or HIV-infected individuals

Diagnosis

- Suspect HEV infection in patients presenting with acute hepatitis and recent travel to endemic areas
- Anti-HEV IgM signifies acute disease, although IgG suggests clearance of a previous HEV infection
- Measure HEV RNA titer in immunocompromised or posttransplant individuals
  - Anti-HEV testing can be unreliable in this cohort

Treatment

- **Often a mild disease course where supportive care is sufficient**
- Ribavirin 600 to 800 mg daily for 3 to 6 months associated with viral clearance in immunocompromised patients

Liver Lesions

Overview

- Focal lesions of the liver are found frequently, and often incidentally, during abdominal imaging studies performed for other indications
- High-quality triphasic (arterial, portal, and washout) imaging often the key to diagnosis
- In addition to malignant lesions, there are two broad categories of benign liver lesions: cysts/abscesses or solid lesions

Cysts and Abscesses

- Simple cysts (solitary or a few cysts) are the most common benign lesions of the liver
  - If symptomatic, can consider surgical drainage
- Hydatid cysts are diagnosed by the presence of daughter cysts and positive anti-*Echinococcus* serologies. Cysts may be calcified.
  - Imaging-guided percutaneous drainage is often paired with months of preprocedure albendazole therapy to reduce risk of seeding and/or anaphylaxis
- Hepatic abscesses are associated with fever, right upper quadrant pain, and other systemic signs of infection
  - Pyogenic abscesses are the sequela of biliary tract disease or colonic/intestinal infection
  - Needle aspiration to help guide antibiotic therapy and placement of percutaneous drainage catheter into larger abscesses

- Abscess caused by *Entamoeba histolytica* should be considered in travelers from endemic areas. It is diagnosed using enzyme immunoassay, and responds to metronidazole.

Other Benign Lesions

- Hemangioma
  - Most frequent benign solid lesion of the liver, found in up to 7.5% of the population
    - ~5:1 female:male ratio
    - Presents most commonly between third and fifth decades of age
  - Congenital vascular malformations with no malignant potential
  - Typically asymptomatic. Giant hemangiomas (>4 cm) are uncommon but may cause intermittent discomfort
  - Severe pain is associated with bleeding or infarction
  - Diagnosis made by ultrasound, triphasic CT, or MRI
  - Biopsy is not recommended because of risk of bleeding
- Focal nodular hyperplasia
  - Second most common benign solid hepatic lesion; occurs in 0.8% of the adult population
    - Around 10:1 female:male ratio
    - Frequently found incidentally on abdominal imaging
  - **No risk of malignancy**
  - Not caused by oral contraceptives, but may grow in high estrogen conditions
  - **Characteristic central scar on CT or MRI**
  - Liver biopsy or surgical intervention is usually unnecessary
- Hepatic adenoma
  - Rare benign tumor made up of hepatocytes; progression to HCC uncertain, estimated to be 8%
    - Male gender and size greater than 4 cm increase risk of malignancy
  - **Most often seen in the setting of long-standing (6 months to greater than 5 years) oral contraceptive use in women**
- Can be associated with glycogen storage disease (types I and III), mature-onset diabetes of the young type 3 (MODY3), anabolic steroids, or familial polyposis coli
- Large lesions can cause pain, particularly in the setting of intralesional bleeding, rupture, and subsequent intraperitoneal bleeding
  - Rapid tumor enlargement can occur during pregnancy
- Treatment includes discontinuation of any offending agents (e.g., oral contraceptives, anabolic steroids, etc.)
- Interval imaging studies to monitor changes, particularly malignant degeneration
- **Consider surgical resection for lesions that are symptomatic or larger than 4 cm, because of increased risk of rupture, bleeding, and malignant transformation**

Review Questions

For review questions, please go to ExpertConsult.com.

SUGGESTED READINGS

Chalasani N, Younossi Z, Lavine JE, et al. The diagnosis and management of non-alcoholic fatty liver disease: practice guideline by the American Association for the Study of Liver Diseases, American College of Gastroenterology, and the American Gastroenterological Association. *Hepatology*. 2012;55:2005-2023.

David S, Hamilton JP. Drug induced liver disease. *US Gastroenterol Hepatol Rev*. 2010;6:73-80.

Heneghan MA, Yeoman AD, Verma S, et al. Autoimmune hepatitis. *Lancet*. 2013;382:1433-1444.

Joshi D, James A, Quaglia A, et al. Liver disease in pregnancy. *Lancet*. 2010;375:594-605.

O'Shea RS, Dasarathy S, McCullough AJ. Alcoholic liver disease. *Hepatology*. 2010;51:307-328.

Seeff LB. Herbal hepatotoxicity. *Clin Liver Dis*. 2007;11:577-596.

Trépo C, Chan HL, Lok A. Hepatitis B virus infection. *Lancet*. 2014;384:2053-2063.

HCV Guidance: Recommendations for Testing, Managing, and Treating Hepatitis C. <www.hcvguidelines.org.>

29

Complications of Liver Disease

PO-HUNG CHEN, MD; and JAMES P. HAMILTON, MD

In the previous chapter, a number of acute and chronic causes of liver disease were described. This chapter focuses on the potential sequelae of those disease entities. Morbidity and mortality from cirrhosis can result from numerous processes, including infection, encephalopathy, renal failure, gastrointestinal bleeding, and hepatocellular carcinoma.

Overview of Cirrhosis

- Definitions
  - Hepatic fibrosis is a potentially reversible wound healing response characterized by an accumulation of extracellular matrix made up of collagen fibrils
  - **Cirrhosis is defined by global hepatic fibrosis, nodule formation, and reduced hepatic synthetic function**
- Pathophysiology
  - Chronic hepatic inflammation and injury result in and hepatic stellate cell activation and endothelial cell damage
  - Activated stellate cells produce collagen (fibrosis), with subsequent vascular and organ contractions
- Causes of cirrhosis (Table 30-1)
- Clinical consequences of cirrhosis (Table 30-2)
- Two widely used prognostic measures of cirrhosis severity are the Child-Turcotte-Pugh score (Box 30-1) and the Model for End-Stage Liver Disease (MELD) score (Box 30-2)

Portal Hypertension and Varices

Basic Information

- Definition of portal hypertension
  - Portal vein pressure of greater than 8 mm Hg
  - The most common and morbid consequence of liver disease and cirrhosis
  - Direct portal pressure measurement is highly invasive; indirect estimation using the hepatic venous pressure gradient (HVPG) is preferred
    - HVPG = wedged hepatic venous pressure (WHVP) − free hepatic vein pressure (FHVP)
    - Obtained via catheterization of the hepatic vein
  - HVPG greater than 10 mm Hg is associated with development of varices, 12 mm Hg or greater is associated with complications of portal hypertension (e.g., ascites, variceal hemorrhage)
- Classification of portal hypertension (Fig. 30-1)
  - Postsinusoidal: obstruction distal to hepatic sinusoids

  - Extrahepatic (e.g., inferior vena cava obstruction, Budd-Chiari syndrome, right heart failure)
  - Intrahepatic (e.g., venooclusive disease, alcoholic central hyaline sclerosis)
  - Presinusoidal: obstruction proximal to hepatic sinusoids
    - Prehepatic (e.g., splanchnic arteriovenous fistula, splenic vein thrombosis, portal vein thrombosis)
    - Hepatic (e.g., schistosomiasis, sarcoidosis, myeloproliferative disorders)
  - Sinusoidal (e.g., cirrhosis, acute alcoholic hepatitis)
- Major complication is development of portosystemic collaterals, the most clinically significant of which are gastroesophageal varices (Fig. 30-2) and hemorrhoids
  - Gastroesophageal varices are present in 85% of Child C cirrhotic patients
  - Patients with cirrhosis have an 8% annual risk of developing varices, plus 8% annual rate of progression from small to large varices.
  - Predictors of hemorrhage: size of varices, Child B or C cirrhosis, red "wale" sign seen on endoscopy
  - Gastrointestinal hemorrhage is associated with increased risk for severe bacterial infections (e.g., spontaneous bacterial peritonitis) that predicts early rebleeding and increased mortality
    - Variceal hemorrhage is associated with greater than 20% mortality at 6 weeks

Clinical Presentation

- For a list of clinical manifestations of portal hypertension, see Table 30-2

Diagnosis

- Laboratory studies to evaluate hepatic synthetic function, renal function, and hematologic values. Thrombocytopenia usually develops from splenic sequestration.
- Radiographic studies may aid in the diagnosis and treatment of various related conditions
- Endoscopy is key to the diagnosis of varices. Screening every 1 to 3 years is recommended for patients with cirrhosis. Frequency of screening increases with severity of liver disease.

Treatment

- Primary management of varices
  - Nonselective β-blockers (e.g., propranolol, nadolol) are recommended for the primary prevention of bleeding in small varices with increased risk of bleeding (e.g., Child B and C, red wale marks) and in any medium or large varices

TABLE 30-1	Causes of Chronic or Cirrhotic Liver Disease
Infections	Viral hepatitis (hepatitis B–D, rarely E), *Echinococcus* infections, brucellosis, congenital tertiary syphilis, schistosomiasis
Drugs and toxins	Alcohol, methotrexate, isoniazid, vitamin A, amiodarone, perhexilene maleate, α-methyldopa, and others
Metabolic or genetic diseases	Wilson disease, hereditary hemochromatosis, α₁-antitrypsin deficiency, carbohydrate metabolism disorders, lipid metabolism disorders, amino acid disorders, porphyria
Biliary obstruction	Chronic biliary obstruction, primary and secondary sclerosing cholangitis, primary and secondary biliary cirrhosis, cystic fibrosis, congenital biliary cysts
Vascular abnormalities	Veno-occlusive disease, Budd-Chiari syndrome, inferior vena cava obstruction, cardiac disease, hereditary hemorrhagic telangiectasias
Miscellaneous	Autoimmune hepatitis, nonalcoholic steatohepatitis, granulomatous liver disease, sarcoidosis, amyloidosis, polycystic liver disease

TABLE 30-2	Clinical Consequences of Cirrhosis
Synthetic defects	Decreased production of procoagulants, albumin, and fibrinogen
Renal	Sodium retention Hepatorenal syndrome Acute tubular necrosis Renal tubular acidosis
Endocrine	Impotence Hypogonadism Anovulation Euthyroid-sick syndrome Hepatic osteodystrophy
Cardiopulmonary	Hypotension Portopulmonary hypertension Hepatopulmonary syndrome
Oncologic	Hepatocellular carcinoma Cholangiocarcinoma
Musculocutaneous	Spider telangiectasis Palmar erythema Jaundice Dupuytren contracture Muscle cramps
Portal hypertension	Portosystemic encephalopathy Variceal hemorrhage Ascites Spontaneous bacterial peritonitis Hepatic hydrothorax Splenomegaly Portal vein thrombosis

---

BOX 30-1 | *Child-Turcotte-Pugh Score*

Based on Five Clinical Parameters of Liver Disease:

Parameter	1 Point	2 Points	3 Points
Bilirubin (mg/dL)	<2	2 to 3	>3
Serum albumin (g/dL)	>3.5	2.8 to 3.5	<2.8
INR*	<1.7	1.7 to 2.3	>2.3
Ascites	None	Mild/moderate (or diuretic responsive)	Tense
Encephalopathy	None	Grade 1 or 2	Grade 3 or 4

Class A, Total of 5 to 6 points; Class B, 7 to 9 points; Class C, 10 to 15 points.
*Original Child-Turcotte classification incorporated nutritional status. In 1972, Pugh et al replaced it with international normalized ratio and designated point values (1 to 3) for each parameter.

30

- Not recommended for small varices without increased risk of bleeding, or as primary prophylaxis to prevent the development of varices
- Serial endoscopic variceal ligation (EVL) performed for primary prevention of bleeding in medium or large esophageal varices, particularly if a patient cannot tolerate β-blockers
- General management of acute variceal hemorrhage consists of intravascular volume resuscitation, maintaining hemoglobin no higher than approximately 8 g/dL (to avoid unwanted portal pressure elevation), somatostatin analogues (to reduce splanchnic blood volume), and short-term prophylactic antibiotics

- Urgent endoscopic evaluation and therapy
- Transjugular intrahepatic portosystemic shunt (TIPS) for uncontrolled or recurrent variceal hemorrhage despite endoscopy
- Balloon tamponade can be an effective but temporary (less than 24 hours) control of hemorrhage
- After recovery from acute variceal hemorrhage, secondary prophylaxis using nonselective β-blockers and serial EVL is recommended. If bleeding still recurs, then consider TIPS (Fig. 30-3)
  - Goal is to lower HVPG to less than 12 mm Hg or at least 20% below baseline levels
- TIPS increases the risk of hepatic encephalopathy, and it is contraindicated in patients with congestive heart

Based on the values of serum creatinine (SCr), total bilirubin (tbili), and international normalized ratio (INR).

Formula

MELD Score = 9.6*ln(SCr [mg/dL]) + 3.8*ln(tbili [mg/dL]) + 11.2*ln(INR) + 6.4

General Rules

- Minimum value for any variable is 1
- Maximum value for SCr is 4, which is also assigned to patients on dialysis
- Maximum MELD score is 40 for organ allocation purposes
  An online calculator is available at: http://optn.transplant.hrsa.gov/resources/MeldPeldCalculator.asp?index=98

MELD, Model for end-stage liver disease; UNOS, United Network for Organ Sharing.

failure, severe pulmonary hypertension, multiple liver cysts, or uncontrolled sepsis
- Also strongly discouraged in patients with significant hepatic dysfunction (e.g., MELD score greater than 18)

Ascites

Basic Information

- Ascites is the most common of the major complications of cirrhosis
  - Approximately 50% of newly cirrhotic patients develop ascites over the following 10 years
  - After development of ascites, mortality is 15% in 1 year and 44% in 5 years
  - Mortality at 1 year after developing refractory ascites (see later) is approximately 50%
- Most frequent cause in the Western world is cirrhosis (85%), followed by peritoneal carcinomatosis and heart failure. Other etiologies include tuberculous peritonitis, nephrotic syndrome, pancreatitis, and Budd-Chiari syndrome.
- Pathogenesis in cirrhosis includes elevated hydrostatic pressure from sinusoidal/portal hypertension, renal sodium retention secondary to sympathetic activation of renin-angiotensin-aldosterone system, and reduced oncotic pressure caused by hypoalbuminemia (Fig. 30-4)

Clinical Presentation

- Patients may complain of early satiety, increased abdominal girth, weight gain, or respiratory distress
- Physical examination can reveal abdominal distention, bulging flanks, shifting dullness (most sensitive), fluid wave (least sensitive), or ballotable liver/spleen. Findings can be insensitive when less than 1500 mL of fluid is present or if the patient is obese.
- General stigmata of cirrhosis are often present, including spider angiomata and palmar erythema

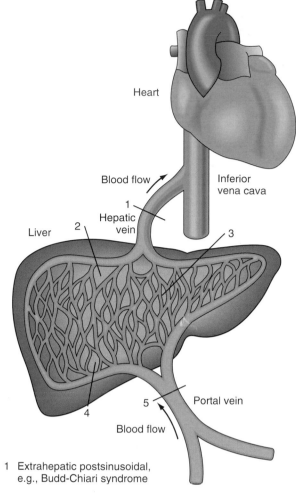

1 Extrahepatic postsinusoidal, e.g., Budd-Chiari syndrome

2 Intrahepatic postsinusoidal, e.g., venoocclusive disease

3 Sinusoidal (e.g., cirrhosis)

4 Intrahepatic presinusoidal (e.g., sarcoidosis, schistosomiasis)

5 Extrahepatic presinusoidal (e.g., portal vein thrombosis)

FIGURE 30-1 Classification of portal hypertension. (From Boon NA, Colledge NR, Walker BR. *Davidson's Principles and Practice of Medicine.* 20th ed. New York; Churchill Livingstone: 2006: Fig. 23.19.)

Diagnosis

- Abdominal ultrasound with Doppler can detect small amounts of intraperitoneal fluid and evaluate for portal vein thrombosis or Budd-Chiari syndrome
- **Diagnostic paracentesis with ascitic fluid analysis is indicated in all patients with new-onset ascites and most patients with ascites who are admitted to the hospital**
  - Considered safe even among cirrhotic patients with coagulopathy. Routine use of fresh frozen plasma and/or platelets before paracentesis is not recommended.
  - Routine ascitic fluid testing includes cell count with differential, total protein, and albumin

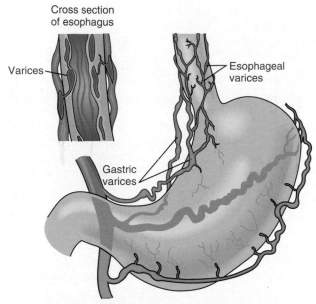

FIGURE 30-2 Esophageal and gastric varices. (From Johns Hopkins Medicine Health Library. http://www.hopkinsmedicine.org/healthlibrary/conditions/adult/digestive_disorders/portal_hypertension_22,PortalHypertension/.)

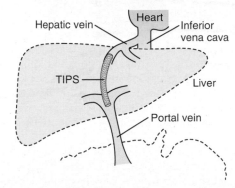

FIGURE 30-3 Transjugular intrahepatic portosystemic shunt (TIPS). A stent is placed from the right hepatic vein into the portal vein, allowing for decompression of the portal system. (From Boon NA, Colledge NR, Walker BR. *Davidson's Principles and Practice of Medicine.* 20th ed. New York; Churchill Livingstone: 2006: Fig. 23.24B.)

- ▪ If infection suspected, also order gram stain, culture, and sensitivity
- ▪ Serum-ascites albumin gradient (SAAG)
  - ▪ SAAG = serum albumin − ascitic albumin
  - ▪ SAAG 1.1 g/dL or greater predicts portal hypertension with 97% accuracy
  - ▪ Ascitic total protein is usually low in cirrhosis
  - ▪ If ascitic total protein greater than 2.5 g/dL and SAAG greater than or equal to 1.1 g/dL, consider a cardiac etiology. If ascitic total protein greater than 2.5 g/dL and SAAG less than 1.1 g/dL, the differential is peritoneal carcinomatosis and tuberculous peritonitis.

Treatment

- ▪ Appropriate management is based on the cause of ascites. The remainder of this section applies to ascites caused by cirrhosis.

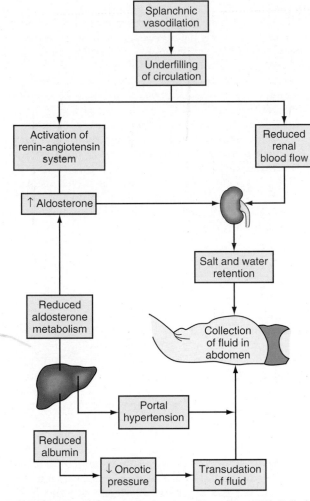

FIGURE 30-4 Pathogenesis of ascites. (From Boon NA, Colledge NR, Walker BR. *Davidson's Principles and Practice of Medicine.* 20th ed. New York; Churchill Livingstone: 2006: Fig. 23.12.)

- ▪ **Restrict dietary sodium to less than 2 g/day**
- ▪ Fluid restriction is only needed if there is severe hyponatremia (serum sodium less than 125 mmol/L)
- ▪ Complete alcohol cessation in patients with alcoholic liver disease
- ▪ Avoid or use with caution certain medications
  - ▪ Nonsteroidal antiinflammatory drugs (NSAIDs) may reduce urinary sodium excretion and induce azotemia
- ▪ **Typical starting diuretic regimen is spironolactone 100 mg and furosemide 40 mg taken orally once a day**
  - ▪ Spironolactone blocks the action of aldosterone on mineralocorticoid receptors in the distal tubule and collecting duct of the kidney nephron, resulting in an inhibition of sodium reabsorption and potassium excretion
  - ▪ Loop diuretics (e.g., furosemide) inhibit the reabsorption of sodium, potassium, and chloride in the ascending limb of the loop of Henle
  - ▪ Goals of diuretic therapy: 24-hour urinary sodium greater than 78 mmol, spot urine sodium/potassium ratio greater than 1, or maximum weight loss of 0.5 kg/day (1.0 kg/day in patients with edema)

30

- Monitor for side-effects, including electrolyte disorders, dehydration, hypotension, and renal injury
- Refractory ascites is defined as persistent ascites despite adequate sodium restriction and maximum-dose diuretics (i.e., spironolactone 400 mg/day and furosemide 160 mg/day), or intolerance of diuretic therapy
  - **Serial large-volume (i.e., 5 L or greater) paracenteses (LVP) may be necessary. Albumin infusion of 6 to 8 g/L of ascites removed may reduce postparacentesis circulatory collapse and improve survival**
  - TIPS in carefully selected patients can offer superior control of ascites compared with serial LVP
  - Liver transplantation should be considered in patients with refractory ascites

Spontaneous Bacterial Peritonitis

Basic Information

- Present in approximately 10% of hospitalized patients with cirrhosis, spontaneous bacterial peritonitis (SBP) is the most important potential sequela of ascites
  - Mortality is 10% to 20% during the same hospitalization, and is predicted by worsening renal function
  - Approximately 70% recurrence rate within 1 year of infection
  - Median survival is 9 months after development of SBP
- **Risk factors for SBP include upper gastrointestinal hemorrhage, ascitic fluid protein concentration less than 1 g/dL, and a previous episode of SBP**

Clinical Presentation

- Suspect SBP in cirrhotic patients with worsening jaundice, encephalopathy, or renal failure
- Fever, chills, and generalized abdominal pain can be seen; 33% of patients with cirrhosis and SBP will not have a fever or leukocytosis

Diagnosis

- **Diagnosis is made when ascitic fluid polymorphonuclear (PMN) cell count is 250/mm³ or higher. PMN count greater than 1000/mm³ suggests bowel perforation.**

Treatment

- **Cefotaxime and ceftriaxone are the empiric antibiotics of choice**
- **Albumin infusion, 1.5 g/kg body weight on day 1 of diagnosis and 1.0 g/kg on day 3**
- Follow-up paracentesis is not essential in many cases, but should be performed after 48 hours if recently exposed to β-lactam antibiotics or if clinical response to treatment is atypical
- Long-term prophylaxis with a fluoroquinolone or trimethoprim-sulfamethoxazole is indicated in patients who recover from an episode of SBP
- Ceftriaxone 1 g daily or norfloxacin 400 mg twice daily for 7 days can reduce bacterial infections in cirrhotic patients (with or without ascites) with hemodynamically significant gastrointestinal hemorrhage

Hepatorenal Syndrome

Basic Information

- Hepatorenal syndrome (HRS) is a class of renal failure that occurs in advanced liver disease and portal hypertension
- Hallmarks are oliguria, azotemia, and reduced urinary sodium excretion.
- Seen in up to 10% of patients hospitalized with liver failure
- Proposed pathogenesis involves severe splanchnic and peripheral vasodilation resulting in reduced effective circulatory volume and compensatory stimulation of sympathetic nervous and renin-angiotensin-aldosterone systems
- Risk factors include cirrhosis, alcoholic hepatitis, acute liver failure, recent large-volume paracentesis, infection, bleeding, overdiuresis, nephrotoxic agents (e.g., NSAIDs and contrast dye), and orthostatic hypotension

Clinical Presentation

- HRS is classified into two types:
  - Type 1: Rapid (less than 2 weeks) progressive impairment of renal function, defined as doubling of initial serum creatinine to more than 2.5 mg/dL or creatinine clearance less than 20 mL/min
  - Type 2: Less rapid, more insidious progression
- There is frequently a precipitating event (e.g., bacterial infection)
- Progressive oliguria, azotemia, reduced urinary sodium excretion, hyponatremia, and hypotension are characteristic. Urinalysis is usually normal.

Diagnosis

- HRS is conventionally diagnosed after excluding other causes of kidney failure
- Proposed diagnostic criteria are shown in Box 30-3

Treatment

- **No established effective medical therapies are available.** Albumin infusion, midodrine, and octreotide are commonly used with modest benefit.

BOX 30-3	*Diagnostic Criteria for Hepatorenal Syndrome*

Cirrhosis with ascites
Serum creatinine >1.5 mg/dL
No improvement in serum creatinine (≤1.5 mg/dL) after 2+ days of diuretic withdrawal and volume expansion using 1 g/kg/day (up to 100 g/day of intravenous albumin)
Absence of shock
No current or recent exposure to nephrotoxic agents
No proteinuria >500 mg/day, microhematuria >50 RBC/hpf, or abnormal renal ultrasonography

RBC, Red blood cell; hpf, high power field.

- Renal replacement therapy can be used as a bridge to liver transplantation

Hepatic Encephalopathy

Basic Information

- Defined as neurologic or psychiatric disturbances associated with acute or chronic liver insufficiency and/or portosystemic shunting
  - West Haven Criteria (WHC) severity grading for hepatic encephalopathy (HE) (Table 30-3)
  - Overt HE spans from disorientation/asterixis to coma, corresponding to WHC grades 2 to 4
  - Covert HE includes minimal and grade 1 HE
- Prevalence of overt HE is 10% to 14% at the time when cirrhosis is initially diagnosed
- Complex pathogenesis not yet fully delineated, but key requirements are hepatocellular failure and portal-systemic shunting
  - Failure of liver to clear intestinal toxins (e.g., ammonia), which then accumulate in the systemic circulation, eventually migrating into the brain
  - Ammonia forms glutamine in astrocytes, causing cellular swelling, which precipitates cerebral edema and impairs cognition
- There are numerous precipitating factors for HE (Box 30-4)

Clinical Presentation

- Wide range of neurologic and psychiatric manifestations (Table 30-3)
- Motor symptoms may include asterixis, hyperreflexia, abnormal Babinski reflexes, and extrapyramidal signs (e.g., parkinsonism)
  - Asterixis is not specific to HE

Diagnosis

- Overt HE is diagnosed primarily by clinical criteria in a patient with acute or chronic liver disease and/or portosystemic shunting
- Minimal HE can be diagnosed using neuropsychometric and/or neurophysiologic testing performed by experienced examiners

- **Elevated serum ammonia level alone is neither sensitive nor specific for HE.** However, a normal value should prompt reassessment for alternate diagnoses.
- Electroencephalography can show general background slowing (nonspecific), initial increasing then decreasing amplitude, and triphasic waves (associated with severe HE)
- Computed tomography (CT) and magnetic resonance imaging (MRI) generally do not provide direct diagnostic value, but are used to rule out other etiologies of mental status changes. HE in acute liver failure can cause cerebral edema that can be seen on CT.

Treatment

- General supportive measures include fluid/electrolyte maintenance, pressure-sore prevention, aspiration precautions
- **Eliminate or treat precipitating factors**; 80% to 90% of cases may improve with this step alone
- **Lactulose (a nonabsorbable disaccharide) is first-line therapy for treatment of overt HE**
  - Titrate dosing to maintain 2 to 3 bowel movements daily
  - Numerous mechanisms have been proposed, including (1) prebiotic promotion of "beneficial" intestinal flora; (2) osmotic laxative effect to decrease intestinal transit time and reduce the production/absorption of ammonia; (3) inhibition of intestinal glutaminase to reduce metabolism of glutamine to ammonia; and (4) stool acidification that results in a net entry of circulating ammonia into the colon to balance the pH change
  - Mostly based on anecdotal experience; existing placebo-controlled trials are severely underpowered
- **Rifaxamin (an antibiotic) can be added to lactulose to reduce recurrence of overt HE**
  - Has activity against intestinal flora, including urease-producing organisms that promote ammonia production
  - Few adverse drug effects because of minimal (less than 0.4%) systemic absorption
  - Insufficient data to support its use alone without lactulose, or its efficacy in shortening the duration of existing overt HE

TABLE 30-3	Stages of Hepatic Encephalopathy (West Haven Criteria)
Grade	**Clinical Description**
0	Normal mental function clinically and on neuropsychological testing
Minimal	Abnormal results on neuropsychological tests without overt clinical manifestations
1	Hypersomnia or insomnia, euphoria or anxiety, short attention span, irritability
2	Lethargy, inappropriate behavior, dyspraxia, disorientation, asterixis
3	Somnolence, gross confusion, responsive to noxious stimuli
4	Coma, no response to noxious stimuli

BOX 30-4	Precipitating Factors for the Development of Hepatic Encephalopathy

(Bleeding and infection most common)
Azotemia
Constipation
Dehydration
Drugs (benzodiazepines, narcotics, sedatives, diuretics)
Electrolyte and acid-base derangements (hypokalemia, hyponatremia, alkalosis)
Gastrointestinal bleeding
Infection
Liver-related (acute hepatitis, progression of chronic disease, portosystemic shunts, portal vein thrombosis)
Malnutrition

30

- Metronidazole, vancomycin, paromomycin, and neomycin are other antibiotics that have been reported to improve HE
  - Worse side-effect profile compared with rifaximin
- **Chronic protein restriction is unnecessary and likely even deleterious**
  - For patients truly intolerant of dietary protein, can supplement with oral branched chain amino acids to reach target daily protein intake
- Routine treatment of minimal and covert HE is currently not recommended
- Routine primary prophylaxis post-TIPS is not recommended

Pulmonary Manifestations of Cirrhosis and Portal Hypertension

- 50% to 70% of cirrhotic patients undergoing evaluation for liver transplantation report dyspnea
  - Most common causes are primary cardiopulmonary disorders, such as congestive heart failure or chronic obstructive pulmonary disease
- Pulmonary disorders related to liver disease
  - Parenchymal lung disease
    - Fibrosing alveolitis and pulmonary granulomas (primary biliary cirrhosis)
    - Panacinar emphysema (α_1-antitrypsin deficiency)
  - Pleural space disease
    - Hepatic hydrothorax
    - Elevated hemidiaphragms secondary to ascites or hepatomegaly
  - Pulmonary vascular abnormalities
    - Hepatopulmonary syndrome
    - Portopulmonary hypertension
    - Bronchial varices
- Hepatic hydrothorax
  - Develops in 5% to 10% of cirrhotic patients with ascites
  - Ascitic fluid enters the pleural space via defects in the diaphragm
  - Affects the right chest in 85%, left chest in 13%, and both sides in 2%
  - Can become infected (i.e., spontaneous bacterial empyema)
  - First-line therapy consists of sodium restriction and diuresis. Therapeutic thoracenteses as needed.
    - Chest tubes may precipitate rapid deterioration and are contraindicated
  - Consider TIPS in medically refractory cases
- Hepatopulmonary syndrome (HPS)
  - Affects 5% to 30% of cirrhotic patients
  - Vasodilation and/or angiogenesis within pulmonary capillary bed, resulting in right-to-left shunt and impaired oxygenation of venous blood
  - **Clinical presentation includes hypoxemia, platypnea (difficulty breathing upon sitting up), and orthodeoxia (decreased oxygen saturation when changing from a lying to a sitting position)**
  - Differential diagnosis includes hereditary hemorrhagic telangiectasia (also known as

Osler-Weber-Rendu syndrome) and cavopulmonary anastomoses
  - Screen via arterial blood gases in patients with abnormal room air pulse oximetry (95% or lower in our center). Characteristics of HPS include alveolar-arterial oxygen gradient 15 mm Hg or greater or partial pressure of oxygen (PaO_2) less than 80 mm Hg while on room air
  - Transthoracic echocardiography with agitated saline is diagnostic with appearance of bubbles in the left atrium after 4 to 5 beats. Technetium-99m-labeled macroaggregated albumin lung perfusion scan with shunt fraction greater than 6% also useful. Angiogram of chest should be performed to evaluate for macroscopic intrapulmonary shunts that could be embolized.
  - Decreased diffusing capacity for carbon monoxide (DLCO) on pulmonary function tests
  - Liver transplantation is the only successful therapy. Patients with PaO_2 less than 60 mm Hg may be eligible for increased transplant priority.
    - Preoperative PaO_2 50 mm Hg or less predicts poor post-transplant survival, and in certain transplant centers may exclude patients from consideration
- Portopulmonary hypertension (PPHTN)
  - Pulmonary artery hypertension (defined as mean pulmonary artery pressure [mPAP] greater than 25 mm Hg and capillary wedge pressure less than 15 mm Hg) in the setting of portal hypertension
  - Underlying mechanism is poorly understood
  - **Clinical presentation can include dyspnea with or without exertion, peripheral edema, syncope, chest pain, and jugular venous distention**
  - Initial screening is with transthoracic echocardiography. If estimated pulmonary artery systolic pressure is 40 mm Hg or greater, then consider cardiology consultation for right heart catheterization
  - Medical treatment is similar to primary pulmonary hypertension, including diuretics for volume management and vasodilators to improve pulmonary hemodynamics
    - Caution with β-blockers because of potential for cardiac depression
    - Avoid anticoagulants (increased risk of bleeding) and calcium channel blockers (may worsen portal hypertension)
  - Moderate to severe PPHTN (mPAP 35 mm Hg or greater) despite medical therapy is a contraindication to liver transplantation

Hepatocellular Carcinoma

Basic Information

- Hepatocellular carcinoma (HCC) is the fifth most common cancer and the third highest cause of cancer death worldwide
  - Wide geographic variation in incidence rates, generally following the prevalence patterns of chronic liver diseases, especially chronic viral hepatitis

- Highest annual incidence rates in Eastern Asia, Southeast Asia, and sub-Saharan Africa. China alone accounts for more than 50% of all cases worldwide.
- In the United States, age-adjusted HCC incidence rates are highest among immigrants from Asian countries (particularly Korea and China)
- Risk factors for development of HCC include cirrhosis, chronic hepatitis B (with or without cirrhosis), aflatoxin, alcohol and tobacco use, obesity, and diabetes mellitus
  - **Cirrhosis (of any etiology) is the most important risk factor for HCC**
  - In most cohorts, rates of HCC are 2 to 4 times higher in men than women
  - Older age (or longer disease duration) also increases HCC risk in cirrhotic patients
- **Chronic hepatitis B is the most common cause (more than 50%) of HCC worldwide**
  - Risk of HCC is 100 times higher in hepatitis B carriers (approximately 1000 times higher with cirrhosis) compared with noncarriers
- Fibrolamellar HCC is a rare variant with characteristic histopathologic and clinical appearances
  - Usually occurs in patients younger than 25 years of age without typical HCC risk factors

Clinical Presentation

- Symptomatic disease is typically advanced, signifying poor prognosis
  - May present with weight loss, jaundice, ascites, and/or variceal bleeding
  - Abdominal pain is the most common symptom
- Examination may reveal a right upper quadrant abdominal mass and/or a bruit over the liver
- **Paraneoplastic syndromes associated with HCC**
  - Hypoglycemia caused by increased serum concentration of insulin-like growth factor II (IGF-II)
  - Erythrocytosis caused by erythropoietin production by tumor cells
  - Hypercalcemia attributed to production of parathyroid hormone-related peptide
  - Hypercholesterolemia caused by impaired cholesterol uptake in HCC cells
  - Feminization caused by HCC converting circulating androgens to estrogens

Diagnosis

- Routine HCC screening is recommended for individuals at increased risk for developing HCC
  - All patients with cirrhosis (regardless of etiology)
  - Asian male hepatitis B carriers older than age 40, or female carriers older than age 50
  - African hepatitis B carriers older than age 20
  - Any hepatitis B carrier with family history of HCC
- **Abdominal ultrasonography every 6 months is the recommended surveillance practice**
  - Many providers also monitor serum α-fetoprotein every 6 months
- Masses found on screening ultrasonography warrant additional evaluation

- Lesions less than 1 cm should be followed by ultrasound every 3 months for 2 years, at which point, if there is no lesion growth, standard 6-month interval screening can be resumed
- Lesions greater than 1 cm should undergo either dynamic CT or MRI. If findings are inconclusive, obtain the other imaging modality. If still inconclusive, then consider biopsy.
- Biopsy is not necessary if a lesion fulfills radiologic criteria for diagnosis

Treatment

- Referral to a multidisciplinary team of specialists is recommended
- Surgical resection is reasonable for noncirrhotic or well-compensated cirrhotic (i.e., Child A) patients with a solitary tumor
  - 5-year survival greater than 70%, but greater than 70% HCC recurrence rate
- **Liver transplantation is an option for patients with small HCCs that fall within the Milan criteria: 1 tumor 2 to 5 cm, or 2 to 3 tumors each 1 to 3 cm.** Contraindications include tumor vascular invasion and extrahepatic spread
  - 5-year survival greater than 70% with less than 15% HCC recurrence rate
  - Preoperative locoregional therapy (e.g., chemoembolization) can delay tumor progression while awaiting transplantation
- Consider locoregional and/or systemic therapy for nonsurgical candidates
  - For HCC less than 2 cm, ethanol injection or radiofrequency ablation offers 70% survival at 5 years
  - For larger or multifocal HCC without vascular invasion or extrahepatic spread, transarterial chemoembolization (TACE) is first-line therapy
    - Contraindicated in advanced liver disease (Child C) because increased risk of liver failure and death, and lack of improvement in survival
  - Radioembolization with yttrium-90 microspheres is an alternative for multifocal disease
- Sorafenib may be considered in patients with preserved liver function (Child A)
  - An oral multikinase inhibitor
  - Only Food and Drug Administration-approved chemotherapy for HCC
  - Adverse effects include blistering rash, diarrhea, and fatigue
- Other systemic chemotherapy, octreotide, interferon, and tamoxifen have not shown survival benefits and are not recommended

Liver Transplantation

Basic Information

- Indications for liver transplantation may include:
  - Acute liver failure
  - Decompensated cirrhosis
  - Inherited metabolic disorders with debilitating extrahepatic features
  - HCC using strict selection guidelines (Milan criteria)

30

TABLE 30-4	*Contraindications to Liver Transplantation*
Absolute Contraindications	**Relative Contraindications**
Active extrahepatic malignancy (except neuroendocrine tumors)	Ongoing alcohol or illicit substance abuse
Unstable cardiopulmonary disease	Untreated HIV
	BMI >40 or <18.5 kg/m²
Uncontrolled sepsis	Age >70 years
Severe, irreversible neurologic disease	Advanced renal disease (requires combined liver/kidney transplantation)
AIDS	Portal vein thrombosis
Severe psychological or social dysfunction	

AIDS, Acquired immunodeficiency syndrome; BMI, body mass index; HIV, human immunodeficiency virus.

- ■ Polycystic disease
- ■ Budd-Chiari syndrome (hepatic vein thrombosis)
- ■ Contraindications to liver transplantation (Table 30-4)
- ■ Donors may be deceased or living
  - ■ More than 90% of transplanted livers in the United States originate from deceased donors
  - ■ Living donation eliminates recipient wait time, but is associated with 0.25% to 1% donor mortality and 14% to 21% donor morbidity
- ■ **Prioritization on the liver transplant waiting list takes into account mortality risk as determined by the MELD score**
  - ■ Except for status 1a patients (acute liver failure, primary graft dysfunction, or hepatic artery thrombosis within 1 week of transplantation) who are prioritized above all others
- ■ The MELD score estimates 90-day mortality risk for patients on the liver transplant waiting list (see Box 30-2)
- ■ Patients with certain disease processes (e.g., HCC, hepatopulmonary syndrome) are granted exceptional MELD points to more accurately reflect their medical urgency
- ■ Complex local-regional-national organ distribution algorithms are constantly being reevaluated and modified by the Organ Procurement and Transplantation Network
- ■ The 5-year survival rate is now close to 80% at well-established liver transplantation centers, and the 1-year survival rate exceeds 85%

Review Questions

For review questions, please go to ExpertConsult.com.

SUGGESTED READINGS

Garcia-Tsao G, Sanyal AJ, Grace ND, et al. Prevention and management of gastroesophageal varices and variceal hemorrhage in cirrhosis. *Hepatology.* 2007;46:922-938.

Rodríguez-Roisin R, Krowka MJ. Hepatopulmonary syndrome—a liver-induced lung vascular disorder. *N Engl J Med.* 2008;358:2378-2387.

Runyon BA. Management of adult patients with ascites due to cirrhosis: an update. *Hepatology.* 2009;49:2087-2107.

Salgia R, Singal AG. Hepatocellular carcinoma and other liver lesions. *Med Clin North Am.* 2014;98:103-118.

Vilstrup H, Amodio P, Bajaj J, et al. Hepatic encephalopathy in chronic liver disease: 2014 Practice Guideline by the American Association for the Study of Liver Diseases and the European Association for the Study of the Liver. *Hepatology.* 2014;60:715-735.

BOARD REVIEW

Nephrology

Acid-Base Disorders and Renal Tubular Acidosis

STEPHEN D. SISSON, MD

Acid-Base

Acid-base disorders are extremely common in clinical medicine and can be seen in numerous disease states. The lungs and kidneys help maintain acid-base equilibrium (in the lungs via CO_2, in the kidneys via bicarbonate; Fig. 31-1). **The body never fully corrects for a single acid-base disorder, except perhaps for respiratory alkalosis. When evaluating acid-base status, begin by looking at the serum pH to decide if acidemia or alkalemia is present** (pH <7.35 indicates acidemia; pH >7.45 indicates alkalemia). Then look at the partial pressure of carbon dioxide ($PaCO_2$) and serum bicarbonate to see which one (or both) is consistent with the pH, to determine if the primary disorder is respiratory or metabolic. **Note that a normal pH does not exclude an acid-base disorder; for instance, with a coexisting metabolic acidosis and metabolic alkalosis, the pH may be normal.**

Metabolic Acidosis

Basic Information

- Primary defect in metabolic acidosis is decreased serum HCO_3^-
- Calculation of the anion gap is used to help narrow differential diagnosis
  - Anion gap calculated as $Na^+ - (Cl^- + HCO_3^-)$
  - **The normal anion gap is 12 ± 2** and is made of phosphates, sulfates, organic acids, and negatively charged plasma proteins
- When metabolic acidosis develops, determining whether the anion gap is elevated, normal, or low will narrow the differential diagnosis

Metabolic Acidosis with Increased Anion Gap

- **The differential diagnosis of the most common causes of an anion gap acidosis is remembered by the mnemonic MUDPILES (Box 31-1)**
- Besides a thorough history and physical examination, **evaluation of serum ketones, serum lactate, toxicology screen, and salicylate level should be considered**

Metabolic Acidosis with Normal Anion Gap

- Also referred to as a non–anion gap acidosis, although an anion gap is present but normal

- In this group, the increased anion is chloride (Cl^-); therefore, the anion gap does not change
- **The mnemonic for the most common causes of a normal anion gap acidosis is DURHAM (Box 31-2)**
- **Calculation of the urine anion gap may be helpful in evaluating normal anion gap metabolic acidosis** to differentiate renal tubular acidoses (RTAs) from other causes of normal anion gap metabolic acidosis
  - Normal kidney response to acidosis is to excrete acid in the form of NH_4^+, which is balanced by increases in urine chloride, so urine chloride is a marker of urine acid excretion. In type 1 or type 4 RTA, NH_4^+ excretion does not occur, and urine chloride is low
  - **Formula for urine anion gap: Urine (Na + K − Cl)**
    - In a normal patient (without RTA) with metabolic acidosis, the sum of this equation is less than 0
    - If normal anion gap metabolic acidosis exists, and urine anion gap is greater than 0, type 1 or type 4 RTA is likely

Metabolic Acidosis with Decreased Anion Gap

- Low anion gap acidoses are less commonly seen
  - **May be caused by hypoalbuminemia, multiple myeloma, ingestion of bromide**
  - The acid-base disorders in these diseases are of little clinical consequence

Investigation of Coexistent Anion Gap and Normal Anion Gap Metabolic Acidoses

- **An anion gap acidosis and a normal anion gap acidosis may coexist**
- To determine if the metabolic acidosis is caused by more than one process, compare the increase in the anion gap with the decrease in HCO_3^-
  - In pure anion gap metabolic acidosis, the decrease in HCO_3^- equals the increase in the anion gap
  - **If the HCO_3^- decreases significantly more than the anion gap increases, then a coexisting normal anion gap metabolic acidosis is present**
  - Expressed as the *delta-delta equation* or the corrected bicarbonate:

    Change (Δ) in anion gap = change (Δ) in HCO_3^-

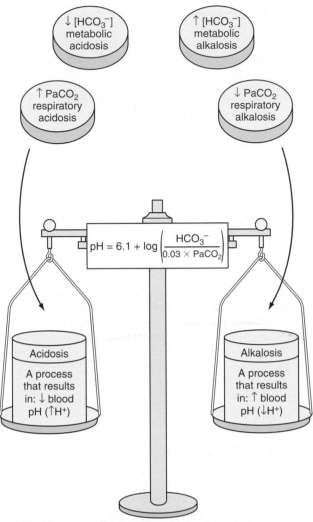

FIGURE 31-1   Acid-base disorders. (From Baynes JW, Dominiczak MH: *Medical biochemistry*, ed 2, St. Louis, Mosby, 2004, Fig. 22-5.)

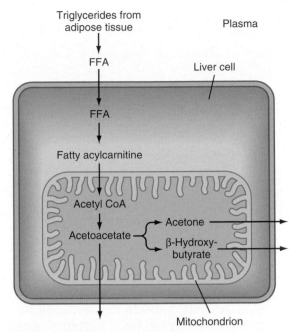

FIGURE 31-2   Pathogenesis of metabolic acidosis in ketogenesis. Acetoacetate, acetone, and β-hydroxybutyrate pass into the bloodstream, producing acidosis. CoA, Coenzyme A; FFA, free fatty acids. (From Kumar P, Clark M. *Clinical medicine.* 5th ed. Philadelphia; Saunders: 2005. Fig. 19-12.)

BOX 31-1	*Differential Diagnosis of Metabolic Acidosis with Increased Anion Gap*

M: Methanol
U: Uremia
D: Diabetic ketoacidosis (Fig. 31-2) or alcoholic ketoacidosis; drugs*
P: Phosphate, paraldehyde, pyroglutamic acid, or propylene glycol
I: Ischemia, isoniazid (rare), or iron toxicity (rare)
L: Lactate (L- and D-)
E: Ethylene glycol
S: Starvation or salicylates

*For example, metformin, nucleoside reverse transcriptase inhibitors.

- Note that the actual values of the HCO_3^- and anion gap are not compared, but rather the change in each of these values from their baseline (baseline HCO_3^- is 24 mEq/dL; baseline anion gap is 12)

Osmolar Gap

- **Metabolic acidosis is occasionally caused by the ingestion of toxic compounds that are osmotically active (e.g., methanol, ethylene glycol, toluene)**

BOX 31-2	*Differential Diagnosis of Metabolic Acidosis with Normal Anion Gap*

D: Diarrhea
U: Ureteral diversion
R: Renal tubular acidosis
H: Hyperalimentation
A: Addison disease, acetazolamide, ammonium chloride
M: Miscellaneous (chloridorrhea, amphotericin B, toluene,* others)

*Toluene initially results in an anion gap metabolic acidosis, but as it is cleared, a hyperchloremic normal anion gap acidosis develops.

- May be investigated in the clinically appropriate setting by calculating the difference between the measured osmolality and the calculated osmolality; in normal host, difference between measured and calculated osmolality is less than 10
- If this difference is greater than 10 (i.e., measured osmolality more than 10 units higher than estimated osmolality), there are extraosmotically active compounds in the blood; compare clinical picture with signs and symptoms of suggested toxin, including methanol (associated with papilledema and retinal hemorrhages), ethylene glycol (associated with calcium oxalate crystals in the urine), and toluene (presents first with anion gap metabolic acidosis, then metabolized resulting in **normal anion gap metabolic acidosis**)
  - Later in the course, methanol and ethylene glycol ingestions result in a normal osmolar gap with ongoing metabolic acidosis
  - Isopropyl alcohol ingestion also results in an osmolar gap, although no acid-base disorder is associated

31

- Written mathematically, the osmolar gap is calculated as:

Osmolality (measured) − osmolality (calculated)

Where

Osm(calc)
= $[2 \times Na] + [blood\ urea\ nitrogen/2.8] + [glucose/18]$

- The normal osmolar gap is less than 10

Clinical Presentation

- Respiratory compensation in patients presenting with metabolic acidosis
  - The body compensates for metabolic acidosis by creating respiratory alkalosis (hyperventilation)
  - $PaCO_2$ may be predicted by the following equation (Winter formula):

$$PaCO_2 = [1.5 \times HCO_3^- + 8] \pm 2$$

  - Equation only valid when the primary disorder is metabolic acidosis; do not use this equation when the primary disorder is not a metabolic acidosis
  - If the measured $PaCO_2$ is not close to what is predicted, a second disorder coexists
    - If the $PaCO_2$ is less than predicted, second disorder is respiratory alkalosis
    - If the $PaCO_2$ is higher than predicted, second disorder is respiratory acidosis

Metabolic Alkalosis

Basic Information

- **The primary defect in a metabolic alkalosis is an increase in the serum HCO_3^-, implying either a gain of HCO_3^- or a loss of acid**
  - **Examples of HCO_3^- gain**
    - Administration of sodium bicarbonate ($NaHCO_3$), baking soda, or medication formulations that include citrate or lactate
  - **Examples of acid loss**
    - Gastric losses, such as vomiting or nasogastric suction
    - Renal causes (e.g., side effects from diuretics), as well as administration of nonresorbable anions (e.g., IV penicillin or carbenicillin)
    - Mineralocorticoid excess states

Clinical Presentation

- The presence of a metabolic alkalosis always implies that two events have occurred: initiation of the alkalosis and maintenance of the alkalosis
  - The initiating factors are the gain of HCO_3^- or loss of acid described previously
  - The kidneys are always responsible for the maintenance of alkalosis; maintenance of alkalosis by the kidney is favored by:
    - **Volume depletion:** The kidney responds to volume depletion by increasing Na^+ resorption in exchange for acid secretion

- **Chloride depletion:** Urine Cl− is low in volume depletion, leading to ongoing renin-angiotensin-aldosterone system stimulation and acid secretion. Low urine Cl− impairs the renal secretion of HCO_3^-.
- **Hypokalemia:** Hypokalemia stimulates renal ammoniagenesis and net acid secretion
- **Mineralocorticoid excess:** Mineralocorticoids stimulate renal hydrogen ion (H^+) excretion; examples include hyperaldosteronism (Conn syndrome; Fig. 31-3), Cushing disease, and Bartter and Gitelman syndromes

Diagnosis and Evaluation

- **Measurement of spot urine Cl− is helpful in evaluating the cause of the metabolic alkalosis (Box 31-3)**
- Respiratory compensation in primary metabolic alkalosis
  - **Response to metabolic alkalosis requires respiratory acidosis; response is therefore limited**
  - In general, the $PaCO_2$ rises 0.5 to 1 mm Hg for every 1-unit increase in serum HCO_3^- from a baseline of 24 mmol/L
  - The maximum $PaCO_2$ in compensation is 55 to 60 mm Hg

Respiratory Acidosis

Basic Information

- **The primary defect in respiratory acidosis is an increase in $PaCO_2$**
- Whereas the lungs can respond rapidly to a metabolic challenge, the kidneys cannot respond immediately to a challenge from the lungs
  - **Respiratory processes (both acidosis and alkalosis) have an acute compensatory phase, in which plasma buffers help maintain pH; and a chronic phase, in which the kidney participates**
  - The acute response takes minutes to hours, whereas the chronic response takes 3 to 5 days
- Prediction of pH and HCO_3^- in respiratory acidosis
  - **Acute respiratory acidosis: For every 10 mm Hg increase in $PaCO_2$, pH decreases by 0.08, and serum HCO_3^- increases by 1**
  - **Chronic respiratory acidosis: For every 10 mm Hg increase in $PaCO_2$, pH decreases by 0.03, and serum HCO_3^- increases by 3 to 4**

Differential Diagnosis

- Differential diagnosis of respiratory acidosis is shown in Box 31-4

Respiratory Alkalosis

Basic Information

- **The primary defect in respiratory alkalosis is a decrease in $PaCO_2$**

35-year-old male

- Mild polyuria
- Blood pressure 188/104 mm Hg

Plasma biochemistry
- Na 144 mmol/L (132–144)
- K 3.1 mmol/L (3.3–4.7)
- HCO₃⁻ 29 mmol/L (21–27)

Lying at 0900 hr
- Renin activity <0.5 (0.4–1.5)
- Aldosterone 850 pmol/L (30–440)

Standing at 1200 hr
- Renin activity <0.5 (1–2.5)
- Aldosterone 750 pmol/L (110–860)

A

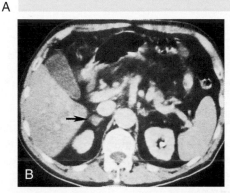

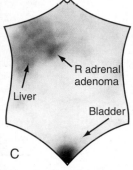

R adrenal adenoma
Liver
Bladder

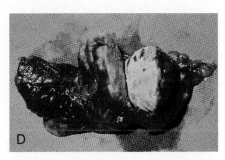

B   C   D

FIGURE 31-3 Conn adenoma causing metabolic alkalosis. **A,** Note hypernatremic, hypokalemic metabolic alkalosis. **B,** Computed tomographic appearance of right adrenal adenoma *(arrow).* **C,** Unilateral uptake of radiolabeled cholesterol in right adrenal gland. **D,** Pathologic specimen following surgical excision. (From Haslett C, Chilvers ER, Boon NA, et al. *Davidson's principles and practice of medicine.* 19th ed. New York; Churchill Livingstone: 2002. Fig. 16.19.)

BOX 31-3	*Differential Diagnosis of Metabolic Alkalosis*

Causes of a saline-responsive alkalosis (urine chloride <10 mEq/L)
- NG suction
- Vomiting
- Diuretics
- Posthypercapnia

Causes of a saline-resistant alkalosis (urine chloride >10 mEq/L) are further divided according to BP:
- With elevated BP: primary aldosteronism (Conn syndrome), Cushing disease, congenital adrenal hyperplasia, Liddle syndrome, licorice ingestion (enzymatically inhibits degradation of cortisol), renal artery stenosis, renal failure plus alkali administration
- With normal BP: hypomagnesemia, severe hypokalemia, Bartter and Gitelman syndromes, NaHCO₃ administration (milk-alkali syndrome), congenital chloride diarrhea

BP, Blood pressure; NG, nasogastric.

BOX 31-4	*Differential Diagnosis of Respiratory Acidosis*

Chest Cavity
Neurologic disorders (e.g., amyotrophic lateral sclerosis)
Muscular disorders
Kyphoscoliosis (severe)
Pleural effusion
Pneumothorax

Central
Sedation or narcotics
Respiratory center hypofunction (infection, ischemia, infarction)
Obstructive sleep apnea

Lung/Airways
Pneumonia, pulmonary edema, bronchospasm or laryngospasm
Chronic obstructive pulmonary disease
Mechanical obstruction (foreign body/tumor)

31

- As with respiratory acidosis, there are acute and chronic phases to respiratory alkalosis
  - **Acute respiratory alkalosis: For every 10 mm Hg decrease in PaCO₂, HCO₃⁻ decreases by 2**
  - **Chronic respiratory alkalosis: For every 10 mm Hg decrease in PaCO₂, HCO₃⁻ decreases by 5; maximum compensation of HCO₃⁻ is 15**
  - Although many use the same estimates of pH change seen in respiratory acidosis (i.e., acutely for each 10 mm Hg decrease in PaCO₂, pH increases 0.08), the pH changes in respiratory alkalosis are less predictable
  - In respiratory alkalosis the body can return the pH to normal

Differential Diagnosis

- Differential diagnosis of respiratory alkalosis is shown in Box 31-5

- Note that sepsis and salicylate toxicity result in both metabolic acidosis and respiratory alkalosis (Fig. 31-4)

Renal Tubular Acidosis

See Table 31-1 for the characteristics of renal tubular acidosis.

Basic Information

- The kidney contributes to the acid-base equilibrium of the serum by either excreting acid or excreting or resorbing HCO_3^- as needed
- If the kidney does not appropriately excrete acid or resorb HCO_3^-, acidosis will develop
- Because a renal tubular defect is responsible when this acidosis occurs in the setting of a normal GFR, these disorders are termed *renal tubular acidoses*

TYPE 1 RENAL TUBULAR ACIDOSES

Basic Information

- **Distal nephron defect in H^+ secretion, resulting in severe acidosis and an inability to acidify urine below a pH of 5.5, even with an acid challenge**

BOX 31-5	*Differential Diagnosis of Respiratory Alkalosis*

Systemic
Sepsis
Salicylates
Liver failure
Hyperthyroidism
Pregnancy
High-altitude residence
Hypotension
Severe anemia

Central
Ischemia or cerebrovascular accident
Tumor
Infection
Progesterone
Anxiety
Fever

Pulmonary
Reactive airways (i.e., early in asthma exacerbation)
Pulmonary embolus
Restrictive lung disease (early)
Hypoxemia (e.g., pneumonia, pulmonary edema)

- Potassium conservation in most patients with type 1 RTA is typically impaired, and **hypokalemia often accompanies this disorder**
- Causes may include
  - Congenital autosomal dominant disorder (most common cause of type 1 RTA) and autosomal recessive (associated with sensorineural deafness)
  - Genetic disorders (sickle cell, Ehlers-Danlos, Wilson disease)
  - Autoimmune diseases (Sjögren syndrome, systemic lupus erythematosus, rheumatoid arthritis)
  - Medications such as amphotericin, lithium, and high doses of salicylates
  - Urinary tract obstruction

Clinical Presentation

- **Clinical manifestations include nephrocalcinosis, hypercalciuria and calcium phosphate stones**
  - Hyperparathyroidism and low vitamin D levels may develop, leading to rickets in children and osteomalacia in adults

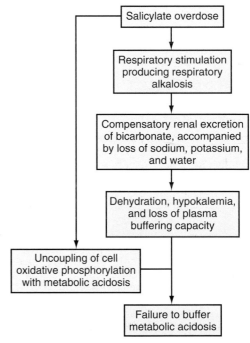

FIGURE 31-4 Salicylate overdose results in metabolic acidosis and respiratory alkalosis. (From Waller D, Renwick A. *Medical pharmacology and therapeutics*. 2nd ed. Philadelphia; Saunders: 2005. Fig. 53-9.)

TABLE 31-1	*Characteristics of Renal Tubular Acidoses*		
	Type 1	**Type 2**	**Type 4**
Basic defect	Distal defect in H^+ secretion	Proximal tubular defect in HCO_3^- resorption	Hyporeninemic hypoaldosteronism
Serum potassium	Low	Low to normal	High
Able to acidify urine to pH <5.5	No	Yes	Yes
Responds to NaHCO₃	Yes	No	Yes

- Other clinical manifestations are related to associated diseases

Diagnosis

- **Diagnosis is made on clinical grounds and confirmed by ammonium chloride (NH_4Cl) administration, which will result in worsening systemic acidosis without drop in urine pH below 5.5**
  - Urine anion gap is 0 or greater

Treatment

- **Treatment consists of combination potassium citrate, sodium citrate, and $NaHCO_3$,** which is titrated until the serum HCO_3^- and urine calcium excretion normalize

TYPE 2 RENAL TUBULAR ACIDOSES

Basic Information

- **A proximal renal tubular defect in HCO_3^- resorption leading to a mild acidosis**
- **Able to acidify urine below a pH of 5.5 with an acid challenge**
- Low level of proximal tubular HCO_3^- resorption does occur, which prevents severe acidosis
  - There is no defect in distal renal H^+ secretion
  - Because potassium often complexes with HCO_3^-, **hypokalemia is common with type 2 RTA**
  - Calcium resorption is also typically impaired, but not as severely as in type 1
- **Commonly seen in conjunction with defective resorption of other molecules, such as glucose and amino acids (as seen in Fanconi syndrome)**
- Other causes: carbonic anhydrase inhibitors, outdated tetracycline, vitamin D deficiency, light chain nephropathy, lead and mercury toxicity

Diagnosis and Evaluation

- Diagnosis is suggested on clinical grounds
  - Administration of NH_4Cl results in normal acidification of urine because acid excretion is normal in type 2 RTA
  - **Administration of $NaHCO_3$ results in alkaline urine despite systemic acidosis because adequate renal HCO_3^- resorption does not occur**
  - Urine anion gap is less useful in evaluation, as it may be normal (less than 0) when serum HCO_3^- is below the renal resorption threshold

Treatment

- Address the underlying cause, if possible
- If necessary, can try very high doses of HCO_3^-

TYPE 4 RENAL TUBULAR ACIDOSES

Basic Information

- **Type 4 RTA is an acquired diffuse renal defect in H^+ secretion, resulting in mild normal anion gap acidosis**

- **Able to acidify urine below a pH of 5.5 with an acid challenge**
- Mechanism in type 4 RTA is not completely understood; the majority of patients with type 4 RTA have low levels of renin and aldosterone (referred to as *hyporeninemic, hypoaldosterone* states)
- **A distinguishing feature is the coexisting inability of the kidney to excrete potassium, leading to high serum potassium (types 1 and 2 RTAs are usually hypokalemic)**
- **Causes include diabetes (the most common cause);** mineralocorticoid deficiency (including Addison disease); therapy with nonsteroidal antiinflammatory drugs, heparin, or angiotensin-converting enzyme inhibitors

Diagnosis and Evaluation

- Diagnosis usually made on clinical grounds
  - Administration of NH_4Cl results in some acidification of urine because limited renal acid secretion occurs; urine pH declines to below 5.5
- Urine anion gap is greater than 0

Treatment

- A low-potassium diet and loop or thiazide diuretic for the hyperkalemia and alkali for the metabolic acidosis can be administered
- Another option is treatment with a mineralocorticoid (e.g., fludrocortisone), although fluid retention and worsening hypertension may result

Review Questions

For review questions, please go to ExpertConsult.com.

SUGGESTED READINGS

Adrogué HJ, Madias NE. Management of life-threatening acid-base disorders (Part 1). *N Engl J Med.* 1998;338:26-34.

Adrogué HJ, Madias NE. Management of life-threatening acid-base disorders (Part 2). *N Engl J Med.* 1998;338:107-111.

Batlle DC, Hizon M, Cohen E, et al. The use of the urinary anion gap in the diagnosis of hyperchloremic metabolic acidosis. *N Engl J Med.* 1988;318:594-599.

Berend K, de Vries APJ, Gans ROB. Physiological approach to assessment of acid-base disturbances. *N Engl J Med.* 2014;371:1434-1445.

Kraut JA, Madias NE. Serum anion gap: its uses and limitations in clinical medicine. *Clin J Am Soc Nephrol.* 2007;2:162-174.

Kraut JA, Madias NE. Differential diagnosis of nongap metabolic acidosis: value of a systemic approach. *Clin J Am Soc Nephrol.* 2012;7:671-679.

Narins RG, Emmett M. Simple and mixed acid-base disorders: a practical approach. *Medicine.* 1980;59:161-187.

Rodriguez-Soriano J. Renal tubular acidosis: the clinical entity. *J Am Soc Nephrol.* 2002;13:2160-2170.

Rose BD. Renal tubular acidosis. In: Rose BD, ed. *Clinical physiology of acid-base and electrolyte disorders.* 5th ed. New York: McGraw Hill; 2001.

31

Electrolyte Disorders

C. JOHN SPERATI, MD, MHS

The maintenance of proper electrolyte concentrations is crucial to normal organ function and regulation of body volume. Alterations in the balance between electrolyte and water content may change electrolyte concentrations, osmolality, body volume status, and cellular function.

Osmolality and Tonicity

- Osmolality: Concentration of particles (osmoles, Osm) dissolved in 1 kg of solution
- Tonicity: Concentration of *effective* osmoles
- Only *effective* osmoles (substances that do not freely cross cell membranes) induce a water shift
  - Predominant effective osmole: sodium
  - Ineffective osmole (does not induce fluid shift): urea, glucose
    - Glucose may become an effective osmole and contribute to tonicity during states of insulin deficiency (e.g., diabetic ketoacidosis)
- Water moves between body compartments along tonicity gradients from an area of lower tonicity to an area of higher tonicity
- The body attempts to regulate osmolality (and hence tonicity) *primarily* via retention or excretion of water, not osmoles (i.e., sodium, Na$^+$)

Sodium and Water Balance

Sodium

- As the major extracellular cation, Na$^+$ is the predominant solute contributing to osmolality and tonicity
  - Na$^+$ is actively pumped from the intracellular to the extracellular space
  - Na$^+$ leaves the body primarily through urinary excretion, which is tightly regulated
- Osmolality may be estimated using the following equation: Osmolality = [2 × serum Na$^+$] + [blood urea nitrogen (mg/dL)/2.8] + [glucose (mg/dL)/18]
- Tonicity (effective osmolality) may be estimated under most conditions as 2 × serum Na$^+$
- Osmolar gap greater than 10 mOsm/kg consistent with presence of unmeasured osmoles
  - Defined as: (measured osmolality) − (estimated osmolality)
  - Consider organic acid ingestion such as ethylene glycol and methanol

Aldosterone

- Mineralocorticoid produced in the zona glomerulosa of the adrenal glands
- **Major actions are to stimulate Na$^+$ reabsorption and potassium (K$^+$) secretion in the renal collecting tubule. Hydrogen (H$^+$) secretion is increased because of the electronegative lumen generated by Na$^+$ reabsorption.**
- Aldosterone release is stimulated by:
  - Hyperkalemia
  - Angiotensin II
- The renin-angiotensin-aldosterone axis modulates Na$^+$ retention and excretion to regulate total body volume (and hence blood pressure)

Water

- Total body water (TBW) represents 60% of body weight in men and 50% in women
  - TBW is distributed:
    - Intracellular ⅔
    - Extracellular ⅔
    - Interstitial ¾ of extracellular
    - Intravascular ¼ of extracellular
- Water losses occur via the kidney, gastrointestinal tract (GI) tract, skin, and respiratory tract
  - Renal water excretion is tightly regulated via concentration or dilution of urine
  - 500 to 1000 mL/day lost through skin and respiratory tract (referred to as *insensible losses*)
- Thirst is an essential mechanism for preventing and correcting a water deficit
  - Stimulated by hypovolemia and an elevated serum osmolality

Antidiuretic Hormone (Vasopressin)

- **Antidiuretic hormone (ADH) is the principal hormone regulating osmolality**
  - ADH increases water reabsorption from the collecting duct lumen back into the circulation
  - ADH present: concentrated urine, smaller urine volume
  - ADH absent: dilute urine, larger urine volume
- ADH release from the posterior pituitary is stimulated by:
  - Increases in plasma osmolality as small as 1%
  - Pain; nausea; medications such as antidepressants, antipsychotics, nonsteroidal antiinflammatory drugs, opiates/opioids, and barbiturates

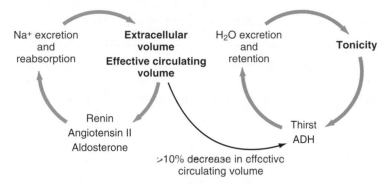

FIGURE 32-1 Regulation of body fluid compartments and osmolality. The renin-angiotensin-aldosterone pathway regulates body volume, although antidiuretic hormone (ADH) regulates osmolality via excretion/retention of water. A greater than 10% decrease in effective circulating volume will stimulate a nonosmotic release of ADH.

- Greater than or equal to 10% decrease in effective circulating volume
- See Fig. 32-1

HYPONATREMIA

Basic Information

- Serum Na^+ concentration less than 135 mEq/L
- Most common electrolyte disturbance in hospitalized patients
- **Can occur with low, normal, or high total body Na^+**
  - **Hyponatremia requires the presence of too much water relative to the quantity of total body Na^+**

Clinical Presentation

- Not all hyponatremia is symptomatic (see later information on iso-osmolar hyponatremia)
- Signs and symptoms of **hypoosmolar hyponatremia** are caused by swelling of the central nervous system (CNS)
  - As plasma tonicity falls, water shifts intracellularly until a tonicity gradient no longer exists
- Signs and symptoms of **hyperosmolar hyponatremia** are caused by dehydration of the CNS
  - As plasma tonicity rises, water shifts extracellularly
- Signs and symptoms: See Table 32-1

Diagnosis and Evaluation

- Fig. 32-2 shows an algorithm for the differential diagnosis of hyponatremia
- Determine osmolality:
  - Normal (280 to 295 mOsm/kg)
    - Pseudohyponatremia: Hyperlipidemia and hyperproteinemia can cause an artifactual decrease in measured serum Na^+ when using an indirect ion-selective electrode. The true serum Na^+ concentration is normal when measured by a direct ion-selective electrode.
    - Iso-osmolar infusions of mannitol, sorbitol, glycine, etc. that do not contain Na^+ result in dilutional hyponatremia without change in tonicity
    - Asymptomatic; exclude before pursuing evaluation of hyponatremia
  - High (greater than 295 mOsm/kg)

TABLE 32-1	Signs and Symptoms of Hyponatremia	
Mild [Na+] 125 to 135 mEq/L	**Moderate [Na+] 120 to 125 mEq/L**	**Severe [Na+] <120 mEq/L**
Anorexia Apathy Restlessness Nausea Lethargy Muscle cramps	Agitation Disorientation Headache	Seizures Coma Areflexia Cheyne-Stokes respirations Incontinence Death

- Osmotically active particles pull water into the extracellular space, creating a dilutional hyponatremia
- At risk for cerebral dehydration
  - Examples: glucose (diabetic ketoacidosis), hyperosmolar infusions of mannitol, maltose, or sorbitol
  - For every 100-mg/dL increase in glucose above 100, serum Na^+ decreases approximately 1.6 to 2.4 mEq/L
- Low (less than 280 mOsm/kg)
  - Characteristic of most cases of hyponatremia
  - At risk for cerebral edema
- Determine volume status
  - Findings suggestive of hypovolemia
    - Hypotension, tachycardia, dry mucous membranes, skin tenting, absence of edema
  - Findings suggestive of hypervolemia
    - Edema, elevated jugular venous pressure, crackles, S_3 heart sound, pulmonary edema on chest x-ray
  - Evaluate urine indices, if necessary
    - Can be seen in hypovolemia or hypervolemia (congestive heart failure, cirrhosis)
      - Urine Na^+ less than 10 mEq/L
      - Fractional excretion of sodium (FE_{Na}) less than 1%: [(urine Na^+ × serum creatinine)/(serum Na^+ × urine creatinine)] × 100
      - Urine osmolality greater than serum osmolality
    - Suggestive of euvolemia or recent diuretic use
      - Urine Na^+ greater than 20 mEq/L

32

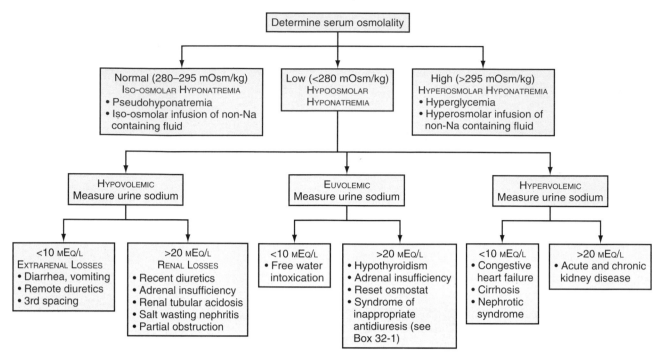

FIGURE 32-2 Differential diagnosis of hyponatremia.

- Special consideration: syndrome of inappropriate antidiuresis (SIAD)
  - Must exclude known stimuli of ADH release before labeling *idiopathic*
  - Must be clinically euvolemic
  - Urine sodium greater than 20 mEq/L
  - Urine osmolality greater than serum osmolality
  - Causes of SIAD are listed in Box 32-1 (medications, pulmonary disease, and CNS disease are major causes)

Treatment

- Treat underlying cause
  - Hypovolemic hypoosmolar: isotonic saline
  - Hypervolemic hypoosmolar: fluid restriction, diuresis, dialysis
  - Euvolemic hypoosmolar: Fluid restriction; consider use of V_2 receptor antagonists; address any contributing medical condition
- V_2 receptor antagonists (referred to as *vaptans*)
  - Block the V_2 ADH receptor in collecting duct
  - Only for use in euvolemic (SIAD) and potentially hypervolemic disorders
  - Results in aquaresis without significant natriuresis
  - Hyponatremia will recur with discontinuation of drug if underlying cause not addressed
  - Must be initiated or reinitiated in a hospitalized setting. Therapy should be limited to no more than 30 days because of risk of hepatotoxicity
  - Patients should not be fluid-restricted while receiving a V_2 receptor antagonist
  - Demeclocycline is an older therapy to antagonize ADH action that is rarely used
- Severe CNS symptoms (e.g., seizure, obtundation)
  - Raise Na^+ concentration with 3% saline until symptoms abate

BOX 32-1	*Causes of Syndrome of Inappropriate Antidiuresis*

Idiopathic
Pulmonary disease
Ectopic ADH production (e.g., small cell carcinoma of lung)
Infections: meningitis, encephalitis, abscess, VZV
Vascular: subarachnoid hemorrhage, CVA, temporal arteritis
Severe nausea/vomiting
Drugs
  Ecstasy ingestion (aggravated by copious fluid intake), SSRIs, SNRIs, narcotics, NSAIDs, desmopressin, oxytocin, cyclophosphamide, chlorpropamide, tricyclic antidepressants, antipsychotics
HIV
Prolactinoma
Waldenström macroglobulinemia
Shy-Drager syndrome
Delirium tremens
Exercise-induced (e.g., marathon runner)

ADH, Antidiuretic hormone; CVA, cerebrovascular accident; HIV, human immunodeficiency virus; NSAIDs, nonsteroidal antiinflammatory drugs; SNRIs, serotonin-norepinephrine reuptake inhibitors; SSRIs, selective serotonin reuptake inhibitors; VZV, varicella-zoster virus.

  - 4 to 6 mmol/L increase in Na^+ concentration should suffice
  - 100-mL bolus of 3% saline infused over 10 minutes. Can be repeated twice if necessary.
- Mild to moderate CNS symptoms
  - Raise Na^+ concentration with 3% saline at 1 mL/kg/hr
- Rate of correction is usually proportional to rate at which hyponatremia developed

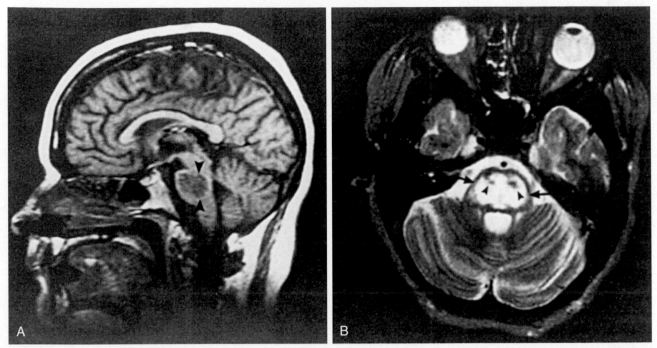

FIGURE 32-3   Central pontine myelinolysis (**A**, *arrowheads*) indicate low signal intensity on T1-weighted imaging. **B**, *Arrows* indicate high signal intensity on T2-weighted imaging; *arrowheads* demonstrate normal corticospinal tracts in a patient who presents with serum Na^+ 99 mEq/L corrected to 125 mEq/L in 24 hours. (From Goetz CG. *Textbook of clinical neurology.* 2nd ed. Philadelphia; Saunders: 2003; and Hart BL, Eaton RP. Images in clinical medicine—osmotic myelinolysis. *N Engl J Med.* 1995;333:1259.)

- Chronic hyponatremia (longer than 24 to 48 hours): Raise Na^+ concentration 0.5 to 1 mEq/L/hr and no more than 10 to 12 mEq/L in 24 hours and 18 mEq/L in 48 hours
  - Limit correction to less than 8 mEq/L in 24 hours if at high risk for osmotic demyelination syndrome
- Acute hyponatremia (less than 24 to 36 hours): Can raise 1 to 2 mEq/L/hr usually without the need for 3% saline unless severe CNS symptoms are present
- Rapid correction can result in cerebral dehydration and irreversible osmotic demyelination of the CNS (i.e., central pontine myelinolysis; Fig. 32-3). Malnourished, alcoholic, and cirrhotic patients may be at particular risk.
- Effect of 1 L of infused solution on Na^+ concentration can be estimated by $\Delta Na^+ = (Na^+_{infusate} - Na^+_{serum}) / (TBW + 1)$, where TBW = weight (kg) × 0.6 (if male), 0.5 (if female)

HYPERNATREMIA

Overview

- Serum Na^+ concentration greater than 145 mEq/L
- **Thirst is the major defense against the development of hypernatremia**
  - Usually requires impaired access to water
  - If free access to water is present, consider impaired thirst mechanism
- Most cases occur in hospitalized patients
- Classic outpatient presentation: elderly nursing home resident with underlying infection

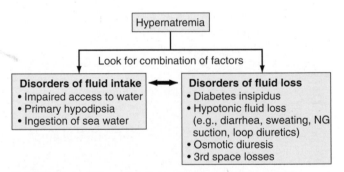

FIGURE 32-4   Differential diagnosis of hypernatremia. NG, Nasogastric.

Clinical Presentation

- Signs and symptoms are because of dehydration of the CNS
- Unlike hyponatremia, hypernatremia exhibits both increased osmolality and increased tonicity
- As serum osmolality/tonicity rises, water moves from inside cells of the CNS into the extracellular space along the osmolal gradient
- **Patients may experience restlessness, irritability, lethargy, muscle twitching, hyperreflexia, spasticity, and, in severe cases, intracranial hemorrhage**

Diagnosis and Evaluation

- Differential diagnosis of hypernatremia is shown in Fig. 32-4

32

- Special consideration: diabetes insipidus (DI)
    - Insufficient ADH action leads to polyuria and electrolyte-free water loss
        - Central: lack of pituitary ADH production
        - Nephrogenic: renal resistance to ADH action
    - High-normal to high serum Na^+ concentration with low urine osmolality (less than 300 mOsm/kg)
    - Differential diagnosis: Rule out polyuria because of:
        - Primary polydipsia
        - Diuretics
        - Osmotic diuresis (e.g., hyperglycemia)
    - Major causes of DI include:
        - Central
            - Idiopathic, pituitary tumor or apoplexy, infiltrative disorders (e.g., sarcoidosis, histiocytosis X, granulomatosis with polyangiitis), anoxic injury
        - Nephrogenic
            - Lithium, demeclocycline, foscarnet, ifosfamide, hypercalcemia, hypokalemia, Sjögren syndrome
        - Pregnancy (placental production of vasopressinase)

Treatment

- Address underlying cause
- **Overly rapid correction can result in cerebral edema**
- If hypovolemic, first correct circulatory needs with isotonic saline
- To calculate free water deficit:
Free water deficit
$$= TBW \times [(\text{serum sodium concentration}/140) - 1]$$
- Decrease serum Na^+ concentration approximately 0.5 mEq/L/hr and no more than 12 mEq/L in 24 hours
- Diabetes insipidus
    - Desmopressin is useful for central etiologies
    - Thiazide diuretic and low-solute diet may decrease polyuria in nephrogenic DI
    - When using lithium, concomitant amiloride or triamterene can limit severity of DI

Potassium Disorders

POTASSIUM BALANCE

- K^+ is the major intracellular cation
    - Intracellular K^+ is maintained at a high concentration by the 3Na-2K-ATPase pump
    - 95% to 98% of total body K^+ is stored intracellularly
- 80% of K^+ excretion occurs via the kidney, with the remainder in the stool and sweat
    - Renal K^+ secretion increased by aldosterone
    - Increased Na^+ and water delivery to the distal nephron increases K^+ secretion
- Disorders of K^+ concentration occur via:
    - Gain or loss in total body K^+ stores
    - Shifts between intracellular and extracellular compartments
- Changes in the electrical potential of cellular membranes lead to the major signs and symptoms

HYPOKALEMIA
Basic Information

- Serum K^+ concentration less than 3.5 mEq/L
- May result from increased excretion, intracellular shifting, inadequate dietary intake, or lab artifact (spurious)
- In the absence of intracellular shifting, **hypokalemia implies low total body K+**
- Most commonly results when K^+ losses exceed intake
    - Rarely may result simply from inadequate daily intake

Clinical Presentation

- May result in fatigue progressing to muscle weakness and arrhythmia, followed by tetany or rhabdomyolysis at K^+ less than 2.5 mEq/L and then paralysis when less than 2 mEq/L
- Cardiac conduction is affected, resulting in T wave flattening, the development of U waves, and arrhythmias (e.g., atrial tachycardia, atrioventricular dissociation, ventricular tachycardia, and ventricular fibrillation; Fig. 32-5)
    - Risk of arrhythmia is increased in the presence of high concentrations of digoxin
- Hypokalemia may increase the risk of osmotic demyelination when correcting hyponatremia
    - **If neurologically stable, correct hypokalemia before correcting hyponatremia**

Diagnosis and Evaluation

- Differential diagnosis of hypokalemia is shown in Fig. 32-6 through 32-8
- Evaluate for spurious hypokalemia, intracellular shift, and inadequate intake
    - Spurious hypokalemia caused by increased uptake after venipuncture when leukocytosis greater than 100,000 cells/mm³ is present
    - Intracellular shift caused by insulin, β_2-receptor stimulation, or alkalosis
    - Classic example of intracellular shifting is hypokalemic periodic paralysis
        - Autosomal dominant inheritance: mutations in CACNA1S (Ca^{2+} channel) or SCN4A (Na^+ channel)

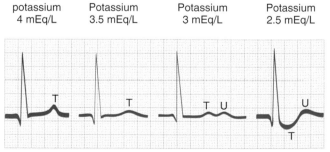

Normal potassium 4 mEq/L	Potassium 3.5 mEq/L	Potassium 3 mEq/L	Potassium 2.5 mEq/L

FIGURE 32-5 Electrocardiogram of patient with hypokalemia. Note flattening of T waves and prominent U waves. (From Goldberger AL. *Clinical electrocardiography: a simplified approach.* 6th ed. St. Louis; Mosby: 1998.)

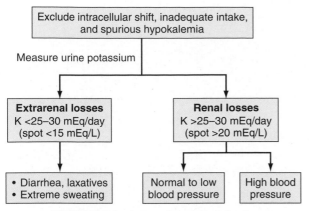

FIGURE 32-6 Approach to hypokalemia.

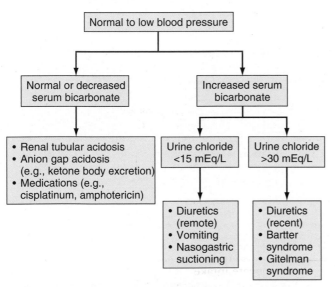

FIGURE 32-7 Renal K⁺ loss with normal to low blood pressure.

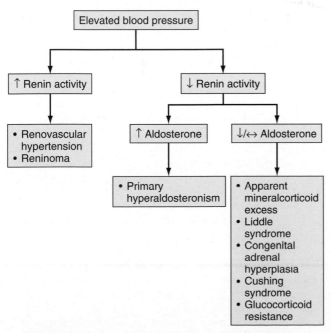

FIGURE 32-8 Renal K⁺ loss with elevated blood pressure.

- Onset in childhood to adolescence
- Attacks last for minutes to days and are of longer duration than in hyperkalemic periodic paralysis
- Acquired form may be seen in thyrotoxicosis, particularly in Asian males
- If hypokalemia results from increased potassium loss from the body, differentiate renal from extrarenal mechanism:
  - Renal K⁺ wasting
    - Consider in context of presence or absence of hypertension
    - Urine K⁺ excretion greater than 25 to 30 mEq/day or spot concentration greater than 15 to 20 mEq/L in the presence of normal urine output
    - Spot index requires urine osmolality greater than plasma osmolality
  - Extrarenal K+ wasting
    - Most commonly caused by diarrhea
    - Urine K+ excretion less than 25 to 30 mEq/day or spot concentration less than 15 mEq/L in the presence of normal urine output
    - Spot index requires urine osmolality greater than plasma osmolality

Treatment

- Investigate and treat underlying cause
- Nature of treatment determined by degree of hypokalemia and presence or absence of symptoms
- Patients at increased risk of arrhythmia (e.g., digoxin therapy, coronary artery disease) merit more aggressive treatment
- In patients with total body potassium depletion, serum K⁺ concentration of 3 mEq/L represents loss of approximately 200 to 300 mEq of K⁺
  - K⁺ concentration 3 to 3.5 mEq/L: Prevent further K⁺ loss and consider oral repletion
  - K⁺ concentration less than 3 mEq/L: Intravenous (IV) K⁺ repletion with cardiac monitoring should be considered
- **Hypomagnesemia and hypocalcemia may render correction of hypokalemia more difficult and should be addressed before K⁺ repletion**
- In patients with impaired renal function, IV K⁺ repletion can lead to unpredictable serum concentrations and should be used with caution

HYPERKALEMIA

Basic Information

- Serum K⁺ concentration greater than 5.5 mEq/L
- May result from decreased excretion, extracellular shifting, excessive dietary intake, or lab artifact (spurious)
- Rarely caused by excess intake alone, as normally functioning kidneys have a substantial excretory capacity

Clinical Presentation

- Mild elevations (5.5 to 6 mEq/L): Usually asymptomatic
- Greater than 6.5 mEq/L: Progressive weakness, muscle aches, areflexia, paresthesias, electrocardiogram (ECG) changes

32

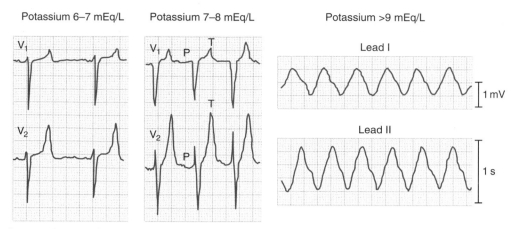

FIGURE 32-9 Electrocardiogram changes in hyperkalemia. The first panel demonstrates peaked T waves, which worsen as the P waves begin to disappear in the second panel. A sine wave configuration is shown in panel 3, as seen in a patient with severe hyperkalemia. (From Goldberger AL. *Clinical electrocardiography: a simplified approach.* 6th ed. St. Louis; Mosby: 1998.)

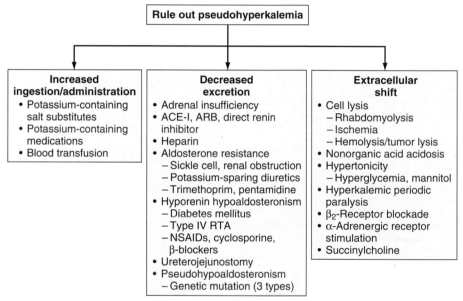

FIGURE 32-10 Differential diagnosis of hyperkalemia. ACE-I, Angiotensin-converting enzyme inhibitor; ARB, angiotensin receptor blocker; NSAIDs, nonsteroidal antiinflammatory drugs; RTA, renal tubular acidosis.

- Greater than 7 mEq/L: Paralysis, respiratory failure, life-threatening arrhythmias
- ECG changes are **not** a sensitive marker for presence or severity of hyperkalemia (Fig. 32-9)
  - 6 to 7 mEq/L: peaked T waves (sharply tented, height greater than 10 mm, best seen in V2-V4)
  - 7 to 8 mEq/L: widening of QRS complex, prolonged PR interval with flattening of P wave
  - Greater than 8 mEq/L: atrial standstill, progressive QRS widening and fusion with T wave to form sine wave pattern, ventricular tachycardia and fibrillation

Diagnosis and Evaluation

- Differential diagnosis of hyperkalemia is shown in Fig. 32-10
- Evaluate for pseudohyperkalemia and extracellular shift
  - Pseudohyperkalemia may occur with:
    - Hemolysis during venipuncture
    - Prolonged application of tourniquet or fist-clenching

- Leukocytosis greater than 100,000 cells/mm^3 or thrombocytosis greater than 500,000 cells/mm^3
  - Plasma K$^+$ should be at least 0.4 mEq/L lower than serum
- Familial pseudohyperkalemia (autosomal dominant)
  - K$^+$ efflux occurs as blood cools. K$^+$ concentration normalizes with rewarming of blood sample
- Numerous etiologies of extracellular K$^+$ shift (Fig. 32-10)
  - Mineral acidosis (e.g., HCl) may result in hyperkalemia while an organic acidosis (e.g., lactic acidosis) does not
  - Classic example of extracellular shifting is hyperkalemic periodic paralysis
    - Autosomal dominant inheritance: mutation in SCN4A Na$^+$ channel
    - Onset early in life
    - Attacks more frequent and of shorter duration than with hypokalemic periodic paralysis

- Respiratory and bulbar involvement is rare
- Evaluate for mechanisms of impaired renal excretion
  - Transtubular potassium gradient (TTKG): TTKG = (urine K/serum K) / (urine Osm/serum Osm)
    - Value less than 5 suggests hypoaldosteronism or K^+ secretory defect
      - Urine Na^+ must be greater than 25 mEq/L
      - Urine osmolality must be greater than serum osmolality
    - Poorly validated in routine evaluation of hyperkalemia, and its clinical use is no longer recommended
    - May be most useful when measured before and after fludrocortisone administration to evaluate for mineralocorticoid resistance
  - Hyperkalemia associated with hypertension and metabolic acidosis characterizes pseudohypoaldosteronism type II (Gordon syndrome)

Treatment

- For K^+ greater than 6.5 mEq/L or in the presence of ECG changes, administer IV calcium to decrease myocardial excitability
- **Decrease intake of K^+**
  - Examine medications and dietary factors high in K^+
  - Avoid medications that inhibit K^+ secretion
- Shift K^+ intracellularly
  - Correct hyperglycemia, if present
  - 10 U of regular insulin administered IV with an ampule of 50% dextrose in water ($D_{50}W$) to prevent hypoglycemia
  - IV bicarbonate has little acute effect in the management of hyperkalemia
- Increase K^+ elimination from the body
  - Oral or rectal administration of a K^+ exchange resin, sodium polystyrene sulfonate (SPS). One gram binds approximately 1 mEq K^+ in vivo.
    - SPS is ineffective in patients with prior colectomy
    - SPS that contains sorbitol is associated with intestinal necrosis
      - Avoid if impaired intestinal motility or reduced mesenteric perfusion
  - Loop diuretics may be of utility in a stable patient with mild hyperkalemia
  - Dialysis if severe and life-threatening

Magnesium Disorders

MAGNESIUM (MG²⁺) BALANCE

- 50% to 60% of total body Mg^{2+} is complexed in bone
- 40% to 50% is stored intracellularly with a very small fraction (<1%) present in the extracellular fluid
- The majority of Mg^{2+} reabsorption in the kidney occurs in the thick ascending limb of Henle
  - Parathyroid hormone increases Mg^{2+} reabsorption
  - Loop and thiazide diuretics decrease Mg^{2+} reabsorption
- Disorders of Mg^{2+} concentration occur primarily via gain or loss in total body Mg^{2+} stores

HYPOMAGNESEMIA

Basic Information

- Most commonly results from increased GI or renal loss
  - Present in over 10% of hospitalized patients
- May be exacerbated by inadequate oral intake
- Most common etiologies include loop and thiazide diuretics, diarrhea, proton pump inhibitor therapy, alcoholism/malnutrition, and diabetes mellitus
- Renders correction of hypokalemia and hypocalcemia more difficult

Clinical Presentation

- Mild reductions (greater than 1.3 mg/dL) are often asymptomatic
  - Diagnosis requires high index of suspicion to prompt laboratory testing
- Moderate to severe reductions (less than 1.2 mg/dL) are associated with:
  - Electrolyte abnormalities
    - Hypocalcemia
      - Decreased parathyroid hormone (PTH) secretion and increased bone resistance to PTH action
    - Hypokalemia
      - Both may result from diuretics and/or diarrhea
      - Intracellular Mg^{2+} deficiency stimulates renal potassium secretion
  - Cardiac conduction abnormalities
    - QRS widening and T wave peaking with moderate hypomagnesemia
    - PR prolongation, increasing QRS widening, and T wave flattening with severe depletion
    - Atrial and ventricular tachyarrhythmias, including atrial fibrillation and ventricular tachycardia/fibrillation
    - Potentiates digoxin toxicity
  - Neuromuscular compromise
    - Tetany, seizure, and choreiform movements
    - Vertical nystagmus
    - Respiratory weakness

Diagnosis and Evaluation

- Differential diagnosis of hypomagnesemia is shown in Box 32-2.
- Evaluate for renal versus GI losses
  - History is usually sufficient
  - Renal Mg^{2+} wasting
    - 24-hour urinary Mg^{2+} excretion greater than 10 mg
    - Fractional excretion of Mg^{2+} (FE_{Mg}) greater than 2%
      $FE_{Mg} = [(\text{urine } Mg^{2+} \times \text{serum creatinine})/(\text{serum } Mg^{2+} \times 0.7 \times \text{urine creatinine})] \times 100$
    - Most commonly associated with loop and thiazide diuretic use
    - May be seen with uncontrolled diabetes mellitus
    - Present in Gitelman syndrome and to a lesser extent in Bartter syndrome
  - GI Mg^{2+} wasting
    - 24-hour urinary Mg^{2+} excretion less than 10 mg
    - FE_{Mg} less than 2%

32

Causes of Hypomagnesemia

Renal Loss
Idiopathic
Drugs
    Loop diuretics
    Aminoglycosides
    Amphotericin B
    Foscarnet
    Cyclosporine A, tacrolimus
    Cisplatin
    Epidermal growth factor (EGF) receptor antibodies
        (cetuximab, panitumumab, matuzumab)
Polyuria
Diabetes mellitus
Acute ethanol intoxication
Hypercalcemia
Hyperaldosteronism
Tubulointerstitial disease (e.g., sickle nephropathy)
Genetic
    Gitelman syndrome
    ± Bartter syndrome
    Familial hypomagnesemia with hypercalciuria and
        nephrocalcinosis
    Mutations in parcellin-1, EGF, and others

GI Loss
Diarrhea
Chronic malabsorption (e.g., short-bowel syndrome,
    chronic pancreatitis)
Proton pump inhibitors
Genetic
    Primary intestinal hypomagnesemia

Miscellaneous
Postparathyroidectomy ("hungry bone")
Citrate chelation following blood transfusion
Acute pancreatitis
Treatment of diabetic ketoacidosis

- Associated with proton pump inhibitor use and
  diarrheal states
- Normomagnesemic magnesium deficiency (intracellular
  deficiency) should be considered in refractory
  hypokalemia or hypocalcemia

Treatment

- Investigate and treat underlying cause
  - Potassium-sparing diuretics (e.g., amiloride,
    triamterene, spironolactone, eplerenone) will
    decrease renal Mg^{2+} excretion

- Continuous cardiac monitoring for symptomatic
  patients or severe hypomagnesemia
- Mild or asymptomatic hypomagnesemia
  - 240 to 1000 mg (20 to 80 mEq) of elemental
    magnesium in divided oral doses
    - Immediate-release preparation
      - Magnesium oxide 400 to 800 mg (20 to
        40 mEq)
        - Diarrhea is common at higher doses
    - Sustained-release preparation
      - Magnesium chloride 2 to 4 tablets
        (approximately 11 to 21 mEq)
      - Magnesium lactate 2 to 4 tablets (14 to 28 mEq)
      - Less diarrhea and better absorption with
        sustained release
- Symptomatic, severe hypomagnesemia, or inability to
  tolerate oral intake
  - IV administration
  - Use **extreme caution** in patients with reduced renal
    function
    - Use smaller doses and frequent reassessment of
      Mg^{2+} concentration
  - 50% of an IV dose may be excreted by the kidneys
    - Smaller, repeated doses are more efficacious

Review Questions

For review questions, please go to ExpertConsult.com.

SUGGESTED READINGS

Agus ZS. Hypomagnesemia. *J Am Soc Nephrol.* 1999;10:1616-1622.
Androgue HJ, Madias NE. Hypernatremia. *N Engl J Med.*
    2000;342:1493-1499.
Androgue HJ, Madias NE. Hyponatremia. *N Engl J Med.*
    2000;342:1581-1589.
Ellison DH, Berl T. The syndrome of inappropriate antidiuresis. *N Engl J
    Med.* 2007;356:2064-2072.
Mandal AK. Hypokalemia and hyperkalemia. *Med Clin North Am.*
    1997;81:611-639.
Nyirenda MJ, Tang JI, Padfield PL, et al. Hyperkalemia. *BMJ.*
    2009;339:1019-1024.
Unwin RJ, Luft FC, Shirley DG. Pathophysiology and management of
    hypokalemia: a clinical perspective. *Nat Rev Nephrol.* 2011;7:75-84.
Verbalis JG, Goldsmith SR, Greenberg A, et al. Diagnosis, evaluation,
    and treatment of hyponatremia: expert panel recommendations. *Am J
    Med.* 2013;126:s1-s42.

Acute Kidney Injury

ADAM R. BERLINER, MD

Acute kidney injury (AKI) (formerly called acute renal failure) may result from a wide array of renal insults in both hospitalized patients and outpatients. A systematic approach that includes a detailed history, focused physical examination, and supporting laboratory or radiologic evaluation is needed to determine the diagnosis. Supportive care, specifically dialysis, may be needed until renal function returns.

Basic Information

- Definition: AKI is deterioration in renal function over a period of hours to days with subsequent inability to clear water, electrolytes, and nitrogenous wastes, and dysregulation of normal acid-base status
- AKI may be oliguric (urine volume <400 to 500 mL/day) or nonoliguric (>400 to 500 mL/day)
- An increase in the level of serum creatinine is the hallmark for diagnosis of AKI, although a single standardized definition of AKI does not exist
  - Commonly used criteria to diagnose AKI include:
    - Greater than 0.3 mg/dL rise in serum creatinine from baseline over 48 hours or a rise of 50% or more in 1 week
    - Urine output less than 0.5 mL/kg/h for 6 hours
- Published RIFLE (Risk, Injury, Failure, Loss, End-stage renal disease) and AKIN (Acute Kidney Injury Network) criteria for defining AKI are more useful for clinical and/or epidemiologic study of AKI rather than for use in clinical care settings
- Categories of AKI (Fig. 33-1)
  - Prerenal: Reduction in effective circulating volume and renal perfusion, or renal artery occlusion (especially bilateral)
  - Intrarenal: Glomerular, tubular, interstitial, or vascular
  - Postrenal: Obstruction of urinary tract or renal veins (especially bilateral)
- General approach to the evaluation of the patient with AKI (see Fig. 33-2)
- General principles for treatment of AKI
  - **Correct any reversible causes**
    - Assess potassium, acid-base status, fluid status, toxin accumulation, and need for dialysis (Table 33-1)
  - **Adjust dosage of renally metabolized/excreted medications and discontinue all potentially nephrotoxic drugs**
    - Avoid angiotensin-converting enzyme (ACE) inhibitors, angiotensin receptor blockers (ARBs), direct renin inhibitors, nonsteroidal antiinflammatory drugs (NSAIDs), aminoglycoside antibiotics,

intravenous iodinated contrast, and intravenous gadolinium
    - Fluid challenge if clinically appropriate

Prerenal Causes of Acute Kidney Injury

Basic Information

- AKI that is caused by reduction of effective circulating volume or decreased renal blood flow
- **Prerenal causes are an extremely common cause (along with acute tubular necrosis) of AKI in the hospital setting**
- Patients can present with severe oliguric renal failure
- Once the effective circulating volume has been restored, renal recovery is the general rule

Clinical Presentation

- **True volume depletion**
  - Prolonged lack of oral fluid intake
  - Gastrointestinal (GI) fluid loss: bleeding, vomiting, diarrhea
  - Urinary fluid loss: diuretics, hyperglycemia (osmotic diuresis), salt-wasting nephropathy, diabetes insipidus
  - Skin loss: fever, diaphoresis, burns
- **Reduction in effective circulating volume or renal perfusion**
  - Congestive heart failure (cardiorenal syndrome)
  - Cirrhosis
  - Nephrotic syndrome
  - Septic or cardiogenic shock
  - Renal artery stenosis, particularly bilateral
- **Hepatorenal syndrome: A poorly understood, relentless worsening of renal function in the patient with advanced liver disease, with no other apparent cause (a diagnosis of exclusion)**
  - Pathophysiology includes dilation of the splanchnic bed vasculature, resulting in a fall in systemic vascular resistance and blood pressure. Reduced renal perfusion occurs via renal arteriolar vasoconstriction in the setting of renin-angiotensin-aldosterone system, sympathetic nervous system, and endothelin stimulation.
- **Medications**
  - Diuretics: volume depletion
  - ACE inhibitor/ARB/direct renin inhibito: Decrease the formation of angiotensin II or block the effects of angiotensin II, thus resulting in efferent arteriolar

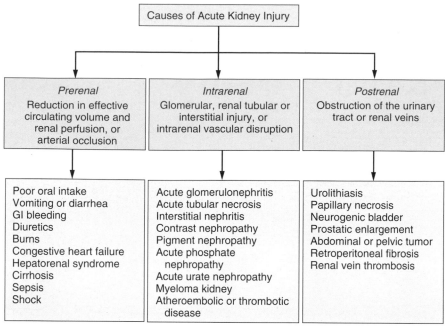

FIGURE 33-1 Differential diagnosis of acute kidney injury. GI, Gastrointestinal.

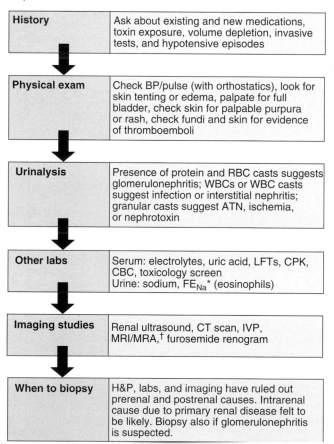

FIGURE 33-2 Initial evaluation of the patient with acute kidney injury. *$FE_{Na} = U_{Na}/P_{Na} \times P_{Cr}/U_{Cr} \times 100\%$. †Gadolinium contraindicated in moderate to severe renal failure because of risk of nephrogenic systemic fibrosis. ATN, Acute tubular necrosis; BP, blood pressure; CBC, complete blood count; CPK, creatine phosphokinase; CT, computed tomography; FE_{Na}, fractional excretion of sodium; H&P, history and physical examination; IVP, intravenous pyelogram; LFTs, liver function tests; MRI/MRA, magnetic resonance imaging/magnetic resonance angiography; RBC, red blood cell; U_{Cr}, urine creatinine; U_{Na}, urine sodium; WBC, white blood cell.

vasodilation and reduced intraglomerular pressure with reduced glomerular filtration rate (GFR)
- NSAIDs: Inhibit the production of vasodilatory prostaglandins, resulting in afferent arteriolar vasoconstriction and reduced GFR
- Calcineurin inhibitors (tacrolimus, cyclosporine): Cause renal artery vasoconstriction, resulting in reduced GFR

Diagnosis

- **Clinical history and physical examination can usually suggest prerenal AKI**
- **BUN/Cr ratio often greater than 20:1** because of increased water and urea reabsorption
- Low urine sodium concentration **(usually less than 20 mEq/L)**
- **Low urine fractional excretion of sodium (FE_{Na} less than 1%; Table 33-2)**
- Urine osmolality greater than 500 mOsm/kg
- Urine Cr/Plasma Cr ratio greater than 40

Treatment

- Volume depletion: **Vigorous intravenous (IV) fluid resuscitation typically improves renal function and urine output within 24 to 48 hours**
- Reduced effective circulating volume: Treat the underlying disease process; **maximize cardiac output**
- **Hepatorenal syndrome is best treated by liver transplantation.** Dialysis may be needed in the interim
  - Midodrine (systemic vasoconstrictor) and octreotide (blocks vasodilator release) may be of some benefit

Intrarenal Causes of Acute Kidney Injury

- Table 33-3 lists intrarenal causes of AKI
- Acute glomerulonephritis and vasculitis are covered in Chapter 34

TABLE 33-1	*Indications for Dialysis*
Indication	**Clinical Scenarios**
Severe metabolic acidosis	AKI; toxic ingestion of aspirin, ethanol, methanol, ethylene/propylene glycol
Electrolyte disturbances	Usually severe hyperkalemia; also severe hypercalcemia/hypermagnesemia
Intoxications	Toxic effects of lithium, isopropyl alcohol
Volume overload	Refractory congestive heart failure/pulmonary edema Anasarca
Uremia	Pericarditis; stupor; seizures; asterixis; platelet dysfunction

AKI, Acute kidney injury.

TABLE 33-2	*Use of Fractional Excretion of Sodium in Acute Kidney Injury*	
AKI		**Fe$_{Na}$* (%)**
Prerenal causes of AKI because of hypovolemia		<1
Prerenal causes of AKI because of decreased effective circulating volume		<1
Acute tubular necrosis, from any cause		>2
Hepatorenal syndrome		<1
Caveat: Fe$_{Na}$ can be >1% with prerenal AKI in patients with preexisting chronic kidney disease because of impaired ability to reabsorb sodium. Can be <1% with glomerulonephritis, iodinated intravenous contrast administration, and rhabdomyolysis		

*Fe$_{Na}$ = U$_{Na}$/P$_{Na}$ × P$_{Cr}$/U$_{Cr}$ × 100%.
AKI, Acute kidney injury; Fe$_{Na}$, fractional excretion of sodium; P$_{Cr}$, plasma creatinine; P$_{Na}$, plasma sodium; U$_{Cr}$, urine creatinine; U$_{Na}$, urine sodium.

TABLE 33-3	*Intrarenal Causes of Acute Kidney Injury*	
Disorder	**Suggestive Features**	**Treatment**
Acute glomerulonephritis	Hypertension; fluid retention; hematuria; proteinuria	Differs based on underlying cause of glomerulonephritis
Acute tubular necrosis	Recent hypotensive event or surgery; recent exposure to nephrotoxin	Supportive care until renal function returns
Contrast nephropathy	Appropriate clinical setting, such as recent (<48 h) intravascular iodinated contrast exposure	Prevention; supportive measures until recovery of renal function
Interstitial nephritis	New medication addition; Fever; skin rash; WBC casts in urine; eosinophilia and eosinophiluria	Discontinue offending drug; corticosteroids
Pigment nephropathy	High serum CPK (typically >10,000 IU/L); pigmented casts, hemoglobinuria, but no RBCs in urine	IV hydration; alkalinize urine to pH >6.5
Acute phosphate nephropathy	Recent administration of oral phosphorus containing laxative or enema	Supportive measures
Acute Urate Nephropathy	Tumor lysis syndrome, serum uric acid >12 to 15 mg/dL, concurrent hyperkalemia and hyperphosphatemia	IV hydration with sodium chloride, uric acid lowering, supportive dialysis
Myeloma cast nephropathy	Known myeloma with heavy Bence-Jones proteinuria	IV hydration, urine alkalinization, chemotherapy
Renal artery atheroembolic disease	Recent (days to weeks) cardiac/aortic surgery or angiography; low serum complement; eosinophilia; eosinophiluria; cholesterol crystals on renal or skin biopsy	Supportive measures, but prognosis poor
Renal artery thromboembolic disease	Flank pain, hematuria; atrial fibrillation/flutter or severe LV dysfunction	Supportive measures, anticoagulation
Thrombotic microangiopathy (TTP, HUS, DIC)	Microangiopathic hemolytic anemia, elevated LDH, decreased haptoglobin, thrombocytopenia, AKI, hematuria	Supportive measures, plasmapheresis for TTP, consideration of plasmapheresis and/or complement inhibition for HUS depending on etiology

AKI, Acute kidney injury; CPK, creatine phosphokinase; DIC, disseminated intravascular coagulation; IV, intravenous; HUS, hemolytic-uremic syndrome; LDH, lactate dehydrogenase; LV, left ventricular; RBC, red blood cell; TTP, thrombotic thrombocytopenic purpura; WBC, white blood cell.

33

Acute Tubular Injury (See Fig. 33-3 and Table 33-4)

Basic Information

- **An extremely common cause of AKI in the hospital setting (along with prerenal AKI)**
- Results from ischemic or toxic injury to renal tubules
- Damaged tubular cells accumulate in tubular lumen resulting in occlusion, in addition to reactive arteriolar vasoconstriction
- Injury commonly most severe in early proximal tubule and medullary tubular segments

Clinical Presentation

- Appropriate clinical setting, such as ischemic event or exposure to nephrotoxin, precedes deterioration in renal function

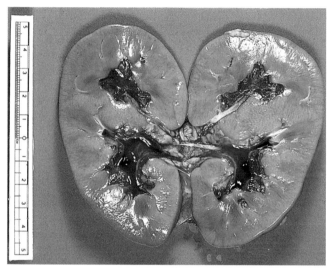

FIGURE 33-3 Acute tubular necrosis. In acute tubular necrosis, kidneys are swollen and pale, particularly in the renal cortex. (From Stevens A, Lowe J: *Pathology.* 2nd ed. St. Louis: Mosby; 2000, Fig. 17.23.)

TABLE 33-4	*Common Drug-Induced Causes of Acute Tubular Injury*
Antimicrobials	Aminoglycosides, fluoroquinolones, vancomycin, colisthemate, acyclovir, tenofovir, amphoterecin B
Radiocontrast	Intravascular iodinated radiocontrast
Hemodynamic injury	NSAIDs, ACE inhibitors, ARBs, calcineurin inhibitors
Chemotherapeutic agents	Cisplatinum, ifosfamide, cyclophosphamide
Hyperosmolar agents	IVIg, hetastarch
Miscellaneous	Cocaine, synthetic cannabinoids, aristolochic acid, lead

ARBs, Angiotensin II receptor blockers; IVIg, intravenous immunoglobulin; NSAIDs, nonsteroidal antiinflammatory drugs.

- **Clinical course (Fig. 33-4): Typically worsens, then usually resolves over 1 to 3 weeks**

Diagnosis

- **BUN/Cr ratio is normal,** usually less than 20 : 1
- Urinalysis shows **muddy brown granular casts and epithelial cell casts**
- **High urine sodium concentration (usually >40 mEq/L)** is caused by tubular injury and decreased sodium reabsorption
- High urine fractional excretion of sodium (**FE_{Na} >2%; see Table 33-2**)
- Urine osmolality less than 350 to 450 mOsm/kg
- **Urine Cr/Plasma Cr ratio less than 20 : 1** (measure of tubular water reabsorption)

Treatment

- **Supportive care** until renal function returns. May require dialysis.
- Loop diuretics do not alter the course or prognosis of renal failure
- Avoid nephrotoxins and minimize fluid overload

Interstitial Nephritis (Table 33-5)

Basic Information

- Results from the infiltration of the interstitial space by inflammatory cells (Fig. 33-5)
- Process usually initiated by **allergic reaction to medication**
- Diagnosis requires a high index of suspicion, as classic findings of pyuria, rash, and eosinophilia may be absent
- β-Lactam antibiotics and cephalosporins are common
- NSAIDs are associated with:
  - Either pure interstitial disease or additional glomerular disease **(minimal change disease or membranous glomerulonephritis)**

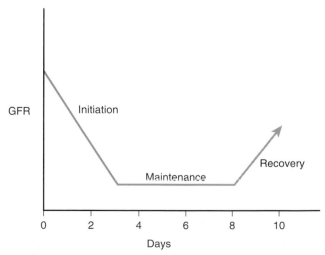

FIGURE 33-4 Time course of acute tubular injury. Fall in glomerular filtration rate (GFR) is often accompanied by a decline in urine output until GFR recovers. Renal replacement therapy may be required during this time.

TABLE 33-5	*Common Causes of Interstitial Nephritis*
Drugs	Antibiotics (β-lactams, fluoroquinolones, rifampin, sulfonamides, vancomycin, macrolides), proton pump inhibitors, NSAIDs, allopurinol, thiazide diuretics, HIV antiretrovirals, lithium
Infections	*Staph* or *Strep* spp., *Brucella*, HIV, CMV, hantavirus, TB, schistosoma, toxoplasma
Systemic disease	SLE, Sjögren syndrome, sarcoidosis, rheumatoid arthritis, tubulointerstitial nephritis with uveitis, IgG4-related systemic disease, atheroembolic disease, lymphoma/leukemia

CMV, Cytomegalovirus; HIV, human immunodeficiency virus; IgG4, immunoglobulin G4; NSAIDs, nonsteroidal antiinflammatory drugs; TB, tuberculosis; SLE, systemic lupus erythematosus.

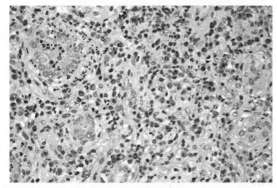

FIGURE 33-5 Drug-induced interstitial nephritis with prominent eosinophilic and mononuclear cell infiltrate. (From Kumar V, Fausto N, Abbas A. *Robbins and Cotran: pathologic basis of disease.* 7th ed. Philadelphia: Saunders: 2005, Fig. 20-44.)

- NSAIDs can also cause **acute ischemic renal injury (hemodynamic change), analgesic nephropathy, or papillary necrosis**
- **Urine sediment may not contain significant eosinophils and microscopic hematuria is common**
- **Proton-pump inhibitors** are an increasingly recognized cause of interstitial nephritis
- Common nondrug causes include infections and autoimmune diseases

Clinical Presentation

- Acute worsening of renal function after starting a new medication
- **Fever and skin rash are NOT common**

Diagnosis

- Diagnosis is often made based on clinical presentation
- Hematuria, pyuria, and urinary white blood cell casts may be present

- Mild proteinuria (usually less than 1.5 g/day)
- Eosinophilia and eosinophiluria are NOT sensitive for diagnosis and their absence does not exclude the diagnosis
- Gold standard for diagnosis is kidney biopsy

Treatment

- Discontinuation of suspected offending agent(s)
- Corticosteroids may be useful, particularly if started early

Contrast-Induced Nephropathy

Basic Information

- **Intravascular iodinated contrast agents cause renal arteriolar vasoconstriction (ischemic insult) and direct renal tubular toxicity**
- Individuals at greatest risk include those with:
  - Kidney disease with estimated glomerular filtration rate (eGFR) less than 60 mL/min
  - Diabetes mellitus
  - Poor renal perfusion: heart failure, dehydration, or liver failure
  - High doses of contrast agent and those receiving low- osmolar or high-osmolar contrast
- Magnetic resonance gadolinium contrast media in high concentrations may also be associated with nephrotoxicity
- Use of gadolinium in the setting of advanced renal failure and/or liver failure may result in nephrogenic systemic fibrosis

Clinical Presentation

- Acute rise of serum blood urea nitrogen and creatinine occurs within 24 to 48 hours of IV contrast exposure
- Creatinine **(Cr) peaks within 7 days and usually returns to baseline within 10 days**
- Renal failure is usually reversible unless baseline renal function is poor

Diagnosis

- Clinical diagnosis based on history of exposure in appropriate time period

Treatment

- No specific therapy; supportive measures only
- Maintain renal perfusion with IV hydration, but be wary of volume overload
- Avoid repeated contrast exposure
- **Best treatment is prevention**
  - **Minimize** IV contrast volume
  - Use **nonionic, isoosmolar contrast**
  - **IV hydration with isotonic fluid (either sodium chloride or sodium bicarbonate) before and after contrast administration** in high-risk patients
- N-Acetylcysteine (600 to 1200 mg orally twice daily on the day-before and day-of contrast exposure) has questionable efficacy but is still

widely used given lack of toxicity and potential benefit
- Statins may lower the risk of injury
- Postcontrast hemodialysis to remove contrast has no proven benefit

Pigment Nephropathy

Basic Information

- Acute renal tubular toxicity from heme pigment (ferrihemate) of myoglobin or hemoglobin
- Ferrihemate also cause renal arteriolar vasoconstriction → ischemia
- **Obstruction of renal tubules** by **myoglobin** casts (**hemoglobin** too large to be substantially filtered at glomerulus into tubules)

Clinical Presentation

- Patient often notes cola- or red-colored urine because of presence of myoglobin or hemoglobin
- Occurs **with rhabdomyolysis** (myoglobin) or **massive hemolysis** (hemoglobin)
    - Common causes of rhabdomyolysis:
        - Extreme exercises, trauma, seizures, ischemia
        - Skeletal muscle toxins (cocaine, heroin, statins),
        - Infections, electrolyte abnormalities (hypokalemia), inflammatory myopathies
- Release of intracellular electrolytes from muscle or red blood cells results in **hyperkalemia, hyperphosphatemia, and hyperuricemia**
- In rhabdomyolysis, sequestration of fluid and calcium into injured muscles leading to **volume depletion and hypocalcemia**

Diagnosis

- AKI associated with rhabdomyolysis; **renal injury often associated with creatine phosphokinase (CPK) greater than 5,000 to 10,000 IU/L**
- Hyperkalemia, hyperphosphatemia, and hypocalcemia also common and support the diagnosis
- Urinalysis reveals dipstick heme and pigmented casts (but no red blood cells), with myoglobin or hemoglobin in the urine

Treatment

- **IV hydration** is important to increase urine flow rate for rapid clearance of ferrihemate
- Though unproven, **urine alkalinization to pH above 6.5** may help prevent release of ferrihemate from myoglobin and decrease precipitation of myoglobin casts
- Recovery often occurs, but dialysis may be needed until renal function returns

Acute Phosphate Nephropathy and Acute Urate Nephropathy

Basic Information

- AKI caused by deposition of either calcium-phosphate (PN) or uric acid crystals (UN) in the renal tubules and interstitium

Clinical Presentation

Phosphate Nephropathy

- AKI with history of antecedent administration of phosphorus-containing oral bowel preparation for surgery or colonoscopy, or enema
- Risk factors include preexisting renal disease, female gender, use of ACE-I or ARB

Urate Nephropathy

- Because of excessive release of uric acid in patients with hematologic malignancies or myeloproliferative diseases (occasionally solid tumors), usually after treatment with radiation or chemotherapy

Diagnosis

Phosphate Nephropathy

- Serum phosphorus often acutely elevated
- Clinical history of antecedent phosphorus-containing bowel purgative or enema

Urate Nephropathy

- Severe hyperuricemia (uric acid more than 15 mg/dL), usually accompanied by hyperkalemia, hyperphosphatemia, and hypocalcemia
Urine uric acid : creatinine ratio more than 1 mg/mg
Urate crystals in urine
Renal biopsy shows characteristic PN or UN crystal deposition throughout the tubules and interstitium

Treatment

- Supportive care, IV hydration
- Prevention:
    - (PN) choose non–phosphorus-containing products
    - (UN) pretreatment with allopurinol or uricase before chemotherapy or radiation
        - Urinary alkalinization with sodium bicarbonate is discouraged unless concomitant metabolic acidosis exists

Myeloma Kidney

Basic Information

- AKI caused by excess filtered clonal immunoglobulin light chains (Bence-Jones proteins) via direct tubular toxicity and/or obstruction by light chain casts

Clinical Presentation

- AKI in multiple myeloma patient with high level of Bence-Jones proteinuria, often in setting of superimposed volume depletion or IV contrast administration

Diagnosis

- Appropriate clinical history
- High serum free light chain levels or high 24-hour monoclonal proteinuria
- Urine dipstick may be negative in the presence of increased urinary protein (nonalbumin)
- Renal biopsy can confirm obstructing light-chain casts

Treatment

- Supportive care and treatment of underlying plasma cell dyscrasia

- IV hydration ± urinary alkalinization
- Plasmapheresis in conjunction with chemotherapy may be beneficial but is unproven

Renal Artery Thromboembolic Disease

Basic Information

- AKI results from
  - Cholesterol atheroemboli to medium or small renal arteries, or
  - Thrombotic emboli usually in patients with intracardiac thrombi (e.g., atrial fibrillation; severe left ventricular dysfunction)

Clinical Presentation

- Atheroembolic
  - Occurs spontaneously (especially in patients with peripheral arterial disease on anticoagulants) or following cardiac/aortic manipulation via catheter or surgery
  - Renal function may worsen acutely or subacutely and continues to worsen over several weeks
  - Physical findings may include cyanosis, gangrene of toes or feet, and livedo reticularis (Fig. 33-6)
  - If pancreatic or mesenteric emboli also occur, abdominal pain/bowel ischemia may result
- Thromboembolic
  - Occurs after myocardial infarction or with atrial arrhythmias, resulting in arterial obstruction and renal infarction
  - Renal function acutely worsens, particularly with bilateral disease
  - Physical findings may include flank pain and hematuria
  - Lactate dehydrogenase often elevated

Diagnosis

- Appropriate clinical history
- Laboratory findings in cholesterol atheroembolic disease can include **eosinophilia, eosinophiluria, and hypocomplementemia**

- Cholesterol crystals may be present in affected organs (Fig. 33-7)
- Decreased renal perfusion on ultrasonography if thromboembolic arterial occlusion is severe

Treatment

- Supportive care only; prognosis is poor
- Consider anticoagulation with thromboembolic disease
- Interventional thrombectomy for complete renal arterial occlusion only beneficial if performed immediately after occlusion

Postrenal Causes of Acute Kidney Injury

Basic Information

- Group of disorders resulting from physical obstruction (Fig. 33-8) of the ureters (e.g., obstructing nephrolithiasis, malignancy, retroperitoneal fibrosis), bladder (e.g., prostatic hyperplasia, clots, tumors), or renal veins (e.g., renal vein thrombosis, see Chapter 34)

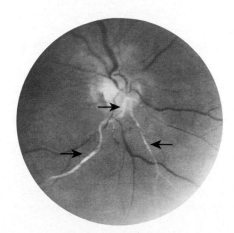

FIGURE 33-7 Cholesterol emboli *(arrows)* noted in the funduscopic exam. (From Swash M. *Hutchison's clinical methods.* 21st ed. Philadelphia: Saunders; 2002, Fig. 12.14.)

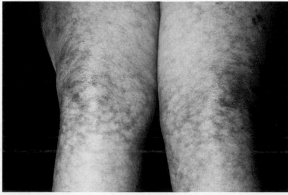

FIGURE 33-6 Livedo reticularis. Note the characteristic "fishnet stocking" pattern of the rash. (From Haslett C, Chilvers ER, Boon NA, et al. *Davidson's principles and practice of medicine.* 19th ed. New York: Churchill Livingstone; 2002, Fig. 20.48.)

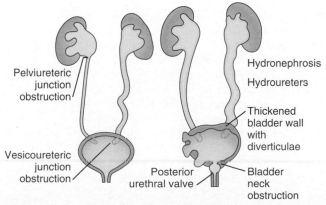

FIGURE 33-8 Postrenal causes of acute kidney injury include any obstruction along the urinary outflow tract. (From Lissauer T, Clayden G. *Illustrated textbook of paediatrics.* 2nd ed. St. Louis: Mosby; 2001, Fig. 16-6a.)

33

Clinical Presentation

- If onset sudden, patient will often note flank pain
- **If bilateral ureteral obstruction is complete, anuria results**
- **Partial obstruction may result in oliguria or seemingly paradoxical polyuria (obstruction transmitted to the distal renal tubules impairs water reabsorption → increased urine output)**
- Physical examination may note abdominal or pelvis mass from hydronephrosis, obstructing tumor, or distended bladder

Diagnosis

- **Ultrasound is the test of choice to determine the presence of ureteral obstruction** because of high sensitivity and specificity, low cost, and safety (noninvasive, no radiation)
- IV pyelography (computerized tomography [CT] or plain film) defines the location of obstruction and anatomy of the ureters; however, one must consider the potential toxicity of IV contrast along with poor visualization of the kidneys with low GFR (Fig. 33-9)
- Noncontrast CT is able to diagnose hydronephrosis and is useful in determining extrinsic mass, hematoma, or stones
- Nuclear medicine furosemide renogram can provide functional status of the kidneys and avoid risk of IV contrast; however, anatomic visualization is poor
- Renal vein thrombosis is most commonly diagnosed by ultrasound, magnetic resonance venography, or venogram

Treatment

- The most effective treatment is determined by the location of the obstruction. **Emergency relief of the obstruction is indicated if AKI or urosepsis is present.**
  - Obstruction distal to the bladder (e.g., bladder neck; urethral stricture) can be relieved by an indwelling urethral catheter or a suprapubic catheter
  - Upper urinary tract obstruction can be relieved by either a percutaneous nephrostomy tube or ureteral stent
- Recovery of renal function is less likely with longer duration of the obstruction
- Postobstructive diuresis: Watch for polyuria with loss of water, sodium, potassium, and other electrolytes
  - Etiology is volume expansion, osmotic diuresis caused by urea accumulation, tubular damage, and accumulation of natriuretic factors before relief of obstruction
- Replacement fluid should be half-normal saline initially and adjusted according to serum electrolyte changes

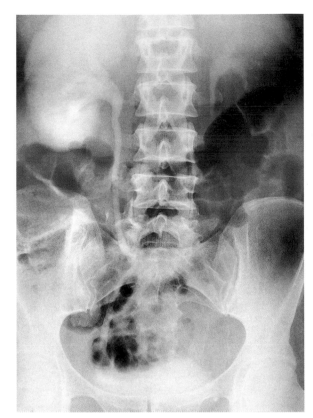

FIGURE 33-9 Unilateral urinary outflow tract obstruction. This patient has an obstructing kidney stone at the lower end of the right ureter. This image, taken 2 hours after contrast injection, demonstrates persistent contrast in the right kidney and collecting system as compared with that on the left. (From Haslett C, Chilvers ER, Boon NA, et al. *Davidson's principles and practice of medicine.* 19th ed. New York: Churchill Livingstone; 2002, Fig. 14.38.)

Acknowledgment

This chapter was adapted from chapters by Hyung M. Lim, MD, written for previous editions of the *Johns Hopkins Internal Medicine Board Review.*

Review Questions

For review questions, please go to ExpertConsult.com.

SUGGESTED READINGS

Abuelo JG. Normotensive ischemic acute renal failure. *N Engl J Med.* 2007;357:797-805.

Brenner BM, Rector FC. *The kidney.* 9th ed. Philadelphia: Elsevier Saunders; 2012.

Perazella MA. Diagnosing drug-induced AIN in the hospitalized patient: a challenge for the clinician. *Clin Nephrol.* 2014;81:381-388.

Wilson FP, Berns JS. Tumor lysis syndrome: new challenges and recent advances. *Adv Chronic Kidney Dis.* 2014;21:18-26.

Glomerular Disease

TARIQ SHAFI, MBBS, MHS; and DEREK M. FINE, MD

Glomerular disease includes a group of disorders in which the glomerular filtration barrier is altered. The resultant change in filtration may be accompanied by proteinuria (in nephrotic disorders) or hematuria (in nephritic disorders), or both. Familiarity with the causes of nephrotic and nephritic disorders will guide the history, physical, and laboratory examination of patients presenting with abnormal urinary sediment.

Basic Information

- *Glomerular disease* **refers to disorders of the glomerular filtration barrier that occur either as a primary disorder or as a result of other diseases, toxins, or infections**
- **The glomerular filtration barrier may be affected such that proteinuria results; if the proteinuria is greater than 3.5 g/24 hours (nephrotic-range proteinuria), a nephrotic syndrome may result**
- **If glomerular filtration barrier is affected so that hematuria results (often accompanied by proteinuria), the disorder is classified as nephritic (glomerulonephritis [GN])**
- Additional clinical features typically accompany nephrotic and nephritic disorders (see following)
- Significant overlap may exist among nephrotic and nephritic disorders

Nephrotic Syndrome

Basic Information

- General features of nephrotic syndrome
  - **Defined by the presence of**
    - **Proteinuria (more than 3.5 g/24 hours)**
    - **Hypoalbuminemia (less than 3.5 g/dL)**
    - **Hyperlipidemia**
    - **Edema**
- Blood pressure is variable depending on the underlying disease
  - Often normal in minimal change disease
  - Frequently elevated in focal segmental glomerulosclerosis (FSGS)
- **Urinary loss of anticoagulant proteins (e.g., protein C, protein S, antithrombin III) may result in a hypercoagulable state**
  - **Renal vein thrombosis** may occur with any cause of nephrotic syndrome but is **most common with membranous**
  - Renal vein thrombosis often presents as sudden-onset worsening of kidney function, worsening proteinuria, hematuria, and/or flank pain

- Loss of immunoglobulins may result in immunodeficiency and predisposes to infection

Clinical Presentation

- Features of specific nephrotic disorders; all may be idiopathic or related to secondary causes (Table 34-1)
  - **Minimal change disease**
    - Rapid onset; patient may be normal one day and have edema the next
    - Glomerular filtration rate (GFR) remains normal
      - **Massive proteinuria common (more than 4 g/24 hours)**
      - **Pathologic hallmark is normal-appearing glomeruli on light microscopy with generalized loss of podocyte foot processes on electron microscopy (Fig. 34-1)**

Secondary causes include Hodgkin lymphoma, thymoma, nonsteroidal antiinflammatory drugs (NSAIDs), bee stings, and lithium
  - **Focal segmental glomerulosclerosis (FSGS)**
    - Classic FSGS common in African Americans
    - Slow onset with progressive decrease in GFR if untreated
    - Creatinine may be normal initially, but if elevated at presentation indicates a poorer prognosis
    - Primary/idiopathic FSGS often presents with hypoalbuminemia and greater than 3.5 g/24 hours proteinuria
      - Secondary/postadaptive FSGS often has normal albumin and less than 3 g/24 hours proteinuria
      - Many secondary etiologies, including diabetes, sickle cell, obesity, and hyperfiltration
    - Human immunodeficiency virus (HIV)-associated nephropathy (HIVAN) presents with a collapsing variant of FSGS
      - Characterized by a very rapid onset of renal failure (over months) with massive proteinuria
      - Collapsing FSGS may occasionally be seen in non–HIV-infected patients (e.g., parvovirus infection, pamidronate)
  - **Membranous**
    - **The most common cause of idiopathic nephrotic syndrome in adults**
    - **Associated with antibody against phospholipase A$_2$ (PLA$_2$) receptor**
    - **Slow onset with loss of GFR usually over years**
    - **Spontaneous remission in one third of patients**
    - Creatinine often normal; if creatinine deteriorates rapidly, consider renal vein thrombosis
    - Proteinuria varies from subnephrotic to massive (more than 20 g/24 hours)

TABLE 34-1	*Diagnosis of Causes of Nephrotic Syndrome*		
Cause	**Typical Age of Onset**	**Associated Diseases**	**Pathologic Findings**
Minimal change disease	<12 years or mid-60s	NSAIDs Lymphoma Bee sting	Light microscopy: Normal Immunofluorescence: Normal Electron microscopy: Diffuse podocyte foot process effacement
Focal segmental glomerulosclerosis (FSGS)	Early teens to mid-30s	Hyperfiltration (seen in morbid obesity; may result from nephron loss because of other causes) HIV (collapsing variant) Heroin nephropathy	Light microscopy: Focal and segmental glomerulosclerosis Immunofluorescence: May show nonspecific IgM deposition Electron microscopy: Foot process effacement Collapsing variant seen on light microscopy in those with HIV
Membranous	Mid-30s to mid-60s	Adenocarcinoma (breast, bowel, lung) Hepatitis B Systemic lupus erythematosus NSAIDs	Light microscopy: Thickened capillary loops Immunofluorescence: Deposition of immunoglobulin and complement Electron microscopy: Subepithelial immune complex deposition
Membranoproliferative glomerulonephritis	Idiopathic: 8 to 16 years Secondary: More common in adults	Type I: Hepatitis C Chronic hepatitis B Endocarditis Idiopathic Dense deposit disease (DDD) / Type II Complement mutations Nephritic factors	Light microscopy: Glomerular lobulation, capillary wall thickening and mesangial expansion Immunofluorescence Type I: C3, early complement components, IgG deposits DDD: C3 Electron microscopy Type I: Subendothelial electron-dense deposits DDD: Dense "ribbon-like" deposits along basement membrane

HIV, Human immunodeficiency virus; IgG, immunoglobulin G; IgM, immunoglobulin M; NSAIDs, nonsteroidal antiinflammatory drugs.

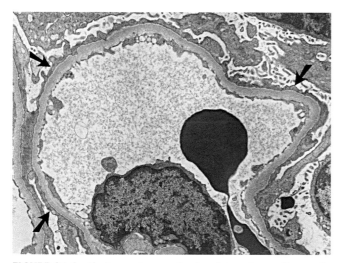

FIGURE 34-1 Electron micrograph of a glomerular capillary wall from a patient with minimal change glomerulopathy, showing extensive foot process effacement *(arrows)* and microvillous transformation (magnification ×5000). (From Brenner BM. *Brenner and Rector's the kidney.* 7th ed. Philadelphia: Saunders; 2004, Fig. 28-4.)

- Secondary causes include malignancy, NSAIDs, systemic lupus erythematosus (SLE), hepatitis B infection, and others (Table 34-1) Secondary causes of nephrotic syndrome
  - **Diabetes**
    - Diabetic nephropathy is the most common cause of nephrotic-range proteinuria

- May initially manifest microalbuminuria (30 to 300 mg albumin/24 hours), which then progresses to albuminuria (more than 300 mg/24 hours), and potentially to nephrotic-range proteinuria
- Renal function declines upon development of overt proteinuria
  - Average time to end-stage renal disease (ESRD) after onset of proteinuria is 10 years
  - Progression to ESRD may be delayed by angiotensin-converting enzyme (ACE) inhibitors or angiotensin receptor blockers
- Diabetic nephropathy rarely develops before 10 years' duration of diabetes
- Type 1 diabetics with nephropathy
  - 95% also have retinopathy
  - The absence of retinopathy should prompt consideration of a nondiabetic etiology of proteinuria/nephropathy
- Type 2 diabetics with nephropathy
  - 50% to 75% have retinopathy
  - Nephropathy in the absence of retinopathy is common, but should still prompt consideration of other causes of nephropathy
  - If retinopathy is present in patients with type 2, almost 100% have nephropathy
- **All diabetic patients with proteinuria should be evaluated for other systemic diseases (e.g., hepatitis B and C, SLE, and monoclonal gammopathy), as up to 20% have a nondiabetic cause of proteinuria**

- Clinical scenarios in which to consider renal biopsy in diabetics
  - Presence of proteinuria with less than 10 years' duration of diabetes
  - Presence of significant hematuria or red blood cell (RBC) casts on urinalysis
  - Absence of retinopathy in patients with type 1 diabetes and possibly type 2 diabetes
  - Any clinical or laboratory evidence of other systemic disease
- Amyloidosis
  - Systemic disease with extracellular deposition of amyloid in various organs (see Chapter 56)
  - Most common is AL amyloid (primary amyloidosis) with deposits of light-chain immunoglobulin
  - Secondary (AA amyloid) associated with chronic inflammatory or infectious states
  - Multiple other amyloidogenic proteins exist (e.g., transthyretin, lysozyme, β_2-microglobulin)
  - AL amyloid is caused by plasma cell dyscrasia with overt multiple myeloma in 20% of cases
    - 90% have monoclonal light chains (Bence Jones proteins) in urine or blood
    - Proteinuria is the consistent feature with associated renal insufficiency
    - Nephrotic syndrome in patient older than 50 years; should have high index of suspicion for AL amyloid
    - Generally poor prognosis, but may respond to chemotherapy

Diagnosis

- **Serologic evaluation: autoantibodies to nuclear antigens (ANA), hepatitis B surface antigen, hepatitis C antibody, serum and urine protein electrophoresis, HIV antibody, complement levels**
- **Glomerular amyloid will result in albuminuria (dipstick positive proteinuria), although light chain cast nephropathy will not**
- **Kidney biopsy needed in most patients**
  - Urgent biopsy needed if creatinine is rising quickly
  - Diabetics with consistent time course (>10 years' disease) and retinopathy with no other systemic disease or serologic abnormalities may not require biopsy for diagnosis
  - Nephrotic patients with amyloid diagnosed by biopsy of other organ (e.g., heart, skin, or bone marrow) may not need kidney biopsy

Treatment

- When nephrotic syndrome is secondary to a systemic disease, treat the underlying disorder
- Additional renoprotective measures:
  - Strict blood pressure control (<130/80 mm Hg)
  - Use of ACE inhibitors or angiotensin receptor blockers
  - Aggressive control of cardiovascular risk factors
  - Improved glycemic control in individuals with diabetes
- Treatment of idiopathic causes of nephrotic syndrome is described in Table 34-2

TABLE 34-2	*Treatment of Idiopathic Nephrotic and Nephritic Disorders*	
Disorder	**Treatment**	**Response**
Minimal change disease	Corticosteroids Cyclosporine or cyclophosphamide or mycophenolate mofetil for relapse	Children respond within 2 weeks Adults respond in 4 to 8 weeks, but often relapse
Focal segmental glomerulosclerosis (FSGS)	Corticosteroids + ACE-I Cyclosporine or mycophenolate mofetil may be added to steroids	40 to 60% Response takes 4 to 13 months
Membranous	ACE-I for all patients Low risk for progression (proteinuria <4 g/day + creatinine clearance >80 mL/min): Observation with close follow-up Moderate risk for progression (persistent proteinuria between 4 g/day and 8 g/day + creatinine clearance >80 mL/min): Corticosteroids ± cytotoxic agents High risk for progression (persistent proteinuria >8 g/day and/or abnormal or declining creatinine clearance): Corticosteroids + cytotoxic agents	Variable, dependent on prognostic indicators One third remit spontaneously without treatment; treatment decisions should be based on persistent proteinuria on 24-h urine collections
Membranoproliferative glomerulonephritis	Corticosteroids ± cytotoxic agents Antiplatelet agents (aspirin; dipyridamole) may slow disease progression	Spontaneous remission in <10% Prolonged course of slowly deteriorating renal function is common

ACE-I, Angiotensin-converting enzyme inhibitor.

Nephritic Disorders

Basic Information

- General features of nephritic disorders (GN)
- **Nephritic disorders are commonly associated with systemic diseases; immunoglobulin A (IgA) nephropathy is the most common cause worldwide**
- **Patients typically present with deteriorating renal function, mild to moderate proteinuria, hypertension, and an active urine sediment (RBCs and RBC casts in the urine; Fig. 34-2)**

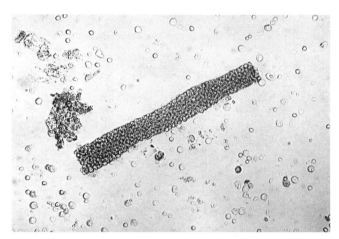

FIGURE 34-2 Red cell casts typically seen in acute glomerulonephritis. (From Noble J, Greene HL, Levinson W, et al. *Textbook of primary care medicine.* 3rd ed. St. Louis: Mosby; 2000, Fig. 144-6.)

- Hypocomplementemia suggests lupus nephritis, postinfectious GN, membranoproliferative GN, or cryoglobulinemic GN
- Patients may report dark urine
- Blood pressure is typically elevated; peripheral edema may be seen (which may progress to include ascites or pleural effusions)
- Urine output may be normal or oliguric

Clinical Presentation

- A search for a systemic, infectious, or postinfectious cause should be undertaken
- Systemic diseases associated with GN
  - Frequently present with rapid-onset renal insufficiency in the setting of immune dysregulation
  - The role of complement in evaluation of GN is shown in Fig. 34-3
  - The role of immune serologies is shown in Fig. 34-4
  - Immunofluorescence (IF) of the kidney biopsy sample is essential in defining the underlying process:
    - Immune complex GN (immune complexes seen on IF)
    - Pauci-immune GN (limited immune staining, hence the term *pauci*-immune)
    - Anti-glomerular basement membrane (GBM) disease (linear IgG staining of the GBM)
  - SLE: A secondary cause of proliferative or membranous GN (see Chapter 45)
  - **Henoch-Schönlein purpura (HSP)**
    - Manifestations include purpura (Fig. 34-5), arthralgias, abdominal pain, and renal involvement
    - Commonly follows upper respiratory infection

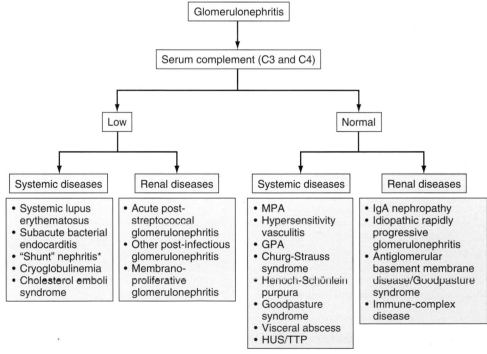

FIGURE 34-3 Role of complement levels in diagnosis of the patient with glomerulonephritis. *Refers to infection of a ventriculoatrial shunt. GPA, Granulomatosis with polyangiitis; HUS/TTP, hemolytic uremic syndrome/thrombotic thrombocytopenic purpura; IgA, immunoglobulin A; MPA, microscopic polyangiitis. (Modified from Madaio MP, Harrington JT. The diagnosis of acute glomerulonephritis, *N Engl J Med.* 1983;309:1299–1302.)

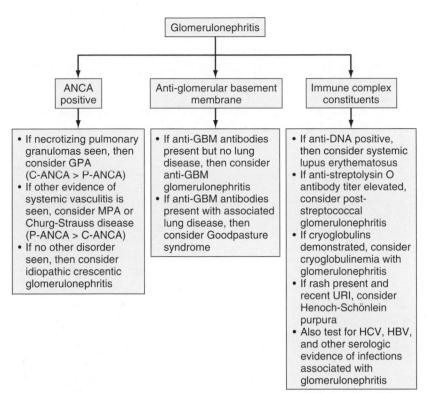

FIGURE 34-4 Role of immune serologies in evaluation of the patient with glomerulonephritis. ANCA, Antineutrophil cytoplasmic antibody; C-ANCA; cytoplasmic antineutrophil cytoplasmic antibody; GBM, glomerular basement membrane; GPA, granulomatosis with polyangiitis; HBV, hepatitis B virus; HCV, hepatitis C virus; MPA, microscopic polyangiitis; P-ANCA, perinuclear antineutrophil cytoplasmic antibody; URI, upper respiratory infection. (Modified from Falk RJ. ANCA-associated renal disease, *Kidney Int.*1990;38:998–1010.)

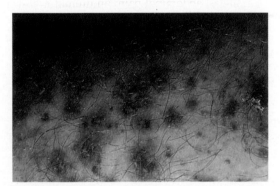

FIGURE 34-5 Typical rash (palpable purpura) on the lower extremities seen in Henoch-Schönlein purpura. (From Goldman L, Bennett JC, Ausiello D. *Cecil textbook of medicine.* 22nd ed. Philadelphia: Saunders; 2004, Fig. 475.4.)

- IgA deposition seen in renal mesangial cells (looks exactly like IgA nephropathy)
- Uncommon in adults; more common in male children
- **Vasculitis** (includes granulomatosis with polyangiitis, microscopic polyangiitis, and Churg-Strauss syndrome; see Chapter 44)
- **Goodpasture syndrome**
  - Results from production of anti-GBM antibodies
  - Defined by presence of both lung and kidney involvement with linear anti-GBM staining on IF
  - Pathology reveals crescent formation in glomeruli; number of crescents relates to severity and prognosis

  - If pulmonary disease is absent, a diagnosis of anti-GBM disease is made
- Infectious diseases associated with GN
  - Endocarditis
  - Hepatitis B and C
  - Less common: syphilis, malaria
- Postinfectious etiologies associated with GN
  - Classic is post-streptococcal GN, but can develop after infection with almost any organism
    - With post-streptococcal GN, patients present with hypertension, oliguria, and elevated antistreptolysin O (ASO) antibody titers 7 to 14 days after throat or skin infection with group A *Streptococcus*
    - Certain strains more likely to cause GN (types 12 and 49)
  - Presentation can be highly variable; from asymptomatic microscopic hematuria to florid nephritic syndrome
  - Postinfectious GN following staphylococcal infection is increasingly being recognized, particularly in diabetics
- **IgA nephropathy (Berger disease)**
  - **Most common cause of GN in adults**
    - **Particularly common in Asians**
    - **Uncommon in African Americans**
  - **Classic presentation is gross hematuria following upper respiratory infection**
  - Others present with persistent, microscopic hematuria long after viral upper respiratory infection has been forgotten; less than 10% have a nephrotic presentation

- Mesangial IgA deposition is seen on biopsy (establishes the diagnosis)
- In contrast to HSP, rash is not seen and course is usually less aggressive
- Membranoproliferative glomerulonephritis (MPGN)
  - Clinical presentation may be nephrotic, nephritic, or mixed
  - **Most often secondary to hepatitis C infection (type I MPGN)**
  - Variable course; from slowly progressive nephrotic syndrome similar to membranous to a rapidly progressive GN as is seen with the necrotizing vasculitides
  - Associated with cryoglobulins when related to hepatitis C (essential mixed cryoglobulinemia–type II cryoglobulins)

Diagnosis

- Clinical presentation and testing for specific diseases (e.g., ASO titer, anti-GBM serology) may be sufficient to diagnose a likely underlying cause
  - Biopsy often still required for definitive diagnosis
- The evaluation and testing differs based on the clinical scenario
- Immunologic testing may also help narrow differential diagnosis (see Figs. 34-3 and 34-4)
- Some diseases manifest with rapidly progressive renal failure and may mimic GN (Box 34-1)

- Renal biopsy should be performed in the following situations:
  - Diagnosis/prognosis remains unclear, particularly with progressive renal insufficiency
  - Rapidly progressive GN
  - More than 2 g/day proteinuria
  - Presence of a systemic disease with potential renal involvement
  - Suspected acute tubular injury not improving after 3 to 4 weeks
  - Course atypical for diabetic nephropathy in a diabetic patient

BOX 34-1	*Diseases That May Present with Rapidly Progressive Renal Failure and Mimic*

Glomerulonephritis
Cholesterol emboli syndrome (transient hypocomplementemia may be seen in 25%)
Thrombotic microangiopathies include HUS, TTP, malignant hypertension, and antiphospholipid antibody syndrome
Scleroderma renal crisis
Myeloma cast nephropathy

HUS, Hemolytic uremic syndrome; TTP, thrombotic thrombocytopenic purpura.

TABLE 34-3	*Treatment of Selected Nephritic Disorders*	
Disorder	**Treatment**	**Response**
Henoch-Schönlein purpura	Supportive care Fluids Pain relief Hospitalize for inadequate oral intake GI bleeding Renal failure Glucocorticoids for severe disease (unproven efficacy, but reasonable)	Excellent prognosis in children; less favorable in adults Roughly one third relapse within 4 mo Acute morbidity: Caused by GI bleeding Chronic morbidity: Chronic kidney disease; 10% develop ESRD
Goodpasture syndrome	Plasmapheresis (to remove anti-GBM antibodies) + corticosteroids + cyclophosphamide Among those with higher creatinine requiring dialysis: Therapy less likely to be beneficial	Prognosis (patient and kidney survival) correlates with number of crescents on biopsy and severity of kidney injury on presentation Relapses are uncommon unless patient is also ANCA-positive
Postinfectious GN	Immunosuppressive therapy generally not helpful Rapidly progressive GN with crescents: Consider pulse steroids (though unproven efficacy)	Prognosis generally quite good Spontaneous resolution usually occurs over 3–4 wk
IgA nephropathy	ACE inhibitors or ARBs to treat hypertension and reduce intraglomerular pressure Corticosteroids may be beneficial in select patients Fish oil (omega-3 fatty acid) use is controversial, but frequently used	Not all patients progress; some have stable course or remit In patients who progress, deterioration is usually gradual Predictors of progression Elevated creatinine at diagnosis Hypertension Proteinuria above 1000 mg/24 hr ESRD eventually develops in 15% by 10 years and 20% by 20 years

ACE, Angiotensin-converting enzyme; ANCA, antineutrophil cytoplasmic antibody; ARB, angiotensin receptor blocker; ESRD, end-stage renal disease; GBM, glomerular basement membrane; GI, gastrointestinal; GN, glomerulonephritis; IgA, immunoglobulin A.

Treatment

- When GN is secondary to a systemic disease or infection, treatment is aimed at the underlying disorder
- Table 34-3 outlines therapy for selected nephritic disorders
- Some patients may require dialysis therapy temporarily or indefinitely

Review Questions

For review questions, please go to ExpertConsult.com.

SUGGESTED READINGS

Introduction to glomerular disease. In: Johnson RJ, Feehally J, Floege J, eds. *Comprehensive clinical nephrology.* 5th ed. Philadelphia: Elsevier; 2015.

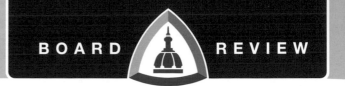
Chronic Kidney Disease and End-Stage Renal Disease

TARIQ SHAFI, MBBS, MHS; PAUL J. SCHEEL JR., MD, MBA; and DEREK M. FINE, MD

Chronic kidney disease (CKD) is a major public health problem in the United States, predominantly because of the increasing prevalence of diabetes and hypertension with resultant renal disease. CKD often leads to end-stage renal disease (ESRD) and the need for renal replacement therapy.

Basic Information

- Definition: **Defined by structural or functional abnormalities of the kidney for 3 months or longer, with implications for health**
- Structural abnormalities of the kidney may include presence of renal cysts or histologic abnormalities
- Functional abnormalities may include albuminuria (albumin excretion rate >30 mg/24 hours or albumin/creatinine ratio >30 mg/g) or abnormal urine sediment
- The 2012 Kidney Disease Improving Global Outcomes (KDIGO) recommend CKD classification based on the cause of CKD, glomerular filtration rate (GFR) category, and albuminuria category
  - Cause: The cause of CKD is based on presence of systemic disease and its location in the kidney (e.g., diabetic glomerulosclerosis or lupus nephritis)
  - GFR category: GFR is categorized as described in Table 35-1
  - Albuminuria category: Albuminuria is categorized as described in Table 35-2
- Epidemiology
  - Many patients with CKD progress to ESRD
  - Prevalence increases with age
  - Estimated ESRD prevalence in the U.S. in 2011 was over 500,000, with an annual incidence of greater than 110,000
- Etiology
  - Diabetes (approximately 40%)
  - Hypertension (approximately 25%)
  - Glomerulonephritis (approximately 10%)
  - Genetic or congenital (e.g., polycystic kidney disease; approximately 3%)
  - Urologic (approximately 2%)

Clinical Presentation

- Usually asymptomatic until the late stages of renal failure
- **Onset of symptoms is usual indication for initiation of dialysis**
- **Early symptoms: anorexia, nausea, lethargy, fatigue**

- **Late symptoms: pruritus, mental status changes caused by encephalopathy, volume overload, chest pain from pericarditis, neuropathy**
- Metabolic abnormalities often seen
  - Anemia
  - Secondary and tertiary hyperparathyroidism (associated with hypocalcemia, hyperphosphatemia, and metabolic bone disease)
  - Metabolic acidosis
  - Hyperkalemia
- Physical examination findings
  - Asterixis (indicative of encephalopathy)
  - Pericardial friction rub
  - Signs of volume overload
  - Uremic fetor: foul-smelling breath similar to urine or fish
  - Pallor
  - Calcific uremic arteriolopathy (also known as calciphylaxis): Skin and fat necrosis with calcification and thrombosis of small arterioles (Fig. 35-1) most commonly seen in patients with ESRD
    - Usually in the setting of a high calcium × phosphorus product
    - Violaceous, indurated skin lesions that may ulcerate
    - Predilection for the lower extremities and trunk

Diagnosis

- Evidence of structural or functional abnormalities of the kidneys for 3 or more months
  - Diagnose by estimated or actual GFR, not serum creatinine (Cr) levels
  - CKD can manifest as proteinuria or abnormal urine sediment of kidney origin (e.g., red blood cell casts) with normal GFR
- **CKD is underdiagnosed if serum Cr is used as sole measure**
- **Need to use GFR estimation equations**
  - Chronic Kidney Disease Epidemiology Collaboration (CKD-EPI) equation is recommended for GFR estimation (available at www.kidney.org)
- Other features consistent with CKD
  - Small kidneys on renal ultrasound (normal kidney size is 10 to 12 cm; kidneys are smaller in women)
  - Presence of manifestations of CKD: anemia, secondary hyperparathyroidism, acidosis

- Rule out reversible causes in any patient with renal insufficiency
  - Obstruction and prerenal causes (see Chapter 33)
  - Treatable glomerular disease (see Chapter 34)
  - Atherosclerotic renal vascular disease (Box 35-1)

Treatment

- Prognosis of CKD
  - Patients with reduced GFR or increasing albuminuria are at higher risk of progression to CKD or death
  - KDIGO recommends timely referral for planning renal replacement therapy in patients with progressive CKD in whom the risk of kidney failure within 1 year is above 10% to 20% as indicated by Table 35-3
  - **Also consider nephrology referral for:**
    - Unexplained proteinuria or hematuria suggestive of glomerulonephritis
    - Rapid decline in GFR (more than 15 mL/min/1.73 m^2 per year)
    - Allows for early intervention (Fig. 35-2)
  - **Delay progression of CKD**
  - **Angiotensin-converting enzyme (ACE) inhibitors and angiotensin receptor blockers (ARBs)**
    - Mechanism: Decrease intraglomerular pressure and hyperfiltration
    - Problem: Reduce GFR and may lead to elevation of serum creatinine and potassium
    - Creatinine rise is 20% or less: Continue therapy as there is long-term benefit in preservation of GFR
- Manage hypertension:
  - Hypertension is a very important risk factor for progression of CKD and decline in GFR
  - Adequate control of blood pressure reduces rate of decline in GFR

- KDIGO Guidelines recommend the following for adult CKD patients:
  - BP goals:
  - Less than 140/90 mm Hg if urine albumin excretion less than 30 mg/24 hours
  - Less than 130/80 mm Hg if urine albumin excretion 30 mg/24 hours or higher
  - ACE inhibitor or ARB in diabetic adults with CKD and urine albumin excretion 30 mg/24 hours or higher and in all patients with CKD if urine albumin excretion 300 mg/24 hours or higher
  - Atenolol is cleared by the kidney; therefore, use with caution or consider switching to a nonrenally cleared β-blocker such as metoprolol
- Manage hyperkalemia
  - Attempt to maintain ACE inhibitor or ARB therapy
  - Exclude renal artery stenosis
  - Dietary potassium restriction (major culprits include bananas, cantaloupe, oranges, potatoes, tomatoes)
  - Add a potassium-depleting diuretic (thiazide-type or loop diuretic)
  - Eliminate potassium-sparing diuretics (triamterene, amiloride, spironolactone, or eplerenone)
  - Switch nonselective β-blocker to β$_1$-selective and/or reduce dose (unless essential for other reasons)
  - Correct metabolic acidosis

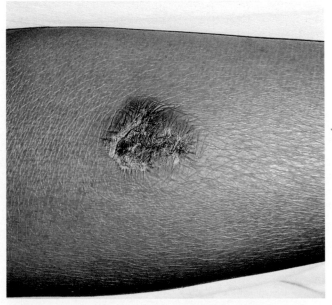

FIGURE 35-1 Typical skin lesion of calciphylaxis. (From Dharmadhikari A, Sukkar A, Mani S. Cases from the Osler Medical Service at Johns Hopkins University. *Am J Med.* 2003;114:765–767, Fig. 1.)

TABLE 35-1	GFR Categories	
GFR Category	**Description**	**GFR (mL/min/1.73 m²)**
G1	Normal or high	≥90
G2	Mildly decreased	60–89
G3a	Mildly to moderately decreased	45–59
G3b	Moderately to severely decreased	30–45
G4	Severely decreased	15–29
G5	Kidney failure	<15

TABLE 35-2	Albuminuria Categories		
Albuminuria Category	**Description**	**Albumin Excretion Rate (mg/24 hours)**	**Albumin-to-Creatinine Ratio (mg/g)**
A1	Normal or mildly increased	<30	<30
A2	Moderately increased	30–300	30–300
A3	Severely increased	>300	>300

Common in patients with evidence of atherosclerotic disease in other vascular beds (20% of these patients)
45% to 50% of renal artery stenosis patients will have bilateral disease

Consider if Any of the Following are Present

New-onset hypertension after age 50 years
Newly difficult-to-control hypertension (requiring >2 medications) in known hypertensive patient
Unexplained increase in creatinine in patient with suspected vascular disease (e.g., CAD, PVD, smoker, diabetic)
Hypotension or worsening creatinine after initiation of ACE inhibitor
Flash pulmonary edema without evidence of cardiac cause

Diagnosis

Renal angiography (gold standard)
CT angiogram (best in those who can tolerate IV contrast)
Magnetic resonance angiography (less invasive, >90% sensitivity and specificity)
Doppler ultrasound (accuracy is very user-dependent)

Treatment

ACE inhibitor or ARB, statin, and aspirin are first-line therapy
Stop smoking
Angioplasty and endovascular stenting—not superior to medical management except in selected cases and should not be routinely employed

Outcomes

Typically a progressive disease
Stenting does not slow progression of CKD except perhaps in selected cases of bilateral disease
Stenting may improve blood pressure control in selected patients already on maximal medical therapy

ACE, Angiotensin-converting enzyme; ARB, angiotensin receptor blockers; CAD, coronary artery disease; CKD, chronic kidney disease; CT, computed tomography; GFR, glomerular filtration rate; IV, intravenous; PVD, peripheral vascular disease.

- Potassium binding resins (caution: risk of bowel necrosis) or fludrocortisone (caution: salt and water retention leading to worsening hypertension) can be considered in highly selected patients
- Manage metabolic acidosis
  - Metabolic acidosis is a risk factor for CKD progression
  - Correction of total CO_2 to greater than 22 mEq/L may slow CKD progression
  - Diets enriched with fruits and vegetables and lower in protein generate less acid
  - Can supplement with sodium citrate, sodium bicarbonate, or calcium citrate (often limited by total calcium dose)
- Consider dietary protein restriction
  - Mechanism: Reduced protein intake may decrease intraglomerular pressure and metabolic demands on kidney
    - Diets higher in fruits and vegetables generate less acid. Metabolic acidosis is a risk factor for CKD progression
  - Conflicting efficacy data from trials
  - Recommendation (largely opinion-based): Decrease protein intake to 0.8 g of protein/kg of body weight/day if GFR is less than 30 mL/min/1.73 m^2
  - If patient is placed on protein-restricted diet, must have close follow-up of nutritional status to avoid malnutrition
- Manage glycemia in patients with diabetes mellitus and CKD
  - Goal hemoglobin A_{1c} (HbA_{1c}) is 7%
    - Lower A_{1c} not associated with slower CKD progression and increases risk of hypoglycemia
  - Modify other cardiovascular risk factors (e.g., tobacco use, hypercholesterolemia)
- Manage hypercholesterolemia
  - Statins are associated with reduced cardiovascular (CV) events in patients with CKD
    - Statins likely do not slow CKD progression

TABLE 35-3 *Risk of Chronic Kidney Disease Progression*

				PERSISTENT ALBUMINURIA CATEGORIES		
				A1 Normal or Mildly Increased <30 mg/g	**A2** Moderately Increased 30–300 mg/g	**A3** Severely Increased >300 mg/g
GFR categories (mL/min/1.73 m^2)	G1	Normal or high	≥90	1 if CKD	1	2*
	G2	Mildly decreased	60–89	1 if CKD	1	2*
	G3a	Mildly to moderately decreased	45–59	1	2	3*
	G3b	Moderately to severely decreased	30–44	2	3	3*
	G4	Severely decreased	15–29	3*	3*	4*
	G5	Kidney failure	<15	4*	4*	4*

Numbers in cells refer to frequency of monitoring per year.
*Consider referral to nephrology.
GFR, Glomerular filtration rate; Green, low risk if no chronic kidney disease; Yellow, moderately increased risk; Orange, high risk; Red, very high risk.
From Summary of recommendation statements. *Kidney Int Suppl.* 2013;3(1):5–14.

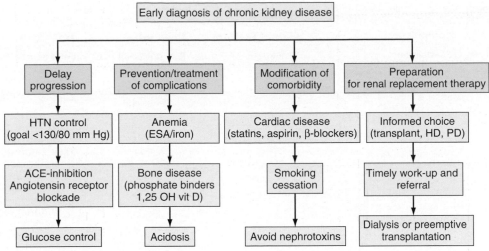

FIGURE 35-2   Management of chronic kidney disease. ACE, Angiotensin-converting enzyme; ESA, erythropoiesis-stimulating agent; HD, hemodialysis; HTN, hypertension; PD, peritoneal dialysis; 1,25-OH-vit D, 1,25-dihydroxyvitamin D.

- Statins are of unproven benefit in ESRD
- Aspirin should be considered in patients at sufficient risk for CV events
- Prevent and treat complications of CKD
  - Anemia, metabolic bone disease, acidosis, and volume overload (see Table 35-4)
    - Studies suggest increased risk of cardiovascular events (especially stroke) with normalization of hemoglobin (more than 13 g/dL)
    - Consider iron repletion in all patients and consider starting erythropoiesis-stimulating agents (ESAs) if hemoglobin is below 9 g/dL
      - ESA use does not slow CKD progression
  - Other endocrine complications
    - Decreased GFR leads to prolonged half-life of insulin
    - Patients with progressive renal failure need a downward titration of insulin and sulfonylurea dosing to avoid hypoglycemia
- Avoid nephrotoxins and adjust medication doses appropriately for kidney function (Table 35-5)
  - Many manufacturers recommend dosing based on creatinine clearance estimated by Cockcroft-Gault equation
  - Avoid additional nephrotoxic agents
  - Iodinated radiocontrast
    - Risk of acute renal failure 20% to 90%
    - Patients with diabetes at highest risk
    - Choose alternative imaging modality if possible
      - Gadolinium-based contrast agent contraindicated in those with estimated GFR less than 30 because of risk of nephrogenic systemic fibrosis (NSF)
        - If use is essential, use low dose of a macrocyclic (more stable) agent (e.g., gadoteridol)
    - If radiocontrast use unavoidable:
      - Ensure adequate hydration with isotonic saline or sodium bicarbonate
      - Minimize contrast volume
      - Utilize nonionic, iso-osmolar contrast

  - N-Acetylcysteine 600 to 1200 mg twice a day for 24 hours before procedure and day of the procedure may reduce incidence of acute kidney injury in high-risk groups
  - Statin therapy may reduce the risk of contrast nephropathy
- Avoid volume depletion
  - Tolerated poorly in this patient population
  - May lead to worsening of CKD secondary to acute tubular injury
  - Low threshold for intravenous (IV) fluids for hydration
- Vaccinate
  - Age-appropriate Advisory Committee on Immunization Practices (ACIP) recommendations
  - Specifically:
    - Annual influenza vaccination
    - Hepatitis B series
    - Pneumococcal vaccine-naïve
      - 13-valent pneumococcal conjugate vaccine (PCV$_{13}$) followed by 23-valent pneumococcal polysaccharide (PPSV$_{23}$) at least 8 weeks later
      - Repeat PPSV$_{23}$ in 5 years
    - Previous vaccination with PPSV23
      - Administer PCV$_{13}$ 1 year or more after last PPSV$_{23}$ dose
- **Renal transplantation**
  - Preferred treatment of ESRD
  - Every patient with ESRD should be considered a candidate for transplantation until proven otherwise
  - Contraindications to transplantation
    - Metastatic or untreated cancer
    - Recent malignancy (time varies according to cancer type)
    - Active infection
    - Severe psychiatric disease
    - Active or unstable coronary artery disease or refractory congestive heart failure
    - Nonrenal organ failure for which the patient is not a transplant candidate (e.g., lung, liver)
    - Persistent substance abuse
    - Unresolved psychosocial problems

TABLE 35-4	*Manifestations of Chronic Kidney Disease*			
Manifestation	**Mechanism**	**Clinical Features**	**Diagnosis**	**Treatment**
Anemia	EPO deficiency	Onset: GFR 25–50 mL/min Early: Asymptomatic Late: Decrease in functional capacity and quality of life, left ventricular hypertrophy	Rule out other causes of anemia Reticulocyte count Peripheral smear, iron studies Hemoccult stool EPO levels *not* useful	**Goal hemoglobin:** >9 g/dL to avoid transfusion **STEP 1: Assess iron status:** Inadequate iron stores if ferritin <100, TSAT <20% IV iron if stores inadequate with oral iron **STEP 2: Consider erythropoiesis-stimulating agents (erythropoietin alfa or darbepoetin alfa) if hemoglobin <9 g/dL and iron replete** Caution: patients with cancer Monitor hemoglobin weekly until "in range," then monthly Avoid hemoglobin >11 g/dL Follow ferritin and TSAT at least quarterly in CKD, monthly in ESRD
Metabolic bone disease	**Low 1,25-dihydroxyvitamin D** (poor conversion from 25-hydroxyvitamin D) **High phosphate** (low excretion) **Low calcium** (caused by low vitamin D) ↓ All lead to secondary hyperparathyroidism (high intact PTH) ↓ Renal osteodystrophy	Onset: GFR 25 to 40 mL/min Usually asymptomatic Bone pain—late manifestation Risk of fractures	High iPTH High phosphate Low calcium	**Goal iPTH:** Controversial. KDIGO: 2–9 times upper limit of normal for the lab K/DOQI goals: CKD III: 35–70 pg/mL CKD IV: 70–110 pg/mL CKD V or ESRD: 150–300 pg/mL **Goal serum phosphorus** 2.7–4.6 mg/dL (CKD III, IV) 3.5–5.5 mg/dL (CKD V or ESRD) **Restrict dietary phosphorus** <800–1000 mg/day **Phosphate binders** Calcium-based Calcium carbonate Calcium acetate Non–calcium-based (if high calcium × phosphorus product [>72]) Sevelamer Lanthanum carbonate **Check 25-vitamin D levels if iPTH is above goal (CKD III–V):** If <30 ng/mL: Supplement with ergocalciferol (caution if serum phosphorus ≥4.6 mg/dL or albumin-corrected serum calcium ≥10.2 mg/dL) **Goal serum calcium:** 8.4–10.2 mg/dL Vitamin D analogues Calcitriol Paricalcitol Doxercalciferol **Calcimimetics** Cinacalcet

TABLE 35-4	*Manifestations of Chronic Kidney Disease* (Continued)			
Manifestation	**Mechanism**	**Clinical Features**	**Diagnosis**	**Treatment**
Acidosis	Inability of kidney to excrete acid load	Chronic acidosis can result in hypercatabolism with poor nutritional status Calcium mobilization from the bone—exacerbation of osteoporosis	Low serum bicarbonate	**Goal serum bicarbonate** >22 mEq/L Start therapy if serum bicarbonate <18 mEq/L **Sodium** citrate 10 mL 3 times daily *or* **Sodium** bicarbonate 650 mg 3 times daily Monitor bicarbonate to avoid alkalosis

Volume overload	Inability of kidney to excrete water and salt	CHF
		Lower extremity edema
			Physical exam
			Chest radiograph
				Sodium restriction <2 g/day (<87 mEq on a 24-h urine collection)
				Fluid restriction <1500 mL/day
				Diuretics
				  Loop—increase dose until maximum; twice-daily dosing
				  Thiazide—add to regimen if patient unresponsive to loop diuretic to overcome distal sodium retention

Hyperkalemia	Inability of kidney to excrete potassium load	Usually asymptomatic
		May cause paralysis or respiratory failure
		Cardiac arrhythmias
			High serum potassium
			ECG changes
			  Peaked T waves
			  Flat or absent P wave
			  Wide QRS complex
			  Sine waves
				Acute
				Calcium gluconate, insulin/glucose, β-agonist, diuretic, dialysis
				Long-term
				Dietary restriction (high-potassium foods include orange, potato, tomato, banana, cantaloupe, and many others)
				Loop or thiazide diuretic
				Correct concurrent acidosis (see earlier)
				Consider discontinuation of β-blockers

CHF, Congestive heart failure; CKD, chronic kidney disease; ECG, electrocardiogram; EPO, erythropoietin; ESRD, end-stage renal disease; GFR, glomerular filtration rate; iPTH, intact parathyroid hormone; K/DOQI, National Kidney Foundation Kidney Disease Outcomes Quality Initiative; PTH, parathyroid hormone; RTA, renal tubular acidosis; TSAT, transferrin saturation.

- Sources of organs
  - Living related: usually best antigen match with recipient
  - Living unrelated: less well matched than related but healthier than deceased
  - Deceased donor: cold ischemic time may result in cell death and antigen release
- Refer to transplantation center for evaluation when GFR less than 30 mL/min/1.73 m^2
- Patients can be listed for deceased donor transplant when GFR less than 20 mL/min/1.73 m^2
- Treatment goal for suitable candidate is to receive a transplant before need for dialysis
- Prognosis: 5-year survival is 80% for deceased donor, 85% for living unrelated donor, and 90% for living related donor
- **Dialysis**
  - 90% of patients are candidates for either hemodialysis (HD) or peritoneal dialysis (PD)
- If therapy prescribed and monitored correctly, PD may equal HD in effectiveness
- Dialysis initiation: Usually based on combination of GFR and presence of symptoms of kidney failure; typically less than 10 to 15 mL/min/1.73 m^2
- Absolute dialysis indications (ideal goal is to avoid these manifestations)
  - Uremic encephalopathy
  - Uremic pericarditis
  - Volume overload not responsive to diuretics
  - Hyperkalemia despite medical management
  - Severe metabolic acidosis despite medical management
  - Life-threatening poisoning by a dialyzable toxin
- Prognosis for dialysis patients is poor in general
  - Median 5-year survival: 36% (1 in 3 dialysis patients will survive for 5 years after starting dialysis)

TABLE 35-5	*Drugs to Use with Caution in Chronic Kidney Disease*	
Drug Name	**Side Effect**	**Mechanism**
Gadolinium-based contrast agents	Nephrogenic systemic fibrosis	Poor clearance with extended half-life and deposition of free gadolinium in tissues. Avoid if GFR <30 mL/min. Macrocyclic agent (gadoteridol) safer than linear agents (gadodiamide or gadopentetate) if exposure is essential.
Iodinated intravenous contrast dye	AKI	Afferent vasoconstriction and acute tubular injury
Phosphate-containing bowel preps or enemas	Phosphate deposition in kidneys (phosphate nephropathy) or high anion gap acidosis	Poor clearance with renal failure
Aminoglycosides	AKI	Tubular toxicity
Atenolol	Bradycardia	Decreased renal clearance
Gabapentin	Altered mental status and other CNS toxicities	Decreased renal clearance
NSAIDs and COX-2 inhibitors	AKI	Reduced prostaglandin-induced afferent vasodilation
Sulfonylureas	Hypoglycemia (glyburide worse than glipizide)	Decreased renal clearance
Metformin	Lactic acidosis (avoid in CKD patients with GFR <30 mL/min; hold before contrast studies)	Mitochondrial toxicity
Magnesium-containing medications	Hypermagnesemia	Decreased clearance of magnesium
Meperidine	Seizure	Low clearance of toxic metabolite normeperidine
Sucralfate	Aluminum toxicity	High aluminum content with decreased clearance in renal failure, especially ESRD
Potassium supplements or potassium-sparing diuretics	Hyperkalemia	Absorption or retention of potassium
Probenecid	Decreased solute clearance	Inhibits tubular transporters responsible for waste secretion

AKI, Acute kidney injury; CKD, chronic kidney disease; COX-2, cyclooxygenase-2; ESRD, end-stage renal disease; GFR, glomerular filtration rate; NSAIDs, nonsteroidal antiinflammatory drugs.

- Most common cause of death: Cardiovascular disease (usually sudden cardiac death), followed by infection
- Patients who start dialysis with a catheter have the worst prognosis
- Peritoneal dialysis (PD)
  - PD is performed at home by the patient with or without the help of a partner
  - Can be automated peritoneal dialysis (APD) done over 12 to 13 hours at night or continuous ambulatory peritoneal dialysis (CAPD) performed throughout the day
  - Major risk is peritonitis; occurs at a rate of 0.5 episodes per patient per year
  - Preparing patient for PD
    - Electively repair ventral and inguinal hernias
    - PD catheter placement 4 to 6 weeks before initiation of therapy
- Hemodialysis (HD)
  - HD can be done at home by selected patients but is typically done in a dialysis unit

- Procedure: Dialyze 3 times per week for 3 to 5 hours each treatment
- Requires access to bloodstream (following options in order of preference):
  - Arteriovenous fistula (AVF)
  - Arteriovenous graft (AVG)
  - Dual-lumen catheter
- AVF preferred given lowest risk of infection, superior longevity, and high blood-flow rates
- AVF may take 2 to 8 months to mature, and multiple attempts may be necessary to achieve desired result
- Once a patient chooses HD as modality of renal replacement therapy
  - Refer patient to vascular surgeon 6 to 12 months before the anticipated need for dialysis to allow for AVF maturation
  - Phlebotomy and blood pressure measurement should be performed on dominant arm, reserving nondominant arm for dialysis access
    - Preferably use hand veins for phlebotomy

Review Questions

For review questions, please go to ExpertConsult.com.

SUGGESTED READINGS

Clinical evaluation and management of chronic kidney disease. In: Johnson RJ, Feehally J, Floege J, eds. *Comprehensive clinical nephrology.* 5th ed. Philadelphia: Elsevier; 2015.

Inker LA, Levey AS. Staging and management of chronic kidney disease. In: Gilbert SJ, Weiner DE, eds. *Primer on kidney diseases.* 6th ed. Philadelphia: Elsevier; 2014.

Kidney Diseases Improving Global Outcomes. KDIGO 2012 Clinical Practice Guidelines for the Evaluation and Management of Chronic Kidney Disease. <http://kdigo.org/home/guidelines/ckd -evaluation-management/>.

Perazella MA. Current status of gadolinium toxicity in patients with kidney disease. *Clin J Am Soc Nephrol.* 2009;4:461-469.

Post TW, Rose BD. Overview of the management of chronic renal failure. Available at: <www.uptodate.com/contents/overview-of-the -management-of-chronic-kidney-disease-in-adults>.

The National Kidney Foundation Kidney Disease Outcomes Quality Initiative (NKF KDOQI). Available at: <www.kidney.org/professionals/ KDOQI>.

Selected Topics in Nephrology

Sumeska Thavarajah, MD; Michelle M. Estrella, MD, MHS; and Michael J. Choi, MD

Hematuria and nephrolithiasis are among the most common clinical problems in nephrology. The differential diagnosis and associated conditions for both hematuria and nephrolithiasis can be narrowed by a stepwise approach to the clinical presentation.

Hematuria

Basic Information

- **Microscopic hematuria**
  - Typically discovered on urinalysis in the **asymptomatic** adult
  - **Increasing incidence with age;** some series show 2% to 18% of those older than 50 years have microscopic hematuria
  - **More than 3 red blood cells (RBCs) per high-power field**
  - Urine dipstick testing is highly sensitive for microscopic hematuria but is not specific. **Heme positive testing in the absence of RBCs suggests myoglobinuria, intravascular hemolysis, povidone-iodine administration, or the presence of oxidizing agents**
- **Gross hematuria**
  - Less common than microscopic hematuria
  - **Presenting symptom in up to 85% of patients diagnosed with bladder cancer and 40% of those with renal cell carcinoma**
  - **Pseudohematuria is the presence of red urine without blood. It may be seen after ingestion of certain foods (e.g., beets, rhubarb) or medications (e.g., phenazopyridine, phenothiazines) or may result from other medical diseases (e.g., porphyria)**
- **General approach to the evaluation of the patient with hematuria**
  - History: Important details include timing, associated symptoms, social and family history (Table 36-1)
  - Laboratory evaluation: Important details include associated abnormalities in urine (e.g., protein, white blood cells [WBCs]) and appearance of RBCs (Table 36-2)
  - The differential diagnosis of hematuria may be divided into glomerular and nonglomerular causes (Fig. 36-1). Depending on the clinical picture, several radiologic studies may be of diagnostic use (Table 36-3). The general approach to the work-up of hematuria is summarized in Fig. 36-2.

- **Patients on anticoagulation who develop hematuria should undergo urologic evaluation.** Excessive anticoagulation resulting in glomerular bleeding is usually a diagnosis of exclusion.
- **The incidence of urinary tract malignancies increases with age.** Those older than 55 years or those with risk factors for bladder or renal malignancy should be referred for urologic evaluation.

Nonglomerular Causes of Hematuria

- **Extrarenal disorders**
  - **The most common causes of hematuria are urinary tract infections and nephrolithiasis**
  - Benign prostatic hyperplasia, endometriosis, and neoplasms of the bladder, prostate, ureters, cervix, and uterus may manifest with either microscopic or gross hematuria
- **Nonglomerular renal disorders**
  - **Autosomal dominant polycystic kidney disease (ADPKD)**
    - Seen in 1 in 500 to 1 in 1000 people
    - Two subtypes: 85% to 95% of cases are *ADPKD1*, located on chromosome 16; the remaining 5% to 15% are *ADPKD2*, located on chromosome 4
    - **Clinical presentation includes gross or microscopic hematuria in 50% of patients, hypertension, flank pain, abdominal distension, and palpable kidneys**
    - **Renal cysts are evident on computed tomography (CT) or ultrasound by age 30 years in those with a positive family history**
    - **Intracranial aneurysms seen in less than 10%; screen for aneurysm if positive family history, symptoms, or high-risk occupation where loss of consciousness would place patient or others at risk**
    - **Other extrarenal manifestations include hepatic cysts, ovarian cysts, mitral valve prolapse, diverticulosis, and hernias**
  - **Exercise-induced hematuria**
    - Usually microscopic; may rarely be associated with **RBC casts**
    - Mechanism unclear, but may be caused by bladder trauma or glomerular ischemia
    - Seen in both contact and noncontact sports
    - Typically resolves with 1 to 3 days of rest

TABLE 36-1 — Historical Details in the Evaluation of the Patient with Hematuria

Historical Details

Timing	Transient
	Can be caused by fever, exercise, CHF. Rule out contamination by menstrual blood
	Initiation of void
	Often implies urethral source
	End of void
	Often implies bladder source
Associated signs and symptoms	Dysuria
	Suggests urinary tract infection
	Flank pain
	Suggests nephrolithiasis or papillary necrosis
	Weight loss, fatigue
	Suggests vasculitis or cancer
	Albuminuria
	Suggests glomerular source

Medications

Analgesics	Suggests papillary necrosis
Antibiotics, other	Consider acute interstitial nephritis, especially if other evidence of hypersensitivity

Family/Social History

FH of renal failure	Suggests inheritable kidney disease, such as autosomal dominant polycystic kidney disease, IgA nephropathy, or others
FH of hematuria in men only	Suggests Alport syndrome (especially if associated with deafness)
SH of tobacco use or dye exposure	Suggests bladder cancer

CHF, Congestive heart failure; FH, family history; SH, social history.

TABLE 36-2 — Laboratory Evaluation of the Patient with Hematuria

Urinalysis

Clots

Most likely urologic source

Proteinuria, dysmorphic RBCs, RBC casts

Indicates glomerular source; consider serologic evaluation with ANA, complement, cryoglobulins, ANCA, anti-GBM, ASO, hepatitis serologies, and rheumatoid factor

Pyuria

Suggests infection or interstitial nephritis; consider urine culture and Hansel's stain for eosinophils

Urine Cytopathology

Obtain if bladder cancer suspected

May detect bladder carcinoma in situ missed by cystoscopy

ANA, Antinuclear antibody; ANCA, antineutrophil cytoplasmic antibody; ASO, antistreptolysin O; GBM, glomerular basement membrane; RBC, red blood cell.

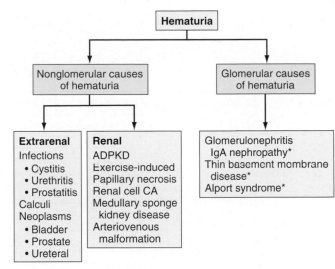

FIGURE 36-1 Causes of hematuria. *Can present with less than 500 mg/day of proteinuria. ADPKD, Autosomal dominant polycystic kidney disease; CA, cancer; IgA, immunoglobulin A.

36

TABLE 36-3 — Imaging Modalities for Evaluation of Hematuria

IVP	Use when nonglomerular cause suggested
	Definitive test for medullary sponge kidney and papillary necrosis
	Superior to ultrasound for detection of stones or cancer in the ureters
	Cannot distinguish between solid and cystic renal masses
	Largely replaced by CT urography
Ultrasound	Use when glomerular cause suspected
	Use when dye allergy or kidney disease present Superior to IVP for ADPKD, renal cell CA, small-bladder CA
	Limited detection of small solid lesions (<3 cm)
CT scan	Superior to IVP for nephrolithiasis
	Better definition of masses
	More expensive than IVP or ultrasound
CT urography	Most sensitive test for hematuria
	Noncontrast CT performed first to evaluate for stones
	If negative, contrast CT is performed with arterial, venous, and delayed imaging with 3D reconstructions

ADPKD, Autosomal dominant polycystic kidney disease; CA, cancer; CT, computed tomography; IVP, intravenous pyelogram.

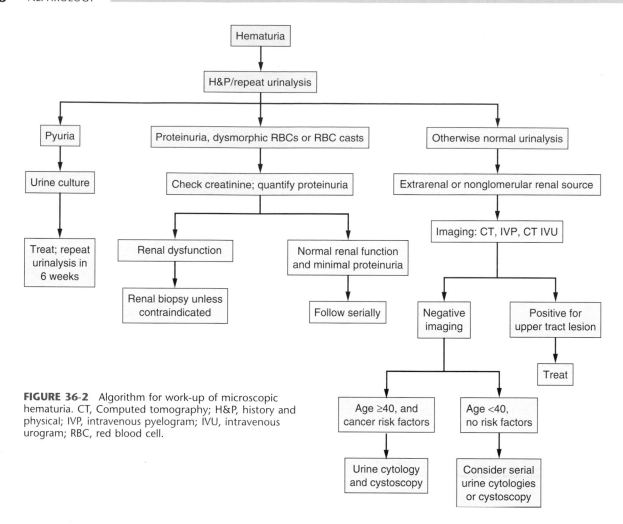

FIGURE 36-2 Algorithm for work-up of microscopic hematuria. CT, Computed tomography; H&P, history and physical; IVP, intravenous pyelogram; IVU, intravenous urogram; RBC, red blood cell.

- **Papillary necrosis**
  - Results from **ischemic damage** to renal papillae
  - **May be precipitated by:**
    - **Sickle cell disease**
    - **Diabetes mellitus**
    - **Heavy use of phenacetin or paracetamol**
    - **Nonsteroidal antiinflammatory drugs**
    - **Urinary tract obstruction**
    - **Tuberculosis**
  - Diagnose by CT urogram or intravenous pyelogram (IVP) (rarely performed)
    - Reveals characteristic changes (Fig. 36-3)
    - Necrotic papillary debris occasionally identified in urine
- **Renal infarction**
  - Thromboembolic event or occlusion of renal artery resulting in renal ischemia and pain
- **Renal trauma**
  - Presents with flank pain and elevated blood pressure
  - Supportive therapy unless evidence of ongoing bleeding

Glomerular Causes of Hematuria

- **The urinalysis serves as an important diagnostic tool in determining a glomerular cause of**

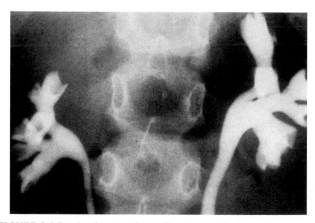

FIGURE 36-3 Grades II and III reflux in a voiding cystourethrographic study from a young boy who presented with recurrent urinary tract infection. Note early clubbing of the calyces and dilation of the ureter on the left side. (From Mandell GL, Bennett JE, Dolin R. *Principles and practice of infectious diseases.* 6th ed. Philadelphia: Churchill Livingstone; 2005, Fig. 66-19.)

hematuria by indicating the presence of proteinuria and/or demonstrating the presence of dysmorphic RBCs and RBC casts

- Dysmorphic RBCs form when RBCs pass through the glomerular basement membrane, resulting in crenated

RBCs (more than 80% dysmorphic RBCs under phase contrast microscopy; Fig. 36-4)
- RBC casts result from RBCs adhering to one another in the presence of Tamm-Horsfall protein, forming a "cast" of the tubule (Fig. 36-5)
- **IgA nephropathy, thin basement membrane disease, and Alport syndrome are the three most common glomerular causes of isolated hematuria**

without significant proteinuria (less than 500 mg/ day) (Table 36-4; see also Fig. 36-1 and Chapter 34)
- **Evidence of systemic illness (e.g., fatigue, arthralgias, hemoptysis, and sore throat) should prompt consideration for collagen vascular disease, other autoimmune disease, postinfectious glomerulonephritis, or viral hepatitis**

Nephrolithiasis

Basic Information

- Epidemiology:
  - 2:1 male:female
  - Approximately 16% of men and 8% of women will have a symptomatic stone by age 70

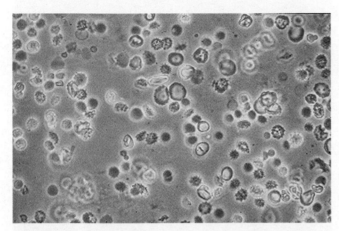

FIGURE 36-4 Dysmorphic erythrocytes as seen under phase-contrast microscopy. These dysmorphic erythrocytes vary in size, shape, and hemoglobin content and reflect glomerular bleeding. (From Johnson RJ, Feehally J. *Comprehensive clinical nephrology*. London: Mosby; 2000, Fig. 4.4.)

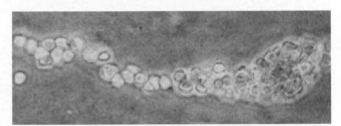

FIGURE 36-5 A cast composed entirely of erythrocytes reflects heavy hematuria and active glomerular disease. (From Johnson RJ, Feehally J. *Comprehensive clinical nephrology*. London: Mosby; 2000, Fig. 4.8B.)

TABLE 36-4	*Glomerular Etiologies of Hematuria Without Proteinuria*		
Disorder	**Diagnosis**	**Associated Findings**	**Treatment**
IgA nephropathy (Berger disease)	Renal biopsy; IgA immune complex deposits in glomerular mesangium Usually seen in young men (M:F 3:1)	Idiopathic form presents as microscopic hematuria or gross hematuria 1–3 days after URI Secondary forms may be associated with cirrhosis, inflammatory bowel disease Increased serum creatinine at diagnosis, >1 g/day proteinuria, hypertension, and scarring on biopsy portend worse prognosis ESRD in 20% after 20 years	ACEI/ARB if proteinuria present Consider corticosteroids if creatinine rising rapidly or if urine protein >1 g/day despite ACEI/ARB Fish oil (controversial) if >1 g/day proteinuria
Thin basement membrane disease (benign familial hematuria)	Familial; autosomal dominant; glomerular basement membrane is half normal thickness	90% present with microscopic hematuria; gross hematuria uncommon. Proteinuria may be present, usually <1.5 g/day	No treatment in most ACEI/ARB in those with proteinuria, as 10% may develop FSGS with progressive CKD
Alport syndrome (hereditary nephritis)	Familial 80% are X-linked because of mutations in COL4A5 Remainder are AD or AR	Microscopic or gross hematuria Proteinuria (late) High-tone sensorineural deafness Lenticonus or cataracts ESRD in majority by age 35	Supportive measures
Warfarin-related nephropathy	AKI associated with INR >3 Renal biopsy reveals tubules obstructed by erythrocytes	Normal baseline kidney function or CKD Microscopic hematuria	Supportive measures Reduction of INR

ACEI, Angiotensin-converting enzyme inhibitor; AD, autosomal dominant; AKI, acute kidney injury; AR, autosomal recessive; ARB, angiotensin receptor blocker; CKD, chronic kidney disease; ESRD, end-stage renal disease; FSGS, focal segmental glomerulosclerosis; IgA, immunoglobulin A; INR, international normalized ratio; M:F, male:female ratio; URI, upper respiratory infection.

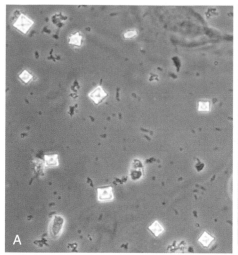
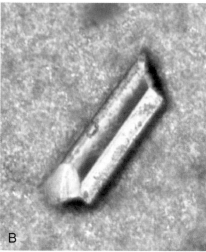
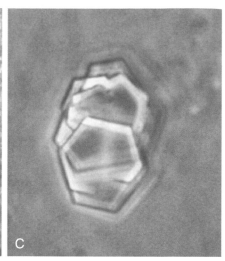

FIGURE 36-6 Representative crystalluria. **A,** Envelope-shaped crystals of calcium oxalate; **B,** Coffin-lid-shaped crystal of struvite (magnesium ammonium phosphate crystals); **C,** Hexagon-shaped crystals of cystine. (From Floege J, Johnson R, Feehally J. *Comprehensive clinical nephrology.* 4th ed. Philadelphia: Elsevier; 2010, Fig. 4.7.)

- There is a 35% to 40% risk of a second stone within 5 years
- Stone types (Fig. 36-6)
  - Calcium-based (oxalate and phosphate): 75% (pure calcium phosphate: 5%)
  - Uric acid: 10% to 12%
  - Struvite: 10% to 20%
  - Cystine: Less than 1%
  - Other (triamterene, indinavir): rare

Clinical Presentation

- Symptoms
  - Typically **severe flank pain radiating to the groin,** often described as worst pain for men, and worst (other than childbirth) for women
  - Some have no pain, with the stone discovered during the evaluation of microscopic or gross hematuria
  - Asymptomatic: incidental finding on abdominal imaging
- **Most commonly caused by idiopathic hypercalciuria**
- **Oxalate crystals can be seen with ethylene glycol poisoning**
- Often seen in the following conditions:
  - Recurrent urinary tract infections
  - Sarcoidosis
  - Distal renal tubular acidosis
  - Primary hyperparathyroidism
  - Intestinal fat malabsorption
  - Low urine volume (e.g., chronic diarrhea, low fluid intake)
  - Diabetes mellitus
  - Obesity
  - Family history of nephrolithiasis

Diagnosis

- **Initial step is to image stone and rule out obstruction (Fig. 36-7)**
  - In the past, IVP was the gold-standard imaging study, but has been largely replaced by **noncontrast stone-protocol CT**

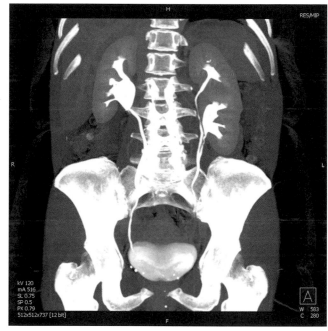

FIGURE 36-7 Computed tomography urogram demonstrating duplicated collecting system of left kidney. (Courtesy Dr. C. John Sperati.)

- IVP and CT urography remain the best for diagnosing medullary sponge kidney disease (anatomic abnormality with outpouching of collecting ducts leading to urinary stasis)
- Urinalysis and culture should be obtained
  - **The presence of WBCs may indicate inflammation without infection**
  - Infected kidney stones need antibiotic treatment and removal
- Strain urine to capture stone for laboratory analysis of its composition
- **Standard initial studies include serum electrolytes, calcium, phosphorus, uric acid ± intact parathyroid hormone**

TABLE 36-5	*Nephrolithiasis: Risk Factors and Treatment*		
Stone Type	**Risk Factors**	**Treatment**	**Comments**
Calcium oxalate	*Hypercalciuria* (urine calcium >300 mg/day in men; >250 mg/day in women) Most common risk factor (e.g., idiopathic, hyperparathyroidism, excess vitamin D)	Low-sodium diet (urine calcium excretion parallels urine sodium excretion) Thiazide diuretics	Envelope-shaped crystals "Idiopathic" most common cause of hypercalciuria
	Hyperoxaluria (urine oxalate >40 mg/day) Fat malabsorption leads to increased colonic absorption of oxalate	Do not restrict calcium intake, as restriction leads to increased intestinal oxalate absorption and increased urinary oxalate excretion	Potatoes, strawberries, spinach, brewed tea, nuts, and chocolate high in oxalate, high-dose vitamin C (>1 g/day)
	Hypocitraturia (urine citrate <320 mg/day in some labs vs <450 mg/day in men and <550 mg/day in women in other labs) Distal RTA, diarrhea	Potassium citrate	
	Hyperuricosuria (<800 mg/day for men and <750 mg/day for women)	Decrease purine intake Allopurinol	
Calcium phosphate	Distal (type 1) RTA, primary hyperparathyroidism Alkaline urine	See hypercalciuria treatment	Pure calcium phosphate stones are uncommon. See hypocitraturia with distal RTA
Uric acid	Acidic urine High urine uric acid (e.g., gout, myeloproliferative disorder)	Potassium citrate if acidic urine Restrict purine intake Allopurinol if hyperuricosuria.	Radiolucent crystals on plain film
Struvite	Urinary tract infection with urease-producing bacteria (e.g., *Proteus*)	Antibiotics Urologic procedure to remove stone	Crystals resemble coffin lids Form staghorn calculi
Cystine	Genetic defect resulting in decreased tubular reabsorption of cystine (urine cystine excretion >400 mg/day)	High fluid intake to decrease urine cystine concentration Alkalinize urine Consider therapy to solubilize crystals with tiopronin, penicillamine, or captopril	Hexagonal greenish-yellow crystals pathognomonic Respond poorly to lithotripsy

RTA, Renal tubular acidosis.

36

- 24-hour urine collection for stone risk profile if:
  - Associated comorbid conditions are present
  - Required stone extraction
  - Recurrent episodes of nephrolithiasis
  - Childhood onset

Treatment

- See Table 36-5 for risk factors and treatment of nephrolithiasis
- Core interventions:
  - Increase fluid intake to ensure urine output more than 2L/day
  - Diet low in animal protein, low in sodium, and normal in calcium intake may reduce recurrent calcium stone formation
- Uncertain if first episode of calcium nephrolithiasis should be extensively evaluated

- **Risk of recurrence after single episode is approximately 35% to 40% over the next 5 years**

Review Questions

For review questions, please go to ExpertConsult.com.

SUGGESTED READINGS

Margulis V, Sagalowsky AI. Assessment of hematuria. *Med Clin North Am.* 2011;95:153-159.
Reynolds TM. Chemical pathology, clinical investigation and management of nephrolithaisis. *J Clin Pathol.* 2005;58:134-140.
Worcester EM, Coe FL. Calcium kidney stones. *N Engl J Med.* 2010;363:954-963.

SECTION SIX

Endocrinology

Diabetes Mellitus

SHERITA H. GOLDEN, MD, MHS

Diabetes is a major health problem. Approximately 8% of the United States population, or 17.9 million individuals, have been diagnosed with diabetes, and it is estimated that 5.4 million individuals have undiagnosed diabetes. Type 2 diabetes accounts for 90% to 95% of cases. Significant complications of diabetes include retinopathy, nephropathy, neuropathy, and cardiovascular disease. Approximately 182,000 deaths per year are related to diabetes and its complications, making it the third largest killer in this country. Whereas death from cardiovascular disease has declined over the past 2 decades, death from diabetes continues to increase.

Diabetes Mellitus

Basic Information

- Diabetes mellitus encompasses several syndromes of altered insulin secretion and/or peripheral resistance that result in hyperglycemia
- Classification of diabetes
  - Type 1 diabetes
  - Type 2 diabetes
  - Gestational diabetes
  - Other specific types
    - Genetic defects: β-cell function, insulin action
    - Disease of exocrine pancreas
    - Endocrinopathies
    - Drug- or chemical-induced
    - Infection-related
    - Other genetic syndromes associated with diabetes
- Pathogenesis of type 1 diabetes mellitus
  - Patients require insulin to prevent hyperglycemia and ketosis
  - Pancreatic β-cell destruction with resulting complete insulinopenia
  - Immune-mediated: Anti-islet cell antibodies and anti-insulin antibodies are humoral markers of islet cell inflammation
  - Idiopathic
- Pathogenesis of type 2 diabetes mellitus
  - Impaired insulin secretion because of β-cell dysfunction
  - Insulin resistance leads to increased hepatic glucose production and decreased peripheral glucose uptake
- Distinguishing between type 1 and type 2 (see Table 37-1)

Clinical Presentation

- Main symptoms include polyphagia, polydipsia, and polyuria

- Type 1 diabetes typically presents in the first two decades of life; however, type 1 diabetes can present in adulthood and is then referred to as latent autoimmune diabetes of adulthood (LADA)
- Type 2 diabetes typically presents after age 40 years
- Acute complications include diabetic ketoacidosis and hyperosmolar hyperglycemic state (Fig. 37-1)
- Chronic complications
  - Nephropathy (see section on diabetic nephropathy)
  - Retinopathy (see section on diabetic retinopathy)
  - Neuropathy (see section on diabetic neuropathy)
  - Cardiovascular disease (see section on cardiovascular disease)
  - Skin manifestations
    - Acanthosis nigricans (Fig. 37-2)
      - Dark, velvety, thickened plaques occurring in flexural areas (axilla, inguinal crease, back and sides of neck)
      - Frequently associated with insulin resistance and obesity; can also be related to underlying malignancy (especially gastrointestinal and lung)
      - Treatment
        - Weight reduction, treatment of the diabetes or underlying disorder
        - For severe, odorous lesions: antibacterial soaps, topical antibiotics
    - Necrobiosis lipoidica (Fig. 37-3)
      - Inflammatory skin condition of unknown etiology; frequently associated with diabetes or impaired glucose tolerance
      - Often asymptomatic lesions; usually occur on the shin
      - Indurated, oval plaques with central atrophy and yellow pigmentation; red-brown margins
      - Treatment is often suboptimal
        - First-line: topical or intralesional steroids
        - For ulcers: cyclosporine, hyperbaric oxygen, infliximab, and others can be tried

Diagnosis and Evaluation

- Four main criteria are used for diagnosis of diabetes (only one of the four is required for diagnosis)
  - Symptoms of diabetes (e.g., polyuria, polydipsia, weight loss, ketoacidosis, hyperosmolarity) plus random plasma glucose greater than 200 mg/dL
  - Fasting plasma glucose126 mg/dL or greater or random plasma glucose greater than 200 mg/dL on two separate occasions

TABLE 37-1	*Distinguishing Between Types 1 and 2 Diabetes Mellitus*	
	Type 1	**Type 2**
Body weight	Lean or normal History of weight loss before presentation	Overweight or obese History of weight gain before diagnosis
Family history	<20% first-degree relatives with diabetes	Strong family history of first-degree relatives with diabetes
Other autoimmune disorders	May be present: Hashimoto thyroiditis, Graves disease, vitiligo, adrenal insufficiency, pernicious anemia	Absent
Glycemic patterns	Greater daily variability Exaggerated hyperglycemic response to stressors and meals	Blood glucose more stable throughout day
Response to oral agents	Nonresponsive	Responsive
Insulin sensitivity	Normal	Very reduced
Islet cell antibodies and/or Glutamic acid decarboxylase (GAD) antibodies	Around 80% have detectable titers at onset	Not present
C-peptide	Very low or undetectable	Detectable or elevated

- Two-hour plasma glucose 200 mg/dL or greater after ingestion of a 75-g glucose load (oral glucose tolerance test [OGTT]) on two occasions
- Hemoglobin A_{1c} (Hgb A_{1c}) 6.5% or greater
- Diagnostic criteria for "prediabetes":
  - Impaired glucose tolerance: 2-hour plasma glucose 140 to 199 mg/dL during OGTT
  - Impaired fasting glucose: fasting plasma glucose 100 to 125 mg/dL
  - Increased risk for type 2 diabetes: Hgb A_{1c} 5.7% to 6.4%

Treatment

- Treatment objective is glycemic control
  - Glycemic control reduces long-term microvascular complications (e.g., nephropathy, neuropathy, and retinopathy) in both type 1 and type 2 diabetic patients
  - **Goals for glycemic control: see Table 37-2**
  - **Insulin therapy is necessary for type 1 diabetic patients**

- Oral agents and/or insulin therapy may be used in type 2 diabetic patients
- Insulin therapy
  - Different forms of insulin are characterized by their duration of action (Table 37-3)
  - **Total daily dosage (TDD) of insulin depends on the type of diabetes, diet, exercise, and degree of insulin resistance**
    - Type 1 diabetes: 0.5 U/kg/day
    - Type 2 diabetes: 0.4 to 1 U/kg/day for patient on only insulin therapy and not on oral agents; daily insulin requirements may be less in patients on insulin-sensitizing agents
  - For both type 1 and type 2 diabetic patients, the insulin regimen should be divided as follows:
    - Determine TDD by multiplying body weight in kilograms by
      - 0.5 to 0.7 U/kg if patient has type 1 diabetes
      - 0.4 to 1 (or more) U/kg if patient has type 2 diabetes
    - Determine the basal insulin requirement
      - 40% to 50% of TDD
      - Options for administration
        - Continuous subcutaneous insulin infusion (CSII) (i.e., insulin pump)
        - Long-acting insulin analogue (glargine or detemir) once daily in the morning or at bedtime
        - Intermediate (neutral protamine Hagedorn [NPH]) twice a day in the morning and at bedtime
    - Determine prandial insulin requirement
      - TDD minus basal insulin dose
      - Split to cover meals
        - Rapid-acting insulin: lispro, aspart, or glulisine
          - Divide into three injections (at start of meal or 15 to 30 minutes before breakfast, lunch, and dinner)
        - Regular: Divide into two injections (before breakfast and dinner)
  - Correction or supplemental insulin
    - Treats hyperglycemia before meals or between meals
    - Corrects hyperglycemia in nil per os (NPO) patient or in patient receiving scheduled nutritional or basal insulin but not eating discrete meals
    - Sliding scale correction dose based on preprandial blood glucose
      - 1 U per 50-mg/dL increment over 180 mg/dL (type 1)
      - 1 U per 30-mg/dL increment over 180 mg/dL (type 2)
- Insulin is the preferable first-line therapy in certain clinical situations
  - Pregnancy: Only insulin is approved for use in pregnancy
  - Polyuria/polydipsia: Indicates severe hyperglycemia that should be rapidly reversed with insulin therapy
  - Ketosis: Indicates insulinopenia
  - Latent autoimmune diabetes of adulthood

37

PROTOCOL FOR MANAGEMENT OF ADULT PATIENTS WITH DKA OR HHS

Complete initial evaluation. Check capillary glucose and serum/urine ketones to confirm hyperglycemia and ketonemia/ketonuria. Obtain blood for metabolic profile.
Start IV fluids: 1.0 L. of 0.9% NaCl per hour.[†]

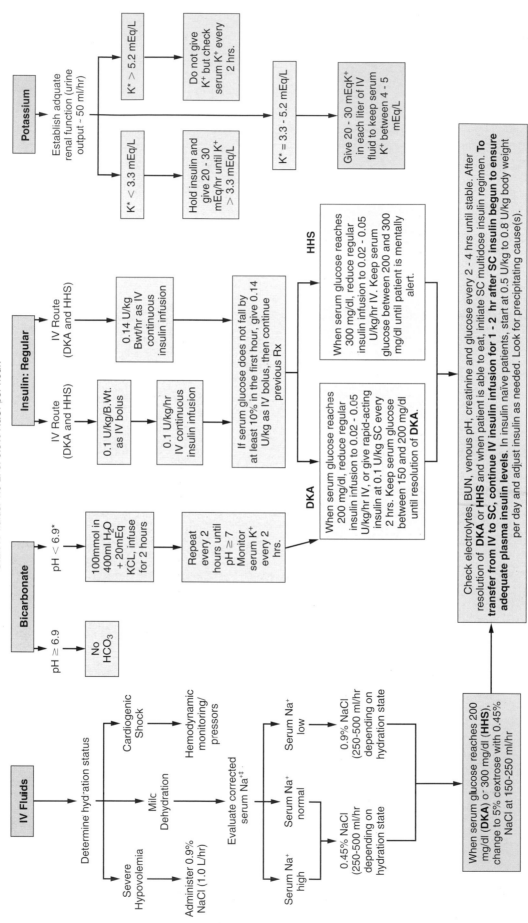

FIGURE 37-1 Protocol for the management of adult patients with diabetic ketoacidosis (DKA) or hyperosmolar hyperglycemic state (HHS). ACTH, Adrenocorticotropic hormone; ARDS, acute respiratory distress syndrome; BUN, blood urea nitrogen; Bwt, body weight; IV, intravenous; KCl, potassium chloride; KPO4, potassium phosphate; L, liter; Na, sodium; NaC, sodium chloride; SC, subcutaneous; U, units.

DKA diagnostic criteria: blood glucose 250 mg/dl, arterial pH 7.3, bicarbonate 15 mEq/l, and moderate ketonuria or ketonemia. HHS diagnostic criteria: serum glucose >600 mg/dl, arterial pH >7.3, serum bicarbonate >15 mEq/l, and minimal ketonuria and ketonemia. †15-20 ml/kg/h; ‡serum Na should be corrected for hyperglycemia (for each 100 mg/dl glucose 100 mg/dl, add 1.6 mEq to sodium value for corrected value). (Adapted from ref. 13.) Bwt, body weight; IV, intravenous; SC, subcutaneous.

*JHH Recommendations: For arterial pH < 7, give 150 mEq of Bicarbonate in 1000 mL of sterile water over 2 hours.

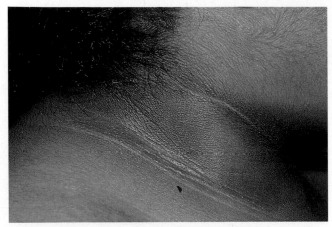

FIGURE 37-2 Acanthosis nigricans occurring in the neck of a patient with severe insulin resistance associated with obesity. (From Besser GM, Thorner M. *Comprehensive Clinical Endocrinology.* 3rd ed. St. Louis: Mosby; 2002: Fig. 36.7.)

TABLE 37-2	*American Diabetes Association Recommended Glycemic Targets for Nonpregnant Adults*
	Glycemic Goals
Preprandial capillary plasma glucose	70–130 mg/dL
Postprandial capillary plasma glucose	<180 mg/dL
Hgb A$_{1c}$	<7%

Hgb A$_{1c}$, Glycosylated hemoglobin A$_{1c}$.

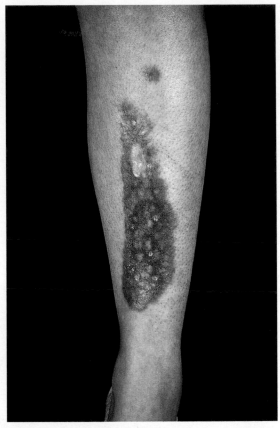

FIGURE 37-3 Necrobiosis lipoidica. (From Swash M. *Hutchinson's Clinical Methods.* 21st ed. Philadelphia: Saunders; 2002: Fig. 8.8.)

TABLE 37-3	*Types of Insulin*		
	Onset of Action	**Peak of Action**	**Duration of Action**
Rapid-acting			
Lispro, aspart, glulisine	5–15 min	1–2 h	3–5 h
Regular	30–60 min	2–4 h	6–8 h
Intermediate-acting			
Neutral protamine Hagedorn	1–3 h	5–7 h	13–18 h
Long-acting			
Glargine	Within 4 hours	Peakless	>24 h
Detemir	Within 4 hours	Peakless	18–24 h

- Suspect in lean individuals presenting in middle age who do not respond to oral agents
- These individuals really have type 1 diabetes presenting later in life and require insulin therapy
- Insulin antibodies (antiglutamic acid decarboxylase and antiislet cell) may be positive within the first year of diagnosis
- Oral antihyperglycemic agents
  - Classes of oral agents: see Table 37-4
  - Multiple factors should be considered in selecting initial oral hypoglycemic agents for patients with type 2 diabetes (Fig. 37-4 gives suggested algorithm)
  - Degree of reduction needed in glycosylated Hgb A$_{1c}$ and/or fasting blood glucose

- Sulfonylureas, biguanides (metformin), and thiazolidinediones all lower Hgb A$_{1c}$ 1 to 2 percentage points on average when used as monotherapy
- Agents targeted at reducing postprandial hyperglycemia, meglitinides, α-glucosidase inhibitors, dipeptidyl peptidase-4 (DPP-4) inhibitors, and sodium-glucose cotransporter 2 (SGLT2) inhibitors are less potent, lowering Hgb A$_{1c}$ 0.5 to 1 percentage point when used as monotherapy
- Body habitus and estimated degree of insulin resistance
  - In obese individuals, insulin resistance is very likely

TABLE 37-4	*Oral Agents for Diabetes Mellitus*		
Therapy	**Mechanism**	**Benefits**	**Precautions**
Metformin	Suppresses hepatic glucose output	No weight gain No hypoglycemia when used as monotherapy	GI side effects: nausea, diarrhea (titrate dose upward slowly to minimize) Contraindicated in renal compromise (Cr ≥1.4 in women; Cr ≥1.5 in men; Cr clearance ≤60) Contraindicated in CHF requiring treatment Discontinuation required before contrast dye studies (may restart in 48 hours if normal renal function) Increased risk of lactic acidosis Older age: Use over age 80 years only if Cr clearance normal Avoid excessive alcohol consumption
Thiazolidinediones Rosiglitazone Pioglitazone	Enhance peripheral muscle sensitivity to insulin	↓ C-peptide and insulin levels No hypoglycemia when used as monotherapy	Monitor LFTs at baseline and every 2 months for first year Contraindicated in active liver disease and/or LFTs >2.5× upper limit of normal Weight gain (~1 to 3 kg) Contraindicated in class III/IV CHF Plasma volume expansion (↓ Hct 3% to 4%) Edema Possible increased MI risk with rosiglitazone Bone fractures
Sulfonylureas Glimepiride Glyburide Glipizide	Increase pancreatic secretion of insulin	Ease of use and familiarity	Weight gain Hypoglycemia Sulfa sensitivity
Metglitinides Repaglinide Nateglinide	Increase pancreatic secretion of insulin	Reduces postprandial hyperglycemia	↓ Compliance caused by multiple daily doses with meals Mild hypoglycemia Use cautiously with liver impairment
Acarbose	Delays glucose absorption by inhibition of pancreatic α-amylase and intestinal α-glucoside	No hypoglycemia as monotherapy Reduces postprandial hyperglycemia	GI: flatulence, cramps, diarrhea Requires multiple dosing with meals Cannot treat hypoglycemia with sucrose
Dipeptidyl Peptidase-4 inhibitors Sitagliptin Saxagliptin Linagliptin	Inhibit breakdown of endogenous incretins, resulting in inhibition of postprandial glucagon release, increased satiety, slowed gastric emptying, and stimulation of glucose-dependent insulin release	No hypoglycemia as monotherapy Reduces postprandial hyperglycemia Weight neutral	Pharyngitis, urinary tract infections, possible pancreatitis; long-term safety not established
Sodium-glucose cotransporter 2 inhibitors Canagliflozin Dapagliflozin	Increase urinary glucose excretion, lower blood glucose, and improve peripheral insulin sensitivity	Weight loss Blood pressure lowering Low hypoglycemia risk	Genital infections, plasma volume depletion; long-term safety not established

CHF, Congestive heart failure; Cr, creatinine; GI, gastrointestinal; Hct, hematocrit; IV, intravenous; LFTs, liver function tests; MI, myocardial infarction.
Modified from Ratner R. *Clinical Endocrinology Update 1999 Syllabus.* Chevy Chase, MD, Washington D.C.: Endocrine Society; 1999.

- Thus, an insulin sensitizer (metformin or thiazolidinedione) would be the preferable therapy
- Because thiazolidinediones can be associated with weight gain and edema, they are not generally recommended as the agent of first choice
- Lean individuals are less likely to be insulin resistant and are more likely to have some β-cell reserve, so a sulfonylurea is a preferable first-line agent
- Contraindications to agents (see Table 37-4)
  - Metformin is contraindicated in renal insufficiency (creatinine 1.4 mg/dL or more in women and 1.5 mg/dL or more in men), treated congestive heart failure, hypoxemia, hypotension, and binge alcohol use, as these conditions increase the risk of lactic acidosis
  - Thiazolidinediones are contraindicated in patients in classes III and IV congestive heart failure and in individuals with active liver disease

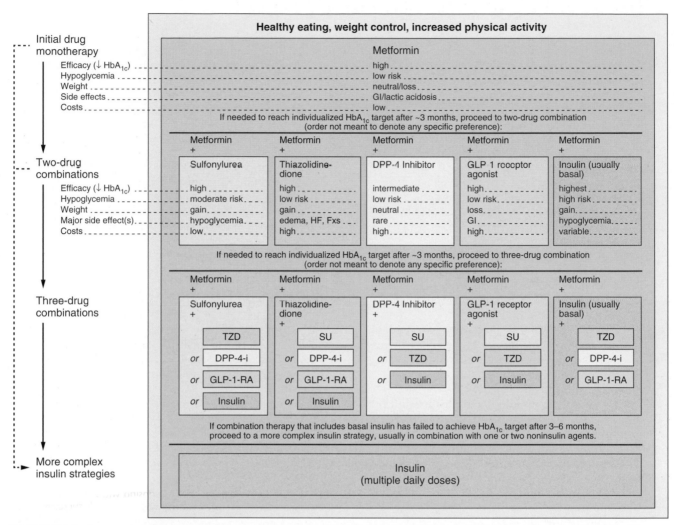

FIGURE 37-4 A suggested algorithm for initiating oral therapy in type 2 diabetes. DPP-4-i, DPP-4 inhibitor; Fxs, bone fractures; GI, gastrointestinal; GLP-1-RA, GLP-1 receptor antagonist; HF, heart failure; SU, sulfonylurea; TZD, thiazolidinedione. (Modified from American Diabetes Association. Standards of Medical Care in Diabetes—2014. *Diabetes Care.* 2014;37:S14-S80.)

- Potential for adverse health risks of hypoglycemia in patients with cerebrovascular or cardiovascular disease
    - Metformin, thiazolidinediones, acarbose, dipeptidyl peptidase 4-intravenous (DPP-IV) inhibitors, and SGLT2 inhibitors do not cause hypoglycemia when used as monotherapy
- Possibility of postprandial hyperglycemia (should be suspected when there is a poor correlation between fasting glucose readings and Hgb A_{1c})
    - Agents that target postprandial hyperglycemia are the meglitinides, acarbose, and DPP-IV inhibitors
- Presence of a coexisting lipid disorder
    - Metformin lowers low-density lipoprotein (LDL) and triglycerides and has no effect on high-density lipoprotein (HDL)
    - Compared with rosiglitazone, pioglitazone resulted in a significant reduction in triglycerides, a greater increase in HDL cholesterol, a smaller rise in LDL cholesterol, and a greater increase in LDL particle size
- Subcutaneous noninsulin glucoregulatory hormone replacement

- The incretins, glucagon-like peptide and glucose-dependent insulinotropic polypeptide, are gut-derived hormones released in response to meals
- Amylin is a β-cell hormone cosecreted with insulin in response to meals
- **The incretin mimetics, exenatide and liraglutide (glucagon-like peptide-1 analogues), and the amylin agonist pramlintide both stimulate glucose-dependent insulin release in response to meals, inhibit glucagon release, and slow gastric emptying in patients with type 2 diabetes when administered by subcutaneous injection**
- Dosages and indications
    - Exenatide
        - Exenatide lowers Hgb A_{1c} by 0.4% to 1% when added to sulfonylurea, metformin, thiazolidinediones, or combination therapy
        - Indicated for patients with type 2 diabetes who have not attained adequate glycemic control on maximal sulfonylurea, metformin, and combination therapy
    - Liraglutide

- Liraglutide lowers Hgb A_{1c} by 0.5% to 1% when used as monotherapy and 0.9% to 1.4% when used in combination with metformin, sulfonylureas, or thiazolidinediones
- Indicated for patients with type 2 diabetes as an adjunct to diet and exercise
  - Pramlintide
    - Pramlintide lowers Hgb A_{1c} by approximately 0.4% when added to insulin alone or insulin in combination with metformin and sulfonylureas
    - Indicated for use in patients with type 1 or type 2 diabetes who have not achieved adequate glycemic control on insulin therapy
    - Mealtime insulin should be decreased by 50% to prevent severe hypoglycemia
  - Adverse event considerations:
    - Subcutaneous incretin-based therapies are associated with nausea and vomiting and are contraindicated in patients with gastroparesis
    - Exenatide and liraglutide may be associated with pancreatitis
    - Liraglutide cannot be used in patients with a personal or family history of medullary thyroid cancer or in patients with multiple endocrine neoplasia-II syndrome
- Combination therapy (see Fig. 37-4)
  - Combination therapy (using multiple modalities) is often required even at an early stage to achieve near normoglycemia
  - Monotherapy fails because of multiple factors
    - Decreasing β-cell function
    - Obesity
    - Noncompliance with treatment
    - Lack of exercise
    - Intercurrent illness
  - Oral agents can be combined and/or used with insulin therapy to improve glycemic control
    - Methods of adding insulin to an established oral regimen
      - NPH, glargine, or detemir insulin at bedtime
      - 70/30 or 75/25 insulin at evening meal

- Dose based on weight and blood glucose, but most patients start with around 10 U/day
- Method of adding oral agents to an established insulin therapy: Continue current insulin dosage initially, then decrease the dose by 15% to 25% if hypoglycemia develops or the fasting blood glucose levels are less than 100 mg/dL
- Exenatide and liraglutide can be added to oral therapy with metformin and/or sulfonylureas in type 2 diabetes
- Pramlintide can be added to insulin therapy in type 1 diabetes and to insulin therapy alone or insulin therapy in combination with sulfonylureas and/or metformin in type 2 diabetes
- Treatment of diabetic ketoacidosis (DKA) and hyperosmolar hyperglycemic state (HHS): see Figure 37-1

Diabetic Nephropathy

Basic Information

- 20% to 30% of patients with type 1 or type 2 diabetes develop evidence of nephropathy, but a smaller fraction progress to end-stage renal disease (ESRD) in type 2 diabetes
- Native Americans, Mexican Americans, and African Americans have higher risk of developing ESRD than do white individuals
- Natural history is summarized in Figure 37-5

Clinical Presentation

- Patients usually asymptomatic until late in course
- Characterized by proteinuria and rising creatinine

Diagnosis and Evaluation

- Urine albumin measurement should be performed annually to screen for diabetic nephropathy after 5 years of disease duration in patients with type 1 diabetes and at diagnosis in patients with type 2 diabetes

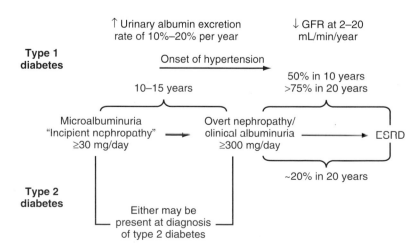

FIGURE 37-5 Natural history of diabetic nephropathy. ESRD, End-stage renal disease; GFR, glomerular filtration rate.

TABLE 37-5	*Definition of Albuminuria*
Category	**Spot Collection (μg/mg creatinine)**
Normal	<30
Increased urinary albumin excretion	≥30

- See Table 37-5 for a definition of albuminuria; two of three specimens collected within a 3- to 6-month period should be abnormal before confirming the diagnosis
- **Factors that may increase urinary albumin excretion over baseline values include exercise within 24 hours, fever, infection, congestive heart failure, marked hyperglycemia, marked hypertension, pyuria, hematuria**
- If initial screening tests are negative, patients should undergo annual screen; whether to continue annual screening after albuminuria has been diagnosed and appropriately treated is less clear

Treatment

- Pharmacologic therapy
  - **Use of angiotensin-converting enzyme (ACE) inhibitors is recommended for all hypertensive and nonhypertensive patients with type 1 diabetes and albuminuria**
  - Angiotensin II receptor blockers (ARBs) are the agents of first choice in hypertensive type 2 diabetic patients with albuminuria
  - Aggressive treatment of hypertension with goal blood pressure of less than 140/80 mm Hg
  - β-Blockers and diuretics are alternatives if ACE inhibitors or ARBs not tolerated or contraindicated
  - Non-dihydropyridine calcium channel blockers should be used as second-line agents
- Behavioral therapy
  - Sodium restriction: Approximately 2000 mg/day
  - Weight loss, moderately intense physical activity (30 to 45 minutes of brisk walking daily), smoking cessation, moderation of alcohol consumption

Diabetic Retinopathy

BASIC INFORMATION

- Diabetic retinopathy is the leading cause of blindness in adults ages 20 to 74 years, and its presence is strongly related to the duration of diabetes
- Factors that increase the risk of retinopathy
  - Hyperglycemia
  - Presence of nephropathy
  - High blood pressure
  - Pregnancy in patients with type 1 diabetes

Clinical Presentation

- Classification of diabetic retinopathy (see Table 37-6 and Figure 37-6)

TABLE 37-6	*Definition of Diabetic Retinopathy*
Nonproliferative	Microaneurysms, increased vascular permeability
Preproliferative	Soft exudates representing ischemic infarcts to the retina (cotton-wool spots), beading of retinal veins, tortuosity of retinal capillaries
Proliferative	Neovascularization (fibrous contraction from previous hemorrhage may lead to retinal detachment)
Rubeosis	Neovascularization of the iris
Macular edema	Suspect if hard exudates in proximity of macula

- Usually asymptomatic unless vitreous hemorrhage occurs (causing visual loss)

Diagnosis and Evaluation

- Ophthalmologic evaluation should be performed starting 5 years after diagnosis of type 1 diabetes and on initial diagnosis of type 2 diabetes (Table 37-7)
- Continue annual screening unless retinopathy warrants more intense follow-up
- Less frequent exams (every 2 to 3 years) can be considered in those with several normal eye exams

Treatment

- Laser photocoagulation therapy to prevent visual loss
  - Panretinal/scatter photocoagulation therapy is treatment to reduce risk of visual loss in patients with high-risk characteristics (neovascularization or vitreous hemorrhage with any retinal neovascularization) and in older-onset patients with severe nonproliferative diabetic retinopathy or less than high-risk proliferative diabetic retinopathy
  - Focal laser photocoagulation surgery for eyes with clinically significant macular edema

Diabetic Neuropathy and Diabetic Foot Disease

- Diabetic neuropathy can take many different forms
- Useful classification
  - Generalized symmetrical polyneuropathies: acute sensory, chronic sensorimotor
  - Focal and multifocal neuropathies: cranial, truncal, focal limb, proximal motor (amyotrophy), coexisting chronic inflammatory demyelinating polyneuropathy (CIDP)
  - Autonomic: cardiac, gastrointestinal, genitourinary
- Chronic sensorimotor distal symmetrical polyneuropathy (DPN) and diabetic autonomic neuropathy (DAN) are the two most common neuropathies
- Distal symmetrical polyneuropathy (DPN)
  - Up to 50% of DPN cases may be asymptomatic, increasing the patient's risk of insensate foot injuries, which can ultimately lead to ulcers and amputations

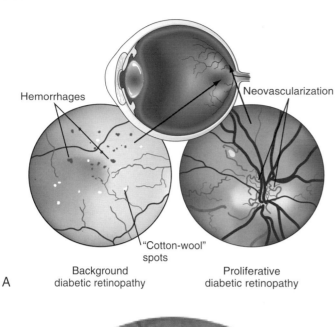

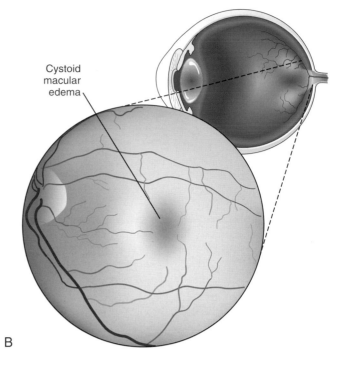

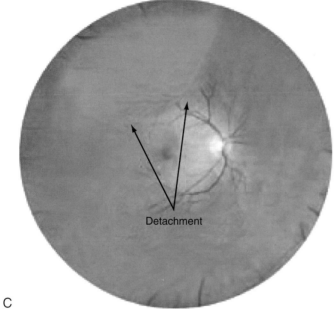

FIGURE 37-6 **A,** Background and proliferative diabetic retinopathy. **B,** Cystoid macular edema. **C,** Retinal detachment.

TABLE 37-7	**Ophthalmologic Examination Schedule**	
Patient Group	**Recommended First Examination**	**Minimum Routine Follow-Up**
≤29 years	Within 3 to 5 years after diagnosis once patient is 10 years or older	Yearly
≥30 years	At diagnosis	Yearly
Pregnancy in patient with preexisting diabetes	Before conception and first trimester	Physician discretion after first trimester

- About 50% of patients have symptoms: Burning pain, electrical or stabbing sensations, paresthesias, hyperesthesia, deep aching pain occurring in the feet and lower limbs; symptoms worse at night
- Diabetic ulcer (Fig. 37-7)
- Patients at increased risk for ulcers and amputations
  - Duration of diabetes 10 years or more
  - Male
  - Poor glucose control
  - Cardiovascular, retinal, or renal complications
  - Peripheral neuropathy with loss of protective sensation
  - Altered foot biomechanics, bony deformity
  - Presence of peripheral vascular disease
  - History of ulcers or amputation

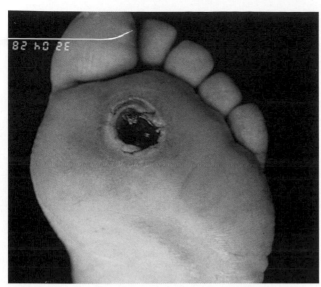

FIGURE 37-7 Stage III ulcer beneath second metatarsal head that extends into metatarsal head with presumptive contiguous osteomyelitis. (From Canale ST. *Campbell's Operative Orthopedics.* 10th ed. St. Louis: Mosby; 2003: Fig. 82-2.)

- Severe nail pathology
- Diagnosis
  - Careful clinical exam with annual screening by examining pinprick, temperature, and vibration perception (using 128-Hz tuning fork), 10-g monofilament pressure sensation at distal halluces, and ankle reflexes
  - Examination in DPN shows loss of vibration, pressure, pain, and temperature sensation, and absent reflexes
  - Signs of peripheral autonomic (sympathetic) dysfunction: Warm or cold feet, distended dorsal foot veins (in absence of peripheral arterial disease), dry skin, calluses in pressure-bearing areas
  - Examine feet for ulcers, calluses, and deformities, and inspect footwear
  - Rule out other forms of neuropathy: CIDP, vitamin B12 deficiency, hypothyroidism, uremia (check B12, thyroid function, blood urea nitrogen, and creatinine)
- Treatment
  - Optimization of blood glucose control and avoiding extreme blood glucose fluctuations
  - Pharmacologic treatment
    - Tricyclic antidepressant drugs: Amitriptyline, imipramine; use limited by anticholinergic side effects, including fatigue and drowsiness
    - Selective serotonin reuptake inhibitors: paroxetine, citalopram
    - Anticonvulsants: gabapentin, pregabalin, carbamazepine, topiramate; use limited by drowsiness
    - Opioid or opioid-like drugs: tramadol, continuous-release oxycodone
    - 5-Hydroxytryptamine and norepinephrine uptake inhibitor: duloxetine
    - Substance P inhibitor: capsaicin cream
  - Podiatry referral to reduce the risk of foot ulcers

- Acute sensory neuropathy
  - Follows periods of poor metabolic control or sudden changes in glycemic control (insulin neuritis)
  - Acute onset of severe sensory symptoms with marked nocturnal exacerbation
  - Few neurologic signs on exam
- Mononeuropathies
  - Focal nerves involved
  - Percent of all diabetic neuropathies
    - Median (5.8%), ulnar (2.1%), radial (0.6%), common peroneal
    - Cranial (0.05%) III, IV, VI, and VII; usually resolve spontaneously
  - Entrapments: median, ulnar, peroneal, medial plantar
  - Spinal stenosis
  - Diagnosis: Electrophysiologic studies useful in identifying conduction blocks at entrapment sites
- Diabetic amyotrophy
  - Occurs in older patients with type 2 diabetes
  - Severe neuropathic pain, unilateral or bilateral muscle weakness, atrophy in proximal thigh muscles
  - Diagnosis: Needs to be distinguished from CIPD and spinal stenosis; CIPD presents with progressive symmetrical or asymmetrical motor deficits, progressive sensory neuropathy despite optimal glucose control, and elevated cerebrospinal fluid protein
- Diabetic autonomic neuropathy (DAN)
  - Cardiovascular autonomic neuropathy (CAN)
    - Associated with morbidity and increased mortality
      - Limits exercise capacity and increases risk of adverse cardiovascular event during exercise
      - May lead to sudden death or silent cardiac ischemia
    - Presentation: Resting tachycardia (heart rate more than 100 beats/min), exercise intolerance, orthostatic hypotension (fall in systolic blood pressure greater than 20 mm Hg on standing)
    - Diagnosis: Three useful tests
      - R-R variation on electrocardiogram (ECG)
      - Valsalva maneuver
      - Postural blood pressure testing
    - Treatment of CAN
      - Graded supervised exercise, ACE inhibitors, and β-blockers for exercise intolerance
      - Mechanical measures, clonidine, midodrine, octreotide to treat postural hypotension
  - Gastrointestinal autonomic neuropathy
    - Presentation: constipation (may alternate with diarrhea), gastroparesis, esophageal enteropathy, fecal incontinence; consider especially in individuals with erratic glucose control
    - Diagnosis: evaluation with gastric emptying study, barium swallow, or referral for endoscopy
    - Treatment
      - Treat gastroparesis with frequent small meals and prokinetic agents (metoclopramide, domperidone, erythromycin)
      - Abdominal pain, early satiety, nausea, vomiting, and bloating treated with multiple approaches:

37

TABLE 37-8	*Cholesterol Targets in Patients with Diabetes*				
	MEDICAL NUTRITION TREATMENT		**DRUG TREATMENT**		
Status	**Initiation Level**	**LDL Goal**	**Initiation Level**	**LDL Goal**	
With CHD, PVD, or CVD	>100 mg/dL	<70 mg/dL	>100 mg/dL	<70 mg/dL	
Without CHD, PVD, or CVD	>100 mg/dL	≤100 mg/dL	≥130 mg/dL	≤100 mg/dL	

CHD, Coronary heart disease; CVD, cerebrovascular disease; LDL, low-density lipoprotein; PVD, peripheral vascular disease.

Antibiotics, antiemetics, bulking agents, tricyclic antidepressants, pancreatic extracts, pyloric Botox, gastric pacing, enteral feeding
- Constipation: high-fiber diet and bulking agents, osmotic laxatives, lubricating agents; prokinetics should be used with caution
- Diarrhea: soluble fiber, gluten and lactose restriction, anticholinergic agents, cholestyramine, antibiotics, clonidine, somatostatin, pancreatic enzyme supplements
- Genitourinary autonomic neuropathy
  - Presentation: erectile dysfunction, retrograde ejaculation, bladder dysfunction (recurrent urinary tract infections, pyelonephritis, incontinence, palpable bladder)
  - Diagnosis: medical and sexual history; psychological evaluation; measurement of hormone levels; measurement of nocturnal penile tumescence; assessment of penile, pelvic, and spinal nerve function; cardiovascular autonomic function tests; and measurement of penile and brachial blood pressure
  - Treatment
    - Erectile dysfunction: sex therapy, psychological counseling, sildenafil, vardenafil, tadalafil, prostaglandin E_1 injection, device, or prosthesis
    - Bladder dysfunction/urinary retention and incontinence: bethanechol, intermittent catheterization

Cardiovascular Disease

Basic Information

- Atherosclerosis accounts for approximately 80% of all diabetic mortality (75% from coronary atherosclerosis and 25% from cerebral or peripheral vascular disease) and more than 75% of all hospitalizations for diabetic complications
- More than 50% of patients with newly diagnosed type 2 diabetes already have coronary heart disease

Clinical Presentation

- Coronary artery disease may present with chest pain and/or silent ischemia
- Peripheral arterial disease may present with claudication or nonhealing extremity ulcers
- Cerebrovascular disease may present as transient ischemic attacks or stroke; carotid bruits on physical exam may indicate underlying cerebrovascular disease.

Diagnosis and Evaluation

- Annual screening for dyslipidemia and hypertension
- Diabetic populations should undergo screening with an exercise stress test
  - Symptomatic
    - Typical or atypical cardiac symptoms
    - Abnormal ECG at rest
  - Asymptomatic
    - History of peripheral or carotid occlusive disease
    - Sedentary lifestyle, age older than 35 years, and plans to begin a vigorous exercise program

Treatment

- Aggressive management of hypertension and dyslipidemia, smoking cessation, and aspirin prophylaxis
- Blood pressure targets in patients with diabetes: see earlier section on diabetic nephropathy
- Lipid targets in individuals with diabetes (see Table 37-8)
- In individuals with a prior history of cardiovascular disease (coronary heart, cerebrovascular, or peripheral arterial disease), treat with statin to achieve LDL reduction of 30% to 40%, regardless of baseline LDL; a lower LDL goal of below 70 mg/dL using a high-dose statin is also an option
- In individuals without a history of cardiovascular disease who are older than 40 years, treat with statin to achieve 30% to 40% reduction in LDL regardless of baseline LDL
- Treatment options for dyslipidemia (see Chapter 3)

Review Questions

For review questions, please go to ExpertConsult.com.

SUGGESTED READINGS

American Diabetes Association. Diagnosis and classification of diabetes mellitus. *Diabetes Care.* 2014;37(suppl 1):S81-S90.

American Diabetes Association. Standards of medical care in diabetes. *Diabetes Care.* 2014;37(suppl 1):S14-S80.

Boulton AJM, Vinik AI, Arezzo JC, et al. Diabetic neuropathies *Diabetes Care.* 2005;28:956-962.

Efendic S, Portwood N. Overview of incretin hormones. *Horm Metab Res.* 2004;36:742-746.

Inzucchi SE, Bergenstal RM, Buse JB, et al. Management of hyperglycemia in type 2 diabetes: a patient-centered approach: position Statement of the American Diabetes Association (ADA) and the European Association for the Study of Diabetes (EASD). *Diabetes Care.* 2012;35:1364-1379.

Tahrani AA, Barnett AH, Bailey CJ. SGLT inhibitors in management of diabetes. *Lancet Diabetes Endocrinol.* 2013;1:140-151.

Thyroid Disease

SWAYTHA V. YALAMANCHI, MD; and DAVID S. COOPER, MD

Thyroid disorders may be broadly classified into two categories: dysfunctional thyroid hormone synthesis and anatomic abnormalities. Although the former category includes hypothyroidism and hyperthyroidism, the latter includes the presence of a goiter, nodules, and cancer. Overlap between these categories may exist in the same patient. Thyroid dysfunction is common, occurring in up to 10% of adults and 20% of women over age 65. Small thyroid nodules may be seen on ultrasound in up to 50% to 75% of middle-aged and older women.

Assessment of Thyroid Function

- Thyroid hormone production is regulated via the hypothalamic-pituitary axis through a negative feedback system involving secretion of thyroid receptor hormone (TRH) from the hypothalamus, thyroid-stimulating hormone (TSH) from the anterior pituitary, as well as thyroxine (T_4) and triidothyronine (T_3) from the thyroid gland
- The thyroid gland primarily secretes T_4, whereas the majority of T_3 production, the bioactive form of thyroid hormone, occurs extrathyroidally (Figure 38-1)
- Thyroid-binding globulin (TBG), prealbumin, and albumin bind T_3 and T_4
  - Multiple conditions may affect TBG levels
  - Free, or nonbound, forms of T_3 and T_4 are biologically active
- **Thyroid dysfunction is most commonly related to *primary* impairment of thyroid hormone synthesis; thus, low and high serum TSH levels usually reflect hyper- and hypothyroidism, respectively**
  - Less commonly, impairment of hypothalamic or pituitary function can result in *central hypothyroidism*, in which the serum TSH is low or low-normal with low free serum T_4
  - Very rarely, *TSH-secreting pituitary adenomas* may occur with resulting inappropriate elevation in both serum TSH and serum free T_4 levels
- Many of the symptoms and signs of thyroid dysfunction are nonspecific; laboratory testing is an important part of the assessment (Table 38-1; Figure 38-2)

Thyrotoxicosis

Basic Information

- *Thyrotoxicosis* is a state of increased tissue exposure to circulating thyroid hormone; it is a syndrome, not a diagnosis

- Lifetime prevalence of thyrotoxicosis is approximately 2% in women and 0.2% in men
- *Hyperthyroidism*, a cause of thyrotoxicosis, refers to excess *endogenous* thyroid hormone synthesis and secretion
- *Subclinical hyperthyroidism* refers to a state of mild thyroid overactivity in which the serum TSH levels are subnormal, but levels of free T_4 and T_3 are within reference range
  - The lower limit of normal for TSH may be lower than established reference ranges in African Americans, leading to possible misdiagnosis of subclinical hyperthyroidism in healthy individuals
  - Low TSH and normal free T_4 are also seen physiologically at the end of the first trimester of pregnancy as a result of increased placental secretion of human chorionic gonadotropin (hCG)
- *Etiology* (Table 38-2)
  - Graves disease, toxic multinodular goiter, toxic adenomas, and thyroiditis account for the majority of cases of hyperthyroidism; less commonly, thyrotoxicosis is because of iatrogenic or drug-related causes such as amiodarone (Table 38-3)

Clinical Presentation

- General symptoms and signs reflect an increased metabolic rate and augmentation of adrenergic activity (Table 38-4; Figures 38-3 and 38-4)
- Manifestations of thyrotoxicosis are quite variable and do not necessarily correlate with circulating thyroid hormone concentrations
- **Apathetic thyrotoxicosis: Classic signs of thyrotoxicosis may be absent in the older individuals, except for weight loss, mental status changes, or atrial fibrillation**
- Most patients with subclinical hyperthyroidism are asymptomatic

Diagnosis and Evaluation

- Thyrotoxicosis often initially suspected on the basis of history and physical examination (see Table 38-2)
- Laboratory studies
  - Confirmation of diagnosis of thyrotoxicosis with suppressed serum TSH and elevated free T_4
    - Rare exception: TSH-secreting adenoma in which serum TSH is inappropriately elevated in the setting of elevated free T_4
    - Measurement of serum T_3 is also helpful because it can be increased in approximately 5% of patients with hyperthyroidism when T_4 levels are still normal (T_3 thyrotoxicosis)

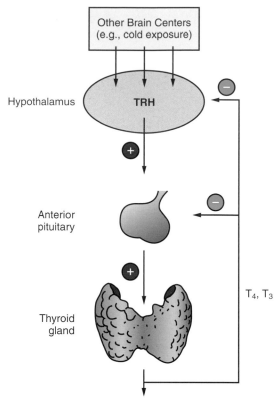

FIGURE 38-1 Hypothalamic-pituitary-thyroid axis. Thyroid hormone synthesis (T_3, T_4) and secretion from the thyroid gland are regulated by a negative feedback system involving thyrotropin-releasing hormone (TRH) from the hypothalamus and thyroid-stimulating hormone from the anterior pituitary. Approximately 20% of circulating T_3 is from direct thyroidal secretion, whereas the remaining 80% is derived from extrathyroidal conversion.

- Laboratory evidence suggestive of Graves disease:
  - Serum T_3:T_4 ratio is increased in Graves disease because the thyroid secretes relatively more T_3 than T_4 compared with the euthyroid state
  - In contrast, in thyroiditis, the serum T_3:T_4 ratio is normal, reflecting the relative concentration of T_3 and T_4 normally present within the thyroid gland
- Circulating antibodies may be present, but are not necessary for diagnosis
  - Thyroid-stimulating antibodies, antithyroperoxidase (anti-TPO) antibodies, and antithyroglobulin antibodies are collectively known as antithyroid antibodies
  - Thyroid-stimulating antibodies stimulate the TSH receptor
  - May be useful in the following circumstances:
    - To confirm diagnosis of Graves disease
    - To stratify risk of neonatal thyrotoxicosis when measured at 22 weeks' gestational age in pregnant women
    - Prognostication in Graves eye disease
- 24-hour radioiodine uptake test (see Table 38-2)
  - Measures uptake of iodine by the thyroid gland
  - Should not be used as a thyroid function test because uptake can also be increased in hypothyroid patients because of elevated TSH

- Uptake will be high in Graves disease because of excessive thyroid hormone synthesis. Conversely, uptake will be low in thyroiditis caused by excessive release, rather than synthesis, of thyroid hormone.
- Thyroid scan should be ordered, along with the uptake in cases when a toxic nodule or toxic multinodular goiter is suspected
- Uptake/scan contraindicated in women who are pregnant or breastfeeding

Treatment

- *Treatment of Graves disease* (Table 38-5)
  - β-Adrenergic blocking agents:
    - Used to control symptoms of palpitations, tremor, heat intolerance, and nervousness
    - Will not treat other symptoms (weight loss, myopathy) and thus not considered to be a primary mode of therapy
    - Best to use a long-acting cardioselective agent (i.e., long-acting propranolol)
  - Antithyroid drugs
    - Both propylthiouracil (PTU) and methimazole (MMI) act primarily to diminish thyroid hormone synthesis by interfering with the intrathyroidal use of iodine
    - **MMI is the drug of choice**
    - PTU, in rare cases, can cause fulminant hepatic failure; its use should be limited to:
      - Patients who experience an allergic reaction with MMI, and in whom surgery or radioactive iodine are not options
      - Pregnant patients during the first trimester
        - Has the potential to cause severe rare congenital defects
        - Switch patients to MMI beginning in the second trimester for the remainder of the pregnancy
      - Patients with life-threatening thyrotoxicosis or thyroid storm because of PTU's ability to quickly inhibit peripheral conversion of T_4 to T_3
    - Common side effects of both medications include rashes, fever, arthralgias, and transient leukopenia
    - Liver dysfunction, which is reversible and seen shortly after initiation of therapy, may also occur
    - **The most serious drug reaction is reversible agranulocytosis (develops in 0.2% to 0.3% of patients, generally within 90 days of starting the medication)**
    - Dose is adjusted to maintain serum free T_4 and total T_3 levels within the normal range
      - Typical starting doses: MMI 10 to 30 mg daily; PTU 100 mg 3 times a day
      - Usually takes 4 to 12 weeks to achieve euthyroid state
      - Serum TSH, however, may remain suppressed for 2 to 3 months after the patient has become euthyroid because of the chronic suppressive effects of the previous hyperthyroidism
    - Remission rate less than 50%
      - Usually treat for 1 to 2 years, then taper or discontinue to see whether a remission has been achieved

TABLE 38-1	*Thyroid Function Tests*	
Test	**Use**	**Comments**
Thyroid-stimulating hormone (TSH)	↑ TSH suggests hypothyroidism and ↓ TSH suggests hyperthyroidism	Very sensitive; normal TSH effectively excludes disease in asymptomatic patients Exceptions: (a) May be ↑ or ↓ in NTI; (b) ↓ in patients on dopamine or high-dose glucocorticoids; (c) normal or ↓ in central hypothyroidism
Total thyroxine (T_4), Triiodothyronine (T_3)	Helpful to quantitate the degree of hormone deficiency or excess T_4 is converted to T_3 in thyroid and peripherally T_3 is active form in tissues	Routine assays measure total T_4 and T_3 levels.
Thyroid-binding globulin (TBG)	>99% of thyroid hormone (T_4 and T_3) is bound to TBG Free fraction (<1%) determines biologic action Must take into account disease states that affect TBG levels when interpreting total T_3 and total T_4 levels.	*Causes of ↑ TBG* Drugs (estrogen, oral contraceptives, tamoxifen, heroin, methadone, 5-fluorouracil) Pregnancy Acute hepatitis Congenital Acute intermittent porphyria
Free T_4 (FT_4)	Direct measurement of free hormone; bypasses interfering effects of disease or drugs on TBG levels	Preferable over total T_4 levels except in pregnancy
Antithyroid Antibodies	*TPO antibody levels*: May be useful if Hashimoto thyroiditis is suspected *Thyroglobulin antibody levels*: May be useful if Hashimoto thyroiditis is suspected, but less sensitive than TPO antibody levels *Thyroid receptor antibody levels*: May be useful if Graves disease is suspected	Checking antibody levels should be reserved for instances in which the diagnosis is unclear from clinical assessment because elevated titers are not necessary for diagnosis
Thyroglobulin	May be helpful in distinguishing causes of hyperthyroidism: levels will be suppressed in the setting of exogenous thyroid hormone intake and elevated in the setting of thyroiditis or autoimmune disease Useful marker to follow in differentiated thyroid cancer after thyroidectomy	Elevated thyroglobulin antibody levels may result in falsely low thyroglobulin levels

The "Causes of ↓ TBG" column for Thyroid-binding globulin (TBG):

Causes of ↓ TBG
Drugs (androgens, glucocorticoids, slow-release nicotinic acid)
Severe illness or malnutrition
Chronic liver disease
Protein-losing states (e.g., nephritic syndrome)
Congenital

NTI, Nonthyroidal illness; TPO, thyroid peroxidase.

- Most likely to achieve remission if initial disease was mild and if thyroid-stimulating antibodies are negative at time of discontinuation
- **If remission achieved, lifelong follow-up is required because (1) remission may not be permanent, and (2) spontaneous hypothyroidism may develop up to decades later**
- Relapse typically occurs in the first 6 months. At that time, another course of drug therapy can be undertaken, or the patient may opt for definitive therapy with radioiodine.
- Radioactive iodine (RAI or ^{131}I):
  - Treatment most often used in the United States for Graves disease
  - The patient should not have received iodinated contrast in the previous 2 months, and urinary iodine concentration measurement may be necessary before proceeding with therapy
  - May have a transient worsening of thyroid function with RAI because of radiation-related thyroiditis or an increase in serum thyroid-stimulating antibodies from thyroid injury
    - **May need to pretreat elderly patients or those with cardiac disease with antithyroid drugs, which will theoretically deplete thyroid hormonal stores**
    - **Antithyroid drugs must be stopped 3 to 7 days before RAI administration to facilitate effective treatment**
  - Approximately 80% of patients will be cured after a single dose; overall cure rate is greater than 95%
    - However, RAI works slowly and euthyroid state may not be achieved for 3 to 6 months with hypothyroidism almost inevitable thereafter
  - No immediate side effects and no evidence of long-term consequences, such as infertility, birth

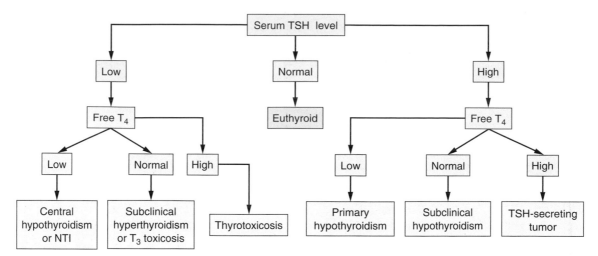

FIGURE 38-2 Sequential thyroid function testing using the serum thyroid-stimulating hormone (TSH) as a starting point. This strategy is useful for screening asymptomatic individuals. If symptoms are present, free thyroxine (FT₄) levels should also be assessed. NTI, Nonthyroidal illness; T₃, triiodothyronine.

defects, cancer, or other neoplasms either in patients or their offspring
- Contraindications to RAI:
  - Absolute contraindications: pregnancy and recent breastfeeding
  - Relative contraindication: moderate to severe eye disease because eye disease may be worsened by RAI; pretreatment with glucocorticoids may be administered to mitigate worsening
- Surgical treatment for Graves disease
  - Cure rate greater than 95%, but rarely used as treatment in the U.S.
  - Reserved for the following patients: those allergic to antithyroid drugs; those who refuse or who have contraindications to RAI; those with concomitant hyperparathyroidism, malignant or suspicious nodule, or very large goiters (latter generally have lower success rates with RAI)
  - Complications may include recurrent laryngeal nerve damage, hypoparathyroidism
- Treatment of Graves ophthalmopathy
  - Local symptoms (irritation, tearing, photophobia) can be managed with artificial tears and lubricating eye ointments
  - Ophthalmology consultation for severe degrees of inflammation, diplopia, severe proptosis leading to corneal exposure, or decreased visual acuity (which is an emergency)
  - May require high-dose glucocorticoids, retro-orbital radiotherapy, and/or surgical decompression of the orbits
  - **As outlined previously, RAI may exacerbate severe ophthalmopathy, especially in smokers**
- Treatment of toxic multinodular goiter (Plummer disease) and solitary toxic nodules
  - These entities are less frequent than Graves disease, but they make up a higher proportion of hyperthyroidism in older individuals
  - Little chance for spontaneous remission

- Antithyroid agents have little role in the management except in preparation for definitive therapy with radioiodine or surgery
- **RAI is the treatment of choice**
  - Surgery is a reasonable therapy in patients with large goiters or malignant nodules
- Treatment of subclinical hyperthyroidism (Figure 38-5)
- In adults older than age 65 years, subclinical hyperthyroidism may predispose to atrial fibrillation; in postmenopausal women, it may be related to osteoporosis
- Recommend treatment in older patients if serum TSH less than 0.1 mU/L. It is also reasonable to treat older patients, women who have osteoporosis, and/or patients who have known heart disease.
- In untreated patients, periodic follow-up is necessary to monitor for the development of overt hyperthyroidism
- Treatment options include antithyroid drugs or RAI

Thyroid Storm

- Represents a rare and severe form of thyrotoxicosis
  - Mortality 10% to 20% with the most important determinant of survival being early recognition and institution of therapy
  - Characterized by fever, severe tachycardia/atrial fibrillation, and altered mental status (agitation, delirium, coma)
  - Clinical features otherwise include more severe features of thyrotoxicosis (see Table 38-3)
  - Diagnosis is clinical; multiple diagnostic scoring systems exist, most notably the Burch and Wartofsky score
  - Often triggered by a precipitating event
  - Conditions associated with a rapid rise in thyroid hormone levels: withdrawal of antithyroid drug,

Etiology	Mechanism	Thyroid Examination	Lab Results	Radioiodine Uptake	Treatment
Graves disease	Stimulatory anti-TSH receptor antibodies	Diffuse goiter	TSH ↓ Normal/↑ FT₄ Normal/↑ T₃ +Antithyroid Abs ↑ thyroglobulin	↑ uptake diffusely	ATDs RAI Surgery
Toxic multinodular goiter or solitary nodule	Activating gene mutations	Nodule(s), usually >3 cm	TSH ↓ Normal/↑ FT₄ Normal/↑ T₃ −TSI/TRAb ↑ thyroglobulin	↑ focal uptake	RAI is the treatment of choice ATDs as temporizing measure Surgery if compressive symptoms or risk of thyroid cancer
Thyroiditis (thyrotoxic phase)	Follicular destruction causing release of stored hormone	Tender goiter in subacute thyroiditis; nontender goiter in "silent" thyroiditis	TSH ↓ Normal/↑ FT₄ Normal/↑ T₃ − Antithyroid Abs ↑ thyroglobulin	↓ uptake	Prednisone
Iodine-induced	Iodine surplus (IV dye or amiodarone-induced thyrotoxicosis type 1)	Nodular or diffuse goiter	TSH ↓ Normal/↑ FT₄ Normal/↑ T₃ − Antithyroid Abs ↑ thyroglobulin	↓ uptake	Withdrawal of offending agent if possible. ATDs, RAI, or surgery in selected cases
Choriocarcinoma	Secretes hCG, a thyroid stimulator	Minimal goiter	TSH ↓ Normal/↑ FT₄ Normal/↑ T₃ − Antithyroid Abs ↑ thyroglobulin	↑ uptake caused by increased thyroid hormone production	Treatment of choriocarcinoma
Pituitary tumor (TSH-secreting)	TSH overproduction	Goiter	TSH normal/↑ Normal/↑ FT₄ Normal/↑ T₃ − Antithyroid Abs ↑ thyroglobulin	↑ uptake	Treatment of pituitary adenoma
Struma ovarii	Ectopic thyroid tissue in ovarian tumor	Normal	TSH ↓ Normal/↑ FT₄ Normal/↑ T₃ − Antithyroid Abs ↑ thyroglobulin	↓ uptake in the region of the thyroid; ↑uptake in the region of the pelvis	Treatment of struma ovarii
Exogenous thyrotoxicosis	Over supplementation with thyroxine	Normal	TSH ↓ ↑ FT₄ (if exogenous T₄ intake) ↑ T₃ (if exogenous T₃ intake) − Antithyroid Abs ↓ thyroglobulin	↓ caused by suppression of thyroid hormone production	Withdraw offending agent
Iatrogenic or factitious	Over supplementation with thyroxine	Normal	TSH ↓ ↑ FT₄ ↑ T₃ − Antithyroid Abs ↓ thyroglobulin	↓ uptake	Withdraw offending agent
Drug-induced	Use of amiodarone, interferon-α, tyrosine kinase inhibitors	Normal	TSH ↓ ↑ FT₄ ↑ T₃ − Antithyroid Abs ↓ thyroglobulin	↓ uptake	Withdrawal of offending agent

Abs, Antibodies; ATDs, antithyroid drugs; IV, intravenous; RAI, radioactive iodine.

TABLE 38-3	*Amiodarone-Induced Thyrotoxicosis*	
Factor	**AIT Type 1**	**AIT Type 2**
Preexisting thyroid disease	Yes	No
Duration of amiodarone therapy before onset of hyperthyroidism	Months	Years
Radioiodine uptake	Low	Very low
Thyroid function tests	$\downarrow$TSH, $\uparrow$T$_4$, normal/$\uparrow$T$_3$	$\downarrow$TSH, $\uparrow$T$_4$, normal/$\uparrow$T$_3$
Color flow Doppler of thyroid	Increased parenchymal blood flow	Normal, decreased parenchymal blood flow
Treatment	Antithyroid drugs; if severe and refractory to therapy, surgery may be a consideration	Prednisone; as with AIT type 1, surgery may be a consideration in refractory disease

AIT, Amiodarone-induced thyrotoxicosis; TSH, thyroid stimulating hormone.

TABLE 38-4	*Clinical Manifestations of Thyrotoxicosis*
Organ System	**Symptoms and Signs**
Constitutional	Weight loss, heat intolerance *Hyperpyrexia (frequently exceeds 40° to 41° C), insensible fluid losses
Cardiovascular	Palpitations, atrial arrhythmias, congestive heart failure, systolic hypertension *Accelerated tachycardia (>130 beats/min), atrial dysrhythmia, heart failure
Respiratory	Dyspnea
Gastrointestinal	Hyperdefecation, increased appetite, nausea, mild transaminase elevation *Vomiting, diarrhea, hepatic dysfunction, jaundice
Musculoskeletal	Proximal muscle weakness, osteopenia, hypercalcuria, hypercalcemia †Extraocular muscle weakness, myasthenia gravis
Neuropsychiatric	Nervousness, anxiety, tremor, insomnia, impaired mentation, delirium, psychosis *Severe agitation, confusion, seizure, coma
Endocrine	Hypomenorrhea, amenorrhea, gynecomastia, decreased libido
Hematologic	†Splenomegaly, enlarged thymus, lymphadenopathy, neutropenia
Ophthalmologic (see Figure 38-3)	†Stare, lid lag, proptosis, diplopia, visual loss
Dermatologic (see Figure 38-4)	Warm, moist, velvety skin; palmar erythema, onycholysis, thinning hair, pruritus, hives, vitiligo †Pretibial myxedema, thyroid acropachy

*Findings seen in thyroid storm.
†Findings seen only in Graves disease.

radioiodine therapy, external beam radiation therapy, overdose of thyroid hormone, contrast dyes, thyroid bed trauma, thyroid surgery
- Conditions associated with an acute or subacute nonthyroidal illness: nonthyroidal surgery, infection, cerebrovascular accident, pulmonary thromboembolism, parturition, diabetic ketoacidosis

Treatment of thyroid storm (Table 38-6)
- **Antithyroid drugs are the mainstay**

Hypothyroidism

Basic Information

- Hypothyroidism is a clinical state in which the circulating levels of thyroid hormone are insufficient for normal cellular function
- Extremely common, especially in women

- Prevalence of approximately 8% in women and 2% in men, more than 80% of which is very mild (subclinical)
- However, physiologic age-related increase in serum TSH may result in falsely high prevalence rates
- **The most common cause of hypothyroidism is to autoimmune-mediated primary thyroid failure (chronic lymphocytic thyroiditis or Hashimoto thyroiditis)**
- **Subclinical hypothyroidism**
  - **Refers to a state of mild thyroid dysfunction in which the serum TSH levels are slightly increased (usually less than 10 mU/L) and the serum levels of free T$_4$ and T$_3$ are normal**
  - Prevalence is up to 15% to 20% in individuals older than age 60 years
  - Causes similar to overt hypothyroidism
  - Note: Slightly elevated serum TSH levels in the elderly (age older than 75 to 80 years) have been associated with a survival benefit

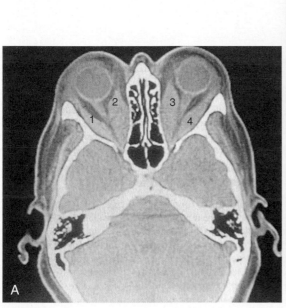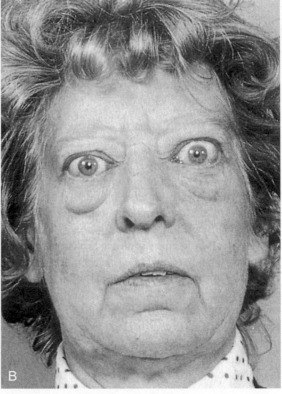

FIGURE 38-3 **A,** Computed tomography scan of orbits showing enlarged extraocular muscles. 1, Right lateral medial rectus muscle; 2, right medial rectus muscle; 3, left medial rectus muscle; 4, left lateral rectus muscle. **B,** Patient with classic features of thyroid-associated ophthalmopathy showing lid retraction, exophthalmos, and periorbital edema. Patients may also have diplopia and strabismus due to edema and fibrosis of the extraocular muscles. (From Souhami R. *Textbook of Medicine.* New York: Churchill Livingstone; 2002: Fig. 17.23B.)

- In this patient population, treatment of subclinical hypothyroidism may be of limited or no clinical benefit
- Mildly elevated serum TSH may be normal
- Recommended to recheck serum TSH because spontaneous normalization may occur

Clinical Presentation

- Symptoms and signs may be nonspecific and overlap with other conditions (Table 38-7; Figure 38-6)
- Development of symptoms depends on the duration of disease, along with individual factors, such as age (older patients have fewer symptoms than younger individuals)
  - Symptomatology may not always correlate with biochemical severity of hypothyroidism
  - Typical patient notes fatigue, mild constipation, cold intolerance, and mild weight gain
  - A weight gain of more than 5 to 10 pounds cannot be attributed to hypothyroidism

Diagnosis and Evaluation

- Laboratory studies
  - **In all forms of hypothyroidism, circulating level of free T_4 will be low**
  - Serum level of T_3 is low as well in severe cases
  - *Primary hypothyroidism:* Serum TSH will be increased (caused by the lack of negative feedback inhibition by thyroid hormone on pituitary TSH secretion)
    - Milder cases: TSH may be only slightly increased (5 to 10 mU/L)

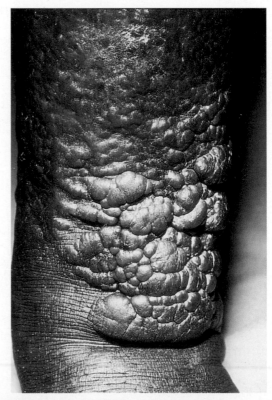

FIGURE 38-4 Chronic pretibial myxedema in a patient with Graves disease and orbitopathy. The lesions are firm and nonpitting with a clear palpable edge. (From Larsen PR, Kronenberg HM, Melmed S, Polonsky KS. *Williams' Textbook of Endocrinology.* 10th ed. Philadelphia: Saunders; 2003: Fig. 82-2.)

38

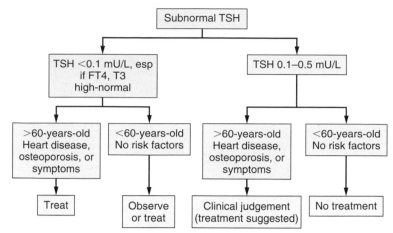

FIGURE 38-5 Management of subclinical hyperthyroidism. If the patient is older than 60 years or younger than 60 years with bone disease, heart disease, or symptoms, treatment is recommended. FT₄, Free thyroxine; TSH, thyroid-stimulating hormone.

TABLE 38-5	*Treatment of Graves disease*			
	Advantages	**Hypothyroidism Frequency**	**Other Disadvantages**	**Cost**
Antithyroid drugs	Nonablative	Low frequency	Not definitive, side effects	+
Radioiodine	Definitive	100%	Fear	++
Surgery	Definitive	100%	Complications, discomfort	+++

TABLE 38-6	*Medical Therapy of Thyroid Storm*
Therapy	**Comments**
1. Inhibition of new thyroid hormone synthesis 　PTU 　Methimazole	*PTU* has additional benefit of inhibition of T₄ → T₃ conversion, but methimazole is the treatment of choice because of adverse reactions associated with PTU
2. Inhibition of hormone release 　Iodine	Iodine should not be initiated until at least 1 hour after ATD administration
3. β-adrenergic blockers 　Propranolol 　Atenolol 　Esmolol	*Propranolol* inhibits T₄ to T₃ conversion at high doses *Atenolol* is cardioselective *Esmolol* allows for expedient dose titration in the ICU
4. Treatment directed against systemic decompensation 　Hydrocortisone 　Supportive care	*Hydrocortisone* treats underlying adrenal insufficiency. Has dual purpose of inhibiting T₄ to T₃ compensation
5. Identification and treatment directed against specific precipitating event.	*Supportive care* includes management of hyperthermia, dehydration, electrolyte imbalances, nutritional deficits and agitation. Aspirin should be avoided as it binds to TBG, increasing FT₄

ATDs, Antithyroid drugs; FT₄, Free thyroxine; ICU, intensive care unit; PTU, propylthiouracil; TBG, thyroxine-binding globulin
Modified from Warnock A. *Endocrine and Metabolic Medical.* Washington, D.C.: Endocrine Press; 2014.

- Severe cases: TSH will be markedly increased (greater than 10 mU/L)
- Positive antibody testing suggestive of autoimmune hypothyroidism, but not necessary for diagnosis
- *Central hypothyroidism* (hypothalamic or pituitary disease): Serum free T₄ is low, and serum TSH levels are low or low-normal
- *Subclinical hypothyroidism:*
  - Free T₄ is still within reference range, but the TSH level is high (usually 5 to 10 mU/L)

- Autoantibodies are not necessary for diagnosis but may be helpful in predicting the likelihood that the patient will develop overt hypothyroidism
- Other causes (Box 38-1).

Treatment

- Synthetic T₄ is the treatment of choice for all forms of hypothyroidism
  - Replacement dose is approximately 1.6 μg/kg/day, which is in the range of 100 to 200 μg/day for the average adult

TABLE 38-7	Clinical Manifestations of Hypothyroidism
Organ System	**Symptoms and Signs**
Constitutional	Weight gain, cold intolerance, fatigue, weakness, hypercholesterolemia Hypothermia* (<90° F or 32.2° C)
Cardiovascular	Bradycardia,* cardiomegaly/ decreased contractility,* pericardial effusion,* hypotension*
Respiratory	Hoarseness, dyspnea, hypoventilation,* sleep apnea, pleural effusion Difficulty protecting airway because of mental status*
Gastrointestinal	Constipation, ileus, macroglossia
Musculoskeletal	Myalgias, arthralgias, nonpitting edema
Neuropsychiatric	Depression, psychosis, carpal tunnel syndrome, delayed reflex relaxation Altered mental status*
Endocrine	Growth failure, menorrhagia, galactorrhea (hyperprolactinemia), precocious puberty, hyponatremia,* hypoglycemia*
Hematologic	Anemia, platelet defect
Dermatologic	Dry skin, pallor, yellowing of skin (carotinemia)

*Clinical features that may be seen in myxedema coma.

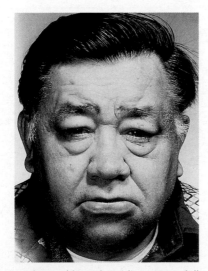

FIGURE 38-6 Advanced hypothyroidism. Note dulled expression, facial puffiness, and periorbital edema. (From Noble J, Green HL, Levinson W, et al: *Textbook of Primary Care Medicine.* 3rd ed. St. Louis: Mosby; 2001: Fig. 97-2.)

- Treatment can be initiated with the full dose in younger patients with goal TSH in low to midnormal range (0.5 to 3 mU/L)
- Replacement dose is 10% to 15% lower in patients older than age 65 years with goal TSH of 4 to 6 mU/L

BOX 38-1	Causes of Hypothyroidism

Associated with Goiter

Chronic lymphocytic (Hashimoto) thyroiditis
Silent (postpartum) thyroiditis (transient)
Subacute thyroiditis (transient)
Iodine deficiency (not seen in North America)
Goitrogenic drugs (lithium, iodine-containing drugs [amiodarone], antithyroid agents, sunitinib and other multikinase inhibitors [mechanism uncertain])
Congenital biosynthetic enzyme deficiencies

Not Associated with Goiter

Postthyroidectomy
Postablation for hyperthyroidism
Congenital absence of the thyroid
Atrophic thyroiditis (variant of Hashimoto thyroiditis)
Following radiation for head and neck tumors

Secondary Hypothyroidism

Pituitary or hypothalamic dysfunction

Peripheral Thyroid Hormone Resistance

Caused by defective thyroid hormone receptor

- Should start with lower doses (25 to 50 μg/day) in elderly patients who may have underlying coronary disease; titrate the dose up gradually
- Overreplacement in the elderly may predispose elderly patients to atrial fibrillation and postmenopausal women to osteoporosis
- In central hypothyroidism, the TSH level cannot be used as a guide to therapy; in this case, the free T_4 level should be maintained in the upper 50% of the reference range
- **Because of its 7-day half-life, T_4 and TSH blood levels take at least 5 to 6 weeks to reach a steady state, and thus dose adjustments should be made only every 6 weeks**
- It may take weeks to months, however, for some symptoms of hypothyroidism to resolve
- Conditions necessitating thyroxine dose adjustment (Box 38-2)
- Subclinical hypothyroidism (Figure 38-7)
  - Treatment is controversial because patients tend to be relatively asymptomatic
  - High rate of progression to overt hypothyroidism in those patients who have positive antithyroid antibodies (5% to 10% per year)
  - Some untreated patients with TSH levels less than 10 mU/L can revert to a euthyroid state, especially if they are antithyroid antibody negative
  - Treatment may result in an improvement of unfavorable lipid patterns, especially if the TSH level is greater than 10 mU/L
  - Relatively small doses of T_4 (50 to 100 μg/day) are needed

Myxedema Coma

- Medical emergency that typically occurs in patients with long-standing untreated severe hypothyroidism

- Mortality may be as high as 50%
- Often precipitated by stress, such as systemic disease, surgery, and sedative drugs or narcotics; occurs more frequently in the winter months
- Clinical diagnosis characterized by hypothermia and decreased mental status (see Table 38-7)
- Treatment of myxedema coma (Table 38-8)
  - Sedatives and narcotics are contraindicated because all drugs are metabolized slowly and may have prolonged and unpredictable effects
  - Hypoadrenalism should be suspected in patients with hypothyroidism caused by autoimmune thyroiditis or in central hypothyroidism

- If adrenal insufficiency is not treated first, administration of T_4 may precipitate an adrenal crisis caused by increased cortisol clearance and increased metabolism (resulting in increased cortisol requirements)
- Thus, it is reasonable to administer hydrocortisone 100 mg every 8 hours intravenously (IV) for several days with rapid tapering as the clinical picture improves, or ideally, until adrenal insufficiency can be ruled out with an adrenocorticotropic hormone (ACTH) stimulation test

---

BOX 38-2 | *Clinical Situations in Which Thyroxine Doses May Need Adjustment*

Increased Dose

Pregnancy
Malabsorption
Certain drugs that
    Interfere with absorption (sucralfate, aluminum hydroxide, cholestyramine, colestipol, ferrous sulfate, calcium, raloxifene, orlistat)
    Accelerate thyroxine metabolism (phenytoin, carbamazepine, phenobarbital, rifampin, sertraline, imatinib [Gleevec])
    Increase TBG (estrogen)
    Block T_4 to T_3 conversion in the pituitary gland (amiodarone)

Decreased Dose

Advanced age
Androgen therapy (decreases TBG)

T_3, Triiodothyronine; T_4, thyroxine; TBG, thyroid-binding globulin.

TABLE 38-8 | *Approach to Management of Myxedema Coma*

Management

1. Check TSH, FT_4 and random serum cortisol (consider short ACTH stimulation test)
2. Hydrocortisone 50 to 100 mg IV every 6 to 8 hours
3. Administer IV T_4 300 to 600 µg IV followed by daily PO or IV doses of 50 to 100 µg PO or IV daily. Consider T_3 5 to 20 µg IV followed by 2.5 to 25 µg IV or PO daily with concomitant T_4 administration if no clinical response to T_4 alone
4. Supportive measures
   Mechanical ventilation
   Fluid and vasopressor drugs to correct hypotension
   Passive rewarming
   Correction of underlying hyponatremia
   IV dextrose
   Consider empiric antibiotics
   Monitor for arrhythmias

ACTH, Adrenocorticotropic hormone; FT4, free thyroxine; IV, intravenous; TSH, thyroid-stimulating hormone.
Modified from Kasid N, Hennessey J. Myxedema coma. In Matfin GM, eds. *Endocrine and Metabolic Medical Emergencies*. Washington, D.C.: Endocrine Press; 2014: p 104-109.

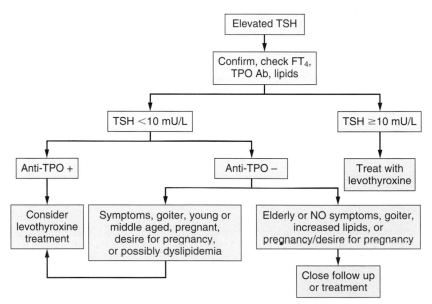

FIGURE 38-7 Management of subclinical hypothyroidism. Treatment is recommended for individuals with TSH 10 mU/L or greater. For individuals with TSH less than 10 mU/L, TPO antibody levels, age, pregnancy status, clinical symptoms/signs, and possibly lipids are important factors in considering whether to initiate treatment. FT_4, Free thyroxine; TSH, thyroid-stimulating hormone; TPO, thyroid peroxidase.

Nonthyroidal Illness

- Nonthyroidal illness (NTI) is a syndrome characterized by changes in thyroid hormone metabolism and protein binding in the setting of severe illness
- Serum TSH may be low or normal in severely ill patients (Figure 38-8)
    - If serum TSH is low (occurs in approximately 20% of hospitalized patients), the diagnosis of hyperthyroidism should not be made in the absence of supporting clinical and laboratory data
    - Completely suppressed serum TSH (<0.05 mU/L), however, is more commonly seen in the setting of hyperthyroidism than NTI
    - If serum TSH is within reference range, the patient is likely euthyroid
    - Elevation in serum TSH may be seen in the recovery phase of illness, although levels greater than 20 mU/L are suggestive of underlying hypothyroidism; if serum TSH is elevated and the patient is not recovering from an illness, the patient likely has underlying hypothyroidism
- Serum T_3 and T_4
    - Serum T_3 will always be low as a result of decreased extrathyroidal conversion from T_4 to T_3
    - In severe disease, T_4 levels may also be low
- Medications that are used in the intensive care unit may contribute to diminished pituitary serum TSH secretion (e.g., high doses of glucocorticoids, dopamine)
- Acute psychiatric illness may result in transient elevations in T_4 with or without low serum TSH concentration
- **Therefore, the diagnosis of thyroid disease can be quite difficult in acutely ill individuals**
- Generally, thyroid function tests should be re-evaluated several weeks to months after recovery

Thyroiditis

- **Thyroiditis refers to a group of diseases characterized by thyroid inflammation (Table 38-9)**
- Refer to Table 38-10 for a summary of the different forms, presentation, diagnosis, and treatment of thyroiditis

Goiter and Thyroid Nodules

Basic Information

- *Goiter* refers to chronic enlargement of the thyroid gland
- *Thyroid nodules* are focal isolated growths in the thyroid gland
    - Prevalence on physical examination of one or more thyroid nodules ranges from 1% to 5%
    - **Frequency of small, nonpalpable nodules that are detected by ultrasound examination is as high as 50% to 75% in older persons, especially women**
    - The major clinical significance of thyroid nodules is the possibility of thyroid cancer, which is present in 5% to 10% of thyroid nodules
- Etiology
    - The cause of goiter and/or thyroid nodules is unknown in most patients
    - Chronic lymphocytic thyroiditis accounts for 10% to 20% of goiters and thyroid nodules
    - Iodine deficiency is the major cause of goiter in the world, but far less common in North America
    - Ionizing radiation and genetic factors are also important in the genesis of thyroid nodular disease

38

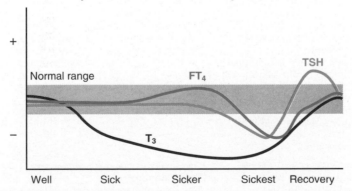

Thyroid Function Tests in Nonthyroidal Illness

FIGURE 38-8 Thyroid function tests in nonthyroidal illness. Thyroid-stimulating hormone (TSH) and free thyroxine (FT_4) levels decline with increasing severity of illness, possibly mediated in part by transient central hypothyroidism in the sickest of patients. TSH suppressive effects of endogenous cytokines such as tumor necrosis factor may play a role as well. Free T_4 levels can occasionally be supranormal and T_3 levels may decline early in illness caused by decreased 5'-deiodination in the setting of critical illness. As recovery from acute illness occurs, free T_4 may decline, although total T_3 and TSH levels may rise, with the latter potentially transiently reaching supraphysiologic levels.

TABLE 38-9	*Types of Thyroiditis*			
Type	**Etiology**	**Clinical Features**	**Diagnosis**	**Treatment**
Chronic lymphocytic thyroiditis (CLT)	Autoimmune	Most patients have symptoms of hypothyroidism Often with firm, nontender goiter Pyramidal lobe may be palpable May have other evidence of autoimmunity	TSH typically high-normal or elevated +antithyroid antibodies	Thyroxine for hypothyroid patients In euthyroid patients, may use higher doses of thyroxine to shrink goiter
Subacute thyroiditis (SAT)	Likely viral More likely to occur if HLA-Bw35 positive	Gradual or acute onset of thyroid pain; may be severe and disabling Pain may radiate to angle of jaw or ear Often preceded by a viral upper respiratory infection May see systemic symptoms, such as fever, night sweats, fatigue, and weight loss On exam, thyroid is very tender, firm, and irregular Course: Pain and hyperthyroidism for 3 to 6 weeks followed by transient hypothyroidism for several months	Acute inflammatory phase: $\uparrow T_4$, $\downarrow$ TSH Radioiodine uptake is low High ESR (>30 mm/hour) or CRP Recovery phase: May see temporary mild $\downarrow T_4$ and $\uparrow$ TSH for 1 to 3 months	Salicylates or other NSAIDs for neck discomfort Severe cases: Glucocorticoids are helpful Treat symptoms of hyperthyroidism with β-blocking drugs Full recovery is the rule
Silent thyroiditis (postpartum thyroiditis when occurs in the postpartum period)	Autoimmune	Symptoms and signs of mild thyrotoxicosis up to 2 to 3 months Usually a firm, nontender goiter Triphasic course (as with SAT) May recur with successive pregnancies May present as postpartum depression	Similar to SAT $\uparrow T_4$ and T_3 but T_3 not as high as seen in Graves disease. T_3 may be normal. Radioiodine uptake is low	Treat symptoms of hyperthyroidism with β-blocking drugs. Glucocorticoids rarely needed for severe hyperthyroidism 25% become permanently hypothyroid
Acute (suppurative) thyroiditis	Bacterial; most commonly *Staphylococcus aureus*, *Streptococcus pyogenes*, *Streptococcus pneumoniae*, and *Enterobacter* spp. Typically preceded by an upper respiratory or pharyngeal infection May also be caused by opportunistic infections in immunocompromised hosts, especially *Aspergillus* and *Pneumocystis*	Anterior neck pain, fever, dysphagia May see erythema over thyroid or jugular venous phlebitis	Thyroid function usually remains normal Leukocytosis Fine-needle aspiration with stains to identify organism	Antibiotics Surgical drainage if abscess develops
Amiodarone-induced thyroiditis (type 2) (Table 38-4)	Occurs in 3% of patients on amiodarone Because of a destructive thyroiditis, leading to excess release of T_4 and T_3 More common in men	Thyrotoxicosis features develop rapidly May have recurrence of atrial fibrillation Thyroid is nontender; not enlarged Usually occurs after 1 to 3 years of therapy	$\uparrow T_4$ and T_3. T_3 may also be normal $\downarrow$ TSH $\downarrow$ Radioiodine uptake Thyroid Doppler ultrasound will demonstrate normal of "low" blood flow similar to euthyroid state	Prednisone 40 mg daily Slow taper over 2 to 3 months

CRP, C-reactive protein; ESR, erythrocyte sedimentation rate; HLA, human leukocyte antigen; NSAID, nonsteroidal antiinflammatory drug; T3, triiodothyronine; T4, thyroxine; TSH, thyroid-stimulating hormone.

TABLE 38-10	*Clinical Features and Therapy of Thyroid Cancer*					
Cancer Type	**% of All Cancers**	**Age at Diagnosis (yr)**	**Rate of Growth**	**Primary Therapy**	**Prognosis**	**Comment**
Papillary	70–80	30–60	Slow	Surgery	Excellent	Radioiodine used as adjunct
Follicular	5-10	50+	Slow	Surgery	Good to excellent	Radioiodine used as adjunct
Medullary	10	50+ (younger if MEN-2)	Moderate	Surgery	Fair to good	RET germline mutation in 20% of cases; produces calcitonin
Lymphoma	<5	50+	Moderate	Radiotherapy, chemotherapy	Good	Seen in association with Hashimoto thyroiditis
Anaplastic	<5	60+	Rapid	Surgery, radiotherapy, chemotherapy	Poor	Often history of goiter or papillary thyroid cancer

MEN, Multiple endocrine neoplasia.

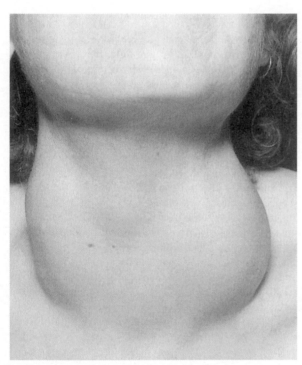

FIGURE 38-9 Dominant left-sided nodule in a multinodular goiter. (From Souhami R: *Textbook of Medicine.* New York: Churchill Livingstone; 2002: Fig. 17.25.)

Clinical Presentation

- Most patients with thyroid nodules and/or goiter are asymptomatic and euthyroid
  - However, a large goiter may cause neck discomfort and pressure, dysphagia, hoarseness, and dyspnea (Figure 38-9)
  - Some multinodular goiters are substernal and may not be readily palpable, but may cause significant airway obstruction or superior vena caval compression (with jugular venous distention and facial edema)
- Benign versus malignant nodules
  - Distinction of benign from malignant thyroid nodule is almost impossible on clinical grounds

---

BOX 38-3	*Clinical Features Suggesting Malignancy in a Thyroid Nodule*

History

Rapid growth
Older male or young child
Childhood neck irradiation
Family history of thyroid cancer

Physical Examination

Firm or rock-hard consistency
Ipsilateral cervical adenopathy
Fixation to surrounding structures

- Certain clinical and sonographic features favor malignancy (Box 38-3)

Diagnosis and Evaluation

- Diffuse or multinodular goiter
  - Laboratory studies: Usually euthyroid (nontoxic goiter), but may be hypothyroid (probable chronic lymphocytic thyroiditis) or hyperthyroid (Graves disease, toxic multinodular goiter, thyroiditis)
  - Thyroid radionuclide scanning: Will provide general information about the size of the thyroid and whether certain areas within the gland concentrate the radioactive tracer (i.e., hyperfunctioning)
  - "Hot" nodules rarely need to be biopsied because these are almost always benign (Figure 38-10)
  - Thyroid ultrasound: Can accurately assess the size of the gland, the overall echotexture of the gland, and the echo characteristics, size, and number of nodules within the gland
- Solitary thyroid nodules (Figure 38-11)
  - Laboratory studies: May be euthyroid (most commonly), hypothyroid (suggestive of chronic lymphocytic thyroiditis), or hyperthyroid (autonomous nodule)
  - Thyroid radionuclide scanning: Useful for identifying hyperfunctioning thyroid nodules

38

- Thyroid ultrasound:
  - Should be performed to evaluate all thyroid nodules to document size/number of nodules and to identify suspicious malignant features
  - Sonographic features including hypoechogenicity, increased blood flow, microcalcifications, and irregular borders have reasonable sensitivity and specificity for malignancy
  - **Fine needle aspiration (FNA) is the procedure of choice in the diagnosis of thyroid nodules (Figure 38-12)**

Treatment

- Diffuse or multinodular goiters: Consider therapy if evidence of thyroid dysfunction (based on thyroid function tests) and/or symptoms/signs of tracheal, esophageal, or recurrent laryngeal nerve compression
  - Thyroid dysfunction: Hypothyroidism is treated with thyroxine therapy; hyperthyroidism is generally treated with radioiodine

- The use of T_4 suppression therapy to reduce the size of the goiter in euthyroid patients is controversial but may be effective in some patients with a nontoxic goiter
- Compressive symptoms: Surgery is usually required for large, obstructive goiters; radioiodine may be used in older patients who are not surgical candidates
- Solitary thyroid nodules:
  - Pharmacologic therapy: Suppression therapy to shrink nodules with T_4 is likely of little use

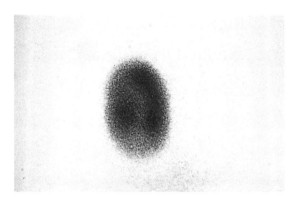

Figure 38-10 Toxic adenoma in the right thyroid (a "hot" nodule) demonstrated with radioiodine uptake scan. Remainder of gland does not take up the isotope because of suppression of thyroid-stimulating hormone. (From Forbes CD, Jackson WF. *Color Atlas and Text of Clinical Medicine*. 3rd ed. St. Louis: Mosby; 2003: Fig. 7.63.)

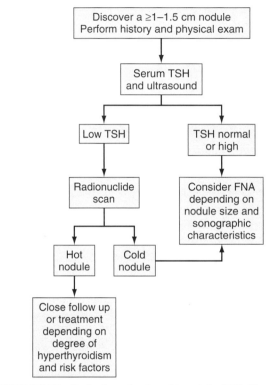

FIGURE 38-11 Evaluation of a thyroid nodule. FNA, Fine-needle aspiration; TSH, thyroid-stimulating hormone.

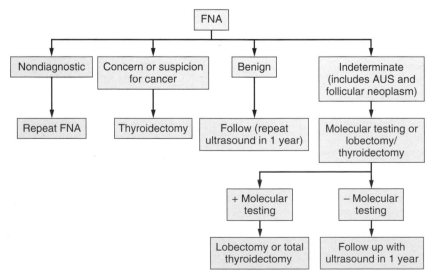

FIGURE 38-12 Management after fine-needle aspiration (FNA) of a thyroid nodule. Individuals with indeterminate thyroid nodules may undergo either molecular testing or surgical intervention with a lobectomy or total thyroidectomy. AUS, Atypia of undetermined significance.

- Radioiodine: Treatment of choice for hyperfunctioning nodules
- Surgical therapy is indicated if the patient is experiencing compressive symptoms, nodule is 4 cm or more, or nodule is suspicious for malignancy on FNA
    - If a biopsy-proven benign nodule, observation and follow-up with ultrasound in 1 year
    - If the nodule enlarges in size with greater than 50% change in volume, should have repeat biopsy

Thyroid Cancer

Basic Information

- Thyroid cancer is a malignancy arising from thyroid follicular cells or C cells
- Rising incidence of thyroid cancer in the U.S., approximately 10 per 100,000 per year presently
- Etiology of most cancers is unknown; ionizing radiation is a risk factor for differentiated thyroid cancer
- Histologic types (see Table 38-10)
    - Differentiated thyroid cancer refers to papillary and follicular thyroid cancer collectively
    - Medullary thyroid cancer (MTC): Approximately 20% of patients belong to kindreds with multiple endocrine neoplasia-2 syndrome, an autosomal dominant condition (see Chapter 41)
    - Thyroid lymphomas, in contrast, may develop from lymphocytes within the thyroid gland, especially in individuals with long-standing Hashimoto thyroiditis

Clinical Presentation

- Patients are usually asymptomatic, and a thyroid nodule is found on routine physical examination or incidentally on imaging done for other purposes

Diagnosis and Evaluation

- FNA required for diagnosis (see Figure 38-12; Table 38-9)

Treatment

- Total thyroidectomy is the primary therapy
- Radioiodine ablation of thyroid remnant after thyroidectomy may be performed as adjuvant therapy in patients with differentiated thyroid cancer with high risk for recurrence
- Serum markers may be helpful for monitoring for disease recurrence
    - Serum thyroglobulin in patients with differentiated thyroid cancer
    - Serum calcitonin useful in patients with MTC
- Factors influencing the prognosis in differentiated cancer include age (better in patients <50 years of age), tumor size, degree of tumor invasiveness, and presence of local or distant metastases

Review Questions

For review questions, please go to ExpertConsult. com.

SUGGESTED READINGS

Bahn R, Burch HB, Cooper DS, et al. Hyperthyroidism and other causes of thyrotoxicosis: Management Guidelines of the American Thyroid Association and American Association of Clinical Endocrinologists. *Endocr Practice.* 2011;17(3):325-333.

Bartalena L, Tanda ML. Clinical practice: Graves' ophthalmopathy. *N Engl J Med.* 2009;360:994-1001.

Biondi B, Wartofsky L. Treatment with thyroid hormone. *Endocr Rev.* 2014;35:433-512.

Bogazzi F, Baralena L, Martino E. Approach to the patient with amiodarone-induced thyrotoxicosis. *J Clin Endocrinol Metab.* 2010;95:2529-2535.

Brent GA. Clinical practice: Graves' disease. *N Engl J Med.* 2008; 358:2594-2605.

Cooper DS. Antithyroid drugs. *N Engl J Med.* 2005;352:905-917.

Cooper DS, Biondi B. Subclinical thyroid disease. *Lancet.* 2012; 379(9821):1142-1154.

Cooper DS, Doherty GM, Haugen BR, et al. Revised American Thyroid Association management guidelines for patients with thyroid nodules and differentiated thyroid cancer. *Thyroid.* 2009;19:1167-1214.

Kasid N, Hennessey J. Myxedema Coma. In: Matfin GM, ed. *Endocrine and Metabolic Medical Emergencies.* Washington, DC: Endocrine Press; 2014:104-109.

McLeod DS, Sawka AM, Cooper DS. Controversies in primary treatment of low-risk papillary thyroid cancer. *Lancet.* 2013; 381(9871):1046-1057.

Warnock A, Cooper D, Burch H. Life threatening thyrotoxicosis. In: Matfin GM, ed. *Endocrine and Metabolic Medical Emergencies.* Washington, DC: Endocrine Press; 2014:110-126.

38

Calcium Disorders and Metabolic Bone Disease

LAILA S. TABATABAI, MD; and DEBORAH E. SELLMEYER, MD

Calcium disorders are common in the inpatient and outpatient setting. Malignancy is the leading cause of hypercalcemia in hospitalized patients. In the outpatient setting, hyperparathyroidism is the leading cause of hypercalcemia. Metabolic bone disease includes a heterogeneous group of disorders. Because of the aging population, osteoporosis is the most prevalent and important of these bone disorders.

Hypercalcemia

Basic Information

- Calcium metabolism
  - Calcium is important for many physiologic processes, including bone matrix mineralization and muscle contraction
  - In the extracellular compartment it circulates in three forms:
    - "Ionized" or the free form: maintained within very narrow limits (45%)
    - Bound to protein (albumin and globulin) (40%)
    - Bound to anions (bicarbonate, phosphate, citrate) (15%)
  - Parathyroid hormone (PTH), produced by the four parathyroid glands, tightly regulates serum calcium levels
    - PTH level is primarily responsive to level of ionized calcium in the blood as well as to the levels of phosphate, magnesium, and 1,25 dihydroxyvitamin D (1,25(OH)$_2$D)
    - PTH actions (via G protein-coupled receptor; Fig. 39-1)
  - Vitamin D
    - A fat-soluble steroid obtained from diet or synthesized in skin in presence of ultraviolet (UV) light
    - Transported to the liver, where it is 25-hydroxylated to 25-OH D
    - Then transported to kidney, where it is 1-hydroxylated (under the control of PTH) to 1,25(OH)$_2$D (calcitriol), the active form
    - Actions of 1,25(OH)$_2$D (see Fig. 39-1)
- Definition of hypercalcemia: An abnormal elevation in the ionized calcium greater than 1.32 mmol/L or total calcium greater than the upper limit of normal for the assay, generally 10.3 to 10.5 mg/dL. The ionized calcium assay can be affected by many factors, including

pH and protein binding; it is generally more variable than the total calcium measurement.
  - Moderate hypercalcemia: levels between 12 and 14 mg/dL; variable clinical manifestations
  - **Severe hypercalcemia: Levels of 14 mg/dL or greater; almost always associated with symptoms and requires immediate treatment**
  - **Calcium is bound to albumin (40%); a "normal" total calcium may actually be high if albumin is low**
    - Formula for correcting the total calcium for low serum albumin: Corrected calcium = total serum calcium + (0.8 * [4 – serum albumin])
  - Acid-base status is also important because alkalosis increases calcium binding to albumin, whereas acidosis decreases it
- Causes of hypercalcemia (Box 39-1; Table 39-1)
  - **The two most common causes are hyperparathyroidism and malignancy, which make up more than 90% of cases**

Clinical Presentation

- The clinical presentation can be variable and often depends on factors other than total calcium level, such as:
  - Age of patient (older patients tend to be more symptomatic)
  - Comorbid conditions
  - Duration of hypercalcemia (longer duration is better tolerated)
  - Rate of increase in calcium concentration (a more rapid increase leads to more severe symptoms)
- Malignancy tends to present most acutely and severely
  - 10% to 20% of cancer patients develop hypercalcemia
  - Associated with a poor prognosis: 50% mortality at 1 month
- Main clinical manifestations of acute hypercalcemia
  - Gastrointestinal (GI): anorexia, nausea, vomiting, constipation (decreased GI motility)
  - Central nervous system: confusion, weakness, lethargy, hyporeflexia, obtundation, coma
  - Cardiovascular: hypertension (may be masked by dehydration), shortened Q-T interval, occasional bradycardia, and first-degree atrioventricular block
  - Renal: polyuria and polydipsia (via interference with antidiuretic hormone action and inhibition of

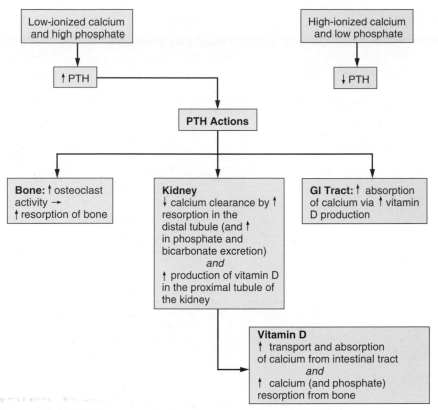

FIGURE 39-1 Actions of parathyroid hormone (PTH). GI, Gastrointestinal.

BOX 39-1	*Causes of Hypercalcemia*

Primary hyperparathyroidism
Malignancy
    Bone metastases
    Humoral hypercalcemia (related to PTHrP)
    Unregulated conversion of 25(OH) vitamin D to
        1,25(OH)$_2$ vitamin D
Granulomatous disease
    Sarcoidosis
    Tuberculosis
Familial hypocalciuric hypercalcemia
Drugs
    Thiazide diuretics (stimulate renal resorption of calcium)
    Lithium (changes "set point" of PTH release)
Vitamin A or D intoxication
Immobilization
Other
    Thyrotoxicosis
    Pheochromocytoma
    Adrenal insufficiency
    Parenteral nutrition

PTH, Parathyroid hormone; PTHrP, parathyroid hormone-related peptide.

sodium resorption), azotemia (dehydration and afferent arteriolar constriction)
- Chronic manifestations of hypercalcemia ("stones, bones, abdominal groans, and psychic overtones"); most commonly associated with chronic hyperparathyroidism
  - Osteoporosis with bone pain
  - Nephrocalcinosis
  - Band keratopathy (deposition of calcium phosphate in sun-exposed cornea; Fig. 39-2)

- Chondrocalcinosis (accumulation of calcium pyrophosphate dehydrate crystals in connective tissues)
- Pancreatitis (calcium deposition in the pancreas)
- Hypertension

Diagnosis and Evaluation

- Often the cause of the hypercalcemia is readily apparent from a good history and physical examination
- **If not, the first step is to distinguish between PTH-mediated and non–PTH-mediated forms of hypercalcemia**
  - **Intact PTH (iPTH) is the test of choice**
  - **Diagnosis often suggested by iPTH level (Fig. 39-3)**

Treatment

- Treatment approach for acute, life-threatening hypercalcemia
  - Rapidity and aggressiveness of treatment depend on absolute calcium level and patient's symptoms
    - **All patients should receive aggressive intravenous (IV) fluids as tolerated**
    - Bisphosphonates including pamidronate and zoledronic acid will have slower onset but will provide more durable response; calcitonin will take effect rapidly, but action is short lived
    - Definitive therapy, however, is to treat the underlying disorder (see Table 39-1)
- **Treatment options for acute, severe hypercalcemia**
  - If severe, acute, symptomatic hypercalcemia is present, institute treatment immediately

TABLE 39-1	Selected Disorders Associated with Hypercalcemia		
Disorder	**Pathophysiology**	**Clinical and Diagnostic Considerations**	**Treatment**
Primary hyperparathyroidism	Oversecretion of PTH by the parathyroid glands Sporadic, solitary adenoma (85%) Hyperplasia of all four glands (10%–15%) Carcinoma (<1%)	Most patients are asymptomatic; high calcium found on routine testing Typical symptoms: fatigue, nausea, constipation Associated with osteoporosis Loss of cortical bone > trabecular bone DXA should include forearm measurement for this reason (higher cortical bone percentage) Advanced form: Osteitis fibrosa cystica (rare) Preoperative sestamibi scan is helpful in localizing adenoma if present If hyperplasia of all four glands present, consider MEN syndromes Follow patients with serum calcium every 6 months and yearly creatinine and DXA	All symptomatic patients should undergo surgery Resection of adenoma, if nodule present Removal of 3½ glands if hyperplasia present Minimally invasive surgery if possible Surgery recommended in asymptomatic patients if: Age <50 years Calcium >1 mg/dL above upper limit of normal Creatinine clearance <60 mL/min Low bone density Difficult periodic follow-up Medical therapy (if not a surgical candidate) Estrogen and raloxifene will decrease serum calcium and decrease bone resorption Cinacalcet: Calcimimetic that binds to calcium-sensing receptor in parathyroid gland ↓ Sensitivity to serum calcium level ↓ PTH secretion FDA-approved indication for severe hypercalcemia
Malignancy	Three mechanisms Bony metastases resulting in local resorption (e.g., breast, multiple myeloma, prostate, lymphoma, thyroid, lung) Humoral hypercalcemia: Mediated by PTHrP; analogy with amino terminus of PTH; usually squamous cell carcinomas (e.g., lung); also renal, bladder, ovarian Conversion of 25(OH) vitamin D to active form (e.g., lymphoma)	More likely to present acutely and severely Can measure PTHrP via sensitive assay	Treat acute, symptomatic hypercalcemia as outlined in text Treat underlying malignancy
Granulomatous diseases	Unregulated synthesis of $1,25(OH)_2$ vitamin D by granuloma-associated macrophages Not sensitive to negative feedback suppression by ↑ calcium	Diseases such as sarcoidosis, tuberculosis, disseminated fungal infections, berylliosis Serum PO_4 often elevated as well; may lead to soft tissue calcification and nephrocalcinosis	Steroids particularly useful Treat underlying disease
Familial hypocalciuric hypercalcemia	Mutation in gene encoding calcium-sensing receptor Kidneys cannot sense calcium level and resorb too much Parathyroid glands also exhibit sensing defect and do not appropriately suppress PTH secretion Autosomal dominant	Clinical manifestations are benign; patients are asymptomatic May have a family history of unsuccessful neck explorations Urine calcium low (<100 mg/24 hours or urinary calcium/creatinine ratio <0.01) PTH usually upper end of the normal range or mildly elevated	No treatment necessary. Important to detect because can be confused with primary hyperparathyroidism and erroneously undergo parathyroidectomy

DXA, Dual-energy x-ray absorptiometry; FDA, Food and Drug Administration; MEN, multiple endocrine neoplasia; PTH, parathyroid hormone; PTHrP, parathyroid hormone-related peptide.

- Saline infusion with diuresis
  - Volume expansion using isotonic saline initially (most patients are severely dehydrated) and delivered at as rapid a rate as patient can tolerate
  - Improves renal blood flow and glomerular filtration rate (GFR) with increased filtration of calcium
  - Once volume is replete, loop diuretic (furosemide) can be added to enhance sodium excretion and protect against volume overload
    - Calcium follows sodium in the proximal tubule; the more sodium excreted, the more calcium excreted

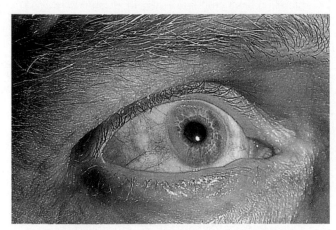

FIGURE 39-2 Ectopic calcification at the lateral and nasal margins of the right cornea (band keratopathy) in a patient with primary hyperparathyroidism. (From Forbes CD, Jackson WF. *Color Atlas and Text of Clinical Medicine.* 3rd ed. St. Louis: Mosby; 2003: Fig. 3.138.)

- Loop diuretics should be used because they also inhibit calcium resorption in the thick ascending limb of the loop of Henle
  - Thiazide diuretics do the opposite and should never be used in hypercalcemia
- Mobilization, if possible (immobility increases bone resorption because of lack of weight bearing)
- Pharmacologic options
  - Bisphosphonates
    - Are the gold standard
    - Bind to hydroxyapatite in bone and inhibit the dissolution of crystals; also inhibit osteoclast activity
    - **Pamidronate or zoledronic acid are drugs of choice; potent and effective**
    - **Calcium level begins to decline within 2 days and hits nadir at 7 days**
    - Adverse effects include transient, mild increase in temperature, myalgias, and transient increase in serum creatinine
  - Calcitonin
    - Inhibits bone resorption and increases renal excretion
    - **Has some analgesic properties and can be effective at relieving bone pain**
    - **Quickest in onset; takes effect within a few hours**
    - Effect is often limited and transient (because of tachyphylaxis)
    - Very safe; patients may have mild nausea, abdominal cramps, and flushing; because of occasional allergic reactions, initial 1-U skin test is recommended

39

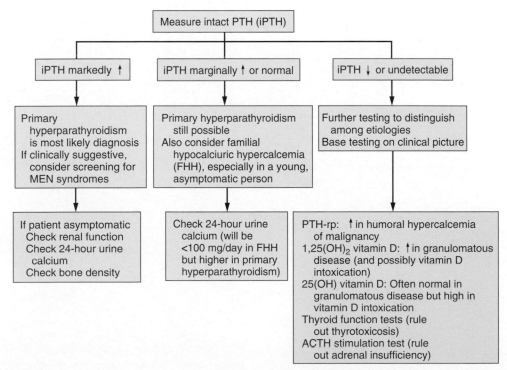

FIGURE 39-3 Approach to the patient with hypercalcemia. ACTH, Adrenocorticotropic hormone; iPTH, intact parathyroid hormone; MEN, multiple endocrine neoplasia; PTH, parathyroid hormone; PTH-rp, parathyroid hormone–related peptide.

- **Glucocorticoids**
  - **Most useful in treating vitamin D-mediated hypercalcemia (i.e., vitamin D intoxication, granulomatous diseases)**
  - **Work via inhibition of 1,25(OH)$_2$D production, decreased intestinal calcium and vitamin D absorption, increased renal calcium excretion**
  - Also useful in certain malignancies involving cytokine release (e.g., some myelomas)
  - Usual dose is prednisone 20 to 40 mg/day
- Treatment of more chronic causes of hypercalcemia (see Table 39-1)

Hypocalcemia

Basic Information

- Causes
  - Defect in action or metabolism of PTH
    - Hypoparathyroidism (after neck surgery, autoimmune, infiltrative diseases)
    - Resistance to action of PTH (pseudohypoparathyroidism)
  - Vitamin D deficiency (often low-normal calcium values) resulting from:
    - Inadequate oral intake
    - GI malabsorptive disorders (celiac disease, pancreatic insufficiency, ileal bypass)
    - End-stage liver or renal disease
    - **May manifest as osteomalacia (Box 39-2)**
  - Large-volume blood transfusions (citrate in transfused blood can bind calcium)
  - Magnesium depletion (decreased PTH release)
  - Acute respiratory alkalosis (increases binding of calcium to albumin)

BOX 39-2 *Osteomalacia*

Main defect: Undermineralized bone
Cause: Usually calcium ± phosphorus deficiency caused by:
  Dietary deficiency
  Gastrointestinal malabsorption
  Decreased vitamin D synthesis (liver disease, inadequate sun exposure, drugs such as phenytoin)
  Phosphorus wasting disorders
Clinical symptoms
  Fatigue
  Diffuse bone pain
  Muscle weakness
Diagnosis
  Laboratory results often reveal low (or low-normal) calcium, significant hypophosphatemia, mildly elevated alkaline phosphatase, low vitamin D levels
  Diagnosis confirmed by bone biopsy (with tetracycline labeling) showing undermineralization
Treatment: Repletion of calcium and vitamin D and phosphorus if necessary
  Calcium: 1000 to 1500 mg by mouth per day in divided doses
  Vitamin D: Often need 50,000 U of ergocalciferol by mouth up to 3 times weekly until symptoms resolve and serum vitamin D levels are normal

---

- Acute pancreatitis (calcium binds to free fatty acids released by lipase)
- Excessive tissue breakdown resulting in calcium binding to excess phosphate (tumor lysis syndrome, rhabdomyolysis)

Clinical Presentation

- Neurologic
  - Numbness, paresthesias (especially perioral), muscle irritability, tetany
  - Chvostek sign (spasm of the facial nerve when tapped)
  - Trousseau sign (carpopedal spasm elicited by inflating blood pressure cuff above systolic pressure; Fig. 39-4)
- Cardiovascular
  - Hypotension with decreased contractility
  - Prolonged Q-T interval on electrocardiogram
- Pulmonary
  - Bronchospasm

Diagnosis and Evaluation

- Measurement of serum calcium (ionized calcium is definitive method), phosphate, magnesium, iPTH, vitamin D levels
  - 25(OH)D is the major circulating form of vitamin D and is the best measure of vitamin D status for most patients
  - 1,25(OH)$_2$D is the active form of vitamin D and should only be measured in certain situations (disorders in the metabolism of 25(OH)D and phosphate, including chronic kidney disease, hereditary phosphate-losing disorders, oncogenic osteomalacia, and chronic granuloma-forming disorders, such as sarcoidosis and some lymphomas)
- Diagnosis often suggested by clinical presentation

Treatment

- Severe cases (symptomatic patients): IV repletion with calcium gluconate or calcium chloride slowly; ensure

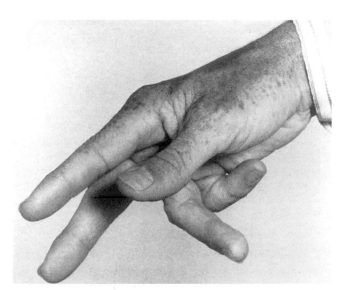

FIGURE 39-4 Trousseau sign (carpopedal spasm). (From Larsen PR, Kronenberg HM, Melmed S, et al. *Williams Textbook of Endocrinology.* 10th ed. Philadelphia: Saunders; 2002: Fig. 26-32.)

magnesium is also replete because this modulates PTH secretion
- Mild cases: Oral calcium carbonate or calcium citrate; usually vitamin D as well, including both vitamin D and, if necessary because of severity or etiology of hypocalcemia, 1,25 dihydroxyvitamin D in the form of oral calcitriol

Osteoporosis

Basic Information

- **Definition: A skeletal disorder characterized by low bone mass, compromised bone strength, and increased risk of fracture**
- Scope of the problem
  - Responsible for 2 million fractures per year
  - Lifetime risk for hip fracture of an average 50-year-old woman: 17.5% (with a 1-year mortality rate of 20%)
- Pathophysiology
  - Bone remodeling is a dynamic equilibrium between bone formation (by osteoblasts) and bone resorption (by osteoclasts)
  - Peak bone mass is achieved by age 30 years and is approximately 30% greater in men than in women
  - Around the fourth or fifth decade, women and men start losing bone at a rate of 0.3% to 0.5% per year
  - Loss is accelerated in women with loss of estrogen at menopause (can lose 3% to 5% per year for up to 5 years after menopause)
  - Pathology reveals distortion in microarchitecture, loss of trabeculae, and microfractures (Fig. 39-5)
- **Risk factors**
  - **Major risk factors**
    - **Older age**
    - **Personal history of a fragility fracture**
    - **Family history of osteoporosis or fracture in a first-degree relative**
    - **Thin body habitus (less than 127 pounds)**
    - **Current smoking**
    - **Current use of glucocorticoid therapy for longer than 3 months**
  - Other risk factors
    - Premature menopause (age younger than 45 years) or hypogonadism
    - Predisposition to falls (vision loss, previous cerebrovascular accident, frailty)
    - Heavy alcohol intake
    - Sedentary lifestyle
    - Dietary deficiencies (calcium, vitamin D)
  - Secondary causes (Box 39-3)
    - **Glucocorticoid use is the most common secondary cause**
      - **Only small doses, equivalent to 5 mg or more of prednisone per day for 3 or more months, are required for bone loss to occur**
    - In men with osteoporosis, consider checking testosterone level (hypogonadism is a fairly common cause)

Clinical Presentation

- Osteoporosis is asymptomatic until a fracture occurs
- Physical examination
  - Routine height measurement: Loss of height (more than 1 inch) may be only clue to vertebral fractures
  - Kyphosis: Decreases thoracic volume and can lead to dyspnea and restrictive lung disease (Fig. 39-6)
  - Look for clues to secondary causes of osteoporosis

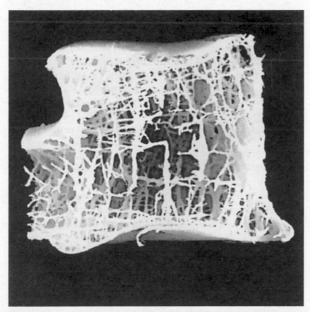

FIGURE 39-5 Cross section of an osteoporotic vertebra showing extensive loss of trabecular bone architecture. (From Larsen PR, Kronenberg HM, Melmed S, et al. *Williams Textbook of Endocrinology.* 10th ed. Philadelphia: Saunders; 2002: Fig. 27-15.)

BOX 39-3	*Select Secondary Causes of Osteoporosis*

Endocrine Disorders
Hyperthyroidism
Hyperparathyroidism
Hypogonadism
Excess cortisol production (e.g., Cushing disease)

Bone Marrow Disorders
Multiple myeloma
Leukemia/lymphoma

Gastrointestinal Diseases
Gastrectomy
Malabsorption syndromes

Connective Tissue Diseases
Rheumatoid arthritis
Osteogenesis imperfecta
Ehlers-Danlos syndrome
Marfan syndrome

Drugs
Glucocorticoids
Anticonvulsants
Cyclosporine
Prolonged anticoagulant use

39

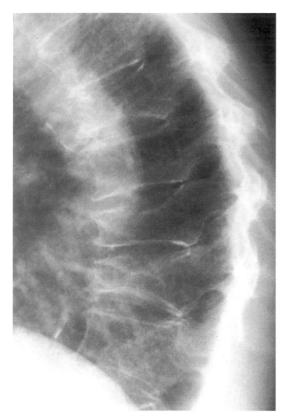

FIGURE 39-6 Radiograph showing radiolucency, compression fractures, and kyphosis in the spine of a patient with osteoporosis. (From Goldman L, Bennett JC, Ausiello D. *Cecil Textbook of Medicine.* 22nd ed. Philadelphia: Saunders; 2004: Fig. 258-4.)

Diagnosis and Evaluation

- Radiography: May see increased lucency of bone
  - Not helpful for detecting early disease; osteopenia not evident until approximately 30% of bone is lost
  - Lateral films useful for visualization of spine compression fractures
- Dual-energy x-ray absorptiometry (DXA)
  - Calculates bone mineral density (BMD) on the basis of tissue absorption of photons from a radionuclide source or x-ray tube
  - Measures BMD both at axial (spine) and at appendicular (hip, radius) sites
  - Low BMD highly correlates with increased risk of fracture
  - Is the gold standard for diagnosis
  - Results expressed as two scores:
    - **T-score: BMD expressed as the number of standard deviations above or below the mean BMD of normal young adults at the age of peak bone mass**
    - Z-score: BMD expressed as the number of standard deviations above or below the mean BMD of adults of the same age and gender
  - **World Health Organization diagnostic criteria for individuals older than age 50 years based on T-scores (see Table 39-2)**
  - **Indications for BMD measurement with DXA scan:**
    - **All postmenopausal women 65 years of age or older and all men 70 years of age or older**

TABLE 39-2	*World Health Organization Criteria for Diagnosis of Osteoporosis*
T-Score	**Assessment**
>−1	Normal bone mineral density
−1 to −2.5	Osteopenia
<−2.5	Osteoporosis

- **Women younger than age 65 years and men younger than age 70 years with one or more clinical risk factors, such as low body weight, previous fracture, high-risk medication use, disease or condition associated with bone loss, previous fragility fracture**
  - Aid in decision regarding hormone therapy
  - Radiologic evidence of osteopenia
  - Before initiating osteoporosis medication
  - Monitoring therapy for osteoporosis
- Biochemical assessment once osteoporosis confirmed by DXA
  - Baseline complete blood count; chemistry panel including calcium, phosphorus, alkaline phosphatase; thyroid-stimulating hormone, 25-hydroxyvitamin D level, 24-hour urinary calcium, PTH, testosterone (in men)
    - Many adults are vitamin D-deficient (minimal sun exposure, dietary insufficiencies)
    - Controversy exists about optimal vitamin D levels with the Institute of Medicine recommending levels greater than 20 ng/mL and the Endocrine Society recommending levels greater than 30 ng/mL
    - If vitamin D-insufficient (level 20 to 29 ng/mL), may need to replete with cholecalciferol
    - If vitamin D-deficient (level less than 20 ng/mL), may need to replete with high-dose ergocalciferol (see Box 39-2 on osteomalacia)
  - Other tests are not routinely ordered unless history, physical, or initial laboratory test results suggest need: serum protein electrophoresis (SPEP), urine protein electrophoresis (UPEP), tissue transglutaminase antibodies, 24-hour urinary cortisol, urine histamine, evaluation for hypercortisolemia

Treatment

- **Treatment guidelines from the National Osteoporosis Foundation (NOF) recommend incorporating other risk factors in addition to BMD; treat if:**
  - **History of a hip or vertebral fracture**
  - **Any T-score is 2.5 or lower**
  - **T-scores are between −1 and −2.5 and the patient also has:**
    - **History of other fragility fracture**
    - **10-year probability of hip fracture is 3% or higher**
    - **10-year probability of any major osteoporosis-related fracture is 20% or greater**
- 10-year probability of both hip and any major osteoporosis-related fracture is calculated using the FRAX algorithm

TABLE 39-3	Recommended Daily Calcium and Vitamin D Intake	
Age (years)	Calcium (mg/day)	Vitamin D (IU/day)
Adults <50	1000	800
Adults ≥50	1200	800

Modified from Cosman F, de Beur SJ, LeBoff MS, et al. Clinician's guide to prevention and treatment of osteoporosis. *Osteoporos Int.* 2014;25:2359-2381.

- FRAX is an online tool developed by the World Health Organization
- Incorporates nine clinical risk factors in addition to BMD
- Tailored to nationality, gender, ethnicity
- All patients with osteoporosis should be prescribed the following:
  - Behavior modification
    - Exercise (particularly modest weight-bearing exercise)
    - Limitation of alcohol intake to moderate levels
    - Smoking cessation, if applicable
  - Calcium
    - Recommended dietary requirements (Table 39-3)
    - Average diet in the United States is deficient (roughly 600 mg/day)
    - Major food sources: milk and dairy products (approximately 300 mg/serving), calcium-fortified foods, tofu, green leafy vegetables, almonds, corn tortillas, beans
    - Calcium supplements are helpful in those with deficient diets
      - Calcium carbonate is better absorbed when taken with meals (presence of acid)
      - Fractional calcium absorption will decrease with higher single doses of calcium so calcium should be provided in divided doses, preferably less than 500 to 600 mg at a time
      - Calcium citrate may be better absorbed in patients with achlorhydria or in those who take histamine$_2$-receptor antagonists or proton pump inhibitors
  - Vitamin D
    - Recommended daily requirements (see Table 39-3)
    - Food sources are limited to fatty fishes and fortified foods
    - Many calcium supplements also contain some vitamin D
- Estrogen
  - At menopause, falling estrogen levels contribute to rapid bone loss
  - Prescribing estrogen will halt bone loss in menopausal women (and result in BMD gain of 3% to 5% in osteoporotic women)
  - The earlier it is started, the bigger the effect on bone density
  - Currently approved only for prevention because of its association with various adverse events and the availability of other options (see later)

- Pharmacologic options for the treatment of osteoporosis (Table 39-4)
  - Therapy must be tailored to individual wants and needs of the patient
  - All approved therapies, except teriparatide, work by inhibiting bone resorption
  - **First-line therapy is often a bisphosphonate because of potency, duration of effect, bone specificity (as opposed to hormonal therapies), and tolerability**
    - IV forms (ibandronate and zoledronic acid) are options for patients who cannot tolerate oral preparations
    - Risks to consider:
      - Osteonecrosis of the jaw (ONJ) linked to IV administration in high doses (particularly in cancer patients); ONJ is rare in osteoporosis patients
      - Long-term, uninterrupted use (5 years or longer) associated with the very rare complication of atypical fractures of the femoral shaft (subtrochanteric or diaphyseal), which present with thigh and groin pain that is worse with weight bearing; x-ray should be obtained to evaluate and bisphosphonates stopped if this occurs
      - Risk of atypical fractures is very low and does not outweigh the benefit of known protection against fractures in individuals at increased risk
    - General approach to bisphosphonate therapy is to provide a 5-year course of medication and then evaluate whether a 1 year or more medication holiday is appropriate
      - On medication holiday, bone density is monitored and the patient should be assessed annually to determine when and if to return to medication
      - Individuals whose femoral neck bone density remains in the osteoporosis range after 5 years or those with a history of vertebral fractures benefit from longer term treatment before considering a medication holiday
  - Raloxifene and calcitonin (see Table 39-4)
  - Teriparatide: a recombinant form of parathyroid hormone
    - Delivered by daily subcutaneous injection
    - Intermittent delivery by injection results in increased bone formation
    - Generally a second-line agent
    - Maximum duration of use is 24 months in an individual's lifetime because of the finding of teriparatide causing osteosarcoma in rats, and therefore, limited duration of use in human fracture studies; there has not been an increased risk of osteosarcoma in humans
  - Denusomab: human monoclonal antibody to receptor activator of nuclear factor-κβ ligand (also known as RANKL)
    - Inhibits development and activity of osteoclasts
    - Injection every 6 months

39

| TABLE 39-4 | *Pharmacologic Options for Osteoporosis Treatment* | | | | |

Medication	Mechanism	Advantages	Prevention of Vertebral Fractures	Prevention of Hip/ Nonvertebral Fractures	Side Effects and Precautions
Raloxifene	Synthetic estrogen receptor agonist and antagonist Inhibits bone resorption	No effect on breast or endometrial tissue (unlike estrogen) Lowers LDL cholesterol	Yes	No	Risk of thromboembolism comparable to estrogen No effect on menopausal vasomotor symptoms
Bisphosphonates (alendronate, risedronate, ibandronate, zoledronic acid)	Structural analogues of inorganic pyrophosphate Bind to hydroxyapatite and inhibit osteoclast activity	Very potent Long half-life: Allows for once-weekly administration (once monthly for risedronate and ibandronate) Zoledronic acid administered IV once yearly	Yes	Yes (for alendronate, risedronate, zoledronic acid)	Poor oral absorption Upper GI irritation—have to take with 8 oz water on empty stomach, then remain upright with no food for 30 min (60 min for ibandronate)
Calcitonin	Naturally occurring peptide Directly inhibits osteoclast activity	Intranasal administration Well tolerated with few side effects Analgesic effect; useful in compression fractures	Yes	Not proven	Limited effectiveness
Teriparatide	Is the amino terminus (1–34) of PTH Subcutaneous administration causes increase in bone remodeling with formation effects greater than resorption effects	First drug to result in bone formation. Large increases in bone mineral density	Yes	Yes	May see transient hypercalcemia Osteosarcoma seen in animal studies; not seen in humans Disadvantage: Daily subcutaneous administration; duration of usage limited to 24 months
Denusomab	Monoclonal antibody to RANK ligand (RANKL) Inhibits osteoclast development and activity	Very potent Long half-life (dosing every 6 months) Well tolerated	Yes	Yes	RANKL plays a role in immune function— 1% increased risk of infections; no opportunistic infections seen

GI, Gastrointestinal; IV, intravenous; LDL, low-density lipoprotein; PTH, parathyroid hormone.

- Monitoring therapy
  - Repeat densitometry is the standard method of follow-up
  - **Reassessment by DXA at 2 years; may be warranted at 1 year in certain patients**
  - **Treatment is probably successful if repeat DXA demonstrates either modest increase in or stabilization of BMD**
    - Regardless of percent increase in BMD, most medications used for treatment decrease fracture risk by approximately 50% because they also improve the quality of the bone
    - A decrease in bone density in treatment indicates the need for evaluation of adherence, effectiveness of absorption of oral bisphosphonate, and presence of a cause of secondary osteoporosis

Paget Disease

Basic Information

- Second most common bone disease; usually manifests after age 40 years
- Pathophysiology: Chaotic osteoclast function with increased bone remodeling (both formation and resorption)
  - Many large osteoclasts with numerous nuclei
  - New bones formed are enlarged, structurally weaker

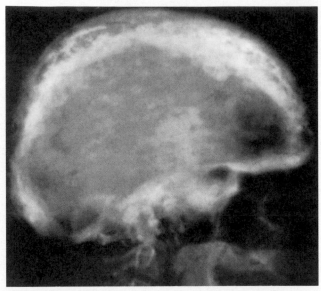

FIGURE 39-7 Radiograph of the skull of a patient with advanced Paget disease showing thickening, disordered new bone formation (cotton-wool patches), and basilar impression. (From Larsen PR, Kronenberg HM, Melmed S, et al. *Williams Textbook of Endocrinology.* 10th ed. Philadelphia: Saunders; 2002: Fig. 27-22.)

- Hypervascularity
- Etiology is unclear; possibly linked to a virus or genetic factors

Clinical Presentation

- **Pattern of bone involvement**
  - **May involve one bone or many bones asymmetrically**
  - **Most common sites: pelvis, lumbar spine, skull, femur, tibia**
- Many patients have no symptoms (more than 90%)
- **Others experience bone pain, skeletal deformities**
  - **Enlarged skull, particularly frontal and occipital areas (Fig. 39-7)**
  - **Bowed lower extremities (Fig. 39-8)**
  - **Increased risk of fracture with minimal trauma, particularly femur, tibia, radius**
  - **Impingement syndromes (e.g., inner ear with hearing loss and vertigo)**
  - Less common and occurring late in course
    - High-output congestive heart failure from numerous vascular shunts
    - Increased risk of osteosarcoma although this is extremely rare
    - Hypercalcemia during immobilization

Diagnosis and Evaluation

- Laboratory studies show an isolated increase in alkaline phosphatase (can be more than 500 U/L)
- Plain films can reveal all three phases of disease; seeing all three is essentially diagnostic
  - First phase: osteoporosis from osteolytic activity
  - Second phase (most commonly seen): mixed phase with both sclerosis and osteolytic activity
  - Third phase: mainly sclerosis with cortical thickening

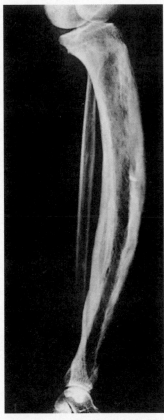

FIGURE 39-8 Paget disease of the tibia. Note the bowing, marked irregularity of the anterior cortex, and flame-shaped lytic lesion of the posterior cortex. (From Larsen PR, Kronenberg HM, Melmed S, Polonsky KS. *Williams Textbook of Endocrinology.* 10th ed. Philadelphia: Saunders; 2003: Fig. 8-14.)

39

- Bone scan: most sensitive test; can identify areas of increased uptake

Treatment

- **Treatment is recommended for:**
  - **All patients with symptoms**
  - **Asymptomatic patients with involvement of the skull, axial skeleton, or weight-bearing long bones (high risk of progression to deformity)**
  - **Asymptomatic patients with alkaline phosphatase greater than 3 times upper limit of normal**
  - **Patients undergoing surgery on sites of active disease because treatment will reduce the hypervascularity in the bone lesion**
- Analgesics for pain
- Bisphosphonates for severe disease
  - First-line therapy
  - Requires higher doses than those used for osteoporosis
  - Oral agents (risedronate, alendronate)
    - Treat until disease in remission , then discontinue drug with close monitoring of the alkaline phosphatase
  - IV agents (pamidronate, zoledronic acid)
    - Single infusion of zoledronic acid provides rapid and sustained response

- Calcitonin is also Food and Drug Administration-approved for Paget disease but is rarely used; causes marked decrease in bone resorption, but disease recurs if drug is stopped
  - Significant bone pain relief, even when used intermittently
  - Some patients develop resistance to drug
- Prognosis is good; disease responds well to treatment with an increase in lamellar bone formation and a decrease in pain
- Disease activity can be monitored with biochemical markers (alkaline phosphatase and C-telopeptide)

Acknowledgment

The authors would like to acknowledge Redonda G. Miller, MD, MBA, for her work on previous editions of this chapter.

Review Questions

For review questions, please go to ExpertConsult.com.

SUGGESTED READINGS

Bilezekian JP, Khan AA, Potts JT Jr, et al. Guidelines for the management of asymptomatic primary hyperparathyroidism: summary statement from the third international workshop. *J Clin Endocrinol Metab.* 2009;94:335-339.

Ettinger B, Black DM, Mitlak BH, et al. Reduction of vertebral fracture risk in postmenopausal women with osteoporosis treated with raloxifene. *JAMA.* 1999;282:637-645.

Liberman UA, Weiss SR, Broll J, et al. Effect of oral alendronate on bone mineral density and the incidence of fractures in postmenopausal osteoporosis. *N Engl J Med.* 1995;333:1437-1496.

McClung MR, Geusens P, Miller PD, et al. Effect of risedronate on the risk of hip fracture in elderly women. Hip Intervention Program Study Group. *N Engl J Med.* 2001;344:333-340.

Pecherstorfer M, Brenner K, Zojer N. Current management strategies for hypercalcemia. *Treat Endocrinol.* 2003;2:273-292.

Ralston SH, Langston AL, Reid IR. Pathogenesis and management of Paget's disease of bone. *Lancet.* 2008;372:155-163.

Rosen CJ. Clinical practice: postmenopausal osteoporosis. *N Engl J Med.* 2005;353:595-603.

U.S. Preventive Services Task Force. Screening for osteoporosis: U.S. Preventive Services Task Force Recommendation Statement. *Ann Intern Med.* 2011;154:356-364.

CHAPTER 40

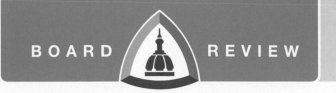
Reproductive Endocrinology

TODD T. BROWN, MD, PhD

This chapter focuses on the reproductive endocrine disorders the internist is most likely to encounter. Common problems for women include amenorrhea and hirsutism. Men may present with symptoms of gynecomastia, impotence, or other features of hypogonadism. Despite their prevalence, patients are often hesitant to discuss these symptoms. Therefore, internists may need to actively inquire about their presence.

Female Reproductive Disorders

FEMALE REPRODUCTIVE PHYSIOLOGY

- Normal menstrual cycle requires cyclic release of gonadotropin-releasing hormone (GnRH) from the hypothalamus, which leads to cyclic secretion of the pituitary gonadotropins: follicle-stimulating hormone (FSH) and luteinizing hormone (LH)
- The ovaries respond to FSH and LH by producing follicles containing ova
- Phases of the normal female menstrual cycle (Fig. 40-1)
  - Follicular phase of menstrual cycle: ovarian follicle development
    - Estrogen predominantly produced by ovary
    - Causes thickening of uterine endometrium
  - Ovulation: LH surge induces release of egg from ovarian follicle
  - Luteal phase: progesterone production by corpus luteum induces maturation of secretory endometrium
  - Menses: decline in estrogen and progesterone results in endometrial shedding

AMENORRHEA

- Oligomenorrhea is defined as infrequent menses (more than 35 days between cycles or fewer than 6 to 8 periods per year)
- Amenorrhea is the absence of menses; may be physiologic or pathologic
  - Physiologic amenorrhea is normal and occurs with pregnancy, lactation, menopause
  - Pathologic amenorrhea can exist in either a primary or a secondary form
    - ***Primary amenorrhea* is defined as the persistent absence of menses by age 16 years**
    - ***Secondary amenorrhea* is the absence of menses for more than 6 months in a patient with a prior history of menses**

PRIMARY AMENORRHEA

Basic Information and Clinical Presentation

- Patients with primary amenorrhea may be grouped into those with and those without secondary sexual characteristics
- Primary amenorrhea with secondary sexual characteristics and normal sexual development
  - Usually indicates presence of ovaries
  - Etiologies include testicular feminization and Müllerian defects
  - **Testicular feminization**
    - **Caused by androgen insensitivity**
    - **XY karyotype**
    - Normal male testosterone levels
    - Physical features: breasts and feminine appearance, absence of axillary or pubic hair, and blind-ending vagina
  - Müllerian defects
    - Usually congenital
    - Physical features: imperforate hymen, abnormal cervix, absence of vagina
- Primary amenorrhea without secondary sexual characteristics or other signs of puberty
  - Etiologies (Table 40-1)

Diagnosis and Evaluation

- Primary amenorrhea with signs of puberty
  - Many causes can be identified on physical examination or ultrasonography and subsequent karyotype if needed
  - If physical examination/ultrasound findings are inconsistent with either testicular feminization or Müllerian defects (i.e., uterus present), then perform withdrawal bleed as described in the section on secondary amenorrhea
- Primary amenorrhea without signs of puberty
  - Check gonadotropin (FSH, LH) levels
    - If elevated, check karyotype to rule out Turner syndrome (Fig. 40-2)
    - If low, perform pituitary magnetic resonance imaging (MRI) to evaluate for hypothalamic-pituitary abnormalities

Treatment

- Primary amenorrhea with signs of puberty
  - For patients with testicular feminization, inguinal testes must be removed at puberty because of risk of malignancy

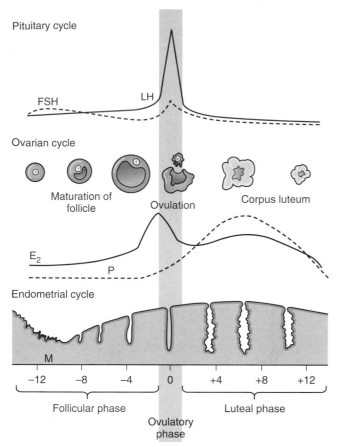

Pituitary cycle

FSH   LH

Ovarian cycle

Maturation of follicle

Ovulation

Corpus luteum

E₂

P

Endometrial cycle

M

−12   −8   −4   0   +4   +8   +12

Follicular phase

Ovulatory phase

Luteal phase

FIGURE 40-1 Hormone levels during the female menstrual cycle. The idealized cyclic changes observed in gonadotropins, estradiol (E_2), progesterone (P), and uterine endometrium during the normal menstrual cycle. The data are centered on the day of the luteinizing hormone (LH) surge (day 0). Days of menstrual bleeding are indicated by M. FSH, Follicle-stimulating hormone. (From Goldman L, Bennett JC, Ausiello D. *Cecil Textbook of Medicine.* 22nd ed. Philadelphia: Saunders; 2004: Fig. 250-1.)

- For patients with Müllerian defects, surgical repair is usually necessary
- Primary amenorrhea without signs of puberty
  - Treat underlying disorder, if possible (see Table 40-1)
  - Hormone replacement therapy
    - Start estrogen and progesterone in young patients to preserve bone density, improve well-being, prevent genitourinary atrophy, and promote breast development; long-term safety of hormone replacement in this setting has not been evaluated
    - Oral contraceptives often used for hormone replacement in young patients
- Patients who desire children should be referred to a reproductive endocrinologist

SECONDARY AMENORRHEA

Basic Information

- Most common causes are physiologic (e.g., pregnancy and menopause)
- **Differential diagnosis of pathologic secondary amenorrhea consists of four main disease states:**
  - **Hyperprolactinemia (e.g., prolactinoma, drugs)**
  - **Anovulatory states (e.g., most commonly polycystic ovary syndrome; Box 40-1)**
  - **Androgen excess (e.g., androgen-secreting tumors)**
  - **Hypothalamic amenorrhea (e.g., physical or emotional stress, anorexia, excessive exercise)**
- Rarely caused by disorders of the outflow tract, such as:
  - Endometrial atrophy from prolonged use of progestins
  - Adhesions and obliteration of the uterine cavity (Asherman syndrome)
  - Endometritis

Clinical Presentation

- **Symptoms and signs of hypoestrogenic state: hot flashes, vaginal dryness, dyspareunia, osteopenia**

TABLE 40-1	Causes of Primary Amenorrhea without Secondary Sexual Characteristics			
Disorder	**Features**	**Diagnosis**	**Fertility**	**Treatment**
Constitutional delay of puberty	Family history of delayed puberty	Family history Difficult to distinguish from GnRH deficiency	Will be present at maturity	Observation and reassurance
Pituitary and hypothalamic disorders	Hypogonadotropic hypogonadism Causes include destructive lesions (tumors) or isolated gonadotropin deficiency (Kallman syndrome)	↓ FSH and LH No change in FSH and LH in response to GnRH stimulation	Variable, depending on underlying disorder	If malignancy, consider surgery or radiation Consider hormone replacement
Turner syndrome (see Fig. 40-2)	45,XO karyotype Physical features include lack of sexual maturation, short stature, webbed neck, shield chest, and valgus deformity of the elbow	↑ FSH and LH XO karyotype	Usually absent unless mosaic of XO and XX cells	Hormone replacement
Gonadal dysgenesis	Absence of ovaries Congenital	↑ FSH and LH	Absent	Hormone replacement

FSH, Follicle-stimulating hormone; GnRH, gonadotropin-releasing hormone; LH, luteinizing hormone.

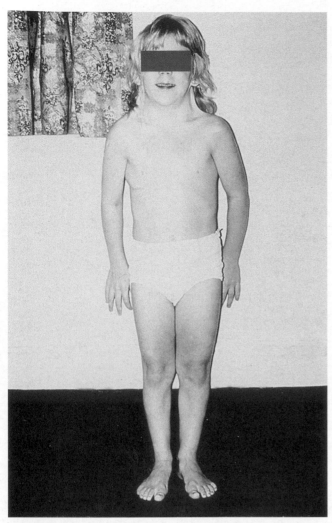

FIGURE 40-2 Girl with Turner syndrome. Note the shield chest, widely spaced nipples, and webbed neck. (From Lowenstein EJ, Kim KH, Glick SA. Turner's syndrome in dermatology. *J Am Acad Dermatol.* 2004;50:767–776: Fig. 1.)

- Findings suggestive of underlying cause
  - Prolactin excess: breast tenderness, galactorrhea
  - Androgen excess: hirsutism, acne, increased muscle mass, clitoromegaly

Diagnosis and Evaluation

- **First step is always to rule out pregnancy**
- Algorithm for evaluation: see Figure 40-3
- Mechanics of inducing a withdrawal bleed with progesterone (see Fig. 40-3)
  - If the endometrium is estrogenized, it should respond to progesterone challenge
  - Give 10-mg medroxyprogesterone daily for 5 to 7 days
  - Withdrawal bleeding should occur within 1 week of completion of progesterone challenge

Treatment

- Treat the underlying disorder (e.g., dopamine agonist for prolactinoma)
- **In women younger than 50 years, oral contraceptives are often used (see treatment of primary amenorrhea)**

BOX 40-1   *Polycystic Ovary Syndrome*

Basic Information

Affects up to 10% of women
Thought to be caused by stimulatory effects of excess insulin on ovarian androgen production

Clinical Features

Amenorrhea, hirsutism, acne, obesity, and insulin resistance

Diagnosis

Is a clinical diagnosis; a diagnostic test with high sensitivity and specificity has not been identified
Ovarian ultrasound (for cysts) and LH:FSH ratio (often increased); do not always distinguish these patients from normal

Treatment

Weight loss

Oral contraceptives if fertility is not desired
Metformin or thiazolidinediones (insulin sensitizers) may restore ovulation and fertility, thus confirming the role of insulin resistance, but oral contraceptives considered first line
Antiandrogens for hirsutism (spironolactone)

FSH, Follicle-stimulating hormone; LH, luteinizing hormone.

- In women older than 50 years, postmenopausal hormone combinations may be used, but benefits versus risks need to be carefully considered
- **In women with normal menopause, postmenopausal hormone therapy (HT) to prevent chronic medical conditions (such as coronary heart disease) is no longer recommended**
  - **Indications for HT: debilitating vasomotor symptoms**
  - Other benefits: preservation of bone mineral density and possible reduced risk of colorectal cancer (but other specific treatments, such as bisphosphonates for osteoporosis, are considered first-line treatments)
  - Risks: Results from the Women's Health Initiative demonstrated that HT increases the risk of breast cancer, stroke, and venous thromboembolic disease and has no benefit in preventing heart disease
  - **If HT started, lowest dose for shortest duration (preferably less than 5 years) is generally recommended; reassessment for continued need should be done at least yearly**
  - Many forms available (oral, transdermal); none are definitively shown to be superior
  - If uterus is present, must administer progestin with estrogen to avoid increased risk of endometrial cancer
    - Cycled if patient desires monthly withdrawal bleeding
    - Continuous if withdrawal bleeding is undesirable (more commonly used in postmenopausal women)
  - Vaginal spotting and bleeding may be a nuisance side effect
    - Usually resolves within 6 months
    - If heavy or first bleeding occurs 6 months after initiating therapy, endometrial biopsy should be performed to rule out hyperplasia or cancer

40

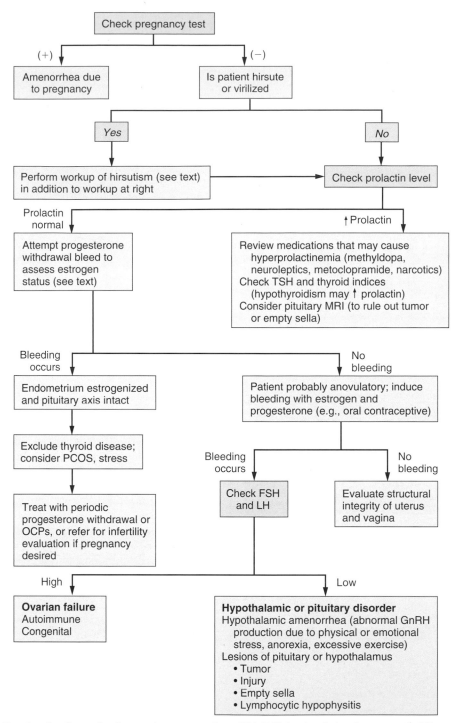

FIGURE 40-3 Algorithm for the diagnosis of secondary amenorrhea. FSH, Follicle-stimulating hormone; GnRH, gonadotropin-releasing hormone; LH, luteinizing hormone; MRI, magnetic resonance imaging; OCPs, oral contraceptive pills; PCOS, polycystic ovary syndrome; TSH, thyroid-stimulating hormone.

HIRSUTISM

Basic Information

- Hirsutism is defined as the presence of terminal (coarse, pigmented) hairs on parts of a woman's body where terminal hairs are considered to be a male secondary sexual characteristic (e.g., face, chest, back, lower abdomen, inner thighs; Fig. 40-4)

- **Virilization refers to signs of more severe androgen excess (e.g., deep voice, clitoromcgaly, frontal balding, enhanced musculature, hirsutism)**
- Hirsutism may occur with or without virilization
- Androgens
  - Testosterone: derived from the ovaries (25%), adrenals (25%), and peripheral conversion from androstenedione (50%)

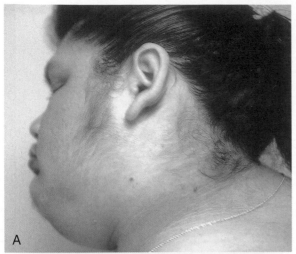

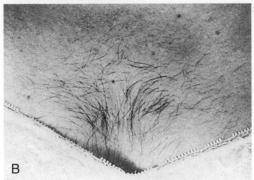

FIGURE 40-4 Examples of hirsutism. Male-pattern hair growth on the face (**A**), and on the chest (**B**). (From Larsen PR, Kronenberg HM, Melmed S, Polonsky KS. *Williams Textbook of Endocrinology.* 10th ed. Philadelphia: Saunders; 2003: Fig. 16-30.)

- ■ Most potent androgen
- ■ Circulates as free (1%) and bound (99%)
- ■ Dihydroepiandrosterone sulfate (DHEA-S) is predominantly derived from the adrenal cortex (95%)
- ■ Causes of hirsutism include ovarian or adrenal causes, drugs, and physiologic (most common; Box 40-2)
  - ■ **Idiopathic familial form (physiologic) is the most common cause overall**
  - ■ **Most common ovarian cause: polycystic ovary syndrome (PCOS; see Box 40-1)**
  - ■ **Most common adrenal cause: congenital adrenal hyperplasia (Box 40-3)**

Clinical Presentation

- ■ History
  - ■ Assess onset, duration, and progression of hair growth
  - ■ Look for symptoms of PCOS: weight gain, acne, diabetes, menstrual irregularities
  - ■ Inquire about family history of hirsutism (suggesting familial form)
  - ■ Inquire about medications that might cause hirsutism (see Table 40-1)
- ■ Physical examination
  - ■ Assess extent of hirsutism (Ferriman-Gallwey score) (Fig. 40-5)

BOX 40-2 | *Causes of Hirsutism*

Ovarian Causes
Polycystic ovary syndrome
Hyperthecosis (rests of ovarian stromal cells that produce testosterone)
Androgen-producing ovarian tumors

Adrenal Causes
Congenital adrenal hyperplasia
Androgen-producing adrenal tumors
Cushing syndrome

Elevated Prolactin
Unclear mechanism

Medications
Androgens (e.g., danazol)
Cyclosporine
Phenytoin

Physiologic Causes
Idiopathic familial
Postmenopausal

BOX 40-3 | *Congenital Adrenal Hyperplasia*

Basic Information
Inherited defects in adrenal cortisol synthesis result in overproduction of other adrenal hormones, including androgens
Late-onset or nonclassic 21-hydroxylase deficiency is the most common form, occurring in 0.1% to 1% of women

Clinical Presentation
Hirsutism begins at menarche
Menstrual irregularities begin in adulthood

Diagnosis
17-Hydroxyprogesterone will be elevated (stimulation with synthetic ACTH may be necessary to elicit the abnormality)

Treatment
Hydrocorticosone will decrease the excess androgen production

ACTH, Adrenocorticotropic hormone.

- ■ Look for signs of virilization (e.g., acne, clitoromegaly, deepened voice, muscle hypertrophy)
- ■ Look for signs of insulin resistance, including acanthosis nigricans (to suggest PCOS)
- ■ Look for signs of Cushing syndrome (e.g., dorsocervical fat pad, striae, proximal muscle weakness)

Diagnosis and Evaluation

- ■ **Sudden onset, rapid course, and/or presence of virilization suggestive of a malignancy**
- ■ Laboratory tests
  - ■ Free and total testosterone
    - ■ Often only free (not total) testosterone is elevated
    - ■ Usually only mildly elevated with PCOS

40

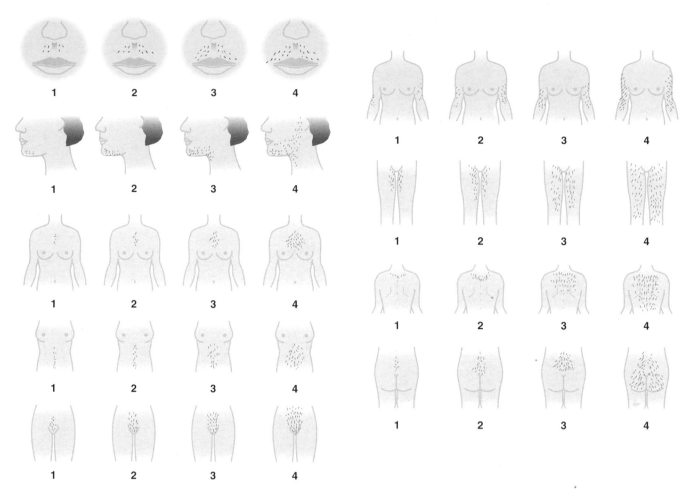

FIGURE 40-5 Ferriman-Gallwey hirsutism scoring system. Each of the nine body areas most sensitive to androgen is assigned a score from 0 (no hair) to 4 (frankly virile), and these separate scores are summed to provide a hormonal hirsutism score. (Modified from Martin KA, Chang RJ, Ehrmann DA, et al. Evaluation and treatment of hirsutism in premenopausal women: an Endocrine Society Clinical Practice Guideline. *J Clin Endocrinol Metab.* 2008;93:1105-1120; Originally appeared in Hatch R, Rosenfield RL, Kim MH, et al. Hirsutism: implications, etiology, and management. *Am J Obstet Gynecol.* 1981;140:815-830.)

- Total testosterone greater than 200 ng/dL raises concern for adrenal or ovarian tumor (DHEA-S helpful to distinguish source)
- DHEA-S
  - If level greater than 500 mg/dL, consider adrenal tumor or late-onset congenital adrenal hyperplasia
- Prolactin (hyperprolactinemia may cause hirsutism)
- 17-Hydroxyprogesterone
  - May be elevated in congenital adrenal hyperplasia
  - Adrenocorticotropic hormone stimulation test may be necessary to elicit elevation
- Imaging
  - Abdominal computed tomography or sonogram if adrenal or ovarian tumors are suspected
  - MRI of the pituitary if prolactin is elevated and no medication is identified as the culprit

Treatment

- Treatment is directed toward correction of the underlying problem (if possible)
- Once terminal hair has developed, it may not disappear, even if abnormal hormone levels resolve

- Oral contraceptives are generally considered the treatment of choice for hirsutism and androgenic symptoms
- Spironolactone is useful for inhibiting effects of androgens on hair follicles but primarily prevents worsening of hirsutism
- **Insulin-lowering medications, such as metformin or pioglitazone, can induce ovulation, decrease hirsutism, and reduce insulin resistance in women with PCOS, but study results have been inconsistent**
- **Oral contraceptives are generally the preferred agents**
- Eflornithine cream may inhibit an enzyme needed for hair growth; often used for facial hair

Male Reproductive and Hormonal Disorders

GYNECOMASTIA
Basic Information

- **Gynecomastia refers to benign growth of glandular tissue of the male breast**

Medications
    ACE inhibitors
    Amiodarone
    Antipsychotics
    Calcium channel blockers
    Diazepam
    Digoxin
    Efavirenz
    HIV nucleoside reverse transcriptase inhibitors
    Ketoconazole
    Omeprazole
    Opiates
    Phenytoin
    Ranitidine
    Spironolactone
    Tricyclic antidepressants
Endocrine disorders
    Hyperthyroidism
    Hypogonadism
    Hormone-secreting tumors
    Chronic systemic illness
    Renal disease
    Hepatic disease
Marijuana
Idiopathic

ACE, Angiotensin-converting enzyme; HIV, human immunodeficiency virus.

- **Considered normal in males at three life stages**
  - **Newborn (first 2 to 3 weeks of life)**
  - **Pubertal (ages 9 to 14 years)**
  - **Elderly (variable)**
- Causes of gynecomastia (Box 40-4)
  - Most causes induce gynecomastia by causing a change in the relative amounts of estrogens and androgens (e.g., the ratio favors estrogen excess)
  - Mechanisms include decrease in androgen or androgen effect or increase in estrogen (exogenous or endogenous)
  - Most common causes in adults are medications and alcoholic liver disease

Clinical Presentation

- Confirm gynecomastia: concentric enlargement of the tissue deep to the nipple
  - May be unilateral or bilateral
  - May be asymmetrical
  - May be associated with pain and tenderness
  - Nipple discharge is rare; if present, consider malignancy
  - Distinguish from obesity by palpating for a ridge of tissue concentric with the nipple
- Assess for sexual dysfunction
- Perform a testicular examination to detect any masses

Diagnosis and Evaluation

- Cause is often clear from history and physical examination
- **Highly consider malignancy if gynecomastia is unilateral, ulcerative, associated with bloody discharge or with axillary adenopathy; in this case, proceed directly to mammography and biopsy**

- Laboratory evaluation (if cause is not clear from the history and physical)
  - Check renal and hepatic function
  - Morning testosterone level (low level suggests hypogonadal cause)
  - FSH, LH
    - High levels associated with primary testicular failure
    - Low levels associated with exogenous steroids or hypogonadotropic hypogonadism
  - Prolactin (prolactinoma), thyroid-stimulating hormone (hyperthyroidism), human chorionic gonadotropin (hCG; hCG-producing testicular tumor), estradiol (estrogen-producing testicular tumor)
- Mammogram: perform if gynecomastia is unilateral or if the mass is not concentric with the nipple

Treatment

- Gynecomastia is primarily a cosmetic problem, although it can be a clue to underlying disease
- Men with gynecomastia may have a slight increase in risk of breast cancer
- **Treatment is aimed at eliminating the underlying cause (e.g., stop any offending medication)**
  - If treatment begins in the first few months after symptoms of gynecomastia appear, chance of regression of the gynecomastia is good
  - **Over time, the enlarged breast tissue becomes fibrotic and is not likely to shrink even if hormones return to normal**
- Options
  - Testosterone replacement therapy for hypogonadal men
  - Antiestrogens (e.g., tamoxifen) may be useful; aromatase inhibitors are ineffective and not recommended
  - Surgery may be performed if gynecomastia does not resolve and is bothersome to the patient

MALE HYPOGONADISM

Basic Information

- **Hypogonadism in men is defined as an inappropriately low testosterone level for age**
  - Normal range for men ages 18 to 29 years is approximately 700 to 1300 ng/dL
  - Declines to approximately 150 to 500 ng/dL for men ages 70 to 79 years
- **Classification of male hypogonadism**
  - **Primary: caused by dysfunction of the testes (hypergonadotropic hypogonadism)**
  - **Secondary: caused by a disorder of the pituitary or hypothalamus that impairs the ability of the pituitary to stimulate testosterone production (hypogonadotropic hypogonadism)**
  - **Testosterone resistance: inability of the target tissues to respond to testosterone**
- Causes of primary and secondary hypogonadism (Box 40-5)
- Most common cause of primary hypogonadism in men is Klinefelter syndrome (Box 40-6; Fig. 40-6)

40

BOX 40-5   *Causes of Male Hypogonadism*

Primary Hypogonadism (Hypergonadotropic Hypogonadism)

Trauma to genital organs
Autoimmune destruction
Mumps orchitis
Medications
    Cyclosporine
    Chemotherapeutic agents
Congenital disorders
    Klinefelter syndrome
    Bilateral anorchia

Secondary Hypogonadism (Hypogonadotropic Hypogonadism)

Chronic illness
Medications
    Opiates
    Glucocorticoids
    Leuprolide
Prolactinoma
Damage to hypothalamus or pituitary
    Radiation
    Tumor
    Trauma
Hereditary
    Hemochromatosis (pituitary iron deposition)
Congenital disorders
    Kallman syndrome

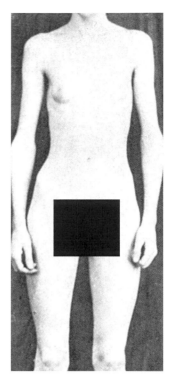

FIGURE 40-6 Klinefelter syndrome. Note the narrow shoulders, long upper body segment, and gynecomastia. (From Ferri FF. *Ferri's Clinical Advisor: Instant Diagnosis and Treatment.* 8th ed. Philadelphia: Mosby; 2006: Fig. 1-133.)

BOX 40-6   *Klinefelter Syndrome*

Basic Information

Incidence of 1 per 1000 live male births
XXY karyotype
↑FSH and LH in response to low testosterone production; promotes estrogen production by the Leydig cells

Clinical Presentation

May be asymptomatic until puberty
Intellect may be subnormal throughout life
Physical examination
    Gynecomastia develops in response to the estrogen
    Variable secondary sexual characteristics ranging from
        no sexual development to normal development
    Infertility
    Testicular exam: During puberty, testes become small
        and firm
    Increased risk of breast cancer, autoimmune disorders,
        varicose veins, germ cell neoplasms

Diagnosis

History and physical
    Upper body segment to lower body segment ratio <1
    High palate
    Above-average arm span
Labs
    Low testosterone
    Elevated FSH and LH
    XXY karyotype is needed to confirm the diagnosis
Treatment
    Androgen replacement

FSH, Follicle-stimulating hormone; LH, luteinizing hormone.

Clinical Presentation

- Symptoms
  - Decreased libido
  - Hot flashes if testosterone loss is sudden
- Signs
  - Sparse facial and body hair
  - Gynecomastia
  - Small penis, prostate, and testes
- Related conditions
  - Infertility
  - Osteoporosis
- **If hypogonadal during adolescence, may have complete failure of sexual maturation**
  - **Absence of growth spurt, high-pitched voice, and upper-to-lower body ratio of less than 1**
  - Consider possibility of:
    - Klinefelter syndrome (see Box 40-5 and Fig. 40-6)
    - Kallman syndrome (congenital lack of development of the olfactory lobes and GnRH-producing cells leading to anosmia; hypogonadotropic hypogonadism; and, occasionally, cleft palate or color blindness)

Diagnosis and Evaluation

- **Low testosterone is diagnostic**
  - **Total testosterone less than 300 ng/dL is generally considered abnormal at any age when accompanied by clinical symptoms**
  - Check a free testosterone level to rule out an abnormality with sex hormone-binding globulin (e.g., human immunodeficiency virus)

- Semen analysis helpful (even if fertility not an issue): if normal, hypogonadism essentially ruled out
- FSH and LH: high in primary hypogonadism, low in secondary hypogonadism
- Other tests should be based on the clinical picture
  - Comprehensive metabolic panel and complete blood counts (to look for undiagnosed chronic disease, such as hepatic or renal failure)
  - Prolactin and brain MRI if pituitary tumor is suspected
  - Estradiol, hCG, and testicular ultrasound if testicular tumor is suspected
  - Iron studies if hemochromatosis is suspected

Treatment

- Treatment of underlying problem if possible
- Androgen replacement with testosterone injection, patch, or gel
  - Contraindication to replacement: history of androgen-dependent tumor (e.g., prostate cancer)
  - **Hematocrit should be monitored regularly given the increased risk of erythrocytosis with testosterone replacement**
  - **Prostate examination and prostate-specific antigen (PSA) testing should be done in men older than 40 years receiving androgen replacement**
  - **Testosterone should be used with caution in men with or at risk for cardiovascular disease because of safety concerns**
- Therapy with FSH and hCG (by injection) may be used in those with hypogonadotropic hypogonadism who desire fertility

ERECTILE DYSFUNCTION

Basic Information

- Definition: inability to attain or maintain an erection to achieve penetration
- Causes
  - Penile disorders
    - Peyronie disease (penile induration): stems from fibrotic plaques of unclear etiology that can result in penile curvature, painful erections, and impotence; treatment is surgical
    - Trauma
  - Nervous system disorders: stroke, spinal cord injury, prostatectomy complicated by nerve injury
  - Vascular disorders
    - Atherosclerotic vascular disease
    - **Leriche syndrome (impotence associated with distal aortic atherosclerosis resulting in claudication of the lower back, buttocks, and thighs)**
  - Endocrine disorders: diabetes, hypogonadism
  - Psychogenic disorders (common in young men)
  - Medications (see Box 40-4 for male hypogonadism), as well as β-blockers, antidepressants, and antipsychotics
  - Substance abuse

Clinical Presentation

- Difficulty with obtaining or maintaining an erection
- May or may not have features of hypogonadism (see previous section)

Diagnosis and Evaluation

- History and physical examination
  - Look for clues to an underlying diagnosis (e.g., presence of peripheral vascular disease, complications of diabetes)
  - **Sudden onset of impotence favors psychogenic cause**
- Check testosterone levels, FSH, LH, estradiol
- Psychiatric evaluation if psychogenic cause suspected

Treatment

- Directed at underlying cause
- **Sildenafil, vardenafil, and tadalafil are phosphodiesterase-5 (PDE-5) inhibitors that prolong vasodilation by nitric oxide and are considered first-line drugs after underlying causes have been investigated**
  - Sildenafil and vardenafil should be taken 1 hour before intercourse; duration of effect is approximately 4 hours
  - Tadalafil has a faster onset of action and longer duration (36 hours)
  - **Warn patients about potential side effects**
    - Color vision changes
    - Headaches
    - Sudden blindness from nonischemic anterior optic neuropathy (case reports)
  - **Avoid in patients on nitrates (may induce hypotension) and those with recent or unstable coronary artery disease**
  - All PDE-5 inhibitors are metabolized by cytochrome P450 isozyme 3A4 (CYP3A4); doses should be reduced when combined with inhibitors of CYP3A4 (erythromycin, ketoconazole, protease inhibitors, and grapefruit juice)
- Other treatment options
  - Vasodilators such as prostaglandin E, papaverine, intraurethral alprostadil
  - Vacuum devices (avoid in patients at risk for bleeding)
  - Penile prostheses (associated with risk of infection)

Review Questions

For review questions, please go to ExpertConsult.com.

SUGGESTED READINGS

Fraser IS, Kovacs G. Current recommendations for the diagnostic evaluation and follow-up of patients presenting with symptomatic polycystic ovary syndrome. *Best Pract Res Clin Obstet Gynaecol.* 2004;5:813-823.

Rosenfield RL. Clinical practice: hirsutism. *N Engl J Med.* 2005;353:2578-2588.

Warren MP, Hagey AR. The genetics, diagnosis and treatment of amenorrhea. *Minerva Ginecol.* 2004;56:437-455.

40

Neuroendocrine and Adrenal Disease

ROBERTO SALVATORI, MD

Protein hormones, most of which are produced or stored in the pituitary gland, and steroid hormones, many of which are produced in the adrenal glands, have profound impact on growth, development, and metabolism. Overproduction or underproduction of single or multiple hormones may result in signs or symptoms that range from minimal to life threatening.

Neuroendocrine Disorders

Overview of the Pituitary Gland and Pituitary Masses

- The pituitary gland includes anterior and posterior parts (Fig. 41-1)
  - Anterior pituitary produces prolactin (PRL), thyroid-stimulating hormone (TSH, also known as thyrotropin), adrenocorticotropic hormone (ACTH), luteinizing hormone (LH), follicle-stimulating hormone (FSH), and growth hormone (GH)
    - ACTH is synthesized as part of a larger protein, pro-opiomelanocortin; any stimulation of ACTH production will result in increased production of pro-opiomelanocortin
  - The posterior pituitary stores antidiuretic hormone (ADH) and oxytocin, which are produced in the hypothalamus
- **Pituitary/sellar masses: Neuroendocrine disorders commonly present in the setting of a sellar mass**
  - Approximately 45% of sellar masses are hormone-secreting pituitary tumors
  - Approximately 45% of sellar masses are non–hormone-secreting pituitary tumors
  - The remainder of sellar masses include craniopharyngiomas, Rathke cleft cysts, meningiomas, metastatic tumors, lymphoma, granulomatous diseases, or the increasingly recognized autoimmune lymphocytic hypophysitis, either primary or secondary to cancer immunotherapy (mainly ipilimumab)
- **Pituitary tumors smaller than 10 mm are referred to as *microadenomas* (Fig. 41-2); tumors 10 mm or larger are referred to as *macroadenomas***
- **Pituitary incidentaloma: a pituitary mass discovered in a patient without endocrine symptoms**

- Prevalence of incidentalomas has increased because of increased use of brain imaging
- Often of no clinical consequence
- **All patients with a pituitary adenoma should be evaluated for hormone hypersecretion syndromes that cannot be excluded by history or physical examination (see later discussion)**
- Incidentally-discovered microadenomas grow in less than 10% of cases
  - If nonsecreting, conservative management with periodic magnetic resonance imaging (MRI) studies at progressively increasing intervals is performed
- **Incidental macroadenomas should also be evaluated for hypopituitarism**
  - **Visual field testing should be performed as well if the adenoma is close to the optic chiasm**
  - Further growth occurs in about 35% of macroadenomas
  - Surgery is indicated if optic chiasm is compressed, if the patient is symptomatic (e.g., otherwise not explainable headaches), or if the tumor is growing

Symptoms Caused by Sellar and Parasellar Masses

- General principles
  - Disorders of the sellar area may present with three classes of signs and symptoms
    - Syndromes of hormone excess (e.g., acromegaly, Cushing disease, hyperprolactinemia)
    - Symptoms of hormone deficit (partial or complete hypopituitarism, discussed in the next section)
    - Compressive symptoms
      - Headaches (typically but not exclusively frontal)
      - Visual changes (typically bitemporal hemianopsia)
      - If cavernous sinus is invaded by expanding tumor, cranial nerve palsies develop (cranial nerves III, IV, VI)
- The clinical presentation will also vary based on the actions of the hormone that is either undersecreted or oversecreted (Table 41-1; see later discussion)
- Pituitary tumors may exist as part of genetic syndromes

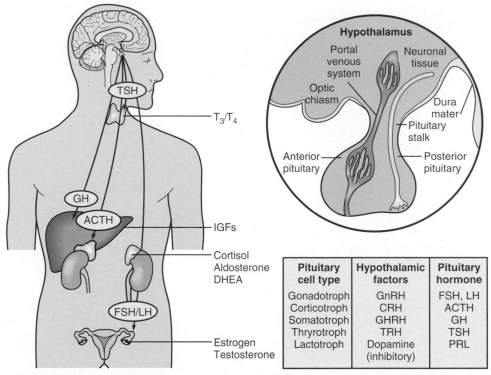

Pituitary cell type	Hypothalamic factors	Pituitary hormone
Gonadotroph	GnRH	FSH, LH
Corticotroph	CRH	ACTH
Somatotroph	GHRH	GH
Thryrotroph	TRH	TSH
Lactotroph	Dopamine (inhibitory)	PRL

FIGURE 41-1 The hypothalamic-pituitary axis. ACTH, Adrenocorticotropin hormone; CRH, corticotropin-releasing hormone; DHEA, dehydroepiandrosterone; FSH, follicle-stimulating hormone; GH, growth hormone; GHRH, growth hormone-releasing hormone; GnRH, gonadotropin-releasing hormone; IGF, insulin-like growth factor; LH, luteinizing hormone; PRL, prolactin; T_3, triiodothyronine; T_4, thyroxine; TRH, thyroid-releasing hormone; TSH, thyroid-stimulating hormone. (From Page C. *Integrated Pharmacology*. 3rd ed. Philadelphia: Mosby; 2006: Fig. 15.2.)

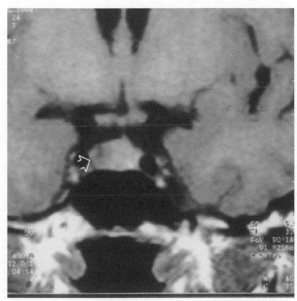

FIGURE 41-2 A magnetic resonance image of a pituitary demonstrating the typical appearance of a pituitary microademona. A hypodense lesion is seen in the right side of the gland with deviation of the pituitary stalk away from the lesion *(arrow)*. After a biochemical diagnosis of Cushing disease, this patient was cured following transsphenoidal hypophysectomy. (From Larsen PR, Kronenberg HM, Melmed S, Polonsky KS. *Williams Textbook of Endocrinology*. 10th ed. Philadelphia: Saunders; 2003: Fig. 14-23.)

- In conjunction with other endocrine tumors; this is known as the multiple endocrine neoplasia (MEN)-I syndrome (Box 41-1)
- As part of the "Carney complex" (autosomal dominant complex of cardiac myxomas, spotty pigmentation of the skin, and various hyperendocrine states, often including GH hypersecretion)
- As the syndrome of familial isolated pituitary adenomas (FIPA) (sometimes isolated familial acromegaly syndrome)
  - May be caused by inactivating mutations in the AIP gene
  - Inheritance is autosomal dominant, but the penetrance is low (about 20%)
  - Tumors are mostly GH-secreting, large and aggressive, typically occurring early in life
- A thorough family history is indicated for all patients diagnosed with a pituitary adenoma
  - **All patients should be asked about personal or family history of hypercalcemia or kidney stones because hyperparathyroidism is the most common feature of MEN-I, with penetrance close to 100% by age 50**
  - All patients should be examined for perioral hyperpigmentation, tumors of the heart, and hyperendocrine states, which may suggest Carney complex

41

TABLE 41-1	*Pituitary Hormones: Key Details*			
Hormone	**Major Actions**	**Secretagogue**	**Inhibitor**	**Deficiency Syndrome**
Prolactin (PRL) Growth hormone	Lactation Linear growth (via insulin-like growth factors)	Thyrotropin-releasing hormone (TRH) Growth hormone-releasing hormone	Dopamine Somatostatin	Inability to lactate Children: dwarfism Adults: loss of bone mass, body composition changes, hypercholesterolemia
Adrenocorticotropic hormone	Release of cortisol from adrenal gland	Corticotropin-releasing hormone	Glucocorticoids	Secondary adrenal insufficiency (no hyperpigmentation or electrolyte disturbances seen)
Thyroid-stimulating hormone	Production and release of thyroid hormones	TRH	Thyroid hormones (thyroxine or triiodothyronine)	Central hypothyroidism (see Chapter 38)
Follicle-stimulating hormone (FSH)	Women: growth of granulosa cells and estradiol production in ovarian follicle Men: stimulates seminiferous tubules to produce sperm	Gonadotropin-releasing hormone (GnRH) GnRH is also known as luteinizing hormone-releasing hormone	Inhibin Estradiol Testosterone (PRL inhibits GnRH release)	Children: delayed puberty Women: amenorrhea Men: impotence, testicular atrophy Kallmann syndrome: gonadotropin deficiency caused by congenital GnRH deficiency
Luteinizing hormone (LH)	Women: stimulates ovarian theca cells to produce androgens; LH surge stimulates ovulation Men: stimulates testosterone production in Leydig cells	Same as FSH	Estradiol Testosterone (PRL inhibits GnRH release)	Same as FSH
Antidiuretic hormone (arginine vasopressin)	Makes collecting ducts in renal tubules permeable to water Stimulates thirst	Increases in osmolality Decreases in volume	Decreases in osmolality	Diabetes insipidus
Oxytocin	Contraction of uterine and breast muscles	Estrogen Suckling	None	None

- As lymphocytic hypophysitis occurs in about 10% of patients treated with the cancer immunotherapy drug ipilimumab, this (and hypopituitarism) should be suspected in symptomatic patients receiving this drug

Pituitary Hormone Excess States

PROLACTINOMA

Basic Information

- PRL is produced by lactotroph cells in the anterior pituitary
- Dopaminergic pathways inhibit PRL production
- Elevations in serum PRL levels may be physiologic (e.g., pregnancy) or pathologic (Box 41-2)
- **Prolactinomas are the most common hormone-secreting pituitary adenomas (see Box 41-2)**

Clinical Presentation

- Elevated PRL levels inhibit gonadotropin secretion (by inhibiting release of luteinizing hormone-releasing hormone) and decrease gonadal responsiveness to gonadotropins (Fig. 41-3)
- **Galactorrhea can be seen in premenopausal women and in postmenopausal women if they are taking hormone replacement, but it is rarely seen in men**
- Menstrual irregularities are common and result in women being diagnosed earlier than men
- Because of the above, women most commonly present with microadenomas
- Men present with decreased libido and erectile dysfunction or visual loss, and are more likely to present with macroadenomas, sometimes very large (giant prolactinomas larger than 4 cm)

Diagnosis

- Exclude other causes of elevated PRL levels, particularly antipsychotic medications (see Box 41-2)
  - If PRL level is greater than 200 ng/mL, prolactinoma is very likely
- Obtain MRI of sella
  - High serum PRL level and pituitary mass by MRI typically used to diagnose prolactinoma

- ■ **A sellar mass in the presence of elevated serum PRL levels, however, is not definitive proof of prolactinoma**
    - ■ **A large, nonsecreting adenoma may cause elevated PRL levels by compressing the pituitary stalk and inhibiting hypothalamic dopaminergic regulation of PRL**
    - ■ **Suspect this if macroadenoma is seen with only moderate elevation of PRL level (i.e., less than 100 ng/mL)**
- ■ If PRL is elevated but the patient has no clinical symptoms, the presence of "macroprolactinemia" must be suspected
    - ■ In this condition, PRL molecules bind to circulating immunoglobulins, causing marked increase in serum half-life, but PRL is not biologically active
    - ■ Macroprolactinemia can be identified by repeating serum PRL measurement after precipitating immunoglobulins with polyethylene glycol
    - ■ Requires no treatment

Treatment

- ■ Normalization of PRL is usually required to normalize menses and to restore eugonadism
- ■ **First-line treatment is with dopaminergic agonists**

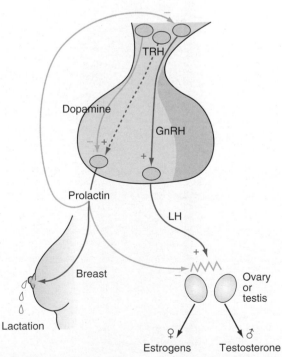

FIGURE 41-3 The control and physiologic effects of prolactin secretion, demonstrating inhibition of luteinizing hormone (LH) secretion and action. GnRH, Gonadotropin-releasing hormone; TRH, thyroid-releasing hormone. (From Kumar P, Clark M. *Clinical Medicine.* 5th ed. Philadelphia: Saunders; 2005: Fig. 18-11.)

41

- Cabergoline and bromocriptine are agents most commonly used
- If medical therapy fails, surgery is performed via transsphenoidal approach
- Radiation used if tumor recurs after surgery (rare)

GROWTH HORMONE-SECRETING TUMORS

Basic Information

- **Excess GH results in gigantism in children, whose epiphyseal bone plates have not closed (Fig. 41-4), or acromegaly in adults (Fig. 41-5)**
- GH acts on tissues both directly and indirectly by stimulating the production of other hormones that stimulate growth (mostly insulin-like growth factor-I [IGF-I])
- Onset of acromegaly is insidious and often missed

Clinical Presentation

- **Most common features are acral growth, excessive sweating, and weakness/fatigue**
  - **Other features may include sleep apnea, arthralgias, vertebral fractures, hypertension, glucose intolerance or diabetes, teeth malocclusion, and carpal tunnel syndrome**

- Incidence of colonic polyps two to three times higher than age-matched controls and may correlate with presence of skin tags
- **Characteristic physical appearance includes coarse facial features with frontal bossing, prognathism, and sonorous voice**
- **Hand, foot, and hat sizes are increased**

Diagnosis

- Because GH levels fluctuate according to a diurnal pattern (and significant overlap exists between normal and abnormal individuals), GH levels alone are not useful to diagnose acromegaly
- **IGF-I levels are more consistently elevated in acromegaly and are the initial test of choice in screening for acromegaly**
- To confirm the diagnosis in dubious cases, a glucose suppression test is performed
  - In normal subjects, a 75-g oral glucose load suppresses GH levels to less than 0.4 ng/mL
  - In acromegaly, a 75-g oral glucose load does not suppress GH levels and may paradoxically increase GH levels
- Brain imaging is typically done after serologic evaluation

Treatment

- Goal of treatment is normalization of IGF-I and reduction of GH levels to less than 2.0 ng/mL, because noncured acromegalic patients have a reduced life expectancy
- **Surgery is initial management in most cases (transsphenoidal approach)**

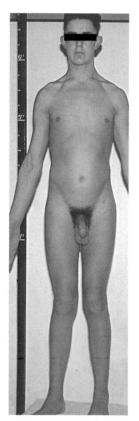

FIGURE 41-4 A 16-year-old patient suffering from gigantism. Growth hormone is raised and bone age is not advanced, indicating that the boy's eventual stature will be abnormally tall. (From Besser GM, Thorner M. *Comprehensive Clinical Endocrinology.* 3rd ed. St. Louis: Mosby; 2002: Fig. 24B.31.)

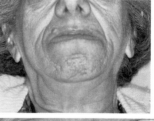
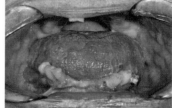
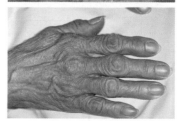

FIGURE 41-5 Acromegaly of the jaw and hand. (From Regezi JA, Sciubba JJ, Jordan RCK. *Oral Pathology: Clinical Pathological Correlations.* 4th ed. Philadelphia: Saunders; 2003: Fig. 15-8.)

- Curative in about 50%; cure less likely with macroadenomas than microadenomas
- **Somatostatin analogues (lanreotide or octreotide) used with postsurgical recurrence, with hormonal response in about 50% of patients**
- Some (20%) may respond to the dopamine agonist cabergoline (particularly if IGF-I is only mildly or moderately elevated)
- GH receptor antagonist (pegvisomant) normalizes IGF-I in 70% to 90% of patients
- Radiation also used with postsurgical recurrence or surgical failure; it requires several years to be effective

HYPERCORTISOLISM
Basic Information

- **Cushing *disease:* hypercortisolism as a result of ACTH-producing pituitary adenoma**
- **Cushing *syndrome*: hypercortisolism from any cause, including pituitary adenoma, adrenal adenoma or carcinoma, ectopic ACTH production, or administration of exogenous glucocorticoids**

Clinical Presentation

- See Figure 41-6 for an example of Cushing syndrome
- Patients present with hypertension, central obesity, moon facies, dorsal fat pad, purple striae on skin, and muscle weakness
- Psychiatric symptoms also common
- Secondary amenorrhea may develop in women, along with hirsutism or other evidence of masculinization
- Osteoporosis also develops in women and men
- Common laboratory abnormalities may include glucose intolerance (or diabetes) and metabolic alkalosis with hypokalemia (in more severe cases)

Diagnosis

- **Diagnosis of hypercortisolism (Fig. 41-7): Begin by measuring 24-hour urine free cortisol or bedtime salivary cortisol or performing a 1-mg overnight dexamethasone suppression test**
- Plasma ACTH levels differentiate between ACTH-dependent (high or normal plasma ACTH) and ACTH-independent (ACTH levels less than 10 pg/mL) types of Cushing syndrome

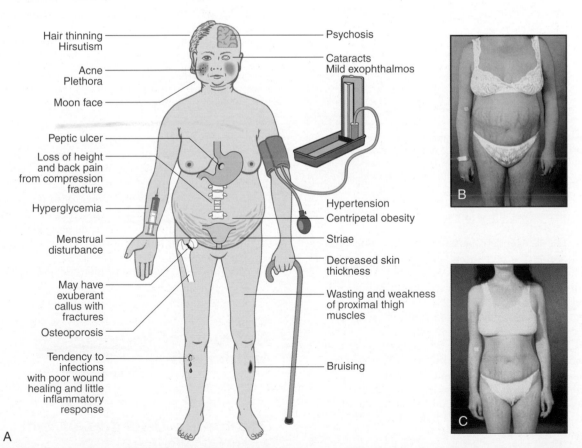

FIGURE 41-6 Cushing syndrome. **A,** Clinical features common to all causes. **B,** A patient with Cushing disease before treatment. **C,** The same patient 1 year after successful removal of an adrenocorticotropic hormone-secreting pituitary microadenoma by transsphenoidal surgery. (From Haslett C, Chilvers ER, Boon NA, et al. *Davidson's Principles and Practice of Medicine.* 19th ed. New York: Churchill Livingstone; 2002: Fig. 16.17.)

41

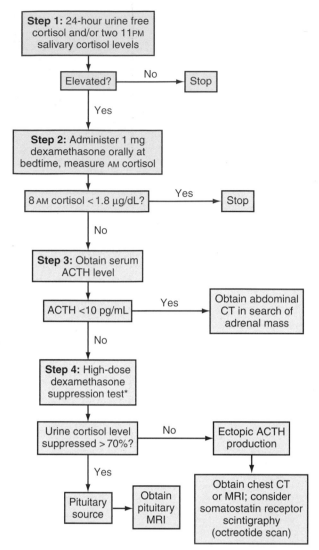

FIGURE 41-7   Evaluation of the patient with suspected hypercortisolism. *Dexamethasone 2 mg every 6 hours for 2 days; collect urine on day 0 and day 2. ACTH, Adrenocorticotropin hormone; CT, computed tomography; MRI, magnetic resonance imaging.

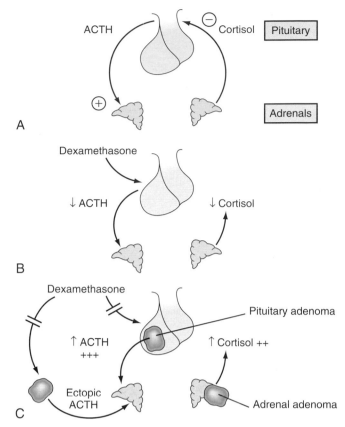

FIGURE 41-8   Dexamethasone suppression test. **A,** Normal feedback mechanism for cortisol production. **B,** Normally, dexamethasone suppresses adrenocorticotropin (ACTH) and hence cortisol production. **C,** In both ACTH-independent (adrenal adenoma) and ACTH-dependent (pituitary or ectopic ACTH) types of Cushing syndrome, dexamethasone has no effect, and cortisol is not suppressed. (From Souhami R. *Textbook of Medicine.* New York: Churchill Livingstone; 2002: Fig. 17.30.)

- If ACTH independent, adrenal imaging is necessary
- Localization of source of ACTH in ACTH-dependent conditions (i.e., pituitary versus ectopic ACTH) requires sequential testing based on the following principles:
  - In normal host, glucocorticoids inhibit ACTH secretion (Fig. 41-8)
  - ACTH-secreting pituitary adenomas are partially autonomous but can be inhibited with high-dose glucocorticoids (e.g., dexamethasone)
- In difficult cases of differentiation of pituitary versus ectopic ACTH, bilateral inferior petrosal sinus sampling is done after administration of corticotropin-releasing factor

Treatment

- For pituitary source: transsphenoidal resection
- For adrenal source: adrenalectomy

- When surgical cure is not obtainable in Cushing disease:
  - Medical treatment can be used with drugs that inhibit ACTH secretion (pasireotide) or cortisol secretion by the adrenal glands (e.g., ketoconazole, metyrapone, mitotane) or block cortisol effect (mifepristone)
  - Pituitary radiation and/or bilateral adrenalectomy is sometimes needed

Syndrome of Inappropriate Antidiuresis

See Chapter 32.

Uncommon Disorders of the Anterior Pituitary

- Pituitary hyperthyroidism, caused by a TSH-producing adenoma, is rare

- Gonadotropin-secreting (i.e., LH, FSH) tumors typically present as macroadenomas and may be asymptomatic
  - Many nonfunctioning macroadenomas may actually produce nonbiologically active gonadotropins (e.g., α subunits of gonadotropins)

Pituitary Hormone Insufficiency States

Basic Information

- **Hypopituitarism is most commonly caused by pituitary macroadenoma, with destruction or compression of normal pituitary cells**
  - **With pituitary tumors/mass effect, GH typically is affected first, followed by gonadotropins, then TSH; ACTH is usually affected last**
  - Order may change with other causes of hypopituitarism (e.g., radiation or lymphocytic hypophysitis)
- Other causes of hypopituitarism include pituitary apoplexy (infarction); inflammation of the pituitary (lymphocytic hypophysitis, typically but not exclusively in postpartum women, or caused by cancer immune-therapy); central nervous system radiation; surgery; head trauma (single or multiple repeated traumas); or replacement of the pituitary or hypothalamus with infectious, granulomatous, or malignant disease (when pituitary metastases are present, often diabetes insipidus occurs)
- Clinical manifestations depend on which hormone or combination of hormones is affected (Fig. 41-9) and to what extent they are affected (see Table 41-1)
- **Pituitary apoplexy: the acute development of pituitary insufficiency, most commonly from sudden hemorrhage or infarction of the pituitary gland**
  - **Most commonly (approximately ⅔) occurs in patients with previously undiagnosed pituitary tumor**
  - **Sudden headache is always present, and visual deficit, ophthalmoplegia (cranial nerves III, IV, or VI may be affected), and altered mental status may occur**
  - Most dangerous result is acute lack of ACTH and therefore acute secondary adrenal insufficiency (see following section on adrenal insufficiency)
- **Sheehan syndrome: pituitary infarction caused by blood loss during or immediately after childbirth; classic presentation is a new mother who is unable to produce milk**

PROLACTIN DEFICIENCY

Basic Information

- Usually occurs in the setting of other pituitary hormone deficiencies, indicates extensive destruction of pituitary tissue

Clinical Presentation

- Asymptomatic in men
- Women will note lack of lactation (i.e., with pregnancy)

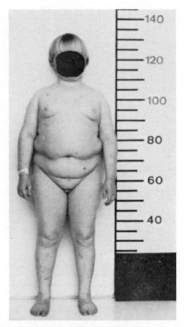

FIGURE 41-9 A 20-year-old man with idiopathic hypopituitary dwarfism and deficiencies of gonadotropins, thyrotropin, corticotropin, and growth hormone, who had a history of arrested hydrocephalus. Note the extreme atrophy of the genitalia, absence of body hair, and apparent gynecomastia associated with obesity. (From Yen SCC, Jaffe RB. *Reproductive Endocrinology.* 2nd ed. Philadelphia: Saunders; 1986: Fig. 24-52.)

Diagnosis

- Low serum PRL level in the appropriate clinical scenario

Treatment

- There is no treatment for PRL deficiency

GROWTH HORMONE DEFICIENCY

Basic Information

- Patients with panhypopituitarism have a 99% likelihood of being GH deficient

Clinical Presentation

- Symptoms of GH deficiency depend on the age of onset
  - In children, stunted growth occurs
  - In adults, symptoms of GH deficiency are usually overshadowed by other manifestations of pituitary insufficiency but include a decreased sense of well-being, decreased muscle mass, increased fat mass, osteopenia, and an abnormal lipid profile (increased total and low-density lipoprotein cholesterol)

Diagnosis

- To diagnose GH deficiency, a low serum IGF-I is typically seen, but this is not sensitive or specific (unless in setting of panhypopituitarism)
- Large overlap exists in serum IGF-I between GH-deficient and normal subjects, particularly in male patients older than 40 years

41

- If IGF-I is normal but suspicion is high, testing of GH reserve by insulin-induced hypoglycemia or glucagon is used

Treatment

- Although in the past GH deficiency in fully grown adults was not treated, adult patients with severe GH deficiency should be considered for GH replacement therapy to improve muscle mass, bone density, quality of life, and lipid profile

ACTH DEFICIENCY

ACTH deficiency is known as secondary adrenal insufficiency and is discussed in the section on adrenal insufficiency that follows.

Central Hypothyroidism

Basic Information

- A rare cause of hypothyroidism
- As with other disorders noted, most commonly occurs in association with other causes of pituitary insufficiency

Clinical Presentation

- Patient presents with the typical signs and symptoms of hypothyroidism, often milder than primary hypothyroidism (see Chapter 38)

Diagnosis

- **Diagnosed by low serum free thyroxine levels in the setting of low (or inappropriately normal, or even mildly elevated) TSH level**

Treatment

- **Treatment is repletion with thyroxine, adjusted to symptoms and serum free thyroxine (T$_4$) levels**
- **TSH cannot be followed for medication dosing in individuals with central hypothyroidism**
- **In patients with central hypothyroidism, never replace thyroid hormone before assessing adrenal function because pharmacologically induced euthyroidism may trigger adrenal crisis (thyroid hormones accelerate cortisol catabolism)**

Central Hypogonadism

Basic Information

- Central hypogonadism, or secondary hypogonadism, is caused by insufficient production of LH and/or FSH
- Occurs by itself or with other features of hypopituitarism
  - **Kallmann syndrome (Fig. 41-10): lack of GnRH secretion resulting in central hypogonadism**
  - **Additional features may include neurosensory hearing loss, red-green color blindness,**

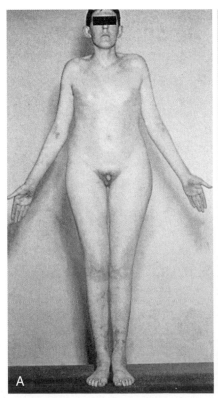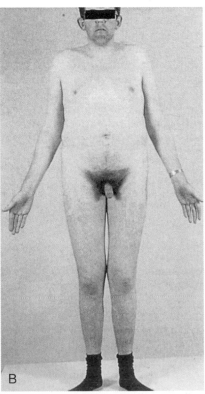

FIGURE 41-10 Grossly eunuchoid 31-year-old man with Kallmann syndrome. **A,** Before androgen replacement. **B,** After 2 years of androgen replacement. (From Souhami R. *Textbook of Medicine.* New York: Churchill Livingstone; 2002: Fig. 17.36.)

urogenital tract abnormalities, and lack of sense of smell

Clinical Presentation

- **Determined in large part by the age of onset of secondary hypogonadism**
  - **Prepubertal boys and girls will fail to develop secondary sexual characteristics**
  - **In adults, infertility and decreased sexual drive are common (in both men and women), as well as amenorrhea (women)**
  - Men whose hypogonadism started before puberty may have eunuchoid body habitus (arm span greater than height; lower body segment longer than upper body segment); and gynecomastia

Diagnosis

- Diagnosed by low sex hormone levels in setting of low (or inappropriately normal) LH and FSH levels

Treatment

- In men, treatment is with testosterone, titrated to normal serum levels
  - If fertility in men is desired, human chorionic gonadotropin (hCG; LH equivalent) and FSH can be administered as intramuscular injections
  - May take several months of therapy to reach normal sperm count
- In women, treatment is with estrogen and progesterone replacement
  - If fertility is desired, hCG and FSH can be administered under the care of a reproductive endocrinologist

Diabetes Insipidus

Basic Information

- **Neurogenic diabetes insipidus (DI): lack of production and release of ADH from posterior pituitary**
  - **Caused by either hypothalamic disease (e.g., sarcoidosis, tuberculosis, craniopharyngioma) or following neurosurgery; pituitary adenomas usually do not cause DI unless there has been a surgical damage**
  - Rare forms include familial DI, traumatic DI, or idiopathic DI
- **Nephrogenic DI: lack of renal response to ADH (no disorder of posterior pituitary implied)**
  - May be congenital or acquired
    - Acquired form may result from hypercalcemia, hypokalemia, or medications (e.g., lithium; nephrogenic DI may persist after discontinuation of lithium)

Clinical Presentation

- **Patients present with impaired renal conservation of water and production of dilute urine**
  - **Polyuria, polydipsia, and sometimes hypernatremia result**

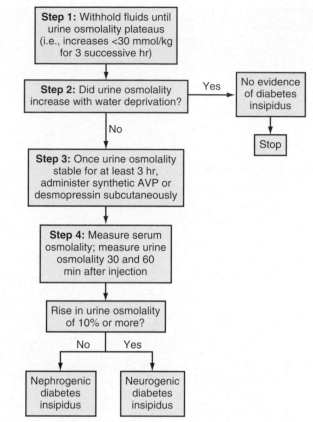

FIGURE 41-11 Water deprivation test. *AVP,* Arginine vasopressin.

Diagnosis

- Suspect if increased serum osmolarity present, or in an individual who produces high volume (may be up to 16 L) of inappropriately diluted urine
- Water deprivation test is test of choice in dubious situations (Fig. 41-11)

Treatment

- Treatment of neurogenic DI is deamino-D-arginine vasopressin (a synthetic vasopressin analogue, administered either intranasally or orally)
- Always be cautious not to overtreat for danger of hyponatremia
- Thiazide diuretics are used for treatment of nephrogenic DI to reduce intravascular volume and polyuria

Adrenal Disease

OVERVIEW OF THE ADRENAL GLAND

- The adrenal glands are the major site of synthesis and secretion of steroid hormones
- **There are three categories of steroid hormones produced in the adrenal glands**
  - **Glucocorticoids, such as cortisol**
  - **Mineralocorticoids, such as aldosterone**
  - **Adrenal androgens, such as dehydroepiandrosterone (DHEA)**
- Major actions of adrenal hormones are shown in Table 41-2

41

TABLE 41-2	*Adrenal Hormones: Key Details*		
Hormone	**Secretagogues**	**Inhibitor**	**Major Actions**
Cortisol	ACTH	Cortisol inhibits CRH release (and thus ACTH release) in negative feedback loop Exogenous steroids also inhibit CRH release	Increases serum glucose levels Opposes insulin Stimulates hepatic gluconeogenesis Creates catabolic protein state Stimulates protein breakdown Stimulates mobilization of amino acid precursors from muscle, bone, skin, and connective tissue Inhibits protein synthesis Opposes inflammatory response Opposes increased vascular permeability and other actions of inflammatory mediators Decreases eosinophils and T cells Mobilizes polymorphonuclear lymphocytes
Aldosterone	Renin-angiotensin system activation Hyperkalemia ACTH	Sodium	Stimulates sodium retention, impacting extracellular fluid volume Stimulates potassium excretion
DHEA	ACTH	Inhibitors of ACTH release	Stimulates secondary sexual characteristics in men (or virilization in women)

ACTH, Adrenocorticotropic hormone; CRH, corticotropin-releasing hormone; DHEA, dehydroepiandrosterone.

- Adrenal incidentalomas: increases in imaging of abdomen result in incidental detection of adrenal mass in 4% to 7% of scans in persons older than 50 years
  - Most adrenal incidentalomas (67% to 94%, depending on the case series) are nonhypersecretory adrenal adenomas
  - Clinically significant incidentally discovered masses may be hormonally active, malignant, or both
    - In absence of clinical signs or symptoms of Cushing syndrome or hyperaldosteronism (see later discussion), no further biochemical investigation for these disorders is indicated
    - Follow-up imaging always needed
    - If any signs or symptoms of hormone excess are present, further evaluation is needed
  - Pheochromocytoma may be asymptomatic and may be present in the nonhypertensive patient; screening for pheochromocytoma with 24-hour urine total and fractionated metanephrines collection or plasma free metanephrines should always be performed, unless radiologic appearance (very low density by computed tomography [CT], such as less than 10 Hounsfield units) rules it out
  - **Mass size determines management; size greater than 4 cm increases the suspicion for malignancy**
    - **Biopsy cannot differentiate between benign and malignant primary adrenal tumors; therefore, all masses greater than 4 cm in diameter should be removed**
    - If mass is less than 4 cm in diameter and not hormonally active, repeat imaging in 3 to 6 months
      - If no change, imaging repeated annually for 3 years
      - If mass increases in size, surgery should be performed
    - Management is different if patient has known primary cancer that risks spread to adrenals;

fine-needle aspiration biopsy may be performed if metastatic disease is suspected (after pheochromocytoma is ruled out)

Adrenal Hormone Excess States

CORTISOL EXCESS (CUSHING SYNDROME)
- See earlier section

ALDOSTERONE EXCESS
Basic Information

- **Most common cause is a bilateral adrenal hyperplasia, followed by functional adrenal adenoma (Conn syndrome; Fig. 41-12)**

Clinical Presentation

- **Patients present with hypertension (caused by sodium retention), metabolic alkalosis, and hypokalemia**
- Hypokalemia is not invariably present; may be unveiled by the use of diuretics, therefore lack of hypokalemia does not exclude the diagnosis
- Hypokalemia may result in muscle weakness

Diagnosis

- Potassium should be normalized before evaluating for hyperaldosteronism because hypokalemia suppresses aldosterone secretion
- If the patient is taking a potassium-wasting diuretic, it must be discontinued, and potassium supplementation should be given
- **Initial screening may be performed with serum aldosterone-plasma renin ratio**
  - If ratio (aldosterone in ng/dL and plasma renin activity in ng/mL/hour) is less than 20, hyperaldosteronism is effectively ruled out

35-year-old man

- Mild polyuria
- Blood pressure 188/104 mm Hg

Plasma biochemistry

- Na 144 mmol/L (132–144)
- K 3.1 mmol/L (3.3–4.7)
- HCO₃⁻ 29mmol/L (21–27)

Lying at 0900 hr
- Renin activity <0.5 (0.4–1.5*)
- Aldosterone 850 pmol/L (30–440*)

Standing at 1200 hr
- Renin activity <0.5 (1–2.5†)
- Aldosterone 750 pmol/L (110–860†)

A

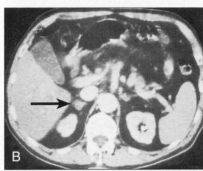
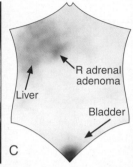
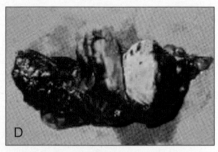

FIGURE 41-12 Conn syndrome. **A,** Characteristic biochemical results, including hypernatremia, hypokalemia, and metabolic alkalosis. Plasma renin activity is suppressed, and aldosterone levels are elevated. Reference ranges provided for supine* and standing† positions. **B,** Right adrenal adenoma *(arrow).* **C,** Uptake of radiolabeled cholesterol in right adrenal gland. **D,** Pathologic specimen of the right adrenal gland shown in **C.** (From Haslett C, Chilvers ER, Boon NA, et al. *Davidson's Principles and Practice of Medicine.* 19th ed. New York: Churchill Livingstone; 2002: Fig. 16.19.)

- If ratio is greater than 20, the next step is to demonstrate nonsuppressible levels of aldosterone in presence of sodium load
  - 2 L of normal saline administered over 4 hours
  - If aldosterone levels do not suppress to less than 8 ng/dL, hyperaldosteronism is present
  - Alternatively, 24-hour urine aldosterone can be measured during oral salt loading (with simultaneous measurement of urinary sodium)
  - Next step is to pursue adrenal imaging to differentiate adrenal adenoma from bilateral adrenal hyperplasia
  - In patients older than 40 years, adrenal vein sampling is always recommended to determine the source of excessive aldosterone, given higher prevalence of bilateral hyperplasia and adrenal incidentalomas

Treatment

- If hyperaldosteronism is caused by a functional adrenal adenoma (i.e., Conn syndrome), treatment is surgical excision of adenoma
- If hyperaldosteronism is caused by bilateral adrenal hyperplasia, treatment is with a potassium-sparing diuretic (e.g., spironolactone or eplerenone)

ADRENAL ANDROGEN EXCESS

Basic Information

- DHEA and DHEA sulfate are the most common adrenal androgens that may be found to be elevated
- Adrenal androgens may be produced because of adrenal tumors, congenital adrenal hyperplasia (CAH), and Cushing syndrome
  - In the most common form of CAH (21-hydroxylase deficiency; Fig. 41-13), cortisol synthesis is impaired, with overproduction of 17-hydroxyprogesterone and androgens
  - Mineralocorticoid production may also be impaired, resulting in hypoaldosteronism
- Androgen synthesis is intact, resulting in their overproduction

Clinical Presentation

- Classic (complete) forms of CAH present in infancy with hypoadrenalism, electrolyte abnormalities, and ambiguous genitalia (in females)
- Nonclassic (incomplete) forms may present in late childhood or young adulthood
- **Men are typically asymptomatic from overproduction of adrenal androgens**
- **Women present with signs and symptoms of androgen excess (Fig. 41-14), including:**
  - **Hirsutism (i.e., hair growth in a male pattern, such as on the chest, face, or back)**
  - **Virilization (e.g., clitoromegaly)**
  - **Oligomenorrhea, amenorrhea, infertility**
  - **Acne**

Diagnosis

- Clinical manifestations typically prompt evaluation of androgen, cortisol, electrolytes, and ACTH levels
- Bilateral adrenal enlargement may be noted on imaging in cases of CAH; an adrenal mass is seen in case of androgen-producing tumor
- **If congenital adrenal hyperplasia suspected, 17-hydroxyprogesterone levels (the cortisol precursor that cannot be further metabolized) will be elevated in the most common form (21-hydroxylase deficiency)**
- Adrenal androgen excess often associated with Cushing disease; less commonly it is associated with adrenal adenomas

41

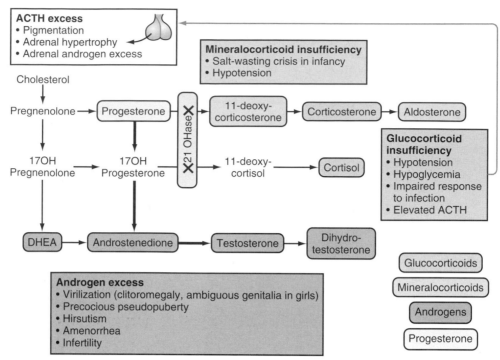

FIGURE 41-13 Congenital adrenal hyperplasia resulting from 21-hydroxylase (21 OHase) deficiency. Note how the enzyme defect results in mineralocorticoid and glucocorticoid deficiency while causing androgen excess. 17OH, 17-Hydroxy; ACTH, adrenocorticotropin hormone; DHEA, dehydroepiandrosterone. (From Haslett C, Chilvers ER, Boon NA, et al. *Davidson's Principles and Practice of Medicine.* 19th ed. New York: Churchill Livingstone; 2002: Fig. 16.21.)

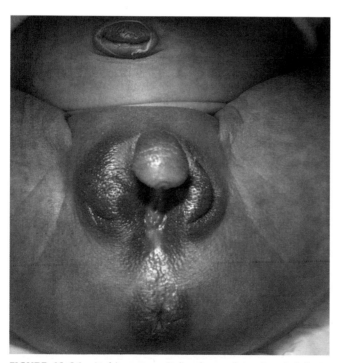

FIGURE 41-14 Ambiguous genitalia of a newborn female infant with virilizing congenital adrenal hyperplasia. An enlarged clitoris (phallic-like structure), genital hyperpigmentation, empty labioscrotal folds, and a single perineal opening into a urogenital sinus were present. (From Shah BR, Laude TA. *Atlas of Pediatric Clinical Diagnosis.* Philadelphia: Saunders; 2000: Fig. 8-14.)

Treatment

- If caused by adrenal tumor, treatment is excision of tumor
- If caused by Cushing syndrome, treatment is focused on treatment of Cushing syndrome
- **Congenital adrenal hyperplasia is treated with glucocorticoid and mineralocorticoid replacement (the latter not always needed) as in adrenal insufficiency (see later discussion)**

PHEOCHROMOCYTOMA

Basic Information

- Most pheochromocytomas occur in the adrenal medulla, where catecholamines are produced and stored
- Rarely, pheochromocytomas develop from the wall of the urinary bladder or in the retroperitoneal space
- Pheochromocytoma may occur as part of MEN-IIA or IIB syndrome (see Box 41-1) and is also seen with von Hippel-Lindau disease, neurofibromatosis, or in succinyl dehydrogenase gene mutations (familial paraganglioma syndromes, or FPGL)
- The inheritance pattern of FPGL depends on the gene involved; most families show traditional autosomal dominant inheritance, but exclusive paternal transmission of the phenotype may occur
- Most pheochromocytomas produce both norepinephrine and epinephrine
- Epinephrine-only secreting tumors are rare and are usually seen in the presence of a MEN-II syndrome resulting in an early clinical phenotype characterized by attacks of palpitations, nervousness, anxiety, and

headaches rather than hypertension seen with sporadic or other hereditary tumors

Clinical Presentation

- **Release of catecholamines results in clinical manifestations**
  - **Most common manifestation is hypertension**
  - **Headache, diaphoresis, tachycardia, and anxiety are also common manifestations**
  - Less common are orthostatic hypotension, polycythemia, and congestive heart failure
- **Symptoms classically described as paroxysmal, caused by episodic release of catecholamines from tumor**
  - Pressure on abdomen or urination (if tumor in bladder wall) can precipitate symptoms
  - Paroxysms more common early in disease; larger tumors lead to more sustained elevations in blood pressure and symptoms

Diagnosis

- **Diagnosis made by collection of 24-hour urine sample for total and fractionated metanephrines**
- **Yield may be increased in the intermittently symptomatic patient by initiating the urine collection at the onset of a paroxysm**
- Other tests used include 24-hour urine collection for vanillylmandelic acid (specific but not sensitive) or measurement of plasma free metanephrines
- Once diagnosed, pheochromocytoma must be located
  - Imaging of abdomen with CT or MRI is the first step, with attention to adrenal glands (Fig. 41-15)
    - **90% of pheochromocytomas are located in the adrenal glands; those external to the adrenal glands are usually elsewhere in the abdomen (including the bladder)**
  - If initial imaging of abdomen is negative, further localization is done, usually with iodinated metaiodobenzylguanidine (MIBG) scan

- If a pheochromocytoma is suspected to be malignant, MIBG scan should be performed before surgery to detect metastatic disease

Treatment

- Treatment consists of surgical excision of tumor
  - **Because surgery can precipitate hormone release, preventive treatment with the α blocker phenoxybenzamine is given for a few weeks before surgery at the maximally tolerated dose**

Adrenal Hormone Deficiency States

ADRENAL INSUFFICIENCY

Basic Information

- **Adrenal insufficiency may occur because of failure of the adrenal glands (primary adrenal insufficiency) or pituitary disease (secondary adrenal insufficiency)**
  - Autoimmune primary adrenal insufficiency is often associated with other autoimmune disorders (e.g., hypothyroidism, vitiligo)
  - Other causes of primary adrenal insufficiency include infection (e.g., tuberculosis), surgical excision, and bilateral hemorrhage of the adrenal glands
    - **Hemorrhagic destruction of the adrenal glands is described in disseminated meningococcal infection (Waterhouse-Friderichsen syndrome), as well as with anticoagulation or lupus anticoagulant**
- **Secondary adrenal insufficiency is much more common than primary adrenal insufficiency and is most often caused by suppression of the hypothalamic-pituitary-adrenal axis by the prolonged (3 weeks or longer) administration of exogenous steroids**

Clinical Presentation

- Clinical manifestations of adrenal insufficiency differ based on whether or not the cause is primary or secondary adrenal insufficiency
  - With primary adrenal insufficiency, the hypothalamus will respond by increasing CRH production, resulting in increased production of pro-opiomelanocortin (the ACTH precursor) and increased serum levels of ACTH
  - **Because of increased production of pro-opiomelanocortin (which contains melanocyte-stimulating hormone) in primary adrenal insufficiency, skin and mucous membrane hyperpigmentation results;** skin hyperpigmentation does not occur in secondary adrenal insufficiency
  - **With primary adrenal insufficiency, mineralocorticoid deficiency is also seen with hyponatremia and hyperkalemia**
  - Hyponatremia is less common with secondary adrenal insufficiency and is seen more often if concomitant central hypothyroidism is present
- Clinical manifestations shared by all patients with adrenal insufficiency include weakness, hypotension, nausea, vomiting, diarrhea, and weight loss

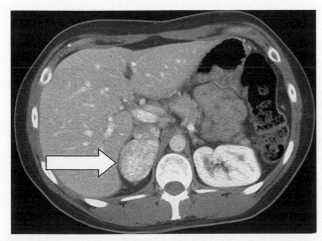

FIGURE 41-15 A computed tomography scan of the abdomen with intravenous administration of a contrast agent demonstrating peripartum discovery of pheochromocytoma *(arrow).* (From Goldman L, Ausiello D. *Cecil Textbook of Medicine.* 23rd ed. Philadelphia: Saunders; 2008: Fig. 246-2.)

41

- **Acute adrenal insufficiency, which is a medical emergency, can be precipitated in patients with chronic adrenal insufficiency who are exposed to stress (e.g., surgery, infection, gastroenteritis) or by rapid destruction of the adrenal glands (such as with hemorrhage) or pituitary apoplexy**

Diagnosis

- **In primary adrenal insufficiency, plasma ACTH levels will be elevated; whereas, in secondary adrenal insufficiency, plasma ACTH levels will be low (or inappropriately normal)**
  - ACTH levels are used in conjunction with other tests to determine presence of primary or secondary adrenal insufficiency
- A random morning cortisol measurement may be insufficient to diagnose partial adrenal insufficiency because normal levels overlap with levels seen in mild adrenal insufficiency
  - However, if a patient is under significant stress (e.g., hypotensive or in the intensive care unit [ICU]) and a random cortisol (taken any time of day) is less than 15 μg/dL, the patient should be considered to be adrenally insufficient (unless serum albumin is less than 2.5 g/dL, as serum cortisol binding capacity is reduced)
    - **All patients diagnosed with adrenal insufficiency based on a low serum cortisol while in the ICU should be restudied after the acute problem is solved**
  - A very low serum morning cortisol level (less than 3 μg/dL) in an ambulatory patient is presumptive evidence of adrenal insufficiency

- Gold-standard test of adrenal function is insulin-induced hypoglycemia or insulin tolerance test
  - Test performed by administering insulin (0.1 to 0.15 U/kg) intravenously (IV), with measurement of cortisol levels during symptomatic hypoglycemia
    - A normal response is considered to be a peak cortisol level greater than 18 μg/dL
  - ITT contraindicated in presence of coronary artery disease, seizure disorder, or age above 60 years
- Most commonly used test is ACTH stimulation test
  - Administer ACTH (cosyntropin) 250 mg IV or intramuscularly
  - Measure serum cortisol just before injection and 60 minutes following injection
  - **If cortisol level is 18.5 μg/dL or more at either measure, patient does not have adrenal insufficiency**
  - If cortisol levels stay below 18.5 μg/dL, adrenal insufficiency is present, and results are combined with ACTH levels, as described previously, to determine cause

Treatment

- Adrenal insufficiency: treatment differs based on cause of adrenal insufficiency (e.g., primary versus secondary) as well as whether or not adrenal insufficiency is acute or chronic (Fig. 41-16)
- Usual dose is hydrocortisone 10 to 12.5 mg/m^2/day
- Oral dose is usually divided into 10 to 15 mg in the morning and 5 to 10 mg later in the day to mimic normal cortisol secretion pattern
- The lowest dose that improves the patient's symptoms should be used

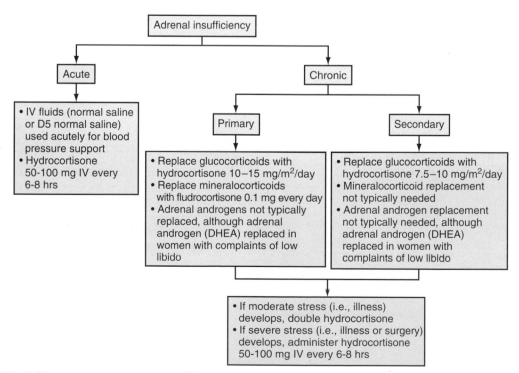

FIGURE 41-16 Treatment of adrenal insufficiency. D5, 5% Dextrose; DHEA, dehydroepiandrosterone; IV, intravenous.

- Dose should be increased during intercurrent illnesses
- All patients should wear a medical alert bracelet or necklace stating their adrenal insufficiency status
- **Mineralocorticoid (fludrocortisone 0.05 to 0.2 mg/day) is used only in primary adrenal insufficiency**

HYPOALDOSTERONISM

Basic Information

- Most common presentation is hyporeninemic hypoaldosteronism
  - Common in patients with renal insufficiency and in those with long-standing diabetes
  - Results in type IV renal tubular acidosis (see Chapter 31)
  - Other causes of hyporeninemic hypoaldosteronism include angiotensin-converting enzyme inhibitors, nonsteroidal antiinflammatory drugs, cyclosporine, and heparin
  - Acquired immune deficiency syndrome may also be associated with hyporeninemic hypoaldosteronism
- Hypoaldosteronism also occurs in patients with primary adrenal insufficiency and congenital adrenal hyperplasia (see earlier discussion)
  - Rare causes include isolated enzyme defects in synthesis of aldosterone and are usually diagnosed in children

Clinical Presentation

- **Hyperkalemia is the major clinical feature of patients with hypoaldosteronism**

Diagnosis

- First step is to exclude obvious causes of hyporeninemic hypoaldosteronism (noted previously)
- With these causes excluded, major differential is between hyporeninemic hypoaldosteronism, adrenal insufficiency, congenital adrenal hyperplasia, or rare enzyme defect
  - After patient is upright for 3 hours, check plasma renin activity, serum aldosterone, and serum cortisol levels
    - With hyporeninemic hypoaldosteronism, plasma renin activity and aldosterone levels will be low; cortisol will be normal
    - With adrenal insufficiency, plasma renin activity will be high; serum aldosterone and cortisol will be low

- Further evaluation of the patient with suspected adrenal insufficiency or congenital adrenal hyperplasia is discussed previously

Treatment

- Treatment may or may not be given, based on the cause of hypoaldosteronism and presence or absence of symptoms
- Hypoaldosteronism in the presence of adrenal insufficiency is treated with fludrocortisone (see Fig. 41-16)
- Hypoaldosteronism from hyporeninemic hypoaldosteronism may be treated with fludrocortisone
- If hypertension or fluid retention is present and prevents treatment with fludrocortisone, potassium-wasting diuretics and a low-potassium diet may be used

Review Questions

For review questions, please go to ExpertConsult.com.

SUGGESTED READINGS

Beckers A, Aaltonen LA, Daly AF, Karhu A. Familial isolated pituitary adenomas (FIPA) and the pituitary adenoma predisposition caused by mutations in the aryl hydrocarbon receptor interacting protein (AIP) gene. *Endocr Rev.* 2013;34:239-277.

Carroll TB, Findling JW. The diagnosis of Cushing syndrome. *Rev Endocr Metab Disord.* 2010;11:147-153.

Dekkers OM, Pereira AM, Romijn JA. Treatment and follow-up of clinically nonfunctioning pituitary macroadenomas. *J Clin Endocrinol Metab.* 2008;93:3717-3726.

Gordon RD, Laragh JH, Funder JW. Low renin hypertensive states: perspectives, unsolved problems, future research. *Trends Endocrinol Metab.* 2005;16:108-113.

Kargi AY, Merriam GR. Diagnosis and treatment of growth hormone deficiency in adults. *Nat Rev Endocrinol.* 2013;9:335-345.

Kennan S, Remer EM, Hamrahian AH. Evaluation of patients with adrenal incidentalomas. *Curr Opin Endocrinol Diabetes Obes.* 2013;20:161-169.

Loh JA, Verbalis JG. Disorders of water and salt metabolism associated with pituitary disease. *Endocrinol Metab Clin North Am.* 2008;37:213-234.

Mathioudakis N, Salvatori R. Pituitary tumors. *Curr Treat Options Neurol.* 2009;11:287-296.

Melmed S, Colao A, Barkan A, et al; for the Acromegaly Consensus Group. Guidelines for acromegaly management: an update. *J Clin Endocrinol Metab.* 2009;94:1509-1517.

Molitch ME. Management of incidentally found nonfunctional pituitary tumors. *Neurosurg Clin North Am.* 2012;23:543-553.

Salvatori R. Adrenal insufficiency. *JAMA.* 2005;294:2481-2488.

Torino F, Barnabei A, De Vecchis L, et al. Hypophysitis induced by monoclonal antibodies to cytotoxic T lymphocyte antigen 4: challenges from a new cause of a rare disease. *Oncologist.* 2012;17:525-535.

Young WF Jr. Adrenal causes of hypertension: pheochromocytoma and primary aldosteronism. *Rev Endocr Metab Disord.* 2007;8:309-320.

41

SECTION SEVEN

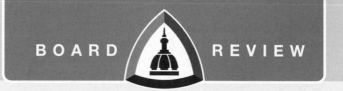

Rheumatology

Arthritis

ALLAN C. GELBER, MD, MPH, PhD

The term *arthritis* encompasses a broad spectrum of disorders that in their aggregate are the leading cause of disability in the United States. More than 60% of the population can expect to develop some form of arthritis in their lifetime.

Approach to the Patient with Joint Symptoms

Basic Information

- Strictly speaking, arthritis refers to joint inflammation, but is often used more commonly to denote more than a hundred musculoskeletal conditions, both inflammatory and degenerative in etiology
- It is important to distinguish true arthritis from conditions that mimic other joint disorders (Box 42-1)

Clinical Presentation

- A careful history and detailed physical examination should be directed at answering the following five key diagnostic questions:
  - **Is the process truly articular?**
  - **Is the process inflammatory or mechanical?**
  - What is the pattern of joint involvement?
  - Are there extraarticular manifestations?
  - Who is the host?
- Historical and clinical features that suggest an articular process
  - Symptoms (pain) localized to the joint(s)
  - Physical findings (swelling, erythema, heat, tenderness) localized to the joint(s)
  - Painful range of motion of the joint
  - Restricted range of motion of the joint
- Historical and clinical features that suggest an inflammatory process
  - **Morning stiffness lasting longer than 60 minutes that improves over the course of the day (versus joint pain that worsens in the evening in mechanical processes)**
  - Gel phenomenon (stiffness after prolonged inactivity)
  - Symptoms improve with use (versus worsening with use in mechanical processes)
  - **Joint swelling, erythema, heat, or tenderness**
  - Active constitutional manifestations (e.g., fever, malaise, anorexia or unintentional weight loss)
- Onset of joint involvement can be
  - Acute onset (e.g., microcrystalline) versus insidious onset (e.g., osteoarthritis [OA])

- Episodic (e.g., microcrystalline) versus migratory (e.g., disseminated gonococcal [GC] infection and acute rheumatic fever) versus additive (e.g., rheumatoid arthritis [RA])
- Number of joints involved
  - Monoarticular: single joint (e.g., microcrystalline and septic)
  - Oligoarticular: four or fewer joints (e.g., human leukocyte antigen [HLA]-B27-associated arthritis)
  - Polyarticular: five or more joints (e.g., RA)
- Pattern of joint involvement
  - **Symmetrical (e.g., RA) versus asymmetrical (e.g., HLA-B27-associated spondyloarthritis)**
  - Axial (e.g., HLA-B27 associated spondyloarthritis) versus peripheral (e.g., RA)
- Relevant extraarticular features
  - Constitutional symptoms and signs (i.e., presence of a fever)
  - Mucocutaneous (e.g., photosensitive and other cutaneous eruptions, alopecia, mucosal aphthous ulcers, and Raynaud phenomenon)
  - Ocular (e.g., conjunctivitis, episcleritis, scleritis, keratitis, and uveitis)
  - Renal (e.g., glomerulonephritis, interstitial nephritis, renal tubular acidosis, and nephrolithiasis)
  - Neurologic (e.g., focal central and peripheral nerve disease, seizures, and cognitive and psychiatric disorders)
  - Pulmonary (e.g., nodules, infiltrates, interstitial fibrosis, pulmonary embolism and hypertension, alveolar hemorrhage, bronchiolitis, and pleuritis)
  - Gastrointestinal ([GI]; e.g., inflammatory bowel disease [IBD] and autoimmune liver disease)
  - Hematologic
    - Anemia (e.g., anemia of chronic disease and hemolytic anemia)
    - Leukopenia (e.g., neutropenia in Felty syndrome and lymphopenia in systemic lupus erythematosus [SLE])
    - Thrombocytopenia (e.g., SLE and antiphospholipid antibody syndrome)
- Relevant host factors include age, gender, race, comorbidities, occupational exposures, and family history

Diagnosis and Evaluation

- Judicious use of laboratory, synovial fluid, and imaging studies serves to test and confirm the diagnostic hypothesis, to assess the severity and prognosis of the disease process, and to guide therapy

BOX 42-1	*Processes that Mimic Arthritis*

Bursitis	Myositis
Tendinitis	Vasculitis
Fasciitis	Neuropathy
Enthesitis	Thyroid disease
Periostitis	Parathyroid disease
Fibromyalgia	Cellulitis

- Obtain relevant laboratory studies as indicated
  - Kidney and liver function, calcium, protein, and albumin
  - Complete blood count with leukocyte differential
  - Urinalysis
  - Erythrocyte sedimentation rate and C-reactive protein
  - Thyroid function tests
  - Autoantibodies/serologies
  - Infectious work-up (if indicated)
- Obtain and evaluate synovial fluid as indicated
  - Check synovial fluid leukocyte cell count, Gram stain and culture, and polarized microscopy for crystals
  - White blood cell (WBC) count
    - If less than 200/mm³, considered normal
    - If between 200/mm³ and 2000/mm³, abnormal but noninflammatory
    - If greater than 2000/mm³, inflammatory
    - If greater than 100,000/mm³, presumptively septic
- Obtain relevant imaging studies
  - Conventional radiography is the starting point in imaging studies because of easy availability, low cost, and high resolution, but may reveal only nonspecific soft tissue swelling in early inflammatory disease
  - Computed tomography (CT) is widely available and a good choice for assessment of the spine
  - Magnetic resonance imaging (MRI) has replaced CT in many situations (e.g., disk herniation, sacroiliac joints, osteonecrosis, synovitis and erosions and soft tissue processes/meniscal injuries/rotator cuff pathology)
  - Arthrography (e.g., evaluation for rotator cuff tears)
  - Angiography (e.g., evaluation for vasculitis)
  - **Both mechanical and inflammatory joint disease cause increased tracer uptake so that nuclear medicine scans have a limited role in the evaluation of arthritis**
  - Ultrasound is useful in differentiating thrombophlebitis from pseudothrombophlebitis (ruptured Baker cyst), with an expanding role in the assessment of synovitis, tendonitis, and erosive joint disease

Osteoarthritis

Basic Information

- **Prototypical and most prevalent mechanical (noninflammatory) joint disorder**
- One third of individuals 65 years and older have radiographic evidence of knee OA

BOX 42-2	*Risk Factors for Osteoarthritis*

Advanced age
Female gender
Developmental
Collagen polymorphisms
   Types II, IX, and XI
Obesity
Trauma
   Acute and repetitive
   Meniscal and ligamentous injury and prior surgeries
     (i.e., knee OA)
Neuropathy
Inflammatory arthritis
Osteonecrosis
Paget disease
Endocrine/metabolic
   Acromegaly
   Alkaptonuria
   Chondrocalcinosis
   Hemochromatosis

OA, Osteoarthritis.

- **Primarily a disease of degenerative cartilage, with secondary bony changes**
- There are a variety of risk factors for OA (Box 42-2)

Clinical Presentation

- Typically presents insidiously in middle-aged or elderly patients
- Most commonly seen in hands (e.g., first carpometacarpal, proximal interphalangeal [PIP], and distal interphalangeal [DIP] joints), weight-bearing peripheral joints (e.g., hips and knees), and spine (e.g., cervical and lumbar levels)
- **Joints ache and are painful, worsening with use and at the end of the day**
- Rest and nocturnal pain may be seen with severe disease
- Patients may experience minimal morning stiffness and gelling
- No constitutional or other extraarticular manifestations with primary OA
- Clinical presentation and patterns may vary
- Hands
  - First carpometacarpal joint
  - Interphalangeal joints (often familial and affects primarily older women; Fig. 42-1)
    - **Bouchard nodes represent bony enlargement of the PIP joints**
    - **Heberden nodes represent bony enlargement of the DIP joints**
  - Erosive OA
    - Affects the DIP and PIP joints
    - Characterized by recurrent flares of pain, swelling, and tenderness
    - Joint destruction occurs, leading to nonuniform joint space loss and joint deformity
    - May be associated with microcrystalline disease and can be confused with RA
- Hip
  - Symptoms often localize to the groin and anterior thigh

42

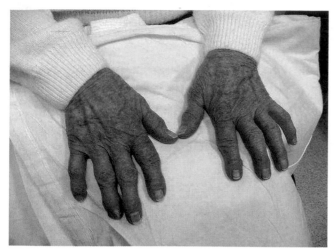

FIGURE 42-1 Osteoarthritis of the hands with Heberden nodes (distal interphalangeal joints) and Bouchard nodes (proximal interphalangeal joints). (Courtesy Don R. Martin, MD.)

- Distinguish from trochanteric bursitis (pain over the lateral aspect of the hip)
- Symptoms provoked by use (e.g., weight-bearing) and internal rotation
- May be associated with congenital malformations (e.g., hip dysplasia, slipped capital femoral epiphysis, and Legg-Calvé-Perthes disease)
- Knee
  - All three joint compartments may be affected (e.g., medial tibiofemoral, lateral tibiofemoral, and patellofemoral)
- Spine
  - Characterized by pain, stiffness, and (sometimes) radicular symptoms
  - Most commonly affects the lower cervical and lumbar spine
- Diffuse idiopathic skeletal hyperostosis (DISH)
  - **Most common in elderly men**
  - Variant of OA with axial and peripheral skeletal manifestations
  - Radiographic diagnosis (Fig. 42-2) characterized by:
    - Flowing calcification or ossification along the anterolateral aspect of at least four contiguous vertebrae
    - Relative preservation of the intervertebral disk space at the involved levels (in contrast to classic OA)
    - Absence of apophyseal or sacroiliac joint involvement (in contrast to ankylosing spondylitis [AS])

Diagnosis and Evaluation of Osteoarthritis

- Clinical presentation highly suggestive in classic cases
- History characterized by:
  - Insidious onset
  - Worsening symptoms with activity
  - Absence of inflammatory manifestations
- Physical examination reveals:
  - Variable pattern of joint involvement as detailed previously
  - **Bony hypertrophy**

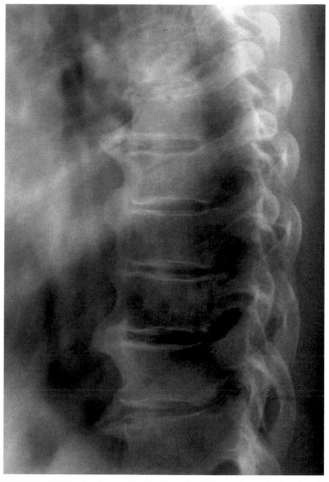

FIGURE 42-2 Radiographic findings in diffuse idiopathic skeletal hyperostosis with flowing ossification along the anterolateral aspect of at least four contiguous vertebral bodies and relative preservation of the disk spaces. (From Harris ED, Budd RC, Genovese MC, et al, eds. *Kelley's Textbook of Rheumatology.* 7th ed. Philadelphia: Saunders; 2005: Fig. 51-66.)

- - Bony deformity
  - Joint line tenderness
  - **Crepitus**
  - Limited joint mobility or laxity/pseudolaxity
  - Muscle (disuse) atrophy
- Laboratory findings
  - Renal and hepatic function normal unless impairment results from drug toxicity
  - Normal erythrocyte sedimentation rate (aside from age-associated changes)
  - Seronegative (aside from age-associated changes)
  - **Synovial fluid is noninflammatory with less than 2000 WBCs/mm³**
- Radiographic findings
  - Symptoms and radiographic findings may be discordant (e.g., significant symptoms or functional limitation with minimal radiographic findings, and vice versa)
  - May be normal in early disease
  - Radiographic hallmarks include:
    - **Osteophytes (bony spurs)**
    - Joint space narrowing (often asymmetrical; Fig. 42-3)

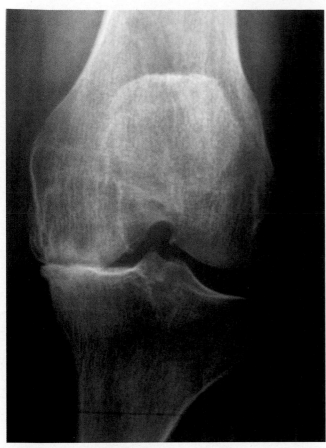

FIGURE 42-3 Radiographic findings in osteoarthritis of the knee, with asymmetrical narrowing of the medial joint space. (From Harris ED, Budd RC, Genovese MC, et al, eds. *Kelley's Textbook of Rheumatology.* 7th ed. Philadelphia: Saunders; 2005: Fig. 92-1.)

- Subchondral bone sclerosis (or eburnation)
- Subchondral cysts

Treatment

- Principles
  - Provide symptomatic relief
  - Maintain and maximize function
  - Minimize medication-associated toxicity
- Nonpharmacologic treatment
  - Patient education, weight loss (if overweight), exercise (low-impact, conditioning, and range of motion, aquatic and resistance exercises), occupational therapy, physical therapy, and assistive devices (e.g., cane, splint, brace)
- Pharmacologic treatment
  - Topical therapy
    - Capsaicin (depletes substance P in sensory nerve endings)
    - Methylsalicylate
    - Diclofenac sodium/naproxen topical gel
  - Oral therapy
    - Acetaminophen (considered first-line oral pharmacologic therapy)
    - Nonsteroidal antiinflammatory drugs (NSAIDs)
      - Therapeutically equivalent, although individual responses may vary

- **Nonselective cyclooxygenase (COX)-1 and -2 inhibitors reduce pain and improve function, but carry significant potential for GI and other toxicities (e.g., renal insufficiency)**
  - Selective COX-2 inhibitors may be safer with respect to GI toxicity and do not block platelet activity, but have been associated with increased risk for cardiovascular and cerebrovascular morbidity and mortality and are not more effective. Only celecoxib remains available in the United States.
  - Other pure analgesics such as tramadol
  - Opioids and duloxetine are options for patients who fail initial medical therapy
  - Glucosamine and chondroitin sulfate may provide symptomatic relief in some patients, but the results of clinical trials vary (see Chapter 70)
  - **There is no role for systemic corticosteroid therapy**
  - Intraarticular therapy
    - May provide temporary relief of symptoms when topical and oral regimens are ineffective or not tolerated
    - Joint aspiration may provide temporary relief when a moderate effusion is present
    - Corticosteroid injections may be particularly helpful in patients who have signs of joint inflammation
    - Hyaluronan injections have demonstrated modest efficacy, but individual responses are quite variable
  - Surgical treatment
    - Arthroscopic débridement is indicated when internal derangements (e.g., meniscal tears) cause joint catching, locking, instability, or pain
    - **Total joint replacement is indicated in patients with symptoms and functional impairment that are unresponsive to medical intervention**
    - Tidal irrigation of joints has not been demonstrated to be effective

Prevention

- Diagnosis and treatment of risk factors for OA may result in prevention of articular damage
- **The relative risk of developing knee OA is higher in obese individuals, so weight loss may have a major role in prevention of disease**

Rheumatoid Arthritis

Basic Information

- **Prototypical and most common inflammatory arthritis**
- Peak incidence in patients aged 30 to 60 years
- Female-to-male ratio 3 : 1
- Familial predisposition, with HLA-DR4 association and amino acid motif QKRAA shared epitope susceptibility
- Smoking is a risk factor for RA
- Twofold to fourfold increased risk of cardiovascular disease in patients with RA

42

■ **Associated with long-term disability and increased mortality**

Clinical Presentation

■ **Additive, symmetric polyarthritis affecting both small and large joints**
  ■ Wrists, metacarpophalangeal (MCP), and PIP joints are prominently involved; DIP joints spared
  ■ Shoulders, elbows, hips, knees, ankles, and feet are commonly involved
  ■ Cervical spine (atlantoaxial joint) may be involved; lumbar spine is spared
  ■ Joint pain, swelling, erythema, heat, and tenderness may develop acutely or insidiously
  ■ Morning stiffness lasts more than 1 hour; gel phenomenon present after inactivity
■ **Fatigue, fever, and weight loss may be present, reflecting systemic nature of the disease**
■ Classic joint deformities associated with RA
  ■ Ulnar deviation and subluxation of the fingers at the MCP joints, with radial deviation at the wrist
  ■ Swan neck deformity (hyperextension of the PIP and flexion of the DIP joints; Fig. 42-4)
  ■ Boutonnière deformity (flexion of the PIP and hyperextension of the DIP joints; Fig. 42-5)

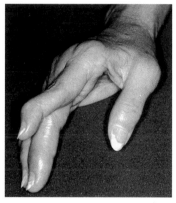

FIGURE 42-4 Swan neck deformity in advanced rheumatoid arthritis. (From Harris ED, Budd RC, Genovese MC, et al, eds. *Kelley's Textbook of Rheumatology.* 7th ed. Philadelphia: Saunders; 2005: Fig. 33-6.)

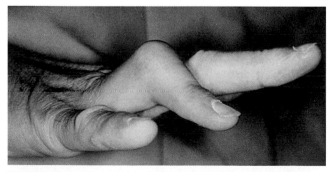

FIGURE 42-5 Boutonnière deformity in advanced rheumatoid arthritis. (From Townsend CM, Beauchamp RD, Evers BM, et al. *Sabiston Textbook of Surgery.* 17th ed. Philadelphia: Saunders; 2004: Fig. 73-17.)

■ **Extraarticular manifestations**
  ■ Rheumatoid nodules
    ■ **Most common extraarticular manifestation in RA (occurs in 25% of patients)**
    ■ Typically appear on extensor surfaces and pressure points (e.g., forearm, olecranon process and Achilles tendon) but may also affect internal organs
    ■ **Associated with rheumatoid factor (RF) seropositivity and more severe disease**
    ■ Nodules are not specific for RA and can occur in other rheumatic diseases
    ■ Histology marked by central necrosis, surrounded by palisading fibroblasts, and a collagenous capsule with a chronic inflammatory infiltrate
    ■ **Methotrexate can worsen nodulosis, even as inflammatory joint disease improves**
  ■ Ocular
    ■ Episcleritis, scleritis, and scleromalacia perforans (ophthalmologic emergency)
    ■ Keratoconjunctivitis sicca (secondary Sjögren syndrome)
  ■ Pulmonary
    ■ Pleural disease (effusions exudative and pleural fluid glucose typically low)
    ■ Interstitial lung disease with fibrosis and honey-combing
    ■ Bronchiolitis obliterans (also known as cryptogenic organizing pneumonia)
    ■ Pulmonary nodules: single or multiple
      ■ Nodules may cavitate and pleural nodules cause bronchopleural fistulae
      ■ **Caplan disease (nodules with underlying RA and pneumoconiosis)**
  ■ Cardiac
    ■ Pericarditis and effusions are common but rarely symptomatic
    ■ Constrictive pericarditis, myocarditis, and conduction defects develop rarely
  ■ Hematologic
    ■ Anemia caused by iron deficiency (NSAID-associated GI loss) and chronic disease
    ■ **Felty syndrome (RA associated with splenomegaly, neutropenia, and leg ulcers)**
    ■ Thrombocytosis or thrombocytopenia
    ■ Twofold increased risk of non-Hodgkin lymphoma
  ■ Neurologic
    ■ Atlantoaxial (C1-C2) instability and subluxation may produce cervical myelopathy
    ■ Peripheral neuropathy
    ■ Compressive neuropathy associated with synovitis (e.g., carpal tunnel syndrome)
    ■ Ischemia associated with vasculitis (e.g., mononeuritis multiplex)
  ■ Rheumatoid vasculitis
    ■ Leukocytoclastic vasculitis, cutaneous ulcers, visceral involvement, and mononeuritis multiplex
    ■ **Associated with long-standing, destructive, nodular, seropositive disease**

Diagnosis and Evaluation

- Clinical presentation highly suggestive in classic cases
- History characterized by:
  - Acute or subacute onset
  - Inflammatory and constitutional symptoms
- Physical examination reveals:
  - Synovitis
  - Symmetrical polyarthritis as detailed previously
  - Subcutaneous nodules
- Laboratory findings
  - Renal and hepatic function normal unless the result of drug toxicity
  - Normochromic normocytic anemia
  - Elevated sedimentation rate and C-reactive protein
  - RF
    - Immunoglobulin (Ig)M autoantibody directed against the Fc fragment of IgG
    - IgM-RF is 60% to 80% sensitive but low specificity for RA
    - **RF is also seen in a wide variety of other rheumatic diseases (Sjögren syndrome, juvenile arthritis, SLE, and cryoglobulinemia) and nonrheumatic diseases (interstitial lung disease, endocarditis, tuberculosis [TB], hepatitis, and malignancy)**
    - Prevalence increases with age
  - Anti-cyclic citrullinated peptide (anti-CCP) antibodies
    - Anti-CCP antibody is 68% to 80% sensitive and 98% specific for RA
    - Anti-CCP is more likely to be present in early RA than is RF
    - **Predictive of more aggressive, erosive disease**
  - Synovial fluid inflammatory with leukocyte count greater than 2000 WBCs/mm³
- Radiographic findings (Fig. 42-6)
  - May reveal only soft tissue swelling in early disease, but with advanced disease show
  - Periarticular osteopenia
  - Uniform joint space narrowing
  - **Joint margin erosions (hallmark of RA) most commonly seen in carpal bones, ulnar styloid, MCPs, and MTPs**
  - Atlantoaxial (C1-C2) instability and subluxation
- 1987 criteria for the classification of RA (Table 42-1)
  - Developed to classify patients for study purposes
  - Requires four of the seven criteria to classify patient with RA
  - May still consider the diagnosis of RA if two or more criteria are present
- 2010 RA classification criteria (see Table 42-1)
  - Designed to address criticism of 1987 criteria for their lack of sensitivity in early disease
  - This new classification system redefines the current paradigm of RA by focusing on features at earlier stages of disease that are associated with persistent and/or erosive disease
  - Intent of criteria is to prioritize the need for earlier diagnosis and prompt institution of effective disease-modifying therapy, and thereby to prevent or

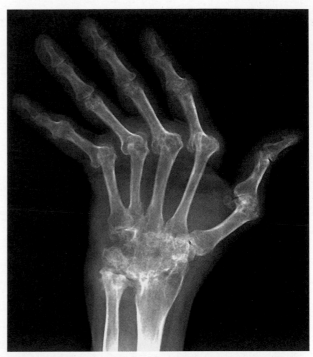

FIGURE 42-6 Radiographic findings in rheumatoid arthritis of the hand: advanced erosive carpal arthritis and subluxation/ulnar deviation across all metacarpophalangeal joints. (From Harris ED, Budd RC, Genovese MC, et al, eds. *Kelley's Textbook of Rheumatology.* 7th ed. Philadelphia: Saunders; 2005: Fig. 51-6.)

minimize future joint damage, associated disability, and long-term morbidity

Treatment

- **Untreated, RA can cause joint destruction and disability, beginning in the first year of disease**
- Principles of treatment
  - Provide symptomatic relief
  - Prevent joint destruction
  - Maintain and maximize function
  - Decrease RA-related morbidity and mortality
  - Minimize medication-associated toxicity
- Pharmacologic treatment
  - **Disease-modifying antirheumatic drugs (Table 42-2)**
    - Disease-modifying antirheumatic drugs (DMARDs) alter the course of RA, reduce joint destruction, and improve long-term outcomes
    - **Early and aggressive treatment with DMARDs to control RA is the standard of care**
    - Treat-to-target approach to induce remission or low disease activity is the new treatment paradigm in RA
    - **Methotrexate remains the initial anchoring therapy in RA**
    - If disease is not adequately controlled by one DMARD, another DMARD is added (combination therapy)
    - **Combination therapy is more effective than monotherapy**
    - If traditional DMARD combination does not achieve target, biologic DMARD is added

42

TABLE 42-1	*Classification Schemes for Diagnosing Rheumatoid Arthritis*

1987 American Rheumatism Association*	**2010 American College of Rheumatology/ European League Against Rheumatism†**	
Criteria 1–4 must be present for 6 weeks RA diagnosis requires 4 of 7 criteria fulfilled	Classification criteria for RA (score-based algorithm: add score of categories A–D; *a score ≥6/10 is needed for classification of a patient as having definite RA*	
		Score
1. Morning stiffness (≥1 hr)	A. Joints (0–5)	
2. Swelling of ≥3 joint areas (simultaneously)	1 large joint	0
3. Swelling of hand joints (wrist, MCP, or PIP joints)	2–10 large joints	1
4. Symmetrical arthritis	1–3 small joints (large joints not counted)	2
5. Rheumatoid nodules	4–10 small joints (large joints not counted)	3
6. Serum rheumatoid factor	>10 joints (at least 1 small joint)	5
7. Radiographic changes (consistent with RA)	B. Serology (at least 1 test is needed for classification)	
	High titer >3× upper limit	
	Negative RF *and* negative ACPA	0
	Low-positive RF *or* low-positive ACPA	2
	High-positive RF *or* high-positive ACPA	3
	C. Acute-phase reactants (at least one test result is needed for classification)	
	Normal CRP *and* normal ESR	0
	Abnormal CRP *or* abnormal ESR	1
	D. Duration of symptoms	
	<6 weeks	0
	≥6 weeks	1

*From Arnett FC, Edworthy SM, Bloch DA, et al. The American Rheumatism Association 1987 revised criteria for the classification of rheumatoid arthritis. *Arthritis Rheum.* 1988;31:315–324.
†From Aletha D, Neogi T, Silman AJ, et al. An American College of Rheumatology/European League Against Rheumatism Collaborative Initiative 2010 Rheumatoid Arthritis Classification Criteria. *Arthritis Rheum.* 2010;62:2569–2581.
ACPA, Anti-citrullinated protein antibody; CRP, C-reactive protein; ESR, erythrocyte sedimentation rate; MCP, metacarpophalangeal; PIP, proximal interphalangeal; RA, rheumatoid arthritis; RF, rheumatoid factor.

- Time to achieve maximal beneficial effect varies from 8 weeks to 6 months for different DMARDs, but a good trial is at least 3 months long for any DMARD
- Gold, D-penicillamine, azathioprine, cyclophosphamide, and cyclosporine are rarely used anymore
- NSAIDs
  - Analgesic and antiinflammatory effects reduce pain and improve function
  - **NSAIDs are not disease-modifying**
  - No role in long-term management of RA
- Corticosteroids
  - Antiinflammatory effect helps to control symptoms and maintain function
  - **Most effective as "bridging therapy" while DMARDs take effect**
  - Used for short-term treatment for RA flares, but long-term use should be avoided if possible
- Nonpharmacologic treatment
  - Patient education, exercise (low-impact, conditioning, range of motion, and yoga), occupational therapy, physical therapy, and assistive devices (e.g., cane, walker)
- Surgical treatment
  - Synovectomy may be rarely indicated when synovitis fails to respond to medical therapy
  - Joint replacement is indicated when joint destruction occurs despite medical therapy, and the resultant pain is no longer responsive to medical management

Gout

Basic Information

- **Intensely inflammatory arthritis caused by deposition of monosodium urate crystals**
- Peak incidence in patients aged 50 to 70 years
- More common in men but incidence rises in women after menopause (uric acid rises after menopause)
- Hyperuricemia results from increased production (10%) and diminished excretion (90%; Box 42-3) of uric acid
  - Limit of solubility of uric acid is approximately 7 mg/dL
  - Primary hyperuricemia caused by polygenic factors
  - Secondary hyperuricemia caused by familial or acquired conditions

Clinical Presentation

- Asymptomatic hyperuricemia
  - Found at some point in about 5% of adult Americans
  - **More than 75% of individuals remain asymptomatic**
- Acute gout
  - Acute onset of intense joint pain, swelling, erythema, and heat
  - Fever (systemic manifestation of inflammation) may be present
  - 50% of patients present with first metatarsophalangeal joint involvement (podagra)
  - **75% to 90% of patients develop podagra at some point in their course**
  - Gout may also affect the ankles, midfoot, knees, wrists, shoulders, and hands

TABLE 42-2	*Disease-Modifying Antirheumatic Drugs*		
DMARDs	**Indication**	**Toxicity/Precautions**	**Monitoring**
Traditional	**DMARDs**		
Methotrexate (MTX)	First-line DMARD Used as monotherapy or in combination with other DMARDs	Stomatitis, nausea, diarrhea, hepatitis, hepatic fibrosis, myelosuppression, interstitial pneumonitis, and teratogenic; requires folate supplementation	Creatinine, LFTs, and CBC monthly until dose stable, then every 2–3 months Effective contraception required
Sulfasalazine	Used as monotherapy or in combination with other DMARDs	Nausea, hepatitis, renal, G6PD-associated anemia, myelosuppression, and oligospermia	Initial G6PD; LFTs and CBC monthly ×3, then every 3 months
Leflunomide	Used as monotherapy or in combination	Stomatitis, nausea, diarrhea, hepatitis, myelosuppression, and teratogenic	LFTs/CBC monthly until dose stable, then every 2–3 months Effective contraception required
Hydroxychloroquine (adjunct therapy)	Not used alone, always in combination	Nausea, rash, and retinal damage (rare)	Eye exam every 6–12 months
Biologic	**DMARDs**		
Anti-TNF therapy Etanercept Adalimumab Infliximab Golimumab Certolizumab	Typically first-line biologics Used if traditional DMARDs fail or are not tolerated	Injection-site and infusion reactions; avoid in patients with active or chronic infections, congestive heart failure or multiple sclerosis; reactivation of tuberculosis	Baseline PPD Monitor CBC and chemistries for cytopenias/transaminitis (rare) No live vaccines during treatment
Abatacept	Inhibitor of T-cell costimulation	Avoid in patients with active or chronic infections; increased adverse respiratory effects in patients with COPD	Baseline PPD; no live vaccines during treatment
Rituximab	Anti-CD20 monoclonal antibody	Avoid in patients with active or chronic infections; infusion reactions common; monitor immunoglobulin levels	Reported cases of PML in RA patients Hepatitis B reactivation reported
Tocilizumab	Monoclonal antibody against the interleukin-6 receptor	Associated with increases in lipid e.g., total cholesterol, triglycerides, LDL cholesterol, and/or HDL cholesterol. Can cause neutropenia, transaminitis and gastric/diverticular perforations Avoid use with hepatic impairment	Baseline PPD; be vigilant for increased susceptibility to severe infections; CBC, chemistries and lipid panel monitored during therapy
Tofacitinib	Oral Janus kinase inhibitor	Elevation in both low-density and high-density lipoprotein cholesterol levels, elevation in serum creatinine, and with reductions in neutrophil counts; avoid use with severe hepatic insufficiency; gastric and diverticular perforations reported	Baseline PPD; be vigilant for increased susceptibility to severe infections, including herpes zoster and malignancies

CBC, Complete blood count; COPD, chronic obstructive disease; DMARD, disease-modifying antirheumatic drugs; G6PD, glucose-6-phosphate dehydrogenase; HDL, high-density lipoprotein; LDL, low-density lipoprotein; LFTs, liver function tests; PML, progressive multifocal leukoencephalopathy; PPD, purified protein derivative; TNF, tumor necrosis factor; RA, rheumatoid arthritis.

- Attacks are usually monoarticular or oligoarticular (two to three joints); rarely polyarticular until late in the disease course
- **Early attacks are self-limited and will resolve over 3 to 10 days, even without treatment**
- Intercritical gout
  - Asymptomatic period between acute attacks
  - May be years in duration
  - Uric acid levels are generally persistently elevated
- Chronic (tophaceous) gout (Fig. 42-7)
  - After years of recurrent attacks, joints develop persistent pain, swelling, and deformity
- Extraarticular disease
- Tophi
  - Deposits of monosodium urate crystals in soft tissue
  - Typically found in the synovium and subchondral bone, on the pinna of the ear, and over extensor surfaces (e.g., forearm) and pressure points (e.g., Achilles tendon)
  - Typically appear after years of repeated episodes of acute gout
  - **May be confused with rheumatoid nodules**
- Renal disease
  - Parenchymal urate nephropathy associated with tumor lysis syndrome (acute) and comorbid conditions (chronic)

BOX 42-3 *Causes of Hyperuricemia*

Increased Production

Hypoxanthine-guanine phosphoribosyltransferase deficiency
Glycogen storage diseases
Increased purine intake
Increased nucleic acid turnover
  Myeloproliferative disorder
  Tumor lysis syndrome
  Hemolytic disorder
  Psoriasis
Accelerated adenosine triphosphate degradation
  Tissue hypoxia
  Sustained exercise
Ethanol

Reduced Excretion

Intrinsic renal disease
Drugs
  Diuretics
  Low-dose aspirin
  Cyclosporine
  Ethambutol
  Pyrazinamide
Ketoacidosis and lactic acidosis
Dehydration
Hyperparathyroidism
Lead nephropathy
Ethanol

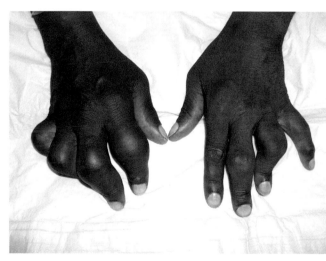

FIGURE 42-7 Chronic tophaceous gout involving the hands. (Courtesy Don R. Martin, MD.)

- Nephrolithiasis risk 50% with serum uric acid greater than 13 mg/dL or urinary uric acid excretion greater than 1100 mg/day

Diagnosis and Evaluation

- **Clinical presentation highly suggestive in classic cases**
- History characterized by:
  - **Acute onset, exquisite pain, and sensitivity in the involved joint**
  - Intermittent nature with asymptomatic intercritical phase
  - Inflammatory manifestations

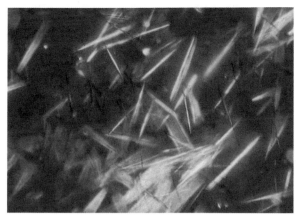

FIGURE 42-8 Polarized light microscopy demonstrating the strongly negative birefringence of needle-shaped uric acid crystals. (From Forbes CD, Jackson WF. *Color Atlas and Text of Clinical Medicine.* 3rd ed. St. Louis: Mosby; 2003: Fig. 3.13.)

- Physical examination reveals:
  - Intensely inflammatory arthritis
  - Tophi may be present
- Laboratory findings
  - **Serum uric acid level elevated more than 80% of the time during acute gout, but can be normal**
  - Arthrocentesis (joint aspiration), with synovial fluid examination both under polarized microscopy and in microbiology culture, to confirm a diagnosis of gout and to rule out septic arthritis, respectively
    - Synovial fluid inflammatory with leukocyte count greater than 2000 WBCs/mm^3, and as high as 100,000/mm^3
  - **Crystals are needle-shaped, negatively birefringent, and may be intracellular (Fig. 42-8)**
    - Crystals may be found in asymptomatic joints (during intercritical period)
- Radiographic findings
  - May reveal only soft tissue swelling in early disease, but with advanced disease will show joint margin erosions with overhanging edges ("parrot's beak"; Fig. 42-9)
  - Uric acid is radiolucent

Treatment

- Acute attack
  - NSAIDs
    - Effective and rapid, especially if started early
    - Indomethacin has traditionally been used, but there is no evidence that one NSAID agent is superior to another
  - Corticosteroids
    - Administered as an oral taper, parenteral infusion, or intraarticular injection
    - Effective when NSAIDs are contraindicated
    - Must first rule out infection before intraarticular injection
    - Carry risk of "rebound" arthritis after taper
  - Colchicine
    - Effective when started early during acute attack, but potential for significant toxicity with

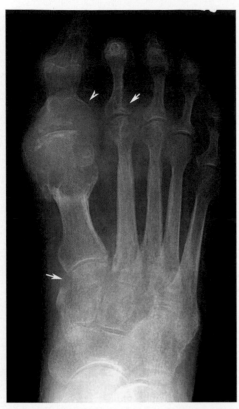

FIGURE 42-9 Radiographic findings in tophaceous gout with extensive bony destruction of the first metatarsophalangeal joint. *Arrows* indicate erosions; *arrowhead* shows overhanging edge ("parrot's beak"). (From Harris ED, Budd RC, Genovese MC, et al, eds. *Kelley's Textbook of Rheumatology.* 7th ed. Philadelphia: Saunders; 2005: Fig. 51-28.)

underlying renal insufficiency (myelosuppression, myopathy, and neuropathy)
- Indications for uric acid-lowering therapy (ULT)
  - Any patient with established gout and
  - Tophus or tophi by exam or imaging
  - Frequent acute gout attacks (more than 2 attacks/ year)
  - Chronic kidney disease stage 2
  - Past urolithiasis
  - **Do not start ULT during acute gout or without prophylaxis, as a change in the uric acid concentration (up or down) may precipitate an acute gout attack**
  - Xanthine oxidase inhibition (e.g., allopurinol, febuxostat)
    - Blocks xanthine oxidase enzyme in production of uric acid
    - Adjust dose for renal function
    - **Lower dose of azathioprine and mercaptopurine by 75% when used in conjunction with allopurinol**
    - Titrate dose to uric acid level of less than 6 mg/dL
    - Adverse effects include fever, rash, hepatitis, and leukopenia
    - Before initiation of allopurinol, consider HLA–B*5801 testing in selected patients (e.g., Koreans with stage 3 or worse chronic kidney disease, and Han Chinese and Thai irrespective of renal

function); these groups are at heightened risk to develop allopurinol hypersensitivity syndrome
- Uricosuric agents (e.g., probenecid and sulfinpyrazone) have limited usefulness in setting of renal impairment
  - Use in patients with reduced uric acid excretion, but glomerular filtration rate greater than 50 mL/ min is needed
  - If used in patients with high excretion, may lead to stone formation
  - **Must have no history of nephrolithiasis**
  - Must maintain daily fluid intake of more than 2 L to avoid stone formation
  - Must avoid low-dose salicylates
  - Prophylaxis with ULT
    - **Recommended to reduce the acute attacks of gout in early ULT**
    - Colchicine 0.6 mg once or twice daily or low-dose NSAIDs with proton pump inhibitor (PPI)
    - Continue prophylaxis for at least 6 months
- General health and life-style measures for patients with gout
  - Avoid high-purine diet and high-fructose corn syrup-sweetened sodas
  - Limit beef, pork, seafood, and alcohol
  - Encourage low-fat or nonfat dairy products
  - Avoid medications that can exacerbate hyperuricemia such as thiazide diuretics

Calcium Pyrophosphate Dihydrate Deposition Disease

Basic Information

- **Inflammatory arthritis caused by deposition of calcium pyrophosphate dihydrate (CPPD) crystals**
- Incidence increases with age; 50% of population has chondrocalcinosis by 80s
- Most cases are idiopathic, but some are associated with other underlying diseases (Box 42-4)

Clinical Presentation

- Acute (pseudogout)
  - Inflammatory arthritis of large joints
  - **Knees involved in 50% of cases**
  - Wrists, MCP joints, hips, shoulders, elbows, and ankles also affected
  - Resembles an acute gout attack with monoarticular inflammation
  - Attacks may be recurrent

BOX 42-4 *Diseases Associated with Pseudogout*

Osteoarthritis	Wilson disease
Gout	Amyloidosis
Hemochromatosis	Hypomagnesemia
Hypothyroidism	Hypophosphatemia
Hyperparathyroidism	

42

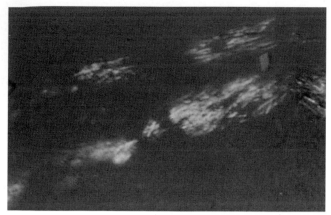

FIGURE 42-10 Polarized light microscopy demonstrating the weakly positive birefringence of rhomboidal crystals of calcium pyrophosphate dihydrate. (From Forbes CD, Jackson WF: *Color Atlas and Text of Clinical Medicine.* 3rd ed. St. Louis: Mosby; 2003: Fig. 3.14.)

- Subacute (RA-like) presentation is uncommon
- Chronic (OA-like) presentation is generally more destructive than is typical of OA

Diagnosis and Evaluation

- History characterized by:
  - Varied onset and course
  - Inflammation often less intense than in gout
- Physical examination reveals:
  - Varied patterns and intensity of disease
- Laboratory findings
  - Synovial fluid inflammatory with leukocyte count greater than 2000 WBCs/mm³ in acute arthritis
  - **Crystals are rhomboid-shaped and positively birefringent (Fig. 42-10)**
- Radiographic findings
  - Chondrocalcinosis (Fig. 42-11)
    - Linear calcifications in cartilage
    - Most commonly found in the wrist, symphysis pubis, and knee

Treatment

- Acute
  - NSAIDs
  - Corticosteroids
  - Colchicine
- Chronic
  - NSAIDs
- Prophylaxis
  - Chronic administration of low-dose colchicine or NSAIDs may be effective
  - No CPPD-lowering agents are currently available

Seronegative Spondyloarthropathies

Overview

- Four diseases grouped together by overlapping clinical features and molecular evidence of a common etiology
  - AS
  - Enteropathic arthritis

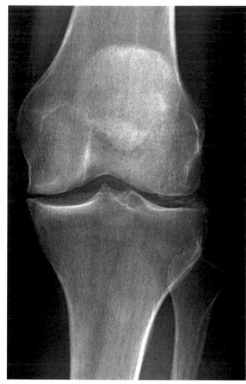

FIGURE 42-11 Radiographic findings of linear calcification of the hyaline cartilage and lateral meniscus in calcium pyrophosphate dihydrate deposition disease. (From Harris ED, Budd RC, Genovese MC, et al, eds. *Kelley's Textbook of Rheumatology.* 7th ed. Philadelphia: Saunders; 2005: Fig. 51-30.)

- Psoriatic arthritis
- Reactive arthritis
- Common clinical features
  - Enthesopathy (inflammation at the site of ligamentous and tendinous insertion to bone)
  - Inflammatory back disease/sacroiliitis
  - Mucocutaneous manifestations
  - Inflammatory eye disease
  - IBD
  - HLA-B27 genetic association
  - RF-seronegative

ANKYLOSING SPONDYLITIS

Basic Information

- Inflammatory arthritis that predominantly affects the axial skeleton
- Affects 0.5% to 1% of whites; less common in blacks
- Peak incidence in in patients aged 20 to 40 years
- Male-to-female ratio is 5:1

Clinical Presentation

- **Presents with insidious onset of low back or buttock stiffness**
- Symptoms typically inflammatory (e.g., worse in the morning; improve with use)
- **Typically begins as sacroiliitis, progressing to the lumbar spine and cephalad, resulting in vertebral body fusion**
- Thoracic spine disease may present as chest pain

- Extraaxial disease
  - Limb-girdle joints (e.g., shoulders and hips) commonly affected
  - Peripheral joints affected less commonly and usually asymmetrically
  - Enthesopathy (e.g., Achilles tendinitis and plantar fasciitis)
  - Anterior uveitis
  - Aortitis and aortic valve insufficiency
  - Pulmonary fibrosis (apical lung fields)
  - Subclinical colitis

Diagnosis and Evaluation

- Clinical presentation highly suggestive in classic cases
- History characterized by:
  - Localization of symptoms to sacroiliac joints and lumbar spine
  - Inflammatory manifestation
  - **Anterior uveitis may be initial manifestation**
- Physical examination reveals:
  - Sacroiliac and lumbar spine tenderness
  - Loss of lumbar lordosis
  - Loss of lumbar spine range of motion
  - **Schober test measures lumbar spine distraction with flexion (less than 5 cm abnormal)**
- Chest expansion is limited in patients with thoracic involvement
- Laboratory findings
  - Inflammatory markers may be elevated
  - **90% of patients are HLA-B27 positive; nearly 100% of those with uveitis or aortitis**
  - **However, HLA-B27 is nondiagnostic, as 6% to 8% of the general white population is positive**
- Radiographic findings
  - Symmetrical sacroiliitis (e.g., iliac margin sclerosis and fusion; Fig. 42-12)
  - Early findings include squaring and sclerosis of the corners of the vertebrae
  - Later findings include ossification of the anterior longitudinal ligament and bridging syndesmophytes resulting in "bamboo spine" (Fig. 42-13)
  - Typical radiographic findings may take months or years to become apparent
  - CT and MRI are sensitive for early sacroiliitis

Treatment

- Pharmacologic
  - NSAIDs: first line of treatment for spinal disease
  - Analgesic and antiinflammatory effects relieve pain and stiffness
  - Regular NSAIDs use my slow radiographic damage in AS
  - Indomethacin has traditionally been used, but there is no evidence that one NSAID is superior to another
- **TNF inhibitors improve quality of life and function in AS patients**
  - To date, little evidence to support slowing of spinal fusion with anti-TNF agents
  - Etanercept and infliximab Food and Drug Administration (FDA) approved for this indication
- Sulfasalazine and methotrexate have little effect in spinal disease but used for peripheral arthritis
- Nonpharmacologic
  - Tailored exercise and stretching program recommended for AS

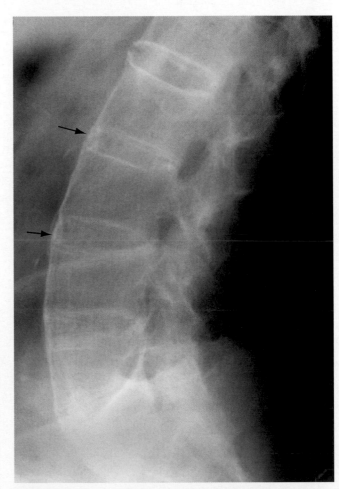

FIGURE 42-13 Radiographic findings of syndesmophytes in ankylosing spondylitis, with bony bridging *(arrows)* extending from the edge of one vertebral body to the next. (From Harris ED, Budd RC, Genovese MC, et al, eds. *Kelley's Textbook of Rheumatology.* 7th ed. Philadelphia: Saunders; 2005: Fig. 51-56.)

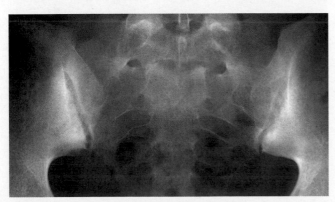

FIGURE 42-12 Radiographic findings of sacroiliitis in ankylosing spondylitis with both erosions and sclerosis along the iliac sides of the sacroiliac joints. (From Harris ED, Budd RC, Genovese MC, et al, eds. *Kelley's Textbook of Rheumatology.* 7th ed. Philadelphia: Saunders; 2005: Fig. 51-54.)

- Physical therapy to maintain posture and prevent progressive thoracic kyphosis and loss of mobility
- Breathing exercises to maintain chest wall expansion

ENTEROPATHIC ARTHRITIS

Basic Information

- Inflammatory arthritis associated with IBD: Crohn disease or ulcerative colitis
- Peripheral arthritis occurs in 10% to 20% of patients with IBD; spondylitis in 10%
- Male-to-female ratio is 3:1 in those with spondylitis

Clinical Presentation

- Axial skeletal disease clinically indistinguishable from AS
- Peripheral joint disease most commonly affects the knees, ankles, and feet
- **Peripheral joint disease activity correlates with GI disease activity; axial skeletal disease is independent**
- Extraaxial disease
  - Anterior uveitis
  - Oral aphthous ulcers
  - Erythema nodosum
  - Pyoderma gangrenosum

Diagnosis and Evaluation

- Clinical presentation highly suggestive in classic cases
- History characterized by:
  - Coexistence of IBD and arthritis
- Physical examination reveals:
  - Manifestations of IBD
  - Inflammatory axial or peripheral joint disease
  - Consider occult IBD in cases of "typical" articular pattern (e.g., isolated knee arthritis in young adult) without otherwise symptomatic GI involvement
- Laboratory findings
  - Inflammatory markers may be elevated
  - 50% of patients with spondylitis are HLA-B27 positive
- Radiographic findings are indistinguishable from AS

Treatment

- **Treat underlying IBD medically or surgically as indicated**
- NSAIDs must be used cautiously as they may provoke flare of bowel inflammation
- Corticosteroids may be used for short periods
- Methotrexate, sulfasalazine, and leflunomide effective for peripheral arthritis
- TNF inhibitors effective in treatment of both axial and peripheral arthritis

PSORIATIC ARTHRITIS

Basic Information

- Inflammatory arthritis associated with psoriatic skin disease
- At least 15% of patients with psoriatic skin disease are affected
- Male-to-female ratio is 1:1

Clinical Presentation

- **Psoriasis may precede (70%), present with (15%), or follow (15%) onset of arthritis**
- Patterns of joint involvement (not mutually exclusive)
  - Peripheral
    - Symmetrical polyarticular (30% to 50%; may be clinically indistinguishable from RA, but RF-negative)
    - Asymmetrical oligoarticular (30% to 50%; "classic" spondyloarthropathy pattern)
    - Distal interphalangeal joints (25%) (frequently associated with nail changes)
    - **Arthritis mutilans (5%) (highly destructive)**
  - Axial (5%)
    - Sacroiliitis (may be asymptomatic or asymmetrical)
    - Spondylitis (may be discontinuous)
  - Enthesitis
    - Dactylitis ("sausage digit"; Fig. 42-14)
- Extraarticular disease
  - Nail pitting, onycholysis, and "oil drop" sign (yellow-orange discoloration of the nail)
  - Anterior uveitis, aortitis, and pulmonary fibrosis are rare

Diagnosis and Evaluation

- Clinical presentation highly suggestive in classic cases
- History characterized by coexistence of psoriasis and arthritis
- Physical examination reveals:
  - Manifestations of psoriatic skin disease (e.g., at scalp, knees, elbow, umbilicus, intergluteal cleft)
  - Inflammatory axial or peripheral joint disease
- Laboratory findings
  - Inflammatory markers may be elevated
  - 50% of patients with spondylitis are HLA-B27 positive

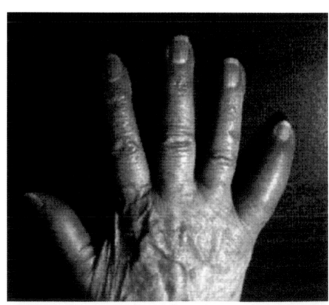

FIGURE 42-14 "Sausage digit" (dactylitis) of the fifth finger in psoriatic arthritis. (From Harris ED, Budd RC, Genovese MC, et al, eds. *Kelley's Textbook of Rheumatology.* 7th ed. Philadelphia: Saunders; 2005: Fig. 71-S169.)

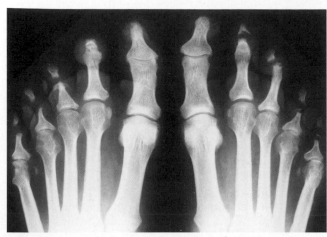

FIGURE 42-15 Bony resorption and osteophyte formation involving the phalanges in psoriatic arthritis creating "pencil-in-cup" changes. (From Harris ED, Budd RC, Genovese MC, et al, eds. *Kelley's Textbook of Rheumatology.* 7th ed. Philadelphia: Saunders; 2005: Fig. 72-9.)

- Radiographic findings marked by both bony destruction and proliferation
  - Erosive arthritis
  - Osteolysis
  - Sacroiliitis
  - Ankylosis
  - Spondylitis
  - Enthesopathy
  - Periostitis
  - **"Pencil-in-cup" deformity** (i.e., erosion of the distal end of an interphalangeal joint with bony proliferation at the proximal end of the affected joint; Fig. 42-15)

Treatment

- Treat underlying psoriasis as indicated
- Methotrexate effective for both skin and joint disease
- Leflunomide effective for psoriatic arthritis
- TNF inhibitors: all anti-TNF agents FDA approved for treatment of skin psoriasis and arthritis
- Ustekinumab: anti-IL 12/23 therapy approved for treatment of skin and joint disease
- Apremilast: phosphodiesterase 4 inhibitor was recently approved to treat psoriatic arthritis
- NSAIDs
  - Analgesic and antiinflammatory effects relieve pain and stiffness
- Systemic corticosteroids may provoke flare of skin disease during steroid taper

REACTIVE ARTHRITIS

Basic Information

- Sterile inflammatory arthritis occurring following a genitourinary or enteric infection
- Reiter disease (arthritis, conjunctivitis, and history of urethritis or enteritis) is the classic triad phenotype
- Etiologic agents: *Chlamydia, Campylobacter, Salmonella, Shigella,* and *Yersinia*

- Typically affects young males
- Male-to-female ratio is 9 : 1
- Epidemiologic association with human immunodeficiency virus/acquired immune deficiency syndrome (HIV/AIDS)

Clinical Presentation

- **Manifestations typically appear 2 to 4 weeks after genitourinary or enteric infection**
- Patterns of joint involvement
- Peripheral
  - Lower extremity oligoarthritis (particularly knees, ankles, and feet)
- Axial
  - Sacroiliitis (may be asymmetrical)
- Enthesitis
  - Achilles tendinitis
  - Plantar fasciitis
  - Dactylitis ("sausage digit")
- Extraarticular disease
  - Inflammatory eye disease (i.e., conjunctivitis or uveitis)
  - Mucocutaneous manifestations
  - Oral aphthous ulcers
  - Circinate balanitis
  - Keratoderma blenorrhagicum (clinically and histologically indistinguishable from psoriasis)

Diagnosis and Evaluation

- Clinical presentation highly suggestive in classic cases
- History characterized by:
  - **Classic triad of arthritis, conjunctivitis, and history of recent urethritis or enteritis**
  - Partial triad raises possibility of forme fruste
- Physical examination as detailed previously
- Laboratory findings
  - Inflammatory markers may be elevated
  - 50% to 80% of patients are HLA-B27 positive; 90% of those with uveitis or sacroiliitis
  - **Urethral swab or urine nucleic acid detection probe may be positive for *Chlamydia trachomatis***
  - Stool cultures are usually negative for enteric infections
- Radiographic findings
  - Sacroiliitis
  - Erosions or spurring at insertion of Achilles tendon into plantar fascia (Fig. 42-16)

Treatment

- Disease is usually self-limited, lasting 3 to 12 months
  - Up to 50% of patients may experience relapse (possible reinfection)
  - 15% of patients may experience chronic, destructive, and disabling disease
- NSAIDs
  - Their analgesic and antiinflammatory effects relieve pain and stiffness
- Doxycycline (3-month course) may be beneficial in patients with persistent disease
- Sulfasalazine may be beneficial in patients with persistent disease

42

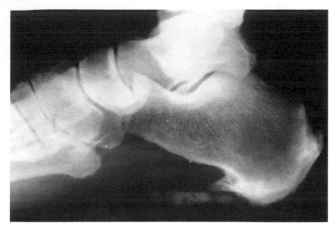

FIGURE 42-16 Calcaneal spur formation at the plantar fascial insertion in reactive arthritis. (From Harris ED, Budd RC, Genovese MC, et al, eds. *Kelley's Textbook of Rheumatology*. 7th ed. Philadelphia: Saunders; 2005: Fig. 71-6.)

- Methotrexate has been used in patients whose disease is refractory to other measures

Septic (Pyogenic/Nongonococcal) Arthritis

Basic Information

- Intensely inflammatory and rapidly destructive arthritis associated with bacterial joint infection
- Populations at risk
  - Chronically ill (e.g., diabetes mellitus, chronic renal failure, and malignancy)
  - Elderly
  - Immunosuppressed (e.g., HIV infection, immunosuppressant medications)
  - Diseased or prosthetic joints
- Routes of infection
  - Direct inoculation
  - Local extension from an adjacent process
  - Hematogenous spread
- Etiology
  - Common agents
    - *Staphylococcus aureus* (approximately 40%)
    - Group A *Streptococcus* (approximately 30%)
    - Gram-negative bacteria (approximately 30%)
  - Injection-drug users may become infected with *Pseudomonas*
  - **Sickle cell anemia associated with *Salmonella* infection**
  - **Prosthetic joints are susceptible to infection with *Staphylococcus epidermidis***
  - Animal bites and scratches may cause *Pasteurella multocida* joint infections

Clinical Presentation

- Most patients present with a monoarticular arthritis
- Oligoarthritis or polyarthritis may be seen with bacteremic route of infection
- **Injection-drug users may present with sternoclavicular, sacroiliac, or disk space infections**

- Both systemic (fever/chills) and local (joint pain, swelling, erythema, and heat) manifestations
- Distinguish primary cellulitis from skin inflammation attributable to an underlying septic joint

Diagnosis and Evaluation

- Clinical presentation highly suggestive in classic cases
- History and physical findings as in preceding discussion
- Laboratory findings
  - **Prompt synovial fluid analysis is critical if there is a concern for septic arthritis**
    - Arthrocentesis for cell count, Gram stain, and culture
    - Highly inflammatory, often with greater than 75,000 WBCs/mm³ (predominantly neutrophils); 60% to 80% of patients have positive Gram stain
  - **Synovial fluid leukocyte count greater than 100,000 cells/mm³ is attributed to presumptive septic arthritis until proven otherwise**
  - **Approximately 80% of patients have positive synovial fluid culture**
  - Approximately 50% of patients have positive blood culture
- Radiographic findings
  - May reveal only soft tissue swelling in early disease
  - Joint space narrowing and bony erosions indicate severe and advanced disease
  - CT and MRI may detect fluid in deep joints (e.g., hip and sacroiliac joints)

Treatment

- **Drainage is essential in the management of infected joints**
  - Repeated needle aspiration is adequate for easily accessible joints without loculation (e.g., knee)
  - Arthroscopy or arthrotomy is required if repeated aspirations do not clear the infection
  - Arthrotomy is indicated as the initial mode of drainage for the hip
- Antibiotics
  - **Broad-spectrum antibiotics must be promptly administered (after arthrocentesis) and continued until the results of the Gram stain and culture are available**
  - Host risk factors (as detailed previously) are taken into consideration with empirical coverage

Disseminated Gonococcal Infection

Basic Information

- GC infection is responsible for most cases of septic arthritis in young adults
- Female-to-male ratio is 3:1; women are more likely to have asymptomatic GC infection
- Congenital complement deficiency is a risk factor

Clinical Presentation

- **May present as migratory arthritis or tenosynovitis, with or without rash**

- **May also present as purulent arthritis most commonly involving the wrist, knee, or ankle**
- Systemic manifestations (fevers and chills) may be present
- Macular, papular, or pustular rash may be present on the trunk or extremities, including palms and soles

Diagnosis and Evaluation

- Clinical presentation highly suggestive in classic cases
- History characterized by:
  - Sexually active young adult
  - Pharyngeal, urethral, cervical, and anal symptoms may be present but are frequently absent
- Physical findings as in the previous discussion
- Laboratory findings
  - Synovial fluid analysis
    - Arthrocentesis for cell count, Gram stain, and culture
    - Inflammatory synovial fluid with greater than 2000 WBCs/mm^3
    - **Gram stain usually negative**
    - Culture positive in less than 50% of cases
  - Blood and skin lesion cultures are rarely positive
  - **Culture pharynx, urethra, cervix, and anus as potential sources of infection**
- Radiographic findings
  - May reveal soft tissue swelling

Treatment

- Repeated needle aspiration may be necessary, but arthroscopy and arthrotomy are rarely needed
- Sensitive to third-generation cephalosporins
- **Recommendation to treat for concomitant *Chlamydia trachomatis* coinfection**

Viral Arthritis

Basic Information

- Common agents
  - Parvovirus B19
  - Rubella virus
  - Hepatitis B and C viruses
  - HIV
- Both children and adults affected

Clinical Presentation

- **May present as migratory arthralgias/arthritis or polyarthritis**
- Most commonly affects the wrists, hands, and knees
- Frequently symmetrical
- Rash may be present
- Hepatitis-associated arthritis may precede icterus
- **RF may be positive and can mimic RA**

Diagnosis and Evaluation

- There may be a history of recent vaccination or exposure to sick contacts

Treatment

- **Most viral arthritides are self-limited and are best managed supportively**

- Parvovirus may occasionally cause a chronic arthropathy

Lyme disease

See also Chapter 16.

Basic Information

- Multisystem inflammatory disease caused by the tick-borne spirochete *Borrelia burgdorferi*
- 90% of cases reported from eight states (N.Y., N.J., Conn., R.I., Mass., Pa., Wis., and Minn.)

Clinical Presentation

- Early localized disease (fewer than 30 days after infection)
- Fever, malaise, headache, arthralgias, myalgias, and erythema migrans (50% to 90%)
- Early disseminated disease (weeks to months after infection)
  - Cardiac (e.g., heart block) and neurologic (e.g., Bell palsy)
- Late disseminated disease (months to years after infection)
  - Cutaneous, neurologic, fibromyalgia-like, and articular (monoarthritis; chronic knee arthritis in 10%)

Diagnosis and Evaluation

- **5% of the population has false-positive enzyme-linked immunosorbent assay (ELISA)**
- Confirmation by Western blot

Treatment

- Arthritis treated with:
  - Doxycycline (100 mg PO twice daily × 14 to 21 days)
  - Amoxicillin (500 mg PO three times daily × 21 to 30 days)
  - Ceftriaxone (2 g IV once daily × 14 to 28 days)

Tuberculous Arthritis

Basic Information

- Develops in only a small percentage of cases of TB

Clinical Presentation

- Chronic granulomatous arthritis
  - Monoarticular
  - Usually involves the hips, knees, or ankles
  - Chronic joint pain and swelling
  - Usually not associated with active pulmonary TB
- Poncet disease (tuberculous rheumatism; rare)
  - Symmetrical polyarthritis
  - Seen in conjunction with active disseminated infection

Diagnosis and Evaluation

- Chronic granulomatous arthritis
  - Acid-fast stain and culture of synovial fluid may be false negative

42

- Synovial biopsy may demonstrate granulomatous inflammation
- Synovial tissue culture is usually positive
- Poncet disease
  - Acid-fast stain and mycobacterial culture are negative

Treatment

- Six to 9 months of combination antituberculosis therapy

Review Questions

For review questions, please go to ExpertConsult.com.

SUGGESTED READINGS

Firestein GS, Budd RC, Gabriel SE, et al. *Kelley's Textbook of Rheumatology.* 9th ed. Philadelphia: Elsevier Saunders; 2013.

Hochberg MC, Silman AJ, Smolen JS, et al. *Rheumatology.* 6th ed. Philadelphia: Elsevier Saunders; 2015.

Klippel JH, Stone JH, Crofford LJ, et al., eds. *Primer on the Rheumatic Diseases.* 13th ed. Atlanta: Arthritis Foundation; 2007.

Levine SM, Gelber AC. Infectious monoarthritis. In: Cheng A, Zaas A, eds. *The Osler Medical Handbook.* Philadelphia: Mosby; 2003.

Gelber AC. In the clinic. Osteoarthritis. *Ann Intern Med.* 2014;161(1):ITC1-ITC16.

CHAPTER 43

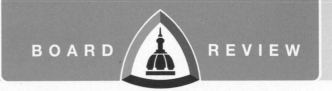
Office Orthopedics

KARIM R. MASRI, MD; and JOHN A. FLYNN, MD, MBA, MED

Office orthopedics covers a broad spectrum of disorders, many of which are not primarily articular and are variously characterized as "regional, soft tissue, or musculoskeletal pain syndromes."

These disorders are common, occur in isolation or as part of a systemic process, involve any of the articular or periarticular soft tissues, cause pain, and may cause progressive functional disability.

In addition, few, if any, specific diagnostic laboratory tests apply to these disorders, with the diagnosis depending instead on a detailed history and physical examination.

Shoulder

Figure 43-1 illustrates normal shoulder range of motion.

Basic Information

- **Shoulder pain is one of the most common musculoskeletal complaints**
- In patients younger than 40 years, symptoms are often caused by acute (e.g., sports-related) injuries
- In older patients, symptoms are more likely caused by chronic, degenerative changes of the rotator cuff
- Tables 43-1 and 43-2 compare the most common shoulder disorders and the common maneuvers used in diagnosis

Elbow

LATERAL EPICONDYLITIS ("TENNIS ELBOW")

Cause

- Repetitive wrist extension and forearm rotation

Clinical Presentation

- Lateral elbow pain

Diagnosis and Evaluation

- Tenderness over lateral epicondyle
- Pain elicited by resisted wrist extension and forearm supination (Fig. 43-2)

Treatment

- Rest
- Nonsteroidal antiinflammatory drugs (NSAIDs)
- Bracing
- Physical therapy

- **Corticosteroid injections (helpful in short-term symptom relief but high rate of recurrence and not better than placebo over long term)**

MEDIAL EPICONDYLITIS ("GOLFER'S ELBOW")

Cause

- Repetitive wrist flexion and forearm rotation

Clinical Presentation

- Medial elbow pain

Diagnosis and Evaluation

- Tenderness over medial epicondyle
- Pain elicited by resisted wrist flexion and forearm pronation (see Fig. 43-2)

Treatment

- Same as for lateral epicondylitis

ULNAR NEUROPATHY

Cause

- Trauma to the ulnar nerve as it traverses the elbow joint

Clinical Presentation

- Posteromedial forearm and fourth and fifth digit and paresthesias

Diagnosis and Evaluation

- Tenderness with percussion over the cubital tunnel
- Decreased sensation in the ulnar nerve distribution

Treatment

- Modification of activity
- NSAIDs
- Splinting
- Surgery is sometimes required for decompression

RADIAL NEUROPATHY

Cause

- Compression of the motor branch of the radial nerve as it traverses the elbow joint between radial head and supinator

Clinical Presentation

- Proximal forearm ache and possible paresthesias radiating to dorsal radial surface of hand and forearm

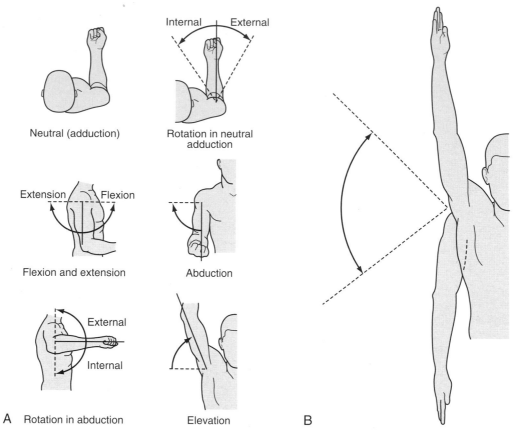

FIGURE 43-1 **A** and **B,** Normal shoulder range of motion. (From Swash M. *Hutchison's Clinical Methods.* 21st ed. Philadelphia: Saunders; 2001: Fig. 10.30.)

TABLE 43-1	*Common Disorders of the Shoulder*			
	Rotator Cuff Tendinitis	**Rotator Cuff Tear**	**Adhesive Capsulitis**	**Bicipital Tendinitis**
Cause	Overuse Inflammatory diseases such as RA	Trauma Recurrent rotator cuff tendinitis RA	Prolonged shoulder immobilization	Overuse
Clinical presentation	Anterolateral shoulder pain	Anterolateral shoulder pain	Shoulder pain Loss of motion	Anterior shoulder pain
Diagnosis and evaluation	Pain with abduction < resisted abduction Internal and external rotation Lateral palpation **Positive "impingement test"***	Same as rotator cuff tendinitis Positive "drop test"† with full-thickness tear	Painful and limited active and passive motion	Tenderness over bicipital groove Positive "speed test"‡ Positive "Yergason sign"§
Treatment	Rest NSAIDs Physical therapy Steroid injection	Orthopedic evaluation for repair	Physical therapy Steroid injection Possible orthopedics referral	Rest NSAIDs Physical therapy Steroid injection

*Relief of pain after injection of the subacromial bursa.
†Unable to maintain active shoulder abduction.
‡Pain with resisted shoulder flexion.
§Pain with resisted forearm supination.
NSAIDS, Nonsteroidal antiinflammatory drugs; RA, rheumatoid arthritis.

TABLE 43-2	*Rotator Cuff Maneuvers and Tendinopathies*			
Rotator Cuff Maneuvers*	**Description**		**Rotator Cuff Tendon**	**Function**
Empty can test	Patient abducts shoulder to 90 degrees with thumbs pointing downward Patient then tries to elevate arms against resistance		Supraspinatus	Abduction
External rotation resistance test	Patient flexes both elbows to 90 degrees with both arms at sides Patient then tries to externally rotate arms against resistance		Infraspinatus Teres minor	External rotation
Lift-off test	Patient places the dorsum of his/her hand on the low back Patient lifts the hand off the back against resistance by internally rotating the humerus		Subscapularis	Internal rotation
Supination resistance test	Patient bends elbow to 90 degrees with arm against their body Examiner holds the patient's hand and provides resistance while the patient tries to rotate the arm such that the hand is palm up		Biceps†	Supination

*Images and videos available at http://www.netterimages.com.
†Not a rotator cuff tendon.

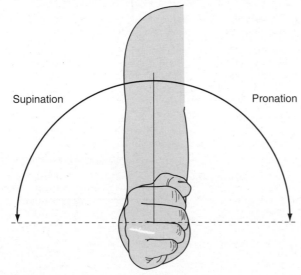

Supination
Pronation

FIGURE 43-2 Forearm pronation and supination. (From Swash M. *Hutchison's Clinical Methods.* 21st ed. Philadelphia: Saunders; 2001: Fig. 10.32.)

Diagnosis and Evaluation

- Reproduction of pain with resisted supination
- Reproduction of pain with elbow flexion while forearm is in supination
- Diagnostic lidocaine injection at lateral epicondyle to differentiate etiology, as symptoms are similar to lateral epicondylitis

Treatment

- Modification of activity
- NSAIDs
- Splinting
- Surgery is sometimes required for decompression

OLECRANON BURSITIS

Cause

- Trauma
- **Infection secondary to overlying cellulitis (most commonly gram-positive bacteria, especially *Staphylococcus aureus*)**
- **Gout and pseudogout**
- Rheumatoid arthritis

Clinical Presentation

- Pain and swelling over olecranon process

Diagnosis and Evaluation

- Inflamed olecranon bursa
- Pain with flexion, but not extension
- **Examination of bursa fluid critical to diagnose infection**

Treatment

- Rest and treatment of the underlying cause
- If gout, see treatment described in Chapter 42
- Drainage and antibiotics for infection

Hand and Wrist

Basic Information

- The hand and wrist are subject to a number of common conditions, many of which may be attributed to overuse or repetitive use (Fig. 43-3)
- Table 43-3 compares the most common disorders of hand and wrist

Hip

Figure 43-4 illustrates normal range of motion in the hip.

43

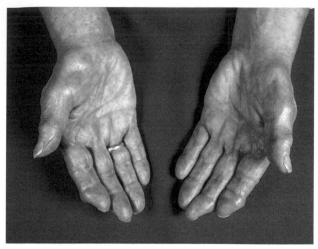

FIGURE 43-3 Thenar eminence wasting caused by carpal tunnel syndrome. (From Swash M. *Hutchison's Clinical Methods*. 21st ed. Philadelphia: Saunders; 2001, Fig. 10.13.)

TROCHANTERIC BURSITIS

Cause

- Overuse
- Inflammatory arthritis
- Trauma
- Associated with obesity

Clinical Presentation

- Deep aching lateral hip pain extending to buttock or lateral knee; not to be mistaken for groin pain, which is suggestive of hip joint pathology (see Chapter 42)
- Painful to lie in lateral decubitus position

Diagnosis and Evaluation

- **Pain on palpation over greater trochanter**
- Pain with resisted hip abduction

TABLE 43-3	*Common Disorders of the Wrist and Hand*				
	Carpal Tunnel Syndrome	**Ulnar Tunnel Syndrome**	**De Quervain Tenosynovitis**	**Trigger Finger**	**Dupuytren Contracture**
Cause	Median nerve compression at wrist	Ulnar nerve compression at wrist	Abductor policis longus and extensor policis brevis tendon inflammation	Inflammation and stenosis of digital flexor tendon	Contracture of palmar fascia
Precipitating factors	Overuse Synovitis Hypothyroidism Amyloidosis Acromegaly Pregnancy	Overuse Trauma Ganglion cyst	Overuse Rheumatoid arthritis	Overuse Rheumatoid arthritis	Heredity Alcoholism Diabetes Epilepsy
Clinical presentation	Numbness and paresthesias in median nerve distribution* Nocturnal exacerbation Wasting of thenar eminence (see Fig. 43-3)	Numbness and paresthesias in ulnar nerve distribution†	Radial wrist pain extending from thumb	Tendon catches with flexion of digit	Unable to fully extend digits
Diagnosis and evaluation	Median nerve Tinel sign‡ Phalen sign§ Abnormal nerve conduction test and electromyography	Ulnar nerve Tinel sign ‡Abnormal nerve conduction test and electromyography	Tender over radial styloid Finkelstein test¶	Pain and palpable "catch" with digit flexion Nodule may be palpable	Flexion deformity of fourth > fifth > third > second digits Palpable thickening of palmar fascia
Treatment	Wrist splint NSAIDs Steroid injection Surgical release	Wrist splint NSAIDs Surgical release	Wrist/thumb splint NSAIDs Steroid injection Surgery	Occupational therapy Steroid injection Surgical release	Surgical excision in extreme cases

*First to third fingers and radial half of the fourth.
†Fifth finger and ulnar half of the fourth.
‡Provoke pain and paresthesia with percussion over nerve at the wrist.
§Provoke pain, paresthesia, and numbness with forced wrist flexion (reversed "prayer position").
¶Provoke pain with forced ulnar deviation of the wrist, with thumb enclosed by fist.
NSAIDS, Nonsteroidal antiinflammatory drugs.

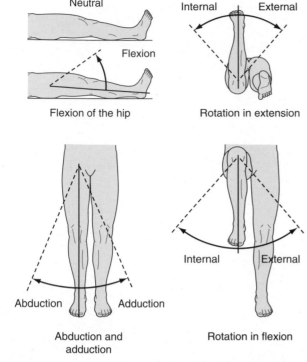

FIGURE 43-4 Normal hip range of motion. (From Swash M. *Hutchison's Clinical Methods.* 21st ed. Philadelphia: Saunders; 2001: Fig. 10.39.)

Right knee, anterior view
(patella removed)

Lateral Femur **Medial**

Lateral femoral condyle

Medial femoral condyle

Lateral collateral ligament

Medial collateral ligament

Posterior cruciate ligament

Medial meniscus

Anterior cruciate ligament

Tibial tuberosity

Fibula Tibia

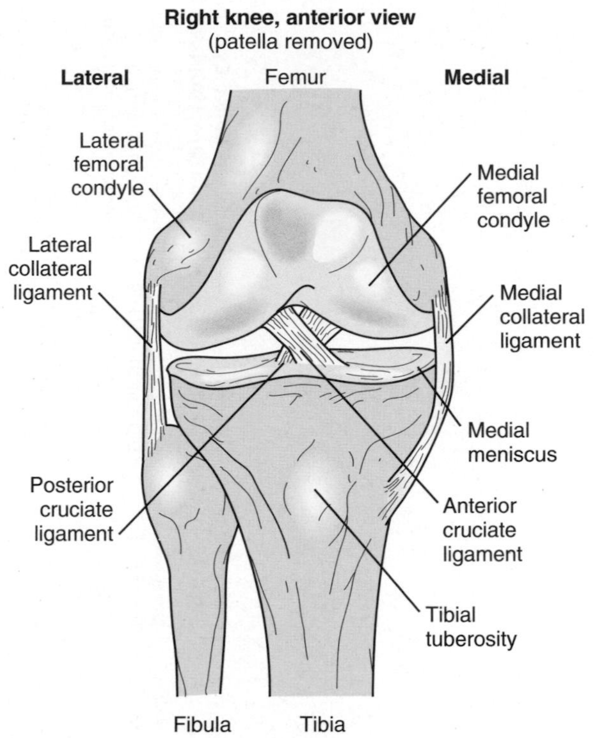

FIGURE 43-5 Anterior view of the knee demonstrating the anterior and posterior cruciate ligaments. (From Gosling J, Willan PLT, Whitmore I, Harris PF. *Human Anatomy: Color Atlas and Text.* 4th ed. St. Louis: Mosby; 2002: Fig. 6.78.)

Treatment

- Rest
- NSAIDs
- Steroid injection
- Physical therapy

MERALGIA PARESTHETICA

Cause

- Entrapment of lateral femoral cutaneous nerve
- Associated with obesity, pregnancy, diabetes, and tight clothing

Clinical Presentation

- Numbness and paresthesias over anterolateral thigh

Diagnosis and Evaluation

- **Anterolateral thigh sensory deficit**
- Tender over inguinal ligament

Treatment

- NSAIDs
- Treat underlying condition

Hip and Knee

ILIOTIBIAL BAND SYNDROME

Cause

- Overuse of iliotibial band (e.g., running)

Clinical Presentation

- Pain over lateral thigh above the joint line of the knee

Diagnosis and Evaluation

- Tender over lateral femoral condyle when flexing or extending the knee

Treatment

- Restrict exacerbating activities
- NSAIDs
- Physical therapy
- Steroid injection

Knee

See Figure 43-5 for ligaments of the knee joint.

Basic Information

- The knee, by virtue of its weight-bearing status, is subject to a variety of disorders
- Table 43-4 compares the most common disorders
- McMurray test (to evaluate meniscal tears)
    - Flex the knee as much as possible
    - Medial meniscus evaluated by externally rotating the foot and extending the knee
    - Lateral meniscus evaluated by internally rotating the foot and extending the knee

43

TABLE 43-4   *Common Disorders of the Knee*

	Chondromalacia Patellae	Meniscal Injury	Collateral Ligament Injury	Anterior Cruciate Ligament Injury	Posterior Cruciate Ligament Injury	Prepatellar Bursitis	Anserine Bursitis	Ruptured Baker Cyst (Pseudothrombophlebitis)
Cause	Patellofemoral cartilage degeneration	Trauma	Overuse Trauma	Twisting injury to knee with foot planted	Hyperextension injury to knee	Overuse Trauma Infection Gout	Overuse Osteoarthritis	One-way flow of knee effusion to gastrocnemius–semimembranosus bursa
Clinical presentation	Anterior knee pain when climbing stairs	Pain Swelling Catching Locking Buckling	Medial or lateral knee pain	Pain Swelling Instability	Pain Swelling Instability	Anterior knee pain Swelling	Anteromedial pain 4–5 cm below joint line	Popliteal fullness Calf pain, swelling, and ecchymosis on rupture
Diagnosis and evaluation	Tender with patellar compression	Tender joint margin Pain with motion Pain with McMurray test	Tenderness over affected ligament Provoke pain with medial or lateral stress in 20° of flexion	Swelling Anterior instability of the tibia at the knee (anterior drawer sign)	Swelling Posterior instability of the tibia at the knee (posterior drawer sign)	Swollen and tender prepatellar bursa Aspirate to diagnose cause	Tender with palpation Pain with knee flexion	Rule out deep venous thrombosis with ultrasound (Fig. 43-6)
Treatment	Quadriceps strengthening exercises NSAIDs Rarely surgery	Rest NSAIDs Physical therapy Possible surgical meniscectomy	Rest Physical therapy Surgery if unstable	Orthopedic evaluation	Orthopedic evaluation	Rest NSAIDs Antibiotic if needed	Rest NSAIDs Steroid injection Physical therapy	Rest Elevation Steroid injection

NSAIDS, Nonsteroidal antiinflammatory drugs.

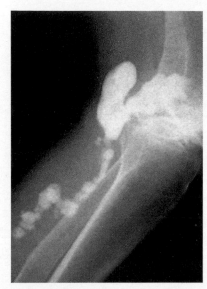

FIGURE 43-6 Arthrogram demonstrating a ruptured Baker cyst. (From Forbes CD, Jackson WF. *Color Atlas and Text of Clinical Medicine.* 3rd ed. St. Louis: Mosby; 2003: Fig. 3.28.)

- A positive test occurs when maneuver provokes pain at the appropriate meniscus; occasionally a click may also be palpated

Ankle

ACHILLES TENDINITIS

Cause

- Overuse, poor training habits, and improper footwear in athletes
- **Fluoroquinolone antibiotics**
- Associated with spondyloarthritis

Clinical Presentation

- Pain along the Achilles tendon

Diagnosis and Evaluation

- Tenderness and thickening along the tendon
- Dorsiflexion of foot is painful

Treatment

- NSAIDs
- Heel lift
- Stretching program
- If underlying spondyloarthritis is detected (ankylosing spondylitis, psoriatic arthritis, reactive arthritis, or inflammatory bowel disease related), treatment is directed at the underlying condition with a rheumatology referral

ACHILLES TENDON RUPTURE

Cause

- Forced dorsiflexion of the foot as the gastrocnemius muscle contracts
- Males affected more than females

Clinical Presentation

- **Tearing and popping sensation in the calf**

Diagnosis and Evaluation

- Swelling of the calf
- Weakness of foot flexion
- Palpation of gap caused by tendon rupture
- Abnormal Thompson test (failure of the foot to plantar flex when squeezing the gastrocnemius muscle)

Treatment

- Orthopedic evaluation and possible repair

TARSAL TUNNEL SYNDROME

Cause

- Posterior tibial nerve entrapment behind the medial malleolus
- Associated with pes planus (flat feet), ganglion cyst, and lipomata

Clinical Presentation

- Burning pain over the medial and plantar aspects of the foot
- Aggravated by activity

Diagnosis and Evaluation

- Posterior tibial nerve (Tinel sign) posterior to the medial malleolus
- Decreased sensation over medial and plantar aspects of the foot
- Nerve conduction study if examination equivocal

Treatment

- Orthotics
- Surgery occasionally necessary

Foot

PLANTAR FASCIITIS

Cause

- Overuse, causing inflammation of plantar fascia
- Heel spur
- Associated with spondyloarthritis

Clinical Presentation

- Heel and posterior foot pain
- Classically, with the first steps of the morning and after prolonged sitting
- Improves with use

Diagnosis and Evaluation

- Tenderness on plantar aspect of heel

Treatment

- Stretching
- Orthotics/night splints to stretch the plantar fascia
- NSAIDs
- Steroid injection
- Rarely surgery

43

MORTON NEUROMA

Cause

- Neuroma formation causing compression of digital nerve in foot

Clinical Presentation

- **Pain and paresthesia most commonly between the third and fourth toes**

Diagnosis and Evaluation

- Tenderness to deep palpation between toes
- Neuroma may be palpable
- Ultrasound/magnetic resonance imaging to visualize the neuroma

Treatment

- Metatarsal bar orthotic
- Steroid injection
- Surgical excision of neuroma

Cervical Spine

Figure 43-7 shows normal cervical spine range of motion.

CERVICAL SPINE STRAIN

Cause

- Overuse
- Poor posture
- Hyperextension injury

Clinical Presentation

- Neck pain and stiffness
- No symptoms or signs of radiculopathy

Diagnosis and Evaluation

- Localized tenderness over cervical musculature
- Absence of neurologic deficits (Table 43-5)

Treatment

- NSAIDs
- Mobilization and supervised physical therapy
- Soft cervical collar (short term only)

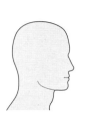
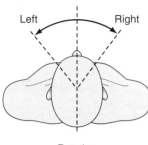

Neutral   Rotation

Flexion and extension   Lateral bending

FIGURE 43-7 Normal cervical spine range of motion. (From Swash M. *Hutchison's Clinical Methods.* 21st ed. Philadelphia: Saunders; 2001: Fig. 10.26.)

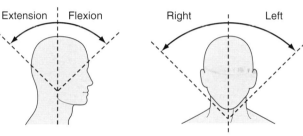

TABLE 43-5	*Cervical and Lumbar Spine Neurologic Examination*		
Nerve Root	**Motor Function**	**Sensory Function**	**Reflex**
C5	Deltoid and biceps (elbow flexion)	Shoulder and lateral aspect of arm	Biceps
C6*	Biceps and wrist extensors	Lateral forearm and thumb	Biceps
C7	Triceps (elbow extension)	Middle finger	Triceps
C8	Finger flexors	Medial forearm and little finger	None
T1	Intrinsic muscles of the hand	Medial aspect of arm	None
L4	Quadriceps (knee extension)	Medial aspect of calf and ankle	Quadriceps (knee)
L5	Tibialis anterior (ankle dorsiflexion)†	Dorsum of foot	None
S1	Gastrocnemius (ankle plantar flexion)‡	Lateral aspect of ankle and foot	Gastrocnemius (ankle)

*May be confused with carpal tunnel syndrome.
†Cannot stand on heels.
‡Cannot stand on toes.

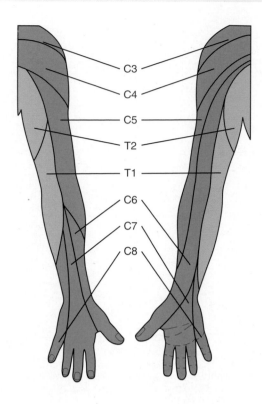

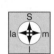

FIGURE 43-8 Cervical nerve root dermatomal distribution in the upper extremity. (From Gosling J, Willan PLT, Whitmore I, Harris PF. *Human Anatomy: Color Atlas and Text.* 4th ed. St. Louis: Mosby; 2002: Fig. 3.6.)

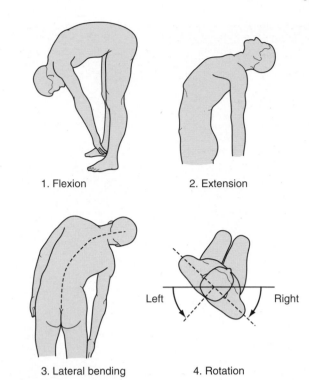

FIGURE 43-9 Normal lumbar spine range of motion. (From Swash M. *Hutchison's Clinical Methods.* 21st ed. Philadelphia: Saunders; 2001: Fig. 10.28.)

Lumbar Spine

Figure 43-9 shows normal lumbar spine range of motion.

Basic Information

- **Low back pain is the most common musculoskeletal complaint in the outpatient setting**
- 80% of the population experience low back pain at some time in their life
- **Low back pain is generally a self-limited condition**
- 50% are better in 1 week
- 90% are better in 6 weeks
- Sciatica can have a more protracted course, but 50% recover in 4 weeks

Clinical Presentation

- Acute low back pain (Box 43-1)
- Spinal stenosis
  - Caused by impingement on lumbosacral spinal cord
  - Associated with degenerative arthritis
  - Pseudoclaudication (nonvascular claudication improving with flexion at the waist)

Diagnosis and Evaluation

- Lumbar spine examination (Fig. 43-10; see also Table 43-5)
- Straight leg raise test
  - Sensitive (more than 90%) but not specific
  - Pain should be radicular
  - Helpful in ruling out sciatica

CERVICAL DISK DISEASE

Cause

- Disk herniation

Clinical Presentation

- Neck pain and stiffness
- Radicular complaints (weakness, numbness, paresthesias along involved nerve root)
- Symptoms worse with straining

Diagnosis and Evaluation

- Symptoms exacerbated with neck compression
- Abnormal neurologic examination (Fig. 43-8; see also Table 43-5)

Treatment

- Initially conservative
- NSAIDs
- Soft collar
- Surgical evaluation for intractable pain or progressive neurologic deficits

43

BOX 43-1 | Low Back Pain

Local Causes

Muscle strain
Lumbar spine osteoarthritis
Degenerative disk disease
Vertebral body infection
Disc space infection
Vertebral body malignancy
Compression Fracture
Spinal Stenosis

Referred/Distant Causes

Ulcer disease
Pancreatitis
Nephrolithiasis
Prostatitis
Aortic dissection
Subacute bacterial endocarditis
Pelvic pathology

Worrisome Findings

Nocturnal pain
   Cancer
   Infection
Writhing pain
   Aneurysm
   Perforated viscus
Evolving neurologic deficits (leg weakness, bowel/bladder
   incontinence)
   Epidural abscess
   Hemorrhage
   Disk herniation
   Cauda equina syndrome
Fever
   Infection

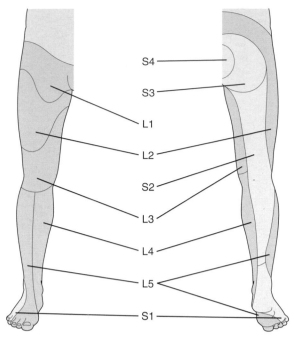

FIGURE 43-10 Lumbar nerve root dermatomal distribution in the lower extremity. (From Gosling J, Willan PLT, Whitmore I, Harris PF. *Human Anatomy: Color Atlas and Text*. 4th ed. St. Louis: 2002; Mosby: Fig. 6.10.)

- Crossed straight leg raise test less sensitive (25%) but more specific (80%)
- Indications for radiographic evaluation
  - Preceding significant trauma
  - Evolving neurologic findings
  - Suggestion of malignancy or infection
  - New onset pain at an older age
  - Persistent pain

Treatment

- Rest
- Heat and cold
- NSAIDs
- Physical therapy
- Surgery may be indicated (e.g., infection, intractable pain, neurologic defects, and spinal stenosis)

Review Questions

For review questions, please go to ExpertConsult.com.

SUGGESTED READINGS

Biundo JJ. Musculoskeletal signs and symptoms: regional rheumatic pain syndromes. In: Klippel JH, ed. *Primer on the Rheumatic Diseases*. 13th ed. Atlanta: Arthritis Foundation; 2008.

Borenstein D. Musculoskeletal signs and symptoms: neck and back pain. In: Klippel JH, ed. *Primer on the Rheumatic Diseases*. 13th ed. Atlanta: Arthritis Foundation; 2008.

Firestein G, et al. Differential diagnosis of regional and diffuse musculoskeletal pain. In: Firenstein G, Budd R, Gabriel S, et al., eds. *Kelley's Textbook of Rheumatology*. 9th ed. Philadelphia: WB Saunders; 2012.

CHAPTER 44

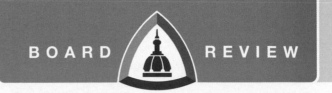
Vasculitis

PHILIP SEO, MD, MHS

The systemic vasculitides (vasculitis) are autoimmune disorders characterized by inflammation of blood vessels. These vasculitides can affect almost any organ system and often lead to significant morbidity. There are at least 20 such disorders, differentiated clinically by: (1) the size of blood vessel typically involved, (2) their predilection for certain organ systems, and (3) characteristic pathologic features. Classifying the vasculitides by the size of the predominant vessels involved is a valuable method of categorizing these diseases: large-vessel vasculitis predominantly affects the aorta and the great vessels; medium-vessel vasculitis predominantly affects the splanchnic vessels; and small-vessel vasculitis affects the capillaries, arterioles, and venules that provide circulation to the lungs, kidneys, and skin. A widely accepted classification scheme based on blood vessel size is depicted in Box 44-1.

Behçet Disease

Basic Information

- **Widest range of blood vessel involvement of all the vasculitides; small, medium, and large vessels, in both the venous and arterial circulations**
- Found most commonly in the regions that once constituted the old Silk Route: Turkey, Iran, China, and Japan
- Associated with human leukocyte antigen (HLA)-B51

Clinical Presentation

- **Classic triad of signs is oral ulcers (Fig. 44-1), genital ulcers, and ocular inflammation**
  - Oral ulcers: by themselves, may be seen in a variety of autoimmune diseases
  - **Genital ulcers: commonly heal with scarring and are virtually pathognomonic of Behçet disease**
  - Ocular inflammation
    - Anterior uveitis: may manifest as a hypopyon (pus in the anterior chamber); asymmetrical pupils may also be present because of synechiae formation between the lens and iris
    - Posterior uveitis: may manifest as retinal vasculitis
  - Folliculitis
  - Erythema nodosum
    - In contrast to erythema nodosum associated with other conditions, nodules may ulcerate and heal with scarring
    - Biopsy often reveals medium-vessel vasculitis rather than septal panniculitis

- **Pathergy: development of sterile pustules at sites of needle stick; only a minority of patients demonstrate the pathergy phenomenon, but when present, this phenomenon is highly suggestive of Behçet disease**
- Superficial and deep venous thrombophlebitis
- Cerebral venous thrombosis
- Aseptic meningitis
- Brainstem involvement: may mimic multiple sclerosis because of its tendency to involve white matter
- Arthritis: typically nondeforming

Diagnosis and Evaluation

- **No specific laboratory or histologic findings are diagnostic**
- Manifestations may occur simultaneously or be separated by several years
- Diagnosis based on physician observation of the various clinical manifestations and recognition of the characteristic constellation of physical findings, guided by the International Criteria for Behçet Disease, which require at least four points, using the following scoring system:
  - 2 points for each of the following: recurrent oral or genital ulcers, eye lesions
  - 1 point for each of the following: skin lesions (including positive pathergy test) vascular manifestations, neurologic manifestations

Treatment

- A variety of regimens have been used, based on the extent and severity of involvement
  - For mucocutaneous disease
    - Colchicine: first-line therapy for oral ulcers; effective only in milder cases; may be used up to 3 times per day, if tolerated
    - Topical glucocorticoids: limited efficacy for oral and genital ulcers
  - For more refractory disease
    - Low-dose systemic glucocorticoids
    - Thalidomide: for mucocutaneous lesions
    - Azathioprine
    - Tumor necrosis factor (TNF) inhibitors
  - For the most serious disease manifestations, including central nervous system (CNS) and uveitis (with risk for blindness)
    - High-dose systemic glucocorticoids
    - Cyclophosphamide

BOX 44-1 *Classification of the Vasculitides*

Predominantly or Exclusively Small-Vessel Vasculitides

Immune complex-mediated
    Cutaneous leukocytoclastic angiitis (hypersensitivity vasculitis)
    Henoch-Schönlein purpura
    Urticarial vasculitis
    Cryoglobulinemia*
    Connective tissue disorders*
    Erythema elevatum diutinum
ANCA-associated disorders
    Granulomatosis with polyangiitis (Wegener granulomatosis)*
    Microscopic polyangiitis*
    Eosinophilin granulomatosis with polyangiitis (Churg-Strauss syndrome)*
Miscellaneous small-vessel vasculitides
    Paraneoplastic
    Infection
    Inflammatory bowel disease

Predominantly or Exclusively Medium-Vessel Vasculitides

Classic polyarteritis nodosa
Cutaneous polyarteritis nodosa
Rheumatoid vasculitis*
Kawasaki disease
Buerger disease (thromboangiitis obliterans)

Predominantly Large-Vessel Vasculitides

Giant-cell (temporal) arteritis
Takayasu arteritis
Cogan syndrome
Behçet disease (can also involve small and medium-sized vessels)

*Common overlap of small- and medium-sized blood vessel involvement.
ANCA, Antineutrophil cytoplasmic antibody.

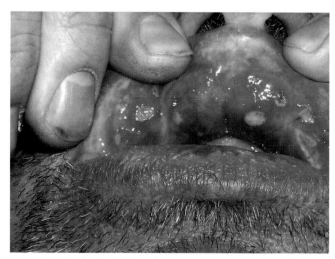

FIGURE 44-1 Aphthous oral ulcers in Behçet disease.

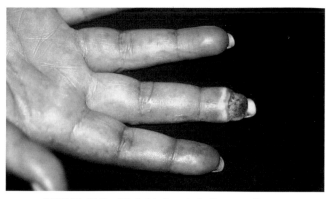

FIGURE 44-2 Digital ischemia in Buerger disease.

Buerger Disease (Thromboangiitis Obliterans)

Basic Information

- Manifestations primarily caused by involvement of medium-sized arteries, but veins may also be affected
- Should not be confused with Berger disease (immunoglobulin [Ig]A nephropathy)

Clinical Presentation

- **Typical patient is a young male smoker with digital infarction, although it may also occur in female smokers**
- **Although patients with Buerger disease may have substantial involvement of the extremities, the internal organs are always spared**
- Does not involve smallest vessels (i.e., capillaries) and is therefore more likely to be associated with digital infarction (Fig. 44-2) than with purpura

Diagnosis and Evaluation

- Superficial thrombophlebitis may be the first sign
- Should be considered high on the differential diagnosis when there is severe digital ischemia involving two or more extremities but no other organ dysfunction
- **Angiography reveals distinctive "corkscrew" collateral vessels in blood vessels at the level of the wrists and ankles**

Treatment

- **Smoking cessation is the only effective form of treatment**
- No form of immunosuppression (including glucocorticoids) provides control or cure
- Continued smoking may result in progression of ischemia and the need for amputation

Eosinophilic Granulomatosis with Polyangiitis (Formerly Known as Churg-Strauss Syndrome)

Basic Information

- Characterized by necrotizing inflammation within small arteries, veins, and capillaries

- Classically described as a clinical triad of asthma, hypereosinophilia, and vasculitis

Clinical Presentation

- **Typical patient presents with the recent onset of allergy or asthma, followed by development of symptoms and signs of vasculitis**
- Asthma associated with eosinophilic granulomatosis with polyangiitis may improve as the vasculitic phase begins
- Typical symptoms and signs include:
  - **Sinusitis: nondestructive, in contrast to Wegener granulomatosis**
  - Wheezing
  - Mononeuritis multiplex: neuropathy involving named motor and sensory nerves, often acute in onset, which manifests as the inability to dorsiflex the foot or to hyperextend the wrist (i.e., footdrop or wristdrop)
  - Cutaneous nodules: necrotizing granuloma over the extensor surfaces of joints

Diagnosis and Evaluation

- In addition to the characteristic clinical features, distinctive diagnostic features include:
  - Fleeting pulmonary infiltrates (30% of cases)
  - **Eosinophilia (up to 60,000 eosinophils/mm^3)**
  - Positive antineutrophil cytoplasmic antibody (ANCA) (50% of cases): These antibodies are against myeloperoxidase (MPO-ANCA), which is associated with a perinuclear staining pattern (p-ANCA) on immunofluorescence
- Biopsy may help confirm the diagnosis

Treatment

- **Usually responds dramatically to glucocorticoids alone**
- Eosinophilia disappears with glucocorticoids; the eosinophilia associated with the idiopathic hypereosinophilic syndromes may be less steroid responsive
- Cyclophosphamide may be required for refractory cases

Cogan Syndrome

Clinical Presentation

- **Typical patient presents with ocular disease (interstitial keratitis) and sensorineural hearing loss**
- Eye and ear disease do not always begin simultaneously, but usually occur within a few months of each other
- Symptoms and signs may include:
  - Ocular manifestations
    - Interstitial keratitis (pain, photophobia, decreased visual acuity, and red eye) is most common
    - Episcleritis
    - Scleritis (Fig. 44-3)
    - Retinal disease
    - Uveitis
  - Sensorineural manifestations
    - Tinnitus
    - Hearing loss

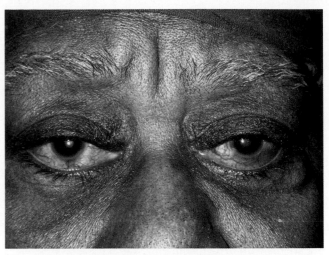

FIGURE 44-3 Scleritis in Cogan syndrome.

  - Vertigo
  - Oscillopsia (objects in visual field oscillate)
- Constitutional symptoms present in 50% of patients
- **10% of patients present with a large-vessel vasculitis mimicking Takayasu arteritis**

Diagnosis and Evaluation

- Diagnosis based on distinctive combination of eye and ear inflammation
- Important to exclude syphilis and acoustic neuromas

Treatment

- Topical glucocorticoids used for interstitial keratitis
- Systemic glucocorticoids required for other manifestations
- Sensorineural hearing loss must be treated promptly and aggressively to avoid permanent hearing loss and may require cyclophosphamide

Cryoglobulinemic Vasculitis (Mixed Essential Cryoglobulinemic Vasculitis)

Basic Information

- **Cryoglobulins are immunoglobulins that precipitate out of serum in cold conditions**
- Cryoglobulinemic vasculitis affects small- to medium-sized arteries, capillaries, and veins

Clinical Presentation

- **Over 90% of patients are infected by hepatitis C virus**
- Symptoms and signs
  - Recurrent purpura
  - Hyperpigmentation that results from repeated bouts of purpura (Fig. 44-4)
  - Brawny induration that mimics venous stasis disease
  - Livedo reticularis
  - Raynaud phenomenon
  - Digital infarction

- Mononeuritis multiplex (e.g., footdrop)
- Glomerulonephritis (seen only with type II cryoglobulinemia)
- CNS vasculitis (rare)

Diagnosis and Evaluation

- Based on clinical presentation and isolation of cryoglobulins (from blood samples kept at body temperature until transport to the lab)
- Classification (and clinical manifestations) based on properties of the cryoproteins (Table 44-1)
- **Hypocomplementemia is a hallmark of cryoglobulinemic vasculitis because the disorder is mediated by immune complex deposition**
  - Pattern of hypocomplementemia is distinctive: C4 levels are decreased out of proportion to C3
- Patients with cryoglobulinemic vasculitis are often initially misdiagnosed as having either rheumatoid arthritis or lupus for the following reasons:
  - **Vast majority are positive for rheumatoid factor (IgM component of mixed cryoglobulins has rheumatoid factor activity)**
  - Majority are antinuclear antibody positive
  - Hypocomplementemia is also commonly seen in lupus

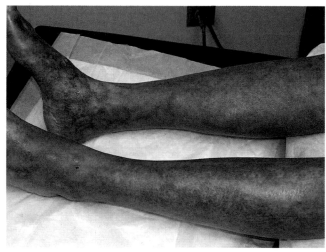

FIGURE 44-4 Hyperpigmentation and ulceration of the legs caused by mixed cryoglobulinemia associated with hepatitis C.

Treatment

- Polymerase or protease inhibitors for hepatitis-C-related cases
- Glucocorticoids and cyclophosphamide (or rituximab) for refractory, organ-threatening cases
- **Plasmapheresis should also be considered in acutely ill patients with severe disease**

Giant-Cell Arteritis (Temporal Arteritis)

Basic Information

- Medium to large arteries of the head and neck are affected
- **Never occurs in people younger than 50 years of age**

Clinical Presentation

- Typical patient is elderly with new-onset headaches and inflamed temporal arteries
- Symptoms and signs:
  - New headaches
  - Jaw claudication (most specific symptom) may manifest itself as pain in the face or throat, particularly with chewing
  - Visual symptoms
    - Possible manifestations include amaurosis fugax, blurriness, or diplopia
    - **Once visual loss occurs in giant-cell arteritis (GCA), it is usually permanent**
  - Large-vessel symptoms (e.g., arm claudication and aortic dissection); symptomatic large-vessel disease occurs in at least 20% of patients with GCA
  - **Polymyalgia rheumatica (50% of cases)**
  - Atypical manifestations include fever of unknown origin; weight loss; nonproductive cough; and nonspecific pains in the neck, throat, or tongue

Diagnosis and Evaluation

- Diagnosis based on typical clinical presentation and these additional findings:
  - The temporal arteries may be abnormal (swollen, tender, nodular) on examination (Fig. 44-5), but

TABLE 44-1	Subtypes of Cryoglobulinemia		
	Type I	**Type II**	**Type III**
Monoclonality of immunoglobulin component?	Yes (usually IgG)	Yes (IgM)	No
Rheumatoid factor activity?	No	Yes	Yes
Clinical syndrome	Hyperviscosity	Vasculitis	Vasculitis
Disease association	Hematopoietic malignancy	Hepatitis C Rheumatic diseases Malignancies Idiopathic	Hepatitis C Rheumatic diseases Idiopathic

IgG, Immunoglobulin G; IgM, immunoglobulin M.

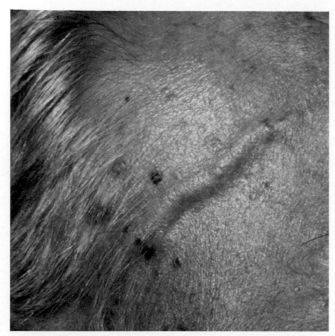

FIGURE 44-5 Inflamed temporal artery in giant-cell arteritis.

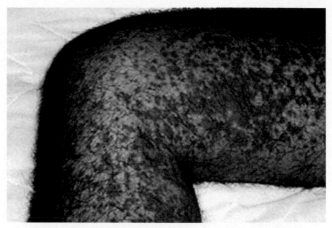

FIGURE 44-6 Palpable purpura in hypersensitivity vasculitis.

arteries are normal in up to one third of biopsy-proven cases
- **Elevated erythrocyte sedimentation rate in the great majority of cases (90% of cases greater than 50 mm/hour)**
- Disruption of internal elastic lamina evident on temporal artery biopsy
  - Giant cells not always present; earliest finding is lymphocytic inflammation in the adventitia
  - Bilateral temporal artery biopsies that do not reveal inflammation have a negative predictive value of 90%
  - **Temporal artery biopsy specimen may be positive for up to 2 weeks or longer after treatment with high-dose glucocorticoids is started**
  - Despite the importance of the temporal artery biopsy, the diagnosis of GCA and the initiation of treatment ultimately remain clinical decisions

Treatment

- Systemic glucocorticoids, initially 1 mg/kg/day
  - **Glucocorticoid treatment should begin at the time the diagnosis is strongly suspected, without awaiting biopsy results**
- Studies of methotrexate efficacy as a steroid-sparing agent give conflicting results
- Flares occur with tapering of medication in at least 25% to 50% of patients
- Glucocorticoids may be tapered off over 1 to 2 years; as many as one third of patients, however, may require chronic low-dose glucocorticoids

Henoch-Schönlein Purpura

Basic Information

- Small arterioles and venules affected
- 90% of cases occur in children

- Majority of cases resolve within a few weeks
- Chronic cases do occur, particularly in adults
- Characterized by IgA deposition in biopsies

Clinical Presentation

- Typical patient is child with recent upper respiratory tract infection, followed by the onset of the typical tetrad of symptoms and signs:
  - Palpable purpura, occasionally with pustular lesions
  - Arthritis
  - Abdominal pain (with or without gastrointestinal [GI] bleeding)
  - Hematuria or proteinuria (renal insufficiency in less than 5% of cases)

Diagnosis and Evaluation

- IgA deposition on tissue biopsy specimen
- Serum and urine protein electrophoresis studies should be performed in chronic cases to exclude IgA paraproteinemia

Treatment

- **Often self-limited illness that requires no therapy**
- Treatment with glucocorticoids needed only in cases of advancing glomerulonephritis or mesenteric ischemia

Hypersensitivity Vasculitis

Basic Information

- A hypersensitivity response to exogenous antigen
- Postcapillary venules affected

Clinical Presentation

- **Typical patient presents with palpable purpura on shins and buttocks (dependent regions)**
- An array of skin lesions may be seen but are not distinctive for hypersensitivity vasculitis:
  - Nonpalpable purpura
  - Palpable purpura (Fig. 44-6)
  - Livedo reticularis
  - Urticaria
  - Erythematous papules or plaques
  - Vesiculobullous lesions
  - Nodules

- Ulceration
- Necrotic lesions
- Vasculitic lesions occur in *crops* (i.e., lesions of approximately same age, corresponding to time of exposure to inciting antigen)
- Hypersensitivity vasculitis usually starts 7 to 14 days after exposure to the offending agent
- In the case of drug-induced hypersensitivity vasculitis, no new lesions appear roughly 3 weeks after removal of the offending agent

Diagnosis and Evaluation

- High index of clinical suspicion necessary
- Impossible to distinguish skin lesions from those of Henoch-Schönlein purpura (HSP) without immunofluorescence testing of biopsy specimens, confirming IgA deposition in HSP
- Important to exclude underlying systemic involvement (e.g., pulmonary, renal, peripheral nerve)

Treatment

- Colchicine or dapsone may be tried for milder cases
- Systemic glucocorticoids may help, although symptoms may rebound with glucocorticoid taper
- Leg elevation and compression stockings may be helpful

Microscopic Polyangiitis

Basic Information

- Small- and medium-sized arteries and veins affected (distinct from polyarteritis nodosa [PAN], which involves only medium-sized arteries)

Clinical Presentation

- **Typical patient presents with pulmonary-renal syndrome**
  - Alveolar hemorrhage caused by pulmonary capillary alveolitis, and rapidly progressive, crescentic glomerulonephritis caused by necrotizing
- More common than Goodpasture syndrome as cause of pulmonary-renal syndrome
- Typical symptoms and signs include hematuria, weight loss, mononeuritis multiplex, fever, and pulmonary hemorrhage

Diagnosis and Evaluation

- **May mimic granulomatosis with polyangiitis (Wegener) clinically, but no granulomatous inflammation evident on pathology**
- Associated with ANCA in most cases (70%), usually directed against MPO that on immunofluorescence staining demonstrates a p-ANCA (perinuclear) pattern (Table 44-2)

Treatment

- Glucocorticoids and cyclophosphamide (or rituximab)
- It is appropriate to use cyclophosphamide (or rituximab) from the outset of treatment in microscopic polyangiitis

Polyarteritis Nodosa

Basic Information

- Medium-sized muscular arteries affected (veins spared)
- **The classic medium-vessel vasculitis**
- May be found in patients chronically infected with hepatitis B

Clinical Presentation

- **Typical patient presents with subacute onset of multisystem inflammatory illness**
- Typical symptoms and signs:
  - Constitutional symptoms
  - Livedo reticularis
  - Cutaneous nodules or ulcers, particularly over distal lower extremities
  - Intestinal angina (abdominal pain after eating)
  - **Mononeuritis multiplex**
  - Hypertension
  - Elevated hepatic transaminases
  - Aneurysms of involved blood vessels (Fig. 44-7)
- Classic PAN spares the lung

Diagnosis and Evaluation

- **Biopsy of affected organ or tissue**
- Blind tissue biopsy rarely useful
- Mesenteric angiogram may reveal aneurysms even in the absence of GI symptoms
- Classic PAN is ANCA-negative (i.e., proteinase-3 [PR-3] and MPO-ANCA assays are negative in this disease)

TABLE 44-2	Correlation between Immunofluorescence and Enzyme Immunoassay in Patients with ANCA-Associated Vasculitis	
Immunofluorescence Pattern	**Enzyme Immunoassay**	**Disease Association**
c-ANCA	Antiproteinase-3 (90%*)	Granulomatosis with polyangiitis
p-ANCA	Antimyeloperoxidase (90%†)	Granulomatosis with polyangiitis Microscopic polyangiitis Eosinophilic granulomatosis with polyangiitis Renal-limited vasculitis

*90% of vasculitis patients who are c-ANCA positive have antibodies to proteinase-3.
†90% of vasculitis patients who are p-ANCA positive have antibodies to myeloperoxidase.
c-ANCA, Cytoplasmic antineutrophil cytoplasmic antibody; p-ANCA, perinuclear antineutrophil cytoplasmic antibody.

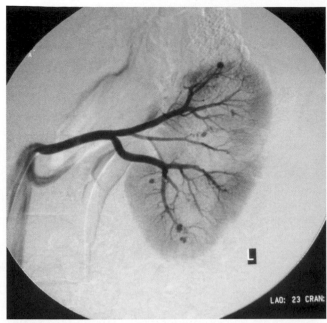

FIGURE 44-7 Angiogram demonstrating renal microaneurysms in polyarteritis nodosa.

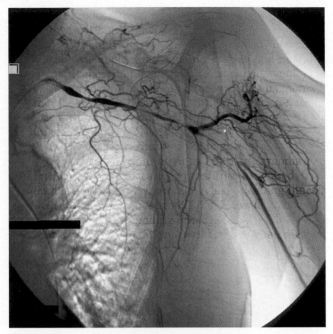

FIGURE 44-8 Angiogram demonstrating subclavian artery narrowing in Takayasu arteritis.

Treatment

- Glucocorticoids
- Cyclophosphamide

Takayasu Arteritis

Basic Information

- Involves large arteries, including the aorta and branches of the aortic arch (Fig. 44-8)

Clinical Presentation

- **Typical patient is a woman younger than 40 years of age**
- Symptoms and signs:
  - Nonspecific constitutional complaints in the prepulseless (inflammatory) stage
  - Extremity or organ ischemia (although loss of digit or limb very rare)
  - Visual disturbance
  - Claudication
  - Intrascapular back pain
  - **Absence of distal pulses in one or more extremities (arms more often than legs)**
  - **Asymmetrical (or undetectable) blood pressures**
  - Hypertension (usually caused by renal artery stenosis)
  - Bruits
    - Subclavian arteries nearly always involved (auscultate for bruits above and below clavicle)
  - Erythema nodosum-like lesions (20% of cases)

Diagnosis and Evaluation

- **Angiography reveals stenoses that are long, smooth, and concentrically tapered (in contrast to short, irregular, and eccentric vascular narrowing caused by atherosclerotic disease)**

- Involves thoracic aorta more than abdominal aorta (10% to 15% of cases affect the latter)
- Collateral circulation in extremities is characteristic, often making mechanical revascularization attempts (stents, balloon dilation, bypass) unnecessary
- Magnetic resonance angiography is potentially useful in making the diagnosis early (thickened aortic wall with edema), before vascular stenosis or aneurysm formation

Treatment

- Glucocorticoids
- Methotrexate
- TNF-inhibition for refractory cases

Granulomatosis with Polyangiitis (Formerly Known as Wegener Granulomatosis)

Basic Information

- Small- to medium-sized arteries, veins, and capillaries affected

Clinical Presentation

- **Typical patient is middle-aged individual with long-standing upper respiratory tract or ear complaints (often lasting months or years), who develops symptoms and signs of a systemic inflammatory illness**
- Symptoms and signs:
  - Skin: palpable purpura and nodules (often over elbows); nodules are identical to eosinophilic granulomatosis with polyangiitis

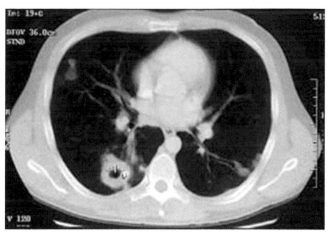

FIGURE 44-10 Computed tomography scan demonstrating nodular and cavitary pulmonary lesions in granulomatosis with polyangiitis.

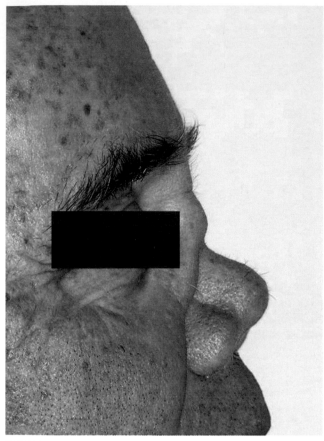

FIGURE 44-9 Saddle-nose deformity in granulomatosis with polyangiitis.

- Eye: episcleritis, scleritis, peripheral ulcerative keratitis, uveitis, and orbital pseudotumor
- Ear: conductive hearing loss caused by serous otitis media or granulomatous inflammation in middle ear; less commonly, sensorineural hearing loss
- Nose: septal perforation and saddle-nose deformity (Fig. 44-9)
- Trachea: subglottic stenosis (can present with stridor)
- Lungs: sodular lesions (with a tendency to cavitate) and pulmonary hemorrhage (Fig. 44-10)
- Cardiac: pericarditis (rare)
- Kidney: segmental, necrotizing crescentic glomerulonephritis; the glomerulonephritis that occurs in ANCA-associated vasculitis is pauci-immune (i.e., characterized by the deposition of few immunoreactants, such as IgG, IgM, C3, within the kidney)
- CNS: chronic meningitis and cranial nerve lesions
- Peripheral nerve: mononeuritis multiplex
- Extremities: arthralgias or myalgias and frank arthritis (often rheumatoid factor positive)

Diagnosis and Evaluation

- Diagnosis based on three histopathologic hallmarks:
  - Granulomatous inflammation
  - "Geographic" (extensive) necrosis
  - Vasculitis
- **Majority of cases associated with cytoplasmic antineutrophil cytoplasmic antibody (c-ANCA)**

pattern on immunofluorescence staining (see Table 44-2) usually caused by antibodies to PR-3
- 10% to 15% of patients with granulomatosis with polyangiitis may demonstrate p-ANCA pattern, typically caused by antibodies to MPO
- PR-3 and MPO-ANCA never occur in the same patient
- Despite rigorous testing, 20% of patients with granulomatosis with polyangiitis may be ANCA negative

Treatment

- Systemic glucocorticoids and methotrexate for limited disease; cyclophosphamide for more severe disease
- **Disease appears to accelerate when serum creatinine begins to rise; detection of renal involvement signals medical emergency that must be treated swiftly**
- ANCA serologies useful in making the diagnosis, but serial testing of ANCA titers not useful in predicting disease flares
- Reflecting dramatic improvements in treatment, there is now 90% survival at 5 years

Review Questions

For review questions, please go to ExpertConsult.com.

SUGGESTED READINGS

Hatemi G, Yazici Y, Yazici H. Behcet's syndrome. *Rheum Dis Clin North Am.* 2013;39:245-261.
Langford CA. Vasculitis. *J Allergy Clin Immunol.* 2010;125:S216-S225.
Ramos-Casals M, Stone JH, Cid MC, et al. The cryoglobulinaemias. *Lancet.* 2012;379:348-360.
Seo P, Stone JH. ANCA-associated vasculitis. *Am J Med.* 2004;117:39-50.
Seo P, Stone JH. Large-vessel vasculitis. *Arthritis Care Res.* 2004;51:128-139.
Seo P, Stone JH. Small-vessel and medium-vessel vasculitis. *Arthritis Care Res.* 2007;57:1552-1559.
Weyand CM, Goronzy JJ. Giant-cell arteritis and polymyalgia rheumatic. *N Engl J Med.* 2014;371:50-57.

Selected Topics in Rheumatology

CAROL M. ZIMINSKI, MD

Clinical presentation is the key element in the diagnosis of rheumatic diseases. The diagnosis of a specific rheumatic disorder is suggested by a particular constellation of what may individually be nonspecific signs and symptoms. The diagnosis is then confirmed by obtaining a detailed history, physical examination, and appropriate laboratory and imaging studies.

Systemic Lupus Erythematosus

Basic Information

- Systemic lupus erythematosus (SLE) is the prototypical autoimmune disease, in which the production of autoantibodies is associated with a multisystem inflammatory process
- Epidemiology and risk factors
  - Incidence greatest from ages 18 to 45 years
  - Female-to-male ratio is 9:1
  - **Four times more prevalent in African American women than in white women**
  - Regulation of the clearance of immune complexes is a common feature of many associated genes
    - Human leukocyte antigen (HLA) associations: DR2 and DR3
    - Congenital deficiency of complement components: C1, C2, and C4
- Pathogenesis
  - **Cardinal feature is the production of autoantibodies directed against nuclear, cytoplasmic, and cell-surface antigens**
  - Process is antigen-driven and T cell-dependent
  - Antigens to which patients with SLE respond are packaged in "blebs" on the cell surface during the process of apoptosis (programmed cell death)
  - Mechanisms of tissue injury involve both immune complex deposition and cell-specific antibodies
    - Most commonly identified immune complex is double-stranded DNA (dsDNA); anti-dsDNA that can form in the circulation and deposit in the kidney, or form in situ
    - Cell-specific antibodies do not usually destroy cells directly but mark cells for premature destruction by the reticuloendothelial system (e.g., hemolytic anemia, leukopenia, and thrombocytopenia)
  - **Most patients who are diagnosed with SLE have at least one autoantibody present before diagnosis, suggesting that SLE is the culmination of compound and complex autoimmune abnormalities that may begin simply, then spread and multiply until manifesting as clinical disease**

Clinical Presentation

- Cutaneous lupus
  - Common presenting feature
  - **Rash occurs at some time in 90% of cases of SLE**
  - Most rashes are photosensitive
  - Types
    - Malar "butterfly" rash (nonscarring) over cheeks and bridge of nose (Fig. 45-1) and sparing the nasolabial folds
    - Discoid lesions (often scarring) (Fig. 45-2)
    - Subacute cutaneous lupus (nonscarring) presents with annular, polycyclic lesions (Fig. 45-3)
    - Bullous lupus (blistering rash) is rare
- Lupus arthritis
  - Episodic and migratory
  - Distribution often symmetrical, similar to rheumatoid arthritis
  - **Rarely erosive or destructive**
  - Jaccoud arthropathy characterized by reversible, nonerosive, "swan neck" deformities
- Lupus nephritis
  - Occurs in one half to two thirds of SLE patients
  - More common in African Americans
  - **Associated with antibodies to native dsDNA and low complements**
  - Diffuse proliferative glomerulonephritis is the most serious form and can lead to rapidly progressive renal failure
- Age effect
  - "Young" SLE manifests with more adenopathy; splenomegaly; and cutaneous, central nervous system (CNS), and renal disease
  - 10% of SLE patients have an onset at 50 years of age or older. Their disease is milder, with more serositis and pulmonary manifestations, but rarely associated with CNS and renal disease.

Diagnosis and Evaluation

- **Diagnosis is clinical but aided by the Systemic Lupus International Collaborating Clinics (SLICC) SLE classification criteria (Table 45-1)**
- Serology (Table 45-2)

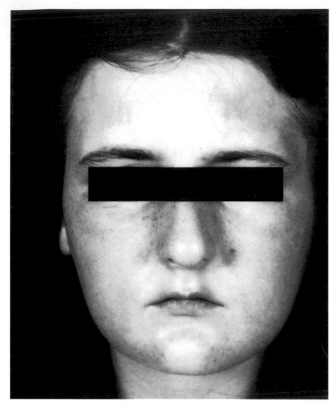

FIGURE 45-1 Malar "butterfly" rash demonstrating the typical distribution over the bridge of the nose and cheeks, sparing the nasolabial folds. (Courtesy Carol M. Ziminski, MD.)

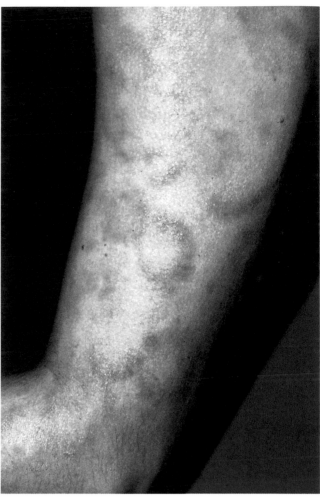

FIGURE 45-3 Subacute cutaneous lupus. The annular polycyclic lesions have an erythematous, slightly scaling border with central clearing. The distribution in light-exposed areas suggests photosensitivity. (Courtesy Carol M. Ziminski, MD.)

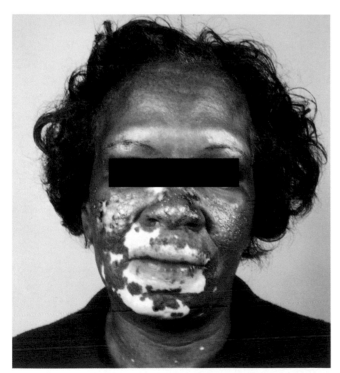

FIGURE 45-2 Discoid lupus lesions typically occur over exposed areas, such as the face or scalp. This patient demonstrates characteristic features including telangiectasias, erythema, follicular plugging, atrophy, and postinflammatory hypo- and hyperpigmentation. (Courtesy Carol M. Ziminski, MD.)

Treatment

- Rationale for treatment
  - Survival is 85% to 90% at 10 years and 68% at 20 years, with treatment
  - 50% have relapsing-remitting course
  - Poor prognostic signs include low socioeconomic status, advanced age, male gender, and increased creatinine at onset
  - Bimodal mortality curve
    - Early deaths caused by active disease (renal and CNS) or infection
    - Late deaths caused by accelerated coronary artery disease are presumably the result of both SLE disease and side effects of corticosteroid therapy
  - Principles
    - **Treat the disease, not the serologic activity**
    - Burden of mortality is linked to cardiovascular disease
    - Use the lowest effective dose of steroids or immunosuppressive therapy for the shortest time necessary

TABLE 45-1	*Clinical and Immunologic Criteria used in the SLICC Classification System*

Clinical Criteria

1. Acute cutaneous lupus, including:
   - Malar rash (do not count if malar discoid)
   - Bullous lupus
   - Toxic epidermal necrolysis variant of SLE
   - Maculopapular lupus rash
   - Photosensitive lupus rash *(in the absence of dermatomyositis)*

   or
   - Subacute cutaneous lupus (nonindurated psoriasiform and/or annular polycyclic lesions that resolve without scarring, although occasionally with postinflammatory dyspigmentation or telangiectasias

2. Chronic cutaneous lupus, including:
   - Classic discoid rash
   - Localized (above the neck)
   - Generalized (above and below the neck)
   - Hypertrophic (verrocous) lupus
   - Lupus panniculitis (profondus)
   - Mucosal lupus
   - Lupus erythematosus tumidus
   - Chilblains lupus
   - Discoid lupus/lichen planus overlap

3. Oral ulcers
   - Palate
   - Buccal
   - Tongue

   or
   - Nasal ulcers
     - *In the absence of other causes, such as vasculitis, Behçet disease, infection (herpesvirus), inflammatory bowel disease, reactive arthritis), and acidic foods*

4. Nonscarring alopecia (diffuse thinning or hair fragility with visible broken hairs)
   - *In the absence of other causes such as alopecia areata, iron deficiency, and androgenic alopecia*

5. Synovitis involving 2 or more joints, characterized by swelling or effusion
   - *or* tenderness in 2 or more joints and at least 30 minutes of morning stiffness

6. Serositis
   - Typical pleurisy for more than 1 day

   or
   - Pleural effusions

   or
   - Pleural rub
   - Typical pericardial pain (pain with recumbency improved by sitting forward) for more than 1 day

   or
   - Pericardial effusion

   or
   - Pericardial rub

   or
   - Pericarditis by electrocardiography
     - *In the absence of other causes, such as infection, uremia, and Dressler pericarditis*

7. Renal
   - Urine protein-to-creatinine ratio (or 24-hour protein) representing 500 mg protein/24 hours

   or
   - Red blood cell casts

8. Neurologic
   - Seizures
   - Psychosis
   - Mononeuritis multiplex
     - *In the absence of other known causes such as primary vasculitis*
   - Myelitis
   - Peripheral or cranial neuropathy
     - *In the absence of other known causes such as primary vasculitis, infection, and diabetes mellitus*
   - Acute confusional state
     - *In the absence of other causes, including toxic/metabolic, uremia, drugs*

9. Hemolytic anemia

10. Leukopenia (<4000/mm³) at least once
    - *In the absence of other causes such as Felty syndrome, drugs, and portal hypertension*

    or
    - Lymphopenia (<1000/mm³) at least once
    - *In the absence of other known causes such as corticosteroids, drugs, and infection*

11. Thrombocytopenia (<100,000/mm³) at least once
    - *In the absence of other known causes such as drugs, portal hypertension, and thrombotic thrombocytopenic purpura*

Continued on following page

TABLE 45-1 *Clinical and Immunologic Criteria used in the SLICC Classification System (Continued)*

Immunologic Criteria

1. ANA level above laboratory reference range
2. Anti-dsDNA antibody level above laboratory reference range (or >twofold the reference range if tested by ELISA)
3. Anti-Sm: presence of antibody to Sm nuclear antigen
4. Antiphospholipid antibody positivity as determined by any of the following:
   - Positive test result for lupus anticoagulant
   - False-positive test result for rapid plasma regain
   - Medium- or high-titer anticardiolipin antibody level (IgA, IgG, or IgM)
   - Positive test result for anti-β2-glycoprotein I (IgA, IgG, or IgM)
5. Low complement
   - Low C3
   - Low C4
   - Low CH50
6. Direct Coombs test *in the absence of hemolytic anemia*

Criteria are cumulative and need not be present concurrently. Proposed classification rule: *Classify a patient as having SLE if he or she satisfies 4 or more of the clinical and immunologic criteria used in the SLICC classification criteria, including at least one clinical criterion and one immunologic criterion, or has biopsy-proven nephritis compatible with SLE in the presence of ANAs or anti-dsDNA antibodies.*
Criteria developed for enrollment of patients in research studies; therefore, they should not be adhered to rigorously for diagnosis in the individual patient.
ANA, Antinuclear antibody; Anti-dsDNA, anti-double-stranded DNA; anti-Sm, anti-Smith; ELISA, enzyme-linked immunosorbent assay; Ig, immunoglobulin; SLE, systemic lupus erythematosus; SLICC, Systemic Lupus International Collaborating Clinics.
From Petri M, Orbai AM, Alarcon GS, et al. Derivation and validation of Systemic Lupus International Collaborating Clinic classification criteria for systemic lupus erythematosus. *Arthritis Rheum.* 2012;64:2677-2686.

- **Chronic steroid use (more than 6 mg/day) associated with greater cardiovascular mortality**
- Minimize morbidity/mortality of SLE and its therapy by aggressively addressing cardiovascular risk factors (high blood pressure, hyperlipidemia, elevated fasting blood glucose levels, cigarette smoking, obesity, lack of exercise) and treating underlying diseases (e.g., coronary artery disease, diabetes, osteoporosis, and osteonecrosis)
- Pharmacotherapy
  - **Hydroxychloroquine is the cornerstone of therapy in all SLE patients**
    - It is protective against renal and CNS flares, and it reduces risk of thromboembolic disease, dyslipidemia, and dysglycemia
  - Cutaneous manifestations: sunscreens, topical steroids, and hydroxychloroquine
  - Arthritis: nonsteroidal antiinflammatory drugs (NSAIDs), hydroxychloroquine, and low-dose steroids
  - Fever and serositis: NSAIDs and low-dose steroids
  - Major organ system involvement (e.g., hematologic, myopathy, renal, and CNS): high-dose steroids and immunosuppressive therapy (mycophenolate mofetil, cyclophosphamide, azathioprine, rituximab, belimumab)
  - In renal disease, use of mycophenolate similar to cyclophosphamide for induction therapy with less toxicity, particularly gonadal toxicity in young females with SLE
- Infections
  - Prednisone (more than 20 mg/day) and other immunosuppressive agents increase risk for fatal infections
  - **50% of fatal infections involve opportunistic organisms (e.g., *Pneumocystis jiroveci* and *Candida*)**

Chronic cutaneous discoid lupus
- Limited to the skin
- Chronic, scarring hyperpigmented lesions
- Antinuclear antibodies (ANA) negative
- **Rarely evolves to systemic lupus**
Drug-induced lupus (see Box 45-1)

Antiphospholipid Syndrome

Basic Information

- Antiphospholipid syndrome (APS) is marked by presence of a specific family of autoantibodies (antiphospholipid antibodies) with hypercoagulable state marked by arterial or venous thromboses, recurrent pregnancy loss, or thrombocytopenia
- Interference with coagulation in vitro contrasts with the thrombotic effect in vivo
- **50% of cases of APS are seen in patients who have no associated diseases ("primary"). Most other cases are seen in patients with SLE ("secondary").**
- Antibodies may be produced transiently after infections (e.g., human immunodeficiency virus [HIV]) or following exposure to certain drugs (e.g., chlorpromazine and procainamide)

Clinical Presentation

- Cutaneous: livedo reticularis (see Fig. 65-37), splinter hemorrhages, leg ulcers, and gangrene
- Hematologic: thrombocytopenia and hemolytic anemia (especially with anticardiolipin immunoglobulin [Ig]M)
- Venous thrombosis: superficial or deep venous thrombophlebitis, retinal vein thrombosis, cerebral venous thrombosis, Budd-Chiari syndrome, and pulmonary hypertension
- Neurologic: transient ischemic attacks, ischemic cerebral infarction, chorea, and transverse myelitis

TABLE 45-2	*Serology in the Rheumatic Diseases*	
Autoantibody	**Disease Association**	**Comment**
ANA	SLE Polymyositis/dermatomyositis Scleroderma CREST syndrome Sjögren syndrome Mixed connective tissue disease Rheumatoid arthritis	Antibody to multiple nuclear antigens (see later) Immunofluorescence: multiple patterns (see later) (+) in 95% to 99% of SLE (+) in 10% to 20% of healthy young women
Antihistone	SLE Drug-induced lupus	Antibody to DNA/protein complex Immunofluorescence: homogeneous
Antinative DNA	SLE	Antibody to double-stranded DNA Immunofluorescence: Rim (+) in 30% of SLE More specific for SLE than ANA, but less sensitive Associated with renal disease
Anti-Smith (Sm)	SLE	Antibody to nuclear ribonucleoprotein Immunofluorescence: speckled (+) in 20% to 30% of SLE More specific for SLE than ANA, but less sensitive
Anti-RNP	SLE Mixed connective tissue disease	Antibody to nuclear ribonucleoprotein Immunofluorescence: speckled 25% of lupus patients
Anti-Ro/La	SLE Subacute cutaneous lupus Neonatal lupus Sjögren syndrome	Antibody to nuclear ribonucleoprotein Immunofluorescence: speckled Associated with photosensitivity and congenital heart block
Anti-Scl 70	Diffuse scleroderma	Antibody to DNA topoisomerase Immunofluorescence: nucleolar (+) in 40% of patients with scleroderma
Anticentromere	CREST syndrome	Antibody to centromere/kinetochore Immunofluorescence: centromere (+) in >50% of patients with CREST
Anti-PM-Scl	Polymyositis/scleroderma overlap	Antibody to nuclear protein Immunofluorescence: nuclear or nucleolar
Anti-Jo-1	Polymyositis Dermatomyositis	Antibody to histidyl-tRNA synthetase Immunofluorescence: diffuse Associated with interstitial lung disease/anti-synthetase syndrome
Anti-SRP	Polymyositis	Antibody to signal recognition particle (cytoplasmic ribonucleoprotein) Associated with resistance to therapy
Anti-Mi-2	Dermatomyositis	Antibody to nuclear protein Immunofluorescence: homogeneous Associated with photosensitivity V (anterior neck/upper chest rash) and "shawl" (posterior neck/shoulder rash) signs

ANA, Antinuclear antibody; DNA, deoxyribonucleic acid; CREST, calcinosis, Raynaud phenomenon, esophageal dysmotility, sclerodactyly, telangiectasia; RNP, ribonucleoprotein; SLE, systemic lupus erythematosus; SRP, signal recognition particle; tRNA, transfer RNA.

- Gynecologic: recurrent pregnancy loss (antiphospholipid antibodies found in up to 10% of women with three or more consecutive pregnancy losses) and late trimester loss

Diagnosis and Evaluation

- **Patients may have antiphospholipid antibodies but not develop the thrombotic manifestations required for the diagnosis of APS**
- Diagnosis is based on the presence of at least one of the following autoantibody types:
  - Biologic false-positive serologic test for syphilis

- Lupus anticoagulant
  - IgM or IgG that prolongs phospholipid-dependent coagulation in vitro by binding to the prothrombin activator complex, impairing conversion of prothrombin to thrombin
  - Assayed by phospholipid-dependent coagulation tests (e.g., activated partial thromboplastin time and Russell viper venom time)
- Anticardiolipin antibodies (ACAs)
  - Directed against the complex of phospholipid and β_2-glycoproteins
  - High-titer ACA IgG is most strongly associated with thrombosis and pregnancy loss

BOX 45-1	*Drug-Induced Lupus*

Many drug associations (e.g., hydralazine, procainamide, sulfonamides, and isoniazid)
Primarily older patients
No CNS or renal disease
ANA (antihistone) (+); antinative DNA (−)
Clinical features improve after discontinuing drug, though ANA may persist for years

ANA, Antinuclear antibody; CNS, central nervous system; DNA, deoxyribonucleic acid.

- Low titers are found in up to 5% of healthy young women

Treatment

- Serologic abnormalities alone
  - **Patient at high risk for thrombotic event (with traditional cardiovascular risk factors) should be treated with low-dose aspirin**
  - Patients with SLE and positive APS antibodies should be treated with hydroxychloroquine plus low-dose aspirin
- Patients with one thrombotic event
  - Warfarin with target international normalized ratio (INR) of 2 to 3 for venous thrombosis
  - Warfarin with INR goal greater than 3 or INR between 2 and 3 plus antiaggregant (e.g., aspirin) for arterial thrombosis
  - Warfarin is not used during pregnancy because of potential teratogenicity
  - Prednisone and aspirin, or subcutaneous heparin and aspirin, have been used successfully in pregnancy with APS
  - Most experts recommend continuing treatment indefinitely in patients with definite APS and thrombosis

Scleroderma and Systemic Sclerosis

Basic Information

- **A multisystem autoimmune disease characterized by vasculopathy, excessive collagen deposition, and tissue fibrosis**
- Epidemiology
  - Usual onset in 20s or 30s
  - Female-to-male ratio is between 3:1 and 4:1
  - More common in African Americans than whites

Clinical Presentation

- Raynaud phenomenon (Fig. 45-4)
  - One of earliest clinical manifestations
  - Classic phases: white (ischemic), leads to blue (cyanotic), leads to red (hyperemic)
  - Primary Raynaud phenomenon
    - Occurs in the absence of another rheumatic disease
    - Symmetric
    - Negative ANA
    - Not associated with ischemic injury such as ulcers, gangrene

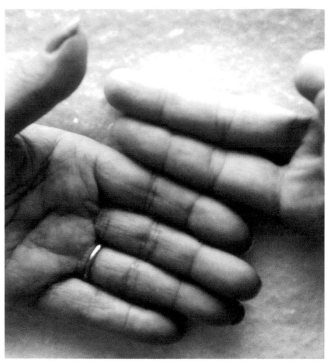

FIGURE 45-4 Raynaud phenomenon manifested by digital cyanosis in a patient with scleroderma. (Courtesy Carol M. Ziminski, MD.)

- Onset: ages 14 to 35 years
- Affects 5% to 10% of young women
- Secondary Raynaud phenomenon
  - Occurs in the setting of another rheumatic disease (e.g., scleroderma or SLE)
  - Should be considered if:
    - Onset in childhood or after age 35 years
    - Patient is male
    - Abnormal nail-fold capillary loops are present (Fig. 45-5)
    - Episodes cause digital tip ulceration or gangrene
    - Positive ANA
- Organ system manifestations (Table 45-3)

Diagnosis and Evaluation

- **Skin changes suggest the diagnosis, but internal organ involvement determines survival**
- Clinical subsets
  - Limited scleroderma (CREST syndrome)
    - **C**alcinosis
    - **R**aynaud phenomenon
    - **E**sophageal dysmotility
    - **S**clerodactyly (Fig. 45-6)
    - **T**elangiectasia
  - Diffuse scleroderma (progressive systemic sclerosis)
    - Scleroderma involving not only the fingers but also the dorsum of the hand proximal to the metacarpophalangeal joints or on forearms, legs, face, and trunk
    or
    - Sclerodactyly associated with either digital pulp pitting (Fig. 45-7) or basilar pulmonary fibrosis
  - Localized scleroderma: morphea and linear scleroderma

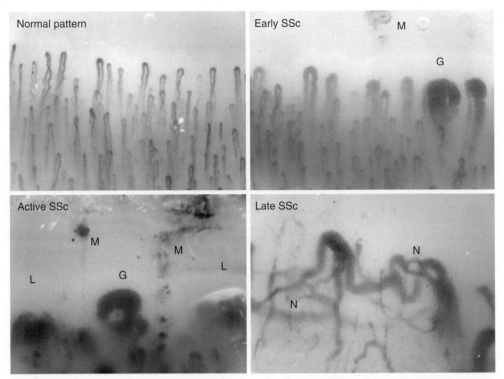

FIGURE 45-5 Nail-fold capillary microscopy showing stages of abnormalities in scleroderma. G, Giant capillaries; L, loss of capillaries; M, microhemorrhages; N, neoangiogenesis; SSc, systemic sclerosis. (From Boin F, Wigley FM. Clinical features and treatment of scleroderma. *Kelley's Textbook of Rheumatology.* 9th ed. Philadelphia: Elsevier; 2013, Fig. 84-4.)

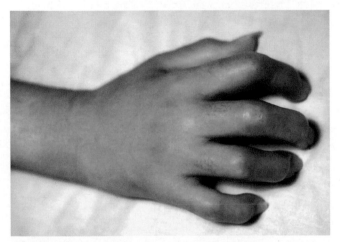

FIGURE 45-6 Scleroderma. Digital flexion contractures caused by thickened, indurated skin (sclerodactyly). (Courtesy Carol M. Ziminski, MD.)

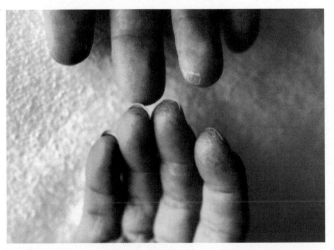

FIGURE 45-7 Scleroderma. Pitting scars on the pulps of the index and middle fingers caused by microvascular disease. (Courtesy Carol M. Ziminski, MD.)

TABLE 45-3	*Organ System Manifestations in Scleroderma*			
Cutaneous	**Gastrointestinal**	**Pulmonary**	**Renal**	**Cardiac**
Early Edematous phase (scleredema); may last several months **Subsequent** Induration and skin tightening; may last several years **Late** Atrophic changes Also telangiectasias, calcification, and pruritis	Esophageal dysmotility, with reflux Gastroparesis, with early satiety Watermelon stomach Small bowel involvement, with pseudo-obstruction Colonic involvement, with wide-mouthed diverticulae	Interstitial pneumonitis with bibasilar interstitial infiltrates Pulmonary hypertension May manifest as cough or dyspnea	Renal crisis presents with malignant hypertension and rapidly progressive renal failure Biopsy reveals transmural microangiopathy (not vasculitis) with intimal proliferation, medial hypertrophy, and adventitial fibrosis	Cardiomyopathy with contraction band necrosis or myocardial fibrosis Pericarditis

- The presence of a tendon friction rub is highly specific (although not sensitive) for the diagnosis of scleroderma
- **Autoantibodies are found in most affected patients: ANA positive in up to 90% of patients (see Table 45-2)**
  - **Anti-Scl 70 antibodies are present in 30% of patients with diffuse scleroderma**
  - **Anticentromere antibodies are present in limited scleroderma**
- Scleroderma renal crisis is a rare complication and associated with early diffuse scleroderma
  - Presents as new-onset hypertension, renal failure, and microangiopathic anemia
  - **Use of angiotensin-converting-enzyme (ACE) inhibitors has improved prognosis in this potentially fatal complication of diffuse scleroderma**
- Interstitial lung disease and pulmonary hypertension are common pulmonary manifestations of scleroderma
  - Bronchoalveolar lavage may identify patients with active inflammatory pulmonary disease, who may benefit from immunosuppressive agents
- Gastroesophageal reflux is a common symptom in scleroderma
- Intestinal involvement can present as malabsorption and ileus

Treatment

- **There is no cure for scleroderma, but many of its organ manifestations can be treated (Table 45-4)**
- In the future, therapy may focus on inhibiting the release of cytokines that induce fibrosis

TABLE 45-4	*Management of Scleroderma*
Manifestation	**Intervention**
Raynaud phenomenon	Cold avoidance Calcium channel blockers
Digital ulcers	Intravenous iloprost (prostaglandin analogue)
Interstitial pneumonitis	Steroids Cytotoxic agents (e.g., cyclophosphamide)
Gastroesophageal reflux	Proton pump inhibitors
GI immotility	Prokinetic agents (e.g., metoclopramide)
GI bacterial overgrowth/malabsorption	Broad-spectrum antibiotics
Pulmonary hypertension	Endothelin receptor antagonist (bosentan) Phosphodiesterase-5 inhibitors (sildenafil, tadalafil) Prostocyclin analogues (epoprostenol, iloprost) Lung transplantation
Renal crisis	ACE inhibitor

ACE, Angiotensin-converting enzyme; GI, gastrointestinal.

- Many of the major advances in management today are directed toward preventing damage to endothelial cells
- **There is no role for systemic steroids except in pneumonitis or myositis**
- Poor prognostic factors include older age, male gender, African American race, the presence of diffuse scleroderma, and early visceral involvement

Polymyositis and Dermatomyositis

Basic Information

- **Immune-mediated inflammatory myopathy affecting striated muscle and resulting in symmetrical proximal (i.e., shoulder and pelvic girdle) weakness**
- Incidence 1 in 100,000
- Bimodal distribution of incidence: ages 10 to 15 years and 45 to 60 years
- Female-to-male ratio is 2:1

Clinical Presentation

- Muscle manifestations
  - Weakness is pathognomonic
    - Proximal and symmetrical weakness
    - May also affect the neck, pharyngeal, respiratory, and trunk muscles, but spares the facial muscles
    - Dysphagia may occur (caused by involvement of striated pharyngeal muscle)
    - Muscle pain (25% of cases)
- Cutaneous manifestations
  - **Heliotrope rash: periorbital edema with violaceous discoloration of eyelids**
  - Erythematous, sometimes scaling rash may occur over face, upper chest (V sign), and upper back ("shawl" sign)
  - **Gottron papules: erythematous or violaceous scaling papules over knuckles (Fig. 45-8)**
  - Mechanic's hand: scaling skin over palms with "dirty" discoloration of creases

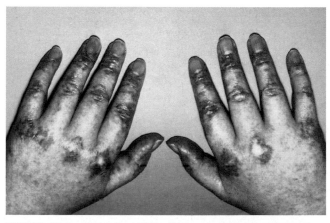

FIGURE 45-8 Dermatomyositis. Gottron papules manifested by a rash accentuated over interphalangeal joints, with variable manifestations including erythematous or violaceous induration, papules, or nodules. (Courtesy Carol M. Ziminski, MD.)

- Calcinosis (especially in children)
- Vasculitis
- Pulmonary involvement with interstitial lung disease occurs in 30% to 50% of patients
- Clinical patterns
  - Polymyositis (PM)
  - Dermatomyositis (DM)
  - Juvenile DM
  - Myositis associated with another rheumatic disease
  - Myositis associated with malignancy

Diagnosis and Evaluation

- **Clinical suspicion based on presentation with symmetrical proximal muscle weakness**
- Elevated muscle enzymes
  - **Creatine phosphokinase is the most specific and sensitive for muscle injury**
  - Aldolase, aspartate aminotransferase, alanine aminotransferase, and lactate dehydrogenase may also reflect muscle inflammation
- Autoantibodies may allow better definition of subsets but may not be widely available (see Table 45-2)
  - Tests are positive for ANAs in 20% to 30% of patients with PM, more frequently in patients who have myositis in the setting of other rheumatic diseases
  - Approximately 30% of patients have antibodies directed against cytoplasmic ribonucleoproteins; found only in myositis and are known as myositis-specific antibodies (anti-Jo 1 is the most well known)
  - Antigens define three subgroups of patients who differ in clinical features and prognosis (Table 45-5)
- Complement system
  - PM: no evidence of complement activation
  - DM: vascular deposition of complement membrane attack complex

- Electromyography (EMG) reveals inflammatory myopathy with short duration, low-amplitude, and polyphasic potentials, and irritative features
- Muscle biopsy may confirm the diagnosis
  - Negative in up to 30% of cases, but abnormal EMG supports diagnosis of myositis in appropriate clinical setting
  - PM: inflammatory cell infiltrate found between muscle fibers, with varying stages of muscle fiber necrosis and regeneration, but vessels spared
  - DM: inflammatory cells surround the small endomysial vessels
- Magnetic resonance imaging adds important dimension and is noninvasive
  - T1-weighted images provide excellent anatomic detail, useful in assessing changes resulting from damage and chronicity
  - T2-weighted images with fat suppression or short tau inversion recovery sequences identify edema, which is indicative of active inflammation
- Differential diagnosis
  - Drugs: colchicine, penicillamine, "statins," corticosteroids, and zidovudine
  - Endocrine: hypothyroidism
  - Malignancy-associated: perform age-appropriate cancer screening
  - Neuromuscular: muscular dystrophies and myasthenia gravis
  - Inclusion body myositis (Box 45-2)
  - Infections
    - Viral: Coxsackie virus, influenza, and HIV
    - Parasitic: *Trichinella*
    - Protozoan: *Toxoplasma*
  - Other: electrolyte disorders and metabolic myopathies

TABLE 45-5	*Syndromes Associated with Myositis-Specific Autoantibodies*	
Autoantibody	**Clinical Features**	**Prognosis**
Aminoacyl-tRNA synthetases (anti-Jo-1, PL-7, and others)	Acute onset Interstitial lung disease Arthritis Hyperkeratotic rash ("mechanic's hands") HLA-DR3, -DR52	Variable Significant mortality
Signal recognition peptide	Hyperacute onset Cardiac involvement Onset in autumn More prevalent in black women	Poor, 5-year mortality rate 75%
Components of histone acetylase complexes (Mi-2)	Dermatomyositis Shawl sign of rash Cuticular overgrowth	Good

HLA, Human leukocyte antigen; tRNA, transfer RNA.

BOX 45-2	*Inclusion Body Myositis*

Basic Information

Unique subset of the inflammatory myopathies
Typical patient is a man older than 50 years

Clinical Presentation

Weakness may be both proximal and distal, and less symmetrical
Typical course is chronic, with slow progression over years, or even decades

Diagnosis and Evaluation

Consider in setting of atypical distribution of weakness
Mild elevation in creatine phosphokinase (up to 5× normal)
Muscle biopsy specimen reveals characteristic rimmed vacuoles with inclusions and occasional ragged red fibers

Treatment

Poor response to steroids

Treatment and Management

- **High-dose steroids (80% response)**
- Methotrexate, mycophenolate mofetil, and azathioprine useful as steroid-sparing agents
- Intravenous immune globulin (IVIg) is used successfully in dermatomyositis as second-line agent
- **In dermatomyositis, evaluate to rule out age-associated malignancies, particularly breast and ovarian cancer in women**

Polymyalgia Rheumatica

Basic Information

- **Clinical syndrome marked by proximal limb-girdle muscle pain and stiffness**
- **May be a prodrome for late-onset rheumatoid arthritis**
- **May be associated with giant-cell arteritis (see Chapter 44)**
- Epidemiology
  - Rarely diagnosed at ages younger than 50 years
  - Female-to-male ratio is 2:1
  - Predominantly whites (especially patients of northern European descent)

Clinical Presentation

- Proximal limb-girdle pain and morning stiffness in the appropriate host
- Constitutional manifestations include fever, malaise, and weight loss

Diagnosis and Evaluation

- **Examination reveals muscle tenderness but no true muscle weakness**
- Laboratory features
  - Elevated erythrocyte sedimentation rate
  - Elevated C-reactive protein
  - Normochromic normocytic anemia
  - Elevated platelets

Treatment

- Steroids
  - Treatment of choice
  - Low-dose (10 to 20 mg of prednisone daily)
  - Rapid and dramatic symptomatic improvement is characteristic
  - Taper guided by symptoms

Fibromyalgia Syndrome

Basic Information

- **Chronic syndrome marked by multifocal musculoskeletal pain and fatigue, in the setting of a noninflammatory physical examination and laboratory studies**
- Epidemiology
  - May affect 2% of population
  - Peak age 30 to 50 years
  - 80% to 90% of patients are female

Clinical Presentation

- May include the following:
  - Chronic, diffuse pain
  - Morning stiffness
  - Subjective swelling
  - Raynaud-like symptoms
  - Sleep disturbance
  - Fatigue
  - Headache
  - Dry mouth
  - Paresthesias
  - Irritable bowel syndrome
  - Urinary urgency
  - Dysmenorrhea
  - Anxiety
  - Depression

Diagnosis and Evaluation

- Criteria for the diagnosis of fibromyalgia were approved by the American College of Rheumatology in 2010 (Table 45-6). A patient satisfies diagnostic criteria for fibromyalgia if the following three conditions are met:
  - Widespread pain index (WPI) 7 or greater and symptom severity (SS) scale score 5 or greater (or WPI 3 to 6 and SS scale score 9 or greater)
  - Symptoms have been present at a similar level for at least 3 months
  - The patient does not have a disorder that would otherwise explain the pain
- Consider possible contributing events
  - Physical trauma: physical abuse or motor vehicle accident
  - Emotional trauma: sexual abuse
  - Infections: hepatitis C, Lyme disease, parvovirus, and HIV

Treatment

- Goals
  - Decrease pain
  - Decrease distress
  - Improve sleep
  - Increase energy level
  - Improve function
  - Treat associated symptoms, including anxiety and depression
- Methods
  - Patient education and reassurance
  - Stress reduction
  - Cognitive behavioral therapy
  - **Aerobic conditioning exercise**
  - Tai chi
  - Pharmacologic intervention
    - Low-dose tricyclic antidepressant (e.g., amitriptyline or nortriptyline)
    - Cyclobenzaprine
    - Dual-receptor inhibitors inhibit serotonin and norepinephrine (e.g., venlafaxine, milnacipran)
    - Anticonvulsants (e.g., pregabalin, gabapentin)
    - Serotonin reuptake inhibitors (e.g., fluoxetine)
- Pitfalls in therapy
  - Psychosocial issues not addressed

| **TABLE 45-6** | *Fibromyalgia Diagnostic Criteria* |

Criteria

A patient satisfies diagnostic criteria for fibromyalgia if the following 3 conditions are met:
1. Widespread pain index (WPI) ≥7 and symptom severity (SS) scale score ≥5 or WPI 3–6 and SS scale score ≥9.
2. Symptoms have been present at a similar level for at least 3 months.
3. The patient does not have a disorder that would otherwise explain the pain.

Ascertainment

1. WPI: Note the number of areas in which the patient has had pain over the last week. In how many areas has the patient had pain? Score will be between 0 and 19.

Shoulder girdle, left	Hip (buttock, trochanter), left	Jaw, left	Upper back
Shoulder girdle, right	Hip (buttock, trochanter), right	Jaw, right	Lower back
Upper arm, left	Upper leg, left	Chest	Neck
Upper arm, right	Upper leg, right	Abdomen	
Lower arm, left	Lower leg, left		
Lower arm, right	Lower leg, right		

2. SS scale score:
   Fatigue
   Waking unrefreshed
   Cognitive symptoms
For the each of the 3 symptoms above, indicate the level of severity over the past week using the following scale:
0 = no problem
1 = slight or mild problems, generally mild or intermittent
2 = moderate, considerable problems, often present and/or at a moderate level
3 = severe: pervasive, continuous, life-disturbing problems
Considering somatic symptoms* in general, indicate whether the patient has:
0 = no symptoms
1 = few symptoms
2 = a moderate number of symptoms
3 = a great deal of symptoms
The SS scale score is the sum of the severity of the 3 symptoms (fatigue, waking unrefreshed, cognitive symptoms) plus the extent (severity) of somatic symptoms in general. The final score is between 0 and 12.

*Somatic symptoms that might be considered: muscle pain, irritable bowel syndrome, fatigue/tiredness, thinking or remembering problems, muscle weakness, headache, pain/cramps in the abdomen, numbness/tingling, dizziness, insomnia, depression, constipation, pain in the upper abdomen, nausea, nervousness, chest pain, blurred vision, fever, diarrhea, dry mouth, itching, wheezing, Raynaud phenomenon, hives/welts, ringing in ears, vomiting, heartburn, oral ulcers, loss of/change in taste, seizures, dry eyes, shortness of breath, loss of appetite, rash, sun sensitivity, hearing difficulties, easy bruising, hair loss, frequent urination, painful urination, and bladder spasms.
From Wolfe F, Clauw DJ, Fitzcharles M-A, et al. The American College of Rheumatology preliminary diagnostic criteria for fibromyalgia and measurement of symptom severity. *Arthritis Care Res.* 2010;62:600–610.

- Benefit of exercise undervalued
- Exercise program too rigorous or advanced too quickly
- Tricyclic therapy discontinued prematurely
- Unrealistic expectations for improvement

Review Questions

For review questions, please go to ExpertConsult.com.

SUGGESTED READINGS

Erkan D, Salmon JE, Lockshin MD. Antiphospholipid antibody syndrome. In: Firestein GS, Budd RC, Gabriel SE, et al., eds. *Kelley's Textbook of Rheumatology.* 9th ed. Philadelphia: Saunders; 2013:1331-1341.

Hellmann DB. Giant cell arteritis, polymyalgia rheumatic, and Takayasu's arteritis. In: Firestein GS, Budd RC, Gabriel SE, et al., eds. *Kelley's Textbook of Rheumatology.* 9th ed. Philadelphia: Saunders; 2013:1461-1480.

Nagaraju K, Lundberg IE. Inflammatory diseases of muscle and other myopathies. In: Firestein GS, Budd RC, Gabriel SE, et al., eds. *Kelley's Textbook of Rheumatology.* 9th ed. Philadelphia: Saunders; 2013:1404-1430 e5.

Petri M, Orbai AM, Alarcon GS, et al. Derivation and validation of Systemic Lupus International Collaborating Clinic classification criteria for systemic lupus erythematosus. *Arthritis Rheum.* 2012; 64:2677-2686.

Wolfe F, Clauw DJ, Fitzcharles M-A, et al. The American College of Rheumatology preliminary diagnostic criteria for fibromyalgia and measurement of symptom severity. *Arthritis Care Res.* 2010;62:600-610.

SECTION EIGHT

Hematology

CHAPTER 46

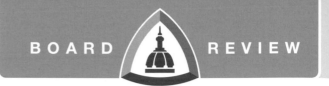

BOARD REVIEW

Anemia

SATISH SHANBHAG, MBBS, MPH; and BIMAL H. ASHAR, MD, MBA

Anemia, a reduction in the quantity of circulating red blood cells (RBCs) or hemoglobin (Hgb), is one of the most common conditions seen by internists. Although patients are often asymptomatic, the presence of anemia is indicative of an underlying disorder. From a laboratory perspective, anemia is somewhat arbitrarily defined by the World Health Organization as an Hgb concentration of less than 12 g/dL in women and less than 13 g/dL in men. Others have proposed slightly different defining values that vary by age and race. If previous Hgb values are available, a significant downward trend should be indicative of anemia regardless of absolute Hgb values. This chapter provides a general framework for approaching patients with anemia to uncover their underlying disorders.

Overview

Basic Information

- Normal erythropoiesis (Fig. 46-1)
  - Regulated by the production of erythropoietin (EPO) in the kidney
    - EPO production increases as a result of hypoxia, as sensed by the kidney
    - EPO then stimulates RBC production by the bone marrow
- Mechanisms of anemia
  - Decreased production of RBCs (hypoproliferation)
  - Increased destruction of RBCs (hemolysis)
  - Acute blood loss (hemorrhage)

Clinical Presentation

- Often asymptomatic when mild or chronic
- When symptomatic, weakness and fatigue are the most common symptoms
- Angina, congestive heart failure, dyspnea, and tachycardia can occur
- **Severity of symptoms is dependent on rapidity of development of anemia, degree of anemia, and ability of the body to compensate**

Diagnosis

- Laboratory evaluation begins with a complete blood count and differential (CBC)
  - Hgb and hematocrit (Hct) values, rather than RBC count, are determinants of the presence of anemia
  - White blood cell (WBC) and platelet counts should be examined to determine the presence or absence of pancytopenia

- Mean corpuscular volume (MCV): serves as an estimate of RBC size
- RBC count: low in most cases of anemia but can be normal or high in some conditions (e.g., thalassemia trait)
- Red cell distribution width (RDW): estimates the degree of variation in red cell size
- Reticulocytes: immature RBCs
  - Correct the reticulocyte count for the degree of anemia as follows:
    - Reticulocyte index = Percent reticulocytes × Patient Hct/normal Hct
    - **A reticulocyte index greater than 2% suggests hemolysis or recovery from acute blood loss**
    - **A reticulocyte index less than 2% suggests a hypoproliferative process or acute blood loss**
- Peripheral smear
  - Can help identify the cause of the anemia, confirm the MCV, and potentially identify mixed disorders (e.g., concomitant iron deficiency and B12 deficiency presenting with a normal MCV)
  - Can be suggestive of specific diagnoses (see Chapter 51)
- Basic approach to anemia (see Fig. 46-2)

Treatment

- Blood transfusions
  - **Not routinely indicated in asymptomatic patients**
  - Transfusion is currently recommended for patients with:
    - Rapid acute blood loss
    - Cardiovascular disease and an Hgb less than 8 g/dL
    - Symptomatic patients with an Hgb between 7 and 9 g/dL
    - Stable patients with an Hgb less than 7 g/dL
  - Can cause a number of immunologic reactions (Table 46-1)
- Erythropoiesis-stimulating agents (ESAs)
  - Can benefit patients with renal failure and Hgb levels less than 10 g/dL, but target Hgb levels should not exceed 11 g/dL
  - Increases quality of life in some patients with anemia of chronic disease (e.g., caused by rheumatoid arthritis [RA])
  - Controversy exists regarding risks and benefits in cancer patients
    - To be considered for symptomatic patients with anemia (Hgb 10 g/dL or less) resulting from

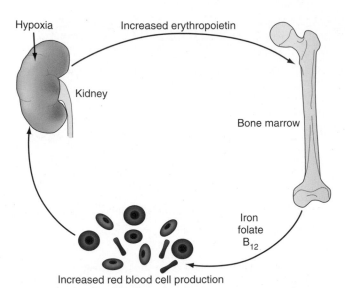

FIGURE 46-1 Regulation of red cell production. (Modified from Hoffman R, Heidrick E, Benz E, et al. *Hematology: Basic Principles and Practice.* 4th ed. Philadelphia: Churchill Livingstone; 2005: Fig. 29-2.)

chemotherapy for malignancies treated with noncurative intent

- Not recommended for patients with anemia caused by a malignancy who are not receiving chemotherapy or for those being treated with curative-intent chemotherapy
- Reduces the need for postoperative transfusion in some patients
- May reduce transfusion requirements in critically ill patients
- Potential adverse effects
  - Hypertension
  - Increased risk of cardiovascular events and death if target Hgb is kept greater than 13 g/dL
  - Arthralgias
  - Thrombosis
  - Seizures (rare)
  - Polycythemia: if Hct not followed closely
  - Aiming for high Hgb goal (greater than 13g/dL) in patients with solid tumors on chemotherapy has been shown to compromise outcomes
  - Iron deficiency can occur if iron levels are not monitored and repleted when necessary
  - Pure RBC aplasia has been reported with older agents, but is not a concern with the newer agents currently available

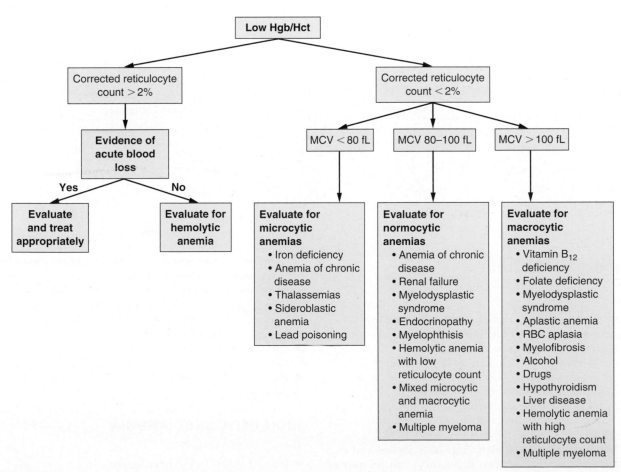

FIGURE 46-2 Basic evaluation of anemia. Hct, Hematocrit; Hgb, hemoglobin; MCV, mean corpuscular volume; RBC, red blood cell.

TABLE 46-1	**Immunologic Blood Transfusion Reactions**
Reaction	**Description**
Febrile nonhemolytic	Fever ± chills 1–6 hr after start of transfusion. Sometimes can be confused with acute hemolytic reactions so transfusion may need to be temporarily halted. Treat with antipyretics

Acute hemolytic	Caused by preformed antibodies in patient's serum that bind and lyse transfused cells
	Most cases are caused by ABO incompatibility
	Can present with fevers and chills with or without flank pain, hypotension, DIC shortly after starting the transfusion
	Management includes:
	    Discontinuing the transfusion
	    Notifying the blood bank
	    Starting IV fluids
	    Obtaining blood for direct antiglobulin test, hemolysis markers, coagulation times, renal function

Delayed hemolytic	Caused by an amnestic response in patients who have previously undergone transfusion and have developed low levels of alloantibodies that go undetected during crossmatch Seen 1–2 wks after transfusion Direct and indirect antiglobulin tests are positive with identification of the antigen. Treatment is supportive.
Anaphylactic	Anaphylaxis and shock seconds to minutes after start of the transfusion Commonly caused by anti-IgA antibodies in patients who are IgA deficient Treat by stopping the transfusion, administering epinephrine, and supporting airway and blood pressure
Urticarial	Can continue transfusion after treating with diphenhydramine
Transfusion-related acute lung injury	Dyspnea, hypoxemia, and pulmonary infiltrates that develop within 6 hr after the end of transfusion of a blood product (commonly plasma) containing preformed antibodies Can cause death in some cases and is treated with adequate supportive care (which may include intubation)
Post-transfusion purpura	Causes severe thrombocytopenia 5–10 days after transfusion of any blood product containing platelet contamination. Treat with IV immune globulin

DIC, Disseminated intravascular coagulation; IgA, immunoglobulin A; IV, intravenous.

TABLE 46-2	**Interpretation of Iron Studies**			
	Serum Iron	**TIBC**	**Transferrin Saturation**	**Ferritin**
Iron deficiency	↓	↑	↓	↓
Anemia of chronic disease	↓	N or ↓	N or ↓	N or ↑
Thalassemia trait	N	N	N	N or ↑
Sideroblastic anemia	N or ↑	N or ↑	N or ↑	N or ↑

N, Normal; TIBC, total iron-binding capacity.

Microcytic Anemia

Basic Approach

- Obtain and interpret iron studies (Table 46-2)
  - Serum iron: not very helpful by itself because there is significant variation in values
  - Total iron-binding capacity (TIBC): Reflects the total amount of transferrin (iron transport protein) available in the blood. It is a measure of aggregate iron-binding sites; elevated if iron is low.
  - Transferrin saturation: normally between 20% and 45%
  - **Ferritin: correlates with total iron stores and is the best marker of iron deficiency; can be normal in iron deficiency if there is concomitant inflammation; even with inflammation, level is usually less than 100 mg/L**
  - Soluble transferrin receptor level: measure of tissue iron; levels typically go up in iron deficiency but do not change in anemia of chronic disease
- Look at the peripheral smear
- Consider Hgb electrophoresis if studies suggest thalassemia or other hemoglobinopathy
- Bone marrow biopsy with iron staining: gold standard if etiology unclear

IRON-DEFICIENCY ANEMIA
Basic Information

- Present in 2% of the population
- Etiologies

- **Blood loss is the most common cause (especially with menstrual losses)**
- Decreased iron intake
- Increased iron use (e.g., with EPO therapy, chronic hemolysis with hemoglobinuria)
- Malabsorption
  - From partial gastrectomy or after gastric bypass surgery: Iron deficiency develops in a significant percentage of patients
  - From malabsorption syndromes (e.g., celiac sprue) if the disease affects the proximal small intestine where iron is absorbed

Clinical Presentation

- Fatigue
- Sore tongue, cheilosis
- Brittle nails or koilonychias ("spoon nails")
- Pica: desire to eat unusual substances (e.g., ice, clay, starch)

Diagnosis

- **Iron studies classically show reduced iron, increased TIBC, reduced transferrin saturation, and reduced ferritin**
- Peripheral smear should show hypochromic, microcytic cells (Fig. 46-3)
- Evaluation of iron-deficient patients
  - Search for evidence of blood loss (e.g., uterine bleeding, gastrointestinal [GI] bleeding, genitourinary [GU] bleeding)
    - If there are no clinical signs or symptoms suggesting a potential cause, start with GI evaluation (esophagogastroduodenoscopy [EGD]/colonoscopy)
    - If EGD and colonoscopy are negative, small bowel capsule endoscopy may be helpful
    - Consider malabsorption if the evaluation for blood loss is negative

Treatment

- Transfusions: only if there is hemodynamic compromise or acute hemorrhage
- Oral iron
  - Oral preparations vary in the amount of elemental iron per tablet (i.e., ferrous sulfate typically has 65 mg elemental iron per 325-mg pill while ferrous

gluconate may have between 28 and 36 mg of elemental iron per 325-mg pill)
- Most patients can tolerate only 1 to 2 divided doses per day because of GI side effects
- Vitamin C administration (250 mg before taking iron) may improve absorption
- Should see reticulocytosis within 7 days
- Correction of anemia in about 6 to 8 weeks if dose is adequate, but repletion of body iron stores usually takes 6 months
- **If anemia does not improve, consider noncompliance, malabsorption, incorrect diagnosis, coexisting disease (e.g., anemia of chronic disease), or continued blood loss**
- Parenteral iron
  - May be indicated in refractory cases or where absorption is a concern
  - Four formulations currently available for use:
    - High-molecular-weight (HMW) iron dextran (intravenous [IV] or intramuscular [IM]) has high rates of anaphylaxis
    - Low-molecular-weight iron dextran is easy to use because total dose can be given in one infusion and does not carry high infusion reaction risk like HMW iron dextran
    - Ferric gluconate (IV) and iron sucrose (IV): need repeat infusions (over weeks) to deliver total dose, but side effects and risk of anaphylaxis are lower
    - Ferumoxytol and ferric carboxymaltose are newer iron formulations where large doses can be administered with low infusion reaction risk but are more expensive

ANEMIA OF CHRONIC DISEASE

Basic Information

- **Most cases are actually normocytic, not microcytic**
- Etiologies
  - Malignancy
  - Chronic infections (e.g., osteomyelitis, tuberculosis, acquired immune deficiency syndrome [AIDS])
  - Chronic inflammatory disorders (e.g., RA, systemic lupus erythematosus [SLE], ulcerative colitis)
  - Congestive heart failure
- Mechanisms
  - Decreased RBC survival
  - Impaired EPO production
  - Impaired marrow response to EPO
  - Impaired mobilization of iron (i.e., increased iron uptake and retention within the reticuloendothelial system)

Clinical Presentation and Diagnosis

- Iron studies (see Table 46-2)
- Peripheral smear usually shows normocytic, normochromic cells but can be microcytic in 30% to 40% of cases
- **MCV is rarely less than 75 fL**
- Bone marrow biopsy may be helpful if the diagnosis is unclear; it should reveal normal to increased iron stores
- Soluble transferrin receptor (sTfR) level may help distinguish pure anemia of chronic disease from anemia

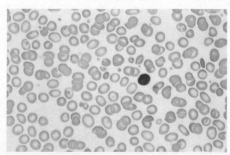

FIGURE 46-3 Iron-deficiency anemia. Hypochromic, microcytic blood cells (smaller than the lymphocyte in the center). (From Goldman L, Bennett JC, Ausiello D. *Cecil Textbook of Medicine.* 22nd ed. Philadelphia: Saunders; 2004: Fig. 167-1.)

of chronic disease with concomitant iron deficiency in patients with normal ferritin levels

- If the sTfR/log ferritin (sTfR/log ferritin index) is greater than 2, iron deficiency probably coexists with anemia of chronic disease
- If the sTfR/log ferritin index is less than 1, iron deficiency is likely not present with anemia of chronic disease

Treatment

- Treat the underlying disorder (if possible)
- Transfusion rarely indicated because anemia is usually not severe
- EPO/darbepoietin has been shown to increase quality of life and reduce the need for transfusion in some patients with anemia of chronic disease, but it is very costly and may be harmful in some cases when the Hgb goal is set high
  - Goal is to not exceed Hgb values of 11 g/dL

THALASSEMIA

Basic Information

- Defined as a decrease in production of one of the two globin chains
  - Normal Hgb A has two α and two β chains ($\alpha_2\beta_2$)
  - In β-thalassemia, there is partial or complete suppression of β-globin chain synthesis, resulting in a relative excess of α-globin chains
  - In α-thalassemia, there is suppression or absence of α chains, resulting in a relative excess of β chains
- Seen predominantly in people of African, Asian, or Mediterranean descent
- There are a number of genetic variations classified clinically as:
  - β-Thalassemia
    - β-Thalassemia major: presents in the first year of life; patients are transfusion dependent
    - β-Thalassemia intermedia: regular transfusions not necessary until second, third, or fourth decade or stressors such as pregnancy; can develop iron overload independent of transfusions
    - β-Thalassemia minor (β-thal trait): causes mild anemia and significant microcytosis
  - α-Thalassemia
    - Hydrops fetalis and Hgb Barts: usually fatal in utero
    - Hgb H: significant anemia, hemolysis, splenomegaly are usually diagnosed in late childhood
    - α-Thalassemia trait (α-thalassemia minor): causes mild anemia and significant microcytosis
    - Asymptomatic carrier (α-thalassemia minima): no significant anemia

Clinical Presentation and Diagnosis

- Most cases of clinically severe anemia present in childhood
- Patients with thalassemia trait are commonly asymptomatic
- Several clues may be present that can help distinguish thalassemia trait from iron-deficiency anemia (Table 46-3)

TABLE 46-3	Clues to Differentiating Thalassemia Trait from Iron-Deficiency Anemia	
	Thalassemia Trait	**Iron Deficiency Anemia**
RBC count	N or ↑	↓
MCV	Lower than would be expected with iron deficiency	↓
RDW	N	↑
Ferritin	N or ↑	↓
Bone marrow iron	N	↓

MCV, Mean corpuscular volume; N, normal; RBC, red blood cell; RDW, red cell distribution width.

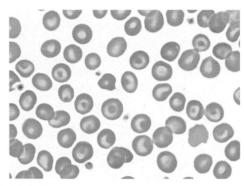

FIGURE 46-4 β-Thalassemia trait. Hypochromic, microcytic red blood cells with frequent targeting. Mild anemia. (From McPherson RA, Pincus MR. *Henry's Clinical Diagnosis and Management by Laboratory Methods.* 21st ed. Philadelphia: Saunders; 2006: Fig. 31-27.)

- Peripheral smear can show basophilic stippling, microcytosis, and target cells (Fig. 46-4)
- Hgb electrophoresis can be helpful in some cases
  - Normal: Hgb A ($\alpha_2\beta_2$) 97%; Hgb A$_2$ ($\alpha_2\delta_2$) 2% to 3%; Hgb F ($\alpha_2\gamma_2$) 0% to 1%
  - **β-Thal trait: increased Hgb A$_2$ and Hgb F**
  - α-Thal trait: Hgb electrophoresis is typically normal

Treatment

- Thalassemia trait: none indicated
- β-Thalassemia intermedia, β-thalassemia major, and Hgb H:
  - Chronic transfusion
  - Splenectomy
  - Treatment for iron overload
  - Management of complications, including leg ulcers, pulmonary hypertension, gallstones, aplasia

SIDEROBLASTIC ANEMIAS

- Consist of inherited or acquired defects that result in impaired heme biosynthesis
- **Characterized by iron-positive granules surrounding the nucleus of RBCs (ringed sideroblasts) in the bone marrow**

- Hereditary sideroblastic anemia
  - Most cases are X-linked and present in childhood
  - Usually presents with a fairly stable anemia
  - **Iron overload develops in all patients because of increased absorption of iron**
  - Iron studies show an increased transferrin saturation and ferritin level
  - Genetic studies should help confirm the diagnosis
  - Anemia responds to pyridoxine in most cases
  - Need to treat iron overload with phlebotomy or chelation
- Acquired idiopathic sideroblastic anemia
  - Usually occurs in older individuals
  - Anemia is usually normocytic or macrocytic
  - Iron studies reveal overload
  - Risk of transformation to acute leukemia
  - **Considered one of the myelodysplastic syndromes (MDSs) (see Chapter 50)**
  - Usually does not respond to treatment with pyridoxine
- Reversible sideroblastic anemia
  - Can be caused by a number of different precipitants, including alcohol, isoniazid, and chloramphenicol
  - Anemia improves with removal of the drug
- Lead poisoning
  - Some causes include ingestion of lead-based paint, ingestion of contaminated dietary supplements, consumption of moonshine from lead-lined stills, and inhalation of fumes
  - **Clinical manifestations include microcytic anemia, autonomic and motor neuropathy, and abdominal pain**
  - Diagnosed by finding elevated blood lead levels
  - Treat with edetate disodium (EDTA) chelation

Normocytic (Nonhemolytic) Anemia

- Basic approach
  - Can result from a number of different processes (see Fig. 46-2)
  - Clues to the diagnosis may be present in the history, physical, and other laboratory tests
    - The presence of pancytopenia suggests a primary bone marrow disorder
    - An elevated creatinine level suggests the possibility of anemia caused by renal insufficiency or failure
    - The presence of cancer, infection, or other inflammatory disorder suggests the presence of anemia of chronic disease

ANEMIA OF CHRONIC DISEASE

See the previous discussion of anemia of chronic disease in the Microcytic Anemia section.

ANEMIA OF RENAL INSUFFICIENCY OR FAILURE

- Usually manifests when creatinine clearance falls to below 50 mL/min
- **The primary abnormality is relative EPO deficiency**

- Uremia can also contribute to anemia by decreasing RBC survival
- Folate deficiency, aluminum overload, and hyperparathyroidism (causing bone marrow fibrosis) can all potentially contribute to anemia
- Treatment
  - Standard of care is now subcutaneous or IV ESA: EPO or darbepoietin
  - ESAs can potentially delay the progression of renal disease in patients with renal insufficiency and anemia
  - **Goal is to maintain Hct between 30% and 33% (Hgb between 10 and 11 g/dL)**
  - Iron therapy is indicated for functional iron deficiency where typically transferrin saturation is less than 20% despite ferritin levels that can be normal to high from concomitant inflammation between 100 and 800 ng/mL

APLASTIC ANEMIA

- Characterized by pancytopenia and severe reticulocytopenia
- Fanconi anemia (short stature, café-au-lait spots, GU abnormalities, microphthalmia, mental retardation, and skeletal abnormalities seen in association with aplastic anemia) is the most common congenital form
- Most acquired cases are idiopathic, but a number of other causes have been described (Box 46-1)
- Usually occurs between the ages of 15 and 25 years, with a second peak after age 60 years
- Thought to be an autoimmune disease
- Bone marrow is hypocellular with fat replacement of bone marrow elements (Fig. 46-5)
- Cytogenetic studies may help to distinguish from hypocellular MDS (i.e., abnormalities can be seen in MDS but not in aplastic anemia)
- Is associated with future development of myelodysplasia and paroxysmal nocturnal hemoglobinuria in 10% to 15% of patients

---

BOX 46-1	*Causes of Aplastic Anemia*

Drugs
    Antiepileptic drugs (e.g., carbamazepine, phenytoin,
       valproic acid)
    Chemotherapeutic agents
    Chloramphenicol
    Gold
    Nifedipine
    Sulfonamides
    Phenylbutazone
Chemicals (e.g., benzene, insecticides)
Radiation
Viruses
    Parvovirus B19
    Non-A, non-B, non-C hepatitis
    HIV, Epstein-Barr virus, cytomegalovirus
Connective tissue disease
Paroxysmal nocturnal hemoglobinuria

HIV, Human immunodeficiency virus.

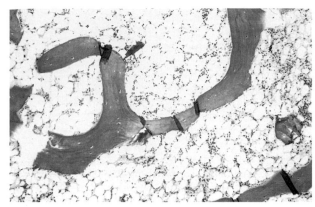

FIGURE 46-5 Bone marrow biopsy from a patient with aplastic anemia. (From Kumar V, Fausto N, Abbas A. *Robbins and Cotran's Pathologic Basis of Disease.* 7th ed. Philadelphia: Saunders; 2004: Fig. 13-27.)

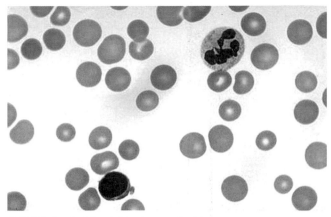

FIGURE 46-6 Megaloblastic anemia. Macrocytes, macro-ovalocytes, and a hypersegmented neutrophil.

- Treatment
  - Withdraw the offending agent (if identified)
  - Support with transfusions as needed; mild forms of disease may not need definitive treatment immediately
  - **Bone marrow transplantation (BMT) is the treatment of choice in all patients under the age of 45 years with severe aplastic anemia when there is a human leukocyte antigen-matched donor**
  - Immunosuppression with antithymocyte globulin plus cyclosporine plus corticosteroids is used when BMT is not possible

PURE RED CELL APLASIA

- Characterized by selective absence of RBCs in the marrow
- Can be idiopathic or associated with a number of conditions:
  - Thymoma
  - Lymphoproliferative disease (e.g., chronic lymphocytic leukemia [CLL], large granular lymphoma, chronic myelogenous leukemia)
  - Collagen vascular disease
  - Drugs (similar to aplastic anemia)
  - EPO
    - Can induce antibodies to EPO, resulting in anemia but occurrence is very rare
  - Parvovirus B19
    - Usually a transient process in normal hosts
    - Can cause severe transient aplastic crisis in patients with underlying hemolytic disorders
    - Can cause chronic aplasia in immunodeficient patients
- CBC reveals anemia with normal WBC and platelet counts
- Bone marrow reveals few or absent erythroid precursors
- **Computed tomography scan should be ordered to look for thymoma in all idiopathic cases**
- Treatment
  - Initial treatment is supportive with transfusions, if needed

- Cases caused by parvovirus infection may respond to IV immune globulin
- Cases caused by thymoma may respond to tumor removal
- Immunosuppressive drugs are used in refractory cases (e.g., corticosteroids, cyclosporine, cyclophosphamide)

Macrocytic Anemia

- Basic approach
  - Confirm that the anemia is hypoproliferative (reticulocyte index less than 2%)
  - Consider the two basic types of macrocytic anemia: megaloblastic and nonmegaloblastic
  - The history and physical examination can suggest certain etiologies
    - Use of certain medications (e.g., methotrexate, hydroxyurea, zidovudine, phenytoin, triamterene, imatinib, sunitinib)
    - Alcohol use
    - History of GI surgery (i.e., gastrectomy, ileal resection)
    - Signs or symptoms of liver disease
    - Signs or symptoms of hypothyroidism
  - Clues on the peripheral smear
    - Macroovalocytes: suggestive of megaloblastic anemias (Fig. 46-6)
    - Hypersegmented neutrophils (more than five to six lobes) suggest megaloblastic anemias (see Fig. 46-6)
      - Can appear before macrocytosis or anemia
    - Target cells: can be suggestive of liver disease
    - Pseudo Pelger-Huët anomaly: hyposegmented neutrophils suggestive of myelodysplasia
  - Laboratory evaluation
    - **A very high MCV (greater than 110 fL) is suggestive of vitamin B_{12} or folate deficiency**
    - Vitamin B_{12} and folate levels
    - Liver function tests
    - Thyroid-stimulating hormone

- Bone marrow examination is necessary if etiology is unclear or if MDS is being considered

MEGALOBLASTIC ANEMIA

- Characterized by abnormal nuclear maturation of red cell precursors (megaloblasts) in the bone marrow
- Causes include vitamin B_{12} deficiency, folate deficiency, MDSs (occasionally), and chemotherapy

VITAMIN B_{12} (COBALAMIN) DEFICIENCY

Basic Information

- Vitamin B_{12} is absorbed in the terminal ileum
- Parietal cells in the stomach secrete intrinsic factor that facilitates absorption
- **Deficiency usually takes years to develop**
- Most cases result from food-cobalamin malabsorption whereby stomach acids are unable to cleave vitamin B_{12} bound to food
- Numerous other causes exist (Table 46-4)

TABLE 46-4	*Etiologies of Vitamin B_{12} Deficiency*
Pernicious anemia	Autoimmune disease that results in achlorhydria and the absence of intrinsic factor Associated with other autoimmune processes (e.g., vitiligo, hypothyroidism, Addison disease) Associated with increased risk of gastric cancer Antiintrinsic factor antibodies are specific but not sensitive for the diagnosis Antiparietal cell antibodies are sensitive but not specific for the diagnosis
Gastrectomy	Can result in intrinsic factor deficiency Can cause impaired ability to cleave cobalamin from food
Atrophic gastritis	Thought to be a major cause of subclinical deficiency in elderly patients Results in inability to cleave cobalamin from food Can be associated with *Helicobacter pylori* infection
Intestinal disorders (e.g., ileal resection, Crohn disease, celiac disease, tropical sprue, bacterial overgrowth syndromes)	Look for other signs of malabsorption Can coexist with iron deficiency
Pancreatic insufficiency	Look for signs of chronic pancreatitis
Diet	Strict vegans have decreased intake of vitamin B_{12}
Medications (e.g., metformin, proton pump inhibitors)	Cause impaired intestinal absorption

Clinical Presentation

- Symptoms of anemia are nonspecific
- **Neurologic symptoms may be present before anemia develops**
  - Symmetrical paresthesias
  - Ataxia, spasticity
  - Memory loss, irritability, dementia
- Asymptomatic patients may present with only laboratory abnormalities
  - Pancytopenia
  - Elevated lactate dehydrogenase and indirect bilirubin caused by destruction of cells within the bone marrow

Diagnosis

- Peripheral smear may show macroovalocytes and hypersegmented neutrophils
- Serum vitamin B_{12} level is the standard diagnostic test, but it might not accurately represent true tissue levels in some patients
- Metabolic testing may be useful in patients who present with clinical evidence of deficiency and borderline serum levels (200 to 300 pg/mL)
  - Methylmalonic acid: Elevated levels are highly sensitive and specific for vitamin B_{12} deficiency in patients with normal renal function; this elevation is not seen in folate deficiency
  - Homocysteine: Elevated levels are very sensitive but not specific for B12 deficiency; elevations are also seen in folate deficiency
  - Antibody testing for the diagnosis of pernicious anemia (see Table 46-4)
  - The Schilling test can be done if a cause for the deficiency is not evident (Table 46-5) but is rarely necessary

Treatment

- IM vitamin B_{12} injections are usually the initial treatment of choice for pernicious anemia
- Oral vitamin B_{12} can be equally effective in raising serum levels
  - Must be given in very large doses (1 to 2 mg/day) in patients with pernicious anemia
  - Lower oral doses (250 µg/day) may be sufficient to treat food-cobalamin malabsorption
  - Consider the risk of noncompliance if choosing the oral route
- Hematologic abnormalities should normalize within 2 months
- Neurologic abnormalities improve within 6 months

FOLATE DEFICIENCY

- **Can develop rapidly (within months)**
- Causes
  - Nutritional deficiency
  - Alcoholism
  - Malabsorption (e.g., celiac sprue, tropical sprue)
  - Excess demands (e.g., pregnancy, chronic hemolytic states)
  - Drugs that interfere with folate metabolism (e.g., methotrexate, phenytoin, trimethoprim)

TABLE 46-5	Schilling Test

Stage I: Oral radioactive free B$_{12}$ is given, followed by intramuscular unlabeled B$_{12}$ to saturate tissue receptors and displace bound radiolabeled B$_{12}$. A 24-hr urine is then obtained to look for absorbed oral B$_{12}$. If <9% of the administered oral dose is found in urine, the test is considered abnormal.

Stage II: Oral radioactive B$_{12}$ plus oral intrinsic factor is given, followed by intramuscular unlabeled B$_{12}$. A 24-hr urine is again obtained. Excretion should correct to >9% if the problem is an intrinsic factor deficiency (e.g., pernicious anemia).

Stage III: Done if the first two stages are abnormal. A gluten-free diet (to diagnose celiac sprue), administration of antibiotics (to diagnose bacterial overgrowth), or administration of pancreatic enzymes (to diagnose pancreatic insufficiency) is done before repeating stage I.

Test Interpretation

Condition	Stage I	Stage II
Normal	Normal	
Dietary deficiency (veganism)	Normal	
Inadequate dissociation of cobalamin from food* (e.g., atrophic gastritis)	Normal	
Pernicious anemia	Low	Normal
Gastrectomy	Low	Normal
Ileal resection/malabsorption	Low	Low
Bacterial overgrowth of the ileum	Low	Low
Pancreatic insufficiency	Low	Low

*A modified version of stage I of the test can be done to diagnose food-cobalamin malabsorption. This test uses radiolabeled B$_{12}$ bound to food rather than free B$_{12}$. Patients with food-cobalamin malabsorption should have abnormally low urine B$_{12}$ excretions.

- Pancytopenia, elevated lactate dehydrogenase (LDH), and elevated bilirubin can occur
- The peripheral smear will be identical to that seen in vitamin B$_{12}$ deficiency
- Red cell folate levels may more accurately measure true tissue status because normal serum folate levels are a reflection of short-term intake
  - It is reasonable to use serum folate levels as an initial screen for deficiency since the test is less expensive and readily available
- Treat with oral folic acid (1 to 2 mg/day is usually sufficient)
- Rarely seen in the United States now with routine dietary folate supplementation

MYELODYSPLASTIC SYNDROMES

- Peripheral smear can have ovalocytes, and dysplastic-looking neutrophils with hypogranulation and Pelger-Huët-like abnormalities. Bone marrow usually does not show megaloblastic changes.
- Vitamin B$_{12}$ and folate levels should be normal
- See Chapter 50 for diagnostic and treatment information

CHEMOTHERAPEUTIC AGENTS

- Hydroxyurea and azathioprine are examples
- Peripheral smear should not show hypersegmented neutrophils

NONMEGALOBLASTIC MACROCYTIC ANEMIA

- Alcohol is the most common cause and may affect RBCs through several different mechanisms (Box 46-2)

BOX 46-2	Effect of Alcohol on Red Blood Cells

Macrocytosis without anemia can occur with regular intake of as little as a half-bottle of wine per day
Anemia may result from a number of different mechanisms
    Direct toxic effect on the bone marrow
    Iron deficiency caused by gastrointestinal bleeding
    Folic acid deficiency
    Liver disease causing splenic sequestration hemolysis
    Liver disease resulting in acanthocyte (spur cell) formation and hemolysis

- Hypothyroidism, multiple myeloma, liver disease, aplastic anemia, drugs, and MDS may also present with macrocytic anemia

Hemolytic Anemia

Basic Approach

- Defined as the premature destruction of RBCs
- Occurs by two different mechanisms:
  - Extravascular hemolysis: RBCs are prematurely removed from the circulation by the liver and spleen (most cases)
  - Intravascular hemolysis: RBCs lyse in the circulation
- Laboratory studies
  - **Reticulocyte index is greater than 2%**
  - Indirect bilirubin is elevated
  - LDH is elevated
  - Haptoglobin is low or absent; haptoglobin binds free Hgb and is then taken up by the reticuloendothelial system; during hemolysis the rate of haptoglobin

catabolism exceeds the liver's ability to produce it, resulting in a low or absent level

- Urine hemosiderin: present in intravascular hemolysis only
- Urine Hgb: present in severe intravascular hemolysis; urine dipstick test is positive for blood but no RBCs seen on microscopic examination
- Direct antiglobulin test (direct Coombs test; Fig. 46-7)
  - Useful in diagnosing immune hemolytic anemia (greater than 95% sensitivity) where there is antibody coating a patient's RBCs

- Done by mixing the patient's erythrocytes with antihuman globulin (which contains antibody to immunoglobulin G [IgG] and C3)
- If agglutination occurs, the test is positive and the diagnosis of immune hemolysis is made
- **Once a positive test is found, further testing is done to determine whether IgG and/or C3 are coating the patient's erythrocytes**
- Indirect antiglobulin test (indirect Coombs test)
  - Useful to detect antibodies present in a patient's serum
  - Helpful in detecting alloantibodies that were induced by prior transfusion or by fetal transfer of RBCs to the mother
- The peripheral smear can assist in developing a systematic approach to patients (Fig. 46-8)

IMMUNE HEMOLYTIC ANEMIA

- Autoimmune hemolytic anemia (a positive direct antiglobulin [Coombs] test)
  - Warm-antibody autoimmune hemolytic anemia
    - Autoantibodies optimally reactive at 37° C
    - **Almost always has IgG identified on red cell surface (Table 46-6)**
    - May also have C3 identified
    - Most cases are idiopathic
    - Can be a complication of an underlying disease
      - Lymphoproliferative disorder: CLL, lymphoma
      - Collagen vascular disease: SLE, RA
      - Ulcerative colitis
      - Congenital immunodeficiency
    - Findings include anemia, reticulocytosis, splenomegaly, and microspherocytosis
    - Rarely, patients may have separate antibodies directed at platelets causing concomitant thrombocytopenia (Evan syndrome)
    - Treatment
      - Initial: support with blood transfusions plus prednisone 1 mg/kg/day with or without IV immunoglobulin G (IgG)

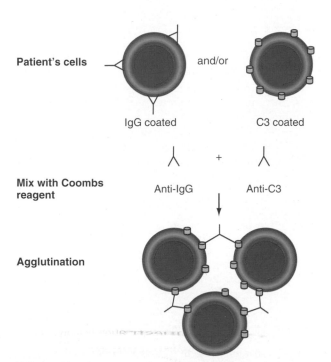

Patient's cells   and/or

IgG coated   C3 coated

Mix with Coombs reagent   Anti-IgG   +   Anti-C3

Agglutination

FIGURE 46-7 Direct antiglobulin (Coombs) test. IgG, Immunoglobulin G.

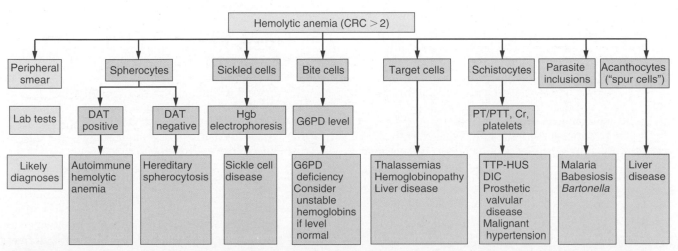

FIGURE 46-8 Basic approach to hemolytic anemia. Cr, Creatinine; CRC, corrected reticulocyte count; DAT, direct antiglobulin test; DIC, disseminated intravascular coagulation; G6PD, glucose-6-phosphate dehydrogenase; Hgb, hemoglobin; PT/PTT, prothrombin time/partial thromboplastin time; TTP-HUS, thrombotic thrombocytopenic purpura–hemolytic uremic syndrome.

TABLE 46-6	*Interpretation of Antiglobulin Tests in Immune Hemolytic Anemia*		
Condition	**DAT-IgG**	**DAT-C3**	**IAT**
Warm Ab	+	±	± No specific Ab
Cold agglutinin	−	+	± No specific Ab
Drug: methyldopa	+	−	± No specific Ab
Drug: PCN, ceph	+*	−	± No specific Ab
Drug: quinine, sulfa	−	+	± No specific Ab
Delayed transfusion reaction	+	±	+ With alloantibody found

*Positive only during exposure to drug.

Ab, Antibody; ceph, cephalosporins; DAT, direct antiglobulin (Coombs) test; IAT, indirect antiglobulin test; IgG, immunoglobulin G; PCN, penicillin.

- Splenectomy: if refractory to prednisone
- Immunosuppressives and/or cytotoxic agents: if refractory to splenectomy and prednisone
- Cold agglutinin syndrome
    - **Caused by an immunoglobulin M (IgM) complement-fixing antibody that binds to C3 on the red cell surface at low temperatures (4° C)**
    - Patients may have worsening of hemolysis and acrocyanosis when exposed to the cold
    - Direct antiglobulin (Coombs) test is positive for C3
    - Associated with a number of infections
        - *Mycoplasma* pneumonia self-limited hemolysis can occur 5 to 10 days after recovery from infection
        - Infectious mononucleosis (Epstein-Barr virus)
    - Also associated with lymphoproliferative disorders and monoclonal gammopathy
        - Disease may be mild and chronic
        - Reticulocytosis may be minimal
    - Diagnosed by IgM cold agglutinin antibody titers
        - Low titers (less than 1:32) can be found in normal serum
        - **Most patients with disease have titers in excess of 1:1000 at 4° C**
    - Treatment is usually supportive, but rituximab, chemotherapeutics, and immunosuppressives have been used
- Paroxysmal cold hemoglobinuria
    - Very rare disorder historically associated with tertiary syphilis
    - Most cases in adults are autoimmune
    - Caused by IgG (Donath-Landsteiner) antibody that can induce hemolysis (and often hemoglobinuria) with cold exposure
    - Direct antiglobulin test can be positive with anti-C3 during episodes of hemolysis but negative between episodes
    - Initial treatment is with prednisone
- Drug-induced hemolytic anemia
    - Drug-independent autoantibody induction
        - Presents identically to warm-antibody hemolytic anemia
        - Seen with methyldopa, procainamide, ibuprofen
        - Red cells coated with IgG but not C3
        - Hemolysis decreases weeks after cessation of drug

- Drug-dependent drug adsorption
    - Antibody is directed against the drug and the membrane protein to which it is attached
    - Direct antiglobulin test is positive for IgG during the period of drug administration
    - Seen most commonly with cephalosporins and high-dose penicillin
- Drug-dependent immune complex
    - Drugs loosely bind to RBC membrane with formation of antibodies reacting to both drug and membrane components
    - Results in stimulation of complement cascade
    - Direct antiglobulin test is positive for C3 but not IgG
    - Seen most commonly with cephalosporins, quinine, quinidine, sulfa drugs
- Nonimmunologic protein adsorption
    - Hypothesized that drug induces change in RBC membrane properties
    - Associated with prolonged exposure to high-dose cephalothin, although other drugs have been implicated as well
- Transfusion-related hemolysis (see Table 46-1)

NONIMMUNE HEMOLYTIC ANEMIA (DIRECT COOMBS' TEST NEGATIVE)

- Inherited nonimmune hemolytic anemia
    - RBC membrane disorders
        - Hereditary spherocytosis
            - More common in patients of northern European ancestry but occurs in all racial groups
            - Clinical manifestations include anemia, splenomegaly, and jaundice
            - Disease severity can range from mild (no anemia) to death in utero
            - Gallstone formation is common
            - Aplastic crises can develop during viral infections (e.g., parvovirus)
            - The mean corpuscular Hgb concentration (MCHC) is commonly elevated
            - Diagnosis is suspected in patients with clinical evidence of hemolytic anemia, spherocytes on peripheral smear (Fig. 46-9), and a negative direct antiglobulin test
            - An abnormal osmotic fragility test confirms the diagnosis (hemolysis occurs at progressively diluted salt concentrations)

46

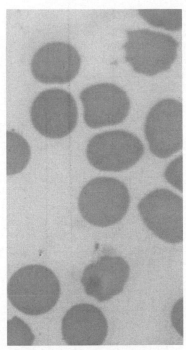

FIGURE 46-9 Hereditary spherocytosis. (From Stevens A, Lowe J. *Pathology.* 2nd ed. St. Louis: Mosby; 2000, Fig. 15.23.)

- ■ Treat with supportive care (e.g., transfusions) and folic acid
- ■ Splenectomy (with or without cholecystectomy) is the treatment of choice in symptomatic patients
- ■ Hereditary elliptocytosis
  - ■ Similar in presentation to spherocytosis
  - ■ More than 75% of cells are elliptical
- ■ RBC enzyme defects
  - ■ Glucose-6-phosphate dehydrogenase (G6PD) deficiency
    - ■ G6PD helps protect Hgb from oxidation on exposure to a drug or toxin that results in the generation of free radicals
    - ■ The World Health Organization has classified different G6PD variants based on the magnitude of enzyme deficiency and the severity of hemolysis (from class V, which is not clinically significant, to class I, most severe)
    - ■ Drugs that have been implicated include primaquine, sulfa drugs, dapsone, and nitrofurantoin
    - ■ Favism is the acute hemolysis seen in some patients with G6PD deficiency after ingestion of fava beans
    - ■ Patients present with an acute hemolytic reaction of varying severity 2 to 4 days after exposure to a drug
    - ■ Infections and diabetic ketoacidosis can also trigger hemolysis
    - ■ Can see "bite" cells on peripheral smear
    - ■ Can also see Heinz bodies (precipitated Hgb) with a reticulocyte stain
    - ■ **Diagnosis is made by measuring the level of the G6PD enzyme, but this may be normal**

TABLE 46-7	*Clinical Manifestations of Sickle Cell Disease*
Organ System	**Type of Complication**
CNS	Stroke Subarachnoid hemorrhage
Eye	Retinopathy Hyphema

Lung	Acute chest syndrome
	   Most common cause of death in adults
	   Patients present with fever, chest pain, and an infiltrate on chest radiography
	   Treat with antibiotics and oxygen
	   Exchange transfusion indicated if there is progressive hypoxemia
	Fat emboli
	Restrictive lung disease
	Pulmonary hypertension/cor pulmonale

Heart	MI CHF (rare)
Renal	Nephrotic syndrome Hypertension Chronic renal failure Hyposthenuria Hematuria Hyperuricemia
Urologic	Priapism
Bone	Joint effusions Avascular necrosis
Skin	Hyperpigmentation Leg ulcers
Liver/GB	Acute/chronic liver disease Gallstones
Infectious disease	Pneumonia (*Streptococcus pneumoniae, Haemophilus influenzae*) Osteomyelitis (*Salmonella* spp., *Staphylococcus aureus*) Urinary tract infection Sepsis
Heme	Chronic hemolytic anemia Splenic sequestration crisis Acute aplastic crisis

CHF, Congestive heart failure; CNS, central nervous system; GB, gallbladder; MI, myocardial infarction.

when there is active hemolysis (levels are high in young reticulocytes)
- ■ Treatment is supportive and avoidance of the offending agent
- ■ Sickle cell disorders (SS, Sβ-thal, SC)
  - ■ Characterized by a chronic hemolytic state in which vasoocclusion is caused by a deformity of RBCs
  - ■ Sickle trait rarely has clinical implications
  - ■ Hgb SC disease is usually milder than Hgb SS disease
  - ■ Functional asplenia results from SS disease
  - ■ Most common presentation is acute pain crisis but can affect virtually every organ system (Table 46-7)

- The most life-threatening complications include acute chest syndrome, stroke, and infections
- **Pulmonary hypertension occurs in about 30% of adults with sickle cell disease and is a strong predictor for near-term mortality**
- Hgb electrophoresis establishes the diagnosis
- Treatment
  - Pain crises: hydration and analgesics (avoid meperidine); transfusion usually not needed despite severity of anemia caused by chronic compensation
  - Acute chest syndrome: antibiotics, oxygen, simple or exchange transfusion
  - Stroke: exchange transfusion
  - Hematopoietic cell transplantation may be potentially curative, but criteria for this option are still being developed
- Prevention of complications
  - Vaccination: pneumococcal, *Haemophilus influenzae* type b, *Meningococcus*, influenza
  - Folate may be necessary to keep up with cell turnover
  - Regular retinal examinations
  - **Hydroxyurea: Has been shown to decrease the incidence of acute chest syndrome, decrease the number of pain crises, decrease transfusions, and possibly decrease mortality**
  - Preoperative transfusion to an Hgb level of 9 to 11 mg/dL can improve outcome in surgical patients
- Acquired nonimmune hemolytic anemia
  - Splenomegaly (sequestrational hemolysis)
    - Can lead to destruction of normal RBCs
    - Causes include lymphoproliferative disorders, myeloproliferative disorders, inflammatory diseases, infection, portal hypertension, and hemolytic anemia
  - March hemoglobinuria
    - Intravascular hemolysis with hemoglobinuria
    - Seen after prolonged physical activity
    - Anemia is usually not present
  - Microangiopathic hemolytic anemia
    - Cardiac hemolysis
      - Occurs in about 10% of patients with mechanical aortic valve replacements
      - Severity of the anemia is variable but can cause significant hemoglobinuria
      - Hemosiderin can be detected in the urine
      - Schistocytes seen on peripheral smear
      - Need to watch for iron deficiency because of Hgb loss in urine
      - **New-onset (or worsening) hemolysis in a patient with a prosthetic valve warrants an evaluation with an echocardiogram to assess for perivalvular leak and valve failure**
    - Thrombotic thrombocytopenic purpura-hemolytic uremic syndrome (see Chapter 47)

- Disseminated intravascular coagulation (see Chapter 48)
- Direct toxic effects on RBCs
  - Infections
    - Parasites: malaria, *Babesia*, *Bartonella*
    - *Clostridium welchii*: produces a phospholipase that can lead to membrane rupture
  - Snake and spider bites
  - Copper: seen in Wilson disease
- Paroxysmal nocturnal hemoglobinuria
  - Caused by an acquired mutation of the X-chromosome gene *PIGA*
  - Ultimately found in 10% to 20% of patients with aplastic anemia
  - Mutation results in impaired synthesis of glycosyl phosphatidylinositol-anchored proteins (GPI-APs)
  - Clinical presentation includes hemolytic anemia (intravascular), venous thrombosis (particularly at unusual sites), and/or deficient hematopoiesis
  - Some patients may also develop esophageal spasm and/or erectile dysfunction from a deficiency in nitric oxide during hemolytic episodes
  - Laboratory features
    - Normocytic anemia usually; can be microcytic if iron deficiency develops from loss of Hgb in the urine
    - Hemoglobinuria: present only intermittently
    - Hemosiderinuria: present in virtually all patients
    - Leukopenia and thrombocytopenia: usually mild but can develop into aplastic anemia
  - Diagnosis
    - Flow cytometry is the test of choice, with demonstration of deficiency of GPI-APs CD55 and CD59
  - Treatment
    - Supportive care with iron, folate, and blood transfusions
    - Humanized monoclonal antibody against complement protein C5 (e.g., eculizumab) reduces the need for transfusion, ameliorates (but does not eliminate) the anemia, and improves quality of life
      - Does not affect the underlying stem cell disorder
      - Treatment is lifelong
      - **Increases the risk of *Neisseria meningitides* infection, so need to vaccinate before therapy begins**
    - Anticoagulation if thrombosis is present
    - BMT can be considered if a donor is available and severe disease is present despite eculizumab

Review Questions

For review questions, please go to ExpertConsult.com.

SUGGESTED READINGS

DeLoughery TG. Microcytic anemia. *N Engl J Med.* 2014;371: 1324-1331.

Parker CJ. Bone marrow failure syndromes: paroxysmal nocturnal hemoglobinuria. *Hematol Oncol Clin North Am.* 2009;23:333-346.

Piel FB, Weatherall DJ. The α-thalassemias. *N Engl J Med.* 2014;371: 1908-1916.

Sawada K, Hirokawa M, Fujishima N. Diagnosis and management of acquired pure red cell aplasia. *Hematol Oncol Clin North Am.* 2009; 23:249-259.

Steinberg MH. In the clinic. Sickle cell disease. *Ann Intern Med.* 2011; 155:ITC31–15.

Swiecicki PL, Hegerova LT, Gertz MA. Cold agglutinin disease. *Blood.* 2013;122:1114-1121.

Yawn BP, Buchanan GR, Afenyi-Annan AN, et al. Management of sickle cell disease: summary of the 2014 evidence-based report by expert panel members. *JAMA.* 2014;312:1033-1048.

Platelet Disorders

SOPHIE M. LANZKRON, MD, MHS

Platelet disorders may result in life-threatening consequences. They may be caused by an isolated defect in the platelet's role in clot formation or may be evidence of systemic disease. A stepwise approach in the evaluation of a patient with a suspected platelet disorder is essential to make the diagnosis and initiate treatment.

BASIC INFORMATION

- Normal platelet function requires four steps to result in clot formation: activation, adhesion, aggregation, and secretion (Fig. 47-1)
- Platelet dysfunction can be categorized as caused by quantitative defects (i.e., the number of platelets), qualitative defects (i.e., how well they function), or both
  - Quantitative assessment of platelets is performed by machine counters and by visualization of the peripheral smear
    - **Automated tests identifying thrombocytopenia should be confirmed with visual inspection of a peripheral smear**
  - Bleeding complications may be associated with thrombocytosis if the platelets produced are dysfunctional or if there is an acquired von Willebrand factor (vWF) deficiency
  - Qualitative assessment for defects in platelet function is evaluated by obtaining a bleeding history, bleeding time, platelet function analyzer (PFA-100), and aggregometry (see later discussion)

Clinical Evaluation

- The medical history
  - Clues in the history suggestive of platelet dysfunction include the following:
    - **Bleeding that is limited to superficial sites such as skin or mucosa (hemarthroses are uncommon with platelet disorders and usually represent defects in the clotting cascade)**
    - **Bleeding that starts immediately after trauma or surgery**
    - Excessive menstrual bleeding
    - Other family members with bleeding histories suggest an inherited platelet disorder
    - Many medications may result in thrombocytopenia or dysfunctional platelets; medication (and toxin) exposure should be reviewed in any patient with a suspected platelet disorder
    - Disorders of platelet excess (e.g., thrombocytosis) are most commonly reactions to other illnesses (e.g., acute hemorrhage, iron deficiency, infection),

which should be sought in the history (see later discussion)
- Physical examination
  - **Clues in the physical examination suggestive of platelet dysfunction include the following:**
    - **Petechiae**
    - **Mucosal bleeding**
    - Splenomegaly (may suggest an underlying bone marrow process or liver disease that may be causing platelet abnormalities)

Laboratory Evaluation

- Peripheral blood smear (Fig. 47-2)
  - Great importance for evaluating both qualitative and quantitative deficiencies in platelets
  - Used to confirm platelet number
    - Spuriously low platelet counts may occur as a result of interaction between ethylenediaminetetraacetic acid (EDTA) and platelet glycoproteins, leading to platelet aggregation; repeating the platelet count drawn in a citrated (rather than an EDTA) tube will verify that the platelet count is normal
  - Used to evaluate platelet morphology
    - Both the size of platelets and the presence of platelet granularity may aid in the diagnosis
    - Many disorders can produce large platelets, but platelets that approximate the size of red blood cells (RBCs) are seen almost exclusively in the context of inherited platelet disorders
- Bleeding time
  - Reflects quantitative and qualitative platelet disorders as well as some vascular defects that are related to interactions with platelets
    - **Bleeding time does not involve the clotting cascade**
      - The most common technique is the Ivy technique, in which a blood pressure cuff is inflated to 40 mm Hg and a small, standardized incision is made in the forearm with a lancet; filter paper or cotton is used to absorb blood at regular intervals, and the time until cessation of bleeding is recorded
    - **Bleeding time is not useful in predicting bleeding risk, does not predict excessive surgical bleeding, and cannot predict bleeding risk in patients who have ingested aspirin**
  - Patients with uremia often have a bleeding diathesis and platelet dysfunction; no controlled study has demonstrated that patients with uremia and

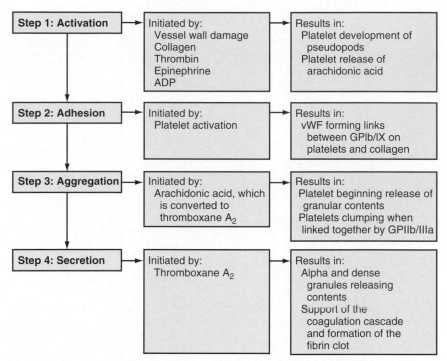

Step 1: Activation	→	Initiated by:
		    Vessel wall damage
		    Collagen
		    Thrombin
		    Epinephrine
		    ADP
			→	Results in:
				    Platelet development of
				        pseudopods
				    Platelet release of
				        arachidonic acid

Step 2: Adhesion	→	Initiated by:
		    Platelet activation
			→	Results in:
				    vWF forming links
				        between GPIb/IX on
				        platelets and collagen

Step 3: Aggregation	→	Initiated by:
		    Arachidonic acid, which
		    is converted to
		    thromboxane A_2
			→	Results in:
				    Platelet beginning release of
				        granular contents
				    Platelets clumping when
				        linked together by GPIIb/IIIa

Step 4: Secretion	→	Initiated by:
		    Thromboxane A_2
			→	Results in:
				    Alpha and dense
				        granules releasing
				        contents
				    Support of the
				        coagulation cascade
				        and formation of the
				        fibrin clot

FIGURE 47-1 Steps in normal platelet function. ADP, Adenosine diphosphate; GP, glycoprotein; vWF, von Willebrand factor.

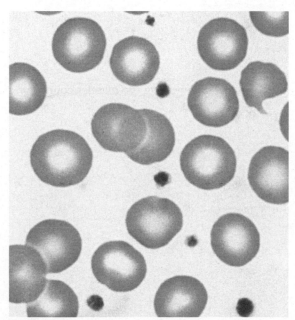

FIGURE 47-2 Normal platelets in a normal peripheral blood smear. (From Young B, Stevens A, Heath JW, et al. *Wheater's Functional Histology.* 5th ed. Philadelphia: Churchill Livingstone; 2006: Fig. 3.10.)

prolonged bleeding time have more surgical bleeding than those with normal bleeding time
- The PFA-100 is an in vitro test that evaluates platelet function
  - It is now being used in lieu of a bleeding time as it is more convenient and less invasive
  - **As with the bleeding time, the PFA-100 has not been shown to predict bleeding risk**

- Classic platelet aggregation assays
  - Platelet-rich plasma or whole blood is exposed to adenosine diphosphate, epinephrine, collagen, and ristocetin; the patterns of aggregation suggest specific platelet defects
- Ristocetin activity
  - Ristocetin is an antibiotic that induces platelet agglutination in the presence of vWF
  - This test is abnormal in patients deficient in vWF (i.e., patients with von Willebrand disease) or in the receptor for vWF (glycoprotein Ib/IX; i.e., Bernard-Soulier syndrome)
- **Laboratory tests for liver disease, hepatitis C, human immunodeficiency virus (HIV), and pregnancy should be ordered as all of these can manifest as thrombocytopenia**

Inherited Disorders of Platelets

Basic Information
- **Inherited platelet disorders are rare**
- There are four major inherited platelet disorders (Table 47-1)
- Glanzmann thrombasthenia and Bernard-Soulier syndrome are autosomal recessive
- Gray platelet syndrome (Fig. 47-3) and storage pool disease are of poorly defined inheritance patterns, in part because of their heterogeneous nature

Clinical Presentation
- Bleeding abnormalities may be present at birth or may become evident later in life
- Aspirin may exacerbate bleeding abnormalities

TABLE 47-1 *Inherited Platelet Disorders*

Platelet Disorder	Defect	Bleeding Time	Aggregation with Ristocetin?	Confirmatory Test	Treatment	Notes
Glanzmann thrombasthenia	Platelets lack functional GP IIb/IIIa receptor (needed to bind fibrinogen and cross-link platelets)	Prolonged	Yes	Flow cytometry, demonstrating absence of receptor	Local measures to stop bleeding; ε-aminocaproic acid. If severe bleeding, transfuse platelets (at risk of developing IIb/IIIa antibodies)	Platelets are normal in quantity and appearance
Bernard-Soulier syndrome	Platelets lack GP Ib/IX complexes (needed to bind subendothelial vWF)	Markedly prolonged	No	Flow cytometry, demonstrating absence of receptor	Local measures; ε-aminocaproic acid; platelet transfusion	Thrombocytopenia common
Gray platelet syndrome	Deficiency of α granules	Prolonged	Yes	Electron microscopy demonstrates absence of α granules	DDAVP; ε-aminocaproic acid; platelet transfusions rarely needed	Large, pale platelets Thrombocytopenia
Storage pool disease	Deficiency of dense granules	Normal or prolonged	Yes	Electron microscopy confirms absence of dense granules	DDAVP; ε-aminocaproic acid; cryoprecipitate; platelet transfusions rarely needed	First wave of platelet aggregation occurs, but second wave does not

DDAVP, Desmopressin; GP, glycoprotein; vWF, von Willebrand factor.

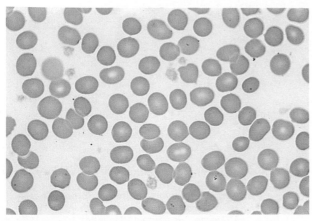

FIGURE 47-3 Gray platelet syndrome. (From Lewis SM, Bain BJ, Bates I. *Dacie and Lewis Practical Haematology.* 10th ed. Philadelphia: Churchill Livingstone; 2006: Fig. 5-97.)

- **Common early manifestations include easy bruising, gingival bleeding, and epistaxis**
- **Menorrhagia with menarche is also common**
- Bleeding with trauma may be severe and life threatening
  - Exception: Patients with gray platelet syndrome or storage pool disease often have only mild bleeding manifestations

Diagnosis

- **Bleeding time is prolonged in all these disorders, except some mild forms of storage pool disease**
- Ristocetin aggregation
  - Absent in Bernard-Soulier syndrome and von Willebrand disease
  - Present in Glanzmann thrombasthenia
- For other results of diagnostic testing, see Table 47-1

Treatment

- **Treatment is determined by severity of bleeding; mild bleeding episodes are treated with local measures (e.g., compression)**
- **Platelet transfusion should be reserved for major episodes of bleeding because transfusion increases risk of alloimmunization and development of platelet receptor antibodies**
- Aminocaproic acid and tranexamic acid
  - Antifibrinolytic agents
  - Useful for treatment of all inherited platelet disorders
- Desmopressin (DDAVP)
  - Analogue of arginine vasopressin but with no activity on blood pressure or vasoconstriction
  - Through an unclear mechanism, increases plasma levels of factor VIII and vWF
  - Effective for treatment of gray platelet syndrome and storage pool disease

Acquired Disorders of Platelets

Basic Information

- **Acquired platelet disorders more common than inherited platelet disorders**

TABLE 47-2	Common Acquired Platelet Disorders
Category of Disorder	**Examples**
Medication-related	Aspirin, NSAIDs, heparin, penicillin, quinine/quinidine, GP IIb/IIIa inhibitors, clopidogrel/ticlopidine
Medical disease-related	Uremia Liver disease Cardiopulmonary bypass
Hematologic or immunologic disease-related	Paraproteinemia ITP TTP HELLP syndrome Myeloproliferative disorders Myelodysplasia Disseminated intravascular coagulation
Infection-related	HIV, CMV, EBV, hantavirus, *Mycoplasma*, viral hepatitis

CMV, Cytomegalovirus; EBV, Epstein-Barr virus; HELLP, hemolysis, elevated liver enzymes, and low platelet count; GP, glycoprotein; HIV, human immunodeficiency virus; ITP, idiopathic thrombocytopenic purpura; NSAIDs, nonsteroidal antiinflammatory drugs; TTP, thrombotic thrombocytopenic purpura.

- Acquired platelet disorders may result from medications, medical disorders, or hematologic disorders (including immune disorders; Table 47-2). These should all be considered in the history, physical, and laboratory evaluation of the patient with a suspected acquired platelet disorder.

Clinical Presentation

- Clinical presentation varies but typically results in bleeding
- Exceptions include the following:
  - Heparin-induced thrombocytopenia (HIT) type 2 is associated with thrombosis (Table 47-3)
  - Myeloproliferative disorders, in which patients may have bleeding or thrombosis
- Medication-related platelet disorders (Box 47-1; see also Table 47-3) may result in immediate increase in risk of bleeding by deactivating platelets or delayed impact on bleeding risk if pathogenesis includes development of autoantibodies
- Medical disease-related platelet disorders (specifically liver disease; Table 47-4) may result in apparent thrombocytopenia caused by sequestration but no clinical bleeding disorder; other causes are included in Table 47-4
- **Hematologic/immunologic disease-related platelet disorders might be associated with normal numbers of abnormally functioning platelets, decreased platelet counts, or both**
  - Paraproteinemias may cause destruction or dysfunction of platelets
  - Myeloproliferative disorders may be associated with thrombocytopenia or thrombocytosis; one third of these patients have bleeding complications, and one third have thrombosis

47

TABLE 47-3	*Medication-Related Platelet Disorders*	
Medication	**Mechanism**	**Notes**
Aspirin	Irreversibly acetylates COX-1 and COX-2	COX-1 needed for production of thromboxane A_2, which is needed for platelet aggregation Impact present for lifetime of platelet (7–10 days)
NSAIDs	Reversibly acetylate COX-1 and COX-2	Impact present only for half-life of drug
Heparin	HIT type 1: nonimmune-mediated; begins a few days after initiation of heparin and will spontaneously resolve if heparin is continued HIT type 2: immune-mediated development of antibodies against heparin/platelet factor 4 complex; begins 5–10 days after initiation of heparin	Type 2 associated with thrombosis (type 1 is not) Suspect a type 2 process if the platelet count falls by >50% within 5–10 days of heparin initiation **Heparin must be discontinued immediately in HIT type 2** **Anticoagulation with a direct thrombin inhibitor should be started immediately if HIT type 2 is suspected** An earlier onset of thrombocytopenia is possible if there has been exposure to heparin in the prior 3 months Thromboses can present 40 days after heparin exposure Type 2 HIT confers significant risk of in-hospital mortality
Penicillin	Binds covalently to platelet membrane and acts as hapten	Typically occurs on reexposure to drug, with rapid drop in platelets Treated by discontinuing drug
Clopidogrel/ ticlopidine	Induces platelet clumping in the microvasculature and results in TTP Inhibits ADP-induced platelet aggregation	Treated by discontinuing the drug and plasmapheresis Peripheral blood smear is essential for diagnosis Impact present for lifetime of platelet (7–10 days)
GP IIB/IIIa inhibitors	Binds directly to the GP IIb/IIIa receptor, exposing neoantigens that are bound by preformed antibody. Thrombocytopenia occurs rapidly following initiation of the drug.	Treated by discontinuing the drug. Platelets should recover at a rate of about 20,000/day (rate of bone marrow production). Peripheral blood smear should be performed to demonstrate isolated thrombocytopenia without schistocytes May be safely treated with platelet transfusions
Quinine/quinidine, procainamide, gold salts	Induces production of autoantibodies to platelet membrane	Treated by discontinuing drug May require treatment with IVIg or steroids

ADP, Adenosine diphosphate; COX, cyclooxygenase; GP, glycoprotein; HIT, heparin-induced thrombocytopenia; IVIg, intravenous immune globulin; NSAIDs, nonsteroidal antiinflammatory drugs; TTP, thrombotic thrombocytopenic purpura.

BOX 47-1	*Select Medications Associated with Platelet Dysfunction*

Aspirin	β-Lactam antibiotics
Nonsteroidal antiinflammatory drugs	Abciximab
	Heparin
Quinine/quinidine	Dextran
Calcium channel blockers	Lepirudin
Ticlopidine	Alcohol
Clopidogrel	Dipyridamole
Nitroglycerin	Antipsychotics
Nitroprusside	Prostacyclin
Thrombolytic agents	

For a complete list of drugs associated with thrombocytopenia, see Pedersen-Bjergaard U, Andersen M, Hansen PB. Drug-specific characteristics of thrombocytopenia caused by non-cytotoxic drugs. *Eur J Clin Pharmacol.* 1998;54:701–706; and Pedersen-Bjergaard U, Andersen M, Hansen PB. Drug-induced thrombocytopenia: clinical data on 309 cases and the effect of corticosteroid therapy. *Eur J Clin Pharmacol.* 1997;52:183–189.

- Myelodysplasia may result in decreased platelet production or in production of abnormal platelets
- Posttransfusion purpura develops when alloantibodies are produced against platelet surface antigens, resulting in a decline in platelet count 7 to 10 days after RBC transfusion; treatment is with intravenous immune globulin (IVIg)
- Immune thrombocytopenic purpura (ITP), thrombotic thrombocytopenic purpura (TTP), hemolysis/elevated liver enzymes/low platelet count (HELLP syndrome), and disseminated intravascular coagulation (DIC) are described in Table 47-5
- **HIV and hepatitis C can cause thrombocytopenia directly**
  - HIV can infect the stromal cells of the bone marrow, leading to decreased platelet production
  - HIV can also be associated with ITP
  - Hepatitis C appears also to have a direct effect on platelets that is not well understood. Recent literature suggests that clearance of hepatitis C virus

TABLE 47-4 *Medical Disease-Related Platelet Disorders*

Medical Disease	Mechanism	Notes
Uremia	Multifactorial, with uremic toxins causing defect in platelet aggregation	Treatment options include dialysis, DDAVP, cryoprecipitate, or estrogen DDAVP increases release of factor VIII:vWF from endothelial cells Cryoprecipitate includes factor VIII:vWF Mechanism of estrogen not understood; given IV, it can be efficacious in 24 hours Erythropoietin or transfusions should be given to maintain a hematocrit of 30% Dialysis improves platelet adhesion to the vessel wall and can decrease bleeding
Liver disease	Dysfibrinogenemia, not thrombocytopenia, leads to bleeding risk	Sequestered platelets will be available should need arise Platelet transfusion, DDAVP, and cryoprecipitate may be used
Cardiopulmonary bypass	Destruction of platelets in bypass circuit as well as platelet dysfunction from activation of platelets	50% drop in platelets common postoperatively Platelet dysfunction a minor cause of postoperative bleeding Prophylactic administration of platelets preoperatively not indicated
Sepsis	Increased platelet phagocytosis mediated by increased concentration of macrophage colony-stimulating factor	Sepsis can also precipitate DIC
HIV	ITP is a major cause, also direct infection of marrow stromal cells contributing to hematopoiesis	1.7% of patients with HIV and 8.7% of patients with AIDS will be asymptomatically thrombocytopenic Increased risk associated with IVDA, anemia, lower CD4 Treatment is the same as for conventional ITP but with the addition of HAART AZT seems to improve platelet count and so should be considered in selecting a regimen Response to prednisone is 80%–90%
Hepatitis C	Unknown mechanism	Recent research has demonstrated a correlation between clearance of viremia and platelet count recovery

AIDS, Acquired immunodeficiency syndrome; AZT, zidovudine; DDAVP, desmopressin; DIC, disseminated intravascular coagulation; HAART, highly active antiretroviral therapy; HIV, human immunodeficiency virus; ITP, idiopathic thrombocytopenic purpura; IV, intravenously; IVDA, intravenous drug abuse; vWF, von Willebrand factor.

infection can result in resolution of thrombocytopenia.

Diagnosis

- **This group of disorders is distinguished by onset of a new platelet-related bleeding disorder in a patient without a preexisting platelet-related bleeding disorder**
- Diagnosis requires a thorough review of all medications that affect either platelet function or production because medications are a common cause of acquired platelet disorders
  - Because the life of a platelet is 7 to 10 days, exposure to a medication that affects platelet function would have to occur within this time
  - Medications (and toxins) that affect platelet production may have a longer interval between exposure and clinical presentation
- **Evaluation of the peripheral blood smear remains essential in this group of disorders to exclude TTP in any patient with an acquired platelet disorder (Fig. 47-4)**
- Antibodies
  - Antiplatelet antibodies are seen in 80% of individuals with ITP

- Anti-heparin/platelet factor 4 complex antibodies are seen in HIT type 2 and mediate platelet activation, which results in increased thrombosis
- The diagnosis of HIT is confirmed by a positive serotonin release assay (a functional assay that measures heparin-dependent platelet activation)
- Evaluation of the bone marrow may be needed in ITP in elderly patients to exclude myeloproliferative, lymphoproliferative, or myelodysplastic disorders

Treatment

- Treatment is based in part on the presence or absence of immediate complications, including either bleeding or thrombosis; if life-threatening bleeding is present, platelet transfusion should be considered
  - **An exception is patients with thrombocytopenia resulting from TTP; patients with TTP should not receive platelet transfusions; treatment is plasmapheresis**
    - **If plasmapheresis is not immediately available, patients should receive fresh-frozen plasma**
- At times, correction of the underlying disorder (e.g., dialysis in a patient with uremia and dysfunctional

TABLE 47-5	Selected Hematologic or Immunologic Disease-Related Platelet Disorders		
Disease	**Basic Information**	**Diagnosis**	**Treatment**
ITP	Most commonly affects women in second and third decade of life Mechanism is autoantibodies against platelet membrane glycoproteins	Diagnosis of exclusion Antiplatelet antibodies demonstrated in 80% of cases Bone marrow shows normal or increased megakaryocytes May be secondary to HIV, SLE, thyroid disease, CLL, lymphoma, and solid tumors	Corticosteroids 1 to 2 mg/kg/day IVIg in refractory cases or if active bleeding Splenectomy rarely needed Transfuse platelets only if severe thrombocytopenia (platelet count <20,000/mm³) and bleeding Thrombopoietin mimetics can be used in refractory cases
TTP	More common in women, typically in their fourth decade of life; 10%–40% report viral URI in 2 weeks before onset Because of autoantibodies against ADAMTS 13: metalloproteinase that cleaves ultralarge vWF multimers	Pentad of symptoms: microangiopathic hemolytic anemia, thrombocytopenia, neurologic symptoms, fever, renal dysfunction Most have hemolytic anemia, thrombocytopenia, and neurologic symptoms; only 40% have complete pentad Neurologic symptoms may range from headache to coma Renal symptoms may include hematuria or proteinuria, with or without renal insufficiency	Plasmapheresis is treatment of choice; done daily until neurologic symptoms, platelet count, and LDH have been normal for 3 consecutive days 30% will relapse Corticosteroids have a questionable role in treatment Splenectomy reserved for refractory cases
HELLP syndrome	One of several causes of thrombocytopenia in pregnant women Normal pregnancy associated with mild thrombocytopenia (100,000–150,000/mm³) ITP, TTP, and DIC also may be associated with pregnancy	Patient typically presents with right upper quadrant pain Often associated with eclampsia/preeclampsia Hematologic findings include hemolysis and low platelet count	Delivery of fetus is definitive treatment, although abnormalities may persist Some evidence that corticosteroids are effective if delay of delivery desired
DIC	Process may be initiated by infection (especially gram-negative bacteria), obstetric complications, tissue injury, burns, or certain malignancies Generation of thrombin is central to pathogenesis; this allows consumption of fibrinogen, factor V, and factor VIII	Coagulopathy usually overshadowed by symptoms of illness that initiated DIC, but bleeding is major clinical manifestation, with thrombosis less common Common laboratory markers include elevated D-dimer and fibrin degradation products, prolongation of PT and PTT, and low fibrinogen and platelet counts	Treat underlying disorder while initiating aggressive supportive measures Platelet transfusions, cryoprecipitate, and FFP may be used if bleeding predominates, especially if associated with very low fibrinogen or platelet counts Heparin indicated if thrombotic complications predominate

ADAMTS, A disintegrin and metalloproteinase with thrombospondin motifs; CLL, chronic lymphocytic leukemia; DIC, disseminated intravascular coagulation; FFP, fresh-frozen plasma; HELLP, hemolysis, elevated liver enzymes, and low platelet count; HIV, human immunodeficiency virus; ITP, idiopathic thrombocytopenic purpura; IVIg, intravenous immune globulin; LDH, lactate dehydrogenase; PT, prothrombin time; PTT, partial thromboplastin time; SLE, systemic lupus erythematosus; TTP, thrombotic thrombocytopenic purpura; URI, upper respiratory infection; vWF, von Willebrand factor.

platelets) may be all that is needed to correct the bleeding disorder

- Medications that are used to treat platelet disorders include the following:
  - DDAVP: a synthetic form of arginine vasopressin that increases plasma levels of vWF factor and factor VIII
  - Corticosteroids are used in disorders in which an immune component predominates; they are the initial treatment of choice for ITP
  - Rh₀(D) immune globulin (Rh₀GAM) can also be used effectively in Rh-positive patients with ITP and bleeding, inducing splenic sequestration of Rh-positive antibody–coated RBCs, thereby sparing

platelets; caution should be taken in using Rh₀(D) as it can cause significant, even life-threatening hemolysis

  - Thrombopoietin (TPO) mimetics: drugs that mimic the effect of TPO available to treat thrombocytopenia; increase the platelet count in more than 80% of patients with ITP
- Plasmapheresis separates plasma from RBCs via centrifugation so that RBCs can be preserved and plasma discarded
  - Plasmapheresis is essential treatment for TTP but is also used for some paraproteinemias
- Cryoprecipitate is a fraction of plasma that is frozen and then thawed (hence the name); the freeze-thaw

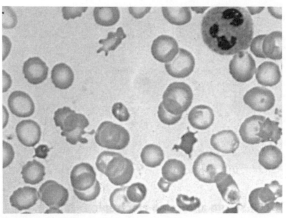

FIGURE 47-4 Thrombocytopenia caused by disseminated intravascular coagulation. Note that platelets are nearly absent. (From Forbes CD, Jackson WF. *Color Atlas and Text of Clinical Medicine.* 3rd ed. St. Louis: Mosby; 2003: Fig. 10.115.)

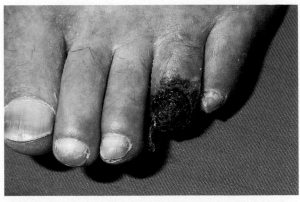

FIGURE 47-5 Thrombocytosis causing vessel occlusion and gangrene. (From Haslett C, Chilvers ER, Boon NA, et al. *Davidson's Principles and Practice of Medicine.* 19th ed. New York; Churchill Livingstone; 2002: Fig. 19.15.)

47

process results in high concentrations of factor VIII, vWF, and fibrinogen
- Cryoprecipitate can be used in patients who have depleted fibrinogen as a result of DIC and can be useful in patients with bleeding from uremia

Thrombocytosis

Basic Information

- **Thrombocytosis is most commonly diagnosed when the platelet count is greater than 600,000/mm³**
- Thrombocytosis may occur either in response to medical illness (i.e., reactive thrombocytosis) or as a clonal disorder
- **Reactive thrombocytosis is much more common than clonal disorders**

Clinical Presentation

- Reactive thrombocytosis may occur in response to infections (e.g., pneumonia, osteomyelitis, tuberculosis) or chronic inflammatory conditions (e.g., vasculitis, rheumatoid arthritis)
  - Other causes of reactive thrombocytosis include iron deficiency, acute hemorrhage, hemolysis, and splenectomy; some nonhematologic malignancies may also be accompanied by thrombocytosis
  - Clinical manifestations of reactive thrombocytosis are rarely seen, and symptoms of the underlying illness predominate
- Clonal thrombocytosis may be caused by an isolated clonal overproduction of platelets (i.e., essential thrombocytosis; Fig. 47-5), but is also commonly seen in polycythemia vera; other clonal disorders include idiopathic myelofibrosis, myelodysplastic syndromes, and chronic granulocytic leukemia
  - Hemorrhagic complications, although mild, are seen in up to 20% of individuals with essential thrombocytosis or polycythemia vera but rarely unless the platelet count exceeds 1,000,000/mm³

- **Thrombotic complications may be venous or arterial and are not predicted by the platelet count (see Fig. 47-5)**
  - Advanced age and previous thrombosis are the greatest predictors of increased risk of thrombosis

Diagnosis

- **As reactive thrombocytosis is by far more common, efforts should be made to exclude infection, chronic inflammation, and iron deficiency (among others) in any patient with thrombocytosis**
- Clonal thrombocytosis is confirmed by associated clinical features and often with cytogenetic markers, including the presence of *JAK2* mutations
  - Rarely, bone marrow aspirate and biopsy are needed
  - Clonal thrombocytosis may be associated with the phenomenon of erythromelalgia (painful erythema, typically of the feet and hands), mediated by platelet thrombi in the peripheral vasculature; aspirin is the treatment of choice for this symptom

Treatment

- Reactive thrombocytosis is treated by treating the underlying illness
- Clonal thrombosis treatment is dictated by the type of clonal disorder
  - Aspirin therapy reduces risk of thrombosis and may be used prophylactically in patients with essential thrombocytosis or polycythemia vera, provided they do not have acquired von Willebrand disease
  - Cytotoxic agents, including hydroxyurea, may be used short term to reduce platelet counts, even when cure is not possible
  - Anagrelide is an agent that prevents the maturation of megakaryocytes into platelets
    - It is used to decrease the platelet count in those with essential thrombocytosis
    - Caution is recommended with use in elderly patients because side effects can include heart failure, myocardial infarction, and pulmonary hypertension
  - JAK2 inhibitors tested in clinical trials in essential thrombocytosis and polycythemia vera have been shown to decrease platelet count

Acknowledgment

The author would like to thank Elizabeth A. Griffiths, MD, for her work on this chapter in previous editions.

Review Questions

For review questions, please go to ExpertConsult.com.

SUGGESTED READINGS

George JN. Platelets. *Lancet.* 2000;355:1531-1539.

George JN, Woolf SH, Rashkob GE, et al. Idiopathic thrombocytopenic purpura: a practice guideline developed by explicit methods for the American Society of Hematology. *Blood.* 1996;88:3-40.

Pedersen-Bjergaard U, Andersen M, Hansen PB. Drug-induced thrombocytopenia: clinical data on 309 cases and the effect of corticosteroid therapy. *Eur J Clin Pharmacol.* 1997;52:183-189.

Pedersen-Bjergaard U, Andersen M, Hansen PB. Drug-specific characteristics of thrombocytopenia caused by non-cytotoxic drugs. *Eur J Clin Pharmacol.* 1998;54:701-706.

Peterson P, Hayes TE, Arkin CF, et al. The preoperative bleeding time test lacks clinical benefit: College of American Pathologists and American Society of Clinical Pathologists position article. *Arch Surg.* 1998;133:134-139.

Warkentin TE, Kelton JG. A 14-year study of heparin-induced thrombocytopenia. *Am J Med.* 1996;101:502-507.

Williams WJ. *Hematology.* New York: McGraw-Hill; 1995.

CHAPTER 48

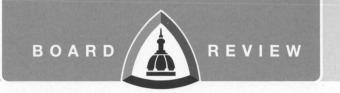
Coagulation Disorders

MICHAEL B. STREIFF, MD

Normal hemostasis is achieved by the cooperative function of coagulation proteins, platelets, and the vessel wall. Qualitative or quantitative abnormalities in any one of these components can precipitate excessive bleeding or thrombosis. Coagulation disorders are fairly common; therefore, internists should be familiar with the components of the hemostatic system, the tests used to evaluate their function, and the most common diseases that affect hemostasis. This chapter focuses on the coagulation system. Platelet disorders are covered in Chapter 47.

Bleeding Disorders

Basic Information

- Bleeding disorders vary in frequency and severity
- Can be categorized as congenital or acquired
- To understand and diagnose these conditions, one needs an understanding of the coagulation cascade (Fig. 48-1)
  - Intrinsic pathway: factors XII, XI, IX, and VIII, prekallikrein, and high-molecular-weight kininogen
  - Extrinsic pathway: factor VII, tissue factor
- Common congenital coagulation disorders include factor deficiencies such as hemophilia A (factor VIII deficiency), hemophilia B (factor IX deficiency), and hemophilia C (factor XI deficiency), as well as von Willebrand disease (vWD) (Table 48-1)
  - **vWD, the most common inherited bleeding disorder, may affect as many as 0.1% of the population**
    - von Willebrand factor (vWF) serves two functions in hemostasis:
      - It mediates the adhesion of platelets to damaged vessel walls
      - It binds to and protects factor VIII from degradation by activated protein C, thus prolonging factor VIII half-life in the plasma
    - Several types of vWD exist:
      - Type I vWD (75% of all vWD) is caused by mutations that result in a quantitative deficiency of functional vWF
      - Type II vWD subtypes (20% to 25%) are caused by mutations that result in the production of a dysfunctional vWF protein
      - Type III vWD (less than 5%) is rare and results in a severe quantitative deficiency of vWF
  - **Bleeding symptoms in vWD patients tend to be in mucosal sites (epistaxis, gum bleeding,**
  menorrhagia, etc.) and mild to moderate in severity; the exception is patients with type III disease, who can develop severe bleeding similar to hemophilia (hemarthroses, etc.)
- **Acquired coagulation disorders include the following:**
  - **Liver disease**
    - **Results in decreased synthesis of all coagulation factors except for factor VIII**
    - Laboratory tests typically show prolongation of the prothrombin time (PT), the activated partial thromboplastin time (aPTT), and the thrombin time (TT) (the last one caused by decreased or dysfunctional fibrinogen)
    - Treatment
      - Plasma for bleeding
      - Recombinant human factor VIIa (rhFVIIa) has been used off-label for life-threatening bleeding refractory to plasma, but it may be associated with an increased risk of thrombotic complications
      - Liver transplantation for definitive long-term management
  - Disseminated intravascular coagulation (DIC) (Box 48-1)
  - Vitamin K deficiency
    - Vitamin K is required for the synthesis of active forms of factors II, VII, IX, and X, as well as the natural anticoagulant proteins C and S
    - Vitamin K deficiency is common with the following conditions:
      - Poor nutrition (especially diets deficient in green, leafy vegetables)
      - Broad-spectrum antibiotics (which kill intestinal bacteria, a significant source of vitamin K)
      - Antibiotics with an *N*-methylthio-tetrazole (MTT) side chain (e.g., moxalactam, cefamandole, cefoperazone), which can interfere with vitamin K metabolism and potentiate the deficiency state
      - Malabsorption (e.g., biliary disease, which interferes with delivery of bile necessary for absorption of fat-soluble vitamins)
    - Vitamin K deficiency is characterized initially by a prolonged PT (factor VII has the shortest half-life of the coagulation factors; factors X and II also influence the PT), then by a prolonged aPTT (reflects factors IX, X, and II deficiency)
  - Coagulation factor inhibitors: antibodies directed against specific coagulation factors

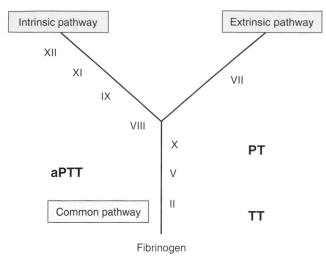

FIGURE 48-1 A simplified view of the coagulation cascade. aPTT, Activated partial thromboplastin time; PT, prothrombin time; TT, thrombin time.

- **Factor VIII inhibitors are the most common inhibitors that result in bleeding**
  - **Develop in 10% to 15% of hemophilia A patients because of chronic exposure to exogenous factor VIII**
  - Rarely occur in nonhemophiliacs (1 : 1,000,000); most common associations are with tumors, pregnancy, drugs, and rheumatologic conditions
  - Inhibitor titer (concentration of the antibody) measured by the Bethesda assay
    - Low-titer inhibitors (fewer than 5 Bethesda units) can be transiently overcome with large doses of factor VIII
    - High-titer inhibitors (more than 5 Bethesda units) require alternative plasma products, such as factor VIII inhibitor-bypassing activity (FEIBA) or rhFVIIa, which can activate the coagulation cascade in the presence of a factor VIII inhibitor
  - Hemophilia B patients have a lower incidence of inhibitor formation (2% to 4%)
- Vessel wall disorders
  - Immune complex-mediated destruction (cryoglobulinemia)
  - Inflammation (infection, vasculitis)
  - Destructive infiltration with proteins (amyloidosis)
  - Defective connective tissue structure (Ehlers-Danlos syndrome, vitamin C deficiency)
- Fibrinolytic disorders can also result in bleeding
  - Fibrinolytic system is responsible for clot digestion and remodeling (Fig. 48-2)
  - Excessive amounts of plasmin (the primary fibrinolytic enzyme) or its activators (tissue plasminogen activator, urokinase) or deficiency of inhibitors (plasminogen activator inhibitor-1, α_2-antiplasmin) can result in bleeding caused by hyperfibrinolysis
  - These are rare disorders characterized by delayed bleeding

Clinical Presentation

- Bleeding history
  - **Easy bruisability is very common and not always pathologic**
  - **More specific indications of a bleeding disorder are excessive bleeding with surgical procedures, an excessive transfusion requirement, a history of reoperation for bleeding, a positive family history of bleeding, and chronic iron-deficiency anemia**
  - A pretest probability model (the bleeding assessment tool) has been demonstrated to be useful in the likelihood of patients having a bleeding disorder (Table 48-2)
  - **Hemarthroses and soft tissue bleeds suggest a coagulation factor deficiency (Fig. 48-3)**
  - **Skin (petechiae) and mucosal (epistaxis, gingival bleeding, menorrhagia) bleeding are more suggestive of vWD or platelet disorders (Fig. 48-4)**
  - Delayed bleeding is typical of factor XIII deficiency or fibrinolytic defects; factor XIII deficiency is also associated with poor wound healing
- Physical examination findings for bleeding
  - Ecchymoses at inaccessible sites suggest a coagulation disorder (Fig. 48-5)
  - Palpable purpura indicates vessel wall inflammation (e.g., vasculitis)
  - Nonpalpable purpura suggests vessel wall disorders, such as scurvy (vitamin C deficiency) or connective tissue disorders (e.g., Ehlers-Danlos syndrome)

DIAGNOSIS AND EVALUATION

- Basic laboratory evaluation
  - PT: measures factors in the extrinsic and common pathways (see Fig. 48-1)
  - International normalized ratio (INR): a method for reporting PT results in patients on vitamin K antagonists (e.g., warfarin) that helps to normalize interlaboratory differences in reagent sensitivity to the effect of warfarin
  - aPTT: measures factors in the intrinsic and common pathways
  - TT: measures fibrinogen function
- Basic coagulation test scenarios
  - Isolated prolonged PT: extrinsic pathway defect (e.g., factor VII deficiency; see Fig. 48-1)
  - Isolated prolonged aPTT: intrinsic pathway defect (e.g., in order of frequency, factor VIII, factor IX, factor XI, factor XII, prekallikrein, or high-molecular-weight kininogen deficiency; the latter two accelerate factor XII activation)
    - Isolated prolonged aPTT (usually markedly prolonged) in the absence of clinical bleeding suggests factor XII, prekallikrein, or high-molecular-weight kininogen deficiency
  - Both PT and aPTT prolonged: common pathway defect (e.g., factor X, factor V, or prothrombin deficiency)
  - Isolated prolonged TT: fibrinogen deficiency or dysfunction, heparin or presence of a heparin-like

TABLE 48-1   *Selected Congenital Bleeding Disorders*

Disorder	Deficiency	Inheritance	aPTT	Laboratory Findings	Clinical Issues	Treatment
Hemophilia A	Factor VIII	X-linked recessive (1:10,000 male births)	↑	Reduced factor VIII level	Mild: factor VIII >5%; bleed after significant trauma Moderate: factor VIII = 1%–5%; bleed after minor trauma Severe: factor VIII <1%; spontaneous bleeding	Factor VIII concentrate
Hemophilia B (Christmas disease)	Factor IX	X-linked recessive (1:50,000 male births)	↑	Reduced factor IX level	Clinically similar to hemophilia A Same severity scale as hemophilia A	Factor IX concentrate
Hemophilia C (Rosenthal disease)	Factor XI	Autosomal-recessive; rare except among Ashkenazi Jews	↑	Reduced factor XI level	Variable severity, but usually mild; bleeding usually in response to trauma	Plasma
von Willebrand disease (vWD)	Quantitative or qualitative defect in von Willebrand factor (vWF)	Autosomal dominant or recessive (1:1000 live births)	Normal or ↑	vWF antigen detects the quantity of vWF protein Ristocetin cofactor activity measures vWF function Factor VIII activity may be low or normal Tests of platelet function (e.g., bleeding time) may also be abnormal	Function of vWF: aids in platelet adhesion and protection of factor VIII from inactivation Types of vWD: Type I: partial deficiency of vWF; 75% of vWD Type II: qualitative defect in vWF Type III: complete deficiency of vWF	DDAVP, which causes the release of preformed vWF multimers from endothelium Factor VIII concentrates that contain vWF (e.g., Humate P)
Factor XIII deficiency	Factor XIII	Autosomal recessive (rare: <1:1,000,000 live births)	Normal	Factor XIII screen Tests for clot solubility in 5 M urea (clot will dissolve because of lack of fibrin cross-links)	Factor XIII is important for cross-linking fibrin strands to make a clot more resistant to fibrinolysis Clinical symptoms include delayed bleeding after trauma or surgery, poor wound healing	Plasma

aPPT, Activated partial thromboplastin time; DDAVP, 1-deamino-8- D-arginine vasopressin.

48

BOX 48-1 Disseminated Intravascular Coagulation

Uncontrolled activation of the coagulation and fibrinolytic cascades caused by excessive tissue factor expression

Exuberant thrombin generation results in excess fibrin clot formation, platelet activation, and secondary fibrinolysis

Consumption of coagulation factors (including fibrinogen) and platelets results in bleeding. If fibrinolysis is inadequate or inhibited, thrombosis may predominate

Causes: infections, neoplasms, snake venom, endothelial disruption, and abnormalities of tissue factor release (e.g., from obstetric complications)

Clinical Presentation

May see bleeding from wounds and venipuncture sites, petechiae, ecchymoses, hematuria, hematemesis, and diffuse bleeding

Thromboembolic phenomena may include pulmonary emboli, necrotic skin lesions, and stroke

Lab diagnosis (suggestive but not diagnostic)

Prolonged aPTT, PT

Low fibrinogen concentration

Elevated D-dimer or fibrin degradation products (most sensitive tests)

Thrombocytopenia and schistocytes on the peripheral blood smear are supportive but nonspecific

Treatment: treat underlying disorder; provide supportive care (plasma, platelets); heparin may be worthwhile if thrombosis predominates (contraindicated if CNS lesions present)

Mortality rate: 50% to 80% in severe cases

aPTT, Activated partial thromboplastin time; CNS, central nervous system; PT, prothrombin time.

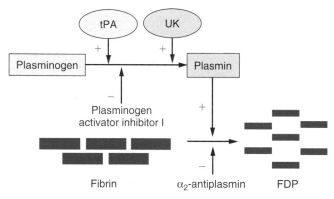

FIGURE 48-2 Regulation of the fibrinolytic system. FDP, Fibrin degradation products; tPA, tissue plasminogen activator; UK, urokinase.

TABLE 48-2 Bleeding Assessment Tool

Symptoms	Assigned Score
Epistaxis	0 = no or trivial 1 = present 2 = packing, cauterization 3 = transfusion, replacement
Cutaneous symptoms	0 = no or trivial 1 = petechiae or bruises 2 = hematomas 3 = medical consultation
Minor wounds	0 = no or trivial 1 = present (1-5 episodes/yr) 2 = medical attention 3 = surgery/blood transfusion
Oral cavity bleeding	0 = no or trivial 1 = present 2 = medical attention 3 = surgery/blood transfusion
Gastrointestinal bleeding	0 = no or trivial 1 = present 2 = medical attention 3 = surgery/blood transfusion
Postpartum hemorrhage	0 = no or trivial 1 = present, iron therapy 2 = blood transfusion, dilatation-curettage, suturing 3 = hysterectomy
Muscle hematomas or hemarthrosis	0 = no or trivial 1 = present 2 = medical attention 3 = transfusion, intervention
Tooth extraction (most severe episode)	0 = no or trivial 1 = present 2 = suturing or packing 3 = transfusion
Surgery (most severe episode)	0 = no or trivial 1 = present 2 = suturing or resurgery 3 = transfusion
Menorrhagia	0 = no or trivial 1 = present 2 = consultation, pill use, iron therapy 3 = transfusion, hysterectomy, dilatation-curettage, replacement therapy

A bleeding score of more than 10 = likely bleeding disorder; a bleeding score of less than 10 = unlikely to have a bleeding disorder.
From Rodeghiero F, Castaman G, Tosetto A, et al. The discriminant power of bleeding history for the diagnosis of type 1 von Willebrand disease: an international, multicenter study. *J Thromb Haemost.* 2005;3:2619–2626: Table 1.

factor (e.g., monoclonal proteins, fibrin degradation products), thrombin inhibitor

- Prolonged PT, aPTT, TT: generally the same considerations as isolated prolonged TT except heparins do not consistently prolong the PT
- Normal PT and aPTT: consider platelet disorders, vWD, factor XIII deficiency, fibrinolytic disorders, and vessel wall disorders

■ **Distinguishing between a factor deficiency and a factor inhibitor**

- ■ **Factor deficiency: The clotting time will correct when 1 part patient plasma is mixed with 1 part normal pooled plasma (NPP; 1:1 mix; Fig. 48-6)**
- ■ **Factor inhibitor: The clotting time fails to correct when 1 part patient plasma is mixed with 1 part normal pooled plasma (see Fig. 48-6)**
  - ■ Weak inhibitors may only be identified in a mix of 3 parts patient plasma with 1 part NPP

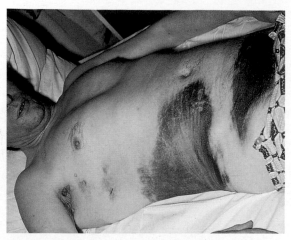

FIGURE 48-3 Massive hematomas in the absence of major trauma suggest a coagulation disorder such as hemophilia or supratherapeutic anticoagulant therapy. (From Forbes CD, Jackson WF. *Color Atlas and Text of Clinical Medicine.* 3rd ed. St. Louis: Mosby; 2003: Fig. 10.104.)

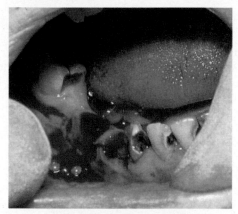

FIGURE 48-4 Hemorrhage after dental extraction is a common presentation of von Willebrand disease. (From Forbes CD, Jackson WF. *Color Atlas and Text of Clinical Medicine.* ed 3. St. Louis: Mosby; 2003: Fig. 10.105.)

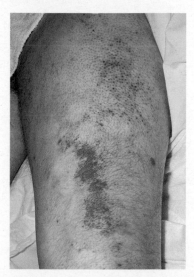

FIGURE 48-5 Ecchymoses and petechiae on the lateral thigh of a patient with septicemia complicated by disseminated intravascular coagulation. (From Mandell GL, Bennett JE, Dolin R. *Principles and Practice of Infectious Diseases.* 6th ed. Philadelphia: Churchill Livingstone; 2005: Fig. 226-7.)

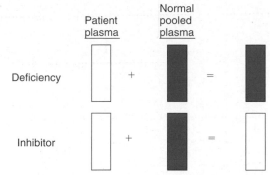

FIGURE 48-6 A mixing study. *Blue* denotes normal clotting activity; *white* denotes abnormal clotting activity.

Treatment

- Goal is to stop bleeding
- Treatment of individual factor deficiencies (see Table 48-1)
- Recombinant products (e.g., recombinant factor VIII concentrate) are preferred because they are less likely to transmit blood-borne infectious agents (e.g., human immunodeficiency virus [HIV], hepatitis B and C)
- 1-deamino-8-D-arginine vasopressin (DDAVP)
  - An analogue of arginine vasopressin that may be administered intravenously or intranasally
  - **Induces factor VIII and vWF release from liver and endothelial cells**
  - **Useful in type I vWD, mild hemophilia A (minor bleeds), and acquired and congenital platelet disorders**
  - Side effects may include flushing, headache, hyponatremia, hypertension, and mild hypotension
  - Doses may be repeated every 12 to 24 hours up to 3 or 4 doses, after which tachyphylaxis develops
- Acquired coagulation disorders: usually treat the underlying cause
  - **Vitamin K deficiency: administer plasma for rapid correction; oral or IV vitamin K (correction begins in 8 to 12 hours) for more gradual but definitive correction**
  - Liver disease: plasma for bleeding; rhFVIIa has been used for life-threatening bleeding unresponsive to plasma; eventual liver transplantation

Thrombotic Disorders

Basic Information

- The procoagulant function of the coagulation proteins is opposed by natural anticoagulants and the fibrinolytic system
- Defects or deficiencies in anticoagulant proteins or excessive function of coagulation proteins predisposes patients to thrombosis (thrombophilia; Table 48-3)
- **Acquired risk factors for venous thromboembolism (VTE): surgery, trauma, cancer, limb paresis or immobility, pregnancy/postpartum, obesity, smoking, estrogen use (including oral contraceptives; see Chapter 21)**

48

TABLE 48-3   *Selected Disorders Leading to Hypercoagulability*

Disorder	Pathogenesis	Importance	Increase in Relative Risk of Thrombosis	Laboratory Findings
Factor V Leiden (activated protein C resistance)	Mutation in the first protein C cleavage site in factor V Prevents down-regulation of factor V activity	Common: 5% of white U.S. population Less common in African Americans and Asians Synergistic with other thrombophilic states (e.g., prothrombin 20210 mutations)	Heterozygotes: 3–5× Homozygotes: 50×	Screening test: activated protein C resistance assay DNA-based test for confirmation
Prothrombin 20210 gene mutation	Mutation beyond the coding region of the prothrombin gene Results in a 25% increase in prothrombin levels	Common: 1%–2% of white U.S. population Less common in African Americans and Asians	2–3×	DNA-based test for mutation
Hyperhomocysteinemia	Homocysteine is a sulfur-containing amino acid produced during methionine metabolism Elevated in folate or vitamin B12 deficiency, homocysteinuria (autosomal recessive inherited enzyme deficiency state associated with dislocated lenses, mental retardation, vascular thrombosis), renal failure Pathophysiology of thrombosis is unclear	Mild hyperhomocysteinemia (15–30 μmol/L) is present in 5%–10% of the general population	2×	Serum fasting homocysteine level >15 μmol/L is considered abnormal
Antiphospholipid antibody syndrome	Antibodies directed at phospholipid-binding proteins Associated with rheumatic disease (SLE, rheumatoid arthritis), neoplasms, drugs (procainamide, phenothiazines), viral infections (HIV), or idiopathic Pathophysiology of thrombosis is unclear	Predisposes to venous *and* arterial thrombosis Recurrence rate of therapy as high as 50% May also see thrombocytopenia and recurrent fetal loss	10×	Prolonged aPTT; no correction with 1:1 mix with normal plasma Prolonged dilute Russell viper venom time Elevated anticardiolipin or β2-glycoprotein 1 antibodies
Antithrombin (AT) III deficiency	In the presence of endogenous or exogenous heparins, AT III binds and inactivates thrombin, factors Xa, IXa, and XIa	Heterozygous deficiency present in 1:2000 to 1:5000	15–20×	Can measure AT III activity in the absence of heparin and acute thrombosis Family studies can be diagnostically useful
Protein C deficiency	In complex with protein S, it inactivates the activated forms of factors V and VIII	Heterozygous deficiency present in 1:250 to 1:500	5–10×	Protein C activity can be measured in the absence of warfarin, vitamin K deficiency, and acute thrombosis Family studies may be helpful
Protein S deficiency	Cofactor of protein C in the inactivation of activated forms of factors V and VIII	Heterozygous deficiency in 1:1000	5–10×	Protein S activity or antigen levels can be measured in the absence of warfarin, acute thrombosis, vitamin K deficiency, inflammation, pregnancy, and estrogen therapy

aPTT, Activated partial thromboplastin time; HIV, human immunodeficiency virus; SLE, systemic lupus erythematosus.

- Identification of acquired risk factors for VTE is important because elimination of removable acquired risk factors reduces thrombotic risk and may allow limited duration of anticoagulation (e.g., 3 months)
- Persistent acquired VTE risk factors (e.g., active cancer) require ongoing anticoagulation as long as the risk factor is present
- "Unprovoked VTE requires consideration of long-term anticoagulation"

Clinical Presentation

- Patients generally have symptoms suggestive of venous thromboembolism
  - Pain, erythema, swelling of an extremity
  - Dyspnea, pleuritic chest pain
- Headache and mental status changes (suggesting cerebral vein sinus thrombosis) and abdominal pain, hepatomegaly, and ascites (suggesting Budd-Chiari syndrome or mesenteric vein thrombosis) are less common presentations

Diagnosis and Evaluation

- Should thrombophilia tests be performed for patients with VTE?
  - No. Thrombophilia testing is rarely useful for determining a patient's risk for recurrent VTE; therefore, these tests should not be ordered for the vast majority of patients with VTE.
  - Thrombophilia test results may be useful for reproductive-age women with a history of triggered VTE (they may warrant prophylaxis rather than observations; but this is based on limited data)
  - If warranted, an initial evaluation for thrombophilia typically includes testing for factor V Leiden, prothrombin gene (20210) mutation, antiphospholipid (antibody) syndrome, antithrombin deficiency, protein C deficiency, and protein S deficiency (see Table 48-3 for details)
  - Antithrombin III activity may be affected by acute thrombosis and heparin therapy
  - Protein C and S activity and antigen levels may be affected by acute thrombosis and warfarin therapy
    - Protein S levels are also reduced by estrogens
    - Protein S total and free antigen tests are preferred by some authorities for diagnosis of protein S deficiency as protein S activity tests are more prone to false positive results caused by preanalytic variables
  - The dilute Russell viper venom time may be affected by warfarin therapy
  - Homocysteine testing is rarely useful for patients with VTE unless significant congenital defects in homocysteine metabolism are suspected, such as homocystinuria
    - If homocysteine testing is performed, blood samples should be drawn after fasting

Treatment

- General principles
  - Modify/eliminate VTE risk factors (e.g., discontinue estrogen therapy)

- Treat patients with symptomatic VTE with anticoagulation
- Do not prescribe anticoagulants to asymptomatic patients (i.e., patients without a history of VTE) with thrombophilia unless they are postpartum, hospitalized, or postoperation, in which case VTE prophylaxis is appropriate
- Consider treating patients with high-risk thrombophilia (e.g., antiphospholipid syndrome, homozygous factor V Leiden, homozygous prothrombin gene mutation, compound heterozygosity for factor V Leiden and the prothrombin gene mutation, antithrombin, or protein C or protein S deficiency) who have had VTE with long-term anticoagulation, although evidence supporting this practice is of modest quality
- Consider treating patients with unprovoked VTE with long-term anticoagulation
- For hyperhomocysteinemia, vitamin supplementation (with folate, vitamins B_{12} and B_6) may lower homocysteine levels, but does not reduce the risk of recurrent thromboembolism
- Anticoagulation options
  - Unfractionated heparin (UFH)
    - Binds to antithrombin III and potentiates its inhibition of thrombin (factor IIa), factor Xa, factor IXa, and factor XIa
    - Quick onset of action (within minutes to hours)
    - Administer intravenously to treat thromboembolism and subcutaneously (5000 U subcutaneously 2 or 3 times daily) to prevent VTE
    - Monitor aPTT
    - **Therapeutic aPTT range should be established using heparin (anti-Xa) levels since the heparin sensitivity of different aPTT reagents varies**
    - Safe during pregnancy (UFH does not cross the placenta)
    - Side effects include bleeding, osteoporosis with prolonged use, and thrombocytopenia (see Chapter 47)
    - Reversal with IV protamine infusion (1 mg/100 U of heparin)
  - Low-molecular-weight heparin (LMWH)
    - Enzymatically/chemically fractionated form of heparin that can be administered subcutaneously in fixed weight-based doses
    - Useful for prophylaxis or treatment
    - Examples: dalteparin, enoxaparin, tinzaparin
    - **Laboratory monitoring of LMWH is usually not necessary; if monitoring is warranted, use the LMWH (anti-Xa) assay**
    - Lower risk of heparin-induced thrombocytopenia
    - LMWH is safe during pregnancy (does not cross the placenta)
    - Partially reversible (60% to 80%) with protamine (1 mg/100 U)
    - **Use with caution in patients with severe renal insufficiency (creatinine clearance less than 30 mL/min)**
    - Use actual body weight for dosing as dose capping may increase the risk of recurrent thrombosis (e.g.,

enoxaparin 150 mg subcutaneously every 12 hours for 150-kg patient)
- Warfarin
  - A vitamin K antagonist that interferes with synthesis of vitamin K-dependent coagulation factors (II, VII, IX, and X), protein C, and protein S
  - Oral bioavailability
  - **Requires at least 96 to 120 hours for onset of antithrombotic effects (reduction in thrombin and factor X levels); therefore, overlap initiation of warfarin with UFH or LMWH to reduce the risk of recurrent VTE**
  - **Monitor with INR**
    - **Standard therapeutic range for venous thromboembolism (VTE), aortic bileaflet mechanical heart valves, atrial fibrillation (INR 2 to 3)**
    - **Mitral bileaflet mechanical heart valves, recurrent VTE (INR 2.5 to 3.5); antiphospholipid syndrome with recurrent thromboembolism (INR 3 to 4)**
  - Contraindicated in pregnancy
  - Many drug interactions (Box 48-2)
  - Avoid use with nonsteroidal antiinflammatory drugs, aspirin, or platelet inhibitors (increase bleeding risk)

| **BOX 48-2** | **Selected Drug Interactions with Warfarin*** |

Drugs That Potentiate Warfarin Effects

Acetaminophen
Allopurinol
Amiodarone
Azole antifungals
Broad-spectrum antibiotics*
Cimetidine
Ciprofloxacin
Clarithromycin
Disulfiram
Erythromycin
Isoniazid
Metronidazole
Norfloxacin
Omeprazole
Phenylbutazone
Propafenone
Quinidine
Sulfa-containing medications (e.g., trimethoprim-sulfamethoxazole)

Drugs That Decrease Absorption of Warfarin

Cholestyramine and other bile acid resins

Drugs That Increase the Hepatic Metabolism of Warfarin

Azathioprine
Barbiturates
Carbamazepine
Phenytoin
Rifampin

*This list is not all-inclusive. The international normalized ratio should be monitored whenever a patient's medical regimen is modified.

- Warfarin reversal
  - INR 4.5 to 10, no bleeding: hold dose, monitor INR closely; restart warfarin at lower dose when approaching therapeutic range
  - INR greater than 10, no bleeding: hold dose, monitor INR closely; consider administration of 2.5 mg oral vitamin K to reduce the INR; restart warfarin at lower dose when approaching therapeutic range
  - Any INR, life-threatening bleeding: reverse warfarin with 5 to 10 mg of IV vitamin K as well as a 4-factor prothrombin complex concentrate (PCC) or a 3-factor PCC plus 2 U of plasma rather than rhFVIIa or plasma alone for rapid INR reversal; monitor INR closely
- Warfarin skin necrosis (Fig. 48-7)
  - A rare hypercoagulable state most commonly seen in association with the use of large loading doses of warfarin (10 mg or more daily) in the absence of concomitant UFH or LMWH anticoagulation
  - Results from the rapid decrease in protein C levels (plasma half-life of 6 to 8 hours) preceding the decline of procoagulant factors II (prothrombin half-life of 72 hours) and X (half-life of 42 hours), which tips the hemostatic balance toward thrombosis
  - Timing: usually within 1 to 10 days of warfarin initiation
  - Histopathology: dermal microvascular thrombosis typically involving the breast, buttocks, or thighs
  - Hypercoagulable states such as factor V Leiden, prothrombin gene mutation, antiphospholipid (antibody) syndrome, antithrombin III, protein C, and protein S deficiencies increase the risk of warfarin skin necrosis
  - Treatment: heparin anticoagulation, protein C concentrate, or plasma; skin grafting in severe cases
- Oral direct thrombin inhibitor
  - Dabigatran etexilate
    - Oral prodrug rapidly converted to oral direct thrombin inhibitor by plasma/intestinal hydrolases
    - Selectively binds to and inhibits thrombin (activated factor II)

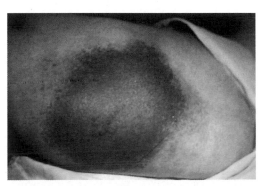

FIGURE 48-7 Warfarin-induced skin necrosis. (From Hoffman R, Benz EJ Jr, Shattil SJ, et al. *Hematology: Basic Principles and Practice.* 4th ed. Philadelphia: Churchill Livingstone; 2005: Fig. 112-19.)

- Rapid onset of action: within 1 to 3 hours of administration
- Half-life of 14 to 17 hours
- Dose: 150 mg bid (twice a day) or 75 mg bid (latter dose used in patients with impaired renal function or drug interaction)
- For acute treatment of VTE, start dabigatran after 5 to 10 days of UFH or LMWH; first dose at the time of discontinuation of UFH or 0 to 2 hours before the next dose of LMWH)
- Advantages: oral administration, no need for routine monitoring, no dietary interactions
- Disadvantage:
  - No antidote available
  - If life-threatening bleeding occurs, consider hemodialysis to accelerate clearance and administration of activated prothrombin complex concentrate (FEIBA 50 U/kg IV)
- Precautions: avoid in patients with creatinine clearance less than 30 mL/min, active cancer, pregnancy, or coadministration with potent p-glycoprotein inhibitors or inducers (see Table 48-4)
- Oral direct factor Xa inhibitors
  - Rivaroxaban
    - Binds selectively to activated factor X
    - Onset of action: 2 to 4 hours
    - Half-life of 7 to 13 hours
    - Dose: 15 mg bid with food for first 3 weeks of VTE treatment, then 20 mg once daily with food
    - Advantages: oral administration, rapid onset of action, can be used for acute treatment of DVT and PE without preceding parenteral therapy (i.e., UFH or LMWH), no dietary interactions, no need for routine monitoring
    - Disadvantage:
      - No antidote available
      - If life-threatening bleeding occurs, consider administration of activated prothrombin complex concentrate (FEIBA 50 U/kg IV)
      - Hemodialysis ineffective for clearance
    - Precautions: avoid in patients with creatinine clearance less than 30 mL/min, active cancer, pregnancy, or coadministration with potent p-glycoprotein inhibitors or inducers and potent inhibitors or inducers of cytochrome P450 enzyme 3A4 (see Table 48-4)
  - Apixaban
    - Binds selectively to activated factor X
    - Onset of action: 1 to 2 hours
    - Half-life of 8 to 15 hours
    - Dose: 10 mg bid for first week of VTE treatment, then 5 mg bid

TABLE 48-4	*New Oral Anticoagulants: Clinically Significant Drug Interactions*	
Anticoagulant	**Potential Drug Interaction**	**Management**
Dabigatran	P-Glycoprotein inhibitors (increase dabigatran levels): amiodarone, azithromycin, captopril, carvedilol, clarithromycin, conivaptan, cyclosporine, diltiazem, dronedarone, erythromycin, felodipine, itraconazole, ketoconazole, lopinavir and ritonavir, quercetin, quinidine, ranolazine, verapamil	Avoid concurrent use of dabigatran and these agents if creatinine clearance (CrCl) <30 mL/min; reduce dose of dabigatran to 75 mg twice daily or avoid use if concurrent use of dronedarone or ketoconazole in setting of moderate renal insufficiency (CrCl 30–50 mL/min)
	P-Glycoprotein inducers (reduce dabigatran levels): avasimibe, carbamazepine, dexamethasone, doxorubicin, nefazodone, paclitaxel, phenytoin, prazosin, rifampin, St John's wort, tipranavir/ritonavir, tenofovir, trazodone, vinblastine	Avoid concurrent administration
Rivaroxaban	Combined p-glycoprotein and strong CYP 3A4 inhibitors (increase rivaroxaban levels): itraconazole, lopinavir/ritonavir, clarithromycin, ritonavir, ketoconazole, indinavir/ritonavir, conivaptan	Avoid use
	Combined p-glycoprotein and moderate CYP 3A4 inhibitors (increase rivaroxaban levels): verapamil, erythromycin, diltiazem, dronedarone	Use with caution
	Combined p-glycoprotein and weak CYP 3A4 inhibitors (increase rivaroxaban levels): quinidine, ranolazine, amiodarone, felodipine, azithromycin	
	Combined P-gp inducers and strong CYP 3A4 inducers (reduce rivaroxaban levels): avasimibe carbamazepine, phenytoin, rifampin, St John's wort	Avoid use
Apixaban	Combined p-glycoprotein and strong CYP 3A4 inhibitors (increase apixaban levels): itraconazole, lopinavir/ritonavir, clarithromycin, ritonavir, ketoconazole, indinavir/ritonavir, conivaptan	Reduce dose to 2.5 mg daily; if already on this dose, switch to alternative anticoagulant
	Combined CYP3A and P-gp inducers (decreased apixaban level): avasimibe carbamazepine, phenytoin, rifampin, St John's wort	Avoid use

Modified from Hellwig T, Gulseth M. Pharmacokinetic and pharmacodynamic drug interactions with new oral anticoagulants: what do they mean for patients with atrial fibrillation? *Ann Pharmacother.* 2013;47:1478–1487.

- ▪ Advantage/disadvantage/precautions: same as rivaroxaban (see earlier)

Review Questions

For review questions, please go to ExpertConsult.com.

SUGGESTED READINGS

Garcia DA, Baglin TP, Weitz JI, et al. Parenteral Anticoagulants American College of Chest Physicians. Antithrombotic therapy for VTE disease: antithrombotic therapy and prevention of thrombosis, 9th ed: American College of Chest Physicians Evidence-Based Clinical Practice Guidelines. *Chest.* 2012;141(suppl 2):e24S-e43S.

Holbrook A, Schulman S, Witt DM, et al. Evidence-based management of anticoagulant therapy: antithrombotic therapy and prevention of thrombosis, 9th ed: American College of Chest Physicians Evidence-Based Clinical Practice Guidelines. *Chest.* 2012;141(suppl 2):e152S-e184S.

Iorio A, Kearon C, Filippucci E, et al. Risk of recurrence after a first episode of symptomatic venous thromboembolism provoked by a transient risk factor: a systematic review. *Arch Intern Med.* 2010; 170:1710-1716.

Kearon C, Akl EA, Comerota AJ, et al. American College of Chest Physicians. Antithrombotic therapy for VTE disease: antithrombotic therapy and prevention of thrombosis, 9th ed: American College of Chest Physicians Evidence-Based Clinical Practice Guidelines. *Chest.* 2012;141(suppl 2):e419S-e494S.

Kitchens CS, Konkle BA, Kessler CM, eds. *Consultative Hemostasis and Thrombosis.* Philadelphia: Saunders; 2013.

Lijfering WM, Rosendaal FR, Cannegieter SC. Risk factors for venous thrombosis—current understanding from an epidemiological point of view. *Br J Haematol.* 2010;149:824-833.

Middeldorp S. Evidence-based approach to thrombophilia testing. *J Thromb Thrombolysis.* 2011;31:275-281.

Yeh CH, Gross PL, Weitz JI. Evolving use of new oral anticoagulants for treatment of venous thromboembolism. *Blood.* 2014;124:1020-1028.

Acute and Chronic Leukemias

KELLY NORSWORTHY, MD; and B. DOUGLAS SMITH, MD

Leukemias arise from the malignant transformation of hematopoietic cells and proliferate primarily in the bone marrow. In general, leukemias are classified as "acute" based on the rapidity of presentation and progression and "chronic," which generally have a more insidious nature. In addition, leukemic cells in acute leukemias are often morphologically poorly differentiated (blasts), whereas chronic leukemias show a more normal differentiation pattern. Finally, leukemias are further classified by the cell of origin being either myeloid or lymphoid. A comparison of the clinical features of the broad leukemia subtypes is seen in Table 49-1. This chapter focuses on three of these subtypes: acute myelogenous leukemia (AML), acute lymphocytic leukemia (ALL), and chronic myeloid leukemia (CML). Chronic lymphocytic leukemia is discussed in Chapter 55.

Acute Myelogenous Leukemia

Basic Information

- Definition: AML is a clonal disorder of a primitive hematopoietic stem cell resulting in excess proliferation of immature cells and suppression of normal hematopoiesis
- Classification of AML was traditionally based on morphology according to the French-American-British (FAB) classification system (Table 49-2). This system has been largely replaced by the World Health Organization (WHO) classification (Table 49-3) that incorporates cytogenetic and molecular markers with the morphologic features of the various AML subtypes.
- Epidemiology
  - Median age at diagnosis: 65 years
  - Approximately 13,000 new cases annually in the United States
- Risk factors
  - Preceding myelodysplastic syndrome (MDS) or myeloproliferative disorder
  - Exposure to DNA-damaging agents
    - Ionizing radiation
    - Chemicals (i.e., benzene)
    - Cytotoxic agents: alkylating agents (cyclophosphamide, chlorambucil, melphalan) and topoisomerase II inhibitors (etoposide, anthracyclines)
  - Genetic factors: Identical twins of leukemic patients have higher rates of leukemia. There is an increased rate of leukemia in patients with Down syndrome,

Bloom syndrome, Fanconi anemia, ataxia-telangiectasia, and Klinefelter syndrome.

Clinical Presentation

- Leukemic cells infiltrate the marrow and suppress normal hematopoiesis, resulting in cytopenias and may also infiltrate other organs (e.g., gums, skin, central nervous system [CNS]) and impact end-organ function
- Most common presenting signs and symptoms caused by decreased production of normal cells:
  - Anemia: pallor, fatigue, and dyspnea
  - Thrombocytopenia: petechiae, hematoma, and bleeding (oral, gastrointestinal)
  - Neutropenia: recurrent infections (sepsis, cellulitis, pneumonia)
- **Leptomeningeal involvement is more common with elevated white blood cell (WBC) count at diagnosis or M4/M5 morphology**
  - Headache and altered mental status are common symptoms
  - Cranial nerve palsies are the most common sign
- **Splenomegaly is uncommon**
- Complications at presentation:
  - Leukostasis because of increased WBC count (may be seen with WBC 35,000 to 50,000/mL, more common with WBC greater than 100,000/mL) results in obstruction of capillaries and small blood vessels, causing widespread ischemic changes such as stroke and/or mental status changes, congestive heart failure, myocardial ischemia, pulmonary congestion and/or hypoxia, and renal failure
  - Tumor lysis syndrome (see Chapter 57)
  - Disseminated intravascular coagulation is seen most commonly with acute promyelocytic leukemia (APL, or M3) and is an oncologic emergency

Diagnostic Evaluation

- Diagnosis depends on identification of myeloblasts in peripheral blood smear or bone marrow preparations
- Peripheral smear may vary from pancytopenia without circulating blasts to marked leukocytosis with blast predominance (Fig. 49-1)
  - **Auer rods: cytoplasmic inclusions of aggregated lysosomes (Fig. 49-2) can be present and are considered pathognomonic for AML**
  - Morphology and immunologic/cytologic markers define the AML subtypes
  - Cytogenetics represent the most important tool for prognostication

TABLE 49-1	Comparison of the Different Types of Leukemia			
	AML	**ALL**	**CML**	**CLL**
Median age at diagnosis (yr)	65	4 (39 in adults)	60	70
Median survival (yr)	1–2	Adults: 2 Children: >10	>10	5
Initial remission rate	60%–70%	90%	90%	90%
WBC count at presentation	High or low	High or low	Elevated with ↑ myeloid cells	Elevated with ↑ lymphocytes
Hemoglobin at presentation	Low	Low	Low or normal	Low or normal
Platelet count at presentation	Low	Low	High or normal	Low or normal
Splenomegaly	Rarely	Common	Common	Common
Adenopathy	Rarely	Common	Rarely	Common
Infection risk	Elevated	Elevated	Normal	Elevated

ALL, Acute lymphocytic leukemia; AML, acute myelogenous leukemia; CLL, chronic lymphocytic leukemia; CML, chronic myeloid leukemia; WBC, white blood cell.

TABLE 49-2	French-American-British Classification for Acute Myeloid Leukemias	
FAB Classification	**Degree of Myeloid Differentiation**	**Associated Cytogenetic Abnormalities**
M0	Undifferentiated	
M1	Minimal differentiation	
M2	With granulocytic maturation	t(8;21)
M3	Acute promyelocytic leukemia	t(15;17)
M4	Myelomonocytic	inv(16), del(16q)
M4Eo	Myelomonocytic with eosinophilia	inv(16), t(16;16)
M5	Monocytic	del(11q), t(9;11)
M6	Erythroblastic leukemia	
M7	Megaryoblastic leukemia	t(1;22)

FAB, French-American-British.

TABLE 49-3	World Health Organization Classification for Acute Myeloid Leukemias	
WHO Classification	**Description**
AML with recurrent genetic abnormalities	AML with t(8;21) AML with inv(16) APL with t(15;17) AML with t(9;11) AML with t(6;9) AML with inv(3) or t(3;3) AML with t(1;22) AML with mutated NPM1 AML with mutated CEBPA
AML with myelodysplasia-related features	Includes patients with preceding MDS or MPD that transforms into AML
Therapy-related AML and MDS	Prior history of chemotherapy ± radiation therapy Often characterized by 11q23 or whole chromosome losses
AML not otherwise specified	
Myeloid sarcoma	Extramedullary leukemia that can occur with or without bone marrow involvement
Myeloid proliferations related to Down syndrome	Myeloid leukemia associated with Down syndrome
Blastic plasmacytoid dendritic cell neoplasm	Derived from precursors of a specialized subset of dendritic cells, plasmacytoid dendritic cells

AML, Acute myeloid leukemia; APL, acute promyelocytic leukemia; MDS, myelodysplastic syndrome; MPD, myeloproliferative disease; WHO, World Health Organization.

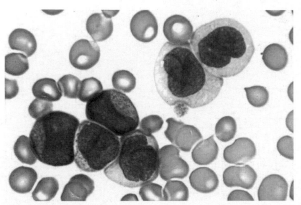

FIGURE 49-1 Acute myelocytic leukemia (FAB AML M4) bone marrow. This category is typified by nearly equal numbers of myeloblasts and monoblasts plus promonocytes. (From Henderson ES, Lister A, Greaves MF. *Leukemia.* 7th ed. Philadelphia: Saunders; 2002: Fig. 11-14.)

TABLE 49-4	*Acute Myeloid Leukemia Cytogenetic Risk Groups*
Risk Status	**Karyotype**
Favorable	inv 16 or t(16;16) t(8;21) t(15;17)
Intermediate	Normal cytogenetics +8 t(9;11) Other nondefined
Poor	Complex (≥3 abnormal clones) −5, −5q, −7, −7q 11q23 inv 3 or t(3;3) t(6;9) t(9;22)—very rare

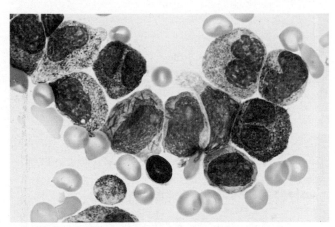

FIGURE 49-2 Bone marrow showing promyelocytes with azurophilic granules. The cell in the center of the field reveals numerous needle-like Auer rods. (From Kumar V, Fausto N, Abbas A. *Robbins & Cotran: Pathologic Basis of Disease.* 7th ed. Philadelphia: Saunders; 2004: Fig. 14-29.)

- Other laboratory features
  - WBC count can be low or high (low WBC count raises suspicion of M3/APL)
    - Spurious abnormalities are related to utilization (oxygen, glucose) by the high WBC count or excessive cell death (potassium) in the phlebotomy tube
  - Blast count may be low or high
  - Hematocrit usually low
  - Platelet count usually low
  - Increased cell turnover can increase serum potassium, phosphate, and uric acid (tumor lysis syndrome)

Prognosis

- Cytogenetic abnormalities are most predictive of prognosis (Table 49-4)
- Molecular markers are also important for prognostication, such as *FLT3-ITD* mutations (poor prognosis) or *NPM1* and *CEBPA* mutations (both associated with better prognosis)
- **Clinical features associated with a worse prognosis include age over 60 years, poor performance**

status, therapy-related AML (secondary to prior chemotherapy), AML arising from another marrow disorder (i.e., MDS or myeloproliferative disease), and WBC count greater than 100,000/mL (hyperleukocytosis)

Treatment

- Hyperleukocytosis at diagnosis is often treated with leukapheresis (temporizing measure) for emergent lowering of counts or with chemotherapy (more longitudinal measure) before full treatment
- Chemotherapy is the mainstay of AML therapy and consists of two parts: induction and consolidation
- Non-APL AML
  - Induction therapy is based on a combination of cytarabine, a pyrimidine antimetabolite (considered the most important and active agent for AML) and an anthracycline (daunorubicin/idarubicin). These agents comprise the classic combination known as "7+3" – 7 days of continuous-infusion cytarabine and 3 days of anthracycline. The goal is to stabilize the patient and restore bone marrow function to a state of morphologic remission.
  - Consolidation: Consists of several additional cycles of intensive cytarabine-based chemotherapy or stem cell transplantation. The goal of consolidation is to *cure* the patient by eradicating remaining microscopic disease.
  - Allogeneic stem cell transplantation (SCT) is potentially curative but is associated with an increased treatment-related mortality compared with traditional chemotherapy. It has traditionally been reserved for younger patients (younger than 60 to 65 years) or those considered incurable by routine chemotherapy (i.e., patients with poor-risk cytogenetics, leukemia related to previous therapy, an antecedent hematologic disorder, or poor-risk molecular markers such as *FLT3-ITD*).
  - Expected that 35% to 40% of patients younger than 60 years and less than 10% of older adults will be alive and free of disease at 5 years; relapse rate declines sharply after 3 to 4 years

49

- New agents undergoing active investigation, particularly in older patients unable to tolerate conventional chemotherapy, include clofarabine (a purine nucleoside antimetabolite), azacitidine/decitabine (demethylating agents used in MDS), and *FLT3* inhibitors in patients harboring the *FLT3-ITD* mutation.
- APL (M3)
  - **APL induction includes the use of all-trans retinoic acid (ATRA) and has resulted in the highest cure rates of the AML subtypes**
  - High-risk patients receive a combination of ATRA and chemotherapy
  - More recently, low-risk patients (WBC 10 or less) are treated with ATRA and arsenic trioxide for induction and consolidation therapy
  - "Retinoic acid syndrome" or "differentiation syndrome" is an important side effect of ATRA (as well as arsenic trioxide), can occur in up to 15% of patients, and is associated with the following:
    - Increasing leukocyte counts
    - Capillary leak
    - Cytokine release resulting in weight gain
    - Respiratory distress
    - Serous effusions (pulmonary/pericardial)
    - Respiratory, cardiac, and/or renal failure
  - Treatment of retinoic acid syndrome consists of prompt initiation of steroids and holding ATRA temporarily for severe cases

Acute Lymphocytic Leukemia

Basic Information

- Definition: ALL is a clonal disorder of a malignant hematopoietic stem cell resulting in excess blasts and suppression of normal bone marrow function
- Epidemiology
  - Most common malignancy in children, but occurs in all ages
  - Median age at diagnosis (in adults): 39 years
  - Approximately 5600 new cases annually
  - Traditional FAB classification system (Table 49-5) and WHO classification system (Table 49-6) are used

TABLE 49-5	French-American-British Classification of Acute Lymphocytic Leukemia
FAB Classification	**Morphology**
ALL L1	Fine to slightly condensed chromatin
ALL L2	Variable nuclear size, moderate cytoplasm
ALL L3 (Burkitt leukemia/lymphoma)	Homogeneous, round nucleus, deeply basophilic, highly vacuolated

ALL, Acute lymphocytic leukemia; FAB, French-American-British.

Clinical Presentation

- Usually acute onset of symptoms (less than 2 weeks) and patients present with fatigue, pallor, bleeding/bruising, or infection
- **Up to 50% will present with fever caused by either pyrogenic cytokine release or true concurrent infection**
- Approximately 50% have lymphadenopathy and splenomegaly
- Anterior mediastinal mass is common, especially with T-cell infiltration of the thymus
- CNS involvement is common in all types of ALL

Diagnostic Evaluation

- Lymphoblasts are seen on peripheral smear and bone marrow preparations (Fig. 49-3) but may be difficult to differentiate from myeloblasts on morphology alone
- Flow cytometry is helpful in distinguishing ALL and AML: pre-B cell ALL expresses B cell markers such as CD19 and CD20, pre-T cell ALL expresses T cell markers such as CD3, and both are distinguished from AML by positivity of TdT (terminal deoxynucleotidyl transferase) and lack of staining for myeloperoxidase
- **Evaluation always includes analysis of cerebrospinal fluid for CNS involvement**

TABLE 49-6	World Health Organization Classification of Acute Lymphocytic Leukemia
WHO Classification	**Description**
Precursor B-cell ALL	t(12;21)(p12,q22) TEL/AML-1 t(1;19)(q23;p13) PBX/E2A t(9;22)(q34;q11) ABL/BCR t(V,11)(V;q23) V/MLL
Precursor T-cell ALL	
Burkitt leukemia/lymphoma	t(8;14), t(2;8), t(8;22)

ALL, Acute lymphocytic leukemia; FAB, French-American-British.

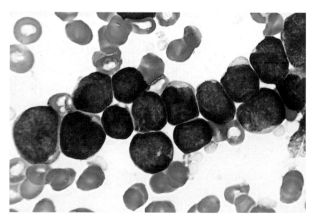

FIGURE 49-3 Acute lymphoblastic leukemia/lymphoma. Lymphoblasts with condensed nuclear chromatin, small nucleoli, and scant agranular cytoplasm. (From Kumar V, Fausto N, Abbas A. *Robbins & Cotran: Pathologic Basis of Disease.* 7th ed. Philadelphia: Saunders; 2004: Fig. 14-5.)

Prognosis

- Generally worsens with increasing age
  - Nearly 90% of children ages 2 to 10 years are long-term survivors with decreased survival rate as age increases
  - Elderly patients with ALL are rarely, if ever, cured. Overall survival for adults is 35% to 40% at 5 years.
- Cytogenetics provide invaluable information on prognosis: hyperdiploidy with best prognosis, hypodiploidy with worse prognosis, and Philadelphia chromosome/t(9;22) with poor prognosis traditionally, but improved with the advent of tyrosine kinase inhibitors targeting *bcr/abl.*
- **Clinical features that affect prognosis include age, initial WBC count, and time to treatment response**

Treatment

- Standard treatment consists of multiple cycles of multiagent chemotherapy plus maintenance therapy for at least 2 years
  - CNS chemoprophylaxis with intrathecal chemotherapy is critical to reduce the chance of CNS relapse
- Salvage chemotherapy for relapsed ALL is rarely effective, and clinical trials are recommended
- Emerging treatment strategies include risk stratification to intensify chemotherapy for patients at highest risk of disease relapse
- Allogeneic SCT is recommended for adults with standard or poor risk features

Chronic Myeloid Leukemia

Basic Information

- Definition: CML is a malignant stem cell disorder characterized by a reciprocal translocation between chromosomes 9 and 22 (t[9;22], the Philadelphia chromosome) that results in a *bcr/abl* gene fusion and a constitutively active tyrosine kinase causing uncontrolled cell proliferation and blocked apoptosis (Fig. 49-4)
- Epidemiology
  - There are three distinct phases of CML: chronic, accelerated, and blast crisis depending on the degree of leukemic blasts versus mature cells
  - **Median age at diagnosis about 60 years**
  - Incidence: 1 to 2 cases/100,000 with slight male predominance

Clinical Presentation

- Chronic-phase patients often present with asymptomatic elevation of peripheral blood counts. When symptomatic, common features include early satiety, left upper quadrant fullness, and fatigue.
- **Splenomegaly on examination present in more than 50% of patients**
- Complete blood count typically shows:
  - WBC count greater than 100,000/mL with left-shifted differential
  - Anemia

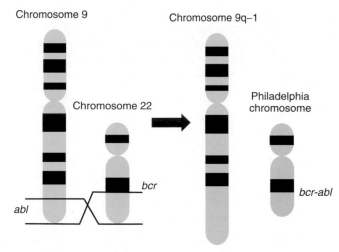

FIGURE 49-4 The Philadelphia chromosome. A reciprocal translocation involving the long arms of chromosomes 9 and 22 results in the production of the Philadelphia chromosome. The t(9;22) translocation results in the fusion of the *c-abl* oncogene on chromosome 9 with the *bcr* gene on chromosome 22. (From Rakel RE. *Conn's Current Therapy 2005.* Philadelphia: Saunders; 2005: Fig. 1.)

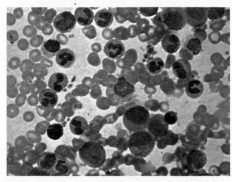

FIGURE 49-5 Chronic myeloid leukemia. Note the abundance of granulocytes at all stages of maturation. (From Forbes CD, Jackson WF. *Color Atlas and Text of Clinical Medicine.* 3rd ed. St. Louis: Mosby; 2003: Fig. 10.77.)

- Thrombocytosis
- Can occasionally see eosinophilia and/or basophilia
- In CML, the mature WBCs are functional and there does not appear to be an increased risk of infection in patients with chronic-phase presentations
- **Anemia, thrombocytopenia, and monocytosis are red flags that you may *not* be dealing with chronic-phase CML**
- Blast crisis may present with constitutional symptoms such as fever, night sweats, bone pain, and symptoms resulting from suppression of normal hematopoiesis (i.e., related to anemia and thrombocytopenia)

Diagnostic Evaluation

- Peripheral smear typically shows a "left-shift" with the presence of virtually all cells of the neutrophilic series, from myeloblasts to bands to mature neutrophils (Fig. 49-5).
- **Diagnosis is established by demonstration of the Philadelphia chromosome by traditional marrow karyotyping or detection by peripheral blood**

49

fluorescence in situ hybridization (FISH) testing; molecular testing for the *bcr/abl* fusion by polymerase chain reaction is the most sensitive test and is used in diagnosis and monitoring response to treatment

Prognosis

- Better for patients younger than age 40, those diagnosed in chronic phase versus accelerated or blast crisis, normal or elevated platelet counts, and mild splenomegaly
- Natural progression of untreated disease moves from a relatively benign chronic phase to fatal blast crisis in 3 to 5 years. Blast crisis is typically myeloid (70%), but can be lymphoblastic (20%) or undifferentiated and carries a very poor median survival of a few months.

Treatment

- Allogeneic SCT remains only known curative therapy, with cure rates as high as 70% reported with human leukocyte antigen-matched donors, and is generally more successful early in the course of disease and/or during chronic phase
  - Graft-versus-leukemia effects are critical for success in CML and are weighed against the potential risks of graft-versus-host disease, which remains the most critical component of morbidity and mortality
- **Medical management: The development of effective tyrosine kinase inhibitors (TKIs) for CML has significantly altered outcomes, so much so that allogeneic SCT is now reserved for patients who have failed medical management or present in blast crisis.**
  - Imatinib mesylate (IM; Gleevec) blocks the activity of *bcr/abl* and was the first TKI to show significant clinical activity in CML
  - Durable, complete hematologic remissions achieved in over 90% of patients
  - Durable complete cytogenetic remissions (FISH negative on peripheral blood) achieved in over 80% of patients
  - TKIs also effective in treating patients with advanced CML (accelerated, blast crisis); however, remissions are often short without additional therapy (i.e., allogeneic SCT)
- Second-generation TKIs dasatinib, nilotinib, and bosutinib were originally developed for IM-resistant CML. More recently, they have shown efficacy and improved time to remission when compared with IM for newly diagnosed patients with CML and are now U.S. Food and Drug Administration approved for use as first-line treatment.
- Several mechanisms of drug resistance exist, the most significant being the *T315I* mutation. In this case, the only effective agent is a third-generation TKI *ponatinib*, an oral pan-*bcr/abl* TKI with potent activity against native and mutated *bcr/abl* and other kinases. Ponatinib has been associated with significant arterial and venous thrombotic events, but is available on a restricted basis for patients with the *T315I* mutation.

Review Questions

For review questions, please go to ExpertConsult.com.

SUGGESTED READINGS

Burns CP, Armitage JO, Frey AL, et al. Analysis of the presenting features of adult acute leukemia: the French-American-British classification. *Cancer.* 1981;47:2460-2469.

Cassileth PA, Harrington D, Appelbaum F, et al. Chemotherapy compared with autologous or allogeneic bone marrow transplantation in the management of acute myeloid leukemia in first remission. *N Engl J Med.* 1998;339:1649-1656.

Ferrara F, Schiffer CA. Acute myeloid leukaemia. *Lancet.* 2013;381: 484-495.

Inaba H, Greaves M, Mullighan CG. Acute lymphoblastic leukaemia. *Lancet.* 2013;381:1943-1955.

National Comprehensive Cancer Network (NCCN) Guidelines: www.NCCN.org.

Schiffer CA. BCR-ABL tyrosine kinase inhibitors for chronic myeloid leukemia. *N Engl J Med.* 2007;357:258-265.

Vardiman JW, Thiele J, Arber DA, et al. The 2008 revision of the World Health Organization (WHO) classification of myeloid neoplasms and acute leukemia: rationale and important changes. *Blood.* 2009;114:937-951.

CHAPTER 50

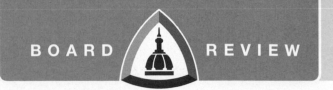
Myelodysplastic Syndrome

KELLY NORSWORTHY, MD; and B. DOUGLAS SMITH, MD

Myelodysplastic syndromes (MDSs) are a complex and heterogeneous group of disorders characterized by ineffective hematopoiesis (in the absence of nutritional deficiencies), dysplasia, cytopenias, and increased risk of infection. In the general population, the incidence is approximately 2 to 10 cases per 100,000 people; however, as age increases, the incidence rises to approximately 50 cases per 100,000 people over age 70.

Basic Information

- Etiology
  - Idiopathic: no known or explained cause of MDS development
  - Secondary: accounts for 20% to 30% of cases. Risk factors include:
    - Exposure to deoxyribonucleic acid (DNA)-damaging agents
    - Benzene
    - Ionizing radiation
    - Tobacco
    - Immunosuppressive therapy
    - Viral infections
    - Treatment-related or chemotherapy-related MDS:
      - Topoisomerase II inhibitors (e.g., anthracyclines, etoposide): associated with 11q23 cytogenetic abnormality; typical onset between 1 and 3 years after chemotherapy
      - Alkylating agents (e.g., cyclophosphamide): associated with unbalanced cytogenetic changes, including abnormalities of chromosome 5 or 7; typical onset is 5 to 7 years after chemotherapy
- Pathophysiology
  - Complete understanding of the MDS pathophysiology has not yet been achieved
  - Inciting genetic event occurs within an early hematopoietic progenitor in a milieu of inflammation with increased levels of cytokines, tumor necrosis factor-α, and interferon-γ
    - Detectable cytogenetic abnormalities are evident in approximately 40% to 70% of patients with primary MDS and greater than 90% of treatment-related MDS
    - **The cytogenetic abnormality predicts outcome**
  - Early MDS: increased levels of apoptosis + increased proliferation → hypercellular bone marrow with peripheral cytopenias
  - Later MDS: apoptosis decreases and proliferation increases → more aggressive disease and possible transformation to acute myelogenous leukemia
- Classifications

- Subtle differences exist among a number of classification systems that have been developed
- Staging systems follow the natural progression of the disease by describing the number of cell lines affected, cellularity of the bone marrow, and percentage of blasts within the bone marrow and blood
  - The French-American-British classification system (Table 50-1) mainly focuses on morphologic descriptions and is less accurate for predicting prognosis for an individual patient
  - The World Health Organization classification system (Table 50-1) focuses more specifically on the biology of MDS and takes into account blast percentage, estimation of degree of dysplasia, and establishment of genetic subclassifications

Clinical Presentation

- Symptoms derive from the bone marrow cell line or lines most affected
  - Anemia can present with fatigue, pallor, dyspnea, or weakness
  - Thrombocytopenia can present with bruising or bleeding
  - Neutropenia can present with infection
- **Red blood cells are typically the first cell line affected, followed by white blood cells, and then platelets**
- Splenomegaly can be seen in some cases, usually in chronic myelomonocytic leukemia

Diagnosis

- Anemia or pancytopenia is typically seen
- The mean corpuscular volume is usually increased, indicating macrocytosis
- Differential diagnosis (Note: Anemia and thrombocytopenia are NOT expected as people age)
  - Vitamin B_{12} or folate deficiency
  - Copper deficiency/zinc toxicity
  - Viral infections (e.g., human immunodeficiency virus, cytomegalovirus)
  - Alcohol abuse
  - Benzene exposure
  - Chemotherapy-induced myelosuppression
  - Aplastic anemia or paroxysmal nocturnal hemoglobinuria (in setting of hypoplastic marrow)
  - Endocrinopathies such as hypothyroidism
- Peripheral blood smear

TABLE 50-1 *Classification Systems for Myelodysplastic Syndromes*

FAB Classification (Morphologic Classification)	WHO Classification (Biologic Classification)
Refractory Anemia (RA) • Cytopenia of one PB lineage • Normocellular or hypocellular BM • <1% PB blasts • <5% BM blasts	1) **Refractory cytopenias with unilineage dysplasia: RA, refractory neutropenia, and refractory thrombocytopenia** 2) **Refractory cytopenias with multilineage dysplasia (RCMD)**
RA with Ringed Sideroblasts (RARS) • Cytopenia, dysplasia, and same blast percentage as RA *plus* • >15% ringed sideroblasts	3) **RARS** 4) **RCMD RS**
Refractory Anemia with Excess Blasts (RAEB) • Cytopenia of two or more lineages • Dysplasia in all three lineages • <5% PB blasts or • 5% to 20% BM blasts	5) **RAEB-1:** 5% to 9% BM blasts, unilineage or multilineage dysplasia 6) **RAEB-2:** 10% to 19% BM blasts, unilineage or multilineage dysplasia 7) **5q– syndrome:** isolated del(5q) cytogenetic abnormality 8) MDS: unclassified
RA with Excess Blasts in Transformation • Same hematologic parameters as RAEB • >5% PB blasts *or* • 21% to 30% BM blasts	Acute myelogenous leukemia: >20% BM blasts
Chronic Myelomonocytic Leukemia (CMML) • Monocytosis in PB • <5% PB blasts *and* • Up to 20% BM blasts	**CMML classified as a MDS/MPN syndrome:** both dysplastic and proliferative features

BM, Bone marrow; FAB, French-American-British; MDS, myelodysplastic syndrome; MPN, myeloproliferative neoplasm; PB, peripheral blood; WHO, World Health Organization.
Modified from Catenacci DV, Schiller GJ. Myelodysplasic syndromes: a comprehensive review. *Blood Rev.* 2005;19:301–319.

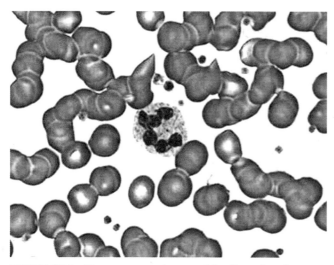

FIGURE 50-1 Hypersegmented neutrophils. (From American Society of Hematology. ASH Image Bank. 2015. Available at imagebank.hematology.org.)

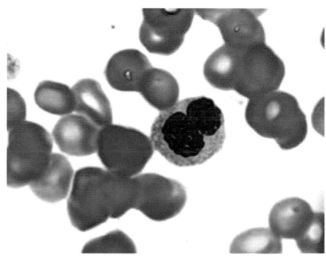

FIGURE 50-2 Pseudo Pelger-Huët cells. (From American Society of Hematology. ASH Image Bank. 2015. Available at imagebank. hematology.org.)

- Hypersegmented (5 to 6 lobes) neutrophils (Fig. 50-1)
- Macrocytosis of red blood cells
- **Presence of pseudo Pelger-Huët cells: hyposegmented "dumbbell"-shaped nuclei of neutrophils (Fig. 50-2)**
- Bone marrow biopsy
  - Required for diagnosis
  - Cellularity: typically normocellular to hypercellular

- **Hypocellular MDS (less than 20% of cases) can occur and can be difficult to distinguish from aplastic anemia or paroxysmal nocturnal hemoglobinuria (PNH). However, because cytogenetic abnormalities are typically seen in MDS and not in aplastic anemia or PNH, chromosome analysis can assist in defining the disorders. Increased CD34+ progenitors also suggest MDS.**

TABLE 50-2	*Revised International Prognostic Scoring System in Myelodysplastic Syndrome*	
	R-IPSS	**Assigned Points**
Percentage marrow blasts	≤2	0
	>2 to <5	1
	5–10	2
	>10	3
Cytogenetics	*Very good:* −Y, del(11q)	0
	Good: normal, del(5q), del(12p), del(20q)	1
	Intermediate: del(7q), +8, +19, i(17q)	2
	Poor: −7, inv(3)/t(3q)/del(3q), complex: 3 abnormalities	3
	Very poor: complex: >3 abnormalities	4
Hemoglobin (g/dL)	≥10	0
	8 to < 10	1
	<8	1.5
Platelets (cells/μL)	≥100	0
	50 to 100	0.5
	<50	1
Absolute neutrophil count (cells/μL)	≥0.8	0
	<0.8	0.5

R-IPSS, Revised International Prognostic Staging System.

TABLE 50-3	*Survival in Myelodysplastic Syndrome based on R-IPSS*	
R-IPSS Score	**Risk Group**	**Median Overall Survival (years)**
≤1.5	Very low	8.8
>1.5 to 3	Low	5.3
>3 to 4.5	Intermediate	3
>4.5–6	High	1.6
>6	Very high	0.8

R-IPSS, Revised International Prognostic Staging System.

- Dysplasia: 1+ cell lines
  - White blood cells: hypogranular, poor maturation, abnormal segmentation of nuclei
  - Red blood cells: binucleate or multinucleate forms, megaloblastic changes, nuclear-cytoplasmic asynchrony
  - Platelets: small, monolobated
- Cytogenetic abnormalities: helpful in determining prognosis
  - **Good prognosis: 20q−, 5q− syndrome, normal, −Y**
  - Intermediate prognosis: trisomy 8, other
  - Poor prognosis: abnormality of chromosome 7, complex cytogenetics
- Prognosis
  - Use the Revised International Prognostic Scoring System (R-IPSS) (Table 50-2)
    - Scoring system that assigns a point scale for three categories:
      - Percentage of blasts within the bone marrow (blasts are usually distinguished by an increase in CD34-positive cells)
      - Cytogenetic abnormalities
      - Degree of cytopenias
    - Calculations based on these categories risk-stratify patients into very-low-, low-, intermediate-, high-, and very-high-risk categories, providing prognostic information (see Table 50-3)

Treatment

- Regardless of stage of disease, there are four major generalizable goals of medical treatment in patients with MDS:
  - Control the symptoms caused by cytopenias and minimize transfusion needs
  - Improve overall quality of life
  - Decrease risk of progression to acute myelogenous leukemia (AML)
  - Improve overall survival
- Supportive care:
  - Careful blood count monitoring with transfusion support
    - Iron overload can occur with repeated transfusions
    - Iron chelation recommended for patients who have had greater than 20 to 30 transfusions; monitor ferritin levels with goal ferritin less than 1000 ng/mL
  - Growth factor support:
    - **Erythropoietin (EPO) effective only when EPO levels are low; response seen in less than 20% of patients**
    - Granulocyte colony-stimulating factor only indicated in setting of repeated infections or in combination with EPO to boost red blood cell response (the combination is especially important for refractory anemia with ringed sideroblasts)
  - Allogeneic stem cell transplantation
    - **Only curative approach to treatment**
    - Best outcome generally seen in younger patients with a matched donor (either sibling or unrelated) and good performance status
      - Numerous studies confirm that nonmyeloablative, or "mini," transplants are feasible in elderly MDS patients with decreased treatment-related mortality (15% to 20%) but at the expense of slightly increased relapse rates
    - Approximately 30% to 50% disease-free survival at 3 years
    - Treatment-related mortality can be as high as 30+% with standard myeloablative transplants
  - Medical management
    - Numerous new agents approved by the U.S. Food and Drug Administration for the treatment of MDS in recent years

50

- Hypomethylating agents (azacitidine or decitabine): traditionally studied in higher-risk patients (intermediate and high IPSS risk score)
  - Overall response rate is approximately 40% to 60% (includes complete response, partial response, and hematologic improvement)
  - Trilineage responses are common and expected, with transfusion independence rates ranging from 40% to 60%
  - Azacitidine shown to delay time to AML and prolong overall survival in Phase III studies
- Lenalidomide is a thalidomide analogue with immunomodulatory effects found to have significant activity in MDS patients with 5q− syndrome
  - **5q− syndrome: a syndrome that typically occurs in older women characterized by anemia, bone marrow findings of small hyposegmented megakaryocytes, and less than 5% blasts**
    - Treatment is typically supportive care only as transformation to acute leukemia rarely occurs
  - Best responses seen in those patients with anemia only, 5q− abnormality, and low or intermediate IPSS risk score
    - Goal of therapy is to decrease or eliminate transfusion requirements
- Conventional chemotherapy (cytarabine based)
  - High-dose chemotherapy targets the abnormal clonal cells
  - Positive results often short lived and toxicity is high

- Overall survival not improved by intense chemotherapy, but this is sometimes needed for those patients with high blast percentage to bridge them to stem cell transplant
- Other items under active investigation include histone deacetylase inhibitors, such as valproic acid and entinostat in combination with hypomethylating agents, and immunotherapy with agents such as ipilimumab

Review Questions

For review questions, please go to ExpertConsult.com.

SUGGESTED READINGS

Bejar R, Steensma DP. Recent developments in myelodysplastic syndromes. *Blood*. 2014;124:2793-2803.

Bennett JM, Catovsky D, Daniel MT, et al. Proposals for the classification of the myelodysplastic syndromes. *Br J Haematol*. 1982;51:189-199.

Kantarjian H, O'Brien S, Ravandi F, et al. Proposal for a new risk model in myelodysplastic syndrome that accounts for events not considered in the original International Prognostic Scoring System. *Cancer*. 2008;113:1351-1361.

Ma X. Epidemiology of myelodysplastic syndromes. *Am J Med*. 2012;125:S2-S5.

Malcovati K, Hellström-Lindberg E, Bowen D, et al. Diagnosis and treatment of primary myelodysplastic syndromes in adults: recommendations from the European Leukemia Net. *Blood*. 2013;122:2943-2964.

National Comprehensive Cancer Network Guidelines for Myelodysplastic Syndromes. Available at: <www.NCCN.org>.

CHAPTER 51

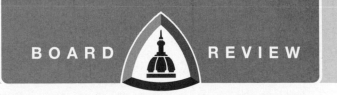
Blood Smear and Bone Marrow Review

GABRIEL GHIAUR, MD, PhD

Evaluation of a peripheral blood smear (PBS) is an inexpensive and rapid powerful diagnostic tool that should be part of the armamentarium of any internist. The evaluation of a PBS should be considered in all cases in which a complete blood count (CBC) with automated differential reveals any abnormalities. Findings obtained from this evaluation save time and resources by narrowing the differential diagnosis and directing further testing, including bone marrow (BM) evaluation (Tables 51-1 and 51-2).

Peripheral Blood Smear

- Develop a routine so that no findings are overlooked
- Relies on pattern recognition; thus, experience improves accuracy
- Be aware of artifacts induced by poor slide preparation/stain
- Identify the correct area of the smear for your suspected diagnosis
  - Feathered edge to evaluate white blood cell (WBC) morphology in a patient with very low WBCs
  - Thick edge to evaluate for parasites
  - **Subfeathered edge (red blood cells [RBCs] barely touch one another) for most applications**
- Examine the smear at low (10×), high (40×, 45×), and oil-immersion (100×) magnifications
- Gather information about all the cellular elements of the blood as well as unusual particles
  - RBC (Fig. 51-1):
    - Distribution. **Rule out artifact of preparation!**
      - Rouleaux formation (Fig. 51-2): increased plasma protein→ multiple myeloma
      - Clumps of RBC: cold agglutinins
    - Size: correlates with the mean corpuscular volume on the CBC
      - *Normocytic*: the size of a lymphocyte nucleus
        - *Microcytic*: may suggest iron deficiency
        - *Macrocytic*: B$_{12}$/folate deficiency, liver insufficiency
      - Relatively uniform: correlates with normal red cell distribution width
        - *Anisocytosis*: variations in cell size
    - Shape
      - *Poikilocytosis*: variation in cell shape
        - Ovalocytes, elliptocytes: inherited abnormalities

- Spherocytes: autoimmune hemolytic anemia or inherited
- Macro-ovalocytes: B$_{12}$/folate deficiency
- Tear drops: extramedullary hematopoiesis, liver disease
- RBC fragments (schistocytes): microangiopathic process (thrombotic thrombocytopenic purpura, disseminated intravascular coagulopathy [DIC], hemolytic-uremic syndrome)
- Sickle cells: sickle cell disease (also called *sickle cell anemia*)
- Target cells: sickle cell disease, thalassemia, liver or splenic disorders
- *Bite cells*: glucose-6-phosphate dehydrogenase deficiency
- Irregular membranes:
  - **Rule out artifact of preparation**
  - Burr: renal insufficiency
  - Spur: liver disease
- Chromasia (amount of hemoglobin) versus chromatophilia (discoloration)
  - Hypochromic (increased central pallor, low mean corpuscular hemoglobin concentration [MCHC]): iron deficiency
  - Hyperchromic (absent central pallor, high MCHC): spherocytosis
  - *Polychromatophilia* suggests increased numbers of reticulocytes (lilac tinged, slightly bigger). Not a substitute for "reticulocyte count"; a supravital stain that identifies RNA.
- Inclusions (abnormal materials inside RBC): **Rule out dirty slide/dust**
  - DNA material:
    - Nucleated RBC: stress erythropoiesis, myelophthisis
    - Howell-Jolly bodies (nuclear remnants) (Fig. 51-3): hyposplenism or asplenism
  - Hemoglobin precipitates:
    - Heinz bodies
  - Granules:
    - Basophilic stippling (ribosomal precipitates) (Fig. 51-4); lead poisoning
    - Pappenheimer bodies (iron granules) (Fig. 51-5); sideroblastic anemia
  - Parasites:
    - Malaria, babesiosis

TABLE 51-1	Abnormalities on Peripheral Blood Smear: Red Blood Cells		
Findings on PBS	**Appearance**	**Differential Diagnosis**	**Further Testing***
Hypochromic, microcytic		Iron deficiency Thalassemia Anemia of chronic disease	Iron studies; Hgb electrophoresis
Target cells		Hemoglobin C Liver disease Thalassemia	Hgb electrophoresis; studies of liver function
Basophilic stippling		Hemolysis Lead poisoning Thalassemia	Coombs test; lead levels; Hgb electrophoresis; reticulocyte count
Sickle cells		Sickle cell syndromes	Hgb electrophoresis
Burr cells		Renal disease	Studies of renal function
Acanthocytes		Liver disease Abetalipoproteinemia	Studies of liver function; lipid profile
Schistocytes		Microangiopathic hemolytic anemia (e.g., TTP, DIC) Malignant hypertension Prosthetic heart valve	See Chapter 46
Spherocytes		Autoimmune hemolytic anemia Hereditary spherocytosis	See Chapter 46
Macrocytes		Vitamin B_{12} deficiency Folate deficiency Myelodysplastic syndrome Liver disease Hypothyroidism	Serum vitamin B_{12} and RBC folate levels; TSH; liver function tests; BM examination

TABLE 51-1	*Abnormalities on Peripheral Blood Smear: Red Blood Cells (Continued)*		
Findings on PBS	**Appearance**	**Differential Diagnosis**	**Further Testing***
Teardrops, nucleated RBCs, bizarre forms	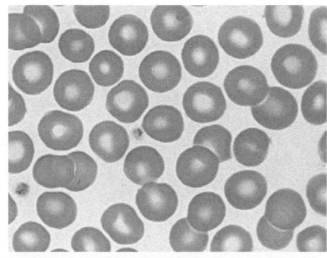	Myelofibrosis Marrow infiltration (e.g., tumor, tuberculosis)	BM examination; splenomegaly suggests extramedullary hematopoiesis
Bite cells		G6PD deficiency Unstable hemoglobinopathy	Enzyme assays; drug history; Heinz body preparation; heat stability test
Parasite inclusions		Malaria (shown) Babesiosis	Thick and thin blood smear remains gold standard for diagnosis of malaria; polymerase chain reaction and antibody testing now available for babesiosis

*See also Chapter 46.

BM, Bone marrow; DIC, disseminated intravascular coagulopathy; G6PD, glucose-6-phosphate dehydrogenase; Hgb, hemoglobin; RBC, red blood cells; TSH, thyroid-stimulating hormone; TTP, thrombotic thrombocytopenic purpura.

FIGURE 51-1 Normal red blood cell. Evenly distributed, size of a lymphocyte nucleus, round and smooth contour, central pallor approximately ⅓ of total diameter, no cytoplasmic inclusions. (From Rodak BF. *Hematology: Clinical Principles and Applications.* 2nd ed. St. Louis: Elsevier; 2003.)

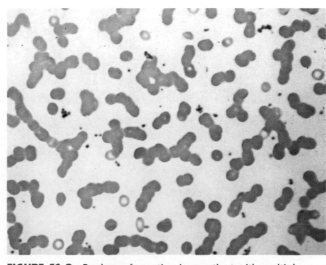

FIGURE 51-2 Rouleaux formation in a patient with multiple myeloma. The occasional normal distribution of red blood cells seen on this smear makes this less likely to be caused by preparation artifact. (From Samuels MA. Neurology of hematology. In Schapira A, ed. *Neurology and Clinical Neuroscience.* St. Louis: Mosby; 2007: Fig. 115-4.)

- WBCs
  - Polymorphonuclear neutrophil (PMN): 3- to 4-lobed nucleus and pink, sandy cytoplasm (granules are too fine to be distinguished by light microscopy)
    - Nuclear abnormalities:
      - Hypersegmented nucleus (>5): B_{12} deficiency, folic acid deficiency
      - Hyposegmented nucleus (2): (pseudo) Pelger-Huët anomaly → inherited disorder or myelodysplastic syndrome (MDS) (decreased granularity)
      - Barr body (nuclear protrusion) (Fig. 51-6)→ X inactivation
  - Granulation:
    - Hypogranulation: MDS
    - Hyper/toxic granulation (dark/blue): infection
    - Döhle body
  - Immature forms (Fig. 51-7): bands, metamyelocytes, myelocytes are rare. Increased

TABLE 51-2	*Abnormalities on Peripheral Blood Smear: Platelet and Leukocyte Disorders*		
Findings on PBS	**Appearance**	**Differential Diagnosis**	**Further Testing**
Thrombocytopenia		Idiopathic thrombocytopenic purpura (if RBC fragments present, suspect microangiopathic hemolytic anemia)	BM examination if patient >50 years old, other cytopenias present, or any other abnormality seen on the PBS; immature platelet fraction (typically high if destructive cause)
Leukopenia with hyposegmented PMNs		Myelodysplastic syndrome Stress, infection Pelger-Huët anomaly	BM examination with cytogenetics/FISH if myelodysplastic syndrome suspected
Leukopenia with hypersegmented PMNs		Vitamin B_{12} deficiency Folate deficiency	Serum B_{12} and RBC folate levels
Lymphocytosis with normal-appearing lymphocytes		Chronic lymphocytic leukemia	Flow cytometry
Lymphocytosis with cell membrane projections		Hairy cell leukemia	Flow cytometry
Lymphocytosis with open nuclei/nucleoli		Activated lymphocytes (e.g., seen in viral infection)	Clinical correlation and viral serologies as appropriate; flow cytometry to rule out leukemia/lymphoma
Leukocytosis with wide range of immature forms		Reactive BM (i.e., leukemoid reaction) Chronic myelogenous leukemia Myeloproliferative neoplasm	Clinical correlation and BM examination (with additional studies) as appropriate
Immature cells (blasts)		Leukemia	BM examination with flow cytometry; cytogenetics/FISH/PCR (see Chapter 49)
Blasts with Auer rods		Acute myeloid leukemia	BM examination with flow cytometry; cytogenetics/FISH/PCR (see Chapter 49)

BM, Bone marrow; FISH, fluorescent in situ hybridization; PCR, polymerase chain reaction; PMNs, polymorphonuclear neutrophils; RBC, red blood cell.

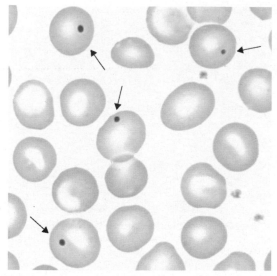

FIGURE 51-3 Howell-Jolly bodies. (From Carr J, Rodak B. Inclusions in erythrocytes. In: *Clinical Hematology Atlas.* St. Louis: Saunders; 2009: Fig. 12-1.)

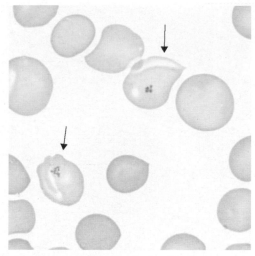

FIGURE 51-5 Pappenheimer bodies. (From Carr J, Rodak B. Inclusions in erythrocytes. In: *Clinical Hematology Atlas.* St. Louis: Saunders; 2009: Fig. 12-3A.)

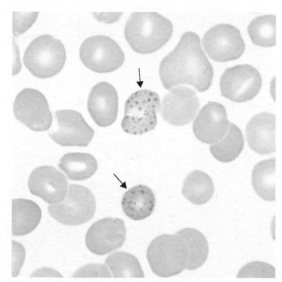

FIGURE 51-4 Basophilic stippling. (From Carr J, Rodak B. Inclusions in erythrocytes. In: *Clinical Hematology Atlas.* St. Louis: Saunders; 2009: Fig. 12-2B.)

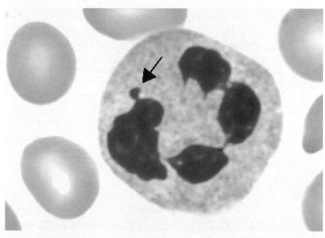

FIGURE 51-6 Barr bodies *(arrow)* in a normal polymorphonuclear neutrophil. (From Carr J, Rodak B. Miscellaneous cells. In: *Clinical Hematology Atlas.* St. Louis: Saunders; 2009: Fig. 23-10B.)

51

immature forms (referred to as *left shift*) → infection, myelophthisis, chronic myeloid leukemia (CML).

- **Steroids cause neutrophilia due to demargination of PMNs but their use does not cause a left shift**
- Lymphocytes (see Fig. 51-7): small nucleus, compact chromatin, and scant cytoplasm
  - Large nucleus with open chromatin (atypical lymphocytes) → viral infection, reactive process
  - Increased cytoplasm and large granules (large granular lymphocytes; Fig. 51-8)→ viral infection, autoimmune
  - "Smudge cells" (Fig. 51-9): mature lymphocytes with disrupted cellular membrane, chronic lymphocytic leukemia

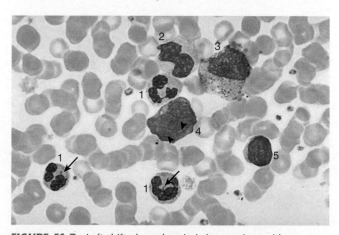

FIGURE 51-7 Left-shifted myelopoiesis in a patient with chronic myeloid leukemia. 1, Polymorphonuclear neutrophil; 2, metamyelocyte/band; 3, promyelocyte/myelocyte; 4, blast (*arrowheads* point toward nucleoli); 5, lymphocyte. Also notice the Barr bodies *(arrows)*, making this more likely to come from a female patient. (From Klatt EC. Hematopathology. In: *Robbins and Cotran Atlas of Pathology.* Philadelphia: Saunders; 2010: Fig. 3-53.)

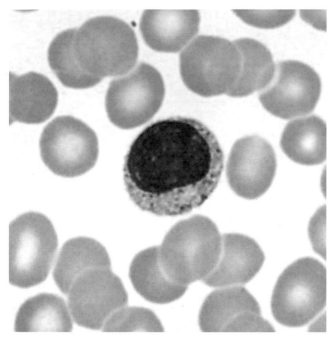

FIGURE 51-8 Large granular lymphocyte. (From Mathur S, Schexneider K, Hutchison R. Hematopoiesis. In: McPherson RA, Pincus MR, eds. *Henry's Clinical Diagnosis and Management by Laboratory Methods.* 22nd ed. Philadelphia: Saunders; 2011:536-556: Fig. 31-32.)

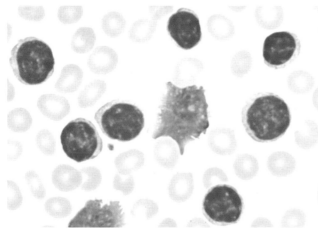

FIGURE 51-9 Mature lymphocytes and smudge cells in a patient with chronic lymphocytic leukemia. (From Turgeon ML. Principles and practice of clinical hematology. *Linné & Ringsrud's Clinical Laboratory Science: The Basics and Routine Techniques.* 5th ed. St. Louis: Mosby; 2007: Fig. 12-51.)

- Eosinophils, basophils, and monocytes are rare
- Blasts (see Fig. 51-7): relatively large cells, with high nuclear/cytoplasm ratio and open chromatin: this is never normal and should prompt evaluation for leukemia. Presence of Auer rods indicates myeloblasts.
- Intracytoplasmic inclusion: bacteria, parasites, phagocytosis nuclear material
  - Platelets
    - Number: 1 platelet per high power field equals approximately 10,000/μL

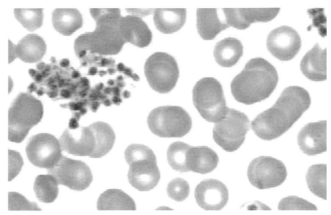

FIGURE 51-10 Pseudothrombocytopenia caused by platelet clumping. The complete blood count would show a spuriously low platelet count. (Courtesy Dr. Gabriel Ghiaur.)

- Distribution: Large clumps of platelets in ethylenediaminetetraacetic acid (EDTA) tubes cause pseudothrombocytopenia (Fig. 51-10) by automated CBC
- Size: approximately 5 to 7 times smaller than an RBC
  - Giant platelets (as large as RBCs): congenital, idiopathic thrombocytopenic purpura (ITP), BM disorder
  - Extracellular parasites: filariasis

Bone Marrow Analysis

- Two components of a BM evaluation:
  - Aspirate (liquid part) → morphology of all cellular elements
  - Biopsy (bony part) → preserves tissue architecture
  - They give nonoverlapping information and both should be ordered
- Bone marrow aspirate:
  - Low-power examination:
    - Cellularity of the specimen **(NOT BM cellularity; obtained from the biopsy)**
    - Presence of spicules (bone/stromal elements)
    - Presence of large cells (megakaryocytes) or clumps of cells (i.e., metastatic disease to the BM)
    - Cellular monotony (i.e., acute leukemia)
    - Macrophage ingesting other cells (hemophagocytic syndrome)
    - Estimation of myeloid to erythroid ratio (M:E ratio)
      - Normal is 3 to 4:1
      - Increased in myeloproliferative processes (CML, polycythemia vera) or in pure red cell aplasia
      - Decreased in agranulocytosis (drug-induced) or in acute/chronic hemolysis
  - High-power examination:
    - A normal BM aspirate slide should have trilineage hematopoiesis (myeloid, erythroid, and megakaryocytic lineage) with full maturation in all lineages and without evidence of dysplasia.

- Myeloid lineage: based on cytoplasm (amount, granules, color) and nuclear (open/close chromatin, nucleoli, folding) features one can identify (i.e., PMN, bands, metamyelocytes, myelocytes, promyelocytes, blasts)
  - Relative to PBS, basophils and eosinophils are easier to identify on BM slides
  - Abundant myelopoiesis with full range of maturation: CML
  - Block in differentiation with increased blasts: acute leukemia
  - Absence of myelopoiesis with normal megakaryocytes and erythropoiesis: drug-induced agranulocytosis
  - Dysplastic changes (lack of appropriate cytoplasmic granularity, unusual nuclear contours) in two or more lineages may indicate MDS
- Erythroid lineage: identify all red cell precursors from RBC to erythroblasts
  - As the cells differentiate, the chromatin becomes more condensed and the cytoplasm changes from dark purple-blue to red. Unmatched nuclear and cytoplasmic maturation = megaloblastoid changes (B_{12}/folate deficiency, MDS, stress erythropoiesis).
  - Karyorrhesis: odd nuclear contour (i.e., "Mickey mouse ears"): dysplasia
  - Some normoblasts can be binucleated or multinucleated
- Plasma cells:
  - Number is better assessed by biopsy but can also be appreciated from the aspirate slide
  - Morphology: Small, binucleated plasma cells can be found in multiple myeloma
- Iron staining: for the evaluation of iron deposits in the BM
  - Gold standard for the diagnosis of iron-deficiency anemia (rarely used anymore)
  - Informative for the diagnosis of MDS (see Chapter 50)
- Bone marrow biopsy:
  - Cellularity: 100 − age = expected cellularity (rule of thumb; doesn't work for extreme ages)
  - Immunohistochemical stain for specific cell population (λ and γ)
  - Special stains for fibrosis (reticulin) or amyloid (Congo red)
  - Stains for infections (fungal, acid-fast, viral antigens)
- **Indications for a BM biopsy and aspirate**
  - Unexplained cytopenias: Young patients with ITP and no other hematologic abnormalities or dysplasia may not need a BM evaluation.
  - Suspected hematologic malignancies (leukemia, MDS, plasma cell disorders, lymphoma)
  - Fever of unknown origin
  - Storage disease
  - Splenomegaly

- Chromosomal abnormalities in neonates
- Donor selection process for stem cell transplant
- When a karyotype is required (cannot be done from peripheral blood)
- **Contraindications:**
  - Coagulation defects → should be corrected before procedure
    - Inherited: hemophilia
    - Acquired: DIC
    - Therapeutic: heparin, warfarin, direct thrombin inhibitors
  - Local infections: skin or osteomyelitis at the site
  - Thrombocytopenia (regardless of number) is not a contraindication for BM biopsy procedure
- Other tests that could be performed from BM and/or PBS:
  - Flow cytometry: used for identification of cellular subsets based on expression of unique markers; can be done from either BM or PBS; almost always a part of BM evaluation
  - Molecular studies (polymerase chain reaction, reverse transcription polymerase chain reaction) can be done from either BM or PBS. Routinely used for the identification of unique transgenes (BCR-ABL → CML, Flt3, CEBPα → AML) that help in diagnosis of hematologic disease. Also used for disease monitoring (mostly PBS).
  - FISH: identifies specific chromosomal abnormalities (i.e., t[9;22] → CML); can be done from either PB or BM and is relatively fast but identifies only targeted abnormalities
  - Classic cytogenetics: needs dividing cells (takes longer, usually done from BM) and identifies abnormalities involving large pieces of genetic material

Acknowledgment

This chapter was adapted from previous editions written by Lawrence Gardner, MD, and Jonathan Gerber, MD, for the second and fourth editions of the *Johns Hopkins Internal Medicine Board Review*. Thomas Kickler, MD, provided valuable feedback on this manuscript.

Review Questions

For review questions, please go to ExpertConsult.com.

SUGGESTED READINGS

Hoffbrand AV, Pettit JE. *Clinical Haematology.* London: Gower Medical Publishing; 1988.
Hoffbrand AV, Pettit JE. *Color Atlas of Clinical Hematology.* 4th ed. London: Mosby; 2010.
Tkachuk DC, Hirschmann JV. *Wintrobe's Atlas of Clinical Hematology.* Philadelphia: Lippincott Williams & Wilkins; 2007.
Zucker-Franklin D. *Atlas of Blood Cells: Function and Pathology.* 2nd ed. Philadelphia: Lea & Febiger; 1988.

51

SECTION NINE

BOARD REVIEW

Oncology

Colorectal Cancer

DAVID COSGROVE, MD, BCh

Colorectal cancer (CRC) is the third most common malignancy seen in both men and women. About 140,000 cases of colon cancer are diagnosed each year in the United States, with 50,000 deaths attributable to the disease on an annual basis.

Basic Information

- Epidemiology
  - Starting at age 40 years, CRC incidence increases with age, with a mean presentation between ages 65 and 70 years
  - Global incidence higher in developed countries
  - Incidence higher in males
  - Third leading cause of cancer deaths in the United States
  - African Americans have a higher incidence of and mortality from CRC than any other ethnic group
- Etiology
  - CRC development proceeds in stepwise fashion from adenoma to invasive carcinoma, with accumulation of oncogenic mutations (Fig. 52-1)
- Classification by location
  - Rectal cancers are those arising below the peritoneal reflection or less than 12 to 15 cm from the anal verge
  - Cancers arising proximal to this area are designated as colon cancers
  - Incidence of CRC by anatomic location (Table 52-1)
- Risk factors
  - Polyposis syndromes are associated with a higher risk of CRC (Table 52-2)
  - **Familial adenomatous polyposis (FAP) increases risk to almost 100% unless prophylactic total colectomy is performed (Fig. 52-2)**
  - Hereditary nonpolyposis colon cancer (HNPCC), also known as Lynch syndromes (Table 52-3), can increase risk by as much as seven times that of the general population
    - Lynch syndromes (autosomal dominant) are associated with *mutHLS* gene complex leading to genetic instability; 4% of CRC cases; extracolonic cancers common in this syndrome (endometrial cancer is the highest incident extracolonic cancer)
    - Usually right-sided lesions
    - Median age 44 years
    - Prognosis not worse than in sporadic tumors
    - Caused by germline mutations of DNA mismatch repair genes (*MLH1*, *MSH2*, *PMS1*, *PMS2*)
    - Total colectomy recommended by some authorities after diagnosis of this syndrome;

most recommend total colectomy after a recurrence
- Risk increases in patients with personal or family history of sporadic CRC or adenoma
- **Sporadic CRC occurs in 80% of cases, with mutations of adenomatous polyposis coli (APC) gene found in 70% of sporadic tumors**
- There is also a higher incidence of CRC in patients with inflammatory bowel disease (IBD), either ulcerative colitis or Crohn disease
  - Risk is associated with duration of IBD, extent of disease, and development of mucosal dysplasia
- Weaker risk factors include environmental, nutritional, and lifestyle factors
  - Increased risk of CRC is associated with higher total calories, animal fat, and protein in diet
  - Lower risk is associated with increased calcium; vitamins A, C, D; folate; and selenium
  - Dietary fiber is currently an area of controversy
  - Diabetes mellitus is an area of controversy
- **Streptococcus bovis bacteremia: Patients who develop this condition have a high incidence of occult CRC**

Clinical Presentation

- Differs depending on the tumor location
- Right-sided lesions commonly produce the following:
  - Vague abdominal aching
  - Abdominal mass
  - Anemia from chronic blood loss (Fig. 52-3)
  - Fatigue
- Left-sided tumors more commonly produce the following:
  - Obstructive symptoms
  - Colicky abdominal pain
  - Changes in bowel habits, with or without rectal bleeding
- Rectal tumors commonly present with the following:
  - Change in caliber of stools
  - Sensation of rectal fullness
  - Urgency
  - Hematochezia, tenesmus
- **Pelvic pain usually indicates local extension into pelvic nerves (later stage of disease)**

Diagnosis and Evaluation

- Screening
  - Because the only definitive cure is via surgical resection, detection at an early stage is imperative

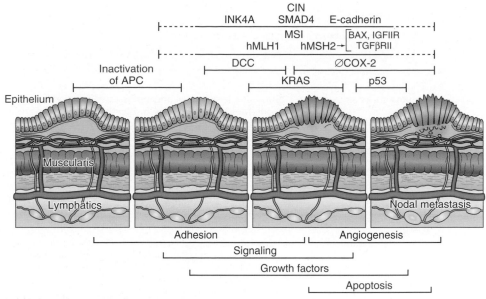

FIGURE 52-1 Adenoma-to-carcinoma sequence and the associated molecular alterations involved in colon cancer development. APC, Adenomatous polyposis coli; CIN, chromosomal instability; DCC, deleted in colorectal cancer; IGF, insulin-like growth factor; MSI, microsatellite instability; TGF, transforming growth factor. (From Abeloff MD, Armitage JO, Niederhuber JE, et al. *Clinical Oncology.* 3rd ed. Philadelphia: Churchill Livingstone; 2004: Fig. 80-3.)

TABLE 52-1	*Location of Colorectal Cancers*
Location	**Incidence (%)**
Cecum	12.5
Ascending colon	9
Transverse colon	11
Descending colon	6.1
Sigmoid colon	23.6
Rectosigmoid junction	8.6
Rectum	22.1

- Current screening recommendations (see Chapter 73)
- Initial diagnostic evaluation for suggested CRC
  - Complete history and physical examination are warranted
  - Preoperative staging includes the following:
    - Complete blood count
    - Liver function tests
    - Renal function studies
    - Urinalysis
    - Serum carcinoembryonic antigen (CEA)
    - Computed tomography (CT) of the chest, abdomen, and pelvis
    - Tumor-node-metastasis (TNM) staging (Table 52-4)

Treatment

- Surgical treatment
  - The primary goal is resection for cure
  - In the setting of known metastatic disease, the need for surgery depends on the presence or risk of obstruction or bleeding

- Types of surgical resections performed also depend on location and extent of tumor. Right, transverse, or left hemicolectomy; wide sigmoid resection; or a low anterior resection with end-to-end anastomosis for proximal rectal cancers may be performed.
- For distal rectal tumors, when unable to spare the sphincter, abdominoperineal resection with permanent colostomy is often necessary
- An alternative procedure for tumors 2 to 5 cm from the anal verge is a coloanal anastomosis
- In selected rectal cancer cases with tumors smaller than 3 to 4 cm, T1, well to moderately differentiated, and without lymphovascular involvement, local excision alone may be performed with a full-thickness negative margin
- Preoperative endorectal ultrasound is an extremely useful tool in defining rectal lesions that are amenable to local excision alone
- Postoperative adjuvant therapy
  - Offered to those at high risk for recurrence because approximately 50% of CRC patients die secondary to metastatic disease
  - For colon cancer
    - The current standard adjuvant chemotherapy regimen in the United States is 5-fluorouracil (5-FU) and leucovorin, with oxaliplatin
    - **Adjuvant chemotherapy has been demonstrated to significantly improve survival in patients with stage III disease**
    - Benefit of chemotherapy in stage II patients is currently unclear, but it is typically offered to patients with high-risk features (T4 lesions, perforation, bowel obstruction, high-grade tumors)
    - Radiation therapy is not routinely used adjuvantly; however, it may be useful in achieving better local control in T4 tumors

52

TABLE 52-2	*Polyposis Syndromes*	
Syndrome	**Inheritance Pattern**	**Clinical Features**
Familial adenomatous polyposis: 1% of CRC cases	Autosomal dominant	Pancolonic adenomatous polyposis by late adolescence; almost all patients will develop CRC unless prophylactic colectomy is performed
Gardner syndrome	Autosomal dominant	Small and large bowel adenomas, extracolonic tumors of soft tissue (desmoid tumors, fibromas, lipomas), bone (osteomas), and ampulla; epidermoid and sebaceous cysts also associated; almost all patients will develop CRC
Turcot syndrome	Autosomal recessive	Bowel polyposis associated with malignant CNS tumors; CRC commonly develops
Peutz-Jeghers syndrome	Autosomal dominant	Hamartomas of the small intestine and colon; also associated with mucocutaneous pigmented lesions of the hands, feet, and mouth; tumors of ovary, breast, pancreas, and endometrium can be seen; rarely transforms to malignancy
Juvenile polyposis	Autosomal dominant	Hamartomas may be limited to the stomach or colon or may be distributed throughout the GI tract; low malignant potential

CNS, Central nervous system; CRC, colorectal cancer; GI, gastrointestinal.

TABLE 52-3	*Lynch Syndromes (hereditary nonpolyposis colon cancer)*
Lynch I	Autosomal dominant, early-onset trait; early development of primarily proximal colon cancers; colon specific
Lynch II	Associated with colonic and extracolonic adenocarcinomas of the ovary, breast, stomach, small bowel, endometrium, pancreas, bile duct, kidney, and urinary tract

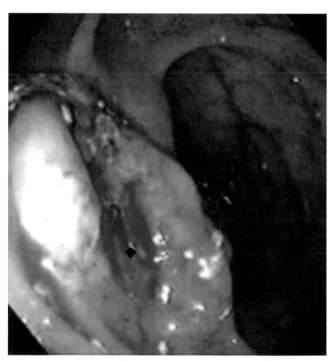

FIGURE 52-3 Colonoscopic view of bleeding carcinoma (with ulceration). Patients may present with evidence of microcytic anemia or with red blood per rectum (hematochezia), depending on tumor site and amount of blood loss. (From Klatt EC. *Robbins and Cotran Atlas of Pathology.* 3rd ed. Philadelphia: Elsevier; 2015: Fig. 7-125.)

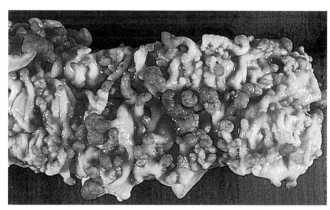

FIGURE 52-2 A segment of a large intestine covered with adenomatous polyps in a patient with familial adenomatous polyposis. The entire colon is covered with hundreds of polyps. (From Skarin AT, ed. *Atlas of Diagnostic Oncology.* 4th ed. St. Louis: Mosby; 2010: Fig. 7.97; and Abeloff MD, Armitage JO, Niederhuber JE, et al. *Clinical Oncology.* 3rd ed. Philadelphia: Churchill Livingstone; 2004; Fig. 80-7.)

TABLE 52-4	*Tumor-Node-Metastasis Staging for Colorectal Cancer*			
TNM Stage	**Primary Tumor**	**Lymph Node Classification**	**Distant Metastasis**	**Duke's Stage**
0	Tis (carcinoma in situ)	N0 (no regional lymph node metastasis)	M0 (no distant metastasis)	—
I	T1 (tumor invades the submucosa)	N0	M0	A
	T2 (tumor invades the muscularis propria)			A
IIA	T3 (tumor invades through the muscularis propria)	N0	M0	B
IIB/C	T4a/b (tumor invades visceral peritoneum/ other organs)	N0	M0	B
IIIA/B/C	T1–T4 (stage III tumors encompass any T stage with N1 or N2 disease)	N1/2 (metastasis in 1–3/≥4 pericolic or perirectal lymph nodes along the course of a named vascular trunk)	M0	C
IV	Any T	Any N	M1 (distant metastasis)	D

TMN, Tumor-node-metastasis.

- For rectal cancer
  - The combination of radiation therapy and 5-FU does increase locoregional control, disease-free survival, and overall survival for patients with stages II and III disease
  - With the preoperative use of combined-modality treatment, locally advanced (T3 or T4) or unresectable cancer may be rendered resectable and sphincter preservation can be achieved
- Recurrence patterns
  - Sites of colon cancer recurrence
    - Liver
    - Peritoneum
    - Other distant sites
  - Rectal cancer commonly associated with locoregional recurrences; in these cases, radiation therapy is important for local control
  - Recurrence evaluation
    - If a patient is found to have only an elevated CEA, colonoscopy and CT scans of chest, abdomen, and pelvis should be performed
    - If imaging is negative, repeat CT scans should be ordered every 3 months
    - If imaging is positive, patients should undergo salvage therapy
- Treatment of local recurrence and metastatic disease
  - Local recurrences
    - Whenever possible, resection is recommended
    - Recurrence to regional or retroperitoneal lymph nodes is associated with poor prognosis
    - Pelvic recurrences may be cured by pelvic exenteration in some patients
  - Recurrences in the liver
    - **If the liver is the only site of recurrence, resection of liver metastases is a viable, and**

potentially curative, treatment option in selected patients
- In the setting of metastatic disease
  - 5-FU–based chemotherapy (preceded by leucovorin) is still the standard systemic palliative treatment, with other cytotoxic agents such as irinotecan and oxaliplatin available. Targeted chemotherapy with epidermal growth factor receptor monoclonal antibodies (cetuximab, panitumumab) or vascular endothelial growth factor monoclonal antibodies (bevacizumab, ziv-aflibercept) can be used in conjunction with chemotherapy in select cases. If these chemotherapy strategies fail, the multikinase inhibitor regorafenib is approved for advanced CRC.
- Palliative radiation therapy for regionally recurrent rectal cancer
  - Can decrease pain and bleeding in 70% to 80% of patients
- Prognosis
  - At diagnosis, 25% of colon cancers have extended through the bowel wall. Of all rectal cancers, up to 60% have extended through the bowel wall or to regional lymph nodes.
  - **The most common site of distant metastasis is the liver**
  - The most commonly affected extraabdominal organ is the lung
  - Stage of disease is the single most significant prognostic factor
  - Other unfavorable clinical prognostic factors include the following:
    - Long duration of symptoms
    - Bowel obstruction or perforation
    - Elevated preoperative CEA level
  - Surveillance after therapy (Table 52-5)

52

TABLE 52-5	*Surveillance of Patients after Treatment for Colon Cancer*
Surveillance Method	**Frequency/Comment**
Colonoscopy	At 1 year after surgery, then every 3 years if no polyps on previous endoscopy
Physical examination, including rectal examination	Every 3 months for 2 years, then every 6 months until 5 years posttherapy (for stage II and III disease)
Fecal occult blood testing	Every 3 months for 2 years, then every 6 months until 5 years posttherapy (for stage II and III disease)
CBC and chemistries	Every 3 months for 2 years, then every 6 months until 5 years posttherapy (for stage II and III disease)
Carcinoembryonic antigen	Every 6 months for 2 years, then annually for 5 years
Chest and abdominal CT	Every 6 months for 2 years, then annually for 3 years in patients who have undergone resection or completed other therapy. Imaging frequency recommendations vary across professional societies, with little survival data to guide interval.

CBC, Complete blood count; CT, computed tomography.

Review Questions

For review questions, please go to ExpertConsult.com.

SUGGESTED READINGS

Aihara H, Kumar N, Thomson CC. Diagnosis, surveillance, and treatment strategies for familial adenomatous polyposis: rationale and update. *Eur J Gastroenterol Hepatol.* 2014;26:255-262.

Andre T, Boni C, Navarro M, et al. Improved overall survival with oxaliplatin, fluorouracil and leucovorin as adjuvant treatment in stage II or III colon cancer in the MOSAIC trial. *J Clin Oncol.* 2009;27:3109.

Benson AB 3rd, Arnoletti JP, Bekaii-Saab T, et al. Colon cancer. *J Natl Compr Canc Netw.* 2011;9:1238-1290.

Brenner H, Kloor M, Pox CP. Colorectal cancer. *Lancet.* 2014;383:1490-1502.

Kemeny N. The management of resectable and unresectable liver metastases from colorectal cancer. *Curr Opin Oncol.* 2010;22:364-373.

Breast and Ovarian Cancer

DEBORAH K. ARMSTRONG, MD

Breast cancer is the most commonly diagnosed malignancy in women, affecting one of every eight women in the United States. It is the second most common cause of cancer deaths in women. Ovarian cancer is less prevalent, affecting 1 out of every 50 to 70 women, but it is associated with high mortality rates because of difficulties in diagnosing early-stage disease. This chapter provides an overview of these two very important malignancies.

Breast Cancer

Basic Information

- Affects 13% of the female population in the United States
  - Less than 1% of breast cancer cases occur in men
- There are significant variations in breast cancer incidence and mortality between countries. This is thought to be caused by variations in genetic, reproductive, environmental, dietary, and social factors.
  - Japan and other Asian countries have the lowest death rates
  - England and Wales have the highest death rates
- A number of breast cancer risk factors have been identified (Box 53-1)
- Genetics of breast cancer
  - **85% to 90% of breast cancer cases appear to be sporadic without an apparent familial or genetic predisposition**
  - Factors suggestive of a familial or genetic inheritance of breast cancer
    - Multiple affected family members
    - Multiple generations involved
    - Early age of onset (before age 50 years)
    - Bilateral disease
    - Triple-negative breast cancer (defined later)
    - Presence of ovarian cancer within the family
    - Male breast cancer in the family
  - Approximately 10% of breast cancers appear to be familial
  - About 18% of breast cancer patients referred for genetic testing will have a germline mutation identified (Table 53-1)
    - The causative gene(s) have not been identified in approximately half of familial breast cancers
  - BRCA mutations
    - Lifetime breast cancer risk in women with a deleterious BRCA mutation is 40% to 85%
    - Lifetime risk of male breast cancer is 6% for BRCA2 carriers

- **The inheritance pattern is autosomal dominant**
- The BRCA genes are not sex-linked, but they are silent in most men
- There is a high penetrance of disease in female carriers
- Certain BRCA mutations are seen more often in specific populations (i.e., three founder mutations in people of Ashkenazi Jewish descent)
- Hormonal prevention with tamoxifen, raloxifene, an aromatase inhibitor, oophorectomy, and mastectomy are all potential prophylactic measures in BRCA-positive patients (see Breast Cancer Prevention section later)
- Breast cancer screening recommendations are controversial in some populations. The American Cancer Society suggests more aggressive screening (Table 53-2) than the U.S. Preventive Services Task Force, which suggests mammography every 2 years for average-risk women ages 50 to 74.
- Pathology
  - Generally classified by the anatomic area of the breast that is affected (ducts versus lobules), by the level of tumor invasion (carcinoma in situ versus invasive carcinoma), and the grade of the tumor cells
    - **Ductal carcinoma in situ (DCIS) is a marker for development of subsequent invasive disease at the same site**
    - **Lobular carcinoma in situ (LCIS) is a marker for development of invasive cancer in either breast, so close surveillance of both breasts is required**
  - Infiltrating (invasive) ductal carcinoma is the most common histologic type of breast cancer

Clinical Presentation and Diagnosis

- Most cases manifest as abnormality on mammogram or as a palpable breast mass
  - Palpable breast mass
    - **Breast imaging (mammogram and/or ultrasound) should be obtained when a breast mass is discovered; however, the absence of a mammographic abnormality does not eliminate the need for tissue diagnosis of a new palpable mass**
  - Tissue diagnosis
    - Fine-needle aspiration does not preserve tissue architecture and is most appropriate for lesions determined by imaging likely to be benign

Known carrier of a deleterious *BRCA1* or *BRCA2* mutation
Personal history of prior breast, endometrial, or ovarian cancer
Family history of breast or ovarian cancer
Increasing age
Nulliparity or late age at first pregnancy (age 30 years or older)
Absence of breast-feeding
Early menarche
Late menopause
Hormone replacement therapy
Prior breast biopsy, especially with documented hyperplasia
Prior radiation to breast area (e.g., mantle radiation for lymphoma)

| TABLE 53-1 | *Germline Mutations in Breast Cancer Patients Referred for Genetic Testing* |

Gene	Contribution to Hereditary Breast Cancer
BRCA1	~8%–9%
BRCA2	~4%–5%
Other genes*	~4%–5%
No mutation identified	82%

*Other genes, in order of frequency: *CHEK2, ATM, PALB2, BRIP1, BARD1, NBN, TP53, CDH1.*

| TABLE 53-2 | *American Cancer Society Breast Cancer Screening Recommendations** |

Age (years)	Examination	Frequency
20 to 39	Breast self-examination	Optional
	Clinical breast examination	Every 3 years
≥40	Breast self-examination	Optional
	Clinical breast examination	Yearly
	Mammography†	Yearly

*Women at increased risk because of family history, genetic risk, or prior breast cancer should have individualized recommendations that may include starting mammography earlier, having additional screening tests such as breast ultrasound or magnetic resonance imaging, or having more frequent exams.
†As long as a woman is in good health.

- **Incisional (core) biopsy maintains tissue architecture of the sample and is the best approach for diagnosis, but the lesion is not completely removed**
  - Excisional biopsy involves complete removal of the lesion
- Mammographic abnormality
  - Risk of the abnormality is stratified based on patient history, exam findings, and imaging characteristics

- A core biopsy of a mammographic abnormality is frequently done by the radiologist with the assistance of imaging

Treatment

- DCIS
  - Requires complete excision (goal of attaining negative margins)
  - May be treated with lumpectomy and radiation therapy (RT) or mastectomy
  - Some low-risk DCIS (small, low-grade, adequate margins) can be observed without the patient undergoing RT
  - Lymph node evaluation not required for pure DCIS without invasion
    - Sentinel node evaluation sometimes done with mastectomy for DCIS in case invasion is ultimately found
  - **Tamoxifen decreases risk of a contralateral cancer and decreases in-breast recurrence after lumpectomy and RT, but it does not improve survival**
- LCIS
  - Treatment ranges from excision with careful surveillance of both breasts, with or without tamoxifen therapy, to bilateral prophylactic mastectomies
  - Lesion excision is recommended to rule out invasion, but negative margins are not required
  - Lymph node evaluation not required for pure LCIS without invasion
- Invasive breast cancer
  - Local control of disease in the breast
    - Removal of the tumor
      - Modified radical mastectomy (MRM): removal of the breast and draining axillary lymph nodes
      - Simple or total mastectomy: entire breast is removed, but axillary contents are not disturbed
      - Lumpectomy or partial mastectomy: Tumor is removed with the goal of attaining pathologically negative margins. Requires subsequent RT for optimal control; therefore, not recommended if RT is contraindicated (pregnant patient, history of prior radiation to the breast) or in multicentric or multifocal tumors.
    - Pathologic evaluation of the regional lymph nodes can be done by sentinel lymph node biopsy. Complete axillary lymph node dissection for a positive sentinel node is not always required, but is done if the information will affect chemotherapy or RT recommendations.
    - RT is used after lumpectomy and for most node-positive patients after mastectomy
    - Choosing between lumpectomy plus RT and mastectomy
      - **Survival is equivalent**
      - More than 80% of patients are good candidates for lumpectomy plus RT; patient preference is a critical element
      - Choice of bilateral mastectomy increasing in frequency even for unilateral disease

- In patients with large tumors, large breast size, or tumors under the nipple, mastectomy may be preferable because of poor cosmetic outcome with lumpectomy
  - Approximately 9% risk of local recurrence in the conserved breast with lumpectomy plus RT (0.5 to 1% per year)
  - Local recurrences after lumpectomy can frequently be salvaged with mastectomy
- Staging (Box 53-2)
- Poor prognostic factors
  - Larger tumor size
  - Axillary lymph node metastases
  - Absent estrogen/progesterone receptor (ER/PR)
  - Poor nuclear grade
  - Elevated measures of proliferation (S-phase fraction, Ki67)
  - Molecular markers such as *HER2/neu* are increasingly used to aid in prognosis and to direct treatment
    - **Tumors that have negative ER, PR, and *HER2/neu* carry an especially poor prognosis and are referred to as "triple-negative" breast cancer**
- Adjuvant systemic therapy
  - Even though 90% of women present with apparently localized disease (i.e., breast and regional lymph nodes), only about 70% will be free of disease 5 years later, despite adequate local therapy

- **Adjuvant therapy is given when no disease is apparent, with the goal of eradicating potential micrometastatic disease and thereby reducing the risk of relapse**
- Important factors to keep in mind with regard to adjuvant therapy:
  - The higher the risk of relapse, the greater the absolute reduction in the risk of relapse with adjuvant therapy
  - The type of adjuvant therapy is based on patient factors (age, comorbidities, menopausal status) and on disease factors (nodal status, hormone receptor status [ER/PR], and *HER2/neu* status) (Table 53-3)
    - In certain clinical situations a genetic profile of the tumor (e.g., oncotype DX) can aid in predicting the relapse risk and the benefit of adding chemotherapy
- Types of adjuvant therapy (hormone therapy, chemotherapy, antibody therapy)
  - Hormonal therapy
    - Used when the tumor expresses ER, PR, or both
    - The highest response rates seen when both receptors expressed
    - Response rate negligible when neither receptor expressed
    - Generally recommended for 5 to 10 years; prolonged tamoxifen treatment for 10 years or sequential use of different agents may extend duration of therapy
  - Premenopausal patients
    - Tamoxifen: mixed ER antagonist/agonist (Box 53-3)
    - Ovarian suppression (OS): inhibition of the pituitary-hypothalamic-gonadal axis with a gonadotropin-releasing hormone analogue (goserelin, leuprolide acetate)
    - The toxic effect of chemotherapy drugs on ovarian follicular cells frequently results in cessation of menses. The closer a woman is to natural menopause, the more likely that amenorrhea will be permanent.
    - Surgical removal of the ovaries
  - Postmenopausal patients
    - Aromatase inhibitors (AIs) (e.g., anastrozole, letrozole, exemestane) are preferred; AIs prevent conversion of androgens to estrogen, thereby suppressing plasma estrogen levels

---

BOX 53-2 *Simplified Staging Schema for Invasive Breast Cancer*

Stage I: small primary tumor (2 cm or smaller), negative nodes, no distant metastases
Stage II: involved axillary lymph nodes *or* large primary (larger than 2 cm), no distant metastases
Stage III: locally advanced disease
  Large tumor and involved nodes
  Matted or fixed axillary nodes
  Tumor with direct extension to the skin or chest wall
  Inflammatory breast cancer: redness, warmth, peau d'orange skin changes
Stage IV: distant metastases; common sites in order of frequency: bone, lung, liver, adrenals, and brain/cerebrospinal fluid

---

53

TABLE 53-3	*Adjuvant Therapy of Breast Cancer*		
	N-Negative	**N-Positive**	**N-Positive and *HER2*-Positive**
Premenopausal			
ER+	Hormone ± chemotherapy	Chemotherapy and hormone Rx	Chemotherapy, Trastuzumab, and hormone Rx
ER–	Chemotherapy	Chemotherapy	Chemotherapy and Trastuzumab
Postmenopausal			
ER+	Hormone Rx	Hormone Rx ± chemotherapy	Chemotherapy, Trastuzumab, and hormone Rx
ER–	Chemotherapy	Chemotherapy	Chemotherapy and Trastuzumab

It is a nonsteroidal antiestrogen when acting on breast tissue

It binds to the estrogen receptor protein and competitively inhibits estrogen action in breast and breast tumors

In some tissues, it acts as a partial estrogen agonist
  Uterus: Estrogenic activity of tamoxifen increases endometrial cancer risk (increase of 1 to 2:1000)
  Bone: increases bone density and delays bone loss
  Cardiovascular: lowers low-density lipoprotein and total cholesterol

Side effects
  Hot flashes and other vasomotor symptoms
  Weight gain
  Thromboembolic disease (rare)
  Increased risk of endometrial cancer (rare)
  Keratopathy and optic neuritis (very rare)

- Tamoxifen can be used for AI-intolerant patients
- Chemotherapy
  - Considered for tumors that are more than 1 cm in size and occasionally for smaller, aggressive tumors
  - **Shown to increase survival for women younger than 70 years old regardless of node or receptor status**
  - The effects of chemotherapy are additive with hormonal therapy when used sequentially; however, they may have antagonistic effects when used together.
  - Breast cancer is responsive to a variety of cytotoxic chemotherapeutic agents, including anthracyclines (doxorubicin, epirubicin), microtubule inhibitors (taxanes [paclitaxel, docetaxel, nab-paclitaxel], ixabepilone), alkylating agents (cyclophosphamide), antimetabolites (5-fluorouracil, capecitabine, gemcitabine), and mitotic inhibitors (eribulin, vinorelbine)
  - Combination multiagent chemotherapy for 3 to 6 months is standard
- Trastuzumab (Herceptin)
  - *HER2/neu* proto-oncogene is overexpressed in 20% to 30% of human breast cancers
  - Cell surface localization of *HER2/neu* allows for therapeutic targeting
  - Trastuzumab: recombinant humanized anti-*HER2* monoclonal antibody
    - Synergistic cardiac toxicity when used with doxorubicin
    - Single-agent activity in *HER2/neu*–overexpressing breast cancer
    - At least additive effects in combination with chemotherapeutic agents
    - **Significantly improves survival when used with adjuvant chemotherapy in patients with *HER-2*–overexpressing tumors**
- Neoadjuvant chemotherapy: given before primary surgery with a goal of reducing tumor size and reducing surgical morbidity. In some cases it can allow breast-conserving surgery instead of mastectomy.

- Response to neoadjuvant therapy is prognostic: Patients with complete pathologic response have better prognosis
- Additional anti-*HER2* therapy with pertuzumab in addition to trastuzumab approved for neoadjuvant treatment of *HER2*-positive breast cancers
- Follow-up after diagnosis and treatment of localized breast cancer
  - Regular history and physical examination
  - Standard blood work: complete blood count, calcium, and liver function testing
  - Yearly mammography
  - Computed tomography (CT), nuclear scanning, and tumor markers are not routinely used for surveillance but can be used for evaluation of specific symptoms or exam findings
- Advanced, metastatic disease
  - Treatment goals for the patient with disseminated breast cancer are to prolong life, improve the quality of life, and palliate symptoms
  - Treatment of advanced disease depends on several factors, including prior therapy, time from diagnosis, sites of metastases, hormone receptor status, and *HER2/neu* status
  - The majority of metastatic breast cancer patients will have some response to chemotherapy
  - Quality of life is improved for some advanced breast cancer patients receiving chemotherapy
  - Response rates are higher for patients who have received no prior chemotherapy or who have had a long treatment-free interval since prior chemotherapy
  - Multiple new agents available for metastatic disease
    - TDM-1 (ado-trastuzumab emtansine[Kadcyla]) is a first-in-class antibody drug conjugate targeting *HER2/neu*-overexpressing metastatic breast cancer
    - Pertuzumab (Perjeta) is a first-in-class antibody that blocks HER dimerization and adds to efficacy of trastuzumab in *HER2/neu*-overexpressing metastatic breast cancer. It is also approved for use in the neoadjuvant setting.
    - Two targeted agents improve response of hormone receptor-positive, *HER2*-negative breast cancer
      - Everolimus (Afinitor): an mTOR inhibitor combined with the AI exemestane
      - Palbociclib (Ibrance): a CDK inhibitor combined with the AI letrozole
  - Patients with lytic bone metastases have decreased skeletal morbidity (bone pain, hypercalcemia, and fractures) with intravenous bisphosphonate therapy

Breast Cancer Prevention

- Bilateral mastectomy prevents greater than 95% of breast cancers. Some breast tissue remains on the chest wall, which is why prevention is not 100%. Preventive mastectomy has significant cosmetic, psychological, social, and sexual impact and is usually reserved for those at highest risk.
- Hormonal chemoprevention
  - Tamoxifen, raloxifene, and the AIs have all been shown to reduce the risk of breast cancer in women at increased risk

- All these drugs have side effects that may be relative contraindications to treatment or may not be tolerated in the prevention setting
- Raloxifene and the AIs can only be used in postmenopausal women

Epithelial Ovarian Cancer

Basic Information

- Cancers of the epithelium of the ovary. Cancers arising from the stromal and germ cells of the ovary are distinct entities.
- Fourth leading cause of cancer deaths in American women
- **High mortality rate because of difficulty in diagnosing localized (early-stage) disease**
- Risk factors
  - Clear-cut cause has not been established for most cases of ovarian cancer
  - Family history
    - Risk of ovarian cancer significantly increased in patients with a familial predisposition (Table 53-4)
    - Patients with *BRCA1* mutations appear to have ovarian cancer onset about 10 years earlier (median age 54 years) than patients with *BRCA2* mutations or sporadic ovarian cancer (64 years)
    - Three inherited genetic mutations currently are associated with an increased risk of ovarian cancer:
      - *BRCA1* is associated with a lifetime risk of 14% to 45%
      - *BRCA2* is associated with a lifetime risk of 10% to 20%
      - Lynch syndrome (also called *hereditary nonpolyposis colorectal cancer* or *familial cancer syndrome*) associated with increased risk of gastrointestinal (GI), ovarian, and endometrial cancers (see Chapter 52)
  - Direct relationship between number of lifetime ovulations and the risk of ovarian cancer
    - Ovulation causes injury to the epithelial surface of the ovary
    - Repeated injury or the process of repairing injury may contribute to malignant transformation
    - **Conditions that cause a relative increase in the number of ovulations (e.g., early menarche,**

TABLE 53-4	*Familial Risk of Ovarian Cancer**
Relationship	**Risk**
One second-degree relative	1:25 (4%)
One first-degree relative (any age)	1:20 (5%)
Age <55 years	1:10 (10%)
Age <45 years	1:5 (20%)
Two first-degree relatives	1:2 (50%)

*Familial ovarian cancer accounts for only 5% to 10% of all cases.

late menopause, nulliparity, and infertility) associated with an increased risk of ovarian cancer
  - Conditions that cause a relative decrease in the number of ovulations (e.g., oral contraceptive use, multiple pregnancies, early pregnancy, and breastfeeding for more than 1 year) associated with a decreased risk of ovarian cancer
  - Recent studies have implicated fallopian tube cells as the cells of origin for many ovarian and peritoneal cancers
- Risk reduction for high-risk patients
  - Oral contraceptives can reduce the risk by more than 50% when used for over 5 years
  - Bilateral salpingo-oophorectomy
    - The degree of risk reduction is estimated to be 90% to 95%
    - Risk of peritoneal cancer remains and is not reduced by removal of the ovaries
    - Oophorectomy results in premature menopause for menstruating women and reduces the risk of breast cancer in these women, but may result in vasomotor symptoms and an increased risk of heart disease and osteoporosis
    - Premenopausal *BRCA* mutation carriers who have undergone prophylactic oophorectomy frequently receive low-dose, short-term hormone replacement therapy to manage hormone withdrawal symptoms without apparent excess risk of breast cancer
  - Close surveillance and screening
- Screening
  - **No ovarian cancer screening techniques have sufficient sensitivity, specificity, or cost-effectiveness to routinely recommend their use for the general population**
  - Screening (with transvaginal ultrasound or cancer antigen 125 [CA 125]) is commonly used in women at high risk for ovarian cancer based on personal or family history

Clinical Presentation

- Specific symptoms are uncommon when disease is localized to the ovary
- Symptoms of advanced disease are vague and are nonspecific for ovarian cancer but are usually present
  - Abdominal fullness or bloating
  - Pelvic heaviness or pressure
  - Pain with intercourse
  - Vaginal bleeding or discharge
  - GI symptoms such as lack of appetite, nausea, vomiting, constipation
- Tumor spread can occur by a number of different mechanisms (in order of decreasing frequency):
  - Local shedding of tumor cells into the peritoneal cavity followed by implantation on the peritoneal surfaces
  - Lymphatic spread to local or distant lymph nodes
  - Hematogenous spread to distant sites (parenchyma of liver, lungs, pleura)
  - Local invasion of bowel or bladder

53

| BOX 53-4 | *Simplified Staging Schema for Ovarian Cancer* |

Stage I: disease limited to the ovaries: 5-year survival, 80% to 90%

Stage II: disease confined to the pelvis: 5-year survival, 60% to 70%

Stage III: disease spread to upper abdomen or regional lymph nodes: 5-year survival, 15% to 30%

Stage IV: distant metastases (liver parenchyma, lung, pleura): 5-year survival, 5% to 10%

Diagnosis

- Not commonly diagnosed by pelvic examination
- Can be found incidentally on ultrasound or CT scan
- Surgical laparotomy necessary for diagnosis, staging, and tumor debulking but laparoscopy and robotic surgery are increasing in use
- CA 125 tumor marker
  - CA 125 common to most ovarian tumors
  - **82% of patients with advanced ovarian cancer have an elevated CA 125, but less than 50% with stage I disease show an elevation**
  - Rising or falling titers correlate with disease in 93% of patients, making it a useful tool for monitoring disease
  - Persistent elevation of CA 125 after treatment strongly associated with residual disease
  - Doubling or an absolute value greater than 100 usually indicates recurrence
  - Even though an elevation of CA 125 may antedate appearance of disease or recurrence, it is not a useful screening tool in unaffected women because of its lack of sensitivity and specificity

Treatment

- Surgery
  - **Aggressive tumor debulking is usually indicated even in advanced disease**
  - Volume of tumor after surgery and before chemotherapy is a major prognostic factor for survival
    - After surgical debulking, patients categorized as:
      - Optimally debulked (1 cm or less postoperative residual disease)
      - Suboptimally debulked (more than 1 cm postoperative residual disease)
- Staging: see Box 53-4
- Chemotherapy
  - Chemotherapy is not used in borderline, low malignant potential, or atypical proliferating tumors

- Use of chemotherapy for stage I invasive ovarian cancer based on risk
  - Patients with well-differentiated stage I tumors have a 5-year disease-free survival rate of over 90% and do not benefit from chemotherapy
  - Chemotherapy justified for patients with high-grade stage I tumors, tumors involving the surface of the ovary, or when there is ascites or positive peritoneal washings
    - Postoperative platinum-based chemotherapy, usually in combination with a taxane
    - Three to six courses standard
- Stage II, III, or IV disease
  - All patients receive systemic, platinum-based chemotherapy
  - Usually receive six courses of treatment
  - Combination of a taxane (paclitaxel or docetaxel) plus platinum (carboplatin or cisplatin) standard
  - Intraperitoneal administration of chemotherapy improves survival in selected low-volume patients
  - Small percentage of patients (10% to 15%) will be cured
  - The addition of bevacizumab (antibody to vascular endothelial growth factor) to chemotherapy improves progression-free survival (prolongs time to recurrence) but does not improve overall survival
- Recurrent ovarian cancer
  - High rate of response to therapy but is generally not curable
  - Noncurative treatment can prolong life
  - A number of chemotherapeutic options available

Review Questions

For review questions, please go to ExpertConsult.com.

SUGGESTED READINGS

Burstein HJ, Prestrud AA, Seidenfeld J, et al. American Society of Clinical Oncology clinical practice guideline: update on adjuvant endocrine therapy for women with hormone receptor-positive breast cancer. *J Clin Oncol.* 2010;28:3784-3796.

Foulkes WD, Smith IE, Reis-Filho JS. Triple-negative breast cancer. *N Engl J Med.* 2010;363:1938-1948.

Gemignani ML, Armstrong DK. Breast cancer. *Gynecol Oncol.* 2014;132:264-267.

Giordano SH, Temin S, Kirshner JJ, et al. Systemic therapy for patients with advanced human epidermal growth factor receptor 2-positive breast cancer: American Society of Clinical Oncology clinical practice guideline. *J Clin Oncol.* 2014;32:2078-2099.

Jelovac D, Armstrong DK. Recent progress in the diagnosis and treatment of ovarian cancer. *CA Cancer J Clin.* 2011;61:183-203.

CHAPTER 54

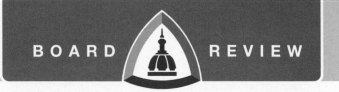
Genitourinary Cancer

MICHAEL A. CARDUCCI, MD; HANS HAMMERS, MD, PhD; and NOAH M. HAHN, MD

Cancers of the genitourinary system are commonly seen in the United States and result in significant morbidity and mortality. Neoplasms of the prostate and testicle are the leading causes of cancer in elderly and young men, respectively. This chapter describes the clinical features of these two cancers, as well as cancers of the bladder and kidney.

Prostate Cancer

Incidence

- Most common cancer for men in the United States
- **One in six lifetime risk for a man to develop invasive prostate cancer**
- Second most common cause of death in men (after lung cancer)

Epidemiology

- The Japanese and mainland Chinese have the lowest rates of invasive prostate cancer; the incidence is highest in Scandinavian countries
- Socioeconomic status appears unrelated to risk

Etiology and Risk Factors

- **Age: Autopsy studies suggest that nearly 60% of men will have prostate cancer by age 80**
- Family history
  - Men with a first-degree relative with prostate cancer have a twofold increased risk; an individual with two first-degree relatives with prostate cancer has a ninefold increased risk
  - Hereditary prostate cancer may account for 5% to 10% of all prostate cancers and tends to develop at a very early age (younger than 55 years)
- Race: African Americans have a 9.8% lifetime risk
- Higher intake of dietary fat may increase the risk of prostate cancer
- Vasectomy, sexual activity, and sexually transmitted disease are not associated with an increased risk of prostate cancer. Some studies have shown a lower risk of prostate cancer with a higher frequency of ejaculation.

Signs and Symptoms

- Early-stage disease
  - **Most are asymptomatic**
  - Some present with bladder outlet obstruction
- Locally advanced disease

- Bladder outlet obstruction causing urinary frequency, urgency, hematuria, or urinary tract infections most commonly seen
- Extension to seminal vesicles may manifest with hematospermia
- Extension to the periphery of the gland and involvement of the neurovascular bundles may manifest as impotence or erectile dysfunction
- Advanced disease
  - Bulky lymph node metastasis can manifest with bilateral lower extremity edema
  - **Men with bony metastases may have localized bone pain or lower extremity neurologic deficits from spinal cord compression**

Screening and Diagnosis

- If prostate cancer is detected early, treatment can be effective and result in limited morbidity
- Controversy exists as to the overall mortality benefit of screening (see Chapter 73)
  - The United States Preventive Services Task Force recommends against screening for prostate cancer
  - The American College of Physicians and the American Cancer Society recommend a shared decision-making approach, with open discussion about the potential risks and benefits of screening
- Digital rectal examination (DRE)
  - 7% to 15% of men older than 50 years will have suggestive results on DRE
  - DRE has 1% to 2% detection rate when used alone
  - A normal DRE does not reduce the odds of clinically significant prostate cancer
- Prostate-specific antigen (PSA)
  - Serine protease specific to prostate tissue, not just cancer
  - **Can be elevated from benign prostatic hypertrophy, acute prostatitis, transrectal needle biopsy, acute urinary retention, prostate surgery, and ejaculation**
  - In general, DRE does not increase serum PSA
  - PSA doubles the detection rate of DRE
  - PSA levels greater than 4 ng/mL are seen in 15% of men older than 50 years; the probability that this PSA level indicates cancer is 20% to 30%
  - **Most men with PSA greater than 10 ng/mL and Gleason grade 7 or higher, are found to have extracapsular disease that is much less likely to be curable**

- Transrectal biopsy
  - Should be done only in those patients who would require therapy, either definitive or palliative
  - Men with PSA values greater than 4 ng/mL or an abnormal DRE suggestive of prostate cancer should consider prostate biopsy
  - Age-specific thresholds and rate of rise of PSA (even with values under 4 ng/mL) may be reason to consider biopsy in younger or high-risk men
  - Side effects of the transrectal biopsy include discomfort, hematuria, hematochezia, and hematospermia
  - **If the biopsy specimen is negative for cancer, the patient should be followed conservatively with serial PSAs and DREs**
    - Consideration for an earlier repeat biopsy depends on the number of cores taken initially and the pretest likelihood of finding cancer
    - If suspicion is high, magnetic resonance imaging (MRI) of the prostate may be used to increase accuracy of sampling

Pathology

- Adenocarcinomas make up the vast majority of tumors, although ductal adenocarcinoma, transitional cell carcinoma, and small-cell neuroendocrine tumors can occur
- Most (70%) occur in the peripheral zone of the gland; only 10% occur in the area surrounding the prostatic urethra
- Histologic grade is summarized using the Gleason system
  - Based on architectural patterns of the tumor
  - A score for each cancer based on the sum of the grade assigned to the most predominant (1 to 5) and secondary (1 to 5) architectural patterns (Fig. 54-1)
  - Gleason grades 2 to 6 are associated with a better prognosis
  - **The risk of developing metastatic disease with a Gleason grade of 8 to 10 is about 43% (17% to 81%)**
- Adenocarcinoma may spread locally to periprostatic fat, seminal vesicles, and regional lymph nodes; hematogenous spread is predominantly to bone, particularly the lumbosacral spine and the axial skeleton

Staging and Prognosis

- Prognosis depends on tumor stage, Gleason score, and pretreatment PSA value
- Table 54-1 summarizes the basic staging for prostate cancer
- **In general, cure is anticipated for men with organ-confined disease and local treatments**
- Men with recurrence despite local treatment can have a long survival
  - Median survival for men with PSA recurrence after local therapy is 13 to 15 years
  - Median survival for men presenting with metastatic disease approaches 7 years

TABLE 54-1	Simplified Staging System for Prostate Cancer

Stage	Description
A	Incidental finding of localized tumor
B	Tumor confined within the prostate capsule
C	Extracapsular disease
D	Disseminated disease to lymph nodes or distant sites

Treatment

- Needs to be individualized; decisions are based on the disease stage and grade, on pretreatment PSA, and on the patient's age and life expectancy
- Physiologic age is of greater importance than chronologic age
- **Patients with short life expectancy (less than 10 years) should probably be observed because there is little evidence to support a prolonged life expectancy with interventions**
- Localized disease (stages A and B): Radical prostatectomy and radiation therapy are effective forms of treatment in the attempt to cure tumors limited to the prostate for appropriately selected patients; comparisons across studies suggest comparable 10-year survival rates with either form of management
  - Radical prostatectomy
    - Most common adverse effects include erectile dysfunction and urinary incontinence
    - Newer surgical techniques (e.g., laparoscopy, robotic-assisted) may decrease the incidence of postsurgical complications but have not been shown to improve mortality
  - Radiation therapy
    - External beam radiation therapy is given over 6 to 8 weeks
    - There is a lower incidence of incontinence compared with prostatectomy
    - Erectile dysfunction, cystitis, and proctitis are the most common adverse effects
    - Brachytherapy, the placing of radioactive seed implants precisely into the prostate, is an alternative to external beam radiation
- Locally advanced disease (stage C): Improved survival may be seen with androgen deprivation (see following discussion) plus radiation
- Advanced disease:
  - First-line therapies include surgical or medical castration (androgen deprivation)
    - Surgical castration
      - Bilateral orchiectomy completely removes testicular androgens permanently
      - It is safe and inexpensive and ensures patient compliance
      - Psychological impact can be severe, so many men choose the chemical option
    - Chemical castration
      - Gonadotropin-releasing hormone (GnRH) agonists (e.g., leuprolide, goserelin, triptorelin,

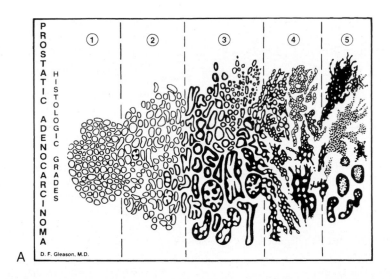

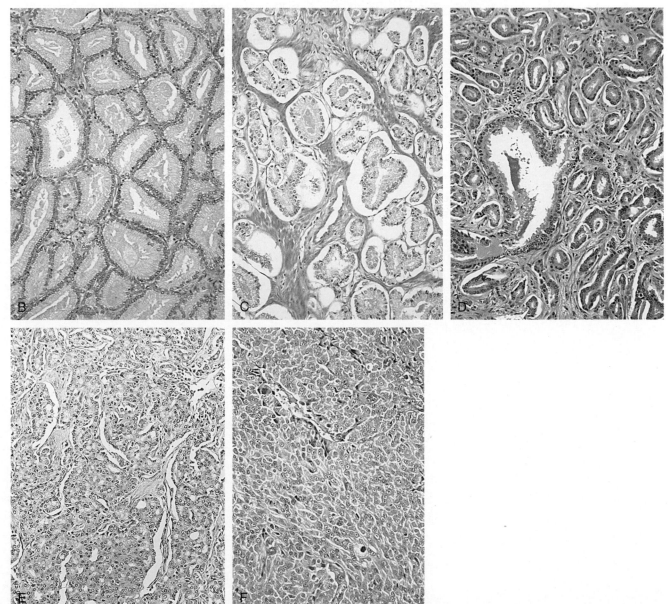

FIGURE 54-1 Gleason scoring system for grading of adenocarcinoma of the prostate. **A,** Schematic of the system. **B** to **F,** Histologic sections showing Gleason patterns 1 through 5, respectively. (From Walsh PC. *Campbell's Urology.* 8th ed. Philadelphia: WB Saunders; 2002: Fig. 86.2.)

54

buserelin, and histrelin) decrease luteinizing hormone (LH), follicle-stimulating hormone (FSH), and testosterone within 3 to 4 weeks of starting therapy
- Antiandrogens (e.g., flutamide, bicalutamide, nilutamide) can be added to GnRH agonists during initiation of therapy to counteract the initial testosterone surge caused by the treatment
- Pure GnRH antagonists (e.g., degarelix) are an alternative to using GnRH agonists, although the latter remains the mainstay of therapy at this time
- **Side effects of androgen ablation**
  - Hot flashes
  - Sexual dysfunction (loss of libido, erectile dysfunction, microgenitalia)
  - Decreased bone and muscle mass
  - Gynecomastia
  - Fatigue
  - Anemia
  - Metabolic syndrome
  - Neurocognitive effects
- Second-line hormonal therapies include the addition and subtraction of antiandrogens, ketoconazole, or estrogens such as diethylstilbestrol
- In men with high-volume metastatic disease, docetaxel given within 4 months of initiating lifelong androgen-deprivation therapy has been shown to improve survival
- **Disease progression (rising PSA, new lesions, or new symptoms) while on androgen ablation (castrate levels of testosterone) defines castration-resistant disease**
  - Docetaxel plus prednisone has been shown to improve survival (median survival 19 months)
  - Cabazitaxel in combination with prednisone is approved for patients with metastatic castration-resistant prostate cancer who have progressed after prior treatment with docetaxel
  - Sipuleucel-T, an autologous cellular immunotherapy for the treatment of castration-resistant prostate cancer, has shown modest improvements in survival when compared with placebo
  - Other treatment options include abiraterone (blocks androgen synthesis) plus prednisone, enzalutamide (novel antiandrogen that blocks translocation of the androgen receptor to the nucleus)
- Treatment of bone metastasis unresponsive to androgen deprivation
  - External beam radiation therapy can reduce pain and fracture risk in patients with isolated painful bony lesions
  - Radium-223 is an α-particle radiopharmaceutical that can be useful in patients with symptomatic multifocal lesions
  - Denosumab, a monoclonal antibody against RANK ligand (RANKL, an osteoclast survival factor), is approved for the prevention of skeletal-related events in men with prostate cancer bone

metastases and for the treatment of bone loss in men receiving androgen deprivation. It has been shown to delay first skeletal-related events in patients with prostate cancer.
- The bisphosphonate zoledronic acid is U.S. Food and Drug Administration (FDA)-approved to reduce skeletal-related events (fractures, cord compression) in men with metastatic, hormone-refractory prostate cancer
- Posttreatment recurrence
  - Men with PSA recurrence after local therapy have a high likelihood of micrometastatic disease
  - Use of androgen ablation in the absence of clinically evident or radiographically evident metastasis is commonplace, although this approach has not been clearly shown to improve survival
  - **Androgen ablation for men with biochemical PSA recurrence and no radiographic metastasis potentially exposes them to the negative aspects of hormonal therapy (see earlier) without known survival benefit**

Urothelial (Bladder, Ureteral, and Renal Pelvis) Cancer

Incidence

- In 2015, an estimated 74,000 cases will be diagnosed and 16,000 deaths will be attributed to cancer of the bladder
- Bladder cancer is much more common than ureteral cancer or cancer of the renal pelvis
- When cancer of the upper urinary tract is diagnosed, there is a 30% to 50% chance of cancer of the bladder developing
- When bladder cancer is diagnosed, there is a 2% to 3% chance of developing cancer of upper urinary tract

Epidemiology

- More common in men (3:1); incidence in women increasing secondary to tobacco use
- Peak incidence in the seventh decade of life
- More common in whites than in African Americans

Etiology and Risk Factors

- Cigarette smoking
- Analgesic abuse, phenacetin use
- Chronic urinary tract inflammation (stones in upper tract, recurrent infections, chronic indwelling catheter in paraplegic patients)
- Occupational exposures (exposure to aryl amines in organic chemicals, rubber, paint, and dyes)
- Balkan nephropathy: a familial nephropathy of unknown cause that results in progressive inflammation of the renal parenchyma, leading to renal failure and multifocal, superficial, low-grade cancers of the renal pelvis and ureters
- *Schistosoma haematobium* infection usually associated with squamous cell carcinoma of the bladder

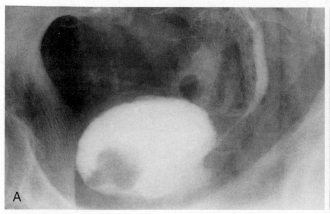 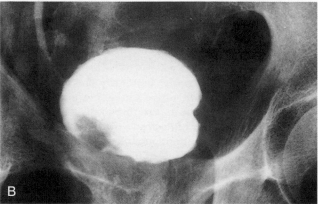

FIGURE 54-2 A and **B,** Excretory urography in a patient with a bladder tumor. Note the filling defect in the right inferior portion of the bladder. (From Bragg DG, Rubin P, Hricak H. *Oncologic Imaging.* 2nd ed. Philadelphia: Saunders; 2002: Fig. 30-1.)

Signs and Symptoms

- Hematuria: usually painless
- Urinary voiding symptoms (e.g., frequency, urgency, or dysuria)
- Vesical irritation without hematuria: common in carcinoma in situ (CIS) of bladder
- Symptoms of advanced disease: pain from metastatic sites, edema of lower extremities, cough or dyspnea from lung metastases

Diagnosis

- **Computed tomography (CT) urogram or excretory urography/intravenous pyelogram (Fig. 54-2) followed by cystoscopy**
- Retrograde pyelography is best for detecting upper tract lesions
- Urine cytology may be helpful; brush biopsies may increase the diagnostic yield
- Biopsies of any lesion must be of adequate size to include bladder wall muscle (muscularis propria)
- CT scan of abdomen: evaluate for local extension and nodal involvement
- Obtain bone scan if bony symptoms are present
- Chest radiograph completes staging evaluation

Pathology

- Urothelial carcinoma: 90% to 95% of all bladder, renal pelvis, ureter, urethra cancers
- CIS
  - Often accompanies higher stages of disease
  - Has high likelihood of progressing to muscle-invasive disease
- Variant histologies
  - Squamous cell carcinoma: 3% to 7% of urinary tract cancers
  - Adenocarcinomas: less than 3% of urinary tract cancers; those arising from the dome of the bladder are urachal in origin
  - Small cell carcinoma: 1% to 2% of urinary tract cancers
  - Plasmacytoid and micropapillary carcinoma: 2% to 3% of urinary tract cancers; tend to be more locally advanced than traditional urothelial carcinomas
- Mixed histologies (urothelial + components of variant histology): approximately 30% of

TABLE 54-2	Simplified Staging System for Bladder Cancer
Stage	**Description**
Tis, Ta	Noninvasive (superficial) carcinoma
T1	Tumor invades lamina propria
T2	Tumor invades muscle
T3	Tumor invades through muscle into perivesicular fat
T4	Invasion of other structures/organs

tumors, exact implications on clinical management unclear

Staging and Prognosis

- Most important prognostic factors are T stage (Table 54-2) and differentiation pattern
- Non–muscle-invasive lesions defined by lack of invasion into bladder muscle wall (muscularis propria)
  - Papillary tumors that involve only the mucosa (Ta) or submucosa (T1) and flat CIS (Tis)
  - Natural history is unpredictable; recurrences are very common
  - Most tumors recur within 6 to 12 months and are the same stage and grade
  - 10% to 15% of non–muscle-invasive cancers develop into invasive or metastatic disease
  - Well-differentiated lesions have a 95% survival rate, whereas high-grade (less differentiated) T1 lesions have a 10-year survival of 50%
- Muscle invasive carcinoma (T2) carries a 5-year survival of 20% to 50%; with regional node involvement and metastatic disease (stage IV), the 5-year survival is 0% to 20%

Treatment

- Localized disease
  - Non–muscle-invasive bladder cancer
    - Surgical approaches
      - Transurethral resection of bladder tumor (TURBT): removes existing tumor; patients require close follow-up

- Laser: not adopted for general use because of limitations of obtaining stage and grade
- Partial cystectomy: Reserved for carefully selected patients. Those with solitary tumors in the bladder dome are best suited.
- **Radical cystectomy: generally not used initially for non–muscle-invasive bladder cancer; indications are unusually large tumors, some high-grade tumors, multiple tumors or frequent recurrences, symptomatic diffuse CIS, prostatic stromal involvement**
  - Intravesical therapy
    - Indications are stage T1 or Tis tumors, multifocal papillary Ta lesions, rapidly recurring superficial disease
    - Agents used: Bacille Calmette-Guérin (BCG), thiotepa, mitomycin, interferon, gemcitabine, docetaxel, valrubicin; BCG has the greatest efficacy
- Muscle-invasive bladder cancer
  - Surgical approaches
    - Radical cystectomy is the gold standard; indicated in patients with muscle-invasive tumors (regardless of grade), diffuse CIS, or recurrent superficial cancers not responding to intravesical therapy
    - Patients can undergo urinary reconstruction with intestinal conduits, continent cutaneous diversions, or orthotopic reconstruction
  - Surgical approaches to ureteral and renal pelvic tumors: nephroureterectomy with resection of cuff of bladder
  - Role of radiation therapy
    - Therapy of choice for patients with clinical condition precluding surgery
    - Addition of chemotherapy as radiosensitizing agent of benefit if patient can tolerate chemotherapy
    - Palliative radiation therapy is quite effective in controlling pain from local or metastatic disease
- Advanced disease
  - Treatment is typically palliative; exception is asymptomatic patients with lymph node-only metastases who have a cure rate of 10% to 20%
  - Cisplatin-based regimens are commonly used; gemcitabine and paclitaxel appear most active as single agents and in combination with cisplatin/carboplatin
  - Median survival is 14 to 20 months depending on prognostic factors, such as performance status, sites of metastasis, and laboratory test results
  - Recent trial data suggest encouraging results with immune checkpoint inhibitors

Renal Cell Carcinoma

Incidence
- Estimated new cases in 2015 were 61,560 (increasing in incidence)
- Estimated deaths in 2015 were 14,080

Epidemiology
- Twice as common in men as in women
- **Most cases diagnosed in fourth to sixth decades of life**
- More common in persons of northern European ancestry

Etiology and Risk Factors
- Sporadic form
  - Etiology unclear
  - Associated with smoking, obesity, and renal dialysis
  - Sporadic renal cell carcinomas of the clear cell type are associated with deletions or hypermethylation on chromosome 3 (location of Von Hippel-Lindau gene)
- Familial form
  - **Von Hippel-Lindau disease: autosomal dominant disease, deletions of short arm on chromosome 3; associated with retinal angiomas, central nervous system hemangioblastomas, and renal cell carcinomas (sometimes bilateral); carries the same prognosis as sporadic disease**
- Signs and symptoms
  - Classic triad of hematuria, flank mass, and flank pain occurs in only 10% of patients and is associated with a poor prognosis
  - Hematuria: more than 50% of patients describe hematuria
  - Normocytic, normochromic anemia, fever, and weight loss are other common manifestations
  - Less common manifestations: paraneoplastic syndromes (polycythemia from excess erythropoietin production, thrombocytosis from increased interleukin [IL]-6, hypercalcemia from release of parathyroid hormone-related peptide), hepatic dysfunction not associated with metastases (Stauffer syndrome)
  - **Varicocele: if acute in onset, right sided, or does not decrease in size in the supine position, consider renal cell carcinoma with obstruction of the venous system**
  - With wide use of CT and ultrasound, renal cell cancer is being diagnosed more commonly as an asymptomatic incidental finding

Diagnosis
- **Standard evaluation includes CT scan of abdomen and pelvis, chest radiograph, urinalysis, urine cytology**
- Contrast-enhanced CT scan differentiates solid from cystic masses; supplies information on nodal or renal vein or inferior vena cava (IVC) involvement
- Venography or MRI: best test to look at IVC involvement
- Evaluation of extraabdominal disease: bone scan if symptoms suggestive; CT of chest if plain film suggestive of metastasis

Pathology
- Tumor cells arise from proximal renal tubular epithelium

TABLE 54-3	*Simplified Staging System for Renal Cell Carcinoma*
Stage	**Description**
I	Tumor ≤7 cm and limited to kidney
II	Tumor >7 cm and limited to kidney
III	Tumor extension outside of kidney but within Gerota fascia or one regional lymph node involved
IV	Tumor extends beyond Gerota fascia or more than one regional lymph node involved or distant metastasis

- Histologic cell types include clear cell, papillary, and chromophobe
- **Clear cell carcinomas are the most common**
- Sarcomatoid variants are more aggressive and associated with a worse prognosis

Staging and Prognosis

- Staging based on tumor size and extension from the kidney (Table 54-3)
- Approximately 30% of patients have metastatic disease at diagnosis
- Five-year survival rates for tumors confined to the kidney are greater than 80%; renal vein involvement does not affect survival
- Before the introduction of approved targeted therapies, patients with metastatic disease had a median 1-year survival rate of 0% to 20%. Survival is improving for patients with metastatic disease.

Treatment

- Surgery
  - Radical nephrectomy is the established therapy for localized disease. Partial, nephron-sparing nephrectomy should be performed when possible.
  - **In the presence of metastatic disease, nephrectomy should be considered to debulk the primary tumor and is associated with a 4-month improvement in survival**
- Radiation therapy to metastatic sites may provide benefit
  - Most commonly used for palliation of bony metastasis
- Systemic therapy of advanced disease
  - Metastatic renal cell carcinoma is relatively resistant to chemotherapeutic agents, although chemotherapy agents such as gemcitabine and capecitabine are used rarely in select patients
  - Immunotherapy and tyrosine kinase inhibitors are the most common approach to therapy
  - Patients with the best response to immunotherapy are those with excellent performance status, lung-only disease, history of nephrectomy, nephrectomy longer than 1 year from treatment, and a long interval history from diagnosis to recurrence and need for treatment
  - At this time, the most effective sequence or combinations of agents have not been defined.

- Clinical trials remain an appropriate first step for patients with metastatic disease.
- IL-2 is FDA-approved treatment for metastatic renal cell carcinoma
  - Response rates range from 15% to 30% (8% are complete, durable responses)
  - Major toxicity is sepsis-like syndrome
- Interferon-α had been used commonly in the past, but has been surpassed by newer targeted agents
- Targeting vascular endothelial growth factor and its tyrosine kinase receptors has demonstrated clinical benefit
  - Sorafenib, sunitinib, and pazopanib are all multitargeted kinase inhibitors that have been approved for advanced metastatic disease
  - Side effects include hypertension, hand-foot syndrome, fatigue, decreased cardiac ejection fraction (sunitinib), liver toxicity, and hypothyroidism
- Mammalian target of rapamycin (mTOR) inhibitors (temsirolimus, everolimus) are also FDA approved

Testicular Cancer

Incidence

- Estimated new cases in 2015 were 8430 (increasing in incidence)
- Estimated deaths in 2015 were 380

Epidemiology

- **Most common cancer in men in the 20- to 34-year age group**
- There is a secondary peak after age 60 years (mostly seminoma)
- Incidence is rare in African Americans

Etiology and Risk Factors

- Previous testicular cancer (500-fold increase in risk)
- Cryptorchidism (20-fold to 40-fold increase in risk)
- High prevalence (90%) have isochromosome 12p
- Association of extragonadal germ cell tumors with Klinefelter and possibly Marfan syndromes
- Association of extragonadal germ cell tumors with hematologic malignancy
- Prior trauma, elevated scrotal temperature, wearing briefs instead of boxer shorts, sleeping with electric blankets, and activities such as horseback and motorcycle riding are not related to development of testicular cancer

Pathology

- **Vast majority are germ cell tumors: seminomas and nonseminomas**
  - Seminoma: 30% of all germ cell tumors
  - Nonseminoma cell types: embryonal, endodermal sinus, teratoma, choriocarcinoma
- Other non-germ cell tumors are rare: Leydig cell tumors, Sertoli cell tumors

54

Presentation

- Most germ cell tumors manifest in the testis (90%)
- Extragonadal (10%) tumors typically manifest in the retroperitoneum, mediastinum, or pineal gland; primary tumor in the testis may be occult
- Classically manifests as an enlargement or mass within testicle
  - Pain and swelling commonly occur
  - An associated hydrocele may be present in 20% of patients
- Gynecomastia (usually bilateral) caused by excess β-human chorionic gonadotropin (β-hCG) production can be seen
- **Inguinal lymphadenopathy is usually not a presenting feature because the regional lymph nodes for the testis are in the retroperitoneum**
- Metastatic spread may present with low back pain (retroperitoneal adenopathy), chest pain, cough, dyspnea, or hemoptysis (mediastinal adenopathy or lung metastases)

Diagnosis

- Testicular ultrasound can easily distinguish extratesticular from testicular abnormalities and solid from cystic lesions
- **All solid intratesticular lesions should be removed by an inguinal orchiectomy. Biopsy or scrotal orchiectomy is contraindicated because it is associated with local spread of tumor cells.**

Staging

- Tumor marker studies should be obtained pre- and postorchiectomy
  - Elevation of β-hCG or α-fetoprotein (AFP) is seen in 80% to 90% of nonseminomatous germ cell tumors
  - Pure seminoma may have elevated β-hCG, but not AFP
  - **Elevated AFP indicates presence of nonseminomatous elements**
  - False-positive β-hCG elevations can be seen with hypogonadism and use of marijuana. AFP may be elevated in patients with liver disease.
  - Lactate dehydrogenase levels may also be elevated in patients with bulky disease and can serve as a useful tumor marker
- CT scan of chest, abdomen, and pelvis should be obtained to search for metastatic sites
- CT of head and bone scan are unnecessary unless symptoms or signs are suggestive of spread to those areas
- Overall staging is based on extent of spread (Table 54-4)

Treatment

- Seminomas
  - Very sensitive to radiation therapy (RT), so very low doses (25 Gy) should be used
    - Acute side effects include nausea, vomiting, diarrhea

TABLE 54-4	*Simplified Staging System for Testicular Cancer*
Stage	**Description**
I	Tumor limited to testis, epididymis, or spermatic cord
II	Tumor extends to but not beyond the regional (retroperitoneal) lymph nodes
III	Disseminated disease

- Late side effects include peptic ulcers, infertility, and second malignancies
- Stage I disease: In compliant patients, observation is preferred after inguinal orchiectomy. Adjuvant RT has been the primary adjuvant approach, with single-dose carboplatin as an alternative.
- Stage II disease: Treat with RT after inguinal orchiectomy for nonbulky disease and with chemotherapy for bulky disease.
- Stage III disease: chemotherapy with bleomycin/etoposide/cisplatin (BEP)
- Nonseminomas
  - Stage I: inguinal orchiectomy with or without retroperitoneal lymph node dissection (RPLND); adjuvant BEP can be considered for patients whose risk for relapse exceeds 50% (e.g., embryonal carcinoma with vascular invasion)
  - Stage II: inguinal orchiectomy followed by RPLND with or without adjuvant chemotherapy (BEP)
  - Stage III: chemotherapy with BEP
- Recurrent disease: treat with salvage chemotherapy

Prognosis

- **Five-year survival of all patients is approximately 95%**
- Cure rates high for disease with minimal-to-moderate spread
- Infertility is common in all stages of testicular cancer, but risk of permanent infertility increases with therapy and stage
- **Sperm banking must be considered in all patients before undergoing therapy for testis cancer**

Review Questions

For review questions, please go to ExpertConsult.com.

SUGGESTED READINGS

Basch E, Loblaw DA, Oliver TK, et al. Systemic therapy in men with metastatic castration-resistant prostate cancer (CRPC): American Society of Clinical Oncology and Cancer Care Ontario Clinical Practice Guidelines. *J Clin Oncol.* 2014;32:3436-3448.

Beer TM, Armstrong AK, Rathkopf DE, et al. Enzalutamide in metastatic prostate cancer before chemotherapy. *N Engl J Med.* 2014;371:424-433.

Clark PE, Agarwal N, Biagioli MC, et al. Bladder cancer. *J Natl Compr Canc Netw.* 2013;11:446-475.

Hayes JH, Barry MJ. Screening for prostate cancer with the prostate-specific antigen test: a review of current evidence. JAMA. 2014;311:1143-1149.

International Germ Cell Cancer Collaborative Group. International germ cell consensus classification: a prognostic factor-based staging system for metastatic germ cell cancers. *J Clin Oncol.* 1997;15:594-603.

Kantoff PW, Higano CS, Shore ND, et al. for the IMPACT Study Investigators. Sipuleucel-T immunotherapy for castration-resistant prostate cancer. *N Engl J Med.* 2010;363:411-422.

Nelson WG, DeMarzo AM, Isaacs WB. Prostate cancer. *N Engl J Med.* 2003;349:366-381.

Park JC, Hahn NM. Bladder cancer: a disease ripe for major advances. *Clin Adv Hematol Oncol.* 2014;12:838-845.

Parker C, Nilsson S, Heinrich D, et al. Alpha emitter radium-223 and survival in metastatic prostate cancer. *N Engl J Med.* 2013;369:213-323.

Rini BI, Campbell SC, Escudier B. Renal cell carcinoma. *Lancet.* 2009;373:1119-1132.

Lymphoma and Chronic Lymphocytic Leukemia

YVETTE L. KASAMON, MD

Leukemia and lymphoma are both hematologic malignancies. Leukemias proliferate primarily in the blood and bone marrow; whereas, lymphomas are characterized by uncontrolled proliferation of cells residing in the lymphoid tissues. Some diseases, like chronic lymphocytic leukemia (CLL), can have features of both.

Classic Hodgkin Lymphoma

Basic Information

- Usually arises from B cells
- Bimodal age distribution (third and seventh decades)
- Subset associated with Epstein-Barr virus infection

Clinical Presentation

- **Patients commonly present with "B symptoms" (fever, weight loss, night sweats) and pruritus**
- Most present with an asymptomatic enlarged lymph node or a mass found on imaging (Fig. 55-1A and B)
  - Nodes are usually painless and rubbery
  - Most common sites are neck and mediastinum
  - Hodgkin lymphoma starts at a single site within the lymphatic system and then progresses to adjacent lymph nodes
  - Alcohol-induced pain is a rare symptom of Hodgkin lymphoma
- **A mediastinal mass in a young person is most often Hodgkin lymphoma**, followed in frequency by non-Hodgkin lymphoma (NHL)
  - Mediastinal masses may be incidental findings or cause chest pain, cough, dyspnea, or superior vena cava syndrome
- Common laboratory findings include:
  - Elevated white blood cell (WBC) count
  - Lymphopenia
  - Thrombocytosis
  - Elevated erythrocyte sedimentation rate

Diagnosis

- Usually diagnosed by lymph node biopsy
  - **Reed-Sternberg cells (giant "owl eye" cells)** are characteristic and are surrounded by a dense inflammatory infiltrate (see Fig. 55-1C)
  - Fine-needle aspiration is usually insufficient because of limited architecture

- Mediastinoscopy may be performed to sample a mediastinal tumor
- Most common subtypes: nodular sclerosis, followed by mixed cellularity
- Lymphocyte-predominant Hodgkin (a rare variant) is not classic Hodgkin
- Staging (Table 55-1) requires computed tomography (CT) of chest, abdomen, and pelvis, preferably with positron emission tomography (PET)
  - Exploratory laparotomy is now rarely performed for staging
  - Bone marrow biopsy is not always necessary; consider especially with B symptoms, cytopenias, or advanced disease
  - PET is a useful adjunct to CT

Prognosis

- Majority are curable
- Adverse prognostic factors include:
  - Age older than 45 years
  - Male gender
  - Stage IV disease
  - Abnormal CBC (WBC 15,000/μL or more, lymphopenia, anemia)
  - Albumin less than 4 g/dL
  - Large mediastinal mass

Treatment

- Treatment is based on staging
  - Stages I and II are usually treated with combination chemotherapy followed by radiation. Some cases may be treated with chemotherapy alone.
  - Stages III and IV are treated with full-course chemotherapy. Radiation may be added afterward to areas of bulky tumor.
  - Doxorubicin, bleomycin, vinblastine, dacarbazine (ABVD) is standard; full-course is 6 to 8 cycles
- Scans are performed during and after treatment to assess remission
- Autologous stem cell transplant is considered for most patients who relapse after first-line treatment
- Sequelae from treatment are common. Treatment toxicities are leading considerations because most Hodgkin lymphoma patients are cured.
  - Pulmonary toxicity from bleomycin can occur, usually during treatment. Patient may be

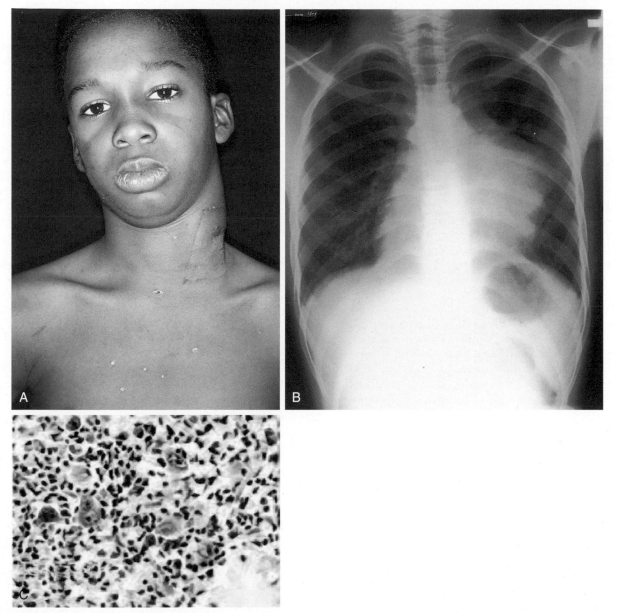

FIGURE 55-1 Hodgkin lymphoma. Most patients present with asymptomatic lymphadenopathy (**A**) or a mediastinal mass (**B**). Multinucleated Reed-Sternberg cells are characteristic pathologic findings (**C**). (**A** and **B**, From Shah B, Laude T. *Atlas of Pediatric Clinical Diagnosis.* Philadelphia: Saunders; 2000: Fig. 7-32; **C**, From Hoffman R, Benz EJ Jr, Shattil SJ, et al. *Hematology: Basic Principles and Practice.* 4th ed. Philadelphia: Churchill Livingstone; 2005: Fig. 74-36.)

TABLE 55-1	*Staging of Lymphoma**
Stage I	Disease in one nodal or one extralymphatic site
Stage II	Two or more nodal areas on same side of diaphragm
Stage III	Nodes on both sides of diaphragm
Stage IV	Disseminated extralymphatic spread

*Stages are designated as: A, absence of constitutional symptoms (unexplained fever >38°C, drenching night sweats, or unexplained >10% weight loss in preceding 6 months) or B, presence of these constitutional symptoms.

asymptomatic, or bleomycin may cause cough, fever, dyspnea, and infiltrates
- Anthracyclines infrequently cause late cardiomyopathy
- Radiation significantly increases the risk of developing other cancers (including lung, breast, thyroid)
- **Mediastinal radiation can also cause cardiac complications, including premature coronary artery disease, constrictive pericarditis, restrictive cardiomyopathy, and valve disease**
- Thyroid function tests should be monitored for hypothyroidism after radiation
- Chemotherapy increases the risk of myelodysplastic syndrome and acute leukemia

Non-Hodgkin Lymphoma

Basic Information

- Incidence
  - **Diffuse large B-cell lymphoma (DLBCL) is the most common NHL, followed by follicular lymphoma**
  - Incidence of lymphoma rises with age
- Histology
  - Most lymphomas arise from B cells
  - Broadly divided into low-grade (indolent) or high-grade (aggressive) lymphomas (Box 55-1)
- Risk factors
  - Altered immunity (human immunodeficiency virus [HIV] infection, organ transplantation, autoimmune diseases, congenital immunodeficiency)
    - Aggressive B-cell lymphoma is an acquired immunodeficiency syndrome (AIDS)-defining illness
  - Infections
    - Epstein-Barr virus (especially in African Burkitt lymphoma and AIDS-related lymphomas)
    - HTLV-1 in adult T-cell leukemia/lymphoma
    - Hepatitis C virus in some low-grade lymphomas
    - *Helicobacter pylori* in gastric mucosa-associated lymphoid tissue (MALT) lymphoma **(H. pylori treatment can eradicate the lymphoma)**
    - Consider antibiotics as first line for low-grade, localized gastric lymphoma that is positive for *H. pylori*, with radiation as second-line treatment
  - Chemical exposure (pesticides)

Clinical Presentation

- Low-grade lymphomas (e.g., follicular lymphomas) manifest subtly
  - Lymph nodes can wax and wane, possibly for years
  - May be discovered incidentally
- More aggressive lymphomas (like DLBCL) usually manifest with firm, enlarging lymph nodes or widespread lymphadenopathy, with or without B symptoms

---

BOX 55-1 | *Examples of Non-Hodgkin Lymphomas*

Indolent
Follicular lymphoma, grade 1 or 2
Marginal zone lymphoma, including mucosa-associated lymphoid tissue lymphoma
Chronic lymphocytic leukemia, small lymphocytic leukemia
Most skin lymphomas

Aggressive
Follicular lymphoma, grade 3B
Diffuse large B-cell lymphoma
Mediastinal large B-cell lymphoma
Peripheral T-cell lymphoma
Mantle cell lymphoma
Burkitt lymphoma*
Acute lymphoblastic lymphoma/leukemia*

*These are highly aggressive.

- **Very high-grade lymphomas (like Burkitt lymphoma) can grow extremely rapidly, usually manifesting with a single large mass in the chest or abdomen and an elevated lactate dehydrogenase (LDH) level**

Diagnosis

- Incisional lymph node biopsy is generally preferable to needle biopsy
- Staging (see Table 55-1) includes chest/abdomen/pelvis CT preferably with PET, and a bone marrow biopsy
- Consider HIV testing in most patients with aggressive NHL

Prognosis

- Stage is relatively poor indicator of outcome, because spread is hematogenous
  - Adverse prognostic features in aggressive lymphomas include:
    - Age older than 60 years
    - Elevated LDH
    - Stage III or IV disease
    - More than one extranodal site
    - Poor performance status
- In AIDS-related lymphomas
  - CD4 count is most important prognostic feature
  - Addition of highly active antiretroviral therapy (HAART) improves survival

Treatment

- Low-grade lymphomas are treatable but usually incurable
  - Many treatment options (e.g., watchful waiting, chemotherapy, monoclonal antibodies such as rituximab, radiation)
  - **No proven benefit to early or aggressive treatment if patient is asymptomatic; consider observation**
  - Transformation to high-grade lymphoma may occur
  - In low-grade follicular lymphoma
    - Median survival is around 8 to 10 years
    - Radiation may cure limited-stage disease
    - Most have disseminated disease at diagnosis
    - Transformation occurs in approximately 40% of patients and is treated like high-grade lymphoma
- Aggressive lymphomas are treated promptly with combination chemotherapy, with or without radiation, and are potentially curable (approximately 50% cure rate in DLBCL)
  - Cyclophosphamide, doxorubicin, vincristine, prednisone (CHOP) is widely used
    - CHOP commonly causes neutropenia. Fever with neutropenia must be treated urgently.
    - Doxorubicin infrequently causes late cardiomyopathy
    - Vincristine commonly causes peripheral neuropathy
    - Chemotherapy increases the risk of myelodysplastic syndrome and acute leukemia
  - Addition of rituximab (monoclonal anti-CD20 antibody) to chemotherapy (e.g., rituximab-CHOP) improves outcomes in B-cell lymphomas

- **Monitor for tumor lysis syndrome caused by rapid cell breakdown**
  - Hyperuricemia
  - Hyperkalemia
  - Hyperphosphatemia
  - Hypocalcemia
  - Acute renal failure
- Spread to the central nervous system (CNS) may occur
  - Usually leptomeningeal disease, rather than a brain mass
  - May be diagnosed by lumbar puncture
  - Risk factors include:
    - HIV infection
    - Extranodal sites, such as bone marrow, sinuses, or testicles
    - High LDH
    - Burkitt lymphoma or lymphoblastic histology
  - CNS lymphoma requires directed therapy
    - Intrathecal chemotherapy, with or without radiation, is the mainstay
    - Most systemic chemotherapies are ineffective
- Autologous stem cell transplant is considered for most patients with relapsed aggressive lymphoma

Chronic Lymphocytic Leukemia

Basic Information

- Most common leukemia in the United States
- Median age of diagnosis is 70 years, with male predominance
- Arises from B cells
- Leading cause of death is infection

Clinical Presentation

- Often asymptomatic at diagnosis
  - Approximately 25% present with **lymphocytosis** found on routine labwork
  - **WBC greater than 50,000/µL can be asymptomatic and not require therapy**
- May also present with lymphadenopathy (usually painless), splenomegaly, anemia, thrombocytopenia, or B symptoms
- **Hypogammaglobulinemia increases infection risk**
- Autoimmune complications may occur, including hemolytic anemia and immune-mediated thrombocytopenia

Diagnosis

- Lymphocytosis in blood
  - At least 5000/µL circulating B cells, with characteristic phenotype
  - **Peripheral smear shows small, mature lymphocytes, some appearing as "smudge cells" (an artifact) (Fig. 55-2A)**
- Lymphocytosis in bone marrow is common (often more than 30% lymphocytes)
- Staging (Table 55-2) based on CBC and presence of enlarged lymph nodes, spleen, or liver
- Small lymphocytic lymphoma is the same disease as CLL, but with more lymphadenopathy than leukemia

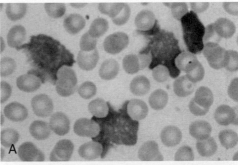
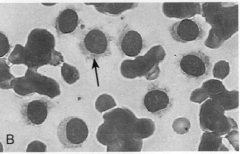

FIGURE 55-2 A, Peripheral blood smear showing "smudge cells" in chronic lymphocytic leukemia. **B,** Lymphocytes with fine surface projections or "hairs" *(arrow)* in hairy cell leukemia. (**A**, From Hoffman R, Benz EJ Jr, Shattil SJ, et al. *Hematology: Basic Principles and Practice.* 4th ed. Philadelphia: Churchill Livingstone; 2005: Fig. 79-5; **B**, from Rodak BF. *Diagnostic Hematology.* Philadelphia: Saunders; 1995.)

TABLE 55-2		*Rai Staging of Chronic Lymphocytic Leukemia*
Risk Group	**Stage**	**Features**
Low	0	Lymphocytosis only (blood or marrow)
Intermediate	I	Lymphocytosis + lymphadenopathy
	II	Lymphocytosis + hepatomegaly or splenomegaly
High	III	Lymphocytosis + anemia (hemoglobin <11 g/dL)
	IV	Lymphocytosis + thrombocytopenia (platelets <100,000/µL)

Prognosis

- Virtually incurable
- Variable natural history
  - Median survival ranges from less than 4 years to more than 20 years, depending on risk factors
- Adverse features include:
  - Rapid lymphocyte doubling time (12 months)
  - Advanced stage at diagnosis
  - Cytogenetics (17p deletion, 11q deletion are unfavorable; isolated 13q deletion is most favorable)
  - Immunoglobulin gene mutation status (unmutated immunoglobulin heavy-chain variable region [*IgVH*] gene is unfavorable)
- **Richter syndrome (transformation to aggressive lymphoma) occurs in approximately 5% and is difficult to treat**

- Suspect if rapid growth in one or more lymph nodes or worsening B symptoms

Treatment

- **Observation is appropriate for early-stage or asymptomatic CLL**
  - No proven advantage to early treatment if asymptomatic
- Indications for treatment
  - Bulky lymphadenopathy or organomegaly
  - Constitutional symptoms (weakness, B symptoms)
  - Bone marrow failure (anemia or thrombocytopenia) from progressive CLL
  - Autoimmune hemolysis or autoimmune thrombocytopenia failing usual therapy
  - Rapidly progressive disease or Richter transformation
- Active drugs include:
  - Purine analogues: fludarabine
  - Antibodies: rituximab, alemtuzumab (Campath; anti-CD52 antibody)
  - Alkylating agents: chlorambucil (commonly used as single agent), cyclophosphamide
  - Other: bendamustine
- **Intravenous immunoglobulin (IVIg) may be given for hypogammaglobulinemia and frequent infection**

Hairy Cell Leukemia

Basic Information

- Rare B-cell leukemia
- Median age of onset 55 years, with strong male predominance
- Indolent course, but progressive

Clinical Presentation

- **Manifests with pancytopenia and massive splenomegaly**
- A "dry" bone marrow tap despite marrow hypercellularity is characteristic

Diagnosis

- Peripheral smear may show small- to medium-sized lymphocytes with hairlike projections (Fig. 55-2B)
- Cells have a specific phenotype

Treatment

- Cladribine (2-CdA) or pentostatin (both purine analogues) usually induces complete remission

Review Questions

For review questions, please go to ExpertConsult.com.

SUGGESTED READINGS

Armitage JO. How I treat patients with diffuse large B-cell lymphoma. *Blood.* 2007;110:29-36.
Borchmann B, Engert A. The past: what we have learned in the last decade. Section title: clinical advances in Hodgkin lymphoma. *Hematology Am Soc Hematol Educ Program.* 2010:101-107.
Freedman A. Follicular lymphoma: 2014 update on diagnosis and management. *Am J Hematol.* 2014;89:429-436.
Hallek M. Chronic lymphocytic leukemia: 2013 update on diagnosis, risk stratification and treatment. *Am J Hematol.* 2013;88:803-816.
Ng AK, Lacasce A, Travis LB. Long-term complications of lymphoma and its treatment. *J Clin Oncol.* 2011;29:1885-1892.

Plasma Cell Dyscrasias

CAROL ANN HUFF, MD

Plasma cell dyscrasias are clonal B-cell disorders characterized by overproduction of monoclonal immunoglobulins (Igs). Patients with plasma cell dyscrasias may present with a number of symptoms, but many are asymptomatic at the time of diagnosis.

Basic Information

- Definition
  - Seven categories of plasma cell dyscrasias (Table 56-1)
  - A characteristic feature of each is the presence of a monoclonal Ig
  - Autoimmune disorders and chronic inflammatory conditions may lead to production of monoclonal Igs; this is not malignant and is distinct from plasma cell dyscrasias. Examples include:
    - Connective tissue diseases (e.g., systemic lupus erythematosus, rheumatoid arthritis, Sjögren syndrome, cold agglutinin disease)
    - Infections (e.g., tuberculosis, endocarditis, hepatitis, human immunodeficiency virus [HIV])
  - **Monoclonal Igs are seen in approximately 1% of adults;** prevalence increases with increasing age
    - Prevalence: IgG > IgM > IgA
- Evaluation of patient with possible monoclonal Ig production (Figs. 56-1 and 56-2)
  - Diagnostic clues to initiate evaluation
    - Asymptomatic individual: elevated total protein; elevated globulin fraction of protein; normochromic/normocytic anemia
    - Symptomatic individual: normochromic/normocytic anemia, recurrent bacterial infections, renal insufficiency, bone pain, pathologic fracture or osteolytic lesion on radiograph, osteoporosis, sensorimotor neuropathy, pyoderma gangrenosum

Multiple Myeloma

Basic Information

- **Second most common hematologic malignancy** (after non-Hodgkin lymphoma [NHL]), resulting in 1% of cancer deaths each year
- Male predominance
- Twice as common in African Americans as whites
- Median age at diagnosis: 68 years
- Median survival after diagnosis is 5 to 7 years and improving

- Poor prognostic indicators include renal insufficiency, elevated β_2-microglobulin, genetic abnormalities including 1q amplification, t[4;14], t[14;16], t[14;20], or p53 deletions detected with fluorescent in situ hybridization (FISH) with or without hypodiploidy, 13q deletion, or a complex karyotype by cytogenetics

Clinical Presentation

- Most common presenting features are hypercalcemia, renal insufficiency, and bone pain
- Presence of one or more of the CRAB (hypercalcemia, renal insufficiency, anemia, or bone disease) criteria is required to diagnose active myeloma
- Figure 56-3 illustrates the clinical manifestations of multiple myeloma

Diagnosis and Evaluation

- Diagnostic criteria for multiple myeloma
  - Smoldering/asymptomatic (Box 56-1)
    - Clonal bone marrow plasma cells 10% or higher
    or
    - Presence of serum and/or urinary monoclonal protein 3 g/dL or higher
  - Active
    - Above criteria with addition of end-organ damage attributable to the underlying plasma cell proliferative disorder, specifically the CRAB criteria
      - **C**alcium greater than 11.5 g/dL
      - **R**enal insufficiency (creatinine greater than 2 mg/dL)
      - **A**nemia (hemoglobin [Hbg] <10 g/100 mL or 2 g/100 mL < normal)
      - **B**one disease (osteopenia or lytic lesions)
- Common complications include the following:
  - Hypercalcemia: present in 25% of patients; results from lytic bone disease; treated with saline hydration, loop diuretics (although now controversial), and bisphosphonates
  - Anemia: normochromic, normocytic with an Hbg value that is at least 2 g/100 mL below the lower limit of normal or an Hbg value less than 10 g/100 mL
  - Renal insufficiency: occurs in 50% of patients; usually progresses insidiously, but acute renal failure may be present
    - Bence Jones proteinuria (may be missed on routine urine dipstick, which detects albumin; sulfosalicylic

TABLE 56-1	*Plasma Cell Dyscrasias*
Disorders	**Disease Definition**
Monoclonal gammopathy of undetermined significance (MGUS)	Overproduction of monoclonal immunoglobulin (<3 g/dL) with <10% clonal plasma cells on bone marrow aspiration and biopsy and absence of end-organ damage (hypercalcemia, renal insufficiency, anemia, bone lesions).
Multiple myeloma	Clonal plasma cells ≥10% in the bone marrow and/or presence of serum and/or urinary monoclonal protein; when there is associated evidence of lytic bone lesions, anemia, hypercalcemia, or renal insufficiency, it is active myeloma. In the absence of associated symptoms, termed smoldering or asymptomatic.
Plasmacytoma	Biopsy-proven solitary lesion with clonal plasma cells and insufficient criteria to diagnose multiple myeloma (see above).
POEMS syndrome	Presence of monoclonal plasma cells; **p**olyneuropathy, **o**rganomegaly, **e**ndocrinopathy, **M** protein, and **s**kin changes
AL amyloidosis	Presence of monoclonal plasma cells creating a syndrome where insoluble proteins deposit in tissues and cause end-organ damage.
Waldenström macroglobulinemia	Immunoglobulin M monoclonal gammopathy with >10% bone marrow lymphoplasmacytic infiltration.
Cryoglobulinemia	Group of disorders associated with overproduction of monoclonal or polyclonal protein production: defining characteristic is that proteins precipitate when cooled and dissolve when heated.

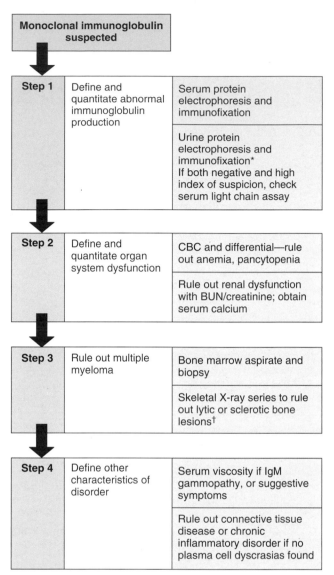

FIGURE 56-1 Evaluation of a monoclonal immunoglobulin. *Spot urine for qualitative assessment: 24-hour collection for quantitative assessment. †Bone scan evaluates for blastic lesions and will be normal in multiple myeloma. BUN, Blood urea nitrogen; CBC, complete blood count; IgM, immunoglobulin M.

acid effectively precipitates light chains), tubular casts, glomerular lesions
- **Avoid intravenous (IV) contrast in patients with known or suspected myeloma unless absolutely necessary**
- Hyperviscosity syndrome: results from elevated serum proteins; symptoms usually not seen until serum viscosity greater than 4 cP (centiPoises) (Box 56-2)
- Neurologic: sensory or sensorimotor neuropathy
- Immunodeficiency: increased risk of recurrent bacterial infections caused by suppression of normal Igs
- Bone lesions: lytic lesions, severe osteopenia, or pathologic fractures (most commonly vertebral compression fractures)
  - To diagnose: obtain skeletal survey to identify high-risk areas and consider prophylactic radiotherapy or surgical pinning of areas at high risk

- Positron emission tomography (PET) scans and spine magnetic resonance imaging (MRI) are more sensitive and should be used in patients with symptomatic bone disease that is NOT detected on plain radiographs and in cases where the skeletal survey is negative to exclude the presence of occult bone disease
- **Bone scan is typically normal in myeloma patients because it only shows blastic lesions**
- Spinal cord compression is a serious complication that can present with pain, lower extremity paresthesias or weakness, urinary retention, and/or fecal incontinence; treatment with IV dexamethasone and radiation therapy and, sometimes, with urgent surgical decompression

- Lenalidomide, bortezomib, and dexamethasone
- Cyclophosphamide, bortezomib, and dexamethasone
- Bone marrow transplantation
  - Autologous: increases survival by 12 to 18 months on average; all patients eventually relapse
  - Allogeneic: potentially curative (25% to 30%) but has greatest toxicities
- Symptomatic management
  - **Bone lesions: bisphosphonates decrease risk of fracture and improve quality of life;** surgical intervention for pathologic fractures; vertebroplasty or kyphoplasty for symptomatic vertebral lesions
  - Anemia: erythropoietin in symptomatic patients who are not hyperviscous
  - Infectious: vaccinate against *Pneumococcus, Haemophilus influenzae,* and influenza; consider prophylactic antibiotics if on long-term corticosteroids, varicella-zoster prophylaxis if on bortezomib

Plasmacytomas

Basic Information

- **Plasmacytomas are proliferations of monoclonal plasma cells forming a mass at extramedullary or osseous sites**
- No evidence of multiple myeloma or end-organ dysfunction (hypercalcemia, renal insufficiency, anemia, or other bone lesions, and no evidence of plasmacytosis on bone marrow biopsy)
- 50% of osseous plasmacytomas develop into overt myeloma; only 15% of extraosseous lesions develop overt myeloma

Clinical Presentation

- Solitary plasmacytoma: single tumor of plasma cells resulting in localized complaints (bone pain, pathologic fracture); no evidence of diffuse plasma cell overgrowth throughout remainder of bone marrow (Fig. 56-4); most common sites are vertebrae, ribs, skull, and pelvis
- Extramedullary plasmacytoma: plasma cell tumor arising outside of the bone marrow; most commonly found in upper respiratory tract (nasal passages, sinuses, nasopharynx, larynx); occasionally described in the lower extremity, gastrointestinal tract, lung, lymph nodes; can be associated with HIV infection

Diagnosis and Evaluation

- Diagnosis made by biopsy, typically when mass or structural abnormality noted on imaging study
- Serum protein electrophoresis (SPEP), urine protein electrophoresis (UPEP), bone marrow aspiration, and biopsy, as well as skeletal survey should be done at diagnosis to rule out extramedullary spread of multiple myeloma; if negative, consider spine MRI and PET scan to exclude occult lesions elsewhere; if truly isolated, follow serially in case of progression to myeloma

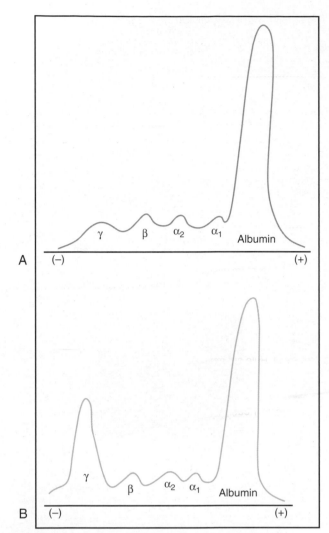

FIGURE 56-2 Serum protein electrophoresis in a normal individual (A) and in an individual with a monoclonal gammopathy (B). (From Waldman SD. *Interventional pain management.* 2nd ed. Philadelphia: WB Saunders; 2001: Fig. 9-1A, C.)

Treatment

- **Treatment of smoldering myeloma considered investigational**
- **For active myeloma:**
  - **Chemotherapy: not curative; should be instituted when patients are symptomatic or demonstrate end-organ dysfunction, as described earlier**
    - Initial treatment decision based on eligibility for stem cell transplantation
      - Transplant-ineligible patients may receive melphalan-containing regimens
        - Melphalan, prednisone, and thalidomide
        - Melphalan, prednisone, and bortezomib
        - Lenaldiomide and dexamethasone
        - Bortezomib and dexamethasone
      - Transplant-eligible
        - Lenaldiomide and dexamethasone
        - Bortezomib and dexamethasone

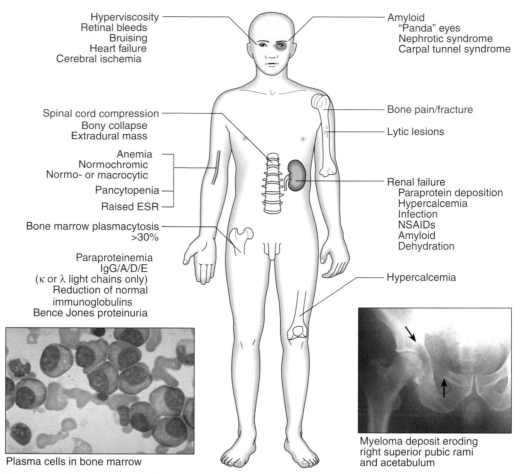

Hyperviscosity
Retinal bleeds
Bruising
Heart failure
Cerebral ischemia

Amyloid
"Panda" eyes
Nephrotic syndrome
Carpal tunnel syndrome

Spinal cord compression
Bony collapse
Extradural mass

Bone pain/fracture

Lytic lesions

Anemia
Normochromic
Normo- or macrocytic

Pancytopenia

Raised ESR

Bone marrow plasmacytosis
>30%

Paraproteinemia
IgG/A/D/E
(κ or λ light chains only)
Reduction of normal
immunoglobulins
Bence Jones proteinuria

Renal failure
Paraprotein deposition
Hypercalcemia
Infection
NSAIDs
Amyloid
Dehydration

Hypercalcemia

Plasma cells in bone marrow

Myeloma deposit eroding
right superior pubic rami
and acetabulum

FIGURE 56-3 Clinical manifestations of multiple myeloma. ESR, Erythrocyte sedimentation rate; Ig, immunoglobulin; NSAIDs, nonsteroidal antiinflammatory drugs. (From Haslett C, Chilvers ER, Boon NA, et al. *Davidson's Principles and Practice of Medicine*. 19th ed. New York: Churchill Livingstone; 2002: Fig. 19.33.)

| BOX 56-1 | *Diagnostic Criteria for Multiple Myeloma* |

Smoldering

M protein ≥3 g/dL and/or clonal plasma cells on bone marrow ≥10%
No evidence of end-organ impairment and asymptomatic

Active

Requires one or more of the following in addition to the criteria for smoldering disease:
Calcium >11.5 g/dL
Renal insufficiency (creatinine >2 mg/dL)
Anemia (hemoglobin <10 g/100 mL or 2 g/100 mL < normal)
Bone disease (osteopenia or lytic lesions)

| BOX 56-2 | *Hyperviscosity Syndrome* |

Symptoms

Neurologic: headache, dizziness, ataxia, paresthesias, somnolence, coma
Visual: diplopia, blurred vision, loss of vision
Cardiac: congestive heart failure, myocardial ischemia
Hematologic: spontaneous bleeding, particularly from nose and gums; GI bleeding described

Physical Findings

Flame-shaped retinal hemorrhages
Papilledema
"Boxcar" formation of RBCs in retinal vessels

Treatment

Plasmapheresis until symptoms resolve (may be needed daily if symptoms persist)
Therapy directed at underlying cause
Caution if RBC transfusion needed, because this will expand volume and worsen symptoms

GI, Gastrointestinal; RBC, red blood cell.

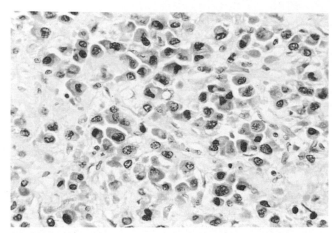

FIGURE 56-4 Bone marrow replaced with plasma cells. (From Stevens A, Lowe J: *Pathology.* 2nd ed. St. Louis: Mosby; 2000: Fig. 15.16.)

Treatment

- Radiation therapy to the involved area; 15% to 25% are disease-free at 10 years

Monoclonal Gammopathy of Undetermined Significance

Basic Information

- Most common plasma cell dyscrasia (3% of population older than age 50 years)
- Asymptomatic premalignant disorder
- Rate of progression of monoclonal gammopathy of unknown significance (MGUS) to myeloma or related malignancy is approximately 1% per year
- **Characterized by overproduction of a monoclonal Ig without other abnormalities;** diagnosis of exclusion, usually made retrospectively, when one demonstrates stability over time in the quantity of M protein and the absence of other findings

Clinical Presentation

- **No symptoms associated with MGUS; diagnosed entirely on laboratory criteria**
- Evaluation: SPEP and immunofixation electrophoresis (IFE); 24-hour UPEP and IFE; complete blood count (CBC) and differential, creatinine, calcium, albumin, serum κ/λ light-chain assay, skeletal survey
- **Bone marrow aspiration, and biopsy recommended for all patients with M protein greater than 1 g/dL and in those with non-IgG paraprotein, regardless of quantification of M protein**

Diagnostic Criteria

- **M protein less than 3 g/dL** (as determined by SPEP)
- Less than 10% plasma cells in bone marrow
- Normal Hgb, creatinine, calcium
- Absence of lytic bone disease
- Asymptomatic

TABLE 56-2	*Criteria for the Diagnosis of POEMS Syndrome*
Major criteria	Polyneuropathy* Monoclonal plasma cell-proliferative disorder (95% are λ)* Sclerotic bone lesions Castleman disease Vascular endothelial growth factor elevation
Minor criteria	Organomegaly (splenomegaly, hepatomegaly, lymphadenopathy) Extravascular volume overload (edema, pleural effusion, ascites) Endocrinopathy (adrenal, thyroid,† pituitary, gonadal, parathyroid, pancreatic†) Skin changes (hyperpigmentation, hypertrichosis, white nails) Papilledema Thrombocytosis, polycythemia
Other signs and symptoms	Clubbing, weight loss, hyperhidrosis, pulmonary hypertension, restrictive lung disease, low vitamin B_{12}, diarrhea, thrombotic diatheses
Possible associations	Arthralgias, cardiomyopathy, fever

*Polyneuropathy and monoclonal plasma cell disorder must be present in all patients; to make diagnosis, at least one other major criterion and one minor criterion are required.
†Endocrinopathy other than isolated thyroid disease or diabetes mellitus is required to meet this criterion (because of the relative frequency of these in the general population).

Treatment/Follow-up

- **Observation alone, without therapy**
- Serial laboratories including SPEP, UPEP, serum κ/λ light chains, CBC and differential, and metabolic panel for creatinine and calcium at least yearly
- Increased risk of progression to myeloma: high monoclonal protein concentration, a non-IgG paraprotein, an abnormal serum-free κ/λ light-chain ratio

POEMS Syndrome

Basic Information

- *Polyneuropathy, organomegaly, endocrinopathy, M protein, and skin changes (POEMS)* **syndrome resulting from overproduction of light chains, usually λ, without significant overgrowth of plasma cells in the bone marrow; many organ systems involved, with characteristic abnormalities**
- Also called osteosclerotic myeloma

Clinical Presentation

Table 56-2 summarizes the clinical presentation of POEMS syndrome.
- Polyneuropathy is an inflammatory demyelinating process with predominantly sensory symptoms
- Organomegaly most common in spleen and liver
- Endocrinopathies seen include hypogonadism and hyperprolactinemia
- M protein is usually λ light chains

- Skin changes include hypertrichosis and thickening of the dermis
- Sclerotic bone lesions
- Elevated vascular endothelial growth factor
- Papilledema
- Thrombocytosis or polycythemia

Diagnosis

- Based on clinical suspicion and constellation of findings (see Table 56-2); neuropathy is typically the most prominent symptom; SPEP/immunofixation/serum-free light-chain assay demonstrating monoclonal protein, typically including λ light chains

Treatment

- Includes radiation therapy to bone lesion if isolated; if diffuse changes, then systemic therapy with corticosteroids, bortezomib- or lenalidomide-based therapy, followed by consideration for high-dose chemotherapy and autologous stem cell transplantation similar to treatment for multiple myeloma

Waldenström Macroglobulinemia

Basic Information

- Also known as lymphoplasmacytic lymphoma
- **A rare lymphoma characterized by bone marrow infiltration of clonal B cells with production of M protein (IgM)**

Clinical Presentation

- **Signs/symptoms commonly related to both tumor infiltration of the marrow and elevated monoclonal IgM**
- Most dangerous complication: hyperviscosity (Fig. 56-5; see Box 56-2) because of high production of IgM

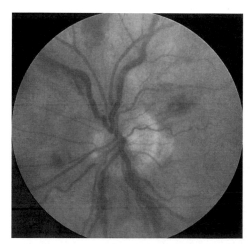

FIGURE 56-5 Waldenström macroglobulinemia (hyperviscosity syndrome). The retina of a patient who presented with blurred vision, headache, and dizziness exhibits gross distention of vessels, particularly the veins, which show bulging and constriction (the "linked sausage" effect), as well as areas of hemorrhage. (From Skarin AT, ed. *Atlas of Diagnostic Oncology.* 3rd ed. Philadelphia: Saunders; 2003: Fig. 15.56.)

- Polyneuropathy and cryoglobulinemia (with digital infarcts) also may be seen because of high production of IgM
- Tumor infiltration causing organomegaly, lymphadenopathy, B symptoms (fevers, night sweats, weight loss)
- Only 25% of patients with IgM monoclonal gammopathy have Waldenström macroglobulinemia; others have MGUS, multiple myeloma, chronic lymphocytic leukemia, NHL, or cold agglutinin disease

Diagnosis

- **Based on presence of IgM and evidence of B-cell lymphoma by pathology**

Treatment

- Plasmapheresis is performed to treat hyperviscosity and its related symptoms
- Chemotherapy: use monoclonal antibody therapy, such as rituximab (anti-CD20) and/or nucleoside analogues (e.g., fludarabine) or alkylating agents (e.g., bendamustine, cyclophosphamide), Bruton's tyrosine kinase (BTK) inhibitors (e.g., iburitinib)
- Some patients develop aggressive lymphoma (Richter transformation)

Cryoglobulinemia

Basic Information

- Group of disorders (3 subtypes) characterized by production of soluble proteins that precipitate on cooling, typically associated with symptoms; often evidence of an underlying clonal disorder (Table 56-3)

Clinical Presentation

- Varies by subtype (see Table 56-3)

Diagnosis

- **Key to detection is proper transport of sample. Must be taken to lab at body temperature (ideally in a warm-water bath); diagnosis requires the demonstration of protein precipitation on cooling of blood.**

Treatment

- Focused on correcting underlying disease
- Plasmapheresis for those symptomatic patients in whom underlying disease is not treatable

Amyloidosis

Basic Information

- Relatively rare
- **Characterized by deposition of insoluble protein in organs and tissues, resulting in organ dysfunction**
- Disease classified by which protein precursor forms the fibril deposits
    - AL amyloidosis: amyloid protein is primarily the variable region of Ig light chains (λ > κ)

TABLE 56-3	The Cryoglobulinemias		
Subtype	Immunoglobulin	Disease Association	Features
I	Presence of isolated monoclonal Ig (usually IgG or IgM, less commonly IgA or free light chains)	Waldenström macroglobulinemia, multiple myeloma	Many patients are asymptomatic; classic symptoms related to hyperviscosity: digital ischemia, Raynaud phenomenon, purpura, livedo reticularis
II	"Essential mixed CG" is a mixture of polyclonal Ig with a monoclonal Ig (usually IgM or IgA); can also have RF activity	Persistent viral infectious; most often hepatitis C or HIV	Membranoproliferative glomerulonephritis, mononeuritis multiplex, vasculitis; classic Meltzer triad of purpura, arthralgias, and weakness
III	Polyclonal Ig	Most often secondary to connective tissue disorders or chronic inflammatory conditions	Treatment directed at primary disorder

CG, Cryoglobulinemia; HIV, human immunodeficiency virus; Ig, immunoglobulin; RF, rheumatoid factor.

TABLE 56-4	Clinical Presentation of Amyloidosis		
Amyloid Subtype	Dominant Protein	Organ Deposit	Symptoms
AL	Immunoglobulin light chains	Heart	Low-voltage ECG Right-sided heart failure with volume overload Echocardiogram shows classic myocardium speckled pattern; orthostatic hypotension
		Kidney	Nephrotic-range proteinuria
		Tongue	Macroglossia
		GI tract	Infiltration of gut with malabsorptive process
		CNS	Peripheral neuropathy, carpal tunnel syndrome
AA	Serum amyloid protein A	Kidney	Most commonly involved with nephrotic-range proteinuria
		Liver, spleen	Organomegaly
Familial	Transthyretin	CNS	Neuropathy with sensory or autonomic insufficiency
		Heart	Conduction abnormalities (see also symptoms of cardiac deposit of AL above)

CNS, Central nervous system; ECG, electrocardiogram; GI, gastrointestinal.

- AL amyloidosis is a plasma cell dyscrasia related to myeloma
- AA amyloidosis: secondary amyloidosis in which the amyloid protein is serum amyloid protein A (an acute-phase reactant produced in response to inflammation)
  - Protein A is not related to a known Ig
  - AA amyloidosis is associated with chronic infections (e.g., tuberculosis, osteomyelitis, bronchiectasis), chronic inflammatory disorders (e.g., rheumatoid arthritis, inflammatory bowel disease, and familial Mediterranean fever)
- Familial amyloidosis: autosomal dominant disorder in which mutant protein (most commonly transthyretin) forms amyloid fibrils
  - Systemic senile amyloidosis: Sporadic disorder characterized by wild-type transthyretin protein deposition in the myocardium leading primarily to late-onset cardiomyopathy and potentially carpal tunnel disease. Survival is generally significantly longer than other causes of amyloid cardiomyopathy.

Clinical Presentation

- Determined by the organs predominantly affected by protein deposition and differs according to amyloid subtype (Table 56-4)

Diagnosis

- **Requires demonstration of deposition of amyloid fibers, typically with a fat pad aspirate; staining with Congo red demonstrates apple green birefringence under polarized light (Fig. 56-6)**
- **Mass spectroscopic analysis of amyloid tissue can be performed to determine amyloid subtype**
- Underlying plasma cell dyscrasias should be ruled out with SPEP/UPEP/serum IFE/urine IFE, bone marrow aspirate/biopsy, CBC and differential diagnosis, chemistry panel, and serum light-chain assay
- Variant transthyretin (familial amyloidosis) should also be ruled out by deoxyribonucleic acid (DNA) testing
- If no plasma cell dyscrasias, transthyretin normal, consider AA amyloidosis

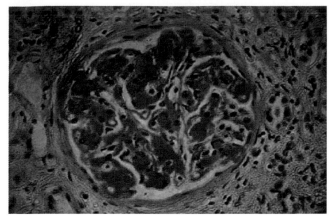

FIGURE 56-6 Amyloidosis. Congo red stain of a glomerulus that is largely replaced by amyloid demonstrates the characteristic birefringence under polarized light. (From Goldman L. *Cecil Textbook of Medicine.* 23rd ed. Philadelphia: Saunders; 2007: Fig. 115-14.)

Treatment

- Directed at the underlying disease, with goal to prevent further deposition of amyloid (resorption of amyloid fibers usually does not occur); management must also focus on control of symptoms from organ dysfunction
- AL: systemic chemotherapy shown to prolong survival; melphalan and prednisone
  - Small studies suggest autologous bone marrow transplantation may improve survival in selected patients

- Prognosis: Median survival is 1 to 2 years, depending on degree of organ involvement; median survival is 6 months if symptomatic cardiac involvement, 21 months with renal involvement
- AA amyloidosis: treat underlying infection or inflammatory disease
- Familial amyloidosis: liver transplantation is curative; often does not reverse the damage
- Senile systemic amyloidosis: supportive care

Review Questions

For review questions, please go to ExpertConsult.com.

SUGGESTED READINGS

Cavo M, Rajkumar SV, Palumbo A, et al. International Myeloma Working Group consensus approach to the treatment of multiple myeloma patients who are candidates for autologous stem cell transplantation. *Blood.* 2011;117:6063-6073.

Dispenzieri A. POEMS syndrome: 2014 update on diagnosis, risk-stratification and management. *Am J Hematol.* 2014;89:214-223.

Kyle RA, San-Miguel JF, Mateos MV, et al. Monoclonal gammopathy of undetermined significance and smoldering multiple myeloma. *Hematol Oncol Clin North Am.* 2014;28:775-790.

Merlini G, Comenzo RL, Seldin DC, et al. Immunoglobulin light chain amyloidosis. *Expert Rev Hematol.* 2014;7:143-156.

Palumbo A, Rajkumar SV, San Miguel JF, et al. International Myeloma Working Group consensus statement for the management, treatment, and supportive care of patients with myeloma not eligible for standard autologous stem-cell transplantation. *J Clin Oncol.* 2014;32:587-600.

Rajkumar V. Multiple myeloma: 2011 update on diagnosis, risk-stratification and management. *Am J Hematol.* 2011;88:57-65.

Richardson PG, Blade J. The comprehensive clinical management of multiple myeloma and related-plasma cell disorders. *Expert Rev Hematol.* 2014;7:1-3.

Selected Topics in Oncology

DAVID COSGROVE, MD

Previous chapters in this section have focused on the diagnosis and treatment of specific types of cancers. This chapter emphasizes other important aspects in the identification and care of oncologic patients. Specifically, the evaluation of patients with cancer of unknown primary, as well as the identification of oncologic emergencies and paraneoplastic syndromes, is emphasized. Although specific chemotherapeutic regimens are generally left to oncologists, basic toxicities and complications of chemotherapeutic agents should be recognized by all internists.

Cancer of Unknown Primary

Basic Information

- 3% to 5% of all patients with newly diagnosed cancers present with primary tumors of unknown origin
- Equal incidence in men and women
- Median age 60 years
- Most common site: lymph nodes
- Typically less than 50% of patients have a primary site identified after work-up
- Cytopathology
  - Helpful in determining the primary tumor site
  - Histology
    - **Adenocarcinoma is the most commonly identified tumor type (60% of cases)**
      - Prostate-specific antigen stain may be helpful in identifying prostate cancer
    - Poorly or undifferentiated carcinoma is seen in about 30% of cases
    - Squamous cell carcinoma is seen in 5% to 10% of cases
    - Specific immunoperoxidase stains may be helpful in suggesting specific causes (Table 57-1)
  - Genetic studies may be helpful in identifying specific cancer subtypes, most commonly lymphomas, sarcomas, and certain other solid tumors

Clinical Presentation

- Depends on site of organ involvement
- Weight loss, fatigue, and malaise are common systemic symptoms
- Lymphadenopathy (cervical, supraclavicular, mediastinal, axillary, retroperitoneal) may be the only clinical abnormality

Diagnosis

- **Avoid the impulse to randomly order tumor markers and imaging studies**

- Start with a thorough history and physical (including gynecologic examination or prostate examination) to guide your evaluation
- Make sure age-appropriate cancer screening is up to date
- Complete blood count (CBC), chemistry profile, liver function tests
- Computed tomography (CT) scan of the chest, abdomen, and pelvis should be ordered routinely. A positron emission tomography/CT scan can be considered, although data on use are lacking.
- Colonoscopy should be considered if clinical symptoms dictate or if screening measures are not up to date
- Mammography for women should be considered if indicated by symptoms or initial work-up, or if screening measures are not up to date
- Order biopsy/tissue sampling of an accessible mass lesion, and special studies (as described previously)
- Specific evaluation measures dictated by location of discovered tumor (Table 57-2)

Treatment

- Directed at the primary site of origin, if discovered
- In cases in which the primary tumor is not identified, treatment is based on tumor histology, location, and most likely primary site (see Table 57-2)
- In cases in which the histology and location do not suggest a specific primary site (most cases), empiric chemotherapy can extend median survival by a few months in select cases

Oncologic Emergencies

SPINAL CORD COMPRESSION

Basic Information

- More than 5% of patients who die from cancer have evidence of spinal cord compression
- The most common primary malignancies include lung cancer, breast cancer, prostate cancer, renal cell cancer, and multiple myeloma
- Compression most commonly caused by extradural metastases involving the spinal cord
- **Any delay in diagnosis and treatment may result in paralysis and incontinence of bowel and bladder that may be irreversible**
- Spinal cord compression may be the initial manifestation of a malignancy

- Most cases (60%) involve the thoracic spine, but compression can occur at the lumbosacral (20%) and cervical (10%) regions as well

Clinical Presentation

- Back pain that continues to increase in intensity is the most common initial finding (90% of cases)
  - Pain can be worsened by movement, coughing, sneezing
  - Radicular symptoms can develop (more common with lumbosacral lesions)
- Progressive motor weakness leading to instability of gait and paralysis is also common
- Sensory loss is seen in over half of patients
- Change in deep tendon reflexes (hyperreflexia or hyporeflexia) and extensor plantar responses may be seen
- Incontinence of stool or urine is usually a late finding

Diagnosis

- History and physical examination should focus on neurologic abnormalities

TABLE 57-1	*Immunoperoxidase Stains*
Tumor Type	**Immunoperoxidase Stain**
Carcinoma	Cytokeratin, chromogranin
Melanoma	S100, HMB45
Sarcoma	Vimentin, desmin
Lymphoma	Leukocyte common antigen
Neuroendocrine	Cytokeratin, synaptophysin, chromogranin

- **Radiologic imaging should be immediately done in all cancer patients who present with persistent back pain with or without radicular symptoms**
  - Plain spinal radiographs may detect vertebral compression fractures or collapse or erosive spinal lesions, but there is a high false-negative rate
  - Magnetic resonance imaging (MRI) is now the test of choice given its widespread availability
    - The entire vertebral column should be imaged, even if symptoms suggest involvement at a specific level, as multiple metastatic deposits are common, and should all be treated
  - CT myelogram is an alternative for patients who cannot lie still for an MRI or who have a contraindication to MRI

Treatment

- Goal is to control pain and preserve neurologic function
- Options are surgical resection or decompression, radiation therapy, and, in some cases, systemic chemotherapy. Urgent surgical, radiation, and medical oncology consults should be obtained.
  - **Surgery, when feasible, has been shown to result in better neurologic outcomes and possibly a survival benefit compared with radiation alone**
- Steroids should be given promptly
  - Initially, high-dose steroid therapy (dexamethasone 96 mg/day) may be given for palliation of pain and improvement of neurologic status, but this regimen may be associated with a higher treatment complication rate than a lower-dose regimen (16 mg/day)
- Surgery
  - Consider in patients who:

TABLE 57-2	*Evaluation and Treatment of Specific Carcinomas*	
Clinical Finding	**Histology/Treatment***	**Evaluation**
Isolated axillary adenopathy in women	Adenocarcinoma	Breast examination Stage II breast cancer Mammogram/breast MRI Estrogen/progesterone receptor studies
Cervical adenopathy and neck mass	Squamous cell carcinoma	Head and neck examination Panendoscopy of the aerodigestive tract CT scan of head and neck area
Inguinal adenopathy	Squamous cell carcinoma	Full gynecologic examination in women Evaluation of prostate and penis in men Rectal examinations Tumor markers (PSA, CA 125)
Bone metastases	Adenocarcinoma or poorly differentiated carcinoma	Physical examination Stage IV prostate cancer or breast cancer X-rays of spine/weight-bearing joints to rule out fracture PSA in men
Mediastinal/retroperitoneal adenopathy in young males	Poorly differentiated carcinoma	Extragonadal germ cell tumor Tumor markers (hCG, AFP, LDH)
Peritoneal carcinomatosis	Adenocarcinoma	Full gynecologic examination in women Colonoscopy

*Empiric treatment if the evaluation failed to confirm the primary site.
AFP, α-Fetoprotein; CA 125, cancer antigen 125; CT, computed tomography; hCG, human chorionic gonadotropin; LDH, lactate dehydrogenase; MRI, magnetic resonance imaging; PSA, prostate-specific antigen.

- Have tumors that are not sensitive to radiation
- Have received prior radiation therapy to the affected area
- Have a predicted survival of more than 6 months
- Need a tissue diagnosis
- Need spinal stabilization
- Chemotherapy should be considered as a primary treatment option only in patients with exquisitely chemosensitive tumors
- Radiation therapy is the mainstay of treatment to control spinal cord compression
- Overall, prognosis is poor; median survival after · diagnosis is less than 6 months

SUPERIOR VENA CAVA SYNDROME

- **Defined as obstruction of blood return to the heart by invasion, compression, or thrombosis of the superior vena cava**
- Most cases are associated with lung cancer (small cell), lymphoma, thymoma, testicular cancer, or breast cancer
- Can also result from venous thrombosis caused by indwelling venous access devices or fibrosing mediastinitis from infections (e.g., histoplasmosis, tuberculosis)
- Signs and symptoms include shortness of breath, facial swelling, fullness of face, cough, arm swelling, and prominent neck and chest veins (Fig. 57-1)
- CT scanning of the chest with contrast or MRI with gadolinium enhancement are the diagnostic modalities of choice
- If the cause is unknown, an evaluation that may include CT-guided biopsy, bronchoscopy, mediastinoscopy, or thoracotomy should be considered
- Treatment with radiation or chemotherapy may be indicated once the tumor type has been identified
- Intraluminal metal stents may provide palliation when cancer is refractory to chemotherapy or radiation
- Thrombolytics and anticoagulation may be necessary for patients with thrombosis

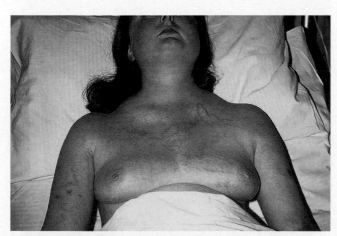

FIGURE 57-1 Superior vena caval obstruction in bronchial carcinoma. Note the swelling of the face and neck and the development of a collateral circulation in the veins of the chest wall. (From Goldman L, Bennett JC, Ausiello D. *Cecil Textbook of Medicine.* 22nd ed. Philadelphia: Saunders; 2004: Fig. 95-6.)

PERICARDIAL TAMPONADE

See also Chapter 8.
- Rarely occurs as the initial manifestation of a cancer
- Seen most commonly in patients with lung or breast cancer, lymphoma, or leukemia
- Cannot assume that all pericardial effusions in cancer patients are caused by metastasis
- Treatment options in symptomatic patients include prolonged catheter drainage, substernal pericardiotomy, pericardiectomy, or injection of a sclerosing agent
- **No need to treat asymptomatic pericardial effusions**

VENOUS THROMBOSIS

- Thromboembolism is the second leading cause of death in patients with malignancy
- Venous thrombosis is seen most commonly with visceral cancers from pancreas, lung, stomach, colon, breast, and ovary
- **Trousseau syndrome refers to migratory thrombophlebitis in the setting of visceral cancers**
- The risk of thrombosis is increased because of release of procoagulants by tumor cells, immobility of patients because of weakness, or obstruction of blood vessels by tumors
- Patients should be treated initially with heparin, then warfarin
- Sometimes the thromboembolism is resistant to warfarin and requires low-molecular-weight heparin therapy or inferior vena cava filter placement
- See Chapter 21 for detailed information regarding deep venous thrombosis and thromboembolism

METABOLIC EMERGENCIES

- Hypercalcemia of malignancy (see Chapter 39)
- Hyponatremia (see Chapter 32)

Paraneoplastic Syndromes

Basic Information

- Defined as conditions that arise as a result of factors produced by cancer cells
- **In some cases, the symptoms of these syndromes may precede the actual diagnosis of malignancy**
- Presence does not necessarily imply a poor prognosis
- Long-term treatment is geared toward the underlying malignancy

NEUROLOGIC SYNDROMES

- A number of specific syndromes have been described that may affect all parts of the nervous system (Table 57-3)
- Antineuronal antibodies may be helpful in diagnosis and in searching for particular neoplasms; however, they may not always be present

RHEUMATOLOGIC SYNDROMES

- Hypertrophic osteoarthropathy (Fig. 57-2)
  - Abnormal proliferation of bone and skin in the extremities

TABLE 57-3 *Selected Neurologic Paraneoplastic Syndromes*

Syndrome	Description	Most Commonly Associated Tumors	Antibody
Encephalomyelitis	Precedes discovery of the tumor in most patients Symptoms vary because it can involve a number of different areas of the nervous system Subacute sensory neuronopathy causing asymmetrical paresthesias is the most common early symptom	SCLC	Anti-Hu (also called antineuronal nuclear antibodies, or ANNA-1)
Cerebellar degeneration	Abrupt onset of dysarthria and ataxia Nystagmus and oculomotor dysfunction can occur	SCLC Ovarian cancer Breast cancer Uterine cancer Hodgkin lymphoma	Anti-Yo Anti-Tr (only in Hodgkin lymphoma)
Limbic encephalitis	Presents with memory loss, mood changes, emotional lability Hallucinations and seizures may occur	SCLC Testicular germ cell tumors Thymoma Hodgkin lymphoma	Anti-Hu Anti-Ta (testicular or breast)
Stiff-person syndrome	Muscle stiffness or rigidity Usually begins asymmetrically Can cause significant pain EMG shows abnormal continuous firing of motor units	SCLC Breast cancer Thymoma Hodgkin lymphoma	Anti-amphiphysin Anti-GAD (breast)
Lambert-Eaton myasthenic syndrome	Presents with proximal weakness that improves with exercise Bulbar weakness not seen (as opposed to myasthenia gravis) EMG shows motor unit potentials whose amplitude increases with exercise Treatment is geared to malignancy but plasmapheresis or immunosuppressives may be helpful	SCLC	LEMS antibody

EMG, Electromyography; GAD, glutamic acid decarboxylase; LEMS, Lambert-Eaton myasthenic syndrome; SCLC, small-cell lung cancer.

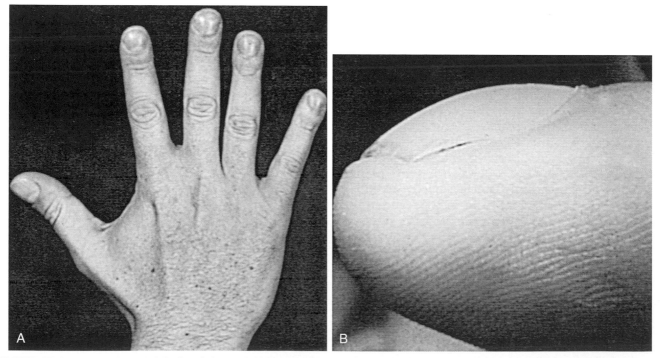

FIGURE 57-2 **A,** Dorsal view of the hand shows clubbing, with widening of the fingertips replacing the normally tapered appearance of the digits. **B,** A lateral view of the index finger demonstrates clubbing with loss of the normal 15-degree angle between the nail and the cuticle because of accentuated convexity of the nail. There is also enlargement of the distal finger pad and shininess of the nail and adjacent skin. (From Harris ED, Budd RC, Genovese MC, et al, eds. *Kelley's Textbook of Rheumatology.* 7th ed. Philadelphia: Saunders; 2005: Figs. 110-2 and 110-3.)

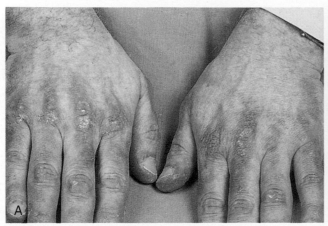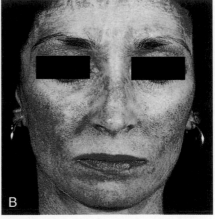

FIGURE 57-3 Dermatomyositis. **A,** Gottron papules of the hands. **B,** Facial rash with periorbital and malar distribution. (From Albert RK, Spiro SG, Jett JR, eds. *Clinical Respiratory Medicine.* 2nd ed. St. Louis: Mosby; 2004: Fig. 48.6.)

- Most commonly associated with adenocarcinoma of the lung but sometimes seen with other lung cancers, lung infections, or conditions that result in right-to-left shunting of blood
- Symptoms include joint pain with or without effusions
- Examination may reveal new digital clubbing
- Radiographs show periosteal new bone formation
- **If the diagnosis is made, the thorax should be imaged to search for lung cancer**
- Dermatomyositis/polymyositis (see Chapter 45)
    - Presents with proximal muscle weakness with or without pain (polymyositis)
    - Dermatomyositis is diagnosed if skin involvement is also present (Fig. 57-3)
    - Associated primarily with ovarian, breast, and lung cancers
    - Tumors usually present within 5 years of the diagnosis
    - Laboratory data reveal increased sedimentation rate and creatine phosphokinase level, and abnormal electromyogram
    - Muscle biopsy confirms the diagnosis

ENDOCRINOLOGIC SYNDROMES

- Carcinoid syndrome
    - Associated with carcinoid tumors of the small intestine, cervix, stomach, rectum, and lung
    - **Usually presents when there is metastasis to the liver**
    - Clinical symptoms include episodic flushing, diarrhea, abdominal pain, and wheezing
    - Fibrosis of the endocardium (predominantly tricuspid valve) is a late complication
    - Diagnose with 24-hour urine for 5-hydroxyindoleacetic acid, or elevated serum or platelet serotonin levels
    - Treat with surgical resection/debulking or liver-directed therapies whenever possible
    - Somatostatin analogues may help control symptoms
- Cushing syndrome
    - Seen predominantly with small-cell lung cancer, pancreatic islet cell tumors, thymic cancer, and bronchial carcinoid

- Usually caused by ectopic secretion of adrenocorticotropic hormones from cancer cells but can rarely occur secondary to ectopic secretion of corticotropin-releasing hormone
- Signs and symptoms include truncal obesity, fatigue, weakness, hypertension, abdominal striae, hyperpigmentation, hirsutism, polyuria, polydipsia
- Laboratory evaluation (see Chapter 41)
- Treatment is geared toward the underlying malignancy
- Ketoconazole, metyrapone, or aminoglutethamide may be used to inhibit steroid production and provide symptomatic relief
- Acromegaly
    - Usually caused by ectopic release of growth hormone-releasing hormone (GH-RH)
    - Associated with bronchial carcinoids, pancreatic islet cell tumors, lung cancer, breast cancer, and colon cancer
    - Signs and symptoms include increasing glove and shoe size, impotence, hypertension, amenorrhea, diabetes
    - Elevated insulin-like growth factor-1, GH-RH, and glucose-suppressed growth hormone levels establish the diagnosis (see Chapter 41)
    - Treat the underlying malignancy
    - Bromocriptine and octreotide may be used to suppress growth hormone secretion from the pituitary
- Hypercalcemia (see Chapter 39)
    - Can be caused by parathyroid hormone-related protein, osteolytic metastases, and tumor production of calcitriol (seen mainly with lymphomas)
    - Most commonly occurs with lung cancer, breast cancer, and multiple myeloma
- Syndrome of inappropriate antidiuresis (see Chapter 32)
    - Caused by ectopic secretion of antidiuretic hormone
    - Most commonly seen with small-cell lung cancer

NONBACTERIAL THROMBOTIC ENDOCARDITIS

- Caused by clotting and platelet activation by procoagulants released by tumors

- Associated primarily with adenocarcinomas (e.g., lung, gastrointestinal [GI] tract)
- Sterile, verrucous lesions are seen, usually on left-sided heart valves
- Clinically may present as embolic stroke, seizure, confusion
- Can be associated with disseminated intravascular coagulation
- Diagnose with echocardiogram and/or cerebral angiogram with negative blood cultures
- Treatment is geared to the underlying malignancy

CUTANEOUS SYNDROMES

See Chapter 65.

Cancer Chemotherapy

Basic Information

- Most cytotoxic drugs are designed to impair cell division
- Selectivity stems from the effect on cells that are more rapidly dividing (i.e., tumor cells)
- Normal cells that rapidly divide are also affected, causing common toxicities (e.g., bone marrow suppression, hair loss, mucosal sloughing)
- Chemotherapy toxicity may be acute or chronic, dose dependent, or idiosyncratic
- Newer classes of agents that are more selectively targeted than classic cytotoxic drugs have been adopted in recent years. These agents typically act on specific cell surface receptors or intracellular proteins to produce their antitumor effect.
  - Monoclonal antibodies target cell surface receptors producing an intracellular effect
  - Small molecule inhibitors target intracellular tyrosine kinases or other proteins to impact signaling pathways

CYTOTOXIC CHEMOTHERAPY TOXICITY

- Acute toxicities are common and include nausea, vomiting, diarrhea, headache, and fatigue
- Delayed toxicities
  - Bone marrow suppression is a common side effect of many agents
  - Some selective toxicities are listed in Table 57-4
- Targeted agents have both on- and off-target effects, but they do not typically produce the same toxicities on rapidly dividing cells as cytotoxic agents

TUMOR LYSIS SYNDROME

- Caused by rapid destruction of a large number of cancer cells
- **Results in hyperuricemia, hyperkalemia, hyperphosphatemia, lactic acidosis, hypocalcemia, and acute renal failure**
- Seen most commonly after treatment of leukemias and lymphomas
- Prevention of renal failure with fluid administration, allopurinol, and sodium bicarbonate should be attempted in high-risk patients (i.e., patients with high

TABLE 57-4	Delayed Toxicity of Selected Chemotherapeutic Agents
Drug	**Toxicity**
Bleomycin	Pneumonitis and pulmonary fibrosis
Cisplatin	Hearing loss, nephrotoxicity, peripheral neuropathy
Cyclophosphamide	Hemorrhagic cystitis
Daunorubicin	Cardiomyopathy
Doxorubicin	Cardiomyopathy
Fluorouracil	Severe diarrhea, oral or gastrointestinal ulcers, palmar or plantar rash
Gemcitabine	Pulmonary fibrosis, peripheral edema
Methotrexate	Oral/gastrointestinal ulcers, pulmonary infiltrates and fibrosis, cirrhosis
Paclitaxel	Peripheral neuropathy
Vincristine	Peripheral neuropathy

tumor burdens, baseline renal dysfunction, baseline hyperuricemia)
- Treatment with intravenous (IV) fluids, loop diuretics, alkalinization of the urine, and allopurinol can by tried initially in patients developing acute renal failure
- Treatment with rasburicase can lower the serum uric acid level rapidly, helping to prevent renal failure
- Hemodialysis may be necessary if the response is inadequate

FEBRILE NEUTROPENIA

Basic Information and Clinical Presentation

- Neutropenia is defined as absolute neutrophil count (ANC) less than 500/mL
- Fever is usually defined as one temperature higher than 38.5° C or three temperatures above 38° C within 24 hours
- Usually occurs as a result of chemotherapy
- Patients may or may not have any localizing symptoms to suggest a source for infection
- Typical etiology is bacterial translocation from the GI tract
- Infectious agents to consider include *Staphylococcus aureus*, *Staphylococcus epidermidis*, *Escherichia coli*, *Klebsiella pneumoniae*, *Pseudomonas aeruginosa*, and fungi

Diagnosis

- History and physical examination
- Inspect rectal area but avoid digital rectal examination because it may introduce infection
- Obtain CBC and calculate ANC
- Obtain chest radiograph or chest CT scan
- Panculture (i.e., blood, urine, sputum, throat, stool [including *Clostridium difficile*])

Treatment

- **Empirical antibiotics should be administered immediately**
- Evaluation usually identifies a primary source of infection in only 20% of patients
- Antibiotic choice depends on hospital practice, but in general should be broad-spectrum unless causal organism is clear
- Possible antibiotic regimens
    - Single-agent therapy: cefepime, cefotetan, imipenem-cilastin, meropenem, ceftazidime
    - Combination therapy: β-Lactam (e.g., piperacillin, ticarcillin) plus an aminoglycoside (e.g., gentamicin, tobramycin) or ciprofloxacin
- In patients with persistent fever, the addition of vancomycin or antifungal drugs (e.g., amphotericin or fluconazole) should be considered

TYPHLITIS

- Necrotizing infection of the cecum and colon
- Symptoms include fever, diarrhea, and right lower quadrant abdominal pain (mimics appendicitis)
- Seen predominantly after treatment for acute leukemia
- Treat with broad-spectrum antibiotics
- Surgery may be necessary

Review Questions

For review questions, please go to ExpertConsult.com.

SUGGESTED READINGS

Chamberlain MC. Neoplastic meningitis and metastatic epidural spinal cord compression. *Hematol Oncol Clin North Am.* 2012;26:917-931.

Ettinger DS, Handorf CR, Aqulnik M, et al. Occult primary, version 3.2014. *J Natl Compr Canc Netw.* 2014;12:969-974.

Pelosof LC, Gerber DE. Paraneoplastic syndromes: an approach to diagnosis and treatment. *Mayo Clin Proc.* 2010;85:838-854.

Picazo JJ. Management of the febrile neutropenic patient: a consensus conference. *Clin Infect Dis.* 2004;39(suppl 1):S1-S6.

Rice TW, Rodriguez RM, Light RW. The superior vena cava syndrome: clinical characteristics and evolving etiology. *Medicine (Baltimore).* 2006;85:37-42.

Varadhachary GR, Raber MN. Cancer of unknown primary site. *N Engl J Med.* 2014;371:757-765.

Wagner J, Arora S. Oncologic metabolic emergencies. *Emerg Med Clin North Am.* 2014;32:509-525.

57

Lung Cancer and Head and Neck Cancer

PATRICK FORDE, MD

Lung cancer is now the most common cause of cancer death in both men and women in the United States, claiming 160,000 lives per year, or about 28% of all cancer-related deaths. Given the well-established relationship between smoking and most types of lung cancer, it also remains the most preventable neoplastic disorder. Although head and neck cancer is less common than lung cancer, its relationship to tobacco use is similar, making it a highly preventable disease. This chapter will serve to highlight the features of these two smoking-related diseases.

Lung Cancer

Basic Information

- **Most common cause of death caused by cancer in both genders**
- Incidence over the past decade has been declining in men but slowly increasing in women
- African American men have highest incidence rates for lung cancer
- Risk factors
  - Tobacco
    - **80% to 85% of lung cancer cases result from cigarette smoking**
    - Risk is dependent upon total lifetime consumption of cigarettes
    - Risk of lung cancer begins to decrease 5 years after smoking has ceased, although the risk always remains higher than that for a nonsmoker
    - Passive or secondhand smoke associated with increased risk (3% to 5% of all lung cancer cases)
    - Smoking cigars may also increase risk, although the association is highly variable
  - Asbestos
    - Increases risk of bronchogenic carcinoma and mesothelioma
    - A potential hazard for a number of occupations, including plumbers, pipefitters, carpenters, electricians, welders, and insulation workers
  - Radon
  - Uranium
  - Ionizing radiation
  - Nickel, chromium
- Screening
  - **The U.S. Preventive Services Task Force (USPSTF) recommends annual screening with low-dose computed tomography (LDCT) in adults aged 55 to 80 years who have a 30 pack-year smoking history**
    - Screening should be stopped (or not started) in people who have not smoked for 15 years or more, have a limited life expectancy, or would not be willing to undergo curative lung surgery
  - Prospective studies of lung cancer screening do not support use of chest radiograph or sputum cytology
- Pathology
  - Non–small-cell lung cancer (NSCLC) (80% to 85% of cases)
    - Adenocarcinoma
      - **Most common type in nonsmokers**
      - Peripheral location
      - Bronchoalveolar carcinoma is a subtype that presents diffusely within the lungs
    - Squamous cell
      - Can be associated with hypercalcemia as a paraneoplastic syndrome (see Chapters 39 and 57)
        - Central location
        - 10% undergo cavitation
      - Large-cell lung cancer; usually peripheral location
  - Small-cell lung cancer (15% to 20% of cases)
    - Small primary tumors, but adenopathy may be bulky
    - Associated with a number of paraneoplastic syndromes, most commonly syndrome of inappropriate antidiuretic hormone (SIADH)
  - Mesothelioma (Box 58-1)

Clinical Presentation

- Cough, dyspnea, and chest pain are the most common presenting symptoms
- Hemoptysis is seen more commonly with central lesions
- Recurrent or unresolving pneumonia caused by obstruction
- Hoarseness: caused by recurrent laryngeal nerve compression
- **Horner syndrome: ptosis, miosis, ipsilateral anhydrosis from sympathetic chain involvement of tumor**
- Paraneoplastic syndromes (see Chapter 57)
- **Shoulder pain: Pancoast tumors (apical tumors locally invading the lower brachial plexus (C8-T2)**

BOX 58-1 *Malignant Mesothelioma*

Most common risk factor is asbestos exposure
Male predominance
Disease manifests 20 to 30 years after initial exposure; usually around age 60 years
Presenting symptoms include dyspnea and chest pain
Chest imaging typically reveals pleural abnormality with a large pleural effusion
Diagnosis is made by thoracentesis and pleural biopsy
Treatment options are limited
Extrapleural pneumonectomy with or without chemotherapy and radiation is one treatment strategy
Prognosis (even with treatment) is currently poor

and chest wall, resulting in shoulder pain and plexopathy) may be missed on chest radiograph

- Poor prognostic factors
  - Weight loss of more than 5% body weight
  - Advanced stage (see following discussion)
  - Poor performance status
  - *K-ras* oncogene mutation (non–small cell)

Diagnosis

- All patients should have a history and physical examination, complete blood count, chemistry profile, liver function tests, and computed tomography (CT) scan of chest and abdomen
- Bronchoscopy
  - 80% to 85% effective in establishing a diagnosis for centrally located tumors
  - Not as effective for peripheral lesions
- CT-guided biopsy is about 90% effective for establishing a diagnosis for peripherally located tumors
- Mediastinoscopy may be used for diagnosis or staging (especially for anterior mediastinal lymph nodes)
- Positron emission tomography (PET) scan is indicated for all patients who may be candidates for definitive chemoradiation or surgery
  - Hypermetabolic tumors enhance on scanning
  - Considered more sensitive than CT for mediastinal disease (Fig. 58-1)
  - Currently recommended to confirm the presence of localized or locally advanced NSCLC
- Bone scan (if PET/CT not indicated/performed) and magnetic resonance imaging of the brain
- Staging
  - NSCLC: tumor-node-metastasis (TNM) staging criteria (Table 58-1)
  - Small-cell lung cancer
    - Limited stage: disease confined to one hemithorax and can be encompassed within a single radiation therapy port
    - Extensive stage: disease spread outside of the preceding area

Treatment

- NSCLC
  - Stages I to IIIa
    - **Surgery is the treatment of choice if performance status is good and postresection**

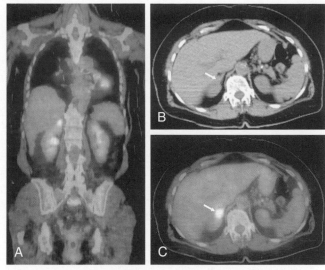

FIGURE 58-1 **A** and **C,** Positron emission tomography/computed tomography (PET/CT) scans demonstrate right adrenal mass *(arrow).* **B,** Less well-delineated mass on CT scan *(arrow).* (From Abeloff MD, Armitage JO, Niederhuber JE, et al, eds. *Clinical Oncology.* 3rd ed. Philadelphia: Churchill Livingstone; 2004: Fig. 75-9.)

TABLE 58-1	*Staging for Non–Small-Cell Lung Cancer*	
Stage	**Description**	**5-Year Survival Rate (%)**
I	Any size tumor with or without extension into visceral pleura, at least 2 cm from carina, no nodal involvement	60 to 80
II	Any size, extension into intrabronchial lymph nodes	40 to 50
IIIa	Any size, extension into parietal pleura, chest wall, or mediastinal pleura, or into hilar or ipsilateral mediastinal lymph nodes	20 to 30
IIIb	Any size, extension into mediastinal structures, contralateral hilar, mediastinal, or supraclavicular lymph nodes	10 to 20
IV	Evidence of distant metastasis	<5

pulmonary reserve is deemed to be adequate (forced expiratory volume in 1 second [FEV$_1$] greater than 0.8 L)

- Adjuvant chemotherapy or radiation may be beneficial for stage II and IIIa disease, but not for stage I disease
- Stage IIIb: definitive radiation therapy with or without chemotherapy
- Stage IV
  - Goal is palliation
  - Chemotherapy prolongs survival
  - Erlotinib, a small-molecule inhibitor of epidermal growth factor receptor (EGFR), is indicated as first-line treatment for patients with advanced

NSCLC with known activating mutations in EGFR
- Crizotinib, a small-molecule inhibitor of anaplastic lymphoma kinase (ALK), is indicated for patients with advanced NSCLC harboring translocations in the ALK gene
- Bevacizumab, a monoclonal antibody targeting vascular endothelial growth factor, is indicated in conjunction with chemotherapy for patients with advanced nonsquamous NSCLC, as long as no contraindication exists
- Small-cell lung cancer
  - Limited stage
    - Combined chemotherapy (platinum-/etoposide-based regimen) plus concurrent radiation
    - Consider prophylactic cranial irradiation for patients with response to chemotherapy
      - Decreases risk of brain metastases and may increase survival
    - Surgical resection may be an option in a small subset of patients after chemoradiation
    - Median survival is 18 months
  - Extensive stage
    - Chemotherapy with platinum/etoposide or platinum/irinotecan
    - Median survival is 9 months

Head and Neck Cancer

Basic Information

- Responsible for as many as 11,000 cancer deaths per year, out of 48,000 cases diagnosed in the United States
- More common in men
- Median age is 60 years
- Can affect the oral cavity, larynx, pharynx, or nasopharynx
- Risk factors
  - Tobacco
    - Dose-response relationship between the occurrence of cancer and duration and amount of cigarette use
    - Secondhand smoke and cigars may also be risk factors
  - Alcohol
    - Increased risk with heavy use (more than 50 g/day)
    - No increased risk with moderate use (less than 19 g/day)
    - Risk is greatly increased in people who drink and smoke cigarettes heavily
  - Prior radiation therapy: increased risk of salivary gland tumors
  - Plummer-Vinson syndrome
    - Characterized by dysphagia, iron-deficiency anemia, and esophageal webs in women
    - Increased incidence of cancer of the hypopharynx and esophagus
  - **Epstein-Barr virus (EBV)**
    - **Strong association with nasopharyngeal carcinoma, which has a high incidence in southern China**
    - Pathology is usually undifferentiated rather than squamous cell type

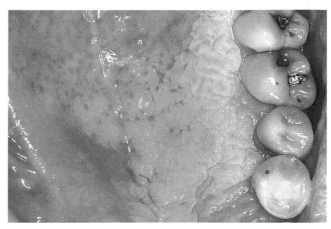

FIGURE 58-2 Leukoplakia of the hard palate. (From Cummings CW, Flint PW, Harker LA, et al. *Otolaryngology: Head and Neck Surgery.* 4th ed. Philadelphia: Mosby; 2005: Fig. 64-5B.)

- Human papillomavirus (HPV)
  - Type 16 most strongly associated with invasive tumors of the oral cavity and oropharynx
  - Presence of HPV may confer a better prognosis
- Pathology
  - Most cancers in the United States are squamous cell carcinomas
  - Precancerous lesions
    - Leukoplakia (Fig. 58-2): hyperkeratosis associated with a low malignant potential (less than 5% of cases)
    - Erythroplakia
      - Red, superficial patches adjacent to normal mucosa
      - Associated with dysplasia
      - Significant malignant potential (40% of cases)
    - Dysplasia
      - Presence of mitoses and prominent nucleoli
      - Can involve entire mucosa (carcinoma in situ)
      - Commonly progresses to invasive cancer
  - Lymphoepithelial: undifferentiated tumors predominantly seen in nasopharyngeal carcinoma because of EBV (see earlier discussion)

Clinical Presentation

- Symptoms vary by the site of the tumor
  - Nasal cavity: epistaxis, ulceration, nasal obstruction
  - Paranasal sinuses: recurrent or persistent sinusitis
  - Nasopharyngeal: mass, eustachian tube dysfunction, serous otitis media
  - Oral cavity, tongue, lips: mass with or without ulceration
  - Laryngeal/glottic: hoarseness, dysphagia, odynophagia, hemoptysis
- Cervical lymphadenopathy may sometimes be the only finding on presentation

Diagnosis

- History and physical examination with emphasis on risk factors and direct visualization of tumor
- **Fiberoptic endoscopy is necessary to assess the extent of the tumor as well as vocal cord mobility**

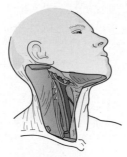

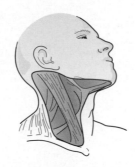

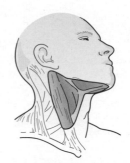

A — Radical neck dissection

B — Modified radical neck dissection: one or more of the nonlymphatic structures are preserved

C — Supraomohyoid neck dissection

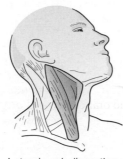

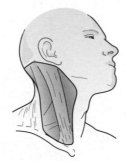

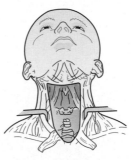

D — Lateral neck dissection

E — Posterolateral neck dissection

F — Anterior compartment neck dissection

FIGURE 58-3 Types of neck dissection. **A**, Radical. **B**, Modified radical: One or more of the nonlymphatic structures are preserved. **C**, Supraomohyoid. **D**, Lateral. **E**, Posterolateral. **F**, Anterior compartment. (From Abeloff MD, Armitage JO, Niederhuber JE, et al, eds. *Clinical Oncology.* 3rd ed. Philadelphia: Churchill Livingstone; 2004: Fig. 71-6.)

- Diagnosis is usually made by direct biopsy of tumor or fine-needle aspiration of a metastatic lymph node
- CT scan of the head and neck aids in the staging process
- Chest CT and panendoscopy (e.g., laryngoscopy, esophagoscopy, bronchoscopy) are helpful for detecting distant metastases and second primary lesions
- PET scan is useful for detecting recurrent tumors in patients who have had surgery and may be useful in detecting occult head and neck cancers

Treatment

- Staging system and treatments vary depending on the primary tumor site
- Primary therapy of squamous cell carcinoma usually includes surgery (possibly neck dissection; Fig. 58-3) and radiation therapy, although the role of chemotherapy continues to expand
  - Early (stages I and II)
    - Goal is for cure with either radiation or surgery
  - Advanced resectable (stages III and IV, without distant metastases)
    - Oral cavity: surgery and postoperative radiation plus chemotherapy
    - Pharynx: definitive concurrent chemoradiation
  - Advanced unresectable

- Treat with chemoradiotherapy
- Prognosis is poor
- Metastatic disease (typically remains localized to head and neck or thorax)
  - Radiation with or without chemotherapy
- Nasopharyngeal cancer is primarily treated with radiation therapy and chemotherapy
- Significant morbidity can be associated with treatment
  - Physical disfiguration
  - Loss of voice or hoarseness
  - Dysphagia or odynophagia leading to malnutrition
  - Xerostomia
    - Artificial saliva can provide temporary relief of symptoms
    - Oral pilocarpine is effective as a treatment and for prophylaxis
  - Osteoradionecrosis of the mandible
  - Fibrosis of neck, pharynx, temporomandibular joint, esophagus
  - Hypothyroidism
- Most tumor recurrences occur within 2 years of the initial treatment
- After 2 years, second primary aerodigestive tumors occur at 3% to 7% per year (field cancerization)
- **Recurrence risk higher in patients who continue to smoke**

58

Acknowledgment

This chapter was based on the chapters by Drs. David Cosgrove and Mark Levis written for previous editions of the *Johns Hopkins Internal Medicine Board Review.*

Review Questions

For review questions, please go to ExpertConsult.com.

SUGGESTED READINGS

Gould MK. Clinical practice. Lung-cancer screening with low-dose computed tomography. *N Engl J Med.* 2014;371:1813-1820.

Huber MA, Tantiwongkosi B. Oral and oropharyngeal cancer. *Med Clin North Am.* 2014;98:1299-1321.

Karam-Hage M, Cinciripini PM, Gritz ER. Tobacco use and cessation for cancer survivors: an overview for clinicians. *CA Cancer J Clin.* 2014;64:272-290.

Molina JR, Yang P, Cassivi SD, et al. Non-small cell lung cancer: epidemiology, risk factors, treatment, and survivorship. *Mayo Clin Proc.* 2008;83:584-594.

Powell CA, Halmos B, Nana-Sinkam SP. Update in lung cancer and mesothelioma 2012. *Am J Respir Crit Care Med.* 2013;188:157-166.

Zandberg DP, Bhargava R, Badin S, et al. The role of human papillomavirus in nongenital cancers. *CA Cancer J Clin.* 2013;63:57-81.

SECTION TEN

BOARD REVIEW

Neurology

Headaches

APRIL S. FITZGERALD, MD

It is estimated that 90% of individuals experience headaches. The most common are tension-type headaches that respond to over-the-counter treatment and therefore do not require patients to seek medical attention. Headaches that do prompt an outpatient visit are most often migraines; however, headaches may also be a symptom of a more ominous illness. Certain characteristics of the headache pattern will help differentiate the type and cause of headaches and can guide the clinical assessment.

Primary Headache Syndromes

Basic Information

- Primary headache syndrome means the headache *is* the disease
  - More common in clinical practice than headaches from a secondary cause
  - By definition has no structural or metabolic cause
- Common primary headache disorders
  - Migraine
    - **P**ounding, **I**ncapacitating, plus **N**ausea (PIN = positive predictive value of 93%)
  - Tension-type
    - Infrequent: headache less than one day per month
    - Frequent: 1 to 14 days per month
    - Chronic: 15 or more days per month
  - Trigeminal autonomic cephalalgias (TACs)
    - Short-lived attacks; unilateral pain in V1 distribution of trigeminal nerve (around eye) with autonomic features
    - **Cluster headache is the most common subtype of TACs**
- History is helpful in determining headache type
  - Ask about pain onset, quality, location, frequency, and associated symptoms (Table 59-1)
  - Consider comorbid medical diseases that might be clues to a possible cause: hypertension, pregnancy, depression, infection, cancer, substance withdrawal, etc.
- Physical exam is important to look for signs of a secondary cause
  - Fever: Could this suggest an infectious cause?
  - Blood pressure: Could this be malignant hypertension and/or bleed?
  - Optic exam: Is there papilledema to suggest increased intracranial pressure?

- Visual fields: Are there field cuts that require neuroimaging?
- Facial tenderness (sinuses, teeth, temporal artery): Could there be a structural etiology or vasculitis?
- Complete neurologic exam: Are there abnormal signs on exam that warrant neuroimaging?

Diagnosis and Evaluation

- Diagnosis is largely history plus physical to rule out secondary cause
- **If the history is consistent with a primary headache syndrome and the physical exam is unrevealing, then central nervous system (CNS) imaging is not necessary**

Treatment

- Migraine (see later section)
- Tension-type headache
  - Nonsteroidal antiinflammatory drugs (NSAIDs) or acetaminophen
  - Some tension headaches may be caffeine-responsive
  - Antianxiety medications or antidepressants if concomitant disorder exists
  - Biofeedback techniques to manage stress and tension (especially in chronic tension-type headache)
  - Limit medication to 2 to 3 times/week to avoid medication-overuse (rebound) headaches
- Cluster headache
  - Abortive therapy
    - 100% oxygen inhalation (7 L/min) at onset of attack
    - Subcutaneous sumaptriptan
    - Dihydroergotamine intravenous (IV) or intramuscular
    - Intranasal lidocaine for anesthesia during attack
  - Preventive therapy (during cluster phase)
    - Calcium channel blockers (verapamil)
    - Lithium
    - Prednisone with taper
    - Valproate

Migraine Headache

Basic Information

- Most common primary headache syndrome
- Pathophysiology is complex, starting in the brainstem and ultimately involving the trigeminal vascular system;

TABLE 59-1	*Clinical Presentations of Primary Headache Syndromes*		
Characteristic	**Migraine Headache**	**Tension-Type Headache**	**Cluster Headache**
Onset (age/sex)	Onset often in adolescence More common in females Family history of migraines	Variable age of onset More common in females	Age 20 to 50 years Male to female ratio 5:1
Frequency	1 to 2 attacks/month, may be more frequent May have hormonal (menstrual) trigger	Infrequent: <1 day/month Frequent: >1 day/month Chronic: daily	*Nightly* or daily for 6 to 12 weeks Circadian association Periods of headache freedom may last months to years
Potential triggers	Stress Change in sleep pattern (too much or too little) Hormonal changes Variations in caffeine intake Foods: chocolate, hard cheese, MSG, nitrates, tyramines	Fatigue Stress	Alcohol (in some)
Location	Unilateral > bilateral Bifrontal in 40%	Bilateral, neck, occipital	100% unilateral Temporal or orbital
Pain characteristics	Crescendo pattern Pulsating Moderate to severe pain Patient retreats to dark, quiet room	Pressure or squeezing Waxing/waning severity Patient may remain active	Quick onset of excruciating pain "Suicide headache" Deep and continuous (nonpulsating) Patient may pace or rock from severity of pain
Duration	4 to 72 hours	Minutes to days	30 minutes to 3 hours Average is 45 to 90 minutes
Associated symptoms	Nausea, vomiting, photophobia, phonophobia ± aura (visual, speech, or motor deficits)	None	Ipsilateral parasympathetic overactivity Ptosis, miosis, lacrimation, conjunctival injection Rhinorrhea, nasal congestion Cheek flushing, facial swelling

MSG, Monosodium glutamate.

abnormal signals cause release of neurotransmitters and dilation of blood vessels, leading to pain and further neural activation
- In migraine with aura subtype, familial hemiplegic migraine, there is an association with mutations in at least three genes that encode for neuron transmembrane channels (i.e., P/Q-type calcium channel, Na^+-K^+ pump)

Clinical Presentation

See Table 59-1 for clinical characteristics
- International Headache Society (IHS) classification scheme for migraine headache:
  - **Migraine without aura. Account for nearly 80% of migraines.** Diagnostic criteria outlined in Box 59-1.
  - Migraine with aura
    - Requires three of four criteria with at least two attacks
      - One or more aura symptoms (visual, sensory, or speech disturbance) are fully reversible
      - At least one aura symptom develops gradually over 5 minutes or longer and/or different aura symptoms occur in succession over 5 or more minutes
      - No aura lasts more than 60 minutes
      - Onset of headache during aura or within 60 minutes of aura termination
    - Underlying cranial disorder must be ruled out

BOX 59-1	*Diagnostic Criteria for Migraine without Aura*

At least five attacks fulfilling the following criteria: untreated headache lasting 4 to 72 hours

Group A (2 of 4):
1. Unilateral headache
2. Throbbing or pulsating pain
3. Moderate to severe pain that inhibits ability to function
4. Pain aggravated by routine physical activity

Group B (1 of 2):
1. Presence of nausea or vomiting
2. Presence of photophobia and phonophobia
Underlying disorders that may cause secondary headaches must be ruled out

- Retinal migraine
  - Monocular blindness with disk edema
  - Peripapillary hemorrhage and slow resolution of vision loss
- Complications of migraine
  - Progression to chronic migraine
  - Infarction
    - Infarction risk is increased in migraine with neurologic aura (other than visual aura)
    - Oral contraceptives and tobacco significantly increase risk.

Diagnosis and Evaluation

- Based on history, physical examination, and classification scheme
- CNS imaging may be warranted for atypical presentations

Treatment

- Therapy for acute migraine attack
  - Basic approach/goals
    - Treat attacks rapidly and consistently
    - Restore patient's ability to function
    - **Choose drug based on severity of headaches**
    - May need to use different approaches for different headaches in same patient
  - Analgesics
    - NSAIDs (e.g., aspirin, ibuprofen, naproxen sodium)
      - Best for mild to moderate headaches
      - Decreased gastric motility may limit effectiveness
    - Metoclopramide (Reglan)
      - Increases gastrointestinal motility and may help as antiemetic
      - Dopamine antagonist and may be used as monotherapy for treatment by IV route
  - Serotonin 5-HT$_{1B/1D}$ receptor agonists ("triptans")
    - **Drugs of choice for moderate or severe migraines or if no response to analgesics**
    - Contraindications: ischemic cardiac or cerebrovascular disease, uncontrolled hypertension, basilar or hemiplegic migraines, ergotamine use
    - Category C drugs for use in pregnancy: inadequate data exist
    - Sumatriptan: subcutaneous form with rapid onset of action
      - Inhaled and oral forms also available: vary in half-life, onset time, tolerability, efficacy, return of headache
  - Ergotamine with or without caffeine
    - Nonspecific serotonin agonist and vasoconstrictor
    - Frequent adverse effects including medication-overuse headache
    - Contraindications: vascular disease, liver disease, pregnancy (potent vasoconstrictor)
  - Dihydroergotamine
    - Available in intranasal form with evidence for efficacy and safety
    - Less vasoactive than ergotamine
  - Combination agents (acetaminophen/dichloralphenazone/isometheptene)
- Preventive therapy for migraine
  - Behavioral modification
    - Avoid "triggers" (e.g., foods, alcohol, caffeine, nicotine, nitrates)
    - Regular sleeping patterns
    - Minimize stress
  - Migraine diary to record patterns of headache and identify possible triggers
  - Consider prophylactic medication in patients who:
    - **Have two or more attacks a month with 3 or more days of disability**
    - Have a contraindication to or have failed acute therapy
    - Require abortive medications more than twice a week
  - Recommendations for use of prophylactic migraine medication
    - Start with low dose and titrate slowly
    - Decrease in headache frequency may be imperceptible the first month
      - For first month, 10% decrease in frequency is considered successful
      - Improvement is cumulative, may take 6 months to reach efficacy
      - Success = 50% reduction in headache frequency
    - After a 6-month period of headache stability, periodically evaluate for taper
- Migraine headache prevention medications
  - Antihypertensives
    - β-Blockers: Metoprolol, propranolol, and timolol have established efficacy. Atenolol and nadolol probably effective.
    - Angiotensin converting enzyme inhibitors: lisinopril probably effective
    - Angiotensin receptor blockers: candesartan probably effective
    - Calcium channel blockers: conflicting evidence regarding efficacy despite their historical use
  - Antiepileptic neuromodulators
    - Valproate and divalproex sodium (teratogenic): Established efficacy. As effective as β-blockers. Side-effect is weight gain.
    - Topiramate (may cause weight loss): Established efficacy. Consider side-effect of weight loss for obese patients.
  - Antidepressants
    - Tricyclics (amitriptyline): probably effective; unrelated to antidepressant activity
    - Selective serotonin reuptake inhibitors: venlafaxine, probably effective
  - NSAIDs: use to prophylax known triggers (e.g., start before menses for for menstrual migraine)
  - Petasites (Butterbur): Small studies suggest effectiveness. Sold as an over-the-counter dietary supplement.
  - Riboflavin (vitamin B$_2$): small studies suggest effectiveness
  - Magnesium: Mixed trial results. May be effective as prophylaxis for patients with low ionized magnesium and migraines with aura.
  - Acupuncture: No more effective than "sham acupuncture" for migraine prevention. However, in studies, both sham and acupuncture groups had fewer headaches than the untreated control group.
  - Botulinum toxin A: No better than placebo for episodic migraine. May offer some benefit for cervicogenic headaches and chronic migraine.

Secondary Headaches

Basic Information

- A secondary headache syndrome means the headache is caused by an underlying pathologic or metabolic condition
  - Less common in clinical practice than primary headaches
  - Often abnormal neurologic exam results
  - **Consider secondary headache even when a patient has a history of primary headaches but the headache pattern changes**

Clinical Presentation

- "Red flags" of secondary headache syndromes (Box 59-2)
- Secondary headache types
  - Subarachnoid hemorrhage (SAH)
    - **Classic "worst headache of life" caused by ruptured intracranial aneurysm**
    - Warning or "thunderclap" headache in 20% to 50% of patients with SAH (severe headache lasting minutes in the days to weeks before major bleed)
    - Headache is severe and develops in seconds
    - Diagnosis
      - Noncontrast computed tomography (CT) scan is first choice (Fig. 59-1)
      - If CT done within 24 hours, blood seen in subarachnoid space in 92% of cases
      - Sensitivity begins to decline 24 hours after bleed
      - Lumbar puncture if head CT negative
        - Xanthochromia is criterion for SAH (red blood cells break down, releasing hemoglobin, which is metabolized to reveal xanthochromia)
        - May be negative if bleed less than 12 hours or more than 2 weeks old
  - Meningeal irritation or meningitis (see Chapter 15)
    - Systemic symptoms, stiff neck, fever
    - Diagnosis made by lumbar puncture
  - Brain tumor
    - Usually other neurologic findings present (seizures, vomiting, papilledema)
      - Worse in morning or if supine
    - Diagnosis made by CNS imaging (magnetic resonance imaging [MRI] is image of choice)
  - Temporal arteritis (see Chapter 44)

BOX 59-2 | *"Red Flags" of Secondary Headache Syndromes*

New-onset headache in absence of headache history
Onset age older than 40 years
Unusually severe headache ("worst of life")
Headaches with progressive course
Significant change in headache pattern over prior 3 months
Precipitation with exercise, Valsalva maneuver, head turning, supine position
Association with seizure or focal neurologic signs
Systemic symptoms (fever, weight loss, jaw pain)

- Vasculitis of large and medium blood vessels
- **Two thirds of patients with giant-cell arteritis have headache with localized temporal pain or jaw claudication**
- Patients are typically older than 50 years
- Other systemic features present (fever, fatigue, weight loss)
- Diagnosis made by temporal artery biopsy
- Other autoimmune illnesses (lupus, vasculitis) may present with headache
- Low-pressure headaches
  - Occur from contraction of subarachnoid space from a cerebrospinal fluid leak or lumbar puncture (Marfan and Ehler-Danlos syndromes predispose to spontaneous leak)
  - Pain is worse with standing and relieved when supine
  - Bedrest, hydration, and analgesics are mainstay of therapy
  - Caffeine (oral or IV) may help relieve the pain
- Subdural hematoma
  - Gradual onset of headache often associated with fall
  - Often seen with elderly patients presenting with headache
  - Diagnosis made with CNS imaging
- Idiopathic intracranial hypertension (previously known as pseudotumor cerebri)
  - Increased intracranial pressure without mass
  - **More commonly presents in overweight young women**
  - Associated with isotretinoin (Accutane), tetracycline, hypervitaminosis A, oral contraceptives

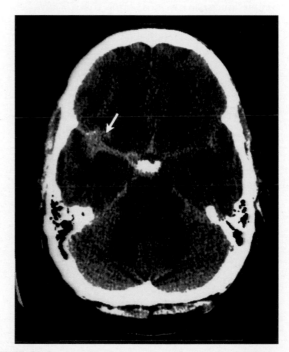

59

FIGURE 59-1 Computed tomography scan of the brain showing a subarachnoid bleed caused by a middle cerebral artery aneurysm *(arrow)*. (From Townsend CM, Beauchamp RD, Evers BM, et al. *Sabiston Textbook of Surgery.* 17th ed. Philadelphia: Saunders; 2004: Fig. 71-1A.)

- Headache pattern similar to tension-type headache
- **Neurologic exam is normal except for papilledema. Can have sixth nerve palsy and possible vision loss.**
  - Diagnosis
    - Patient has normal neuroimaging (MRI or CT) but elevated opening pressure on lumbar puncture without other cause for increased pressure
- Cerebral venous thrombosis
  - Rare cause of headache with increased intracranial pressure
  - CT scan may be normal in 30% of cases
  - Magnetic resonance venogram is gold standard

Chronic Daily Headache

Basic Information

- Can be primary and secondary headaches
- Headache frequency more than 15 days of the month for duration longer than 3 months
- Chronic migraine and medication overuse headaches are common types of chronic daily headache and most common reason for referrals to headache clinics

Clinical Presentation

- Chronic migraine and medication-overuse headache patients are more frequently women and have history of episodic migraines
- Medications implicated in causing medication-overuse headache
  - Overuse of any headache medication for more than 3 months
  - Simple analgesic use more often than15 days per month
  - Combination analgesics, narcotics, ergotamine, triptans more than 10 days per month

Treatment (Medication-Overuse Headache)

- Lifestyle modification (discontinue caffeine; exercise, regular sleep patterns, etc.)

- Stop all medications (taper opioids)
- If severe headache, try NSAIDs or dihydroergotamine (parenteral route)
- Start preventive migraine therapy
- Use of a 30-day course of steroid with taper can reduce headache severity during withdrawal and allow time for preventive therapy to take effect.

Acknowledgment

This chapter was based on the chapter by Dr. Kimberly Peairs written for the third edition of the *Johns Hopkins Internal Medicine Board Review*.

Review Questions

For review questions, please go to ExpertConsult.com.

SUGGESTED READINGS

Detsky ME, McDonald DR, Baerlocher MO, et al. Does this patient with headache have a migraine or need neuroimaging? *JAMA.* 2006;296:1274-1283.

Hainer BL, Matheson EM. Approach to acute headache in adults. *Am Fam Physician.* 2013;87:682-687.

Hale N, Paauw DS. Diagnosis and treatment of headache in the ambulatory care setting: a review of classic presentations and new considerations in diagnosis and management. *Med Clin North Am.* 2014;98:505-527.

Halker RB, Hastriter EV, Dodick DW. Chronic daily headache: an evidence-based and systematic approach to a challenging problem. *Neurology.* 2011;76:S37-S43.

Holland S, Silberstein SD, Freitag F, et al. Evidence-based guideline update: NSAIDs and other complementary treatments for episodic migraine prevention in adults: report of the Quality Standards Subcommittee of the American Academy of Neurology and the American Headache Society. *Neurology.* 2012;78:1346-1353.

Silberstein SD, Holland S, Freitag F, et al. Evidence-based guideline update: pharmacologic treatment for episodic migraine prevention in adults: report of the Quality Standards Subcommittee of the American Academy of Neurology and the American Headache Society. *Neurology.* 2012;78:1337-1345.

Cerebrovascular Disease and Seizure Disorders

RAFAEL H. LLINÁS, MD

Cerebrovascular disease is a common disorder in the United States: 800,000 strokes occur each year. It is the fifth leading cause of medical deaths in developed countries. Stroke can be classified into ischemic disease (80%) and hemorrhagic disease (20%). Mortality from ischemic stroke has been declining in the U.S. because of an increased awareness of and attention to modification of risk factors.

Seizures are electrical events of the brain, with varied clinical manifestations, that can be a cause of significant morbidity. Epilepsy is the chronic recurrence of seizures with a usual onset before age 20 years. Often, the underlying cause of epilepsy is unknown.

Cerebrovascular Disease

Basic Information

- Definitions
  - **Ischemic stroke**: Focal neurologic deficit lasting more than 24 hours because of loss of blood flow to a portion of the brain that results in irreversible cell death (Fig. 60-1)
    - Mechanisms of ischemic stroke
      - Large-vessel disease
        - Carotid atherosclerosis
        - Intracranial atherosclerotic disease
        - Arterial dissection
        - Embolic disease
        - Cardioembolic
        - Atheroembolic disease from atherosclerotic disease
        - Paradoxic emboli from patent foramen ovale or pulmonary right to left shunts
      - Lacunar disease
        - Atherosclerosis of small vessels
        - Lipohyalinosis of small vessels (Fig 60-2)
      - Hypercoagulable states
        - Lupus anticoagulant
        - Adenocarcinoma of the gastrointestinal (GI) tract and pancreas
        - Anticardiolipin antibody syndrome
  - **Transient ischemic attack (TIA):** Transient focal neurologic deficit caused by loss of regional blood flow; lasts less than 24 hours; typically only 10 to 60 minutes
    - Same mechanism as that of ischemic stroke
      - High-risk patients can have 5% stroke risk within 48 hours of TIA

- ABCD score (age, blood pressure, clinical features, duration of symptoms; Table 60-1) is excellent at differentiating low-risk from high-risk patients. Adding diabetes (i.e., ABCD^2; Table 60-3) further differentiates risk.
- Large artery disease most common cause
- **Intracerebral hemorrhage:** Bleeding into the brain parenchyma (Fig. 60-3)
  - Hypertension is major risk factor
  - Central nervous system (CNS) arteriovenous malformations (AVMs)
  - Trauma
  - Cerebral venous occlusion
  - Neoplastic disease
- **Intracranial hemorrhage**
  - Subdural hematoma crescent-shaped low-pressure venous bleeding
  - Epidural hematoma lens-shaped, high-pressure arterial bleeding
- **Subarachnoid hemorrhage (SAH):** Bleeding into the subarachnoid space around the brain
  - Aneurysms most common and life-threatening cause
  - Trauma
  - AVM
- Classification of ischemic cerebrovascular disease (Table 60-2)

Clinical Presentation

- **Ischemic atherosclerotic stroke risk factors are similar to those of coronary artery disease (CAD)**
  - Increasing age
  - Male sex
  - African American
  - Hypertension, diabetes, high cholesterol
  - Smoking
  - Drug abuse (cocaine, amphetamines)
  - Sedentary lifestyle, obesity
  - Family history
- **Embolic stroke risk factors**
  - Cardiac arrhythmias: atrial fibrillation, sick sinus syndrome
  - Dilated cardiomyopathy, including left ventricular aneurysm
  - Valvular disorders, including prosthetic valves, rheumatic heart disease
  - Infective and nonbacterial endocarditis
  - Left ventricular or left atrial thrombus
  - Cardiac myxoma

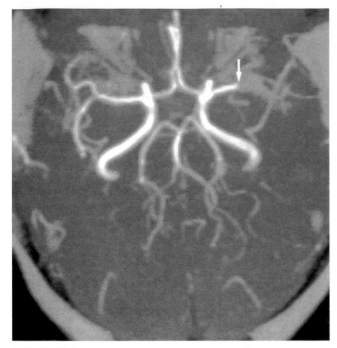

FIGURE 60-1 Magnetic resonance angiogram demonstrating occlusion of the left middle cerebral artery *(arrow),* consistent with a thromboembolic event. (From Forbes CD, Jackson WF. *Color Atlas and Text of Clinical Medicine.* 3rd ed. St. Louis: Mosby; 2003: Fig. 11.34.)

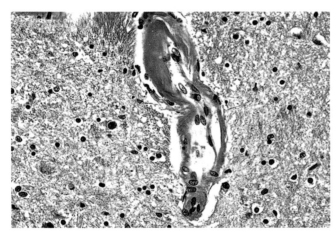

FIGURE 60-2 Lipohyalinosis of a small artery within the white matter. (From Prayson RA: *Neuropathology.* 2nd ed. Philadelphia: Elsevier; 2012: Fig. 2-21.)

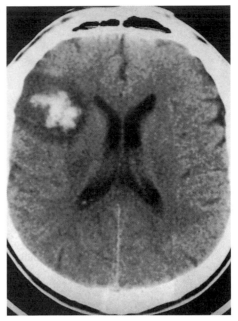

FIGURE 60-3 Hemorrhagic cerebral infarction demonstrated by a noncontrast computed tomography scan. (From Forbes CD, Jackson WF. *Color Atlas and Text of Clinical Medicine.* 3rd ed. St. Louis: Mosby; 2003: Fig. 11.66.)

TABLE 60-1	*Six Point Score Predictive of 7-Day Risk of Stroke*
	Points
Age >60 years	1
Blood pressure: systolic >140 or diastolic >90 mm Hg	1
Clinical Features	
Unilateral weakness	2
Speech disturbance without weakness	1
Duration of Symptoms	
>60 minutes	2
10 to 59 minutes	1
<10 minutes	0

Modified from Rothwell PM, Giles MF, Flossmann E, et al. A simple score (ABCD) to identify individuals at high early risk of stroke after transient ischaemic attack. *Lancet.* 2005;366: 29–36.

- Arial and ventricular septal defects, patent foramen ovale
- **TIAs**
  - Usually last 10 to 15 minutes, most resolve within 1 hour
  - High correlation with future stroke depending on ABCD^2 score (Table 60-3)
  - Predictor of vascular death, especially myocardial infarction
  - Amaurosis fugax is a common presentation
    - Temporary monocular blindness ("shade falling over vision")
  - Secondary to carotid artery atherosclerosis with embolization
- Classic (common) ischemic stroke presentations (see Table 60-2)
- Hemorrhagic stroke (Table 60-4)
  - **Subarachnoid hemorrhage**
    - **Bleeding in the space between the brain and the pia arachnoid**
    - Mortality 50%; prognosis particularly poor for patients who present in coma
    - Often seen in younger patients (age 35 to 65 years)

TABLE 60-2	*Classification of Ischemic Cerebrovascular Disease*		
	Examples	**Clinical Presentation**	**Treatment**
Large artery atherosclerosis	Carotid stenosis (extra- or intracranial) Vertebrobasilar disease	Carotid stenosis Ipsilateral face and hand numbness/weakness Aphasia or dysarthria Amaurosis fugax Vertebrobasilar disease Dizziness Vertigo Ataxia "Drop attack"	For intracranial carotid disease: antiplatelet agent or anticoagulation For extracranial carotid disease: <30%: Antiplatelet agent 50% to 70%: Modest benefit of carotid endarterectomy (CEA) >70% and symptomatic: CEA For vertebrobasilar disease: Antiplatelet agent or anticoagulation
Lacune (small-vessel disease)	Atherosclerosis of small, penetrating vessels Associated with hypertension and diabetes	Pure motor ipsilateral hemiparesis (caused by internal capsule or pons lesion) Pure ipsilateral hemisensory stroke (caused by thalamic lesion)	Antiplatelet agents
Cardiac embolism	Atrial fibrillation Dilated cardiomyopathy Endocarditis	Presentation depends on site of embolization Often occurs at gray-white junction	Anticoagulation for primary or secondary prevention (except for endocarditis—bleeding risk too high) Acute anticoagulation not advised because of bleeding risk
Nonatherosclerotic vasculopathy	Fibromuscular dysplasia (FMD) Arterial dissection Vasculitis	Depends on location FMD more common in women May have systemic symptoms with vasculitis May have neck pain with arterial dissection	Treat underlying cause (i.e., vasculitis) Antiplatelet agent for FMD Antiplatelet agent for anticoagulation for arterial dissection
Hematologic disorders/ coagulopathy	Antiphospholipid antibody Sickle cell disease	Depends on location	Treat underlying cause Consider anticoagulation for antiphospholipid antibodies
Watershed infarction	Caused by hypotension from various causes (e.g., shock)	Bilateral proximal weakness of arms and legs	Volume repletion Treat underlying cause
Other Drug abuse Migraine Venous infarction	Cocaine Sagittal sinus thrombosis	Depends on location	Individualize treatment Consider anticoagulation for cerebral vein thrombosis

60

TABLE 60-3	*7-Day Risk of Stroke Stratified According to ABCD^2 Score at First Assessment in the OXVASC Validation Cohort of Patients with Probable or Definite Transient Ischemic Attack*		
	Patients (%)	**Strokes (%)**	**% Risk (95%CI)**
ABCD^2 Score			
≤1	2 (1%)	0	0
2	28 (15%)	0	0
3	32 (17%)	0	0
4	46 (24%)	1 (5%)	2.2 (0–6.4)
5	49 (26%)	8 (40%)	16.3 (6.0–26.7)
6	31 (16%)	11 (55%)	35.5 (18.6–52.3)
Total	188 (100%)	20 (100%)	10.5 (6.2–14.9)

ABCD^2, Age, blood pressure, clinical features, duration of symptoms, and diabetes; CI, confidence interval.
From Rothwell PM, Giles MF, Flossmann E, et al. A simple score (ABCD) to identify individuals at high early risk of stroke after transient ischaemic attack. *Lancet.* 2005;366(9479): 29–36.

TABLE 60-4	*Hemorrhagic Cerebrovascular Disease*			
	Etiology	**Clinical Presentation**	**Diagnosis**	**Treatment**
Subarachnoid hemorrhage	Berry aneurysm (at bifurcation of vessels in circle of Willis) Trauma (dissecting aneurysm) Atherosclerosis (fusiform aneurysm) Infection (mycotic aneurysm) Arteriovenous malformation (AVM)	Sudden, severe headache: "worst of life" Meningismus Often decreased consciousness Focal neurologic deficits possible Oculomotor palsy (CN III) is clue to posterior communicating artery aneurysm (common location)	CT is most sensitive to blood; >90% accuracy If CT is negative but suspicion high, must perform LP with RBC counts in tubes 1 and 4, as well as spin for xanthochromia MRI relatively insensitive Cerebral angiography to detect underlying aneurysm	Supportive care Nimodipine for associated vasospasm Early surgical clipping of aneurysms in patients with minor deficits Endovascular therapy (coiling of aneurysms)
Intracranial hemorrhage (ICH)	Chronic hypertension (50% to 80% of ICH) Cerebral amyloid angiopathy (older patients with Alzheimer disease) AVM (young patients) Tumor (renal cell, melanoma, glioma, choriocarcinoma) Drugs (cocaine, amphetamines, phenylpropanolamine) Other: vasculitis, coagulopathy, endocarditis, thrombocytopenia	Headache Vomiting Coma Seizures May be sudden onset or gradual progression of symptoms Lobar most common, followed by basal ganglia, thalamus, cerebellum, pons	CT most sensitive to blood MRI with gadolinium to detect underlying AVM, tumor Cerebral angiography if AVM suggested Avoid LP if mass effect from bleed	Control extreme hypertension Ventilation; airway protection Intracranial pressure management: elevate head of bed, avoid hypotonic fluids, possibly mannitol and hyperventilation Surgical evacuation if possible
Subdural hemorrhage	Trauma (often minor in elderly)	Headache Confusion Seizures	CT: concave-shaped bleed, may have mass effect	Supportive care Consider surgical evacuation
Epidural hemorrhage	Trauma	Headache Decreased level of consciousness	CT: lens-shaped bleed between dura and skull, pushing on parenchyma	Often requires urgent surgical evacuation

CN, Cranial nerve; CT, computed tomography; LP, lumbar puncture; MRI, magnetic resonance imaging; RBC, red blood cell.

- Causes, presentation, treatment (see Table 60-4)
- Berry aneurysm is common cause (Fig. 60-4)
- May occur with exertion, during rest, or even in sleep
- **Complications of SAH**
  - Rebleeding: most common in first 2 weeks; 50% mortality
  - Hydrocephalus
  - Vasospasm: cause of late ischemic infarctions
  - Hyponatremia (caused by atrial natriuretic factor)
  - Autonomic dysfunction
- **Intracerebral hemorrhage**
  - Presentation and treatment (see Table 60-4)
- **Subdural hematoma**
  - **Classic "crescent" shape on computed tomography (CT) underlying inner table of the skull (Fig. 60-5)**
  - Often seen in elderly after trauma, particularly if on anticoagulants

- **Epidural hematoma**
  - Often seen with trauma associated with skull fracture
  - Classic "lens" shape pushing on parenchyma by CT
  - High morbidity and mortality
  - Surgical decompression is often required

Diagnosis and Evaluation

- **General diagnostic evaluation: tailor to individual presentation**
  - Brain imaging
    - CT (high sensitivity for blood)
    - Magnetic resonance imaging (MRI) (better for brainstem visualization or lacunar strokes)
  - Vascular imaging
    - Carotid duplex ultrasound
    - CT angiography
    - Transcranial Doppler (ultrasound of intracranial vessels)
    - Magnetic resonance angiography

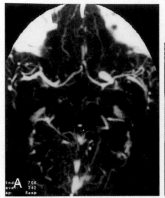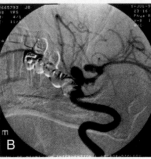

FIGURE 60-4 Proximal left middle cerebral artery aneurysm. Comparison of computed tomographic angiography (CTA) with conventional catheter angiography. **A,** Maximum-intensity projection image from CTA of the circle of Willis shows a berry aneurysm of the M1 segment. **B,** Catheter angiography, submentovertex view following left internal carotid artery injection shows excellent correlation. (From Bradley WG, Daroff RB, Fenichel GM, Jankovic J. *Neurology in Clinical Practice.* 4th ed. Philadelphia: Butterworth-Heinemann; 2004: Fig. 37B.16.)

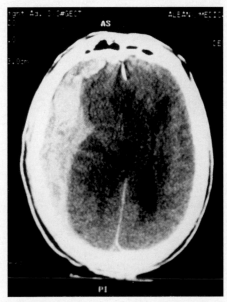

FIGURE 60-5 Head computed tomography scan demonstrating an acute subdural hematoma. (From Ferrera PC, Couciello SA, Marx J, Verdile V. *Trauma Management: An Emergency Medicine Approach.* St. Louis: Mosby; 2001: Fig. 11-2.)

- Cerebral angiography (gold standard)
  - Better anatomic localization of disease
  - Involves dye load
  - **1% risk of stroke with procedure**
- Cardiac evaluation
  - Electrocardiogram (examine rhythm, evidence of old CAD)
  - Echocardiogram: transesophageal preferred over transthoracic for better visualization of atria and aorta
  - Holter monitor: often low yield for arrhythmia
- Other
  - **Hypercoagulable evaluation (especially in young stroke patients; consider**

antiphospholipid antibodies and lupus anticoagulant)

- Toxicology
- Blood cultures
- Vasculitis should be considered only when there is evidence of disease systemically, erythrocyte sedimentation rate and C-reactive protein elevations

- **Differential diagnosis of stroke or TIA**
  - Focal seizure with Todd paralysis (see following discussion)
  - Complicated migraine
  - Brain mass
  - Peripheral vestibular disorder
  - Cardiac arrhythmia

Treatment

- General treatment of ischemic stroke
  - Supportive medical care: Prevent aspiration, deep venous thromboembolism, pressure sores
  - **Recommend against aggressive blood pressure control in the acute setting because this may lower cerebral perfusion**
  - **Aggressively control fever and hyperglycemia (may worsen stroke outcome)**
  - Observe for cerebral edema (peaks typically at 48 hours)
  - **Antiplatelet therapy: Reduces future events by roughly 25%**
    - Aspirin: 81 to 325 mg/day
    - Clopidogrel: 75 mg/day
    - Dipyridamole 200 mg plus aspirin 25 mg sustained-release orally twice daily
  - Anticoagulants
    - **Heparin: no proven benefit and acutely increases bleeding risk**
    - Low-molecular-weight heparinoids: no proven benefit but alternative to intravenous (IV) heparin
    - **Warfarin for secondary prevention of cardioembolic stroke in atrial fibrillation**
    - **New thrombin inhibitors such as dabigatran have been shown to prevent stroke in atrial fibrillation to same degree as warfarin**
      - It is important to remember that the thrombin inhibitors cannot be reversed with fresh-frozen plasma
  - Thrombolytic therapy
    - The U.S. Food and Drug Administration approved use of tissue plasminogen activator (tPA) for acute ischemic stroke in 1996
    - Criteria for use
      - Suggested acute ischemic stroke
      - Administration of tPA can be achieved within 3 hours from onset of symptoms
        - Some benefit may be seen in patients who receive tPA within 4.5 hours
      - No contraindications for thrombolytic therapy (i.e., active GI bleeding and others as with thrombolysis for myocardial infarction)
    - **Exclusions for use of tPA**
      - Time of onset uncertain or more than 3 hours
      - Minor stroke or resolving symptoms

60

- Suggested or witnessed seizure
- Blood pressure greater than 185/110 mm Hg or requiring aggressive treatment
- Early hypodensity or other lesion on CT that would increase risk of bleeding (e.g., tumor)
  - Protocol
    - tPA dose 0.9 mg/kg, maximum dose of 90 mg (10% bolus followed by 60-minute infusion)
    - No invasive procedures for 24 hours
    - Strict blood pressure control to maintain less than 185/110 mm Hg
- Carotid endarterectomy (CEA)
  - Useful for extracranial carotid stenosis
  - Helpful for long-term management and prevention of future events
  - **Indications (based on large trials)**
    - **50% to 70% symptomatic stenosis: Modest benefit from CEA; individualize treatment**
    - **Greater than 70% symptomatic stenosis: CEA superior to medical therapy in patients who are good surgical candidates**
    - **Greater than 60% asymptomatic stenosis: Modest benefit from CEA over medical therapy; individualize treatment**
- Carotid stenting
  - Useful for those patients who are not surgical candidates
  - Head-to-head trials versus CEA show equivalence of outcomes
  - Surgery still preferred treatment for patients who are good surgical candidates. CEA patients have lower rate of stroke and high rate of postoperative myocardial infarction (MI)
  - Carotid stent patients have higher rate of stroke and lower rate of MI
  - Patient selection should depend on cardiac and stroke risks

Seizure Disorders

Basic Information

- Seizures do not necessarily imply epilepsy; they may be caused by a temporary underlying disorder

- **In adults, the most common type of seizure is complex partial (40%), followed by generalized and simple partial seizures**
- The most common cause of epilepsy is *idiopathic* or *cryptogenic*
- Up to 70% of patients can achieve remission; about half of them (35%) can remain seizure-free without medication

Clinical Presentation

- Todd paralysis: A transient (not longer than 48 hours) neurologic deficit (e.g., motor weakness) after a seizure that reflects postictal depression of the involved area
- Classification of seizures (Table 60-5)
  - **Partial seizures: Onset is limited to one cerebral hemisphere**
    - May be motor, sensory, or psychoillusory (i.e., déjà vu)
    - May generalize secondarily
    - Jacksonian march: Focal seizure that begins in motor cortex and spreads to rest of motor area; clinically, clonic movements that spread proximally (usually up a limb)
  - **Primary generalized seizures (grand mal): Involve the cerebral cortex diffusely from the beginning**
    - Tongue biting and incontinence can be hallmarks
    - Can begin with focal seizure activity
    - New seizures in those 50 years and older should raise concern for CNS space-occupying lesion
- Each class of seizures can have varied clinical presentations (see Table 60-5)

Diagnosis and Evaluation

- **Diagnosis depends on the clinical presentation and setting; electroencephalogram (EEG) findings are helpful but not definitive**
- Goals of diagnosis
  - Classify the type of seizure
  - Determine if epilepsy is truly present
  - Identify the underlying cause if possible
- Seizures may have underlying structural causes
  - Hippocampal sclerosis
  - Glial tumors

TABLE 60-5	*Classification of Seizures*	
Class	**Definition**	**Examples**
Simple partial seizure	Normal consciousness	Simple motor (limb jerking) Simple sensory (paresthesias)
Complex partial seizure	Alteration of consciousness	Temporal lobe epilepsy Aura (strange odor, déjà vu, automatisms, lip smacking, agitation, nondirected violence) May be associated with frontal or temporal lobe tumors, herpes encephalitis, hippocampal sclerosis
Generalized seizure	Complete impairment of consciousness	Primary generalized tonic-clonic (grand mal) Secondary generalized tonic-clonic (focal seizure that spreads) Absence (petit mal) Myoclonic (juvenile myoclonic epilepsy) Atonic (Lennox-Gastaut syndrome; drop attack)

- Cavernous malformations
- Encephalitis
- Trauma
- Hemorrhage
- Acute, subacute, or chronic stroke
- **Consider metabolic and other causes of seizure (secondary seizure) in the right clinical setting**
  - Hyperglycemia (often focal seizures)
  - Hypoglycemia
  - Hyponatremia
  - Hypoxia
  - Uremia
  - Meningitis, encephalitis
  - Head trauma
- Drugs that can precipitate seizures
  - Antibiotics such as metronidazole, ciprofloxacin, acyclovir, high-dose penicillin and its derivatives
  - Bupropion
  - Methylphenidate
  - Rapid withdrawal of barbiturates, alcohol, benzodiazepines
- Differential diagnosis of seizures
  - Convulsive syncope
  - Pseudoseizures
    - Also known as psychogenic seizures
    - **Change in behavior not associated with abnormal brain electrical activity**
    - Often helpful to check prolactin 15 to 45 minutes after the event (will be normal in pseudoseizures, elevated in true seizure disorder)
  - Anoxic myoclonus
- Evaluation of new-onset seizures
  - History: focality of onset, aura, family history (may need to talk with witnesses)
  - Brain imaging: MRI with gadolinium enhancement is best to rule out structural abnormalities

- EEG (Fig. 60-6)
  - *Spikes* or *sharp waves* help localize seizure focus and classify seizure type
  - Most useful if obtained during a clinical attack to avoid false negatives
  - EEG in the setting of sleep deprivation enhances seizure detection
  - Video EEG for unusual symptoms or suggested pseudoseizures
- Serum prolactin may be elevated at 45 minutes with partial complex or generalized seizures
- Increased recurrent seizure risk: focal neurologic deficit, brain lesion, abnormal EEG
- First isolated seizure: Recurrence rate is 50% within 2 years if untreated (25% if treated); risk drops to about 20% if physical examination, MRI, and EEG are all normal

Treatment

- General principles
  - New seizure onset
    - **Work-up as in preceding section; hospitalization is usually not necessary**
    - Initiation of drug treatment for first seizure is controversial; must tailor to individual; assessing risk of further seizures is helpful
      - Low risk: normal physical examination, MRI, EEG, no history of brain trauma, and no family history of epilepsy
      - Higher risk (consider drug therapy): two or more of preceding risk factors
  - Seizures that do not need long-term treatment: drug- or alcohol-related, seizures immediately associated with head injury, convulsive syncope
  - Seizures from metabolic causes: Treat the underlying metabolic abnormality

60

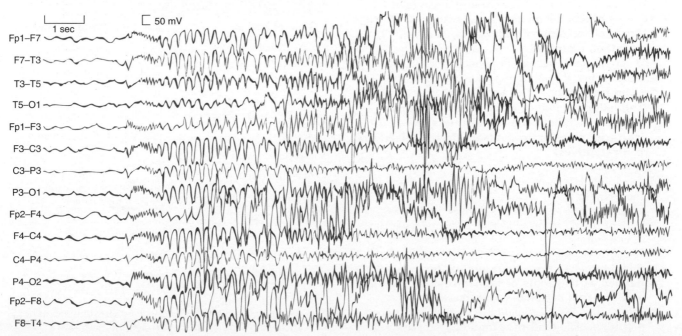

FIGURE 60-6 Electroencephalogram recorded at the onset of a generalized tonic-clonic seizure. (From Goetz B. *Textbook of Clinical Neurology*. 2nd ed. Philadelphia: Saunders; 2003: Fig. 24-7.)

TABLE 60-6	Common Antiepileptic Drugs		
Drug	**Indication**	**Typical Dose**	**Side Effect**
Lorazepam	Rapid treatment of acute seizures Not useful for long-term prophylaxis	0.5 to to 1 mg PO every 6 to 8 hours	Sedation Respiratory compromise
Phenytoin	Partial seizures Generalized seizures	300 mg PO daily	IV dose may cause cardiac arrhythmias Nausea, ataxia, sedation Rash Hypersensitivity (mononucleosis-like) syndrome with rash, fever, lymphadenopathy Gingival hyperplasia Peripheral neuropathy Cerebellar degeneration Osteoporosis Fosphenytoin may be safer but is more costly
Carbamazepine	Partial seizures Generalized seizures Temporal lobe epilepsy	200 mg PO bid or tid	Nausea, ataxia, sedation Rash Leukopenia Aplastic anemia Hyponatremia Osteoporosis
Phenobarbital	Generalized seizures	30 to 120 mg PO daily	Sedation Respiratory depression with IV dosing
Valproic acid (valproate)	Partial seizures Generalized seizures Myoclonic seizures Lennox-Gastaut seizures	500 to 1000 mg PO bid or tid	Nausea Weight gain Birth defects Tremor Thrombocytopenia and platelet dysfunction Hair loss Pancreatitis
Gabapentin	Add-on to other therapy	300 to 900 mg tid	Sedation Ataxia
Levetiracetam	Add-on therapy	500 mg bid	Agitation, exacerbation of psychiatric symptoms

bid, Twice daily; IV, intravenous; PO, orally; tid, three times daily.

- Common antiepileptic drugs (Table 60-6)
- Antiepileptic drugs of choice by diagnosis (Table 60-7)
- **Adverse effects common to most antiepileptic drugs**
  - **Dose-related side effects: ataxia, nausea, sedation, diplopia**
  - Allergic effects (all except phenobarbital): neutropenia, thrombocytopenia, aplastic anemia
  - **Drug interactions: Can be complex, but most antiepileptics induce cytochrome P450 and increase metabolism of other drugs (e.g., warfarin, other anticonvulsant drugs, folate, oral contraceptives)**
- Birth defects
  - All antiepileptics increase birth defects twofold (3% increased to 6%)
  - Valproate considered worst offender
  - Patient should be on folic acid supplements at time of conception
- Surgical treatment
  - **Consider when drug therapy fails (usually defined as two trials of high-dose monotherapy and one trial of combination therapy)**
  - Most common procedure: focal cortical resection
    - Must be able to identify focal epileptogenic region
    - Surgery must not leave patient with significant neurologic deficits

TABLE 60-7	Antiepileptic Drugs of Choice by Diagnosis
Type of Seizure	**Drug of Choice**
Generalized seizure	Phenytoin Carbamazepine Valproate Phenobarbital Levetiracetam
Partial complex seizure	Carbamazepine
Absence seizure	Ethosuxomide
Myoclonic seizure	Valproate
Add-on therapy	Gabapentin Lamotrigine Topiramate Levetiracetam

- Most commonly used for refractory temporal lobe epilepsy
- Treatment of status epilepticus
  - Medical emergency
  - Untreated, a variety of complications may occur, including aspiration, hypertension, cardiac dysrhythmias, lactic acidosis, rhabdomyolysis, hyperpyrexia, and, ultimately, death

- Assess: Give oxygen; obtain IV access; obtain stat chemistry (glucose, calcium, magnesium)
- Give IV normal saline, thiamine 100 mg, and 1 ampule of D50 empirically
- Seizure-specific therapy (in usual order of preference)
  - Lorazepam 2 to 4 mg IV at 2 mg/min (0.05 to 0.2 mg/kg), maximum 8 mg for adults
  - Phenytoin 20 mg/kg IV in 50-mL normal saline at maximum rate of 50 mg/min (e.g., 1000 mg over 20 minutes for an adult), or fosphenytoin 20 "phenytoin equivalents" (PEs)/kg IV at maximum rate of 150 PEs/min (1 g IV over 10 minutes)
    - Monitor for hypotension, arrhythmia
  - Phenobarbital 20 mg/kg IV at 100 mg/min (5 to 10 mg/kg)
    - Monitor for respiratory depression
  - Last resort: pentobarbital coma
    - Potential complications: hypotension, hypothermia, decreased cardiac output

Acknowledgment

I would like to thank Robert J. Wityk, MD, for his work on previous editions of this chapter.

Review Questions

For review questions, please go to ExpertConsult.com.

SUGGESTED READINGS

Grotta JC. Clinical practice: Carotid stenosis. *N Engl J Med.* 2013;369:1143-1150.

International Stroke Trial Collaborative Group. The International Stroke Trial (IST): a randomized trial of aspirin, subcutaneous heparin, both, or neither among 19,435 patients with acute ischemic stroke. *Lancet.* 1997;349:1569-1581.

Jobst BC, Cascino GD. Resective epilepsy surgery for drug-resistant focal epilepsy: a review. *JAMA.* 2015;313:285-293.

Lansberg MG, O'Donnell MJ, Khatri P, et al. Antithrombotic and thrombolytic therapy for ischemic stroke: Antithrombotic Therapy and Prevention of Thrombosis, 9th ed: American College of Chest Physicians Evidence-Based Clinical Practice Guidelines. *Chest.* 2012;141(2 suppl):e601S-36S.

Rothwell PM, Giles MF, Flossmann E, et al. A simple score (ABCD) to identify individuals at high risk of stroke after transient ischaemic attack. *Lancet.* 2005;366:29-36.

Schmidt D, Schachter SC. Drug treatment of epilepsy in adults. *BMJ.* 2014;348:g254.

60

Movement Disorders

SHAWN F. SMYTH, MD; RAINER VON COELLN, DR MED; and
JOSEPH M. SAVITT, MD, PhD

The primary motor pathways from the cerebral cortex to the brainstem and spinal cord (upper motor neuron) and from the brainstem and spinal cord to the muscle (lower motor neuron) control the basics of voluntary muscle contraction. The term *movement disorders* refers to disorders at a higher level of control over movement, such as the speed, timing, gain, accuracy, planning, feedback, and integration of directed movement. The diagnosis of movement disorders depends on the recognition of clinical patterns of movement. Understanding the nature and types of abnormal movements is crucial to the diagnosis of these disorders.

There are two categories of abnormal movements based on whether excessive movement (hyperkinesis) or not enough movement (hypokinesis) is seen. Also addressed in this chapter are other topics in movement disorders that do not neatly fit this distinction.

- **Hyperkinesis is too much movement:**
  - Tremor
  - Chorea, athetosis, and ballism
  - Dystonia
  - Myoclonus
  - Urge to move: tics, restless legs syndrome (RLS), akathisia
- **Hypokinesis is too little movement:**
  - Parkinsonism
  - Parkinson disease
  - Catatonia (often classified as a psychiatric disorder)
  - Apraxia (often classified as a cognitive disorder)
- **Other topics in movement disorders:**
  - Ataxia
  - Drug-induced movement disorders
  - Psychogenic movement disorders

Hyperkinesis

TREMOR

Basic Information

- Definition: Rhythmic oscillations of any body part
- Three types of tremor:
  - **Rest:** Present when the affected body part is completely relaxed
  - **Postural:** Present when the affected body part is held, not moving, against gravity (arms extended, or holding a cup or newspaper)
  - **Kinetic:** Present during motion of a body part (reaching, pouring)

- Intention tremor is a subtype of kinetic tremor that increases in amplitude/intensity at the end of movement (close to target)
- Etiologies
  - Physiologic tremor: normal, very small oscillations usually unnoticed in most people
  - Enhanced physiologic tremor: an increase in physiologic tremor triggered by a substance or condition
    - Medications/toxins: caffeine, antidepressants, β-agonists, others
    - Metabolic: hyperthyroidism, hypoglycemia, liver disease
    - Stress: anxiety, hunger, cold, or fatigue
  - **Essential tremor (ET)**
    - Most common tremor disorder, affecting 10 million Americans.
    - Roughly **50% have a first-degree relative with ET**
    - **Gradual onset** (average is fourth decade of life but can be at any age) and slow progression of a postural and kinetic limb tremor, but can have tremor in the head and voice. Tremor may eventually develop a rest component.
    - Worsens with anxiety, caffeine, lack of sleep, and some medications; **may improve with relatively small amounts of alcohol consumption**
  - **Cerebellar tremor: intention/kinetic tremor more common than postural tremor,** often with coincident ataxia. Can result from degenerative disorders, masses, strokes, multiple sclerosis, medications, toxins, etc.
  - Dystonic tremor, parkinsonian tremor, and psychogenic tremor are discussed in following sections

Diagnosis and Evaluation of Tremor

- History and examination: Define the pattern of tremor
- Determination of etiology: Assess for underlying metabolic and toxic conditions, medications, anatomic lesions, and other identifiable etiologies. Often the determination involves distinguishing ET from parkinsonian tremor (Table 61-1).

Treatment

- Treatment of tremor dependent on cause
  - Enhanced physiologic tremor: **Remove the triggering cause** if known
  - ET

TABLE 61-1	Essential Tremor versus Parkinson Disease-Associated Tremor	
Clinical Feature	**Essential Tremor**	**Parkinson Disease**
Family history	Positive in 50%	Usually negative
Response to alcohol	Tremor attenuates	No obvious effect
When does it occur?	With action	At rest
Speed	Fast (6–10 Hz)	Slow (4–6 Hz)
Appearance	Flexion-extension of wrists	Pill-rolling movement of fingers with pronation, supination of wrist
Location	Hands/arms (bilateral), head/neck, voice	Hands/arms (unilateral), jaw/chin
Associated features	Mild imbalance	Masked face, cogwheel rigidity, bradykinesia, gait impairment

Hz, Hertz (cycles per second).

BOX 61-1	*Pharmacotherapy for Essential Tremor*

First Line:
Propranolol (both short- and long-acting formulations)
Primidone (with or without propranolol)

Second Line:
Other β-blockers (e.g., metoprolol, atenolol)
Anticonvulsants (e.g., gabapentin, topiramate)
Benzodiazepines (e.g., alprazolam, clonazepam, lorazepam)

- Pharmacotherapy: see Box 61-1. Propranolol is the only U.S. Food and Drug Administration (FDA)-approved drug for tremor
- Surgical treatment: for medically refractory and functionally disabling tremors
  - Thalamotomy: A small lesion is made in the thalamus (rarely done now)
  - Deep brain stimulation: implanted brain electrodes connected to a battery pack/pulse generator in the chest, to electrically stimulate the thalamus
- Cerebellar tremor: Sometimes responds to benzodiazepines, carbamazepine, and more traditional ET treatments

DYSTONIA
Basic Information

- Definition: Sustained or intermittent muscle contractions causing abnormal, often repetitive, movements, postures, or both. Movements are often patterned, twisting, and may be tremulous. It is worsened by volitional action and associated with overflow muscle activation.

TABLE 61-2	Subtypes of Dystonia Based on Involved Area
Dystonia Subtype	**Affected Region**
Focal	**Limited Body Region**
Torticollis	Neck muscles
Blepharospasm	Periocular muscles
Spasmodic dysphonia	Vocal cords
Writer's cramp	Hand and forearm muscles
Segmental	**Two Contiguous Regions**
Meige syndrome	Periocular and perioral muscles
Oromandibular	Mouth, jaw, tongue
Hemidystonia	Half of the body
Generalized	Majority of the body

- Most often associated with dysfunction of the neural circuits of the basal ganglia, cerebellum, and cerebral cortex
- Patients may have a sensory trick whereby a sensory stimulus (touching the chin, having a toothpick in the mouth) relieves the dystonia
- Etiologies
  - Inherited diseases: Wilson disease (dysfunction of copper metabolism), *DYT1* gene-associated dystonia, and many other pure and mixed dystonic diseases
  - Ischemia or stroke, including perinatal injury
  - Toxic/metabolic: carbon monoxide, manganese, cyanide poisoning
  - Medications: antipsychotics, antiemetics, levodopa, dopamine agonists, calcium channel blockers, anticonvulsants
  - Infections: viral encephalitis, tuberculosis, syphilis
  - Parkinson disease: often affects the foot
  - Idiopathic: In many cases the cause remains undetermined

Clinical Presentation

- Dystonia may develop at any age
  - **Childhood**-onset cases are more likely to be **genetic,** with progression from focal/segmental to generalized involvement. Often a cause is discovered.
  - **Adult**-onset cases are more likely to be **idiopathic,** with progression in a focal/segmental pattern over weeks or months followed by stabilization (not usually generalized)
- **Dystonias are often categorized according to the body part affected,** with several well-recognized syndromes such as cervical dystonia (neck), blepharospasm (eyelids), spasmodic dysphonia (voice), oromandibular dystonia, and writer's cramp (Table 61-2)
- **Dystonia can be focal (one body region affected), segmental (two or more contiguous regions affected), multifocal (two or more noncontiguous regions affected), or generalized (trunk and two or more other regions affected)**

61

- Dystonic head tremor often mimics essential tremor
- Severity can range from mildly exaggerated normal movements to intermittent contractions and twisting postures, to sustained postures with fixed deformities, severe incapacitation, and even death

Diagnosis and Evaluation

- History and exam: age at onset, manner of progression, family history, region affected, and associated clinical features
- Brain and/or spine magnetic resonance imaging (MRI) is indicated in many cases
- Test for reversible/treatable causes, especially in early-onset cases
  - Wilson disease: Check for increased 24-hour urinary copper excretion, low serum ceruloplasmin, liver biopsy, and Kayser-Fleischer rings by ophthalmologic exam
  - Dopa-responsive dystonia (DRD): Give diagnostic or therapeutic trial of levodopa/carbidopa (Sinemet)
  - *DYT1* gene-associated dystonia:
    - The most common heritable form of generalized dystonia (autosomal dominant but reduced penetrance, so family history may be negative), although other genetic dystonias also exist
      - Consider this gene test for generalized and atypical focal dystonia, in young-onset disease and for those with a family history of dystonia
    - Evidence of successful treatment with deep brain stimulation of the globus pallidus interna
  - Consider Parkinson disease (especially young-onset Parkinson disease) or a parkinsonian syndrome as the cause of the dystonia

Treatment

- **Treat the underlying cause,** if found and if possible, such as in Wilson disease, drug-induced dystonia, and dopa-responsive dystonia
- Symptomatic treatment
  - **For focal dystonia: The most effective treatment is injected botulinum toxin** every 3 to 6 months
    - Used to treat blepharospasm, cervical dystonia, spasmodic dysphonia, foot and hand dystonia
    - When larger regions are involved (hemi- or generalized dystonia), this often is not feasible
  - For more generalized dystonia
    - First: **carbidopa/levodopa** to rule out DRD
    - If unresponsive, then try **anticholinergics, benzodiazepines, baclofen, or tetrabenazine**
    - Surgical procedures are used for medically refractory cases: selective denervation, intrathecal baclofen pump, or deep brain stimulation of the globus pallidus

CHOREA, ATHETOSIS, AND BALLISM

Basic Information

- These three terms refer to a group of movements that exist on a spectrum
  - **Chorea: Involuntary, irregular, abrupt, unpatterned, and unsustained movements** with variable timing and distribution
  - **Athetosis: Involuntary slow and irregular writhing movements** most often affecting the distal limbs
  - **Ballism: Involuntary, large-amplitude, flinging movements,** typically involving proximal muscles that move an entire limb
- These three movements often blend together, with distinctions being the speed and location of movements. The term *choreoathetosis* acknowledges the frequent co-occurrence of chorea and athetosis.
- Anatomy: These movements are most often associated with **dysfunction of neural circuits of the basal ganglia**
- Etiology
  - **Inherited diseases:** usually gradual onset
    - **Huntington disease:** Autosomal dominant inheritance assayed with gene test for triplet nucleotide repeat. Usual onset in adulthood though aged- and childhood-onset can occur. Often worse when inherited from the father (paternal anticipation). Chorea, psychiatric symptoms, and cognitive dysfunction progress over 10 to 20 years until death.
    - Other less common genetic syndromes seen as well
    - Inborn errors of metabolism (mainly in children)
  - Stroke: often to the subthalamic nucleus or another nucleus of the basal ganglia
  - Toxic or metabolic: cocaine intoxication, hyperthyroidism, renal failure
  - Medications (Table 61-3)
  - Infections: toxoplasmosis, syphilis, encephalitis, human immunodeficiency virus (HIV)
  - Autoimmune disorders: lupus, anticardiolipin syndrome, or Sydenham chorea (after rheumatic fever/streptococcal infection)
  - Pregnancy (chorea gravidarum): occurs only during pregnancy
  - Cardiac surgery: postpump chorea, especially in children

Clinical Presentation

- The mildest forms of chorea are **easily overlooked as occasional fidgeting movements**
- Affected individuals often try to mask the abnormal movements by blending them into more purposeful-appearing movements

Diagnosis and Evaluation

- History and exam
- Laboratory evaluation, including thyroid-stimulating hormone (TSH), antinuclear antibodies, antistreptolysin O, anticardiolipin, pregnancy testing, and ceruloplasmin
- Huntington and other gene testing
- Brain MRI

Treatment

- Consider if the movement interferes with daily activities or is significantly embarrassing
- **Antipsychotic medications:** Used with caution, because they can cause tardive dyskinesia (that looks like chorea) and can cause parkinsonism

| TABLE 61-3 | *Drug-Induced Movement Disorders** | | | |

Tremor	Parkinsonism (see Table 61-5)	Choreoathetosis	Acute Dystonia	Tardive Dyskinesia
Stimulants Amphetamine Pemoline Cocaine Caffeine Adrenergics Ephedrine β-Agonists **Anticonvulsants** Valproic acid Lamotrigine Phenytoin **Others** Cyclosporine Amiodarone Thyroxine Lithium	**Dopamine Antagonists** Classical Atypical **Antiemetics** Metoclopramide Prochlorperazine **Cardiovascular** Reserpine α-Methyldopa Calcium channel blockers Amiodarone **Others** Antidepressants Lithium Tetrabenazine	**Stimulants** Amphetamine Pemoline Cocaine Theophylline Adrenergics Ephedrine β-Agonists **Anticonvulsants** **Carbamazepine** Phenytoin **Others** Lithium Oral contraceptives Levodopa	**Dopamine Antagonists** Classical Atypical† **Antiemetics** Metoclopramide Prochlorperazine **Antihistamines** Cimetidine Ranitidine **Antitussives**	**Dopamine Antagonists** Classical Atypical† **Antiemetics** **Metoclopramide Prochlorperazine** **Antidepressants** SSRI/SNRI

*This is a partial list of the most common offenders.
†Exceptions: It is less likely for quetiapine, and extremely rare for clozapine, to cause these movement disorders, compared with the other neuroleptics.
SSRI/SNRI, Selective serotonin reuptake inhibitor/serotonin and norepinephrine reuptake inhibitor.

- **Tetrabenazine:** FDA-approved medication for Huntington disease with less tardive dyskinesia or parkinsonism but risk of depression and suicide
- Chorea from stroke often improves on its own. Chorea from some autoimmune disorders, medications, hormonal imbalance, and other causes may improve with correction of the underlying disorder or withdrawal of the medication.

MYOCLONUS

Basic Information

- Definition: **Involuntary, abrupt, brief, jerky movement of a body part. Often described as "lightning fast."**
- Anatomy: The origin ("generator") of this movement can be the cerebral cortex, subcortical structures (basal ganglia, thalamus, brainstem), or spinal cord
- Classification of myoclonus by etiology
  - Physiologic myoclonus (e.g., when falling asleep; startle reaction; hiccups)
  - Essential myoclonus (idiopathic, possibly genetic)
  - Myoclonic epilepsies (Unverricht-Lundborg disease, myoclonic epilepsy with ragged red fibers, neuronal ceroid lipofuscinoses, sialidosis, and Lafora body disease)
  - Symptomatic myoclonus (the most common form) from a wide variety of underlying conditions:
    - Metabolic encephalopathies (most commonly hepatic or renal encephalopathy), typically with asterixis (wrist flapping)
    - Toxic encephalopathies (cocaine, marijuana, tricyclic antidepressants, levodopa, penicillin, others)
    - Neurodegenerative diseases (Wilson disease, Creutzfeldt-Jakob disease, Huntington disease, corticobasal syndrome, Alzheimer disease, many others)
    - Infectious/Inflammatory (viral encephalitis, malaria, syphilis, Lyme, celiac, Hashimoto encephalopathy, etc.)
    - Posthypoxic myoclonus (Lance-Adams syndrome)
    - Head or spine trauma/tumor
- Further classification of myoclonus
  - Distribution: focal, segmental, multifocal, or generalized
  - Provoking factor: spontaneous or reflex
  - Source: cortical, subcortical, spinal, peripheral
  - Character: arrhythmic (random), rhythmic (regular pattern), or oscillatory (resembling a tremor)

Clinical Presentation

- **Movements can be spontaneous, stimulus-induced, or associated with action**
- Etiology determines the onset, progression, distribution, and character

Diagnosis and Evaluation

- History and exam: Characterize the myoclonus regarding the distribution, spontaneity, triggering factors, and accompanying symptoms
- Laboratory work-up, MRI of the brain and/or spine, lumbar puncture, and/or electrophysiology (electroencephalography [EEG], somatosensory-evoked potentials, electromyography)

Treatment

- Treatment is difficult, and in many cases therapeutic response is incomplete
- **The most common treatments include valproic acid, levetiracetam, and benzodiazepines** (e.g., clonazepam)

61

Disorders with "Urge to Move"

TICS AND TOURETTE SYNDROME

Basic Information

- Definitions
  - **Tics: Sudden, rapid, nonrhythmic, and recurrent movements, preceded by an urge and followed by a sense of relief,** that are usually temporarily suppressible.
  - **Tourette syndrome: multiple motor and at least one vocal tic beginning before age 18** and lasting for at least 12 months
- Etiology
  - **Idiopathic.** Tourette syndrome likely has a genetic component
  - Toxin-induced (cocaine, amphetamine, neuroleptics)
  - Neurodegenerative: Huntington disease, Lesch-Nyhan syndrome, Wilson disease.
  - Vascular: stroke

Clinical Presentation

- Varied, with onset at any age, but more commonly in childhood
- Symptoms may be chronic or have a waxing/waning course, which may remit for years
- **Common simple tics include eye squinting or shoulder shrugging**
- **Complex tics may include neck or shoulder rolling, brief ritualized sequences, utterances of phrases**
- Coprolalia (blurting out of obscenities) only occurs in a minority of patients
- Suppression of a tic is accompanied by a buildup of tension that is released when the tic is expressed
- Tics can closely resemble other movement disorders such as chorea, dystonia, or myoclonus
- **Tics and Tourette syndrome are frequently associated with obsessive-compulsive disorder or attention-deficit/hyperactivity disorder**

Diagnosis and Evaluation

- History and exam
- Not much is needed with regard to ancillary tests except for adult-onset tics (without any previous childhood history), as the movement may be a sign of a neurodegenerative disorder and further investigation may be needed (if medications are excluded)

Treatment

- **Only treat if functionally limiting or significantly embarrassing**
- Antipsychotics in low doses. Atypical antipsychotics are used for severe cases.
- Other medications include tetrabenazine, clonidine, guanfacine, gabapentin, baclofen, topiramate, and botulinum toxin
- Deep brain stimulation may be a future therapy

RESTLESS LEGS SYNDROME

Basic Information

- Definition: **discomforting sensations in the legs, most prominent at rest and in the evening/nighttime, causing an urge to move;** leg movement usually temporarily relieves the discomfort
- Epidemiology: Approximately 5% to 10% of the adult population will have RLS; it is **more common in women**
- Etiology
  - **Primary RLS (approximately 67%): About 50% of these patients have a first-degree relative with RLS**
  - **Secondary RLS (approximately 33%): iron-deficiency anemia, end-stage renal disease, diabetes, pregnancy, peripheral neuropathy, lumbar radiculopathy, autoimmune disorders, vitamin B_{12}, folate, or magnesium deficiencies,** and medications/substances (antipsychotics, antidepressants, alcohol, caffeine, antihistamines, etc.)
  - Pathophysiology: Iron metabolism and dopaminergic transmission may be involved

Clinical Presentation

- Most commonly **begins in early adulthood with slow progression**
- Often unrecognized or misdiagnosed
- Sometimes symptoms are described as vague discomfort, restlessness, irritation, creeping/tingling sensations, or less commonly pain
- Symptom relief by movement: stretching, cycling legs, walking, etc.
- Symptoms can disrupt sleep, which can lead to daytime sleepiness
- In more serious cases, discomfort may appear during any period of rest (sitting to read), at any time of day, and can affect the arms and trunk

Diagnosis and Evaluation

- History and exam: The exam is usually normal in RLS
- Overnight polysomnogram (PSG) may show co-existing periodic limb movements in sleep (PLMS) that are usually asymptomatic. PLMS as an incidental finding on PSG does not require treatment, but may raise suspicion of RLS.
- Other testing: Check for iron deficiency, renal dysfunction, diabetes, peripheral neuropathy, pregnancy
- Also, differentiate from akathisia (see following)

Treatment

- Usually dosed once in the evening
- **Dopaminergic agents:** Lower doses than in Parkinson disease
  - Dopamine agonists: popinirole, pramipexole, rotigotine
  - Carbidopa/levodopa
  - Two problems can occur with dopaminergic medications:
    - Rebound: Symptoms can worsen in the morning when the medication wears off
    - Augmentation: Symptoms occur earlier in the evening and eventually during the day the longer these medications are used
- Nondopaminergic agents
  - Antiepileptic medications: gabapentin, pregabalin, carbamazepine, valproic acid

- Benzodiazepines: These promote sleep if needed, but do not suppress RLS symptoms. Effective for PLMS.
- Opioids: effective in refractory cases

AKATHISIA

Basic Information

- Definition: **An inner sense of restlessness that temporarily improves upon voluntary movement and can be temporarily suppressed by the patient, though anxiety/tension builds during that suppression**
- Etiology
  - Often medication induced: antipsychotics, dopamine-blocking antinausea medications (e.g., metoclopramide, prochlorperazine), antidepressants
  - Sometimes seen in degenerative parkinsonian disorders

Clinical Presentation and Characteristics

- **Restlessness or uneasiness is relieved by movement but does NOT predominate in the legs** and is NOT more common while resting or lying down (as in RLS)
- It is differentiated from anxiety since it is temporarily relieved by movement and is not typically associated with recurrent worry

Treatment

- Remove offending medication, or treat underlying disorder

Hypokinesis

PARKINSONISM

Basic Information

- Definition: A clinical syndrome defined by motor dysfunction, including **bradykinesia** (slowness), **rest tremor**, **rigidity** (stiffness), and **postural instability** (balance and gait dysfunction)
  - Bradykinesia is assessed by rapidly tapping the index finger on the thumb and rapidly opening and closing a fisted hand
  - Rigidity very often has a cogwheel component on passive movement
  - *Parkinsonism* simply defines a collection of symptoms that can have many different etiologies; *Parkinson disease* (PD) refers to a specific disorder that is the most common cause of parkinsonism
- Etiology
  - Primary: PD (see later)
  - Secondary causes are reviewed in Table 61-4
    - Hereditary-degenerative disorders (e.g., Huntington disease; Wilson disease) may cause parkinsonism
    - There are also metabolic (e.g., hypothyroidism) and toxic (e.g., methylphenyltetrahydropyridine [MPTP]; manganese; carbon monoxide) causes of parkinsonism
    - Medication-induced causes are listed in Table 61-5
    - Traumatic brain injury
    - Postencephalitis

Diagnosis

- History and exam: Determine if the syndrome is consistent with PD or if there are atypical features that suggest a different etiology
- Ancillary testing: Brain MRI (if suspected vascular or hydrocephalic changes), TSH, and as needed, genetic testing for Huntington disease or 24-hour urine copper and serum ceruloplasmin for Wilson disease
- Medication trial: **PD also is characterized by a robust and sustained response to dopaminergic medications (especially carbidopa/levodopa), whereas other etiologies have only a partial or short-lived response**
- No clear role for genetic testing of PD-related genes at present, but such testing can provide a diagnosis in

TABLE 61-4	Red Flags for Other Parkinsonian Disorders*	
Parkinsonian Disorder	**Clinical Features (in Addition to Parkinsonism)**	**Brain Magnetic Resonance Imaging**
Progressive supranuclear palsy	Slow saccades, gaze palsies, early falls, dysarthria, midline dystonia	Normal or midbrain and frontal atrophy
Dementia with Lewy bodies	Early dementia, fluctuating alertness, early visual hallucinations	Diffuse atrophy, possibly posterior-predominant
Corticobasal degeneration	Dysarthria, dementia. Asymmetrical stiffness, apraxia, dystonia and slowness of a limb	Normal or asymmetrical cortical atrophy
Multiple system atrophy	Early autonomic dysfunction, dysarthria, cerebellar ataxia	Normal or brainstem and cerebellar atrophy
Normal-pressure hydrocephalus	Prominent gait dysfunction (imbalanced, slow, feet sliding on ground), dementia, urinary incontinence	Enlarged lateral ventricles out of proportion to cortical atrophy
Vascular parkinsonism	Lower body and gait-predominant parkinsonism, cognitive dysfunction /dementia	Extensive patchy or diffuse white matter disease

*Poor response to dopaminergic medications is present in most patients with these disorders.

TABLE 61-5	*Medications Associated with Secondary Parkinsonism*	
Class of Medication	**Drug(s)**	
Cardiovascular drugs	α-Methyldopa Reserpine Calcium channel blockers Amiodarone	
Dopamine antagonists for nausea	Prochlorperazine Metoclopramide	
Dopamine antagonists for psychosis	Typical Antipsychotics Haloperidol Thioridazine Fluphenazine Pimozide Chlorpromazine Perphenazine Atypical Antipsychotics Risperidone Paliperidone Olanzapine Ziprasidone Lurasidone Asenapine Iloperidone Aripiprazole Quetiapine Clozapine*	
Neurologic or psychiatric drugs	Valproic acid Some antidepressants Lithium Tetrabenazine	

*Much less so than the other atypical neuroleptics.

some familial and a small minority of seemingly sporadic cases

Treatment

- Depends on the underlying etiology. If there is a concern for hydrocephalus, refer to a specialist. **Treat vascular risk factors if vascular parkinsonism is suspected.** Correct underlying metabolic changes and remove medications that may be contributing.
- **PD movement-related symptoms respond well to dopaminergic medications** (see following)
- Other forms of parkinsonism may also respond somewhat to dopaminergic medications and therefore may be considered

PARKINSON DISEASE
Basic Information

- Definition: A chronic and progressive movement disorder characterized by bradykinesia, muscle rigidity, rest tremor, and postural instability.
- Pathology: PD is characterized by the progressive degeneration of dopaminergic neurons within the **substantia nigra.** Also seen are the formation of cytoplasmic inclusions (Lewy bodies; Fig. 61-1) and neurodegeneration in other parts of the central nervous system (CNS). Pathology outside the CNS has become more recognized (gastrointestinal tract, salivary glands, skin).
- Most motor symptoms of PD are related to a deficiency in striatal levels of dopamine

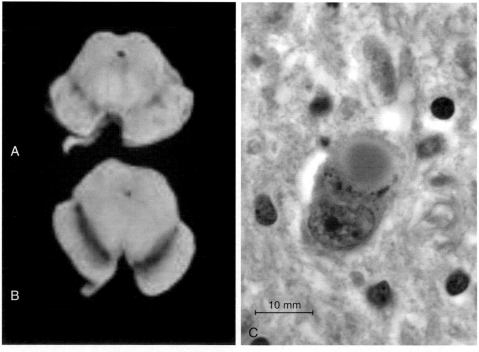

FIGURE 61-1 **A,** Substantia nigra in a patient with Parkinson disease, showing area of depigmentation caused by neuronal loss. **B,** Normal substantia nigra showing typical pigmentation for comparison. **C,** A large neuron *(center)* showing a typical irregular, bean-shaped nucleus and round, homogeneous, pink-staining cytoplasmic Lewy body with surrounding lighter halo. Surrounding the Lewy body are typical brown pigmented granules of substantia nigra neurons.

- Epidemiology/Etiology
  - **Average age of diagnosis is 62 years, and increased age is a risk factor for developing PD,** though 4% to 10% of patients present younger than 40 years
  - **Most cases are idiopathic, but several rare monogenetic forms have been identified** (mutations in genes for parkin, α-synuclein, DJ-1, LRRK2, and others), as well as several "risk genes"
  - Association of PD with environmental risk including chemical exposures has been shown, though the degree of causation is unclear. PD is likely the result of aging, genetic predisposition, and environmental exposure contributing to varying degrees.

Clinical Presentation

- Onset is usually insidious, and progression is lifelong
- PD is characterized by four cardinal motor (movement) symptoms: **bradykinesia,** and often **rest tremor, rigidity,** and **postural instability**. Other motor symptoms may include dysarthria, dysphagia, and dystonia. **It is a common misconception that all PD patients must have a rest tremor.** This leads to a delay in diagnosis in those who lack tremor.
- **Initial manifestations may include a single isolated symptom, making early diagnosis more difficult.** Examples include rest tremor of one hand/arm, stiff or awkward movements of one limb, slow or labored gait, shoulder pain/stiffness, or finding that daily tasks are taking longer to perform.
- **Asymmetry is a key feature distinguishing PD from many other causes of parkinsonism.** Thus it should start in one arm or side, before progressing to the other side and typically remaining worse on the initially affected side.
- Nonmotor symptoms
  - Psychiatric: anxiety, depression, hallucinations, delusions
  - Cognitive: executive or memory dysfunction, and often eventual dementia
  - Autonomic: orthostatic hypotension, constipation, urinary urgency or retention, and sexual dysfunction
  - Other: rapid eye movement (REM) behavior disorder (acting out dreams), RLS, fatigue, decreased olfaction, and mild pain
  - Usually autonomic or cognitive symptoms are absent or mild initially and slowly worsen over time. Hallucinations are usually a late feature unless they are triggered by a dopaminergic medication. Anxiety and depression can occur early.

Diagnosis

- History and exam: **Look for asymmetrical motor features that must include bradykinesia plus one of the other three cardinal motor features of parkinsonism (does not have to include tremor)**
- Assess for any "red flags" that would suggest a different cause of the patient's parkinsonism (e.g., early, prominent dementia; imbalance with falls; autonomic findings; posturing of one limb; eye movement changes may suggest another etiology) (Table 61-4)

- Response to a dopaminergic agent: A medication trial of a dopaminergic agent that provides *significant* and sustained improvement in motor symptoms supports a diagnosis of PD
- Brain imaging (MRI, computed tomography) may be helpful if vascular disease or hydrocephalus is suspected. Should be normal in PD.
- Functional imaging, including radioactive tracers (i.e., DaTscan), may offer additional evidence for disease, but cannot differentiate PD from other degenerative parkinsonian disorders

Treatment

- See Figure 61-2 for a treatment algorithm for PD.
- Symptomatic medication treatments
  - **Carbidopa/levodopa** is the most effective treatment. Levodopa is converted to dopamine in the brain, although carbidopa reduces the peripheral conversion of levodopa to dopamine in the periphery. After several years of disease and treatment, levodopa therapy is typically complicated by dose-to-dose fluctuations in level and duration of response. L-dopa-induced dyskinesia (i.e., drug-induced choreoathetosis) and a reduction in the duration of response (wearing off) requiring multiple drug doses daily also occur over time.
  - **Dopamine agonists:** Pramipexole, ropinirole, and rotigotine patch have longer lasting effects than carbidopa/levodopa, but usually more side effects, especially in the elderly (aged older than 70 years). Apomorphine injections are used to treat "off" times but are limited by nausea, hypotension, and cost.
  - **Monoamine oxidase (MAO)-B inhibitors:** Selegiline and rasagiline provide mild symptomatic benefits and prolong the per-dose benefits of carbidopa/levodopa. It is unclear if they provide neuroprotective effects.

61

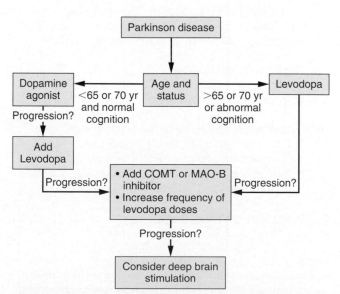

FIGURE 61-2 Algorithm for treatment of Parkinson disease. COMT, Catechol-*O*-methyltransferase; MAO, monoamine oxidase. Other treatment options include amantadine, apomorphine injection, early MAO B inhibitor use, and anticholinergics. See text for details.

- **Catechol-O-methyltransferase (COMT) inhibitors:** Entacapone can be dosed along with carbidopa/levodopa, or manufactured with carbidopa/levodopa, to prolong the effects of each levodopa dose. Tolcapone is similar though hepatic monitoring is required.
  - **Amantadine:** Weak symptomatic benefit and may suppress levodopa-induced dyskinesia and improve fatigue. Use is limited by anticholinergic side effects.
  - **Anticholinergics (benztropine and trihexyphenidyl):** Used for refractory tremor or dystonia, but use is limited by side effects
- Symptomatic nonmedication treatments
  - Exercise: Three to four times weekly with aerobic and strength training improves overall function and might have mild protective effects
  - Yoga, Tai Chi, dancing, walking, and physical therapy: May improve balance and likely reduce the risk of falling. Often improve overall function, independence, and quality of life.
  - Occupational therapy: May improve manual dexterity, optimize activities of daily living, and ensure that driving is safe
  - Speech/swallowing therapy: May aid with dysarthria, hypophonia, and swallowing functions. May be important to avoid aspiration.
- Possible disease-modifying (neuroprotective) therapies
  - Currently, there is no conclusive evidence of disease-modifying effects of any agent, but *possible* such effects are suggested in certain studies for monoamine oxidase B (MAO-B) inhibitors (selegiline and rasagiline), dopamine agonists, and exercise
  - There is current research into possible modifying effects of deep brain stimulation, neurotropic/growth factors, gene therapies, stem cell implantation, calcium channel blockers, antiinflammatories, and cell survival-promoting agents
- Surgical therapies
  - Treatment usually is for medically refractory motor fluctuations (from levodopa) or tremors in PD (not shown to be consistently helpful in other causes of parkinsonism)
  - **Deep brain stimulation**
    - **The most frequent surgical intervention**
    - Involves stimulation of the subthalamic nucleus or the globus pallidus (basal ganglia) via an implantable battery/impulse generator and wire leads that penetrate the skull and brain
    - Improves tremor, wearing off, and dyskinesia
    - Side effects include dysarthria, cognitive changes, and impaired gait, as well as surgical risks

CATATONIA SYNDROMES

Basic Information

- Often considered a psychiatric disorder
- Definition: **A motor and behavioral dysregulation syndrome with difficulty initiating and terminating movement and behavior, despite full physical capability**
- Postures become frozen or oddly positioned, and actions become contrary to intent

- Epidemiology
  - Incidence unknown
  - **It occurs most commonly in the setting of mood and psychotic disorders** and also general medical conditions and neurologic disorders
- Etiologies
  - Often more than one per patient
  - Psychiatric disorders: mood disorders (especially bipolar mania), psychotic disorders
  - Neurologic disorders: cerebral structural damage (stroke, mass, trauma to specific regions), encephalitis, seizures
  - Medical and toxic disorders: Liver dysfunction or postliver transplantation, renal dysfunction, other metabolic dysfunction, hypothyroidism, lupus, HIV/AIDS (acquired immune deficiency syndrome), low iron, vitamin B_{12}, or folate, and drug intoxication (e.g., phenylcyclidine, disulfiram, corticosteroids)

Clinical Presentation

- *Hypokinetic/retarded* **form is the most common:** posturing, rigidity, mutism, staring, repetitive actions, negativism (resistance to commands or examination), waxy flexibility (can position the patient), and stupor
- *Excited* form: similar to an agitated delirium or mania
- *Malignant* form: acute onset, fever, autonomic dysfunction, and with other similarities to neuroleptic malignant syndrome (see section on Drug-Induced Movement Disorders following)

Diagnosis

- History (from family/friends) and exam
- Brain MRI and EEG are typically recommended
- Additional testing for etiologies listed above should be used as indicated

Treatment

- **Supportive care:** intensive nursing care, artificial hydration, or nutrition as needed, deep venous thrombosis prevention, urinary catheterization, and range of motion through physical therapy
- **Address the underlying etiology**
- **Benzodiazepines:** With a test dose of lorazepam 1 to 2 mg intravenously, often within minutes there is lessening of symptoms, but not in all cases. Repeating the same dose every 4 to 12 hours can be used symptomatically.
- **Electroconvulsive therapy:** Can be used under the supervision of a psychiatrist for cases that do not respond to benzodiazepines
- N-methyl-D-aspartate (NMDA) receptor antagonists: Amantadine and memantine have been used successfully when added to lorazepam and electroconvulsive therapy
- Atypical antipsychotics: Data for these agents are uncertain, and some patients will worsen or progress to neuroleptic malignant syndrome when these are used

APRAXIA

Basic Information

- Often considered a cognitive disorder
- Definition: **Dysfunction in performing learned, skilled movements that is not caused by primary neurologic dysfunctions such as weakness, sensory loss, changes in posture or tone, incoordination, or impaired attention, comprehension of the task, or cooperation**
- Apraxia is a higher order motor-cognitive symptom. It is as if all the appropriate pieces are in place, but the patient cannot "put it all together."
- Examples
  - Difficulty using objects appropriately (e.g., picks up toothbrush not knowing what to do with it, or tries to eat with it)
  - Difficulty gesturing, interpreting gestures, or with imitation
  - Difficulty in orienting movements appropriately in relation to other body parts
  - Difficulty in imagining and planning complex movements
- Etiologies
  - Localizes best to the parietal lobes, frontal lobes, and their subcortical connections. Disorders that cause dysfunction in these regions can cause apraxia.
    - **Focal brain damage:** stroke, trauma, masses
    - **Degenerative disorders:** corticobasal degeneration, Alzheimer disease, progressive supranuclear palsy, and other dementias or parkinsonian conditions
  - Other causes of general cognitive dysfunction and/or delirium can cause apraxia within the setting of general brain dysfunction

Diagnosis

- History and exam: Verifying normal basic motor and sensory function on neurologic exam as well as comprehension of tasks is necessary
- Look for additional features of dementia (memory, language, executive function, visuospatial impairments) and signs of parkinsonism that may suggest a particular disorder. Assess for focal neurologic signs that may indicate focal brain damage.
- Have the patient demonstrate how to do specific tasks with imagined objects ("show me how you would brush your teeth as if you were holding a toothbrush") or imitate complex hand postures (interlocking hands in various ways)

Treatment

- **Apraxia is difficult to treat.** Addressing any underlying conditions that can be modified is the first step.
- Strategies from occupational and speech/language therapists to augment each step in the sequence of actions to accomplish daily tasks can be helpful and implemented by patients
- Correctly identifying apraxia as the problem can remove the need to perform further testing or treatments

Other Movement Disorders

ATAXIA

Basic Information

- Definition: **Incoordination arising from dysfunction in timing, rhythm, accuracy, and smoothness of movement (Fig. 61-3).** This is usually caused by

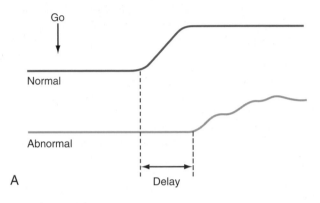

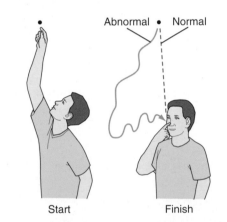

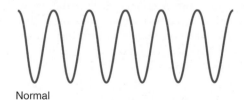

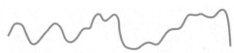

FIGURE 61-3 Typical defects in upper limb ataxia. **A,** Initiation of movement is delayed. **B,** Dysmetria (inaccuracy in range and direction) and kinetic tremor. **C,** Dysdiadochokinesis, an irregular pattern of alternating movements, can be seen in the abnormal position trace. (From Kandel ER, Schwartz JH, Jessell TM, eds. *Principles of Neural Science.* 3rd ed. Norwalk, CT: Appleton & Lange; 1991: Fig. 41-16; Modified from Thach WT, Montgomery EB: Motor system. In Pearlman AL, Collins RC, eds. *Neurobiology of Disease.* 3rd ed. New York: Oxford University Press; 1990:168–196.)

61

abnormalities in the cerebellum or its motor and/or sensory pathways (cerebellar or spinocerebellar ataxia). Sensory ataxia may arise from neuropathy. Ataxic patients may appear to be drunk. The term *ataxia* is often incorrectly applied to movement abnormalities caused by weakness, dystonia, chorea, or poor attention.

- **Dysmetria** ("poorly measured"): **irregular timing or trajectory of targeted movements**
- **Dysdiadochokinesis: breakdown of the normal timing and sequencing of rapid alternating movements** (e.g., rapid succession of pronation and supination)

- Etiology
  - Vascular: **stroke to cerebellum or brainstem**
  - Autoimmune: Includes **celiac disease, anti-glutamic acid decarboxylase (anti-GAD) syndrome, Miller Fisher syndrome**
  - Inherited disorders: **spinocerebellar ataxia** (often autosomal dominant trinucleotide repeat diseases); Friedreich ataxia; ataxia-telangiectasia; others
  - Metabolic/toxic: vitamin E deficiency; hypothyroidism; chronic alcoholism (alcohol often causes trunk/gait ataxia, and may clinically present with combination of cerebellar ataxia and sensory ataxia caused by alcohol-induced length-dependent neuropathy)
  - Medications, especially antiepileptics
  - Infections
  - Tumor/mass, or **paraneoplastic/parainfectious disease**
  - Idiopathic: multiple system atrophy (especially multiple system atrophy-cerebellar subtype, with components of parkinsonism and autonomic dysfunction) and idiopathic late-onset cerebellar ataxia

Clinical Presentation

- May be rapid or slow in onset depending on etiology
- **Common symptoms include imbalance, wide-based gait, falls, dysarthria, eye movement abnormalities, intention tremor, and mistargeting with the limbs** (trouble pouring water, poor handwriting, knocking over objects, etc.)

Diagnosis

- History and exam supplemented with laboratory testing and brain imaging. May included a paraneoplastic work-up in subacute-onset cases.
- Genetic tests can be done if there is a family history or after other testing is unrevealing

Treatment

- If found, treat the underlying cause
- No medication therapies have proven efficacious
- Physical, occupational, and speech therapies play an important role for maximizing function, preventing injury and aspiration, and optimizing an assistive walking device

DRUG-INDUCED MOVEMENT DISORDERS

Basic Information

- Medications can produce side effects that closely mimic "natural" movement disorders, including tremor, ataxia, chorea, dystonia, tics, and parkinsonism (see Table 61-3)
- Drug-induced movement disorders are important to recognize as many are "cured" by eliminating the offending agent

Clinical Presentation

- **Drug-induced tremor: can be postural, kinetic and/or rest tremor**
- Clinical features of drug-induced movement disorders include **ataxia, parkinsonism,** and **chorea**
- Antidopaminergic agents: Antipsychotics, as well as some antinausea medications (metoclopramide and prochlorperazine), cause several types of movement disorders:
  - **Acute dystonic reaction: sudden and forceful abnormal dystonic posturing typically within hours of receiving an offending medication**
  - **Tardive dyskinesia: usually choreoathetosis of the tongue, mouth, and/or face**
  - **Parkinsonism: more often symmetrical rather than asymmetrical,** with or without tremor
  - **Neuroleptic malignant syndrome** (NMS): Characterized by **rigidity, fever, autonomic instability, decreased level of consciousness, and an elevated creatine kinase and white blood cell count**
    - Mortality may be as high as 50%
    - May follow chronic or acute exposure to an offending medication, often after an increase or decrease in dose
    - A partial syndrome that is important to catch early may occur

Diagnosis

- History and exam
- Reviewing the side effects and timing of medications

Treatment

- **Stop the offending medication**, if possible. Depending on the reason for the patient taking the medication, it may need to be tapered.
- Resolution of the movement disorder may occur within hours or be delayed to weeks or months (often similar to the onset)
- **Acute dystonic reactions: Diphenhydramine or benztropine** can speed resolution
- **Tardive dyskinesia can be permanent**. Treatment with tetrabenazine has shown promise in clinical trials.
- **NMS: Hospitalization with supportive care** is often required because the syndrome can be life-threatening. Intravenous fluids, benzodiazepines, dopamine agonists, dantrolene, and antipyretics have been used.

PSYCHOGENIC MOVEMENT DISORDERS

Basic Information

- Also known as *functional* or *nonorganic* disorders
- Definition: **Physical symptoms (resembling movement disorders listed above) that are brought on by psychological mechanisms.** Psychogenic movement disorders (PMDs) encompass a spectrum of mainly three types of psychological phenomena:
  - **Conversion disorder: a subconscious, nonwillful manifestation of a psychiatric disturbance that leads to physical symptoms**
  - **Factitious disorder: When a patient knowingly creates physical symptoms usually to gain the benefit of attention by assuming the sick role**
  - **Malingering: a deliberate production of symptoms for material gain or avoidance** (not strictly considered a psychiatric disorder)
- Epidemiology
  - About 2% to 3% of patients in a movement disorder clinic have PMDs
  - Women are more affected than men
- Comorbid psychiatric symptoms are often present
- Outcomes are poor, with prolonged disability and lack of resolution in at least 50% of patients
- Patients often report a physical injury or event (infections, physical pain, drug reactions) before the onset of symptoms

Clinical Presentation

- **Most common manifestations are tremor, dystonia, gait disorder, and myoclonus**
- Less common manifestations include parkinsonism, chorea, ataxia, and tics
- **Red flags** to suggest a PMD
  - **Acute onset and fast progression** to maximal severity
  - **Waxing and waning course;** temporary complete remissions
  - Symptoms are incongruent with any established organic disease
  - Symptoms are inconsistent over time and regarding involved body parts
  - Symptoms are distractible and increase with attention to the affected body part
  - Association with false neurologic symptoms (e.g., weakness only with certain tasks)

Diagnosis

- **History and careful examination** involving maneuvers to distract the patient
- Look for differences between casual observations of function and function during an examination
- Ancillary work-up, including imaging, electrophysiology, and lab tests, may be necessary depending on the presentation and the diagnostic certainty
- Evaluation by a psychiatrist and/or psychologist to search for other psychiatric comorbidities and possible psychological factors underlying the movement disorder (though they may not be obvious or present)
- **Delivery of the diagnosis in an empathic, accurate, and clear manner is very important** for a patient to accept it and comply with treatment. Acknowledge symptoms as "real and serious," and emphasize that symptoms are not present 100% of the time and therefore normal function is possible and can be "tapped into" more and more over time. Give an unambiguous message that this is an established cause of movement disorders and that additional diagnostic tests are unnecessary.
- Avoid unnecessary work-up, including aggressive and costly procedures, or administration of potentially harmful drugs

Treatment

- **Treatment of psychiatric comorbidity** (i.e., anxiety, depression) and underlying psychological mechanisms, if identified. This may include antidepressants or psychotherapy.
- Stress management and relaxation techniques (e.g., biofeedback, yoga, meditation)
- Physical therapy and occupational therapy can help reestablish healthy patterns of movement
- Early and sustained treatment is important for recovery

61

Review Questions

For review questions, please go to ExpertConsult.com.

SUGGESTED READINGS

Daniels J. Catatonia: clinical aspects and neurobiological correlates. *J Neuropsychiatry Clin Neurosci.* 2009;21:371-380.
Fahn S, Jankovic J, Hallett M. *Principles and Practice of Movement Disorders.* 2nd ed. Philadelphia: Saunders; 2011.
Fink M, Taylor MA. The catatonia syndrome. *Arch Gen Psychiatry.* 2009;66:1173-1177.
Janavs JL, Aminoff MJ. Involuntary movements in general medical disorders. In: Aminoff MJ, ed. *Neurology and General Medicine.* 3rd ed. New York: Churchill Livingstone; 2001:983-1002.
Olanow CW, Schapira AH. Therapeutic prospects in Parkinson disease. *Ann Neurol.* 2013;77:337-347.
Petreska B, Adriani M, Blanke O, et al. Apraxia: a review. *Prog Brain Res.* 2007;164:61-83.
Tolosa E, Koller WC, Gershanik OS. *Differential Diagnosis and Treatment of Movement Disorders.* Boston: Butterworth-Heinemann; 1998.

SUGGESTED WEBSITE

The following website provides useful basic information on many movement disorders for both practitioners and patients: www.movementdisorders.org.

Selected Topics in Neurology

RAFAEL H. LLINÁS, MD

This chapter reviews a selection of central and peripheral neurologic disorders involving the spinal cord, peripheral nerves, and neuromuscular junction and toxic myopathies. Inflammatory myopathies are reviewed in Chapter 45. Localization of neurologic lesions, based on clinical evaluation or imaging studies, is the diagnostic theme.

Spinal Cord

Basic Information

- The spinal column is made up of vertebrae separated by intervertebral disks (Fig. 62-1)
- The spinal cord is found within the spinal canal, beginning at the end of the brainstem and extending to L1
- Below L1 is the "cauda equina," which consists of nerve roots
- Spinal cord circulation
  - The anterior spinal cord is dependent on a single anterior spinal artery
  - The posterior spinal cord is fed by numerous posterior spinal arteries
  - **Spinal stroke preferentially affects the anterior spinal cord**
- Table 62-1 lists the most common entities affecting the spinal cord

Clinical Presentation

- Spinal cord lesions may be categorized by presentation
  - **Upper motor neuron signs (long tract signs): weakness, spasticity, hyperreflexia, and positive Babinski sign (Fig. 62-2)**
  - Sensory signs (anterior or posterior columns or both): sensory level or loss of single modality (pinprick/temperature or light touch/proprioception)
  - Bowel, bladder, and sexual dysfunction signs: urinary overflow incontinence or bladder spasticity and weak rectal tone with fecal incontinence
  - Local root dysfunction: multimodal sensory and motor loss in a dermatomal distribution (Fig. 62-3)
  - Caveats
    - No cranial nerve abnormalities should be present
    - In acute spinal cord trauma, weakness may be the only long tract sign present
    - The sensory level reveals only the lowest level possible for a lesion (e.g., a T10 sensory level may be caused by a cervical lesion)
- Spinal cord lesions may be categorized by location
  - Anterior spinal cord lesions

  - **Loss of pain and temperature sense (lateral spinothalamic tract)**
  - Fine touch, proprioception, and vibration sense are spared
  - May occur with or without motor loss
  - Posterior spinal cord lesions
    - **Loss of fine touch, proprioception, and vibration sense (posterior columns)**
    - Pain and temperature sense are spared
    - May occur with or without motor loss
  - Central spinal cord lesions (Fig. 62-4)
    - Lateral spinothalamic tract and local motor neurons disrupted
    - **Pain and temperature sense lost in "capelike" distribution**
    - Fine touch, proprioception, and vibration sense spared
    - **Lower motor neuron weakness may be evident in the extremities**

Diagnosis and Evaluation

Table 62-2 provides a comparison of spinal cord syndromes

- Anterior spinal cord syndromes are caused by the following:
  - Trauma
  - Rupture of disk, causing compression of the spinal cord (Fig. 62-5)
  - Occlusion of anterior spinal artery causing spinal stroke
  - Primary spinal cord tumors
  - Metastatic cancer
- Posterior spinal cord syndromes are caused by the following:
  - Cervical spondylosis (arthritis and ligamentous hypertrophy)
  - Epidural abscess
  - Vitamin B_{12} deficiency
  - Syphilis
  - Multiple sclerosis
  - Primary spinal cord tumors
  - Metastatic cancer
- Central spinal cord syndromes are caused by the following:
  - Syringomyelia (congenital or posttraumatic)
  - Primary spinal cord tumors
  - Hyperextension injuries that disrupt the central spinal cord gray matter
- Brown-Séquard syndrome
  - Caused by hemisection of the spinal cord
  - Findings depend on where each tract decussates

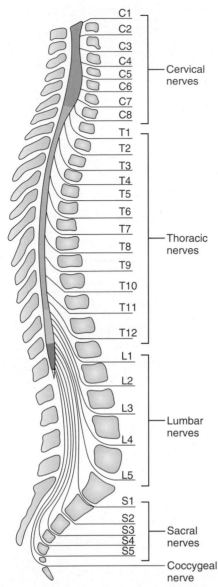

FIGURE 62-1 The spinal column, showing the relationships among the spinal cord, spinal nerves, and vertebral column. (From Crossman AR, Neary D. *Neuroanatomy*. 3rd ed. Philadelphia: Churchill Livingstone; 2006: Fig. 8.3.)

- Motor tract lesions give ipsilateral weakness (motor fibers cross in the brainstem)
- Sensory tract lesions give ipsilateral fine touch, proprioception, and vibration loss (posterior columns cross in brainstem); and contralateral pain and temperature sense loss (spinothalamic tracts cross in the spinal cord through the gray matter)

Treatment
See Table 62-1.

Peripheral Nerves

Basic Information

- The peripheral nerves include the spinal roots, cauda equina, nerve plexus (brachial and lumbar), and named nerves

Clinical Presentations

- Lower motor neuron signs (Box 62-1)
  - **Acute: weakness, multimodal sensory loss, lancinating pain, and loss of reflexes**
  - Chronic: atrophy and fasciculation
  - Not all features need to be present
- Spinal roots (Table 62-3)
- Cauda equina syndrome: bowel and bladder dysfunction, flaccid paralysis of bilateral lower extremities, and saddle anesthesia
- Plexus: unilateral extremity affected without spinal cord signs; all sensory modalities are affected and upper motor neuron signs are absent
- Named nerves
  - **Compression neuropathies commonly present with pain and are caused by repetitive or chronic external compression (Table 62-4)**
  - Inflammatory neuropathies present with motor involvement more than sensory involvement and are caused by demyelination (Table 62-5)
  - Toxic neuropathies commonly present with lancinating pain and are caused by axonal damage (Table 62-6)

Diagnosis and Evaluation

- Electromyography (EMG) and nerve conduction studies (NCSs) are helpful in localizing peripheral nerve lesions
  - **EMG evaluates for myopathy and denervation**
  - **NCSs can differentiate axonal from demyelinating neuropathy**
- Magnetic resonance imaging is the most useful imaging study
- Peripheral nerve lesions have the lengthiest differential diagnosis in neurology, being subject to acute trauma, chronic compression, inflammation, demyelination, and toxic and infectious injury
  - Spinal nerve roots: most commonly caused by compression by intervertebral disk; consider mass lesion
  - Cauda equina syndrome: most common causes are disk herniation, tumor, and epidural hemorrhage
  - Plexus: Pancoast tumors present with brachial plexus lesion and Horner syndrome

Treatment

- Eliminate or correct cause
- Symptomatic treatment with tricyclic antidepressants, gabapentin, and anticonvulsants
- See Tables 62-4 to 62-6

Neuromuscular Junction

Basic Information

- Myasthenia gravis is the prototypical disorder
- **Antiacetylcholine receptor (AChR) autoantibodies block the postsynaptic receptor and block the effect of acetylcholine released from the presynaptic nerve ending to stimulate associated muscle cells**

62

TABLE 62-1 *Diseases Affecting the Spinal Cord*

	Multiple Sclerosis	Vitamin B₁₂ Deficiency	Syringomyelia	Tabes Dorsalis	Epidural Abscess
Basic information	Prototypical demyelinating disease "Transverse myelitis" when it affects the spinal cord Most common presentation "optic neuritis"	Neurologic symptoms develop after prolonged B_{12} deficiency (months to years) Neurologic symptoms occur in most patients with pernicious anemia Anemia need not be present	Central cord cavitation, CSF accumulation and compression Often cervical cord Congenital (e.g., with Arnold-Chiari malformation) or posttraumatic	Onset many years after primary syphilitic infection	Often caused by *Staphylococcus aureus* May occur at any level
Clinical presentation	Two basic forms Chronic-progressive: lesions develop, persist, and progress Relapsing-remitting: lesions develop, resolve, and recur elsewhere	Loss of vibration and proprioception sense Loss of reflexes Mild weakness Mental status change Night blindness	Central cord syndrome (see Table 63-2) Atrophy, fasciculation, and lost reflexes	"Lightning shocks" in abdomen and legs Loss of vibration and proprioception sense Bladder dysfunction	Fever and chills Pain Cord or nerve root compression
Diagnosis and evaluation	Lesions "separated in time and space" Lhermitte sign* MRI with contrast	Vitamin B_{12} (low) Methylmalonic acid (high)	MRI	Argyll Robertson pupil† CSF VDRL (+)	Focal tenderness to percussion over spine Elevated WBC count
Treatment	Acute: steroids Chronic: immune modulators (e.g., interferon beta-1a or beta-1b, and glatiramer acetate)	Vitamin B_{12} injections	Neurosurgical evaluation	IV penicillin	Antibiotics Urgent surgery for cord compression

*Sensation of an electric shock radiating to the arms or legs and provoked by neck movement or cough.
†Pupils react to convergence but not to light.
CSF, Cerebrospinal fluid; IV, intravenous; MRI, magnetic resonance imaging; VDRL, Venereal Disease Research Laboratory; WBC, white blood cell.

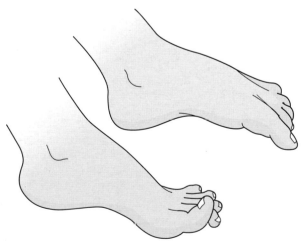

FIGURE 62-2 Babinski sign. The normal adult response to stimulation of the lateral plantar surface of the foot *(top)*. The abnormal adult response *(bottom)*. (From Goetz B. *Textbook of Clinical Neurology.* 2nd ed. Philadelphia: Saunders; 2003: Fig. 15-13.)

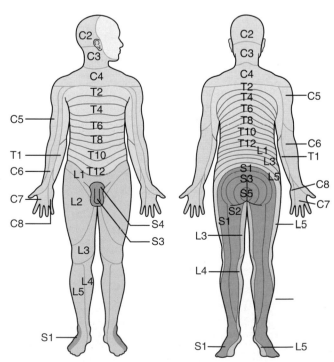

FIGURE 62-3 Dermatome map. (From FitzGerald MJT, Folan-Curran J. *Clinical Neuroanatomy and Related Neuroscience.* 4th ed. Philadelphia: Saunders; 2002: Fig. 11.10.)

TABLE 62-2	*Comparison of Spinal Cord Syndromes*	
	Clinical Manifestations	**Possible Causes**
Anterior	Loss of pain and temperature sensation Motor weakness may or may not be present	Trauma Ruptured intervertebral disk Anterior spinal artery occlusion ("spinal stroke") Primary spinal cord tumors Metastatic cancer
Central	Loss of pain and temperature sensation Lower motor neuron weakness (in lower extremities)	Syringomyelia Primary spinal cord tumors Hyperextension injuries
Posterior	Loss of fine touch, vibratory sensation Loss of proprioception Motor weakness may or may not be present	Cervical spondylosis Epidural abscess Vitamin B_{12} deficiency Syphilis Multiple sclerosis Primary spinal cord tumors Metastatic cancer

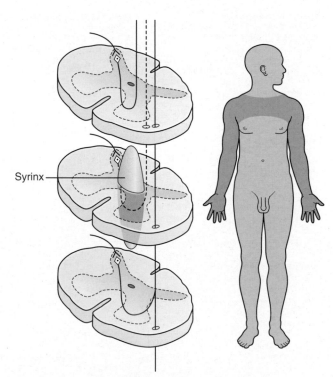

FIGURE 62-4 Central spinal cord lesion (in this case, syringomyelia), showing capelike distribution of analgesia. (From FitzGerald MJT, Folan-Curran J. *Clinical Neuroanatomy and Related Neuroscience.* 4th ed. Philadelphia: Saunders; 2002: Fig. 12.1.1.)

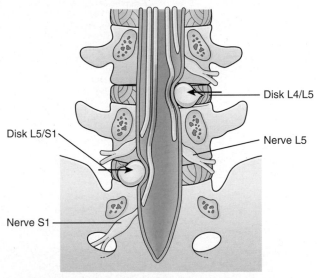

FIGURE 62-5 Nerve compression by rupture of intervertebral disks *(arrows).* (From FitzGerald MJT, Folan-Curran J. *Clinical Neuroanatomy and Related Neuroscience.* 4th ed. Philadelphia: Saunders; 2002: Fig. 11.2.2.)

BOX 62-1	*Upper and Lower Motor Neuron Signs*
Upper Motor Neuron Signs	**Lower Motor Neuron Signs**
Weakness	Weakness
Spasticity	Multimodal sensory loss
Hyperreflexia	Lancinating pain
Positive Babinski sign	Areflexia

Clinical Presentation

- Muscles fatigue and become weak with activity
- **Presents with fatigue with chewing, swallowing disorder, and diplopia**
- **Often associated with other autoimmune disorders or thymoma**
- Can be precipitated or worsened by aminoglycosides, clindamycin, erythromycin, tetracycline, procainamide, quinine, quinidine, β-blockers, and calcium channel blockers (Box 62-2)

Diagnosis and Evaluation

- Neurologic examination is otherwise normal
- Measure AChR antibodies in serum

62

TABLE 62-3	Cervical and Lumbar Root Lesion Presentation		
Root Level	**Weakness**	**Sensory Loss Distribution**	**Reflex Dropped?**
C5	Deltoid	Top of shoulder	None
C6	Biceps	Lateral upper and lower arm, including first finger and thumb	Biceps jerk
C7	Triceps	Medial arm and middle finger	Triceps jerk
C8	Grip strength	Lateral arm and little finger	Triceps jerk
L4	Knee extension	Posterolateral thigh	Knee jerk
L5	Foot dorsiflexion	Top of the foot	Hamstring jerk
S1	Foot plantar flexion	Sole of the foot and lateral foot	Ankle jerk

TABLE 62-4	Compressive Neuropathies		
	Carpal Tunnel Syndrome	**Ulnar Neuropathy**	**Peroneal Neuropathy**
Basic information	Caused by median nerve compression at wrist	Caused by ulnar nerve compression at elbow "funny bone"	Caused by peroneal compression at fibular head
Clinical presentation	Pain, numbness, and paresthesias in first through third fingers and radial half of fourth Weakness of thumb flexion, opposition, and abduction Nocturnal exacerbation	Pain, numbness, and paresthesias in fifth finger and ulnar half of fourth Weakness of finger abductors May resemble C8 radiculopathy	Footdrop Foot inversion spared
Diagnosis and evaluation	Positive median nerve Tinel sign* and Phalen sign† Abnormal EMG/NCS Rule out overuse, synovitis, hypothyroidism, amyloidosis, acromegaly, and pregnancy	Positive ulnar nerve Tinel sign at the elbow‡ Rule out trauma caused by leaning on elbows or repetitive curls	May resemble L5 nerve root, but no sensory abnormalities Usually traumatic May be seen in diabetes
Treatment	Wrist splint, NSAIDs, steroid injection, and surgical release	Splinting, NSAIDs, and surgical transposition of the nerve	Splinting and physical therapy

*Provoke pain and paresthesias with percussion over nerve at the wrist.
†Provoke pain, paresthesias, or numbness with forced wrist flexion (reversed "prayer position").
‡Percussion between medial elbow epicondyle and olecranon process.
EMG, Electromyography; NCS, nerve conduction study; NSAIDS, nonsteroidal antiinflammatory drugs.

- **If the AChR antibodies are negative, measure muscle-specific tyrosine kinase antibodies**
- Deficits improve transiently with edrophonium (Tensilon) test
- **EMG/NCS repetitive stimulation shows fatigue, but is otherwise normal**
- Differential diagnosis includes Lambert-Eaton myasthenic syndrome (see Chapter 57, Table 57-3), botulism, and drug toxicity

Treatment

- Prednisone, mestinon, intravenous immunoglobulin, and thymectomy

Toxic Myopathies

Basic Information

- **Caused by a variety of agents, including alcohol, cimetidine, colchicine, d-penicillamine, heroin, prednisone, and statins**

Clinical Presentation

- **Prolonged, high-dose steroid use is associated with chronic progressive proximal muscle weakness**
- Classic myopathic exam findings with other agents

TABLE 62-5   *Inflammatory Neuropathies*

	Acute Inflammatory Demyelinating Polyneuropathy (Guillain-Barré Syndrome)	Chronic Inflammatory Demyelinating Polyneuropathy
Basic information	Immune-mediated Onset 1 to 3 weeks after respiratory or GI illness, in two thirds of cases Herpesvirus (CMV and EBV) *Campylobacter jejuni* Nonseasonal, nonepidemic	Immune-mediated
Clinical presentation	Longest nerves affected first (presents with leg paresthesias and disordered gait) Motor > sensory Ascending pattern of progression Respiratory failure Bowel/bladder function preserved Dysautonomia Areflexia	Slowly progressive Atrophy and fasciculation Motor > sensory
Diagnosis and evaluation	Elevated CSF protein EMG/NCS normal early in course, except for loss of "F-waves"	EMG/NCS consistent with demyelination ↓ Conduction velocity Partial conduction block
Treatment	IVIg Plasmapheresis	Steroids IVIg Plasmapheresis

CMV, Cytomegalovirus; CSF, cerebrospinal fluid; EBV, Epstein-Barr virus; EMG, electromyography; GI, gastrointestinal; NCS, nerve conduction study; IVIg, intravenous immunoglobulins.

TABLE 62-6   *Toxic Neuropathies*

	Diabetic Neuropathy	Lead Neuropathy	Alcoholic Neuropathy	Critical Illness Neuropathy
Basic information	Caused by hyperglycemia	Caused by lead toxicity	Caused by long-standing alcohol abuse	Associated with: Prolonged stay in ICU Sepsis Exposure to steroids and paralytic agents
Clinical presentation	Distal symmetrical sensory or sensorimotor neuropathy Multimodal sensory loss	Unilateral or bilateral wristdrop (classic) Distal symmetrical sensorimotor neuropathy Abdominal pain	Pain Ataxia	Often difficult to wean from ventilator
Diagnosis and evaluation*	Host presentation	Host presentation Confirmed by serum and 24-hour urine lead measurement	Host presentation	Host presentation Nerve biopsy may be useful
Treatment	Glycemic control Symptomatic	Chelation therapy Symptomatic	Eliminate exposure Symptomatic	Remove offending agents Supportive care

*Axonal changes seen on electromyography/nerve conduction study.
ICU, Intensive care unit.

BOX 62-2   *Medications That Exacerbate Myasthenia Gravis*

Aminoglycosides
Clindamycin
Erythromycin
Tetracycline
Procainamide

Quinine
Quinidine
β-Blockers
Calcium channel blockers

Diagnosis and Evaluation

- **Prednisone myopathy is unique in that it has normal creatine phosphokinase (CPK) levels and is diagnosed by myopathic changes on EMG**
- The other agents cause elevated CPK levels, and the EMG shows myopathic changes

Treatment

- Tapering the steroid dose or changing to a steroid-sparing immunosuppressive is the only effective treatment for steroid myopathy
- Likewise, the other inciting agents must also be stopped

62

Review Questions

For review questions, please go to ExpertConsult.com.

SUGGESTED READINGS

Bradley WG, Daroff RB, eds. *Neurology in Clinical Practice.* 2nd ed. Philadelphia: WB Saunders; 1945.

Collins RD. *Illustrated Manual of Neurological Diseases.* Philadelphia: JP Lippincott; 1962.

Harrison DM. Multiple sclerosis. *Ann Intern Med.* 2014;160:ITC4-2-ITC4-18.

Pasnoor M, Barohn RJ, Dimachkie MM. Toxic myopathies. *Neurol Clin.* 2014;32:647-670.

Spillane J, Higham E, Kullmann DM. Myasthenia gravis. *BMJ.* 2012;345:e8497.

Yuki N, Hartung HP. Guillain–Barré syndrome. *N Engl J Med.* 2012;366:2294-2304.

SECTION ELEVEN

Selected Topics in General and Internal Medicine

Selected Topics in Geriatric Medicine

MIA YANG, MD; and COLLEEN CHRISTMAS, MD

The medical issues facing the elderly include those commonly seen in all adults, but also encompass issues that become increasingly prevalent with advancing age. With aging, people become less resilient and often suffer from several chronic diseases simultaneously. These issues call on special skills when approaching elderly patients. With the aging of the United States population, internists will need to be familiar with the diagnosis and management of health issues common among the elderly. In this chapter, we review four syndromes commonly seen in older adults: urinary incontinence, pressure ulcers, falls, and dementia.

Urinary Incontinence

Basic Information

- Definition: involuntary loss of urine that causes a social, health, or hygiene problem
- Physiology of micturition involves the following:
  - Sympathetic innervation: relaxes bladder and contracts bladder neck and urethra
  - Parasympathetic innervation: contracts bladder (detrusor muscle) for emptying
  - Somatic innervation: leads to voluntary contraction of external urethral sphincter
    - Helpful mnemonic: sympathetics store, parasympathetics pee

Clinical Presentation

Table 63-1 summarizes the types of urinary incontinence.
- **Urge incontinence: the most common cause of incontinence (accounts for 40% to 70% of cases)**
  - **Results from detrusor overactivity, detrusor instability, or detrusor hyperreflexia**
  - **Characterized by a sudden urge and desire to void, a fear of leakage, and ultimately urine loss**
  - May lose small or large amounts of urine depending on sphincter function
  - May result from defects of neurologic inhibition of the bladder (e.g., stroke, foraminal stenosis, central nervous system masses, multiple sclerosis, Parkinson disease, spinal cord injury, dementia) or local bladder irritants (e.g., infection, tumor, stone)
- **Stress incontinence: the second most common cause of incontinence in the elderly**
  - **Characterized by small-volume losses of urine during times of increased intraabdominal**

pressure (e.g., coughing, sneezing, laughing, exercising)
  - Usually seen in women who have lost pelvic support of the urethra, with resultant failure of the urinary sphincter mechanism during periods of increased intraabdominal pressure. Clinical history may reveal multiparity or grand parity (birth of a child weighing more than 4000 g).
  - If seen in men, typically seen in those who have undergone urologic procedures
- **Overflow incontinence: accounts for 10% of urinary incontinence among elderly patients**
  - Typically associated with some form of urinary outflow obstruction (e.g., prostatic enlargement, urethral stricture, or cystocele)
    - Also seen in diabetes mellitus, in part because of neurogenic bladder and in part because of nerve damage to control of detrusor contractility
  - Patients complain of reduced urinary stream, incomplete voiding, frequent or continuous dribbling
  - Most commonly, leakage occurs without warning
- **Functional incontinence: occurs when an individual is unable or unwilling to reach the toilet in time**
  - Associated factors include dementia, depression, physical impairments that impede mobility (e.g., degenerative arthritis, stroke, Parkinson disease), or physical restraints or inaccessible toilets

Diagnosis

- Important historical features in the incontinent patient
  - Frequency, timing, and situations associated with incontinent episodes
  - Volume of urine loss
  - Comorbid medical and psychiatric conditions
  - Medications (Box 63-1)
  - Bladder (or voiding) record: patient or caregiver records continent and incontinent voids over 48 hours; used to diagnose cause, assess effect on daily life, and track response to therapy
- The physical examination in the incontinent patient
  - Abdominal examination for bladder distention
  - Rectal examination for rectal tone, fecal impaction, and, in males, prostatic enlargement
  - In women, pelvic examination for cystocele, uterine prolapse, rectocele, atrophic vaginitis
  - Full neurologic examination, including mental status and mobility assessment

TABLE 63-1   Types of Urinary Incontinence

Type	Pathophysiology	Characteristic of Urine Lost	Common Causes
Urge	Detrusor overactivity	Small to large with brief "warning"	UTI, fecal impaction, CVA, cord injury
Stress	Weak bladder outlet	Small, often with coughing or standing	Weakened pelvic muscles from childbirth
Overflow	Bladder outlet obstruction	Small, frequently dribbling without "warning"	BPH, diabetes, cystocele
Functional	Cannot or will not get to toilet	Can be small but usually large	Dementia, mobility problems, toilet inaccessible

BPH, Benign prostatic hypertrophy; CVA, cerebrovascular accident; UTI, urinary tract infection.

TABLE 63-2   Treatment of Incontinence

Type	Nonpharmacologic	Pharmacologic
Urge incontinence	Pelvic muscle exercises (Kegel exercises) Bladder retraining Scheduled or prompted voiding	Anticholinergics Oxybutinin Tolterodine Imipramine Botox injections
Stress incontinence	Pelvic muscle exercises Biofeedback Surgery Colposuspension Sling procedure Pessaries	α-Adrenergic agonists: pseudoephedrine Anticholinergics: imipramine Estrogen alone of no proven benefit; may be of use in combination with α-adrenergics
Overflow incontinence	Intermittent or chronic catheterization Surgical correction of obstruction	Discontinue medications that exacerbate overflow obstruction
Functional incontinence	Prompted or scheduled voiding Absorbent undergarments Remove barriers to bathroom Bedside commode when appropriate Optimize physical function	None

BOX 63-1   Medications That Exacerbate Incontinence

Sedatives/hypnotics
Diuretics
α-Adrenergic agonists
α-Adrenergic antagonists
Anticholinergics
Narcotics
Alcohol
Calcium channel blockers
Angiotensin-converting enzyme inhibitors and angiotensin receptor blockers

- Laboratory examination in the incontinent patient should include measure of renal function as well as glucose and calcium (which cause osmotic diuresis)
  - Urinalysis as well as urine culture to exclude infection as cause of incontinence
- Postvoid residual: patient voluntarily empties bladder completely, followed by bladder catheterization to measure residual volume in bladder
  - Normal is less than 50 to 100 mL
  - **Postvoid residual of more than 100 mL suggests overflow incontinence either from impaired detrusor contractility (e.g., neurogenic bladder) or outlet obstruction**
- Urodynamic testing: used to assess lower urinary tract function; tests commonly include cystometry, urinary flow measurement, and measurement of urethral pressure (some would add intravenous pyelography and cystourethrography to this list)
  - In majority of cases of incontinence, diagnosis can be made without testing
  - No clear guidelines exist on when to refer for testing
  - May help in the following situations:
    - Failure of the initial treatment plan
    - Confusing or inconsistent history
    - Clarification of the need for surgery

Treatment

See Table 63-2

Pressure Ulcers

Basic Information

- A pressure ulcer results when unrelieved pressure on skin and subcutaneous tissue results in infarction and necrosis

63

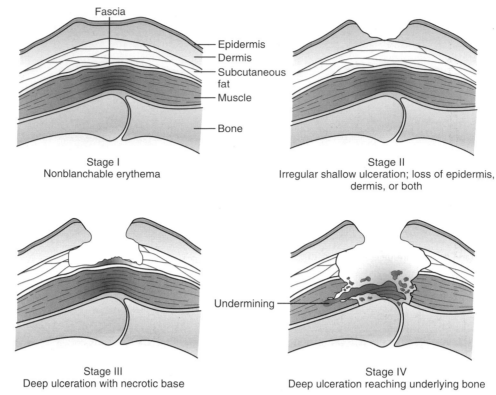

FIGURE 63-1 National Pressure Ulcer Advisory Panel classification of pressure ulcers. (From Bolognia JL, Jorizzo JL, Rapini RP. *Dermatology*. St. Louis: Mosby; 2003: Fig. 106.20.)

TABLE 63-3	*Staging of Pressure Ulcers*
Stage I	Nonblanchable erythema of intact skin
Stage II	Superficial ulcer extending through the epidermis or dermis or both
Stage III	Full-thickness skin loss exposing fat or subcutaneous tissue
Stage IV	Full-thickness skin loss exposing bone, muscle, tendon, or joint capsule

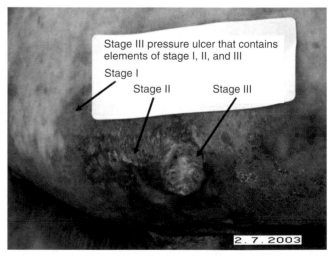

FIGURE 63-2 Pressure ulcer demonstrating stages I, II, and III of ulceration.

- Moisture, friction, and body habitus may contribute to susceptibility and formation of ulcer
- Four stages of pressure ulcers (Table 63-3; Figs. 63-1 to 63-3)
  - Stage I: damage to intact skin; apparent clinically as nonblanchable erythema of intact skin
  - Stage II: partial-thickness skin loss involving epidermis or both epidermis and dermis; clinically apparent as a blister or superficial ulcer
  - Stage III: full-thickness skin loss exposing subcutaneous tissue, with damage to subcutaneous tissue as well; underlying fascia is not affected; clinically apparent as a deep ulcer but without exposure of bone, muscle, or joint capsule
  - Stage IV: full-thickness skin loss extending to and including underlying fascia, including muscle and bone; clinically apparent as a crater with visibly involved underlying structures

Clinical Presentation

- Risk factors have been quantified into clinical prediction rules for likelihood of developing a pressure ulcer
  - **Risk factors predictive of pressure ulcers include poor physical condition, decreased mental status, reduced activity, and incontinence**
  - Other clinical prediction rules add "poor nutritional status" (which is variably defined) and chronic skin moisture as risk factors for pressure ulcers

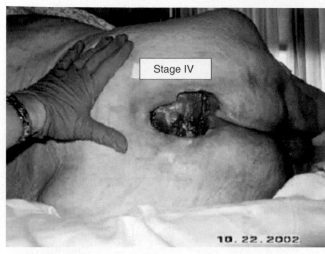

FIGURE 63-3 Stage IV pressure ulcer on the sacrum.

TABLE 63-4	Principles of Pressure Ulcer Management
Ulcer Appearance	**Management**
Infected or necrotic	Sharp or chemical débridement Iodine product (e.g., Iodosorb) Bleach product (e.g., Chlorpactin)
Clean granulating	Supportive environment (e.g., Calginate, hydrogel)
Undermined	Fill tissue space with wick or vacuum device
Epithelializing	Petroleum gauze, collagen
Hypergranulating	Control granulation with salt foam (e.g., Mesalt) or silver nitrate

- Complications of pressure ulcers may accompany clinical presentation and include wound infection (manifesting as purulent drainage, often with foul odor, and surrounding erythema, warmth, and tenderness); osteomyelitis; and sinus tract formation
  - **Pressure ulcers are colonized with bacteria; a positive swab culture does not imply infection**
  - **Osteomyelitis is presumed if bone is grossly visible or can be reached with a probe**

Diagnosis

- Diagnosis based on preceding staging system
- If eschar overlies ulcer, staging cannot be performed

Treatment

Table 63-4 summarizes principles of management, and Table 63-5 provides information on various wound care products
- **Best treatment is identification of individuals at risk and prevention of ulcer development**
  - **Pressure reduction: Turn and reposition immobile patients every 2 hours**
    - Specialized mattresses and beds may decrease risk of ulcer development, although it is unclear if they are superior to vigilant bedside care
    - Avoid friction: Use draw sheets to lift and turn patients; avoid any shearing forces to the skin

TABLE 63-5	Wound Care Products and Indications
Product	**Indication(s)**
Film covering	Stage I ulcer
Foam covering	Noninfected stage II or III ulcer
Hydrocolloid covering	Noninfected stage II ulcer; stage III ulcer with light exudate
Hydrogel	Stage II to IV ulcer with moderate drainage
Alginate	Stage II to IV ulcer with copious drainage

- Nutrition: It is unclear whether nutritional interventions improve pressure sore outcomes. Oral supplementation could play a role.
  - Despite this weak evidence, many authorities advise a diet providing 30 to 35 cal/kg/day and 1.25 to 1.5 g protein/kg/day in undernourished individuals with pressure ulcers
  - If tube feeding is used and causes increased immobility and diarrhea, pressure sore outcomes may be worsened
  - The role of zinc supplementation was unclear; however, new evidence (Cereda et al, 2015) suggests zinc, arginine, and antioxidants help in the healing of pressure ulcers.
  - Vitamin deficiencies should be corrected
- Optimize skin condition: avoid and treat maceration, fungal infection, or contact irritants and relieve pressure
- Débridement: to remove necrotic material and promote healing
  - Mechanical débridement is achieved with scalpel or scissor or wet-to-moist dressings
  - Enzymatic débridement is achieved with collagenases
  - Autolytic débridement is achieved by covering ulcer with synthetic dressing, which allows enzymes in the wound to digest the necrotic but noninfected tissue; should not be used in infected wounds
- **Infection: As noted previously, colonization is common and does not represent infection; swab cultures of the wound base have no clinical utility**
  - Use of topical antibiotics is controversial; they may be toxic to fibroblasts
    - If used, topical antibiotics should be discontinued after 48 hours
  - **Systemic antibiotics are reserved for patients with signs of cellulitis, osteomyelitis, or systemic illness**
  - If a pocket of abscess is identified, culture of purulent contents may be useful in selecting antibiotics

Falls

Basic Information

- A fall represents an individual's unintentional coming to rest on the ground or other lower level without overwhelming intrinsic or extrinsic cause
- **Falls are distinct from syncope; with syncope, loss of consciousness occurs (see Chapter 5)**

63

- Incidence of falls increases with increasing age of patient
- Situational factors that predispose to falling include the type of activity and the environment
  - **70% of falls occur at home**
  - 10% of falls occur on the stairs
  - 50% of falls are associated with environmental hazards (e.g., wet surface, throw rugs)
- In addition to risks associated with trauma, falls are associated with a decline in the ability to perform activities of daily living (ADLs) and an increasing likelihood of nursing home placement

Clinical Presentation

- Among the tasks of the clinician is to differentiate a fall from a syncopal event
  - Evidence of trauma should also raise concern for abuse or neglect
- Otherwise, the clinical presentation is straightforward

Diagnosis

- The events surrounding the fall and other fall history should be reviewed
  - The frequency of falling and the location of falling (e.g., in the home, on the stairs) should be reviewed
    - Look for patterns to falls, such as timing in relation to medications or meals or directions of falling (e.g., falling backward would suggest parkinsonism or falling to one side could suggest footdrop or a subtle weakness on that side)
- Risk factors for falling should be reviewed (Box 63-2)
  - More than one risk factor is typically present in the patient who falls
  - **Medications such as sedatives, antidepressants, and neuroleptics are associated with the greatest risk for falling;** the more medications, the higher the risk of falling
  - Dementia increases the chances of falling fivefold

- Physical examination should include particular attention to cognition and volume status; comprehensive evaluation of neuropsychiatric, cardiovascular, and musculoskeletal systems should be performed
  - Visual and auditory acuity should also be checked regularly
  - Many physicians informally evaluate fall risk with the "get up and go" test, in which they observe the patient rise from a chair and walk while paying attention to the speed and steadiness of the patient's gait

Treatment

- Prevention of falls for at-risk individuals
  - **Exercise and balance training: both have demonstrated effect at reducing falls**
  - **Home modification: improve home lighting, maintain clutter-free passageways, install raised toilet seats, add grab bars in the bathroom, secure loose carpets, add stair rails (Box 63-3)**
  - **Adjust or avoid medications that increase risk of falling, particularly sedating medications**
  - Emerging evidence suggests supplementation with vitamin D may reduce falls in older individuals
  - The ideal dose, formulation, and duration are not yet clear
  - Vitamin D supplementation (median dose in available studies was 800 IU) to prevent falls in community-dwelling adults aged 65 years or older who are at increased risk for falls because of a history of recent falls or vitamin D deficiency is a grade B recommendation in the most recent U.S. Preventive Services Task Force (USPTF) guidelines
  - Evaluate for appropriate assistive devices, such as a cane or walker, in those with imbalance or physical disability
  - Consider a referral to a physical therapist for assessment for assistive devices and for training to improve strength and balance

---

BOX 63-2	*Risk Factors for Falling*

Medications
  Benzodiazepines
  Neuroleptics
  Tricyclic antidepressants
  Antihypertensives
  Diuretics
  Use of four or more medications simultaneously
Sensory impairment
  Visual loss
  Vestibular dysfunction
  Decreased proprioception
Central nervous system disease
  Stroke
  Parkinson disease
  Cognitive disorders
Musculoskeletal disorders
  Arthritis
Depression
Substance abuse
Past history of falling

BOX 63-3	*Home Environmental Modifications to Prevent Falls*

Stairs
Light switch at both ends
Clutter free
Tightly woven carpet or treads
Handrails

Kitchen
Avoid high shelves
Step stool with handrails
Keep floor dry

Living Area
Open pathway
No footstools, low tables, pets
Cords out of pathway
No throw rugs
Cordless phone

Bathroom
Night light
Nonskid rugs
Handrails in tub and toilet
Tub mat, chair

Bedroom
Clutter-free path
Night light
Sit on edge of bed before getting up

Footwear
Low heel, nonskid soles
Appropriate fit
Keep laces tied/Velcro

- Prevention of injury in those at risk of falling
  - Osteoporosis screening and treatment
  - Hip protectors
  - Lifeline or other contact strategy if fall occurs

Dementia

Basic Information

- **Dementia: a syndrome that results in a decline in memory and other cognitive abilities to the point that it interferes with ADLs**
  - Impairment of ADLs is an important distinction; age-related modest decline in intellectual function that does not impair physical function is normal and does not represent dementia
  - **Mild cognitive impairment: a loss of cognition more significant than anticipated from age alone and a precursor to dementia; poorly understood**
- At age 60 years, 1% of the population has dementia
  - The age-related prevalence of dementia then doubles every 5 years
- Once diagnosed, estimates of average survival range from 5 to 9 years, but may be as short as 3 years
- Common causes of dementia
  - **Alzheimer disease is the most common cause of dementia (up to 70% of cases)**
  - Vascular dementia is the second most common cause (10% to 20% of cases)
  - Dementia with Lewy bodies may be more common than previously thought
  - Alcohol-related causes are commonly associated with dementia; one out of five patients with dementia has a significant history of alcohol use
  - Often individuals will have clinical features of more than one type of dementia and will be labeled as having "mixed-type" dementia
- Conditions which may present with or mimic dementia include:
  - Infectious causes (e.g., human immunodeficiency virus, neurosyphilis)
  - Endocrine or metabolic causes (e.g., hypothyroidism, hypercalcemia, vitamin B_{12} deficiency)
  - Neurologic disorders (e.g., Parkinson disease, frontotemporal dementia [formerly known as Pick disease], Creutzfeldt-Jacob disease, subdural hematoma, and normal-pressure hydrocephalus)
  - Vitamin B_1 deficiency (Wernicke encephalopathy)
- **Only 2% of cases of dementia are caused by reversible causes; even when found and treated (e.g., hypothyroidism, syphilis), dementia may not resolve**
  - **Depression may present with impairments of cognition ("pseudodementia") that improve significantly when the depression is adequately treated**

Clinical Presentation

- Family members or caregivers are usually the ones who initially raise concern for dementia

- **A patient who complains of memory problems is more likely to be depressed or under stress than demented**
- **Consciousness is clear in the demented patient; clouded consciousness (especially waxing and waning symptoms) suggests delirium**
- Clinical features vary based on cause of dementia
  - **Alzheimer disease results in a gradual decline in cognitive function over months to years; language skills commonly affected; motor skills typically spared**
  - **Vascular dementia is associated with a stepwise, sudden progression of decline in cognitive function;** the medical history typically uncovers other risk factors for vascular disease such as history of strokes, heart attacks, peripheral vascular disease, and end-stage renal disease
  - **Dementia with Lewy bodies is commonly associated with fluctuations in alertness or cognition, visual hallucinations, and features of parkinsonism such as facial masking**
    - **These patients have exquisite sensitivity to neuroleptic medications**
    - **Abnormal motor signs are common, including rigidity, an extensor plantar reflex, cogwheel rigidity, and gait disturbances**

Diagnosis

- Diagnostic criteria for dementia are listed in Box 63-4
- Assessment of neurocognitive functioning
  - The mini-mental status examination (MMSE), mini-cog, Montreal Cognitive Assessment, or another similar test may be used to provide a quantitative assessment of cognitive impairment and to provide a baseline for comparison over time
    - Age and education level affect score on MMSE
    - For English-speaking individuals with at least an eighth-grade education, a score less than 24 in the appropriate clinical setting suggests the presence of dementia
  - Functional status can also be assessed with standardized tests such as a functional activities questionnaire, which assess high-level activities

---

BOX 63-4 | *Diagnostic Criteria for Dementia*

Part 1: The development of multiple cognitive defects, manifested by both:
Memory impairment
plus
One or more of the following cognitive (or cortical) disturbances:
Aphasia (language disturbance)
Apraxia (impaired ability to carry out motor activities despite intact motor function)
Agnosia (failure to recognize or identify objects despite intact sensory function)
Disturbance in executive functioning (planning, organization, abstraction)
Part 2: The cognitive deficits must cause significant impairment in social or occupational functioning and represent a decline from a previous level of functioning

63

BOX 63-5	*Laboratory Evaluation of the Patient with Dementia**
Complete blood count	Thyroid-stimulating
Electrolytes	hormone
Blood urea nitrogen	Rapid plasma reagin
Creatinine	Human immunodeficiency
Liver enzymes	virus
Calcium	Vitamin B$_{12}$

*Some clinicians would add homocysteine and methylmalonic acid to this list.

(e.g., writing checks and balancing a checkbook, organizing tax records, shopping for groceries)
- Formal neurocognitive testing is recommended when there is sufficient concern for the diagnosis of dementia and, in particular, in individuals with a coexisting mood disorder
- Laboratory examination in the patient with suspected dementia (Box 63-5)
  - Increasing evidence has linked the apolipoprotein E ε4 allele with an increased risk of developing Alzheimer disease
  - Until more medical evidence is available, routine testing for the apolipoprotein E genotype when evaluating a demented patient is not recommended
  - Testing for syphilis recommended if there is a history of prior infection, risk factors for syphilis, or the individual lives in an area with high prevalence of syphilis
- Neuroimaging is now recommended by the American Academy of Neurology in the evaluation of all patients with dementia, although not all authorities agree with this approach and its cost-effectiveness has not been demonstrated
  - Often performed to exclude identifiable causes such as tumors, mass lesions, subdural hematoma, or normal-pressure hydrocephalus

Management

- **Overall goals of therapy are to identify and treat reversible causes of dementia, provide expectant management to caregivers, improve quality of life, and maximize functional performance**
  - Caregiver and family education and counseling improve quality of life and delay the need for nursing home placement by as much as 1 year
- Symptomatic therapy focuses on treating cognitive impairment, mood disturbances, and behavioral disturbances
  - **Pharmacotherapy for cognitive impairment is limited; all share mechanism of cholinergic augmentation by inhibiting cholinesterase**
    - Examples include donepezil, rivastigmine, mematine, and galantamine
    - Best experience is in use in patients with mild to moderate Alzheimer disease; only mematine has been approved for use in moderate to severe Alzheimer disease, though higher-dose donepezil may have some benefit in this stage of disease based on limited evidence

- Modest improvement in cognitive functioning may be demonstrable on neurocognitive testing, but improvement is often not evident to caregiver or clinician and does not prevent disease progression
- The role of estrogen, vitamin E, nonsteroidal antiinflammatory drugs, and 3-hydroxy-3-methylglutaryl coenzyme A reductase inhibitors in the prevention and development of Alzheimer disease has not been defined
- **Mood impairment, most commonly depression, should be anticipated and treated in the patient with dementia**
  - Selective serotonin reuptake inhibitors are preferred
  - The anticholinergic side effects of tricyclic antidepressants should be avoided
- Behavioral therapy should be added if the patient becomes agitated or psychotic (seen in 50% of demented patients)
  - Haloperidol has been the drug of choice for behavioral issues that cannot be managed with redirection alone and if behavior poses a risk to the individual or caregiver; however, note the following:
    - Caution is urged if there is suspicion of Lewy body dementia
    - Some use newer-generation antipsychotics that may have fewer extrapyramidal side effects (e.g., risperidone, olanzapine, quetiapine), but at greater cost and without demonstration of enhanced efficacy
- **All neuroleptic medications have a "black box warning" for increased mortality in patients with dementia; their use should include a careful weighing of risks and benefits given this concern**
  - Benzodiazepines can worsen confusion and should be avoided, particularly in ambulatory patients for whom the risk of falling is markedly increased with this class of drugs

Review Questions

For review questions, please go to ExpertConsult.com.

SUGGESTED READINGS

Boustani M, Peterson B, Hanson L, et al. Screening for dementia in primary care: a summary of the evidence for the U.S. Preventive Services Task Force. *Ann Intern Med.* 2003;138:927-937.

Cereda E, Klersy C, Serioli M, et al. A nutritional formula enriched with arginine, zinc, and antioxidants for the healing of pressure ulcers: a randomized trial. *Ann Intern Med.* 2015;162:167-174.

Cobbs EL, Duthie EH, Murphy JB, eds. *Geriatrics Review Syllabus: A Core Curriculum in Geriatric Medicine.* 5th ed. Malden, MA: Blackwell; 2002.

Courtney C, Farrell D, Gray R, et al. Long-term donepezil treatment in 565 patients with Alzheimer's disease (AD2000 Collaborative Group): randomised double-blind trial. *Lancet.* 2004;363:2105-2115.

Moyer VA, U.S. Preventive Services Task Force. Prevention of falls in community-dwelling older adults: U.S. Preventive Services Task Force recommendation statement. *Ann Intern Med.* 2012;157:197-204.

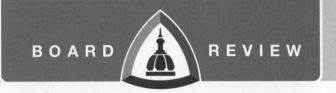
Selected Topics in Women's Health

ASHLEY M. HARRIS, MD, MHS; REDONDA G. MILLER, MD, MBA; and WENDY L. BENNETT, MD, MPH

Internists provide care for women of all ages and often are faced with a variety of disorders specific to women. Familiarity with gynecologic disorders is essential. In addition, pregnant women may have medical complications that require close evaluation and monitoring by the internist. This chapter covers many of these important issues, including cervical cancer screening, contraception, and medical complications of pregnancy.

Cervical Cancer Screening and Treatment

- Epidemiology
  - In the United States, cervical cancer is common, with about 12,000 new cases and 4000 deaths annually
  - From 2001 to 2010, cervical cancer incidence and mortality decreased significantly across all racial groups except American Indian/Alaska Native (incidence has remained stable)
  - Early detection through the Papanicolaou (Pap) smear has greatly reduced mortality
- **Risk factors for cervical cancer**
  - **Human papillomavirus (HPV) infection**
  - **Smoking**
  - **Multiple sexual partners**
  - **Early age of first intercourse**
  - **History of other sexually transmitted infections (STIs)**
  - **Prolonged use of oral contraceptive agents (longer than 5 years vs. never used); risk returns to normal after 10 years**
  - **Immunocompromised state:**
    - **Human immunodeficiency virus (HIV) infection (see Chapter 12)**
    - **Immunosuppressant medications for rheumatologic disorders or organ transplantation**
- **Human papilloma virus**
  - **Cervical cancer and its precursors are caused by oncogenic serotypes of HPV**
  - HPV exposure is common and becoming more prevalent in humans:
    - 75% to 80% of all sexually active adults will acquire genital tract HPV before age 50
    - Most HPV infections are asymptomatic and resolve on their own

- **HPV serotypes 16, 18, 33, 35, and 39 are the most common high-risk serotypes and are associated with high-grade neoplasia and invasive cancer**
  - Serotypes 16 and 18 are found in 70% of all cervical cancers
  - HPV serotypes 6, 11, and 42 are more often associated with low-risk lesions and cause more than 90% of condylomata (genital warts)
  - Cervical cancer in the absence of heterosexual activity is extremely rare
  - Testing for high-risk HPV DNA enhances the sensitivity of cervical cytology screening
    - **HPV cotesting is not recommended for women younger than 30 years, however, because of the high prevalence of transient HPV infection**
- HPV vaccine
  - Two HPV vaccines are approved by the U.S. Food and Drug Administration (FDA)
    - The bivalent HPV vaccine (Cervarix) prevents the HPV serotypes 16 and 18 and related high-grade cervical intraepithelial neoplasia (CIN) and carcinoma in situ
    - The quadrivalent HPV vaccine (Gardasil) prevents four HPV types, 16 and 18, as well as 6 and 11; it also protects against cancers of the anus, vagina, and vulva
      - Only the quadrivalent vaccine is licensed for use in males
  - The vaccines are given in a 3-dose series (0, 2, and 6 months)
  - HPV vaccination is most effective if administered before onset of sexual activity
  - HPV vaccination is recommended for:
    - Females ages 13 through 26 years
    - Males ages 13 through 21 years
    - Males who have not completed the vaccination series
    - Gay and bisexual men
    - Persons with HIV through age 26 years
  - HPV vaccines are not recommended for use in pregnant women
    - If a woman is found to be pregnant after initiating the vaccination series, the remainder of the 3-dose series should be delayed until completion of pregnancy

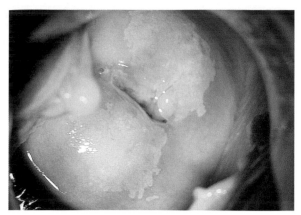

FIGURE 64-1 Cervix demonstrating abnormal epithelium on the anterior and posterior margins, demonstrating the white discoloration after the application of acetic acid. (From Oats J, Abraham S. *Llewellyn-Jones Fundamentals of Obstetrics and Gynaecology.* 8th ed. Philadelphia: Mosby; 2004: Fig. 37.6.)

- Pregnancy testing is not needed before vaccination
- **Vaccination recommended, even if a prior test was positive for high-risk HPV DNA, cervical abnormalities, or genital warts, to protect against the other HPV genotypes**

Clinical Presentation

- The cervical epithelium most often affected by malignant transformation is the transformation zone (where the columnar cells of the endocervical canal are undergoing transformation into the squamous cells of the exocervix) (Fig. 64-1)
- Most women with precursors to cervical cancer are asymptomatic
- Invasive cervical cancer becomes symptomatic at a late stage
  - Abnormal bleeding (menorrhagia, postcoital, or intermenstrual) may occur early in the disease
  - Late-stage symptoms are usually caused by local spread and may include pelvic, leg, or back pain; pedal edema; rectal bleeding; or hematuria
- Physical examination may show evidence of the following:
  - HPV infection: *Condylomata acuminata* or genital warts (verrucous-like lesions) (Fig. 64-2)
  - Invasive cancer: induration, friable tissue, ulceration, exophytic (cauliflower-like) lesions (Fig. 64-3)

Diagnosis and Evaluation

- **Cervical cytology (the Pap smear) is the screening test of choice; screens for both dysplasia and cancer**
  - Involves exfoliative cytology of the uterine cervix
  - Proven to reduce the incidence of squamous cervical cancer and resultant mortality
  - Sensitivity is approximately 70% to 80%; specificity is 90% to 95%
    - Proper interpretation of Pap smear is crucial to avoid unnecessary testing
    - **Many lesions regress over time and do not portend a diagnosis of cancer**

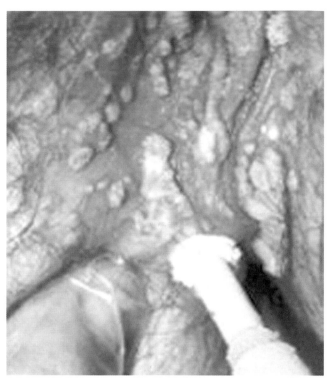

FIGURE 64-2 Genital warts on the vulva of a woman. The warts are associated with human papillomavirus. (From http://en.wikipedia.org/wiki/Genital_warts.)

- **Management of abnormal Pap smears differs significantly in women with HIV infection; see Chapter 12 for details**
  - Technique
    - Perform before bimanual examination
    - Visualize the entire cervix, if possible
    - Remove any discharge carefully before obtaining specimen
    - Small amount of blood is acceptable; large amounts (e.g., menses) may preclude adequate testing
    - Must include cells from the transformation zone to be deemed adequate
    - Conventional brush-and-scrape technique
      - Sample obtained with an endocervical spatula and brush (sequentially)
      - Scrape exterior cervix before endocervical canal
      - Must undergo rapid fixation on slide to avoid air-drying and subsequent artifact
    - Liquid-based sampling
      - Specially designed round brush is inserted into the cervix and rotated clockwise five full rotations
      - Entire brush placed into liquid medium
      - Better sensitivity over conventional technique
      - HPV testing may be performed on the same sample (concurrently or retrospectively)
  - **Pap smear frequency**
  - **Pap smear screening should be initiated in all women at age 21 years**
    - **Testing before age 21 years is not recommended**

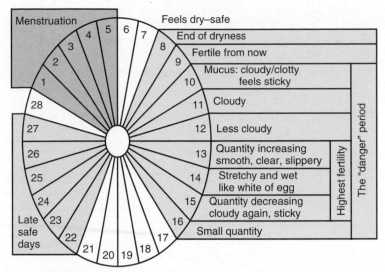

FIGURE 64-3 Periodic abstinence ("rhythm method"), using the mucus (ovulation) method. (From Oats J, Abraham S. *Llewellyn-Jones Fundamentals of Obstetrics and Gynaecology.* 8th ed. Philadelphia: Mosby; 2004.)

- Women are considered high risk (for persistent HPV infection and for high-grade cervical dysplasia) if they have HIV immunosuppression, diethylstilbestrol exposure (high risk of clear cell adenocarcinoma of vagina, which can be detected on Pap smear), history of CIN or HPV-related cancer, or other similar risk factors such as systemic lupus erythematosus (SLE) and organ transplantation
- Guidelines for average-risk women:
  - Pap smears should NOT be performed annually on average-risk women
  - If cytology is performed alone:
    - Women aged 21 to 65, screen every 3 years
  - If cytology is performed with a negative HPV cotest:
    - Women aged 30 to 65, screen every 5 years
  - Do not perform HPV cotesting in women under 30
- Women at high risk (see earlier risk factors) or women with prior abnormal Pap smears require annual Pap smear screening indefinitely at the onset of sexual activity (even if before age 21) with biannual Pap smears for 1 year, followed by annual screening, even if they never have a subsequent abnormal result
- **In women who have undergone hysterectomy without a cervical remnant, Pap smears are no longer required unless the hysterectomy was performed for a high-grade precancerous lesion or for cervical cancer**
- It is reasonable to discontinue cervical cancer screening in women over age 65 who have three or more negative cytology test results in a row and no abnormal test results in the past 10 years
- The Bethesda System provides standard terminology for reporting cervical cytology test adequacy and results (Table 64-1)
  - Descriptions may include the following:
    - Benign cellular changes (e.g., infection)

- Reactive cellular changes (e.g., inflammation)
- Epithelial cell changes
- **Infections found on Pap smear (e.g., *Candida, Trichomonas*) should be treated**
- Squamous metaplasia is a normal finding
- **Consensus guidelines for management of abnormal Pap smears are based on the 2012 American Society for Colposcopy and Cervical Pathology (ASCCP) clinical management guidelines (see Table 64-1)**

Treatment

- Treatment of invasive cervical cancer is based on staging
  - Stage I: confined to the cervix
  - Stage II: extends beyond cervix but not to pelvic sidewall or lower third of vagina
  - Stage III: involves pelvic sidewall or lower third of vagina
  - Stage IV: metastatic disease (beyond pelvis) or involvement of bladder or rectum
- Treatment based on stage
  - Stage I can usually be treated with radical hysterectomy with or without radiation
  - Stages II and III are predominantly treated with radical hysterectomy with or without radiation
  - Stage IV requires radical surgery, usually with radiation, or palliative chemotherapy or radiation
- Prognosis based on tumor size, stage, and nodal involvement
  - Stage I: 78% overall survival
  - Stage IV: 8% overall survival

Contraception

- Half of all pregnancies are unplanned; contraception is important to address for all reproductive-age women, especially those on potentially teratogenic medications

64

TABLE 64-1 *The Bethesda Classification of Pap Smear Results and Management Options*

Pap Smear Result	Risk of High-Grade Lesion (by Histology)	Management Options*
Normal	Essentially none	Continue routine screening
Unsatisfactory cytology		If HPV unknown or negative: repeat in 2 to 4 months If HPV positive and >30 years old: repeat cytology in 2 to 4 months *or* Refer for colposcopy
Normal cytology but absent or insufficient endocervical cells or transitional zone		If <30 years old: routine screening If ≥30 years old and HPV unknown: screen for HPV *or* Repeat cytology in 3 years If ≥30 years old and HPV negative: routine screening If ≥30 years old and HPV positive: repeat cotesting in 1 year *or* Genotype and if 16+ or 18+: colposcopy
Normal cytology but human papillomavirus (HPV)+		HPV genotyping: If 16 or 18, refer for colposcopy If negative, repeat cotesting in 1 year *or* Repeat cotesting in 1 year If HPV+ or ASCUS, refer for colposcopy If HPV negative and cytology negative: repeat cotesting in 3 years
Atypical squamous cells of undetermined significance (ASCUS)	Low	Most common abnormal Pap smear finding Majority are benign on colposcopy Options: Women 21 to 24 years old: repeat cytology in 1 year If ASCUS or more severe: refer for colposcopy If negative, repeat cytology in 1 year Women ≥25 years old: Test for high-risk HPV strains: If positive, refer for colposcopy If negative, repeat Pap smear in 12 months *or* Repeat cytology with HPV cotest in 3 years if ≥30 years old Immunocompromised: colposcopy
ASCUS: cannot exclude high-grade squamous intraepithelial lesion (HSIL), atypical squamous cells: cannot exclude HSIL (ASC-H)		Colposcopy Very high rate of HPV positivity, no need to test
Atypical glandular cells (AGC)	CIN 1, 2, 3: 20% Cervical adenocarcinoma in situ, or cervical adenocarcinoma: 6% May also be related to endometrial hyperplasia or endometrial adenocarcinoma: 2% to 3%	If endometrial subtype: refer for endocervical and endometrial sampling If no endometrial pathology: colposcopy If another subtype (AGC NOS): colposcopy and endometrial sampling if women is ≥35 years old or at risk
Low-grade squamous intraepithelial lesion (LSIL)	15% to 30%	If negative HPV: repeat contesting in 1 year If HPV unknown: colposcopy If LSIL, HPV+: colposcopy
High-grade squamous intraepithelial lesion (HSIL)	70% to 75%	Colposcopy with endocervical assessment *or* Loop electrosurgical excision

TABLE 64-1	*The Bethesda Classification of Pap Smear Results and Management Options* (Continued)	

Pap Smear Result	Risk of High-Grade Lesion (by Histology)	Management Options*
Cervical intraepithelial neoplasia (CIN) Grade 1		After ASCUS or LSIL: repeat cytology in 12 months If same or less, repeat in 12 months If ASC-H or HSIL: colposcopy After ASC-H or HSIL: Inadequate colposcopy: excision Adequate colposcopy: excision, observation with colposcopy, and cytology at 6 months
CIN Grade 2,3		Adequate colposcopy: ablation or excision followed by cotesting at 12 and 24 months Inadequate colposcopy or recurrent CIN 2, 3: diagnostic excisional procedure followed by cotesting at 12 and 24 months; if abnormalities, proceed to colposcopy with endocervical sampling
Adenocarcinoma in situ (AIS)		Hysterectomy (preferred) *or* Excision with close follow-up

*See Chapter 12 for a discussion of management of abnormal Papanicolaou (Pap) smears in women with human immunodeficiency virus.

- Many different forms of contraception are available to women; choice is often based on personal preference
- **Contraceptive efficacy is measured by the Pearl Index (Table 64-2)**
  - Failure rates may be higher in women weighing more than 90 kg; such women should be counseled about potential contraception failure
  - Young women and those at high risk should always be counseled to use condoms in addition to any other form of birth control to protect against STIs
- Specific types of contraception
  - Rhythm method
  - Barrier methods
    - Condoms
      - Latex sheath that fits snugly over the penis during intercourse
      - **Advantages: protection from STIs, easily obtained over the counter**
      - Efficacy greatly enhanced by addition of spermicides, which decrease sperm motility (e.g., nonoxynol-9)
    - Diaphragm
      - Rubber dome-shaped cup that fits over the cervix
      - Inserted manually before intercourse
      - Major disadvantages are inconvenience and required fitting by clinician
  - Hormonal
    - Combination oral contraceptives
      - Most commonly used reversible method of contraception
      - Contain both estrogen and progestin in 21 tablets; remaining 7 tablets contain inert ingredients (to bring on withdrawal bleed)
        - **Estrogen: serves mainly to inhibit ovulation by suppressing pituitary gonadotropin secretion; usually dosed between 20 µg ("low-dose") and 35 µg per tablet**
        - **Progestin: causes changes in cervical mucus and endometrium that hinder fertility**
      - Many different formulations and combinations exist on the market
        - Choice of prescribed formulation often based on patient or doctor familiarity, cost, and/or availability
        - Monophasic pill: constant dose of estrogen and progestin in each tablet
        - Phasic pill: changing dose of progestin (and sometimes estrogen
      - Combination oral contraceptives are highly effective; most common reason for failure is noncompliance
        - If a woman misses 1 or 2 tablets, she should take 1 tablet immediately upon remembering, followed by 1 tablet twice daily until missed tablets are taken
        - If more than 2 tablets are missed, another form of contraception should be used as a backup during that cycle
      - Potential benefits:
        - Improvement in dysmenorrhea, premenstrual symptoms, and benign breast disease
        - Decreased risk of pelvic inflammatory disease (PID) and ectopic pregnancy
        - Decreased risk of ovarian and endometrial cancer
      - Some women experience cessation of menses (not dangerous)
      - **Relative contraindications include:**
        - **History of thromboembolic disease**
        - **Stroke**
        - **Active liver disease**
        - **History of breast or endometrial cancer**
        - **Smokers older than 35 years of age**
    - Third-generation oral contraceptives
      - Contain newer progestins (i.e., norgestimate)

64

TABLE 64-2	Contraceptive Options, Efficacy, and Side Effects	
Technique	**Pearl Index* Typical/Correct Use**	**Possible Side Effects**
Attempting conception	85/85	N/A
Withdrawal	27/4	None
Rhythm	3 to 5 for correct use No data for typical use	None
Spermicidal suppositories or foam	29/18	Local irritation, allergic reactions
Condom	Male: 15/2 Female: 21/5	Skin irritation, latex allergy
Diaphragm	16/6	Pelvic irritation and discomfort, small increase in urinary tract infections
Intrauterine device (IUD) Levonorgestrel IUD Copper IUD	0.2/0.2 0.8/0.6	Menorrhagia, dysmenorrhea, increased risk of salpingitis (leading to possible infertility), uterine perforation
Combination, progesterone only oral contraceptive pills, contraceptive patch, and contraceptive vaginal ring	8/0.3	Breakthrough bleeding (if occurs for >3 months, deserves evaluation) Amenorrhea (not harmful) Headache Worsening migraines Breast tenderness Increase in blood pressure Increased risk of thromboembolism Increased risk of gallbladder disease
Injected progesterone	3/0.3	Breakthrough bleeding, weight gain, acne, loss of bone density with prolonged use
Nexplanon	2/0.9	Breakthrough bleeding, headache, weight gain, acne, breast tenderness
Female sterilization	<1<1	Risk of anesthesia

*Pearl Index is the number of couples out of 100 using a particular method that are likely to be pregnant at the end of a year of usual use. Actual failure rates of the techniques listed are higher than the values shown; usually caused by improper use of the method.

- Fewer side effects
- May improve acne, hirsutism, or polycystic ovary syndrome (PCOS), though evidence that it is more effective for these symptoms than other oral contraceptive preparations is lacking
- May also have a slightly higher thrombosis risk, though evidence is contradictory
  - Drosperinone
    - Has both antiandrogenic and antimineralocorticoid properties
    - Useful in PCOS
    - Reduces hirsutism and acne, but no evidence that it is more effective for these symptoms than other oral contraceptive preparations
    - Watch for hyperkalemia
  - Other dosing and administration options
    - Continuous-use or extended-cycle regimens:
      - Dose oral contraceptive continuously (skipping the 7 placebo pills) to bring on withdrawal bleed every 3 months (or even longer) rather than monthly
      - Benefits include convenience for patient and decreases in premenstrual migraines, premenstrual dysphoric disorder symptoms, endometriosis symptoms, and hyperandrogenism

- **Starting oral contraceptives:**
  - **Quick start method for birth control initiation involves starting birth control on any day during menstrual cycle rather than waiting for day 1 of the cycle and is associated with less unplanned pregnancy**
  - **Pelvic exams are not required for starting hormonal birth control**
- Contraceptive patch
  - Apply patch once weekly for 3 weeks, then remove for 1 week
  - Some patients find it more convenient
  - Minor side effect of local irritation in a few
  - Not contraindicated in women who weigh more than 90 kg, but these women need to be counseled about unpredictable absorption and risk of contraception failure
  - May confer higher venous thromboembolism risk compared with other hormonal methods, but this is controversial
- Combined contraceptive vaginal ring
  - Inserted by patient for 3 weeks, then removed for 1 week
  - If left in for more than 3 but less than 5 weeks, will still inhibit ovulation

- No need to remove during intercourse, but may remove for up to 3 hours if desired
  - Caution patients to watch for spontaneous expulsion
- Progestin-only pill ("mini-pill")
  - Contains small doses of progestin only
  - Has 28 tablets of active hormone; no inert tablets
  - Less efficacious
  - More breakthrough bleeding than with combination pill
  - **Useful for women who have relative contraindications to estrogen (migraines with aura, smokers over age 35), lactating women, and older women with cardiovascular risk factors**
  - **Contraindicated in women with a history of breast cancer**
- Long-acting reversible contraception
  - Injectable progesterone (depot medroxyprogesterone acetate [Depo Provera])
  - Should be administered once every 3 months
  - Higher efficacy than combination oral contraceptive pills, possibly because of better compliance
  - Long-term use associated with reversible losses in bone mineral density
  - Bleeding changes are common with irregular bleeding and amenorrhea
  - Gradual weight gain is common
  - Return to fertility is delayed by several months
- Implants
  - Small, flexible rods or capsules placed under the skin in the upper arm
  - Very effective and, depending on the implant, lasts 3 to 7 years
  - Immediately reversible upon retrieval
  - Do not contain estrogen, so commonly cause bleeding changes
  - Can use during breastfeeding and by women who are unable to use estrogen-containing methods
  - Etonogestrel implant (Implanon)
    - Single rod implant provides effective 3-year contraception
    - Side effects: spotting, irregular menstrual bleeding, headache, weight gain, acne, breast tenderness, emotional lability, and abdominal pain
    - Contraindications:
      - Pregnancy
      - Hepatic tumor or active liver disease
      - Undiagnosed abnormal genital bleeding
      - Breast cancer
      - Hypersensitivity
- Intrauterine devices (IUDs) (Fig. 64-4)
  - Contraceptive device inserted into the lining of the uterus by a gynecologist
  - Precise mechanism not known but likely multifactorial: inhibition of sperm transport caused by cervical mucus changes, spermicidal effects

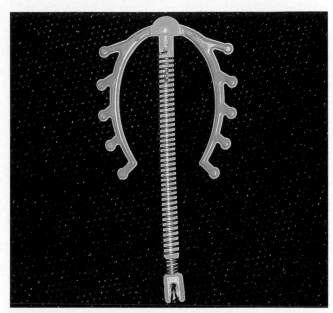

FIGURE 64-4 Copper 375 multiload intrauterine device. (From Oats J, Abraham S. *Llewellyn-Jones Fundamentals of Obstetrics and Gynaecology.* 8th ed. Philadelphia: Mosby; 2004: Fig. 38.9.)

caused by chronic inflammatory changes; implantation inhibition caused by thinning of endometrium; ovicidal effects
- Confers excellent efficacy and convenience
- Underused option in the United States
- Best candidates are women at low risk for acquiring an STI (since infection may require IUD removal) and not planning pregnancy for at least 1 year
- Options
  - Copper-clad T-shaped IUD:
    - Inserted every 10 years
    - Advantages of copper IUD:
      - Avoids hormonal contraception for women who have history of breast cancer or who prefer nonhormonal methods
      - Insertion can be used to provide emergency contraception
    - Disadvantages of the copper IUD:
      - Heavier, longer, or more painful menses
      - No protection against STIs; greater risk of PID if exposed to STI
  - Levonorgestrel-releasing IUD (e.g., Mirena):
    - Inserted every 5 years
    - High rates of amenorrhea
    - No loss of bone mineral density
    - Advantages of levonorgestrel IUD:
      - Reduces dysmenorrhea and menstrual bleeding
      - May decrease endometriosis-related pain and delay recurrence of endometriosis after surgery
      - May protect against STIs and upper tract infection because of thickening of cervical mucus
      - Whereas one third of failures with female sterilization result in an ectopic pregnancy,

64

there is no increased risk of ectopia with the IUD
- However, if a pregnancy occurs while an IUD is in place, that pregnancy is more likely to be ectopic
- Disadvantages of both types of IUDs:
  - Risk of expulsion; higher if inserted soon after childbirth
  - Increased risk of PID (greatest risk in first 20 days after insertion)
  - Uterine perforation at time of insertion
- **Contraindications:**
  - **Severe uterine distortion**
  - **Acute pelvic infection**
  - **Known pregnancy**
  - **Unexplained uterine bleeding**
  - **Current breast cancer**
  - **Copper allergy and Wilson disease for copper IUD**
- Special considerations in adolescents, women with prior STIs, immunocompromised women, and women on anticoagulation
- **Emergency contraception**
  - **Use of a contraceptive within 5 days after unprotected intercourse to prevent pregnancy; the sooner taken the more effective (75% to 80% effective if used within 72 hours of intercourse)**
  - Probably works by preventing or delaying ovulation; thus, it is not an abortifacient and will not work if a woman is already pregnant
  - Many options can be used as emergency contraceptive pills (dedicated products, progestin-only pills, combined oral contraceptive pills)
  - Most common form is 0.75 mg of levonorgestrel given within 72 hours of intercourse and repeated once 12 hours later
  - Alternatively, a single dose of 1.5 mg of levonorgestrel is probably equally effective with fewer side effects, and is available over the counter without age restrictions
  - Patient should expect usual menses within 21 days of treatment
  - Main side effect of hormonal method is nausea and vomiting; consider simultaneous prescription of an antiemetic to take 1 hour before
  - The copper IUD can also be used as emergency contraception if inserted within 5 days of unprotected sex
  - **Contraindications:**
    - **Pregnancy**
    - **Undiagnosed pathologic genital bleeding**
  - Consider STI testing and HIV prevention after unprotected intercourse
- Female and male sterilization
  - Tubal ligation or vasectomy are standard procedures
  - Most effective methods of contraception

Abnormal Uterine Bleeding

- Ovulatory bleeding is usually cyclic and may be caused by:

- Structural abnormalities:
  - Fibroids, polyps, adenomyosis, including malignancy or premalignancy
  - Coagulopathy
    - Most common cause: von Willebrand disease
  - Endometrial infection or inflammation
  - Iatrogenic or medications:
    - Hormonal birth control, copper IUD, anticoagulants, antipsychotic medications, tricyclic antidepressants
- Anovulatory bleeding is irregular because of loss of cyclical hormonal influences on the endometrium (oligoovulation or anovulation) and can be caused by:
  - Abnormalities in ovulation, progesterone production, endocrinopathies (PCOS, hypothyroidism, hyperprolactinemia, obesity, hypothalamic amenorrhea)
  - Often the cause during adolescence and perimenopause
- Evaluation in reproductive-age women
  - Assess site of bleeding: examine to make sure bleeding is not urinary, rectal, or vaginal and is actually coming from the uterus itself
  - Pregnancy test, complete blood count to assess anemia
  - If heavy or prolonged menses:
    - Pelvic ultrasound to evaluate structural causes
    - Testing for bleeding disorder if indicated by history
  - If long history of heavy menstrual bleeding and either postpartum hemorrhage, surgical site bleeding, or dental work-associated bleeding *or* two or more of the following: regular bruising, epistaxis, gum bleeding, family history of bleeding symptoms:
    - Test for von Willebrand disease or other coagulopathies, as indicated
  - If intermenstrual bleeding with normal menses:
    - Pelvic ultrasound and endometrial sampling if recent uterine or cervical procedure or childbirth
    - Biopsy if risk factors for endometrial cancer
  - If irregular bleeding, no regular menses:
    - Serum progesterone
    - Androgen testing for PCOS
    - Prolactin if galactorrhea present or taking antipsychotic medication, tricyclic antidepressant, metoclopramide, or methyldopa
    - Thyroid-stimulating hormone (TSH) if symptoms of thyroid disease
    - Pelvic ultrasound and uterine biopsy/sampling if risk factors for uterine cancer (i.e., family history of hereditary nonpolyposis colorectal cancer syndrome), age, concerning appearance on ultrasound
- Evaluation in postmenopausal women
  - Most common cause of bleeding is atrophic vaginitis
  - Uterine cancer, however, must be excluded with pelvic ultrasound and referral to gynecology for endometrial sampling
- Treatment
  - Medical treatment options for abnormal uterine bleeding caused by ovulatory dysfunction include:

- Progestin therapy (e.g., levonorgestrel-releasing IUD, medroxyprogesterone acetate)
- Combined oral contraception
- Amenorrhea: see Endocrinology section

Benign Breast Disorders

- Benign breast disorders are divided into categories of nonproliferative, proliferative without atypia, and atypical proliferative diseases
- Proliferative diseases may confer an increased risk of development of breast cancer, though an increased risk may be seen in nonproliferative disorders; age at time of biopsy (younger women are at greater risk), histology, and family history influence that risk
- Nonproliferative diseases:
  - Breast cysts
    - Fluid filled-round/ovoid masses; may be painful and can present with sudden onset of pain on enlargement
    - Hormone fluctuations influence breast cysts
    - Common in women 35 to 50 years old
    - Evaluation by ultrasound, mammogram, or magnetic resonance imaging may be needed
    - Low risk of malignancy with simple and complicated cysts
    - **Risk of malignancy with complex cyst varies from 1% to 23%; likelihood increased if thick cyst wall, septations, mix of cystic and solid components, lobulated, or hyperechogenic**
  - Other nonproliferative breast disease: papillary apocrine change, epithelial related calcifications, mild hyperplasia of the usual type
- Proliferative breast lesions without atypia:
  - Fibroadenomas
    - Most common in women 20 to 30 years old
    - Usually located in the upper, outer quadrant
    - Hormone-dependent
    - Confers slightly elevated risk of breast cancer if complex, if adjacent proliferative disease, or if a family history of breast cancer is present
    - Clinical exam: discrete, smooth, homogeneous, mobile, nontender lump
    - Imaging has high sensitivity
  - Usual ductal hyperplasia: a pathologic diagnosis that does not warrant further treatment
  - Intraductal papillomas:
    - Frequently associated with nipple discharge
    - Treatment: excision because of risk of atypia and ductal carcinoma in situ (DCIS)
  - Other breast lesions requiring excision because of risk of premalignancy or malignancy
    - Multiple papillomas
    - Sclerosing adenitis
    - Radial scars
    - Complex sclerosing lesions
- Proliferative with atypia disease:
  - Atypical hyperplasia:
    - Includes atypical ductal and atypical lobular hyperplasia

- Pathologic diagnosis: features of DCIS or lobular carcinoma in situ
- Associated with increased risk of ipsilateral or contralateral malignancy, especially if multifocal
- Treatment: excision
- Monitoring: biannual clinical breast exam, annual mammography
- Risk reduction:
  - Hormonal birth control and hormone replacement are contraindicated
  - Lifestyle changes include weight loss if obese, less than 3 alcoholic drinks per week, smoking cessation
  - Selective estrogen receptor modulators (tamoxifen, raloxifene) may be considered
- Flat epithelial atypia: unclear entity
  - Low risk of recurrence or malignancy
  - Treatment: excision
- Inflammatory breast lesions
  - Mastitis
    - Cellulitis of mammary gland connective tissue
    - Postpartum complication of lactation, often within the first 3 months
    - Clinical presentation: tender, warm, indurated, inflamed area, temperature higher than 38° C
    - Treatment
      - Cold compresses, antiinflammatories
      - Continue breast feeding; important to empty breasts to decrease milk stasis
      - Antibiotics if no response to symptomatic treatment within 48 hours
      - Empiric therapy: cephalexin, dicloxacillin, clindamycin
      - If risk for methicillin-resistant *Staphylococcus aureus*: clindamycin, trimethoprim/sulfamethoxazole, linezolid; vancomycin if severe
      - If abscess present: incision and drainage
      - Imaging if suspicion of abscess or no response to appropriate treatment course
  - Fat necrosis
    - Result of breast trauma, surgery, or radiation resulting in inflammation of adipose tissue
    - Radiologic diagnosis often unclear; may require biopsy
    - Treatment with warm compresses, antiinflammatories

Preconception Care

- Preconception care is recognized as important to promote healthy pregnancy
- The Centers for Disease Control and Prevention (CDC) recommend preconception counseling at all visits in women of childbearing age
- CDC has listed 14 preconception interventions that can improve pregnancy outcomes:
  - Folate supplementation: best outcome if started at least 1 month before conception
  - Immunization: tetanus, measles, mumps, and rubella (MMR), varicella, and hepatitis B vaccine (HBV)

64

- HIV/AIDS screening and treatment
- Management and optimization of chronic conditions:
  - Diabetes
    - Importance of optimal glucose control before conception
    - Risk of congenital abnormalities directly related to glucose level at time of conception
  - Hypothyroidism with need for adequate replacement before conception and increased dosing after conception
  - Obesity reduction with consideration of bariatric surgery for eligible patients
  - Hypertension and avoidance of potentially teratogenic medications (angiotensin-converting enzyme [ACE] inhibitors)
  - Seizure disorder and avoidance of potentially teratogenic medications
- Lifestyle modification screening and counseling
  - Weight loss or gain
  - Smoking cessation
  - Alcohol cessation
  - Avoidance of teratogenic medications such as vitamin A supplements
  - Importance of vitamin D and calcium
- Preconception evaluation of women on certain types of medication:
  - Isotretinoins
  - Warfarin
  - Antiepileptics
  - ACE inhibitors/angiotensin receptor blockers

Medical Issues Related to Pregnancy

HYPERTENSIVE DISORDERS IN PREGNANCY
(Table 64-3)

- **Chronic hypertension**
  - **Definition: blood pressure (BP) greater than 140/90 mm Hg observed before pregnancy or within the first 20 weeks of gestation**
  - Risks: intrauterine growth retardation, cesarean delivery, abruptio placentae, preterm birth, superimposed preeclampsia, and fetal death
  - Treatment
    - Antihypertensive drug therapy in pregnancy has not been proven to improve outcomes, and there is concern about impact of BP-lowering drugs on placental perfusion (resulting in decreased fetal growth)
    - There is no consensus on the treatment of mild (less than 150/100 mm Hg) or moderate (less than 160/110 mm Hg) hypertension in pregnancy
    - Treating mild to moderate hypertension reduces the risk of development of severe hypertension, but does not decrease the risk of preeclampsia, fetal mortality, preterm birth, or small for gestational age infant
    - Treatment of severe hypertension (higher than 160/110 mm Hg)

- Benefit in stroke reduction
- Once the decision to treat is made, avoid large drops in maternal BP because uterine, placental, and fetal perfusion will fall in proportion
- Goal BP: 130 to 150/80 to 100 mm Hg
- Medications
  - **All antihypertensive medications cross the placenta**
  - **Several agents are safe, but no data from large trials on choice**
  - **Methyldopa**
    - **Medication most frequently prescribed during pregnancy**
    - **Drug of choice but poorly tolerated**
  - Clonidine
  - Calcium channel blockers (long-acting nifedipine is commonly used)
  - Combined α-, β-blockers (labetalol is commonly used after methyldopa)
  - Hydralazine
- Medications to avoid:
  - β-Blockers: associated with fetal growth restriction and inadequate neonatal response to hypoglycemia
  - Diuretics: associated with fetal growth restriction and fetal distress if started or increased during pregnancy because the lack of uterine or placental autoregulation puts perfusion of the fetus at the mercy of maternal blood volume
  - **ACE inhibitors, angiotensin receptor blockers, and direct renin inhibitors are absolutely contraindicated in pregnancy because of risk of fetal toxicity**
  - Nitroprusside is contraindicated because of concerns for fetal cyanide poisoning
- Preeclampsia and eclampsia
  - Diagnostic criteria for mild preeclampsia:
    - BP 140/90 mm Hg or higher after 20 weeks with:
      - Proteinuria
      - Thrombocytopenia less than 100K
      - Renal insufficiency
      - Abnormal liver function/transaminitis more than 2 times normal
      - Pulmonary edema
      - Cerebral symptoms (generalized tonic clonic seizures progressing toward coma) or visual symptoms (may include changes in visual field, scotomata, or homonymous hemianopsia)
  - Diagnostic criteria for severe preeclampsia
    - BP 160/110 mm Hg or higher with:
      - Thrombocytopenia less than 100K
      - Impaired liver function, transaminitis more than 2 times normal, or right upper quadrant pain unresponsive to pain medications
      - Renal insufficiency
      - Pulmonary edema
      - Cerebral symptoms
  - Diagnostic criteria for eclampsia:
    - Preeclampsia complicated by seizures that cannot be attributed to another cause
    - Risks

TABLE 64-3	*Hypertensive Complications of Pregnancy*	
Disorder	**Clinical Manifestations**	**Treatment**
Chronic hypertension	Usually asymptomatic, preexisting hypertension diagnosis, or BP 140/90 mm Hg before the 20th week of pregnancy If severe, may have headache, blurred vision, hematuria, pulmonary edema	Nonpharmacologic treatment if woman is low risk for stroke or cardiovascular complications with short time frame of pregnancy Methyldopa is drug of choice, if treating Second-line choices: labetalol, calcium channel blockers
Gestational hypertension	Transient hypertension (>140/90 mm Hg) at later than 20 weeks' gestation, if preeclampsia not present, and BP returns to normal by 12 weeks' postpartum	Nonpharmacologic treatment preferred, close monitoring
Preeclampsia		Delivery of fetus, if possible, is definitive therapy **Antepartum** Bed rest and observation Frequent fetal ultrasonography and surveillance Antihypertensives are of unproven benefit **Intrapartum** Hydration with careful fluid monitoring Seizure prevention: intravenous magnesium sulfate Hypertension: intravenous hydralazine, labetalol, or nitroglycerin; sublingual nifedipine **Postpartum** Need to continue magnesium for 24 to 48 hours
Eclampsia	New-onset seizures or coma in patient with preeclampsia, and no other cause of seizure	Similar to preeclampsia
HELLP syndrome	Hemolysis Elevated liver enzymes (AST and ALT up to 4000 U/L) Low platelet count (as low as 6000/mm^3) **Other symptoms:** Epigastric pain Nausea, vomiting Headache Edema	Delivery is definitive treatment Lab values (AST, ALT, platelets) normalize within 5 days postpartum

ALT, Alanine aminotransferase; AST, aspartate aminotransferase; BP, blood pressure; HELLP, hemolysis, elevated liver enzymes, and low platelet count.

From Report of the National High Blood Pressure Education Program Working Group on High Blood Pressure in Pregnancy. *Am J Obstet Gynecol.* 2000;183:S1–S22.

- Preeclampsia occurs in up to 7% of all pregnancies
- Preeclampsia and eclampsia have increased maternal and fetal morbidity and mortality
  - Maternal: intracranial hemorrhage, abruptio placenta with hemorrhage, renal cortical necrosis
  - Fetal: intrauterine growth retardation, increased mortality
- Women with a history of preeclampsia may have an increased risk of long-term cardiovascular disease, diabetes, and renal disease
- Features associated with preeclampsia:
  - First pregnancy
  - Advanced maternal age
  - Twin gestation
  - History of preeclampsia, superimposed on chronic hypertension, or diabetes, pregestational diabetes, obesity, chronic kidney disease, chronic hypertension
  - Family history of preeclampsia in a first-degree relative

- Management: only "cure" is delivery of the fetus
- **Hemolysis, elevated liver enzymes, and low platelet count syndrome**
  - **Variant of preeclampsia (10% to 15%) in which patients may also develop microangiopathic anemia, thrombocytopenia, or hepatocellular necrosis**
  - Can also develop in pregnant women without preeclampsia
  - May occur antepartum (two thirds of patients) or postpartum (one third of patients)
  - May be difficult to differentiate from hemolytic uremic syndrome and thrombotic thrombocytopenic purpura
  - Unlikely to recur in subsequent pregnancies (only 2% to 6%), but confers an increased risk of preeclampsia more than 20% in subsequent pregnancies
  - Clinical manifestations and management (Table 64-3)
- Postpartum considerations in patient with hypertensive disorder in pregnancy
  - Women with chronic hypertension may develop postpartum complications, such as heart failure,

64

pulmonary edema, and renal failure, especially if there are underlying comorbid health conditions
  - Oral hypertensive medications may be required after delivery to control BP, particularly for women who were hypertensive before pregnancy and who discontinued medications during pregnancy

DIABETES MELLITUS IN PREGNANCY

- Epidemiology
  - Most common medical complication of pregnancy, affecting approximately 7% of pregnancies in the United States
  - Prevalence rates are higher in African Americans, Hispanics, Native Americans, Pacific Islanders, and South and East Asians when compared with white women
- Definitions of diabetes in pregnancy
  - **Pregestational diabetes: type 1 or 2 diabetes diagnosed before or in early pregnancy using standard diagnostic tests and cutoffs**
  - **Gestational diabetes mellitus (GDM): glucose intolerance detected for the first time in pregnancy**
    - Hyperglycemia and insulin levels insufficient to meet insulin demands; pregnancy-induced insulin resistance, which normally occurs in late pregnancy, unmasks (likely chronic) defects in pancreatic β-cell
  - Risk factors for GDM
    - Maternal obesity
    - Increased gestational weight gain
    - Maternal age older than 25 years
    - Member of a high-risk ethnic group
    - Previous GDM
    - Previous delivery of an infant heavier than 9 lbs
    - Parity
    - History of metabolic syndrome, PCOS, or hypertension
    - Family history of diabetes
- Risks associated with GDM
  - **GDM is associated with an increased risk of developing type 2 diabetes later in life (35% to 60% in the 10 to 20 years following pregnancy), so women with a history of GDM should have periodic screening for diabetes and risk reduction counseling (e.g., weight loss)**
  - Diabetes in pregnancy is associated with increased perinatal risks of the following:
    - Fetal macrosomia (defined as birth weight greater than 4000 g)
      - Decreased risk if blood glucose is well controlled
    - Shoulder dystocia
      - Decreased risk if blood glucose is well controlled
    - Cesarean section
    - Other neonatal problems, including respiratory distress syndrome, hypercalcemia, hyperbilirubinemia, and polycythemia
    - Fetal anomalies: primarily cardiac and skeletal
    - Preeclampsia
      - Decreased risk if blood glucose is well controlled

- Screening for GDM
  - Universal or risk factor-based, using a 50-g glucose challenge test between 24 and 28 weeks gestation
  - A positive screen is a serum glucose of 140 mg/dL or greater 1 hour after or more than 120 mg/dL 2 hours after the oral ingestion of 50 g of hyperosmolar glucose, irrespective of prior oral intake
  - If the screen is greater than 200 mg/dL, patient is diagnosed as having GDM
  - If the screen is 140 to 200 mg/dL, a 3-hour glucose tolerance test should be performed (more sensitive and specific)
- Management of GDM
  - Insulin or an oral agent (sulfonylurea or metformin) is usually started for fasting glucose values consistently above 100 mg/dL or values 2 hours postprandial consistently over 120 mg/dL
  - **Goals of glycemic control are a fasting glucose value of 60 to 80 mg/dL and a 2-hour postprandial value less than 120 mg/dL (1-hour value less than 140 mg/dL)**

ASTHMA IN PREGNANCY

- Asthma may worsen, improve, or stay the same during pregnancy; course is unpredictable
- Asthma exacerbations in pregnancy can result in maternal, and thus fetal, hypoxemia, leading to fetal death, prematurity, or low birth weight
- Benefit of continuing pharmacologic therapy for asthma far outweighs the risk
  - Studies show lack of adverse effects for use of albuterol inhaler or inhaled steroids (budesonide and beclomethasone)
  - Oral steroids may confer increased risk of prematurity and low birth weight, and some studies have shown an associated risk of preeclampsia
  - Given these concerns about frequent oral steroid use, prevention of exacerbations is very important

THYROID DISEASE IN PREGNANCY

- Increased incidence of thyroid disease during pregnancy (see Chapter 38)
- During pregnancy, serum thyroid-binding globulin concentration increases, and human chorionic gonadotropin (HCG) stimulates the thyrotropin receptor
- TSH reference ranges are lower in pregnancy because of this HCG cross-reactivity with the TSH receptor
- The following groups should be screened for thyroid disease:
  - Those with a history of thyroid disease, including postpartum thyroid dysfunction
  - Those with other autoimmune disease or a family history of autoimmune thyroid disease
  - Those with history of high-dose neck radiation
  - Those with a goiter
- Thyroid medications are generally safe in pregnancy
- Hypothyroidism in pregnancy
  - Increased risk of miscarriage, fetal neurocognitive deficits, low birth weight
  - Increased risk of anemia, hypertension in pregnancy

- Increased risk of placental abruption, preterm delivery
  - Treatment for hypothyroidism decreases risk of miscarriage, preterm birth, and fetal neurocognitive problems
- Treatment for hypothyroidism does not reduce the risk of hypertension in pregnancy
- Natural and synthetic thyroid hormones (thyroxine, triiodothyronine) do not cross the placenta and can be used during pregnancy
- **Thyroid replacement requirements increase 20% to 40% early in the first trimester; must monitor aggressively to improve fetal outcomes**
- **Goal is to maintain TSH level less than 2.5 mIU/L**
- Hyperthyroidism in pregnancy
  - Increased risk of maternal heart failure, hypertension in pregnancy, and placental abruption
  - Increased risk of fetal goiter, intrauterine growth retardation, preterm delivery, and stillbirth
  - Antithyroid medications (propylthiouracil and methimazole) do cross the placenta and may be teratogenic; radioiodine is contraindicated
  - **Antithyroid therapy is directed at keeping the maternal serum free thyroxine in the upper one third of the normal range; risks of treatment need to be discussed with patient**

DEPRESSION IN PREGNANCY

- Treatment of depression in pregnancy with selective serotonin reuptake inhibitors (SSRIs) is considered generally safe; however, counseling regarding risks and benefits should be undertaken
- Decision to start, continue, or switch antidepressant medication in pregnancy should include severity of prior depression including functional status and suicidality
- Choosing an SSRI
  - Sertraline and citalopram are first line
  - Fluoxetine is no longer first line because of its long half-life and risk of accumulation in fetus/neonate during pregnancy and breast feeding
  - Paroxetine should be avoided because of potential risk of congenital cardiac defects
  - Escitalopram likely safe, but little data to support this
- Serotonin/norepinephrine reuptake inhibitors: concern about contributing to increased risk of preeclampsia
- Atypical antidepressants:
  - Bupropion is probably safe
  - Mirtazapine may be associated with preterm birth

MEDICATIONS IN PREGNANCY

- No medication is proven to be absolutely safe; therefore, pregnant women should limit medication use to true needs and minimize use as much as possible
- FDA classification of drugs regarding safety in pregnancy is as follows:
  - Category A: Controlled studies in women fail to demonstrate risk to fetus in first trimester; unlikely to cause fetal harm
  - Category B: Studies of animal reproduction have not demonstrated risk to fetus, but no controlled studies

in pregnant women or animal studies have shown effect
- Category C: Animal studies have revealed adverse effects in fetus; no controlled studies in women; should be given only if potential benefit justifies risk
- Category D: evidence for fetal risk, but benefits may be acceptable in pregnant women despite risk
- Category X: Studies in humans and animals demonstrate significant fetal risk; contraindicated in pregnancy
- Reasonable treatment for common symptoms in pregnancy (Table 64-4)
- Drugs contraindicated in pregnancy (Box 64-1)
- Vaccines
  - **"Dead" vaccines (using killed virus or bacterial or viral fragments) are considered safe**
    - Examples: hepatitis A vaccine, HBV, influenza (injected), polio (injected), pneumococcal, and meningococcal vaccines
    - Influenza vaccine is indicated for all trimesters because pregnant women have higher risk of complications from influenza
    - Tdap (tetanus-diphtheria-acellular pertussis combined vaccine) is recommended during each pregnancy regardless of prior history of receiving Tdap or Td. Optimal timing to transfer passive antibodies to the infant is between 27 and 36 weeks gestation.
  - Avoid HPV vaccine in pregnancy
- **Only one live attenuated virus vaccine, the oral polio vaccine, is considered safe in pregnancy**

TABLE 64-4	Generally Considered Safe Drug Therapy for Common Pregnancy Symptoms
Symptom	**Drug**
Acne	Topical clindamycin, erythromycin, or benzoyl peroxide
Allergic rhinitis	Topical glucocorticoids and cromolyn Antihistamines, including loratadine, chlorpheniramine, and diphenhydramine
Cough	Guaifenesin and dextromethorphan
Constipation	Docusate sodium, lactulose, and mineral oil
Nausea	Pyridoxine (vitamin B_6) and doxylamine succinate
Gastrointestinal reflux	Calcium carbonate and ranitidine
Pneumonia	Amoxicillin and azithromycin
Urinary tract infection	Nitrofurantoin (avoid in first trimester unless it is the only available agent: associated with neonatal jaundice)
Headache, generalized aches, and pains	Acetaminophen
Thrombophlebitis	Heparin

64

- Although no reported problems are associated with MMR vaccine during pregnancy, it is preferred to withhold until postpartum when it is considered safe
- The varicella-zoster and smallpox vaccines are contraindicated during pregnancy

Menopause

- **Definition of menopause:**
  - **The permanent cessation of menses following loss of ovarian activity**
  - **A clinical diagnosis made after 12 months of amenorrhea**
- **Definition of perimenopause:**
  - **The entire time period from the onset of menstrual irregularity and hormonal fluctuations to menopause**
  - **May be associated with menopausal symptoms such as hot flashes and vaginal symptoms**
  - **Lasts an average of 4 years**
- Median age of menopause is 51 years, with a range of 45 to 55 years; occurs earlier in smokers and nulliparous women

---

BOX 64-1 *Selected Common Medications Contraindicated in Pregnancy*

Antihypertensives

ACE inhibitors (birth defects in first trimester, decreased fetal renal perfusion and death if used in second or third trimester)
Angiotensin receptor blockers (same as ACE inhibitors)
Direct renin inhibitors
Loop diuretics (fetal growth restriction and distress)

Antimicrobials

Tetracyclines (brittle bones and cartilage and yellow teeth)
Fluoroquinolones (arthropathies)

Anticonvulsants

Phenytoin
Carbamazepine
Valproic acid

Other

Warfarin (fetal anomalies and fetal death)
Temazepam

ACE, Angiotensin-converting enzyme.

- An elevated follicle-stimulating hormone (FSH) level can provide supporting evidence, but is not useful for routine diagnosis (FSH fluctuates greatly during the perimenopause)
  - **FSH may be useful in certain situations: women with premature menopause, uncharacteristic clinical presentations, or hysterectomized women without classic symptoms**
- Loss of estrogen at the menopause greatly affects women and affects quality of life
  - Vasomotor symptoms (hot flashes) highly prevalent (75% or more of women in the United States); more frequent at night
  - Genitourinary
    - Vaginal atrophy and fragility can lead to dryness, pruritus, and discharge, as well as painful intercourse
    - Decreased vaginal pH can lead to increased genitourinary infections
  - Loss of bone mineral density (3% to 5% per year during the first 5 years after menopause)
  - Cardiac: decrease in high-density lipoprotein, increase in low-density lipoprotein cholesterol
- Treatment of hot flashes
  - Oral hormone replacement therapy (HRT) with estrogen is the most effective therapy (reduces frequency and severity by >90%) (See HRT section)
  - With the exception of the estradiol ring, topical estrogen formulations do not reach high enough systemic levels to relieve hot flashes
  - Other potential treatments:
    - Layered, cotton clothing
    - Avoidance of known triggers (caffeine, alcohol, warm humid environments, spicy food)
    - Gabapentin, clonidine, and methyldopa have shown efficacy (Table 64-5)
    - SSRIs: Systematic review found that SSRIs resulted in 10% decrease in hot flash frequency and moderate improvement in severity
    - Escitalopram may be more effective, but all SSRIs were more effective than placebo
    - Available selective estrogen receptor modulators are not effective for hot flashes
    - Herbal therapies (soy products, black cohosh) have low efficacy
- Evaluation and treatment of genitourinary symptoms:
  - Appearance: thin, dry, pale mucosa with patches of erythema or petechiae, loss of vaginal ruggae and labial fat pad with decreased distinction between labia majora and minora

---

TABLE 64-5 *Alternatives to Estrogen for Vasomotor Symptoms*

Class	Typical Agents	Side Effects
SSRIs	Sertraline, citalopram, bupropion	GI symptoms, decreased libido
α-Adrenergic agents	Clonidine, methyldopa	Fatigue, dizziness, dry mouth, constipation
Gabapentin		Drowsiness, lethargy
Progestins	Medroxyprogesterone acetate (oral, depot, or transdermal)	Breast tenderness, irritability, depression, headaches, long-term safety

GI, Gastrointestinal; SSRIs, selective serotonin reuptake inhibitors.

- Treatment is aimed at alleviation of symptoms:
  - Long-acting nonhormonal moisturizers (water-, silicone-, and oil-based lubricants, as well as moisturizers)
  - Topical estrogen (delivered intravaginally at a low dose via a cream, ring, or tablet) relieves vaginal mucosal atrophy and subsequent dryness
    - Lower risk profile compared with oral HRT because of low systemic absorption
    - 2006 Cochrane review did not find increased risk of venous thromboembolism
    - Insufficient evidence regarding endometrial hyperplasia or uterine cancer or systemic absorption
  - May require prolonged or recurrent treatment after first 1- to 3-month trial
  - Transdermal or oral HRT is also an option if no response to local administration or if simultaneous hot flashes; can be used in conjunction with locally administered low-dose estrogen preparations
  - There is no evidence to support the use of herbal remedies; randomized clinical trials have shown no effect on genitourinary symptoms from black cohosh, soy, or other products, and there was no change in hormonal levels
- **Hormone replacement therapy:**
  - **Benefits:**
    - **Preservation of bone mineral density**
    - **Improvement in lipid profile**
    - **Potential reduced risk of colorectal cancer**
  - **Risks:**
    - **Women's Health Initiative (WHI) study findings indicate potentially increased risk of breast cancer, coronary artery disease (CAD), cerebrovascular disease (CVD), and venous thromboembolism (VTE)**
    - These findings are difficult to interpret given that women began HRT at different postmenopausal stages/ages
  - Indications for HRT:
    - 2012 Cochrane review found that the risks of HRT outweigh the benefits and recommended against HRT for primary or secondary disease prevention
    - **2012 North American Menopause Society position statement**
      - **Support initiation of HRT *at* menopause to treat menopause-related symptoms (vasomotor, genitourinary symptoms that do not respond to topical formulations) and to prevent osteoporosis among women at high risk of fracture; initiation should occur only in women with a favorable risk profile for CAD, CVD, VTE, and breast cancer**
      - **Estrogen therapy alone has better risk profile and thus can potentially extend duration of use; however, should not be used alone (without progesterone) in women with a uterus**
      - **Estrogen and progestin therapy should not be used beyond 3 to 5 years, given concern for breast cancer**
      - **For women with premature or early menopause with favorable risk profiles, HRT can be given until age 51, the median age of onset of menopause**
  - Many forms available (oral, transdermal); none definitively shown to be superior
  - If HRT started, lowest dose for shortest duration (preferably less than 5 years) generally recommended; reassessment for continued need should be done at least yearly
  - If uterus present, must administer progestin with estrogen to avoid increased risk of endometrial cancer
  - Cycled use if patient desires monthly withdrawal bleeding
  - Continuous use if withdrawal bleeding undesirable (more commonly used in postmenopausal women)
  - Vaginal spotting and bleeding may be a nuisance side effect: usually resolves within 6 months
  - **If heavy or if first bleeding occurs 6 months after initiating therapy, endometrial biopsy should be performed to rule out hyperplasia or cancer**

Review Questions

For review questions, please go to ExpertConsult.com.

SUGGESTED READINGS

Abalos E, Duley L, Steyn DW, et al. Antihypertensive drug therapy for mild to moderate hypertension during pregnancy (Cochrane Review). In: *The Cochrane Library*, Vol. 2. Oxford: Update Software; 2001.

American College of Obstetricians and Gynecologists (ACOG). Gestational diabetes. In: ACOG *Practice Bulletin 30*. Washington, DC: ACOG; 2001.

American College of Obstetricians and Gynecologists. Practice Bulletin No. 140: management of abnormal cervical cancer screening test results and cervical cancer precursors. *Obstet Gynecol*. 2013;122:1338-1367.

American College of Obstetricians and Gynecologists Committee on Practice Bulletins—Gynecology. ACOG Practice Bulletin No. 109: cervical cytology screening. *Obstet Gynecol*. 2009;114:1409-1420.

Committee on Practice Bulletins—Gynecology. Practice Bulletin No. 136: Management of abnormal uterine bleeding associated with ovulatory dysfunction. *Obstet Gynecol*. 2013;122:176-185.

Grimes DA, Raymond EG. Emergency contraception. *Ann Intern Med*. 2002;137:180-189.

Herndon EJ, Zieman M. New contraceptive options. *Am Fam Physician*. 2004;69:853-860.

Kronenberg F, Fugh-Berman A. Complementary and alternative medicine for menopausal symptoms: a review of randomized, controlled trials. *Ann Intern Med*. 2002;137:805-813.

North American Menopause Society. Estrogen and progestogen use in postmenopausal women: 2010 position statement of the North American Menopause Society. *Menopause*. 2010;17:242.

Rossouw JE, Anderson GL, Prentice RL, et al. Risks and benefits of estrogen plus progestin in healthy postmenopausal women: principal results from the Women's Health Initiative randomized controlled trial. *JAMA*. 2002;288:321.

Wright TC, Cox JT, Massad LS, et al. 2001 Consensus guidelines for the management of women with cervical cytological abnormalities. *JAMA*. 2002;287:2120-2129.

64

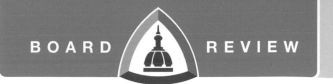
Dermatology for the Internist

MARY SHEU, MD; REBECCA A. KAZIN, MD; and THOMAS B. HABIF, MD

Internal medicine physicians often encounter patients complaining of skin eruptions. Even though some cutaneous diseases may require specialty referral, it is imperative for internists to be able to recognize common dermatologic conditions, serious conditions that may require urgent referral, and cutaneous manifestations that may signify other disease processes.

Common Dermatologic Conditions

ACNE VULGARIS

See Figure 65-1 for an example of acne vulgaris.

Basic Information

- Defined as a chronic inflammation of pilosebaceous units of the face and trunk
- Affects nearly all adolescents with varying severity
- The primary lesion in acne is the microcomedo, which is an accumulation of keratin and sebum within the follicle
- With androgenic stimulation during puberty, sebum production increases, providing the opportunity for *Propionibacterium acnes* to colonize and proliferate within the follicle, resulting in an inflammatory reaction
- Most patients with acne vulgaris do not overproduce androgens; however, they probably have a genetic hyperresponsiveness to androgens
- Acne formation can also be influenced by external factors
  - Oil-based cosmetics
  - Medications (e.g., steroids, phenytoin, lithium)
  - Endocrine disorders (e.g., Cushing disease, polycystic ovary syndrome)
  - Chloracne: severe acne occurring after exposure to halogenated hydrocarbons (e.g., herbicides, Agent Orange)

Clinical Presentation and Diagnosis

- Closed comedone ("whitehead"): further accumulation of sebum within a microcomedo
- Open comedone ("blackhead"): opening of the follicular orifice; follicle is packed with melanin and keratin, exposure to air results in oxidative darkening of sebum
- Inflammatory lesions: rupture of follicular contents resulting in formation of cysts, papules
- Cutaneous nodules and scarring
- **Emotional scarring (often permanent) is quite common; treatment has been shown to improve self-esteem**

Treatment

- Comedonal acne
  - Topical retinoids (e.g., tretinoin, adapalene, tazarotene)
  - Salicylic acid
- Mild comedonal or inflammatory acne
  - Topical retinoids (e.g., tretinoin, adapalene, tazarotene)
  - Topical benzoyl peroxide, clindamycin, erythromycin, or dapsone
- Moderate inflammatory acne
  - Oral antibiotics (antiinflammatory property of antibiotics thought to play major role in action against acne; doxycycline, minocycline usually; may also try erythromycin or trimethoprim-sulfamethoxazole)
  - Hormonal therapy (females only): oral contraceptives or spironolactone (used as an antiandrogen; warn patients about hyperkalemia and teratogenicity)
  - In-office therapies (acne surgery: extraction of comedones; chemical peels with salicylic acid; laser therapy; photodynamic therapy: topical aminolevulinic acid hydrochloride [Levulan] followed by exposure to light source)
- Severe or resistant inflammatory acne
  - Isotretinoin
    - Synthetic vitamin A derivative
    - Common side effects include dry skin and hyperlipidemia
    - Rare side effects include pseudotumor cerebri, myalgias, alopecia
    - **Teratogenicity is a concern; therefore, women of childbearing age must be on two reliable means of birth control during treatment, which should be continued for at least one menstrual period after the drug has been stopped. Patients must be registered in the iPLEDGE program (www.ipledgeprogram.com).**
  - In women with treatment-resistant acne, consider an endocrinopathy (e.g., polycystic ovary disease, Cushing disease)

ACNE ROSACEA

See Figure 65-2 for an example of acne rosacea.

Basic Information

- Chronic inflammatory disorder of the face
- Lesions typically last days to weeks and recur
- Seen predominantly in middle-aged and older adults

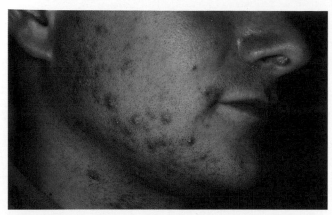

FIGURE 65-1   Acne vulgaris. (From Bolognia JL, Jorizzo JL, Rapini RP. *Dermatology.* St. Louis: Mosby; 2003: 533.)

TABLE 65-1	*Differential Diagnosis of Acne Rosacea*
Disease	**Clinical Differences**
Acne vulgaris	Comedones present Flushing not present Younger age group
Carcinoid syndrome	Rare Flushing is fleeting (lasts only seconds)
Systemic lupus erythematosus	Malar rash that spares the nasolabial folds No papules or pustules Systemic symptoms present
Seborrheic dermatitis	No papules or pustules Background erythema and telangiectasias are usually absent Can occur concurrently with rosacea

- Eye involvement can cause blepharitis, conjunctivitis, iritis, and keratitis
- Hyperplasia of the soft tissues and sebaceous glands of the nose (rhinophyma) can be seen in severe cases (usually in men)
- Can easily be confused with a number of other conditions (Table 65-1)

Treatment

- Topical antibiotics (metronidazole, clindamycin), sulfacetamide/sulfur, azelaic acid, or benzoyl peroxide can be tried initially to reduce inflammation
- Oral antibiotics (e.g., tetracycline, doxycycline, erythromycin, or minocycline; mechanism of action also thought to be antiinflammatory as in acne vulgaris treatment) or topical tretinoin (or both) can be used in cases that do not respond to the preceding treatments. (Note: Topical retinoids have been reported to worsen telangiectasia in some patients.)
- Light-based therapy including intense pulsed light or pulsed dye laser (a series of treatments improves the flushing and telangiectasia)
- Topical brimonidine can reduce flushing and redness

ECZEMA

- Defined simply as an inflammation of the epidermis of the skin
- Can be caused by a number of different conditions (Table 65-2; Figs. 65-3 to 65-6)
- Broadly classified into three categories that define the approach to therapy
  - Acute eczema
    - Presentation: edema, papules, vesicles, bullae, crusting, serous discharge, and scaling can be present
    - Initial treatment: saline compresses or warm-water bath, followed by medium-strength topical glucocorticoids (e.g., triamcinolone 0.1%) and emollients; use only low-potency steroids (e.g., desonide) for facial lesions; topical tacrolimus or pimecrolimus for maintenance
  - Subacute eczema
    - Presentation: erythematous, scaling, and pruritic lesions, but no vesicles, bullae, or serous discharge

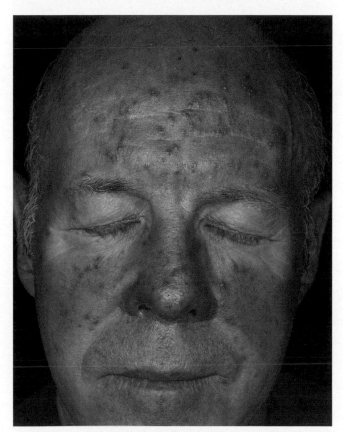

FIGURE 65-2   Rosacea.

Clinical Presentation

- Four subtypes; patients may have one or more than one manifestation: (1) erythrotelangiectatic, (2) papulopustular, (3) rhinophyma and (4) ocular
- Earliest lesions include facial erythema and telangiectasias
- Vascular reactivity (flushing) can be triggered by food (caffeine, alcohol, spicy food, hot beverages), environmental exposure (heat and sun), or emotion (stress)
- Papules, pustules, cysts, and nodules can develop similarly to acne vulgaris, but comedones are not present

65

TABLE 65-2	*Features of Eczematous Eruptions*	
Disease	**Description**	**Treatment**
Atopic dermatitis (see Fig. 65-3)	Patients usually have a history of allergic rhinitis, asthma, or family history of atopy Lesions often involve flexures of neck, wrist, legs, and arms; hands and face can be involved Secondary staphylococcal infections are common	Topical corticosteroids (medium to high potency) plus emollients Oral antibiotics if there is superinfection Topical nonsteroidal antiinflammatory agents (e.g., pimecrolimus, tacrolimus)
Allergic contact dermatitis (see Fig. 65-4)	Caused by a delayed hypersensitivity reaction Most commonly caused by plant exposure (e.g., poison ivy, oak, sumac) Can also be caused by jewelry, cosmetics, and occupational exposures Diagnose by history or patch testing (or both)	Removal or avoidance of irritant Topical corticosteroids plus emollients Oral corticosteroids may sometimes be necessary
Irritant contact dermatitis	Caused by harsh cleansers and acids	Same as above
Dyshidrotic eczema (see Fig. 65-5)	Affects fingers, toes, palms, and soles Small (1-mm) vesicles, scaling, fissures Can be quite pruritic	Can be difficult to treat High-potency corticosteroids plus emollients
Seborrheic dermatitis	Epidermal inflammation in areas populated with sebaceous glands (e.g., scalp, face, ears, and chest) Scaling macules and plaques; can develop crusts or fissures *Pityrosporum* yeast may stimulate inflammation Increased incidence in patients with HIV and Parkinson disease	Scalp: ketoconazole, selenium sulfide, or tar shampoos plus corticosteroid topical solution Face: low-potency corticosteroids and ketoconazole cream
Stasis dermatitis	Erythematous scaling plaques seen in the lower legs in persons with chronic venous insufficiency Can form ulcers Brown hemosiderin hyperpigmentation may also be present	Dermatitis: wet dressings, topical corticosteroids, antibiotics (if needed) Ulcer: wet dressings, leg elevation, compression bandages
Nummular eczema (see Fig. 65-6)	Sharply circumscribed, 1- to 5-cm diameter plaques on the extremities Can resemble tinea corporis but potassium hydroxide prep is negative Secondary staphylococcal infections are common	Topical corticosteroids and emollients Oral antibiotics if there is superinfection Skin should be kept lubricated after treatment to avoid recurrence
Asteotic eczema	Seen in winter in older adults Dry ambient air may predispose to disease Dry, cracked, fissured skin with or without pruritus most commonly seen on the lower legs	Humidify ambient air Tepid baths using oils or oil-based soaps Medium-potency corticosteroid ointment (not cream) plus emollients

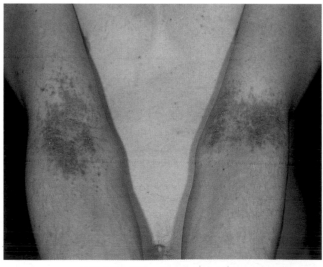

FIGURE 65-3 Atopic dermatitis.

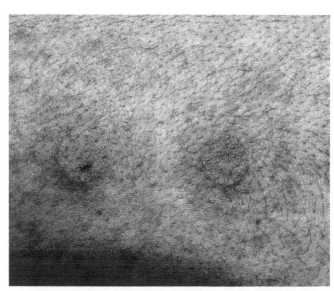

FIGURE 65-4 Contact dermatitis: A 2+ positive patch test.

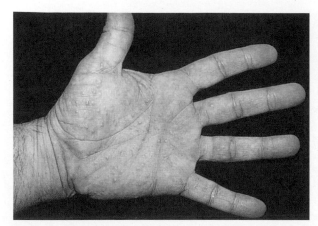

FIGURE 65-5 Dyshidrotic eczema.

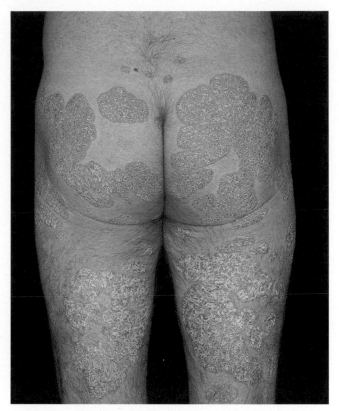

FIGURE 65-7 Chronic plaque psoriasis.

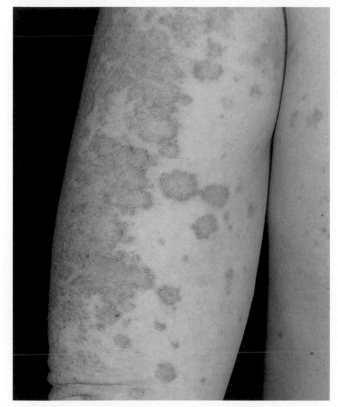

FIGURE 65-6 Nummular eczema.

- Initial treatment: high-potency corticosteroids (e.g., fluocinonide) and emollients; topical tacrolimus or pimecrolimus for maintenance
- Chronic eczema
  - Presentation: scaly thickening of the skin (lichenification); hypopigmentation or hyperpigmentation can occur
  - Treatment: high-potency topical steroids and emollients; topical tacrolimus or pimecrolimus for maintenance
- Refractory eczema may require systemic therapy (i.e., phototherapy, methotrexate, or, rarely, a brief course of cyclosporine; appropriate laboratory monitoring required)

- Subclassification of eczemas can be useful for guiding specific therapy in many instances (see Table 65-2)

PSORIASIS

Basic Information

- A T cell-mediated immune disorder in which CD4$^+$ and CD8$^+$ memory T cells stimulate the hyperproliferation of keratinocytes, causing chronic scaling papules or plaques
- **Average age of onset is in the third decade of life**
- Disease is characterized by periods of exacerbations and remissions
- Disease can be exacerbated by infections, drugs (e.g., lithium, antimalarials, β-blockers, corticosteroid withdrawal), alcohol, or stress

Clinical Presentation

- Skin disease
  - Chronic plaque psoriasis (Fig. 65-7): sharply marginated, erythematous plaques with silvery-white scale, commonly seen on scalp and extensor surfaces of the knees and elbows
  - Guttate psoriasis (Fig. 65-8)
    - Presents as an acute exanthem over the trunk and proximal extremities
    - Lesions are small (less than 1 cm) and scaly
    - **Often follows streptococcal pharyngitis or viral infection**
    - May be self-limited, but in some cases may also herald the beginning of chronic psoriasis

65

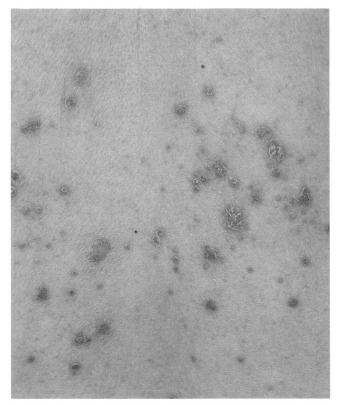

FIGURE 65-8 Guttate psoriasis.

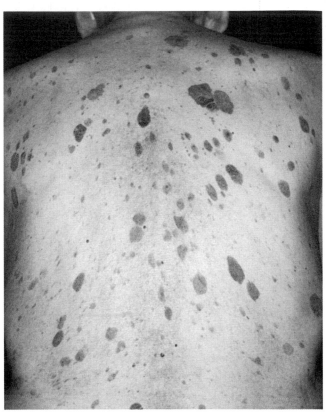

FIGURE 65-9 Seborrheic keratosis.

- Erythrodermic and pustular psoriasis are rare; more severe types can be triggered by tapering of systemic corticosteroids
- Nail findings are seen in 30% of patients with psoriasis
  - Nail pitting, onycholysis (separation of nail from nail bed), and subungual hyperkeratosis can occur
- Arthritis can be seen in up to one third of patients and is more common in patients with psoriatic nail disease (see Chapter 42)

Treatment

- Limited chronic plaque psoriasis: bland emollients with keratolytics, topical corticosteroids, calcipotriene (topical vitamin D derivative), or tazarotene (topical vitamin A derivative)
- Generalized plaque psoriasis: methotrexate, cyclosporine, acitretin, phototherapy (ultraviolet B radiation), photochemotherapy (psoralen plus ultraviolet A radiation), biologics (e.g., alefacept, etanercept, infliximab, efalizumab, ustekinumab)
- Guttate psoriasis: phototherapy plus emollients and midpotency topical corticosteroids
- Erythrodermic and pustular psoriasis: methotrexate, cyclosporine, or acitretin (synthetic retinoid); hospitalization may be necessary
- **Systemic corticosteroid therapy should be avoided in patients with psoriasis as it can lead to erythrodermic or pustular psoriasis, especially upon withdrawal of the systemic steroid**

SEBORRHEIC KERATOSIS

Figure 65-9 illustrates seborrheic keratosis.
- Very common benign epidermal growth that usually occurs after the age of 30
- Start as small papules or plaques with or without pigment
- Grow into fairly large (up to 6 cm) plaques with warty, "stuck on" appearance; variation in pigmentation (e.g., brown, black, gray) can be seen within individual lesions, may contain horn pseudocysts
- Commonly on the face, trunk, and upper extremities (light-exposed areas)
- Lesions may become irritated and resemble atypical pigmented lesions, but do not have a malignant potential
- Once diagnosis is made, therapy is not necessary and considered elective unless the growths are irritated or pruritic
- Lesions can be destroyed with liquid nitrogen, electrocautery, or curettage

PITYRIASIS ROSEA

See Figure 65-10 for an example of pityriasis rosea.
- **Self-limited, exanthematous eruption thought to be related to a viral illness**
- Predominantly seen in children and young adults
- Begins with a 2- to 5-cm oval, reddish pink lesion with a fine scale often found on the back or chest (herald patch)
- Similar smaller lesions then develop along the lines of cleavage of the skin (Christmas tree pattern on the back)

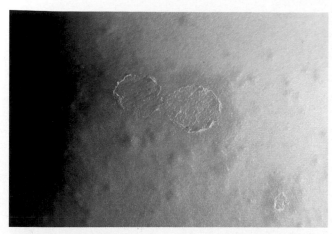

FIGURE 65-10 Pityriasis rosea with herald patch.

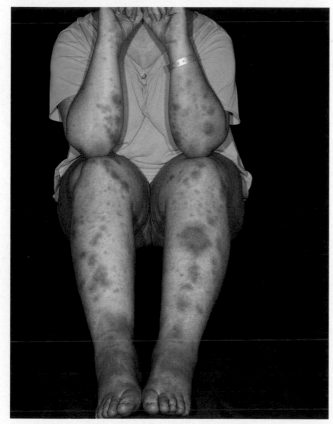

FIGURE 65-11 Erythema nodosum.

- Usually asymptomatic, but occasionally may be pruritic
- Differential diagnosis includes secondary syphilis, drug eruptions, guttate psoriasis, tinea corporis, human immunodeficiency virus (HIV) seroconversion illness
- Usually resolves without treatment in 2 to 3 months; if course is prolonged or pruritus is significant, treatment may include topical steroids or ultraviolet B phototherapy

ERYTHEMA NODOSUM

See Figure 65-11 for an example of erythema nodosum (EN).

Basic Information

- Proposed to be a delayed hypersensitivity reaction to antigens resulting from drugs, infections, or other inflammatory conditions
- More common in women
- Most commonly associated with streptococcal pharyngitis, but a number of other causes have been discovered
  - Sarcoidosis
    - **Löfgren syndrome: hilar lymphadenopathy, EN, and acute polyarthritis**
  - Tuberculosis, histoplasmosis, coccidioidomycosis
  - Hodgkin lymphoma
  - *Chlamydia* infection
  - Inflammatory bowel disease
  - Behçet disease
  - Medications (e.g., omeprazole, sulfonamides, oral contraceptives, hepatitis B vaccine)

Clinical Presentation

- **Erythematous nodules that can develop into bruise-like lesions that can be tender and painful**
- **Commonly seen on the lower extremities**
- Palpation of the subcutaneous tissue is often more sensitive than inspection of the rash
- Fever and arthralgias can accompany the eruption even in idiopathic cases

Diagnosis

- Usually made by clinical examination
- When the diagnosis is unclear, deep incisional biopsy (rather than punch biopsy) will show septal panniculitis with no evidence of vasculitis
- Complete blood count, antistreptolysin O titer, urinalysis, throat culture, intradermal tuberculin test, and chest radiograph should be obtained as part of the initial evaluation of a patient with EN

Treatment

- Rash is usually self-limited and improves with treatment of the underlying disease (if known)
- Nonsteroidal antiinflammatory drugs (NSAIDs), potassium iodide, or systemic corticosteroids may alleviate discomfort

Bacterial Infections of the Skin

See Chapter 15

Viral Infections of the Skin

HERPES SIMPLEX VIRUS TYPE 1

Figure 65-12 illustrates herpes simplex virus type 1 (HSV-1).

- Transmitted from person to person through oral secretions
- More than 90% of the world's population ages 20 to 40 years is seropositive for HSV-1

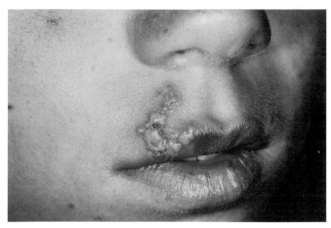

FIGURE 65-12 Herpes simplex virus type 1. (From Bolognia JL, Jorizzo JL, Rapini RP. *Dermatology.* St. Louis: Mosby; 2003:1237.)

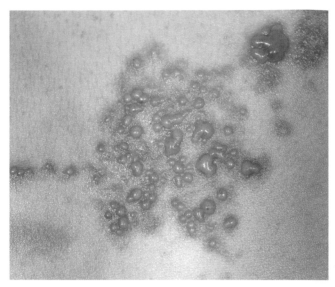

FIGURE 65-13 Herpes zoster.

- **Characterized by the sudden appearance of multiple grouped vesicles with an erythematous base**
- Infection can occur anywhere in the body but is often asymptomatic
  - Oral cavity
    - Primary infection: Exudative pharyngitis is commonly the primary infection and can be associated with fevers, lymphadenopathy, and myalgias
    - Recurrent infections present as vesicles on the lips or in the oral cavity; associated systemic symptoms are usually absent
  - Skin: any site on the skin, including the fingers (herpetic whitlow), and hips or buttocks
  - Other sites include the eye (see Chapter 66), lungs, liver, and central nervous system (CNS) (see Chapter 15)
- **Diagnosis can be made by Tzanck preparation of vesicular fluid, which typically shows multinucleated giant cells; viral culture, immunofluorescence staining, and detection of HSV DNA by polymerase chain reaction may also be useful**
- Treatment of primary infections with oral (or intravenous [IV]) acyclovir may shorten the duration of illness and decrease viral shedding time
- Generalized treatment of all patients with recurrent herpes labialis with acyclovir has not been proven to be beneficial. However, for patients with a distinct prodrome, early administration of oral acyclovir, famciclovir, valacyclovir, or topical penciclovir may be useful.

HERPES SIMPLEX VIRUS TYPE 2
See Chapter 11 for a discussion of HSV-2.

HERPES ZOSTER
Figure 65-13 shows an example of herpes zoster.

Basic Information
- Primary varicella-zoster virus (VZV) infection occurs after inhalation of respiratory droplets and results in a generalized vesicular rash (chickenpox)
- **Primary infection is usually seen in children but can occur in adults and immunocompromised hosts**

- Following primary infection with VZV, latent infection is established in the dorsal root ganglia
- Reactivation of the infection results in a painful, unilateral vesicular rash limited to a restricted dermatomal distribution (herpes zoster, or "shingles")
- At times, neighboring dermatomes can be involved
- Risk factors include advancing age and immune suppression

Clinical Presentation and Diagnosis
- Localized pain and systemic symptoms, including fever, malaise, and headache, may precede the vesicular rash by several days
- Crusting of the vesicular lesions usually occurs within 10 days, at which time the patient is no longer infectious
- A number of complications can result from infection
  - Postherpetic neuralgia: persistence of pain more than 30 days after the rash began
  - Herpes zoster ophthalmicus: can lead to blindness (See Chapter 66)
  - **Ramsay Hunt syndrome (type 2): ipsilateral facial paralysis caused by involvement of cranial nerve VII, ear pain, vesicles in the auditory canal; can lead to significant hearing loss**
  - Encephalitis/meningitis
  - Motor neuropathy
  - Transverse myelitis: more common in patients with HIV

Treatment
- Acyclovir, valacyclovir, or famciclovir can be used
- Starting therapy within 72 hours of appearance of the rash reduces pain and incidence of postherpetic neuralgia
- The addition of prednisone may accelerate healing time
- **Postherpetic neuralgia pain can be severe and require treatment with opioids, tricyclic antidepressants, carbamazepine, gabapentin, pregabalin, or topical lidocaine**

- Shingles vaccine now recommended for disease prevention in patients older than 60 years (see Chapter 73)

MOLLUSCUM CONTAGIOSUM

See Figure 65-14 for an example of molluscum contagiosum.

- A disease caused by a poxvirus spread by direct skin-to-skin contact
- Common in young children and in patients with HIV
- Lesions are usually small (2 to 5 mm), flesh-colored, or white umbilicated papules that can occur anywhere on the body except the palms and soles
- Diagnosis is made by clinical presentation or by histologic examination of a biopsied lesion

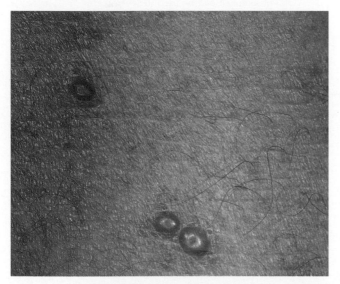

FIGURE 65-14 Molluscum contagiosum.

- Lesions are self-limited in immunocompetent hosts; curettage, cryotherapy, or laser therapy can be used, if needed; topical immune modulators (e.g., imiquimod) may also be effective
- In HIV patients, lesions can be long-lasting and extensive; there may be some improvement from treatment with antiretroviral therapy

Fungal Infections of the Skin

DERMATOPHYTOSIS

See Figure 65-15 for an example of dermaphytosis.

- **Caused by a group of fungi that penetrate the stratum corneum of the skin, hair, and nails**
- Symptoms usually consist of pruritus and burning
- Transmission is usually through direct contact
- Microscopic examination of the lesion with the addition of 1 or 2 drops of potassium hydroxide (KOH prep) usually reveals rod-shaped hyphae with branching
- Classification is based on location of the lesions (Table 65-3)

YEAST INFECTIONS

- Tinea versicolor (Fig. 65-16)
  - Recurrent superficial infection caused by *Pityrosporum orbiculare* (*Malassezia furfur*)
  - Most often seen in young adults
  - More commonly presents during warm, humid weather
  - Lesions are round and scaly; they can be hypopigmented, hyperpigmented, or erythematous
  - Occur predominantly on the trunk
  - **Diagnosis is made by KOH prep showing pseudohyphae and spores ("spaghetti and meatballs")**

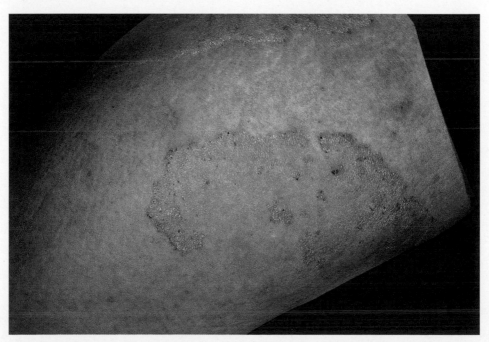

FIGURE 65-15 Dermatophytosis. (From Bolognia JL, Jorizzo JL, Rapini RP. *Dermatology*. St. Louis: Mosby; 2003: Fig. 2-8.)

65

TABLE 65-3	*Dermatophyte Infections*	
Disease	**Description**	**Treatment**
Tinea capitis	Usually occurs in children but can be seen in adults Commonly caused by *Trichophyton tonsurans* Starts as an erythematous, scaly patch on the scalp with broken-off hairs Can cause kerion formation (inflammatory pustular plaques with scarring) and permanent patches of hair loss	Topical antifungals usually not effective Griseofulvin is the treatment of choice Oral itraconazole and terbinafine can also be used Kerion treatment may require the addition of selenium sulfide shampoos and oral anti-staphylococcal antibiotics
Tinea corporis ("ringworm")	Annular, scaling, papular lesions with an area of central clearing on the trunk, limbs, or face The presence of multiple lesions may be a sign of underlying immunosuppression	Topical antifungals (e.g., terbinafine) are usually effective Oral griseofulvin can be used in severe cases
Tinea cruris	Predominantly seen in men Associated with physical activity and sweating ("jock itch") Can occur with tinea pedis Semicircular erythematous, scaly lesion that begins on the thigh and can extend to the perineal area and buttocks Typically does not involve the scrotum	Topical antifungals (e.g., terbinafine) are usually effective Oral griseofulvin can be used in severe cases Groin area should be kept clean and dry to avoid recurrences Treat tinea pedis (if present)
Tinea pedis ("athlete's foot")	Lesions can range from having mild erythema and scales to maceration and bullae between the toes and on the soles of the feet Can be a point of entry of bacteria, causing cellulitis	Topical antifungals (e.g., terbinafine) are usually effective Oral terbinafine or itraconazole can be used in resistant cases
Tinea unguium (onychomycosis)	Signs include white discoloration, crumbly debris from beneath the nail, and thickening of the nail	Topical therapy is generally ineffective Oral terbinafine or itraconazole for 6 to 12 weeks is the most effective treatment Ciclopirox nail lacquer is effective in <10% of patients Efinaconazole 10% nail solution is about 20% effective

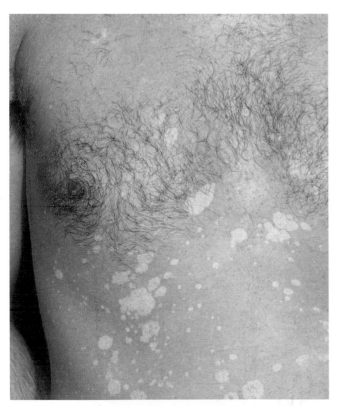

FIGURE 65-16 Tinea versicolor.

- Treatment is with topical antifungals, ketoconazole shampoo, selenium sulfide solution, or oral antifungals (e.g., fluconazole, itraconazole); griseofulvin is not effective
- Patients experiencing frequent recurrences may benefit from prophylactic treatment with selenium sulfide solution, applied every 3 weeks; or oral ketoconazole, once per month
- Mucocutaneous candidiasis
  - Infection generally involving moist skin sites or mucosal surfaces
  - Most cases caused by *Candida albicans*
  - Predisposing factors include increased moisture at the site of the infection, diabetes mellitus (DM), antibiotic therapy, and immunosuppression (e.g., HIV)
  - Infection seen at a number of different sites
    - Oral cavity: whitish plaques on erythematous base (thrush)
    - Vulvovaginitis: thick, creamy vaginal discharge with erythema of the vaginal skin and mucous membrane
    - Balanitis: erosions, scaling, erythema along the penis
    - Diaper candidiasis: erythema and edema caused by incontinence of urine or stool in the elderly

- Interdigital candidiasis: erythema and fissuring between the fingers
- Intertriginous candidiasis: erythema, edema, pustule formation beneath the breasts, in the groin, or around the scrotum
- Paronychial candidiasis: edema and erythema of the nail folds; creamy discharge may be present
- Angular cheilitis: fissures and erythema of the angles of the mouth
- Chronic mucocutaneous candidiasis
  - Characterized by recurrent, severe mucocutaneous candidal infections caused by an underlying T-cell defect
  - Usually presents in childhood
  - Suspect HIV in adult patients presenting with this syndrome
  - Treatment is with topical antifungal agents; long-term therapy may be necessary in patients with chronic disease

Infestations of the Skin

SCABIES

- Caused by infestation with the mite *Sarcoptes scabei*
- Transmission is from person to person by direct contact, although cases of transmission from clothing and bed linens have occurred
- In young adults, transmission commonly occurs during sexual contact
- **Intractable pruritus that is worse at night is the most prominent symptom**
- The primary lesion is usually a small, erythematous papule or vesicle that may be difficult to find
- Threadlike linear ridges that range from 2 to 15 mm in length (burrows) are pathognomonic for the disease
- **Vesicles, papules, and burrows are most commonly found on the hands, wrists, penis, nipples, axillae, and gluteal cleft; usually spares the scalp**
- *Norwegian scabies* describe an extensive scabies infestation involving the hands and feet and elsewhere with asymptomatic thick crusting. There is thick, subungual, keratotic material and nail dystrophy. It occurs in people with neurologic or mental disorders (especially Down syndrome), senile dementia, nutritional disorders, infectious diseases, leukemia, and immunosuppression (e.g., patients with AIDS).
- Diagnosis can be presumed on clinical grounds or confirmed by microscopic examination of the lesion by scraping and applying 2 drops of mineral oil before covering with a coverslip. Identification of the mite, eggs, or feces confirms the diagnosis. Complete blood count may reveal eosinophilia.
- **Treatment with permethrin cream over the entire body (washed off after 12 hours and repeated 1 week later) is usually effective**
- Family members and close contacts must also be treated
- Clothing and linens should be laundered
- Oral ivermectin may be considered to treat difficult cases and the elderly

PEDICULOSIS (LICE)

See Figure 65-17.
- Infestation with the human louse (*Pediculus humanus*)
- Characterized by the location of the infestation
  - *Pediculosis capitis* (head lice)
    - Can be transmitted by hats and brushes
    - Epidemics can occur in schools
  - *Pediculosis pubis* (pubic lice, crabs)
    - Most commonly occurs in young adults
    - Usually transmitted during sexual contact
  - *Pediculosis corporis*: seen in patients with poor hygiene with exposure to others with poor hygiene
- Predominant symptom is itching
- Diagnosed by visualization of nits attached to hair shafts or identification of the louse (usually by microscopy)
- **Treatment is with pyrethrin, permethrin, malthion, or lindane shampoos or lotions. Treatment should be followed by combing to remove all visible nits.**
- Ivermectin is also effective and may be used in cases resistant to topical medication

Benign, Premalignant, and Malignant Neoplasms of the Skin

MOLES

- Common moles (melanocytic nevi) are seen in everyone
  - They are small (<6 mm), tan, or brown macules or papules
  - Develop in childhood, peak in early adulthood, and decline thereafter
- Atypical moles (dysplastic nevi) (Fig. 65-18)
  - Are often larger (>6 mm) than common moles
  - Have irregular borders and variegated color
  - Surface may be complex and variable, with both macular and papular components; a characteristic presentation is a pigmented papule surrounded by a macular collar of pigmentation ("fried-egg lesion")
  - Can continue to appear after age 35 years, in contrast to common moles
  - Associated with an increased risk of melanoma
  - Biopsy often necessary to rule out melanoma
  - Familial atypical mole and melanoma syndrome (dysplastic nevus syndrome)
    - Patients have a large number of melanocytic nevi, often more than 50, some of which are atypical and often variable in size, and a positive family history of melanoma in one or more first- or second-degree relatives
    - Atypical lesions begin during puberty; melanoma often presents before the age of 40 years
    - **Lifetime risk of melanoma approaches 100% for those people with atypical moles from families with two or more first-degree relatives who have cutaneous melanoma**
    - Patients need to perform monthly self-examinations
    - Referral to a dermatologist is often necessary so that appropriate photographs and biopsies can be done at regular intervals (every 3 to 12 months)

65

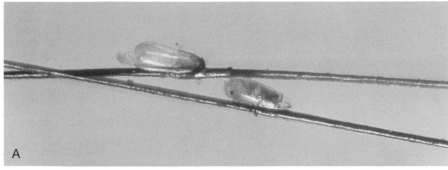

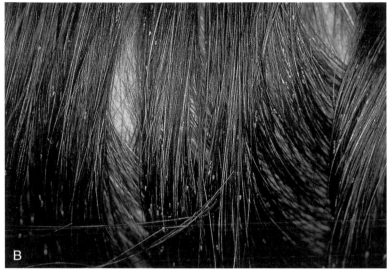

FIGURE 65-17 Pediculosis capitis. (From Bolognia JL, Jorizzo JL, Rapini RP. *Dermatology.* St. Louis: Mosby; 2003:1325.)

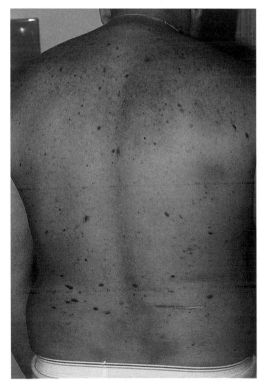

FIGURE 65-18 Atypical nevi. (From Bolognia JL, Jorizzo JL, Rapini RP. *Dermatology.* St. Louis: Mosby; 2003:1779.)

- Evaluation of a mole
  - All pigmented skin lesions should be examined for the following features (ABCDE):
    - **A**symmetry
    - **B**order irregularity
    - **C**olor variegation—variable degrees of black, brown, tan, or blue
    - **D**iameter greater than 6 mm
    - **E**volution: change in appearance or symptoms
  - Excisional biopsy should be considered for any lesion considered to be melanoma

MELANOMA

See Figure 65-19 for examples of melanoma.

Basic Information

- Risk factors (Box 65-1)
- Melanoma subtypes
  - Superficial spreading melanoma
    - Most common type
    - Deeply pigmented macules or papules usually greater than 6 mm in diameter; usually displays one of the ABCDE criteria (see earlier section on Moles)
  - Nodular melanoma
    - Dark black, tan, or brown (rarely amelanotic) dome-shaped papule or nodule

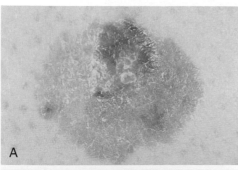

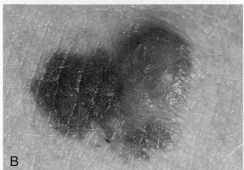

FIGURE 65-19 **A** and **B,** Superficial spreading melanomas.

| BOX 65-1 | *Risk Factors for the Development of Melanoma* |

Sun exposure
Blond or red hair
Freckling on the upper back
Blistering sunburns in childhood
White race
Family history of melanoma
Therapy with psoralen and ultraviolet A radiation for
  psoriasis
Changing pigmented mole
Many (>50) common moles
Atypical mole
History of basal cell carcinoma or squamous cell carcinoma
  of the skin
Immunosuppression (e.g., after organ transplantation)
History of treated melanoma

- Typically do not present with the ABCDEs, making diagnosis difficult
- Acral lentiginous melanoma
  - **Most common type found in African Americans and Asians**
  - Presents in palms, soles, or nail beds
  - Hutchinson sign: pigmented streak in nail with extension onto the nail-fold skin
- Lentigo maligna melanoma
  - Involves sun-exposed skin (usually the face)
  - Irregular pigmented macule that can develop papules within
  - One of the ABCDEs is typically present

Clinical Presentation

- Most melanomas exhibit one of the ABCDEs or have recently changed in size, shape, or color

- Bleeding, inflammation, or a sensory change at the site of the lesion should also suggest the possibility of malignancy
- In patients with numerous moles, an individual lesion that appears different from the others should be thoroughly evaluated
- Metastasis can occur (typically to the brain, liver, or lung)

Diagnosis

- Suggested by the clinical appearance
- Excisional biopsy of the lesion providing full-thickness skin sample that extends to the subcutaneous fat is the preferred diagnostic method
- **Staging is primarily based on tumor thickness**
- Ulceration and mitoses are the next most important histologic determinants of prognosis
- Sentinel lymph node biopsy is used for staging information in melanomas greater than 1.0 mm in depth
- Chest radiograph, liver function tests, and lactate dehydrogenase levels should also be obtained
- Imaging is indicated if metastatic disease is suggested

Treatment

- Excision with adequate margins is the treatment of choice for tumors without evidence of metastasis
- Elective lymph node dissection for patients with clinically enlarged lymph nodes and no evidence of distant disease
- Adjuvant systemic therapies may be employed for more advanced disease

BASAL CELL CARCINOMA

Figure 65-20 provides an example of basal cell carcinoma (BCC).

- **Risk factors include inability to tan, intermittent sun exposure, cumulative sun exposure, fair skin, and older age**
- Usually develop on the head and neck
- A patient typically complains of a red, peeling, eroded or bleeding lesion that may improve and then recur
- Subtypes of BCC
  - Nodular ulcerative
    - Most common type
    - Presents as a well-circumscribed pearly papule with telangiectasias; may ulcerate
  - Superficial
    - Well-circumscribed, erythematous, scaly patch
    - Resembles tinea, psoriasis, or dermatitis
    - Often occurs on non–sun-exposed skin
  - Sclerotic
    - Whitish plaque with sclerosis or fibrosis on palpation
  - Pigmented
    - Similar to nodular but are pigmented
    - Most common form seen in darker skinned individuals
- Metastatic disease is very rare
- Diagnosis is made by clinical appearance or biopsy specimen

65

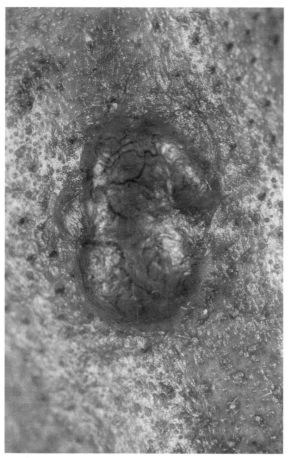

FIGURE 65-20 Basal cell carcinoma.

- Standard treatment options include electrodesiccation and curettage, surgical excision, and radiation
- Superficial BCC may respond to topical treatment with the immune modulator imiquimod
- Mohs micrographic surgery is used for sclerosing BCC and other BCC with poorly defined clinical margins; for tumors in areas of potentially high recurrence, such as the nose or eyelid; and for very large primary tumors and recurrent BCC

ACTINIC KERATOSIS

Figure 65-21 illustrates actinic keratosis.
- Premalignant lesions that develop on sun-exposed skin, usually in people older than 40 years
- **Low but significant risk of transformation to squamous cell carcinoma (SCC)**
- Fair-skinned individuals are more susceptible to developing actinic keratosis
- Presents as erythematous, 2- to 8-mm macules with a whitish scale; or as hyperkeratotic plaques on the face, scalp, back of the hands, arms, chest, upper back, and lower legs
- Diagnosis is usually made by clinical appearance; lesions suggestive of SCC should be biopsied
- There is no way to determine which lesions will progress to SCC
- Patients who are immunosuppressed (especially transplantation patients) are at high risk for the development of SCC from actinic keratosis

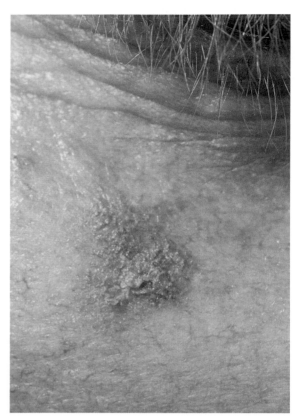

FIGURE 65-21 Actinic keratosis.

- Current treatment modalities include the following:
  - Cryotherapy with liquid nitrogen or surgical curettage is effective for individual lesions
  - Topical 5-fluorouracil, imiquimod, ingenol mebutate, and photodynamic therapy (topical aminolevulinic acid followed by exposure to a blue light source) may be useful in patients with multiple lesions (field therapy)
  - Excision or electrodesiccation and curettage should be performed for thicker or resistant lesions

SQUAMOUS CELL CARCINOMA

See Figure 65-22 for an example of SCC.
- More than half of cases arise from transformation of actinic keratoses
- Chronic exposure to ultraviolet sunlight and increasing age are the more important risk factors
- **Very common in patients after organ transplantation**
- In patients with chronic lymphocytic leukemia, the development of multiple SCCs may be an indication of clinical deterioration and disease progression of the leukemia
- Presents as an erythematous papule, nodule, or plaque with a hyperkeratotic scale; ulceration may also occur
- Clinical variants
  - Bowen disease (SCC in situ): reddish brown plaque that may have pigment or hyperkeratosis; has been associated with chemical exposures and human papillomavirus infection (SCC of the anogenital skin)

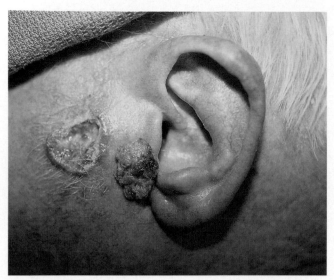

FIGURE 65-22   Squamous cell carcinoma. (From Bolognia JL, Jorizzo JL, Rapini RP. *Dermatology*. St. Louis: Mosby; 2003:1682.)

- Keratoacanthoma: hyperkeratotic nodule with a keratin plug; grows rapidly (over 3 to 6 weeks); most spontaneously regress
- Cutaneous horns: columns of hyperkeratosis on an erythematous base; can grow within an SCC
- 5% to 10% metastasize
- Surgical excision is the treatment of choice

CUTANEOUS T-CELL LYMPHOMA

- Presents as erythematous, scaly plaques resembling psoriasis or eczema on sun-protected sites (i.e., buttock and covered areas of trunk and limbs); most common subtype is *Mycosis fungoides*
- Fulminant lesions may be preceded by months to years by nonspecific scaly lesions that have been diagnosed as other dermatoses
- Significant pruritus, fever, and lymphadenopathy can be present
- **Sézary syndrome (Fig. 65-23) is a leukemic variant characterized by generalized erythroderma, lymphadenopathy, pruritus, and leukocytosis with atypical T cells (Sézary cells) in the peripheral blood**
- Patients can be treated with topical nitrogen mustard, phototherapy, topical or oral retinoids, or radiation therapy

Cutaneous Drug Reactions

Basic Information

- Occur in up to 3% of hospitalized patients
- Antibiotics are responsible for most reactions
- Drug-induced skin eruptions can take many forms (the most common and significant ones are discussed in the following section)

EXANTHEMS

- **The most common acute drug-induced eruption, accounting for 75% of cases**

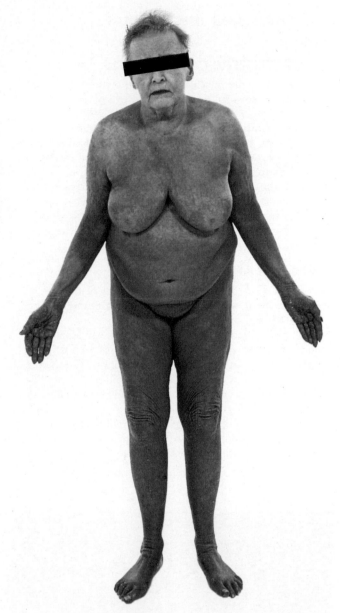

FIGURE 65-23   Sézary syndrome.

- Rash is generalized, pruritic, macular, and papular
- In some cases, exfoliative erythroderma can occur and can be an early sign for the development of toxic epidermal necrolysis (see following discussion)
- Onset of the rash is usually within 2 weeks of beginning drug therapy
- In patients who have been sensitized to the drug (by prior use), the rash typically develops within the first 3 days of therapy
- The most commonly implicated drugs include penicillins, cephalosporins, sulfonamides, quinidine, allopurinol, isoniazid, carbamazepine, and phenytoin
- Cessation of the drug usually leads to resolution of the rash; symptomatic treatment with topical corticosteroids, topical antipruritics, or oral antihistamines can be used

65

URTICARIA AND ANGIODEMA

See Chapter 68

HYPERSENSITIVITY VASCULITIS

- Most commonly implicated drugs include penicillins, cephalosporins, sulfonamides, allopurinol, and phenytoin
- **Clinical findings include palpable purpura, petechiae, fever, arthralgias, and lymphadenopathy that usually begin within 10 days of the initial drug exposure**
- The sedimentation rate may be elevated; complement levels may be low
- Discontinuation of the drug should lead to resolution of symptoms within weeks; systemic corticosteroids may be necessary in severe cases

LICHEN PLANUS

See Figure 65-24 for an example of lichen planus.

- **Can be drug-induced, liver disease-related (e.g., hepatitis C), or idiopathic**
- Implicated drugs include β-blockers, methyldopa, penicillamine, quinidine and quinine, NSAIDs, angiotensin-converting enzyme inhibitors, sulfonylurea agents, carbamazepine, gold, and lithium
- Most lesions occur on the skin or mucous membranes
  - Skin lesions
    - Pruritic, violaceous, polygonal, flat-topped papules with white lacy lines (Wickham striae)
    - Most common site is the flexor aspect of the wrists
  - Mucous membranes
    - Most common presentation
    - Milky-white papules with white lacework on the buccal mucosa
    - Patients with chronic disease may have an increased risk of oral SCC
- Withdrawal of the medication should lead to resolution of the lesions
- In cases that are not drug-induced, topical corticosteroids are first-line therapy
- Resistant disease can be treated with systemic corticosteroids, retinoid therapy, or phototherapy

ERYTHEMA MULTIFORME

See Figure 65-25 for an example of erythema multiforme (EM).

- Cell-mediated cytotoxic skin reaction triggered by infection (usually HSV or *Mycoplasma*) or drugs (e.g., sulfonamides, anticonvulsants, penicillins, or NSAIDs)
- Two basic forms of disease:
  - EM major
    - Affects more than one mucosal surface (usually conjunctiva and oral mucosa)
    - Typical or raised atypical target lesions
    - Epidermal detachment involving less than 10% of body surface
    - Lesions are usually located on the extremities or face
    - Usually associated with drugs
  - EM minor
    - Most are preceded by an HSV infection (a small percentage associated with *Mycoplasma pneumoniae*)
    - Limited or no mucous membrane involvement
    - Bullae and systemic symptoms are seen in some cases
    - Target lesions favor hands, feet, arms, and legs
    - Chronic suppressive acyclovir therapy prevents HSV and EM recurrences

STEVENS-JOHNSON SYNDROME AND TOXIC EPIDERMAL NECROLYSIS

- A spectrum of disease characterized by epidermal necrosis and mucous membrane involvement

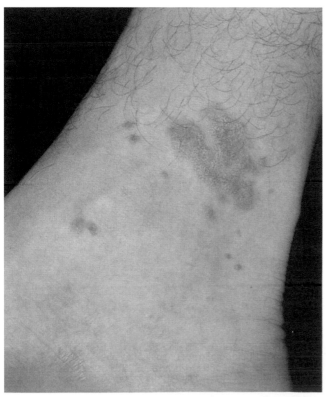

FIGURE 65-24   Lichen planus.

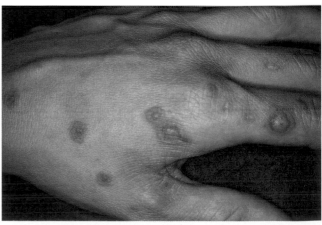

FIGURE 65-25   Erythema multiforme.

- **Stevens-Johnson syndrome (SJS) involves less than 10% of the epidermis, whereas toxic epidermal necrolysis (TEN) involves over 30% of the epidermis. Involvement of 10% to 30% is considered SJS-TEN overlap.**
- Most commonly implicated drugs are sulfonamides, anticonvulsants, allopurinol, penicillins, and NSAIDs
- Lesions usually appear within a few days after the initiation of drug therapy; a prodrome of fever, malaise, and arthralgias can be present
- Skin lesions
  - Begin as tender erythematous macules, followed by formation of blisters that become confluent; the epidermis then begins to slough, leaving areas that resemble burns
  - Nikolsky sign (separation of the outer layer of the epidermis from the basal layer with minimal pressure applied to the skin) may be present
- Mucous membranes
  - At least two mucosal surfaces are involved
- Erythema and sloughing of the lips, buccal mucosa, conjunctiva, or anogenital area can occur
- Complications of the disease include acute renal failure, fluid and electrolyte imbalances, gastrointestinal (GI) hemorrhage, and sepsis
- **Treatment of TEN involves discontinuation of the offending agent, transfer to a burn unit, possible IV immunoglobulin, not corticosteroids**
- Death occurs in 40% of patients with TEN
- Patients with SJS may benefit from oral corticosteroids

HYPERSENSITIVITY SYNDROME

- Also known as DRESS (Drug Rash with Eosinophilia and Systemic Symptoms)
- Usually starts 2 to 8 weeks after initiation of drug therapy
- **Phenytoin, carbamazepine, phenobarbital, sulfonamides, and allopurinol are most commonly implicated**
- **High fever, followed by rash, lymphadenopathy, and internal organ involvement.** Rash may take on various forms and last several weeks; most often present as morbilliform eruption: erythematous papules and macules. Other presentations include pustules, vesicles, bullae, targetoid lesions, or erythroderma.
- Eosinophilia and other hematologic abnormalities (abnormal lymphocyte count, low platelets)
- Internal organ inflammation (liver most common; also can involve kidney, lungs, heart, CNS, GI, endocrine)
- Diagnosis is primarily clinical; laboratory tests can assist: high fever, rash, internal organ involvement, particularly elevated liver function tests, in a patient with exposure to a high-risk medication; eosinophilia is supportive of the diagnosis but not required. Skin biopsy can help in some cases but is not diagnostic.
- Management: prompt withdrawal of the suspected medication and supportive measures; possible role for systemic steroids in severe cases; however, evidence from large trials is lacking. Skin rash may be treated with topical steroids and antihistamines. Maintain fluid and electrolyte homeostasis in patients with widespread skin involvement. Monitor for infections and treat as needed.
- Some studies suggest that a concurrent viral infection (most often HHV-6, among others) may play a role in the development of DRESS
- Be aware of cross-reactivity among anticonvulsants to avoid reexposure. Some evidence of genetic basis for drug hypersensitivity; first-degree relatives should be alerted.

LEVAMISOLE-INDUCED VASCULITIS

- Recently emerging vasculitis caused by levamisole used as a cutting agent in cocaine (estimated 69% of cocaine seized in the United States contains levamisole)
- Purpuric, tender lesions often with a retiform/reticular pattern and central necrosis: most common on ears, nose, cheeks, extremities
- Diagnosis: clinical suspicion warrants screening for cocaine use
- Skin biopsy can be diagnostic: reveals leukocytoclastic vasculitis and thrombotic vasculopathy of small vessels
- Lab abnormalities: neutropenia, elevated erythrocyte sedimentation rate, decreased complement
- Treatment: Discontinuation of cocaine leads to resolution; supportive care; systemic steroids occasionally indicated in severe cases. Beware of increased risk of infection.

Autoimmune Blistering Disorders

Basic Information

- Blisters are fluid-filled skin lesions; small (<0.5 cm) blisters are called vesicles, whereas larger ones are referred to as bullae
- Most acquired forms of disease are autoimmune
- The unifying pathologic abnormality resulting in fluid-filled cavity formation is separation of skin at some level
- One method of classifying these diseases is by their level of tissue disadhesion; some diseases separate within the level of the epidermis; whereas others separate below the epidermis (Table 65-4)

Clinical Presentation, Diagnosis, and Treatment

See Table 65-4.

Cutaneous Manifestations of Internal Disease

CARDIOVASCULAR DISEASE

- LEOPARD syndrome: generalized **l**entigines (brown macules), **e**lectrocardiogram abnormalities, **o**cular hypertelorism, **p**ulmonic stenosis, **a**bnormal genitalia, **r**etardation of growth (dwarfism), and **d**eafness
- LAMB syndrome: generalized **l**entigines, **a**trial myxoma, **m**ucocutaneous myxomas, and **b**lue nevi

65

TABLE 65-4	*Autoimmune Blistering Diseases*			
Disease	**Basic Information**	**Clinical Presentation**	**Diagnosis**	**Treatment**
Subepidermal Blistering Diseases				
Bullous pemphigoid (BP) (Fig. 65-26)	Most common type Typically affects older adults Usually chronic and recurrent Most cases are idiopathic, related to drugs (e.g., diuretics, neuroleptics)	Starts as urticarial eruptions and evolves into crops of tense blisters with urticarial bases The edges of the blister do not extend with gentle manual pressure Often involve the axillae, groin, medial aspects of the thighs, lower legs, and flexor aspects of the forearm Cicatricial pemphigoid is a variant that involves the oral cavity, nasopharynx, or conjunctiva	Skin biopsy showing subepidermal blister with inflammatory cells (including eosinophils) Direct immunofluorescence (DIF) shows linear deposition of IgG and C3 in the epidermal-dermal junction (basement membrane zone)	Disease in some patients is self-limited Corticosteroids (topical or oral) can significantly improve symptoms High risk of complications because of systemic steroid therapy Immunosuppressives may be used
Epidermolysis bullosa acquisita	May be associated with inflammatory bowel disease, rheumatoid arthritis, and SLE	Blisters and erosions induced by minor trauma on the hands and feet Mucosal lesions can be present	Histology is similar to BP DIF and shows IgG at the basement membrane zone NaCl-split skin technique applied to biopsy specimen shows IgG on the dermal side (as opposed to the epidermal side in BP)	Supportive therapy Does not usually respond to immunosuppressives
Dermatitis herpetiformis (Fig. 65-27)	Usually occurs between ages 20 and 50 years Almost all patients have some degree of gluten-sensitive enteropathy (similar to celiac disease) Also associated with a number of other autoimmune disorders Linear IgA dermatosis is a variant associated with medications (e.g., NSAIDs, vancomycin) and not gluten-sensitive enteropathy	Clusters of pruritic, grouped vesicles on the elbows, knees, buttocks, or scalp Mucous membranes usually spared except in cases of linear IgA dermatosis Small-bowel lymphoma in a small number of patients	Histology reveals a subepidermal vesicle with neutrophils and eosinophils in the dermal papillae DIF shows granular IgA deposits at the basement membrane zone	Steroids not helpful Improvement seen with gluten-free diet Dapsone is the treatment of choice

TABLE 65-4	*Autoimmune Blistering Diseases (Continued)*			
Disease	**Basic Information**	**Clinical Presentation**	**Diagnosis**	**Treatment**
Intraepidermal Blistering Diseases				
Pemphigus vulgaris	Usually occurs between the ages of 30 and 60 years Has been associated with myasthenia gravis and thymoma	Begins with painful, nonhealing ulceration of the oral cavity Bullous lesions on the skin usually present months later Bullae are flaccid and rupture easily Pressure placed on the bulla leads to lateral extension of the blister (unlike BP) Nikolsky sign* is positive when done on normal-appearing skin	Histologically there is intraepithelial acantholysis (separation of keratinocytes) Basement membrane is intact DIF reveals deposition of IgG and C3 at the epidermal cell surface Serum antidesmoglein antibodies	Fatal if not treated High-dose systemic corticosteroids initially Long-term steroid use may be needed Adjuvant immunosuppressives can help decrease steroid dose
Drug-induced pemphigus	Associated with penicillamine and captopril	Same as PV or PF	Same as PV or PF	Discontinuation of the drug
Mixed Subepidermal and Intraepidermal Blistering Disease				
Paraneoplastic pemphigus	Associated with lymphomas	Large, tense, bullous lesions on skin Oral and conjunctival involvement can be severe	DIF shows IgG in the intraepidermal layer and C3 involvement of the subepidermal layer	Difficult to treat Steroids are attempted

*Separation of the outer layer of the epidermis from the basal layer with application of minimal pressure to the skin.

BP, Blood pressure; DIF, differential; Ig, immunoglobulin; NSAIDs, nonsteroidal antiinflammatory drugs; PF, pemphigus foliaceus; PV, pemphigus vulgaris; SLE, systemic lupus erythematosus.

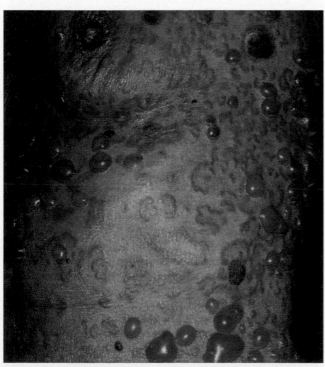

FIGURE 65-26   Bullous pemphigoid.

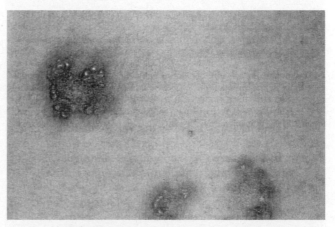

FIGURE 65-27   Dermatitis herpetiformis.

- Pseudoxanthoma elasticum
  - Confluent collections of yellow papules found on the neck, axillae, or other body folds
  - Associated with peripheral vascular disease, stroke, myocardial infarctions, retinal hemorrhages, and GI hemorrhage
- Ehlers-Danlos syndrome
  - Defects in collagen biosynthesis result in hypermobility of joints and hyperelasticity of the skin
  - Associated with abdominal aortic aneurysm and GI hemorrhage

65

PULMONARY DISEASE

- Sarcoidosis (Fig. 65-28) (see Chapter 20)
  - **Lupus pernio: violaceous plaques on the nose, cheeks, and ears**
    - Pathology reveals noncaseating granulomas
    - Course is chronic and requires treatment with intralesional steroids, antimalarials, or methotrexate
  - A number of other cutaneous diseases are seen with sarcoidosis, including EN (see earlier discussion)

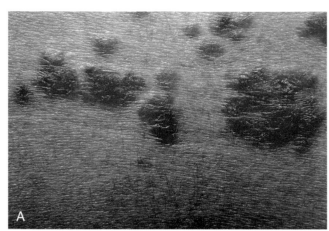
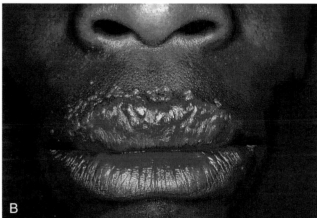
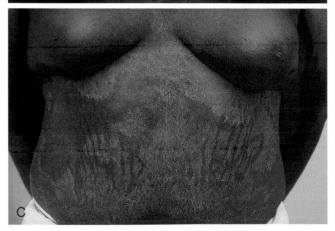

FIGURE 65-28   A to **C,** Cutaneous sarcoidosis. (From Bolognia JL, Jorizzo JL, Rapini RP. *Dermatology.* St. Louis: Mosby; 2003:1457.)

- Yellow nail syndrome: yellow nails, lymphedema, pleural effusions

ENDOCRINE DISEASE

- DM
  - Acanthosis nigricans (Fig. 65-29)
    - Hyperpigmented velvety patches seen predominantly in skin folds such as the axillae, neck, and groin
    - Associated with insulin resistance (type 2 DM)
    - **Also associated with other endocrinopathies (e.g., acromegaly, Cushing syndrome, polycystic ovary, thyroid disease) and GI malignancies**
  - Necrobiosis lipoidica diabeticorum (Fig. 65-30)
    - Multicolored plaques with atrophic centers found on the anterior and lateral aspects of the legs
  - Granuloma annulare
    - Skin-colored or erythematous fine papules that exhibit an annular arrangement
    - Seen on the hands, feet, arms, or legs
    - Diffuse form of granuloma annulare can be associated with DM
  - Stiff hand syndrome
    - Seen in type 1 DM
    - Scleroderma-like tightening of the skin over the hands with limited joint mobility
    - Associated with nephropathy and retinopathy
  - Scleroderma
    - Induration of the skin of the posterior neck and back
    - Usually seen in men with poorly controlled type 2 DM
  - Diabetic dermopathy
    - Hyperpigmented atrophic macules on anterior shins, from trauma

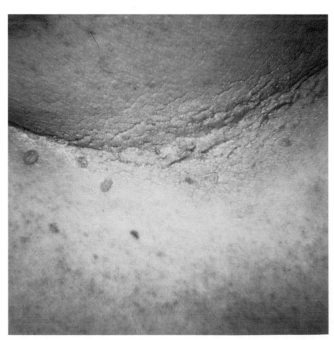

FIGURE 65-29   Acanthosis nigricans.

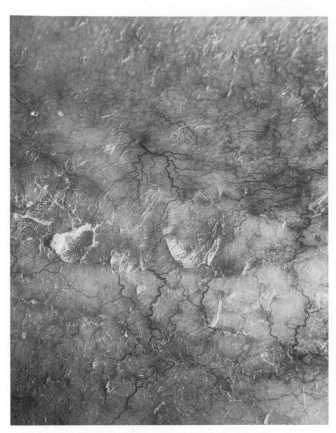

FIGURE 65-30 Necrobiosis lipoidica.

- Bulla diabeticorum
  - Bullae on anterior shins
- Hyperthyroidism
  - Thinning of hair
  - Onycholysis: separation of the nail from the nail bed
  - Pretibial myxedema (if Graves disease): edematous plaques primarily on anterior shins, can also get periorbital myxedema
  - Vitiligo (Fig. 65-31)
    - Depigmentation of skin, with white macules covering small or large amounts of the body surface
    - Can affect the hair and mucous membranes
    - **May be associated with autoimmune disorders (e.g., thyroid disease, type 1 DM, pernicious anemia, and adrenal insufficiency)**
- Hypothyroidism
  - Dull, coarse hair with slow growth
  - Loss of lateral third of eyebrows
  - Dry skin, brittle nails

GASTROINTESTINAL AND LIVER DISEASE

- Inflammatory bowel disease
  - Aphthous stomatitis
  - Pyoderma gangrenosum (Fig. 65-32)
    - Rapidly progressing blue-red ulcers with irregular borders and purulent drainage
    - Can occur at sites of trauma (pathergy)
    - Also seen with inflammatory bowel disease, myeloproliferative disorders, rheumatoid arthritis, and chronic hepatitis; 50% of cases are idiopathic

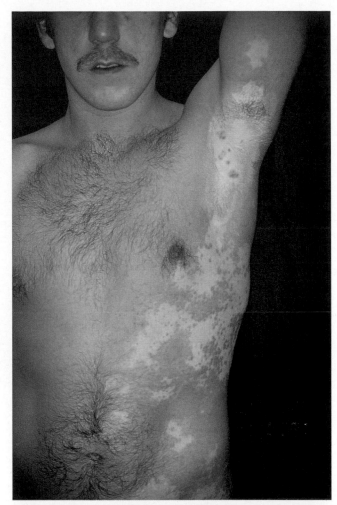

FIGURE 65-31 Vitiligo.

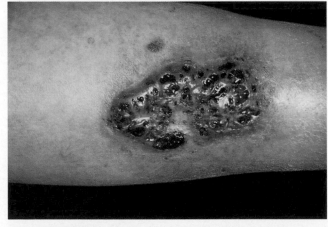

FIGURE 65-32 Pyoderma gangrenosum.

- EN (see earlier discussion)
- Cutaneous Crohn disease
  - Skin lesions with noncaseating granulomas on histology
  - Can take many forms
- Sweet syndrome (febrile neutrophilic dermatosis)
  - Multiple erythematous nodules, most commonly on the head, neck, and upper extremities but can occur anywhere

65

- May be associated with fever, arthritis, arthralgias, myalgias, ocular symptoms, neutrophilic pulmonary alveolitis, sterile osteomyelitis, acute renal failure, aseptic meningitis, and transient involvement of the kidney, liver, and pancreas
    - Also may be associated with infections, malignancy, autoimmune disorders, and pregnancy
- Celiac disease (gluten-sensitive enteropathy)
    - Aphthous stomatitis
    - Dermatitis herpetiformis (see Table 65-4 and Fig. 65-27)
- Hepatitis C infection
    - Porphyria cutanea tarda (Fig. 65-33)
        - Patients may present with fragile skin, vesicles, or bullae (usually on the dorsum of the hands) after minor trauma or sun exposure
        - Hypertrichosis, scleroderma-like induration, hyperpigmentation, and hypopigmentation can all occur as well
        - Also associated with alcohol and drugs (e.g., estrogens)
        - Diagnosis is made by showing elevated uroporphyrin levels
        - Patients who have been diagnosed should be screened for hepatitis C
    - Cryoglobulinemia (see Chapter 44)
    - Lichen planus
    - Pruritus
- Peutz-Jeghers syndrome (Fig. 65-34)
    - **Pigmented macules (freckles) on the lips, oral mucosa, palms, soles, fingers, and toes**
    - Associated with small bowel hamartomas

- Hereditary hemorrhagic telangiectasia (Osler-Weber-Rendu disease)
    - Characterized by telangiectasias on the skin, lungs, GI tract, and CNS
    - Can cause life-threatening bleeding from noncutaneous sites

HEMATOLOGIC DISEASE

- Mastocytosis
    - Cutaneous and visceral infiltration of mast cells
    - **Urticaria pigmentosa: reddish brown macules and papules that can urticate on stroking (Darier sign)**
    - Can cause pruritus, flushing, diarrhea, abdominal pain, and wheezing
    - Diagnosis is made by demonstration of mast cell infiltration on skin biopsy specimen

RENAL DISEASE

- Fabry disease
    - X-linked disorder resulting in deposition of glycosphingolipids in body tissues
    - Causes angiokeratomas (purple papules) on the trunk, extremities, palms, soles, and mucous membranes
    - Also results in paresthesias, renal failure, and cardiovascular disease
- Calciphylaxis (Fig. 65-35)
    - Localized areas of skin necrosis caused by vascular calcification
    - Seen in patients with end-stage renal disease
    - Parathyroidectomy may result in healing
- Nephrogenic systemic fibrosis
    - Thickening and hardening of the skin overlying extremities and trunk caused by fibrosis of the dermis
    - Fibrosis can also affect deeper structures, including muscle, fascia, lungs, and heart
    - Seen exclusively in patients with kidney disease

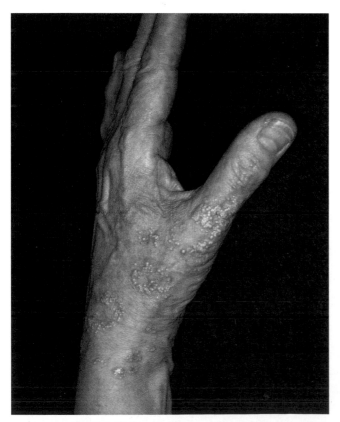

FIGURE 65-33 Porphyria cutanea tarda.

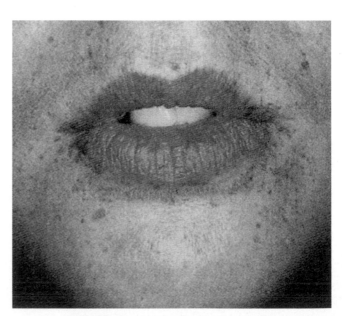

FIGURE 65-34 Peutz-Jeghers syndrome.

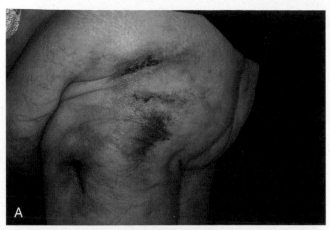

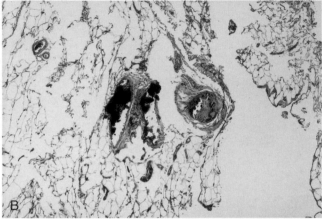

FIGURE 65-35 Calciphylaxis. **A,** Cutaneous. **B,** Histopathology. (From Bolognia JL, Jorizzo JL, Rapini RP. *Dermatology.* St. Louis: Mosby; 2003:694.)

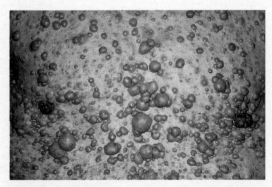

FIGURE 65-36 Neurofibromatosis. (From Bolognia JL, Jorizzo JL, Rapini RP. *Dermatology.* St. Louis: Mosby; 2003:855.)

- **Associated with administration of gadolinium contrast medium for magnetic resonance imaging**
  - Risk is thought to be about 5% after gadolinium exposure in a patient with end-stage renal disease
  - Disease is usually chronic and unremitting
  - No effective treatment at this time

NEUROLOGIC DISEASE

- Neurofibromatosis (Fig. 65-36)
  - Autosomal dominant disease characterized by soft, tan-colored nodules that arise from peripheral nerves

- Cutaneous lesions develop before puberty and increase with age
- Predominantly involves the trunk
- Can be associated with severe pruritus
- **Café-au-lait spots (pigmented patches), axillary freckling, and Lisch nodules (pigmented iris hamartomas) are also seen in most patients**
- Tuberous sclerosis
  - Autosomal dominant disease characterized by skin lesions, mental retardation, seizures, and angiomyolipomas of the kidneys
  - Skin lesions include "adenoma sebaceum" (skin-colored facial papules that are angiofibromas), ash-leaf macules (hypopigmented macules), shagreen patch (connective tissue nevus), and periungual and subungual fibromas

ONCOLOGIC DISEASE

See Table 65-5 for a summary of the dermatologic manifestations of oncologic disease.

RHEUMATOLOGIC DISEASE

- Vasculitis
  - Livedo reticularis (Fig. 65-37)
    - Mottled, blue-purple discoloration in a net-like pattern usually on legs or arms
    - **Can be idiopathic or associated with vasculitis, syphilis, tuberculosis, atheroemboli, or drugs (e.g., amantadine, quinine)**
  - Purpura
    - Caused by extravasation of blood cells into the dermis
    - Nonpalpable purpura and petechiae
      - Primarily caused by thrombocytopenia, disorders of hyperglobulinemia, or disorders of capillary fragility (e.g., amyloidosis, Ehlers-Danlos syndrome, scurvy)
    - Palpable purpura (Fig. 65-38)
      - Seen in vasculitic disorders, embolic disorders (e.g., cholesterol emboli, atrial myxoma, endocarditis), and coagulopathies (e.g., antiphospholipid syndrome)

ITCHING (PRURITUS) IN THE ABSENCE OF A RASH

- Commonly caused by xerosis or xerotic dermatitis ("winter itch")
- Many skin disorders have pruritus as a major finding (atopic dermatitis, infestations such as scabies)
- Localized pruritus without evidence of a rash: notalgia paresthetica (usually located on the upper back)
  - May be a sign of systemic disease (generalized, chronic, and progressive)
  - Biliary/hepatic disease (primary biliary cirrhosis, hepatitis)
  - Renal disease (end-stage renal disease)
  - Lymphoma (Hodgkin lymphoma)
  - Polycythemia vera, myelodysplasia, essential thrombocythemia
  - Thyroid disorder
  - Mastocytosis

TABLE 65-5   *Dermatologic Manifestations of Oncologic Disease (Paraneoplastic Syndromes)*

Skin Disorder	Oncologic Disease(s)	Description
Acanthosis nigricans	Gastric cancer Colon cancer	Velvety hyperpigmentation in axillae, groin, neck Also associated with endocrinopathies (see text)
Acquired ichthyosis	Hodgkin lymphoma Breast, lung, bladder carcinoma	Generalized scaling of the skin, including palms and soles
Bazex syndrome	Squamous cell carcinoma of the pharynx and esophagus Hodgkin lymphoma	Psoriasiform lesions on the hands, feet, ears, and nose
Necrolytic migratory erythema	Glucagonoma	Weeping, eczematous lesions around the mouth, intertriginous areas, flexures, and perigenital area Weight loss, diarrhea, and glossitis also present
Paget disease	Breast: intraduc carcinoma	Breast: erythematous eczematous, and scaly lesions around the nipple
	Extramammary: adnexal cancers, genitourinary cancers, gastrointestinal cancers	Extramammary: erythematous plaques around the vulva, scrotum, or perianal area
Sweet syndrome	Acute myelogenous leukemia	Acute onset of violaceous/erythematous papules or plaques usually on the face, neck, and upper extremities Fever, arthritis, leukocytosis may be present
Tylosis	Esophageal carcinoma	Inherited disorder presenting with yellow, smooth thickening of the palms and soles (palmar-plantar hyperkeratosis)
Tripe palm	Gastric cancer Bronchogenic carcinoma	Velvety thickening of the palms that leads to accentuation of palmar creases

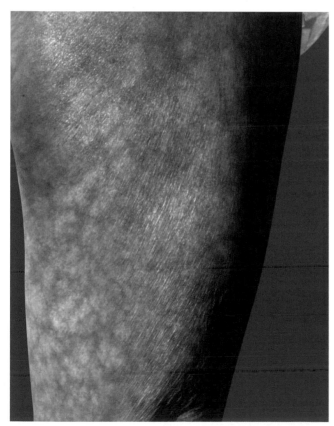

FIGURE 65-37 Livedo reticularis. (From Bolognia JL, Jorizzo JL, Rapini RP. *Dermatology*: St. Louis: Mosby; 2003.)

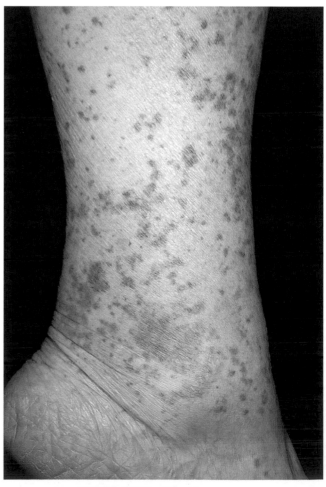

FIGURE 65-38 Palpable purpura.

- Hypereosinophilic syndrome
- DM
- HIV
- Psychogenic pruritus
- Pregnancy-related pruritus

Review Questions

For review questions, please go to ExpertConsult.com.

SUGGESTED READINGS

Bershad S. In the clinic: atopic dermatitis (eczema). *Ann Intern Med.* 2011;155:ITC5-1-ITC5-16.

Habif TB. *Clinical Dermatology.* 5th ed. St. Louis: Elsevier; 2010.

Khan DA. Cutaneous drug reactions. *J Allergy Clin Immunol.* 2012;130:1225-1225.e6.

Nainani N, Panesar M. Nephrogenic systemic fibrosis. *Am J Nephrol.* 2009;29:1-9.

Vary JC, O'Connor KM. Common dermatologic conditions. *Med Clin North Am.* 2014;98:445-485.

Weigle N, McBane S. Psoriasis. *Am Fam Physician.* 2013;87:626-633.

Ophthalmology for the Internist

JAMES P. DUNN, MD

Although most patients with underlying eye disorders are seen regularly by their ophthalmologists, it is imperative that internists recognize ophthalmologic emergencies, ocular manifestations of systemic diseases, and common causes of diminished visual acuity. Timely management and appropriate referral can serve to minimize potential visual loss and other ocular morbidity.

Review of Anatomy and Function

Figure 66-1 shows the cross-sectional anatomy of the eyelids and globe.
- Eyelids
  - Protect the eye
- Conjunctiva
  - Provides lubrication
  - Immunologic functions (conjunctival-associated lymphoid tissue)
- Cornea
  - Most important refractile component of vision
- Anterior chamber and angle
  - Filtration of the aqueous humor through trabecular meshwork
- Lens
  - Responsible for accommodation (focusing for near tasks)
- Uvea (iris, ciliary body, choroid)
  - Produces aqueous humor (ciliary body)
  - Nourishes outer retina
- Retina
  - Converts light to electrical impulses in first stage of visual processing
  - Macula (central retina) much more critical than peripheral retina; the fovea is the center of the macula and subserves central visual acuity
- Optic nerve
  - Connects retinal nerve fibers (approximately 1 million per eye) to the brain
  - The optic disk is nasal to the fovea and is the only visible part of the optic nerve
- Orbit
  - Contains extraocular muscles, adipose tissue, nerves, blood vessels, part of optic nerve

Common Causes of Visual Loss

REFRACTIVE ERROR
- Myopia (nearsightedness): Distance vision is blurred because light rays are focused anterior to the fovea
- Hyperopia (farsightedness): Near vision is blurred because light rays are focused posterior to the fovea
  - In children, accommodation of the ciliary body can overcome mild hyperopia but can induce accommodative esotropia ("crossed eyes")
  - In moderate and severe hyperopia, distance vision is also blurred
- Astigmatism
  - Refraction unequal in different parts of eyeball
  - Cylindrical (toric) lens needed to correct vision
- Presbyopia
  - Age-related diminution in near vision
  - Onset usually noticed around ages 40 to 45 years
- Laser in situ keratomileusis (LASIK) and photorefractive keratectomy (PRK) are used to alter the corneal surface and correct for some refractive errors

CATARACT
Basic Information
- Opacification of the lens of the eye; morphology includes nuclear sclerosis, posterior subcapsular, and cortical
- Most cataracts are age-related (senescent)
- Other causes include steroid use, trauma, diabetes, family history, uveitis, radiation, poor overall nutrition, Wilson disease (sunflower cataract), and prior ocular surgery (especially pars plana vitrectomy)
- Usually bilateral (except for unilateral trauma) with slow progression

Clinical Presentation and Diagnosis
- Symptoms include blurred vision, glare (especially at night), and difficulty with driving, reading, and other visual aspects of daily living
- **No pain or redness except in cases of lens-induced glaucoma or uveitis**
- On examination, visual acuity is impaired; clouding of the lens can often be appreciated with an

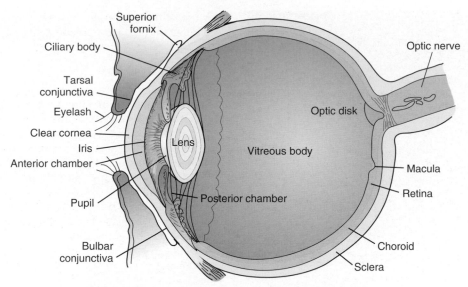

FIGURE 66-1 Cross-sectional anatomy of the eyelids and globe.

ophthalmoscope if slit lamp is unavailable (impairment of normal red reflex and/or difficulty visualizing optic disk and retina)

Treatment

- If refraction does not improve vision, surgery is the only effective treatment
- **Indications for surgery revolve around functional impairment and difficulty with activities of daily living; Snellen acuity (i.e., vision on eye chart) alone is a poor predictor of visual function (or dysfunction)**
  - Uncommonly, cataract surgery is necessary to allow visualization of internal structures of the eye for diagnostic and treatment purposes (e.g., glaucoma, diabetic retinopathy)
  - Cataract surgery reduces the risk of hip fracture within the first year in patients over 65 years of age, presumably from decreased risk of falls
- Standard treatment is phacoemulsification with posterior chamber lens implant (within capsular bag behind the iris)
  - Nearly always performed as outpatient surgery
    - Anesthesia may be general (e.g., in children; in uncooperative or extremely anxious adults), local (e.g., retrobulbar or peribulbar), or topical/intraocular (most common)
    - Surgery performed through peripheral clear cornea using topical or intraocular (intracameral) anesthesia allows patients to remain on anticoagulants such as warfarin or aspirin through cataract surgery; sutureless incisions now common
  - **Intravenous sedation (e.g., midazolam or propofol) is usually required for surgery, but preoperative laboratory testing in otherwise healthy patients is usually unnecessary**
  - Multifocal intraocular lens implants reduce spectacle dependence compared to traditional monofocal implants but cause significantly more dysphotopsias (darkness in the temporal visual field, shimmering or pulsing lights, arc, flare, and central flashes)
- Risk of infection is on order of 0.5% or less (usually within 2 weeks of surgery)
- Patients with good vision in one eye and visual loss from cataract in the fellow eye derive substantial benefit from cataract extraction. Second-eye cataract surgery is an extremely cost-effective procedure when compared with other interventions across medical specialties.

AGE-RELATED MACULAR DEGENERATION

Basic Information

- Two forms of age-related macular degeneration (AMD)
  - Nonneovascular ("dry," atrophic, nonexudative): 90% of cases
    - "Drusen" are deposits of material in the macula that probably represent the accumulation of by-products of photoreceptor metabolism. On ophthalmoscopy, they appear as small, bright yellow objects (Fig. 66-2).
    - "Geographic atrophy" is well-circumscribed area of retinal pigment epithelium or choriocapillaris
  - Neovascular ("wet," exudative): less common, more rapidly progressive
    - Choroidal neovascularization causes retinal pigment epithelial detachment and photoreceptor damage
    - Hypertension and cigarette smoking are risk factors for progression of neovascular AMD
- **Leading cause of legal blindness in patients age 55 years and older in the United States**
- Non-Hispanic blacks over 60 years have a lower incidence of AMD than non-Hispanic whites of the same age
- Two percent of those older than 65 years have vision of 20/200 or less in at least one eye because of AMD; there is a high correlation between severity of AMD in both eyes

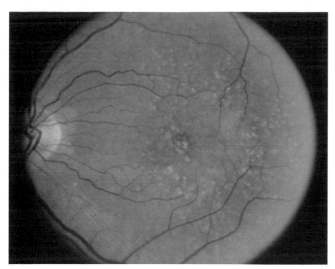

FIGURE 66-2 Drusen in non–neovascular age-related macular degeneration.

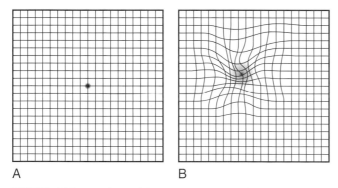

A   B

FIGURE 66-3 Amsler grid for monitoring age-related macular degeneration (AMD). **A,** How it would appear normally. **B,** How it might appear to someone with AMD.

- By 2020, nearly 3 million Americans will have advanced AMD
- Risk factors include increasing age, family history, cigarette smoking, light iris color
- Likely that different genetic (e.g., variants in complement factor H and complement component 3) and environmental factors influence different forms of AMD
- Genotyping may eventually determine which patients will respond best to a given therapy

Clinical Presentation and Diagnosis

- Blurred central vision caused by loss of foveal function
- Distortion of straight lines may be an early presenting complaint
  - Amsler grid has been used to assess progression of disease (Fig. 66-3)
    - The patient covers one eye and focuses the other eye on the center dot of a hand-held copy of the grid; any new distortion in the lines (metamorphopsia) or blind spots (scotoma) suggests progression of disease
- No pain or redness
- Peripheral vision remains intact

- Monitoring of anatomic disease done with retinal photographs, fluorescein and indocyanine angiography, and optical coherence tomography

Treatment

- Nonneovascular AMD
  - **A combination of zinc, vitamins C and E, and beta-carotene (AREDS formula) may reduce the risk of progression from moderate to severe AMD, but has not been shown to reduce the risk of progression of mild to moderate AMD. Additionally, it has no role in primary prevention.**
  - Genetically guided nutritional therapy may eventually replace fixed combinations of zinc and antioxidants
  - Beta-carotene should be avoided in smokers (increased risk of lung cancer)
- Neovascular AMD
  - **Anti–vascular endothelial growth factor (VEGF) agents (bevacizumab, ranibizumab, aflibercept) injected intraocularly (usually monthly) can stabilize AMD and often improve vision, and are now the standard of care for exudative AMD**
  - Bevacizumab is much less expensive than ranibizumab, although systemic adverse effects (stroke, heart attack, hypertension) may be slightly less with ranibizumab compared with bevacizumab
  - Ideal frequency of injections and efficacy of changing from one anti-VEGF agent to another if first agent initially unsuccessful being evaluated in various studies, but lifetime therapy appears necessary, and some patients develop irreversible macular scarring after prolonged anti-VEGF therapy
  - A cumulative effect of high-risk alleles in *CFH*, *ARMS2*, and *VEGFA* may be predictive of a younger age of onset in combination with poor response rates to ranibizumab treatment
  - **Compounding of drugs for intraocular injection may pose risks in terms of drug concentration and purity**
  - Argon laser photocoagulation still used in some cases, but vision loss usually severe because of thermal damage to adjacent retinal tissue
  - Less destructive laser treatments (photodynamic therapy) and intravitreous corticosteroids limited to adjunctive role (e.g., with anti-VEGF agents)
  - Referral to low-vision specialist is highly recommended

Prevention

- Sunglasses or hats to block ultraviolet light possibly helpful
- Control of blood pressure to reduce risk of wet AMD may also be useful
- Cessation of smoking strongly encouraged

Screening

- Comprehensive examination by ophthalmologist recommended every 2 to 4 years for patients ages 40 to 64 years and every 1 to 2 years for patients age 65 years and older

PRIMARY OPEN-ANGLE GLAUCOMA

Basic Information

- **Most common type of glaucoma** (several dozen types overall)
- Some forms are strongly associated with genetic factors (e.g., alterations in *myocilin* gene)
- **Second-leading cause of legal blindness in the United States (and leading cause of legal blindness among African Americans)**
- Primary open-angle glaucoma (POAG) frequently goes undiagnosed
- Definition
  - Slowly progressive optic neuropathy characterized by optic disk cupping
  - Trabecular meshwork is blocked by excess glycosaminoglycan production, decreasing aqueous outflow, but not clinically visible
  - **Elevated intraocular pressure (IOP) and elevated cup-to-disk ratio are risk factors, but not diagnostic of POAG by themselves**
  - Other risk factors include increasing age, African American or Latino heritage (10.3% cumulative probability for African-Americans vs 4.2% for whites), family history, thinner corneas

Clinical Presentation and Diagnosis

- Asymptomatic until late stages, so measurement of visual acuity is not an adequate screening test; a combination of IOP measurement, automated visual field testing, and imaging studies of optic nerve is mandatory
- Central visual loss occurs in end-stage disease
- **No eye pain or redness unless long-standing with corneal edema**
- Rarely causes headache unless IOP is extremely high
- Direct ophthalmoscopy may reveal an enlarged optic cup (cup-to-disk ratio of 0.5 or more is suggestive)
- Screening asymptomatic patients
  - Recommended every 2 to 4 years for patients ages 40 to 64 years, every 1 to 2 years for patients older than 65 years
  - Begin before age 40 years in African Americans

Treatment

- Medical
  - Prostaglandin analogues
  - Aqueous suppressants (topical β-blockers, topical or oral carbonic anhydrase inhibitors)
    - Side effects of oral carbonic anhydrase inhibitors render them poor long-term treatment options
  - Adrenergic agonists (brimonidine, epinephrine derivatives)
  - Cholinergic agonists (e.g., pilocarpine) now used infrequently because of side effects
  - **Need to be aware of potential systemic effects of medications (Table 66-1)**
- Laser therapy (argon laser trabeculoplasty, selective laser trabeculoplasty)
  - Easy to perform with low risk
  - Effect may only be temporary

TABLE 66-1	*Side Effects of Common Ocular Medications*
Drug	**Effects**
β-Adrenergic blocking agents	Bronchospasm Bradycardia Hypotension Fatigue, depression Erectile dysfunction
Corticosteroids	Glaucoma Cataracts Corneal infection
Anesthetics	Poor epithelial healing Corneal melting (with chronic use)
Aminoglycosides	Toxic or allergic keratoconjunctivitis
α-Agonists	Hypotension Dry mouth Dizziness
Oral carbonic anhydrase inhibitors	Fatigue, depression Hypokalemia Acidosis Nausea Aplastic anemia (rare)

- Surgical therapy (trabeculectomy, tube shunt surgery, or canaloplasty) all carry a small but lifetime risk of endophthalmitis

NARROW-ANGLE GLAUCOMA

Basic Information

- One-tenth as common as open-angle glaucoma in the United States
- Seen in Asians and native Alaskan Aleutians more commonly than whites or African-Americans

Clinical Presentation

- **Manifests with pain, redness, halos, and decreased visual acuity because of rapid elevation in eye pressure and corneal edema**
- Headache, nausea, and vomiting are commonly present
- **Attack may be precipitated by mydriatic, sympathomimetic, and hypnotic medications**
  - Warnings about glaucoma risk with these medications apply to narrow-angle, not open-angle, glaucoma

Treatment

- Prostaglandin analogs and carbonic anhydrase inhibitors may temporarily reduce IOP and pain and decrease corneal edema
- Requires urgent referral to ophthalmologist for laser iridotomy (and prophylactic laser treatment in opposite eye)

DIABETIC RETINOPATHY

Basic Information

- Leading cause of blindness in patients ages 20 to 60 years in the United States

66

- **Risk of retinopathy directly related to duration of diabetes in both type 1 and type 2**
  - After 20 years of diabetes, more than 60% of patients with type 2 disease and nearly all patients with type 1 disease have some degree of retinopathy
  - Among diabetics older than 40 years of age, prevalence rates for diabetic retinopathy and sight-threatening retinopathy are 40.3% and 8.2%, respectively
- Level of glycemic control very important
  - Once retinopathy is present, degree of glucose control is a better predictor of progression to more serious disease than is duration of disease
  - Intensive therapy reduces onset and slows progression of retinopathy
  - Gestational diabetes is not associated with development of retinopathy, but pregnancy may exacerbate preexisting retinopathy

Clinical Presentation and Diagnosis

- Screening recommendations
  - Yearly dilated funduscopic examination for all diabetics
  - More frequent examinations if retinopathy is present
- Nonproliferative ("background," "preproliferative") retinopathy
  - Cotton-wool spots, microaneurysms, intraretinal hemorrhages, lipid ("hard") exudates, retinal edema, venous beading, and intraretinal microvascular abnormalities can be seen (Fig. 66-4)
  - 30% of patients blind after 5 years because of ischemia or macular edema
- Proliferative
  - Retinal vascularization caused by elaboration of angiogenic factors
  - 30% of patients blind after 5 years because of vitreous hemorrhage, retinal detachment, or neovascular glaucoma (angle closed by neovascularization)

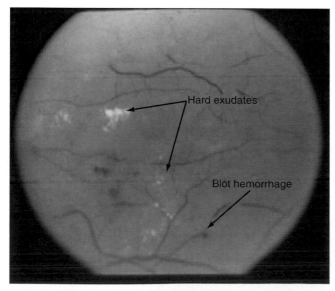

FIGURE 66-4 Nonproliferative diabetic retinopathy.

Treatment

- **Optimal control of diabetes, hypertension, and hyperlipidemia is crucial**
- Grid or focal laser photocoagulation more effective than intraocular corticosteroids for leaking vessels causing macular edema
- Intravitreal injections of VEGF antagonists (bevacizumab, ranibizumab, aflibercept) increasingly used to treat diabetic macular edema (often in combination with focal or grid laser); role in proliferative diabetic retinopathy unclear, but can be especially helpful as short-term therapy in patients with neovascular glaucoma or vitreous hemorrhage requiring surgery to reduce intraoperative bleeding and in diabetics with macular edema to reduce worsening after cataract surgery
- **Panretinal laser photocoagulation proven effective for proliferative retinopathy**
  - Most effective when patient has just reached high-risk proliferative diabetic retinopathy or before vision decreases caused by macular edema
  - Laser photocoagulation may stabilize vision loss but often does not restore vision
- Anti-VEGF agents with or without laser more effective than laser alone for diabetic macular edema
- Sustained-release fluocinolone acetonide intravitreal implant shown to reduce diabetic macular edema and can be considered if other treatments fail; long-term risks include cataract, exposure of implant, infection, and glaucoma
- Surgical treatment (often combined with laser photocoagulation) necessary to remove vitreous hemorrhage and repair retinal detachments

OCULAR INFLAMMATORY DISEASE (UVEITIS AND SCLERITIS)

- "Uveitis" includes inflammation of uveal tract (iris, ciliary body, choroid) as well as retina
  - **Signs/symptoms vary widely, including acute pain and redness (ciliary flush), floaters, blurred or distorted vision, but may be asymptomatic in early disease**
  - Complications include cataract, glaucoma, synechiae (scarring of iris to cornea or lens), hypotony, iris and retinal neovascularization, and retinal detachment
  - May be part of systemic disease or isolated ocular disease
  - Commonly associated systemic diseases include sarcoidosis, seronegative spondyloarthopathy, and juvenile rheumatoid arthritis. May be initial manifestation of systemic disease process such as ankylosing spondylitis.
  - Always consider infectious causes (e.g., syphilis, tuberculosis, herpes viruses) as well
  - Work-up should be parsimonious and based on symptoms, duration, onset (sudden or insidious), careful examination, and through review of systems
- Scleritis usually isolated to sclera but can involve cornea and internal structures of eye as well

- Always consider infectious causes (e.g., syphilis, tuberculosis, herpes viruses) and trauma
- **Signs/symptoms usually include sectoral or diffuse redness and severe, throbbing pain (anterior scleritis) but may be less severe in posterior scleritis or even painless in scleromalacia perforans in older patients with rheumatoid arthritis**
- Commonly associated systemic diseases include rheumatoid arthritis, systemic lupus erythematosus, and granulomatous polyangiitis

Treatment

- Corticosteroids
  - Topical (anterior uveitis)
  - Periocular injections (intermediate/posterior uveitis)
  - Intravitreal injections (intermediate/posterior/ panuveitis)
  - Sustained-release dexamethasone or fluocinolone acetonide implants (intermediate/posterior/panuveitis requiring chronic therapy)
  - Oral (intermediate/posterior/panuveitis, scleritis)
  - Intravenous (severe, vision-threatening disease, usually for 3 days followed by high-dose oral therapy)
- Nonsteroidal antiinflammatory agents
  - Anterior scleritis
  - Generally not helpful for uveitis
- Immunosuppressive therapy
  - Antimetabolites (methotrexate, mycophenolate mofetil, azathioprine)
  - Calcineurin inhibitors (cyclosporine, tacrolimus)
  - Alkylating agents (chlorambucil, cyclophosphamide)
  - Biologics (antitumor necrosis factor agents, interleukin antagonists, rituximab)
  - Use of these drugs requires careful monitoring for toxicity and should be limited to patients with severe, chronic disease unresponsive or intolerant to other therapies

CAUSES OF SUDDEN VISUAL LOSS

- **Usually monocular; patient may not recognize immediately if contralateral eye is normal**
- Can result from a number of different conditions (Box 66-1)

BOX 66-1	*Causes of Sudden Visual Loss*

Transient (Amaurosis Fugax)

Emboli (endocarditis, cholesterol or calcific plaques, cardiac myxoma, platelet-fibrin thrombi)

Vasospasm (migraine, subarachnoid hemorrhage, hypertensive crisis)

Sustained

Optic neuritis (MS, lupus, sarcoidosis)

Anterior ischemic optic neuropathy

Arteritic: associated with giant-cell arteritis

Nonarteritic: associated with advancing age, hypertension

Hemorrhage (neovascular AMD, vitreous hemorrhage in diabetes)

Occipital infarct

AMD, Age-related macular degeneration; MS, multiple sclerosis.

Red Eye

See Table 66-2.

Eye Infections

HERPES SIMPLEX VIRUS

Basic Information and Clinical Presentation

- Major cause of blindness because of keratitis (infection of cornea)
- Usually caused by herpes simplex virus type 1 (HSV-1)
- **Unilateral redness, with a dendritic pattern on fluorescein staining, is pathognomonic (Fig. 66-5)**
- Recurrences frequent
- May also cause acute retinal necrosis

Treatment

- Trifluoridine 1% eye drops or ganciclovir 0.15% gel for 14 days for keratitis
- **Avoid topical corticosteroids (can cause exacerbation of HSV infection)**
- Suppressive oral antiviral therapy (valacyclovir 500 mg/day or equivalent) may help reduce recurrences

HERPES ZOSTER VIRUS

Basic Information

- Herpes zoster ophthalmicus (HZO) can threaten vision if there is vesicular eruption along any branch of the trigeminal nerve (V_1 most commonly affected single dermatome in zoster)
- Ocular complications include keratitis, uveitis, scleritis, acute retinal necrosis, optic neuritis, and extraocular muscle palsies
- Postherpetic neuralgia more common in HZO than with lower extremity zoster
- Widespread use of zoster vaccine may ultimately reduce risk of HZO

Treatment

- Treat with valacyclovir or similar antiviral therapy
  - Most effective if given within 72 hours of outbreak of vesicles

OCULAR COMPLICATIONS OF HUMAN IMMUNODEFICIENCY VIRUS INFECTION

Basic Information and Clinical Presentation

- Noninfectious retinopathy (background human immunodeficiency virus [HIV] retinopathy)
  - **Most common ocular manifestation of HIV infection**
  - Occurs in 50% to 100% of patients with CD4 counts less than 200 cells/mm^3
  - Clinical features: cotton-wool spots, intraretinal hemorrhages
  - Symptoms: none
  - Clinical marker of advanced immunosuppression

66

TABLE 66-2 | *Differential Diagnosis of the Red Eye*

	Allergic Conjunctivitis	Bacterial Conjunctivitis	Viral Conjunctivitis	Corneal Ulcer	Anterior Uveitis	Acute Glaucoma	Anterior Scleritis
Symptoms/ findings	Bilateral, itchy eyes	Prominent discharge; no itching or adenopathy	Itching, preauricular adenopathy	Irregular corneal light reflex	Photophobia with ciliary flush	Headache, nausea, vomiting	Pain can be worse at night
Vision	Usually normal	Usually normal	May be impaired	Impaired	Slightly blurred	Decreased	Normal
Discharge	Watery	Mucopurulent	Watery	Tearing or purulent	Tearing	Tearing	None
Pain	None	Minimal	Minimal	Present	Photophobia	Severe	Severe
Pupil size/ shape	Normal	Normal	Normal	Normal	Miotic or irregular	Mid-dilated	Normal
Pupillary responses	Normal	Normal	Normal	Normal	May be nonreactive	Nonreactive	Normal
Redness	Diffuse	Diffuse	Segmental or diffuse	Localized or diffuse	Ciliary flush*	Diffuse with ciliary flush	Local or diffuse
Management/ comments	Eliminate allergen Topical antihistamines or mast cell stabilizers	Topical antibiotics to cover *S. aureus, S. pneumoniae, H. influenzae*	Supportive Avoid close contact with other people for 7 to 14 days	Associated with trauma, contact lenses, topical steroid use; may require fortified topical antibiotics	Topical corticosteroids† and cycloplegics Systemic work-up usually necessary to assess for rheumatologic disease or sarcoid	Aqueous suppressants Laser Surgical iridectomy	Systemic corticosteroids or NSAIDs Systemic work-up usually necessary to assess for rheumatologic disease or sarcoid

*Ring of injection around the limbus.
†Topical corticosteroids should never be used to treat a red eye without a specific diagnosis because they may cause glaucoma, cataract, or recurrent herpetic keratitis.
NSAIDS, Nonsteroidal antiinflammatory drugs.

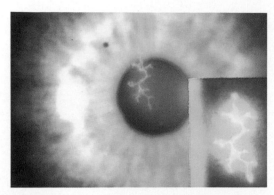

FIGURE 66-5 Dendritic pattern of herpes virus keratitis after fluorescein staining. *Inset* shows pattern after passing through cobalt blue filter. (From Goldman L, Bennett JC, Ausiello D. *Cecil Textbook of Medicine.* 22nd ed. Philadelphia: Saunders; 2004: Fig. 465-10.)

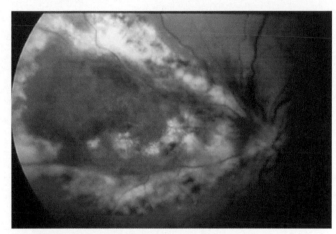

FIGURE 66-6 Cytomegalovirus retinitis in patient with acquired immunodeficiency syndrome (note mixed hemorrhage and necrosis with optic nerve infiltration).

- Need to rule out other causes of retinopathy (e.g., diabetes, hypertension, cytomegalovirus [CMV])
- CMV retinitis
  - **Most common ocular opportunistic infection in acquired immune deficiency syndrome (AIDS)**
  - CD4 count usually less than 50 cells/mm^3
  - Floaters, flashing lights, blind spots (no pain, discharge, or redness) common
    - 15% to 50% of patients are asymptomatic
    - No external signs of inflammation
  - Retinal examination reveals white, fluffy lesions associated with hemorrhage (Fig. 66-6)
  - Some clinicians recommend screening at-risk patients (CD4 count less than 100 cells/mm^3) every 6 months

Treatment

- Systemic
  - Oral valganciclovir (intravenous foscarnet if ganciclovir resistance or intolerance to oral therapy)
  - Reduces morbidity (extraocular disease), mortality, and second-eye involvement
- Local
  - Intravitreous ganciclovir or foscarnet injections (off-label use)

- Effect of highly active antiretroviral therapy (HAART)
  - Reduces risk of ocular complications
  - CMV retinitis in less than 5% of patients versus more than 30% in pre-HAART era
  - In patients responsive and adherent to HAART (CD4$^+$ count consistently higher than 100 cells/mm^3), chronic anti-CMV therapy usually not necessary
  - Immune recovery uveitis (IRU) occurs in minority of eyes with CMV retinitis in patients responsive to HAART
    - Syndrome of uveitis, vitreitis, macular edema, and epiretinal membrane formation
    - Risk factors for IRU unclear

BACTERIAL AND VIRAL CONJUNCTIVITIS

See Table 66-2.

Disease of the Eyelid

BLEPHARITIS

Basic Information and Clinical Presentation

- Noninfectious lid margin inflammation (bacterial superinfection can occur)
- Symptoms: crusting, irritation, chronic redness
- Common in patients with seborrhea, eczema, and rosacea

Treatment

- Warm compresses, lid scrubs; antibiotic ointment (erythromycin, bacitracin) if superinfection suggested; topical azithromycin drops may be helpful on chronic basis

HORDEOLUM

Basic Information and Clinical Presentation

- Internal hordeolum: infection of meibomian gland on the conjunctival side of the eyelid
- External hordeolum (stye): infection of gland and eyelash follicle on skin side of the lid
- *Staphylococcus aureus* is the organism most commonly responsible for infection
- Symptoms: pain, focal lid erythema; globe unaffected; patients often also have blepharitis

Treatment

- Warm compresses, topical antibiotics (e.g., erythromycin)

CHALAZION

Basic Information and Clinical Presentation

- Focal, noninfectious blockage of meibomian gland
- Symptoms: nontender swelling of lid (unless superinfected)
- Upper lid more commonly affected
- Commonly associated with acne rosacea

TABLE 66-3	*Ocular Manifestations of Rheumatologic Disease*	
Condition	**Description**	**Associated Diseases**

Keratoconjunctivitis sicca	Reduced or absent tear production
	Burning sensation in eye
	Photophobia may be present
	Eye(s) may be red
	Symptoms of dry mouth may also be present
	  and are suggestive of Sjögren syndrome
		Primary Sjögren syndrome
		Secondary Sjögren syndrome
		  Rheumatoid arthritis
		  Systemic lupus erythematosus
		  Polyarteritis nodosa
		  Scleroderma

Episcleritis and scleritis	Episcleritis
	  Redness of eye usually limited
	  Painless
	Scleritis
	  Redness more diffuse
	  Painful
		Rheumatoid arthritis
		Systemic lupus erythematosus
		Wegener granulomatosus
		Polyarteritis nodosa
		Relapsing polychondritis
		Seronegative spondyloarthropathies
		Inflammatory bowel disease

Uveitis (see Fig. 66-7)	Pain Redness Photophobia Ciliary flush—ring of injection around limbus	Sarcoidosis (bilateral) Seronegative spondyloarthropathies (unilateral) Behçet disease Lyme disease (bilateral) Syphilis
Keratitis	Inflammation of the cornea May lead to ulceration Vision affected	Systemic lupus erythematosus Wegener granulomatosus Polyarteritis nodosa Syphilis
Anterior ischemic optic neuropathy	Sudden loss of vision	Giant-cell arteritis Systemic lupus erythematosus

Treatment

- Warm compresses; incision and drainage if chronic and bothersome

BASAL CELL CARCINOMA

Basic Information and Clinical Presentation

- Most common eyelid tumor
- Usually occurs on lower lid or medial canthus

Treatment

- Surgical excision preferred to radiation or cryoablation

OCULAR SIDE EFFECTS OF SYSTEMIC THERAPY

Basic Information and Clinical Presentation

- Regular ophthalmic screening indicated in patients taking systemic corticosteroids (glaucoma, cataract), antimalarials (retinopathy), and ethambutol (optic neuropathy)
- Bisphosphonates have occasionally been associated with development of scleritis and uveitis
- Topiramate can cause angle-closure glaucoma

Treatment

- Cessation of drug therapy if possible (e.g., change from oral corticosteroid therapy to steroid-sparing immunosuppressive therapy)
- Cataract surgery for steroid-induced cataract as necessary
- Topical glaucoma therapy for steroid-induced glaucoma; surgery may be necessary in more severe cases

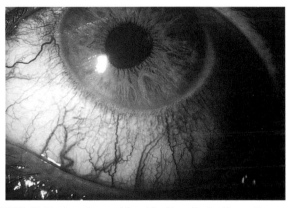

FIGURE 66-7 Anterior uveitis with ciliary flush. (From Henry MM, Thompson JN. *Clinical Surgery.* 22nd ed. Philadelphia: Saunders; 2005: Fig. 36.14.)

Eye in Rheumatologic Disease

See Table 66-3. See Figure 66-7 for an example of anterior uveitis.

Review Questions

For review questions, please go to ExpertConsult.com.

SUGGESTED READINGS

Age-Related Eye Disease Study Group. A randomized, placebo-controlled, clinical trial of high dose supplementation with vitamins C and E and beta-carotene for age-related cataract and vision loss, AREDS report no. 9. *Arch Ophthalmol.* 2001;119:1439-1452.
Arevalo JF. Diabetic macular edema: changing treatment paradigms. *Curr Opin Ophthalmol.* 2014;25:502-507.

Brown GC, Brown MM, Menezes A, et al. Cataract surgery cost utility revisited in 2012: a new economic paradigm. *Ophthalmology.* 2013;120:2367-2376.

Congdon N, O'Colmain B, Klaver CC, et al. for the Eye Diseases Prevalence Research Group. The Diabetes Control and Complications Trial/Epidemiology of Diabetes Interventions and Complications Research Group: retinopathy and nephropathy in patients with type 1 diabetes 4 years after a trial of intensive therapy. *N Engl J Med.* 2000;342:381-389.

Gelston CD. Common eye emergencies. *Am Fam Physician.* 2013;88:515-519.

Marmor MF, Kellner U, Lai TY, et al. Revised recommendations on screening for chloroquine and hydroxychloroquine retinopathy. *Ophthalmology.* 2011;118:415-422.

Martinez-Zapata MJ, Martí-Carvajal AJ, Solà I, et al. Anti-vascular endothelial growth factor for proliferative diabetic retinopathy. *Cochrane Database Syst Rev.* 2014;(11):CD008721.

Miguel A, Henriques F, Azevedo LF, et al. Ophthalmic adverse drug reactions to systemic drugs: a systematic review. *Pharmacoepidemiol Drug Saf.* 2014;23:221-233.

Tseng VL, Yu F, Lum F, et al. Risk of fractures following cataract surgery in Medicare beneficiaries. *JAMA.* 2012;308:493-501.

Psychiatry for the Internist

PAUL S. NESTADT, MD; THOMAS W. KOENIG, MD; and
O. JOSEPH BIENVENU, MD, PhD

Psychological and social problems are pervasive in our society. **An estimated 25% of adults experience some form of mental illness at some time in their lives.** This chapter provides the basic framework for diagnosing and treating a number of common conditions, including disorders of mood, anxiety, somatization, body image, and psychosis. Additionally, issues involving the care of victims of domestic violence will be addressed.

Mood Disorders

DEPRESSION

Basic Information

- Everyone experiences periods in life when he or she feels "depressed"
- Depression is a symptom, not a diagnosis
- "Pathologic depression" refers to a condition that results in limitations to a person's functioning (i.e., social, occupational, or physical)
- **Major depression is seen in up to 15% of all outpatients and inpatients**
- Risk factors for major depressive disorders
  - History of a major depressive disorder in the past
  - Female gender: Major depressive episodes occur in women twice as often as in men
  - Family history of a depressive illness in a first-degree relative
- A pathologic depressive episode can be triggered by a stressful life event, but can also occur without apparent cause
- A number of medical conditions have been associated with depression, including coronary artery disease, stroke, diabetes, human immunodeficiency virus (HIV), cancer, fibromyalgia, chronic fatigue syndrome, dementia, other neurodegenerative disorders such as Parkinson disease, and hypothyroidism (including subclinical disease)
  - Treatment of the underlying medical disorder may lead to improvement in the depressive symptoms in many cases
- A number of medications (e.g., β-blockers, glucocorticoids, opioids, and interferon) and illicit substances have also been associated with depression

Clinical Presentation and Diagnosis

- Can coexist with other mental disorders (e.g., anxiety, somatization)

- The evaluation begins with an assessment of functional impairment and inquiry into the presence of a number of symptoms (Box 67-1)
- **Before making the diagnosis of a primary depressive disorder, inquiry should be made into substance misuse, underlying medical disorders, and medication use**
- Depression can be divided into three main groups: major depression, persistent depression (formerly dysthymia), and atypical depression (see Box 67-1)
  - Grief reactions are normal responses that are not considered depressive disorders, but they may progress to major depressive episodes (Box 67-2)
- **If the diagnosis of major depression is suggested, screening for the possibility of bipolar disorder (see following discussion) is recommended**
- Suicidal or homicidal risk should also be assessed
  - Questioning a patient about suicidality does NOT plant the idea or increase a patient's likelihood of considering suicide, but in fact this screening is necessary to identify at-risk patients
  - Up to 15% of patients with untreated depression commit suicide
  - Epidemiologic studies reveal increased suicide risk in persons with the following characteristics:
    - Previous history of suicide attempt
    - Coexisting anxiety or panic disorder
    - Substance use disorder
    - Age older than 65 years
    - White or Native American
    - Living alone (e.g., single, divorced)
    - A recent stressful life event
    - Family history of completed suicide
  - If suicidal or homicidal ideation is present, an assessment of the patient's plan for such action should be obtained
  - **Patients with an imminent risk of suicide should be immediately referred for emergent psychiatric evaluation**

Treatment

- The first step is an open discussion of and education about depression with the patient, in an effort to minimize reluctance to accepting therapy
  - Emphasizing that clinical depression is a medical illness that affects numerous individuals should assist in such discussions
- Psychotherapy
  - Many different types of therapy (e.g., cognitive, behavioral, interpersonal, and group)

Symptoms and Classification of Depression

Symptoms of a Depressive Episode

Depressed mood
Markedly diminished interest or pleasure (anhedonia)
Significant weight loss or weight gain
Insomnia or hypersomnia
Mental and physical agitation or slowing
Fatigue or loss of energy
Feelings of worthlessness or guilt
Poor concentration or indecisiveness
Recurrent thoughts of death or suicidal ideation

Major Depressive Disorder

Depressed mood or anhedonia must be present
At least five of the nine symptoms of a depressive episode should be present
Symptoms persist for most of the day, every day, for >2 weeks
Seasonal affective disorder is a subclassification used when patients present with recurrent depressive episodes at characteristic times of the year

Persistent Depressive Disorder (Formerly Dysthymia)

Depressed mood >2 years
Symptoms less severe than with major depression
Anhedonia, low self-esteem, and low energy are commonly present

Atypical Depression*

Most common mood disorder
Symptoms persist for most of the day, every day, for >2 weeks
Less than five of the nine symptoms of a depressive episode are seen

*Includes the subcategory minor depression.
Modified from Task Force on DSM-V. *The Diagnostic and Statistical Manual of Mental Disorders.* 5th ed. Arlington, VA: American Psychiatric Association; 2013.

- Effective as the sole mode of therapy for milder presentations of major depression
- For more severe presentations, medications should be combined with psychotherapy
- Medications
  - A number of antidepressant medications are currently available with roughly equivalent efficacy rates (Table 67-1)
  - Many factors should be considered when choosing a specific antidepressant
    - Patient's previous success with a specific medication
    - Coexisting medical conditions
    - Potential drug interactions
    - Cost
    - Anticipated side effects
    - History of response of a family member to a particular agent
  - A response is usually seen within 6 to 8 weeks after a therapeutic dose of antidepressant is attained
    - Initially, patients may not report any improvement in mood or anhedonia, but questioning may reveal improvement in other symptoms, such as energy

Grief and Bereavement Reactions

Are considered normal responses to loss of a person from a close relationship (usually a spouse)
Usually resolves within a few months of the death
In the past, bereavement was considered pathologic if grieving persisted for >2 months, but modern criteria allow the use of clinical judgment based on the individual's history and cultural norms to guide diagnosis
Normal grief is characterized by momentary wellings (pangs) of dysphoria that decrease in frequency and intensity over weeks to months, and a preservation of self-esteem
Complicated grief reactions involve the persistence of symptoms (e.g., preoccupation with thoughts of the deceased, auditory or visual hallucinations of the deceased, difficulty accepting the death)
The risk of major depression is very high (up to 35%) within the first year of the loss of a loved one, and highest with the loss of a child

level, sleep, appetite, anxiety, or ability to concentrate
  - If there has been a partial response to therapy, the medication dosage can be increased, the medication can be changed, psychotherapy can be added, or medication augmentation therapy can be added (see following discussion)
  - If there is absolutely no response to therapy within 8 weeks, another medication should be chosen
- **The duration of therapy is usually 6 to 12 months. Patients with a history of recurrent major depressive episodes should be considered for maintenance therapy.**
- Tapering of medications is usually necessary to prevent the return of depressive symptoms and withdrawal symptoms
- Electroconvulsive therapy (ECT)
  - Typically used for severe depression or cases refractory to other therapies
  - Requires general anesthesia
  - Typically requires 6 to 12 treatments over the course of 2 to 4 weeks
  - Patients usually require antidepressant treatment following a course of ECT to prevent relapse
  - Some patients benefit from "maintenance ECT" when medication trials have failed
- Augmentation therapy
  - Considered when there is a partial response to antidepressant therapy
  - A number of medications have been shown to be useful in conjunction with standard antidepressants (e.g., lithium, triiodothyronine, pindolol, and methylphenidate)

BIPOLAR AFFECTIVE DISORDER
Basic Information

- Refers to the occurrence (and recurrence) of manic or hypomanic episodes, usually alternating with episodes of depression
- Affects 1% of the population

TABLE 67-1	Antidepressant Medications		
Drug Class	**Examples**	**Side Effects**	**Comments**
Selective serotonin reuptake inhibitors (SSRIs)	Escitalopram Citalopram Fluoxetine Paroxetine Sertraline Luvoxamine	Nausea, vomiting, diarrhea Sweating Headache Sedation or agitation Sexual dysfunction Serotonin syndrome*	Widely used because of tolerability and ease of use Also effective for cases of anxiety and panic disorder Can raise levels of many drugs including anticonvulsants, digoxin, warfarin, antiarrhythmics, β-blockers
Serotonin/ norepinephrine reuptake inhibitors	Venlafaxine Desvenlafaxine Duloxetine	Nausea, vomiting, diarrhea Headache Insomnia Hypertension	Activating rather than sedating, so good for "understimulated" patients
Norepinephrine and dopamine reuptake inhibitor	Bupropion	Dry mouth Constipation Dizziness Weight loss Seizures (at high doses)	Also used for smoking cessation Low incidence of sexual dysfunction Activating rather than sedating Avoid in patients with eating or seizure disorders
Norepinephrine and serotonin antagonist	Mirtazapine	Sedation Weight gain Orthostatic hypotension	Low incidence of sexual dysfunction
Serotonin antagonist and reuptake inhibitor	Trazodone Nefazodone	Sedation Orthostatic hypotension Dry mouth Liver damage or failure (nefazodone) Priapism (trazodone)	Low incidence of sexual dysfunction
Serotonin reuptake inhibitor with multimodal serotonin receptor effects	Vilazodone Vortioxetine	Nausea, vomiting, diarrhea Headache Dry mouth Sleep disturbance Sexual dysfunction Serotonin syndrome	New to market, with literature showing equal efficacy to other antidepressants, but variances of side effect profiles still require further research
Norepinephrine/ serotonin reuptake inhibitors (tricyclic antidepressants)	Amitriptyline Imipramine Desipramine Nortriptyline Doxepin	Orthostatic hypotension Dry mouth Blurry vision Constipation Sedation Weight gain Urinary retention Sexual dysfunction QT prolongation and arrhythmias	Need to titrate dose and follow blood levels Should avoid in patients with cardiac disease Can be useful in patients with coexisting illnesses such as insomnia, migraine, panic disorder, neuropathic pain
Monoamine oxidase inhibitors	Phenelzine Tranylcypromine Selegiline Isocarboxazid	Orthostatic hypotension Dry mouth Constipation Sedation Urinary retention Sexual dysfunction Hypertensive crisis with intake of tyramine-rich foods, meperidine, decongestants, SSRIs	Useful for "atypical depression" (hypersomnia, overeating, worsening depression in the evenings, prominent anxiety) Can treat hypertensive crisis with phentolamine

*Serotonin syndrome is a change in mental status, diaphoresis, rigors, hyperreflexia, and tachycardia because of hyperstimulation of brainstem serotonin receptors caused by coadministration of an SSRI and another agent that increases serotonin levels.

- First episode usually occurs in the second or third decade of life, and depression is most common as the index episode

Clinical Presentation and Diagnosis

- **Mania consists of a persistently elevated, expansive, or irritable mood and three of the following lasting at least 1 week:**
  - Inflated self-esteem
  - Decreased need for sleep
  - Flight of ideas or racing thoughts

- Hypertalkativeness, pressured speech
- Distractibility
- Psychomotor agitation, hyperactivity, or increased activity
- Excessive involvement in pleasurable activities (e.g., sexual indiscretions, spending money)
- May involve psychotic symptoms (delusions and/or hallucinations)
- Hypomania is considered an abnormal elevation of mood but not to the extent that it seriously impairs functioning

- Hypomanic episodes must last at least 4 days
- Delusions and hallucinations do not occur in hypomania
- Classification of bipolar disorder
  - Type I: positive history of at least one manic episode, with or without past major depressive episodes
  - Type II: positive history of at least one episode of major depression and at least one hypomanic episode
- Need to evaluate the patient for medical conditions and drug use that may mimic bipolar disorder (e.g., substance misuse, personality disorders, thyrotoxicosis, steroid-induced mania)
- "Mood swings" within the same day do not, on their own, qualify as bipolar disorder

Treatment

- Lithium carbonate
  - Most studied mood stabilizer
  - Also has antidepressant effects
  - Side effects include gastrointestinal (GI) distress (nausea, vomiting, diarrhea), sedation, weight gain, acne, bradycardia, diabetes insipidus (polyuria, polydipsia, hypernatremia), hypothyroidism, renal insufficiency, and benign leukocytosis
  - **A creatinine level, thyroid function tests, electrocardiogram, and pregnancy test (if appropriate) should be obtained before beginning therapy**
  - Drug levels must be monitored
- Anticonvulsants (e.g., carbamazepine, valproic acid) can also be effective; lamotrigine shows promise as a treatment for bipolar depression
- Antipsychotics (e.g., olanzapine, quetiapine, lurasidone) can also be used
- **Antidepressants for bipolar depression should be used cautiously, as they can precipitate a manic or "mixed" state or "rapid cycling"**
- ECT can be helpful during an acute manic episode, as well
- Psychotherapy, with an emphasis on psychoeducation, should be employed in addition to pharmacotherapy in virtually all patients

Anxiety Disorders

GENERALIZED ANXIETY DISORDER

Basic Information

- Characterized by excessive anxiety and worry that result in some degree of functional impairment
- Affects women more than men
- Patients often present first to their primary physician with physical complaints (GI or urinary distress, headaches, or myalgias) that sometimes worsen during periods of stress
- Commonly coexists with substance misuse and other psychiatric disorders (e.g., depression, obsessive-compulsive disorder)

Clinical Presentation and Diagnosis

- Excessive anxiety and worry for more days than not, for at least 6 months

- The patient's worry is difficult or impossible to manage or control and out of proportion to the likelihood of feared negative events
- Three or more of the following must also occur:
  - Restlessness
  - Easy fatigability
  - Poor concentration
  - Muscle tension
  - Sleep difficulties
  - Irritability or edginess

Treatment

- Antidepressant medications (e.g., selective serotonin reuptake inhibitors [SSRIs], tricyclic antidepressants, and dual reuptake inhibitors) can all be effective
- Benzodiazepines can be useful for short-term therapy until antidepressants have taken effect
  - Avoid short-acting agents (e.g., alprazolam) because of the high incidence of dependence
- Buspirone
- Counseling or psychotherapy can be effective as sole therapy or in conjunction with medications

PANIC ATTACKS

Basic Information

- Common problem seen in primary care
- **Most patients present with unexplained somatic complaints (e.g., chest pain, abdominal pain, dizziness, fatigue) rather than the complaint of fear or anxiety**
  - Results in high use of health care resources for doctor visits, laboratory testing, hospitalizations, and specialty referrals
- Seen more commonly in patients with mitral valve prolapse, asthma, and migraine headaches
- Although one third of the population will have at least one panic attack in their lives, only about 5% of the population will develop **panic disorder**
  - Panic disorder is defined as a persistent fear of further attacks or a maladaptive change in behavior to avoid them

Clinical Presentation and Diagnosis

- Presents with an abrupt onset of intense fear that may manifest with somatic or cognitive symptoms
- The *Diagnostic and Statistical Manual of Mental Disorders, Fifth Edition* (DSM-5) criteria for diagnosing a panic attack are presented in Box 67-3
- Attacks commonly occur after a significant life stress
- Panic disorder coexists with other psychiatric conditions (e.g., agoraphobia, major depression, personality disorders, posttraumatic stress disorder, and somatization disorders)
- Need to consider the presence of an underlying medical disorder that may mimic panic attacks (e.g., angina, arrhythmias [especially paroxysmal supraventricular tachycardia], pheochromocytoma, thyroid disorders, anemia, and temporal lobe epilepsy)

Treatment

- **For mild cases that involve infrequent attacks related to stressors, supportive psychotherapy and**

A discrete period of intense fear or discomfort during which four or more of the following occur, reaching a peak within 10 minutes:
Palpitations
Diaphoresis
Shakiness or trembling
Shortness of breath
Sensation of choking
Chest pain or discomfort
Nausea or abdominal distress
Dizziness or lightheadedness
Depersonalization (feeling detached from oneself) or derealization (feelings of unreality)
Fear of losing control
Fear of dying
Paresthesias
Hot flashes or chills

Modified from Task Force on DSM-V. *The Diagnostic and Statistical Manual of Mental Disorders.* 5th ed. Arlington, VA: American Psychiatric Association; 2013.

relaxation techniques may be the only necessary interventions
- A single isolated attack usually does not require treatment
- For more severe cases of panic disorder, with or without phobic tendencies, cognitive behavioral therapy or medications are useful
  - Cognitive behavioral therapy designed to modify maladaptive behavior is equivalent or superior to therapy with medications
  - Effective medications include SSRIs, serotonin and norepinephrine reuptake inhibitors, tricyclic antidepressants, and monoamine oxidase (MAO) inhibitors
- Treatment should be continued for at least 12 months
  - Tapering of medications can be tried thereafter
  - There is a high rate of recurrence after discontinuation of therapy
- For acute treatment of recurrent panic attacks, benzodiazepines (e.g., lorazepam) are useful in the short term but carry the risk of dependence when used long term

OBSESSIVE-COMPULSIVE DISORDER
- Occurs in 2% of the population
- Diagnosed in patients with either obsessions or compulsions (or both; most commonly)
  - Obsessions: Recurrent thoughts, images, or impulses that cause marked anxiety and are perceived as being senseless or intrusive
    - Common examples include the fear of contamination or fear of harm
  - Compulsions: Ritualistic behaviors or mental acts that are often done in response to an obsession to decrease anxiety or avoid a feared consequence
    - Common examples include excessive hand washing or checking

- Has a significant negative effect on activities of daily living, social functioning, occupational functioning, and overall quality of life
- Treatment is psychotherapy with or without medications
  - Effective medications include SSRIs (e.g., paroxetine, fluvoxamine, fluoxetine, sertraline) or clomipramine

PHOBIAS
- One of the most common psychiatric conditions (affect 7% to 9% of population)
- Divided into three basic categories:
  - Specific phobia
    - Fear of objects (e.g., insects, snakes) or situations (e.g., heights, flying, getting blood drawn)
    - Usually responds to behavior therapy (gradual exposure)
    - Benzodiazepines or β-blockers can be used in some cases
  - Social phobia (social anxiety disorder)
    - Fear of social situations (e.g., public speaking)
    - Treated with psychotherapy and medications
    - SSRIs are considered first-line medications
    - Benzodiazepines and MAO inhibitors are also effective
    - β-Blockers may be particularly useful in cases of performance anxiety where somatic sensations (e.g., palpitations) are troubling
  - Agoraphobia
    - Fear or anxiety about being in a place or situation from which escape might be difficult (e.g., being alone when away from home, being in crowds)
    - Often occurs with panic disorder
    - Treatment is similar to that of panic disorder (see earlier discussion)

POSTTRAUMATIC STRESS DISORDER
- Severe response to a traumatic event that involved the **risk of serious injury or death to the patient or someone close to the patient**
- Characterized by intrusive recollections of the traumatic event, avoidance of any situations or activities associated with the event, increased arousal, and emotional detachment
- Results in significant functional impairment
- Because of the complexity of the disorder, most patients should be referred to a psychiatrist
- Treatment is with psychotherapy and medications (e.g., SSRIs)
- Recovery is expected within 1 year in one third of patients and within 10 years in two thirds of patients

Psychotic Disorders

SCHIZOPHRENIA
Basic Information
- A syndrome featuring some combination of delusions, hallucinations, disorganized thought/speech/behavior, and "negative symptoms," such as reduced emotional

| BOX 67-4 | *Psychotic Symptoms* |

Delusions: False beliefs that are held with certainty, often involve the patient personally, and are not generally held in the patient's culture. Persecutory delusions (sometimes referred to as paranoid delusions) are most frequent.

Hallucinations: Involuntary, vivid perceptions without a stimulus. To the patient, these are indistinguishable from true perceptions. Auditory hallucinations are most common, but hallucinations can involve any sensory modality.

Disorganized thinking: Speaking incoherently, tangentially, or jumping between seemingly unrelated topics. Should be severe enough to impair communication.

Grossly disorganized/abnormal motor behavior: Includes agitation, lack of goal-directed behavior, or catatonia. Catatonia is a significant lack of response to the environment, sometimes including repetitive movements, speech, or strange posturing.

Negative symptoms: Most prominently includes diminished emotional expression (flattened affect, monotonous speech, reduced eye contact and gesturing) and avolition (lack of motivation, purpose, socialization). Negative symptoms are seen more in schizophrenia than in the other psychotic illnesses.

expression and motivation, resulting in functional impairment (Box 67-4)

- Affects 0.7% of the population, usually beginning in the early twenties in men and the late twenties in women
- Impaired cognition is common and can be progressive
- Strong genetic contributions are evident, though many patients do not have a family history of schizophrenia
- 20% of cases will attempt and 5% will complete suicide

Clinical Presentation and Diagnosis

- Active psychotic symptoms (see Box 67-4) should be present for at least 1 month, but need to be present at least in diminished form for more than 6 months
- Schizophrenia can be thought of as a diagnosis of exclusion, as psychotic symptoms can also be seen in:
  - 15% to 20% of major depressive episodes
  - 60% of bipolar disorder mood episodes
  - Substance use
  - Delirium
  - Other primary brain diseases (e.g., Alzheimer disease, malignancy)
    - More likely to be smokers and to have medical comorbidity than the general population

Treatment

- Neuroleptic (antipsychotic) medications are first-line treatments
  - Work primarily by blocking postsynaptic dopamine receptors in the mesolimbic system
  - Some effect seen in the first few days, but the full effect can take 2 to 6 weeks
  - Beware of neuroleptic malignant syndrome: confusion, hyperthermia, tachycardia, muscle rigidity, and labile blood pressure

- First-generation (typical) neuroleptics include chlorpromazine, fluphenazine, and haloperidol
  - Side effects include movement abnormalities (extrapyramidal symptoms), sedation, postural hypotension, hyperprolactinemia, and anticholinergic effects (blurred vision, flushing, hyperthermia, dry skin and mouth, urinary retention, ileus/constipation, and tachycardia)
  - Most severe side effects are QTc prolongation (can cause torsades de pointes) and tardive dyskinesia, which is a sometimes irreversible onset of involuntary, repetitive movements, most commonly of the face
- Second-generation (atypical) neuroleptics include aripiprazole, clozapine, quetiapine, olanzapine, and risperidone
  - In addition to dopamine receptors, these also antagonize serotonin receptors
  - Some evidence suggests that they may be more effective for the negative symptoms of schizophrenia
  - **Side effects include fewer instances of movement abnormality, but far greater incidence of metabolic syndrome (weight gain, hyperlipidemia, elevated fasting glucose, and hypertension, sometimes leading to diabetes and cardiovascular disease)**
  - Clozapine (atypical) is the most effective treatment, but it causes agranulocytosis in 1% to 3% of patients, and so regular CBC checks are required
- Patients often benefit from psychiatric hospitalization during illness exacerbations, sometimes brought on by medication nonadherence
- Schizophrenia can be treated but not cured, although there are reports of some patients making full recoveries as they age
- Counseling or psychotherapy is less effective than medication

SCHIZOAFFECTIVE DISORDER

- Affects 0.3% of the population (less common than schizophrenia)
- Patients have mood episodes (depression or mania) with more than 1 psychotic symptom (Box 67-4), but also have psychotic symptoms for at least 2 weeks in the absence of mood episodes
- Sometimes used as a working diagnosis until further illness course reveals itself as either schizophrenia or bipolar disorder
- Treatment consists of neuroleptics and mood stabilizers or antidepressants
  - ECT can be considered for patients with treatment-unresponsive symptoms

Other Psychotic Disorders

- Brief psychotic disorder is defined as hallucinations, delusions, and/or disorganization for up to 1 month
- Schizophreniform disorder is defined as a full schizophrenia syndrome lasting between 1 and 6 months

- Delusional disorder is a rare disorder defined by delusions lasting more than 1 month, usually without other psychotic symptoms or mood abnormalities
  - Average onset is in the fourth decade of life
- All can be treated with neuroleptics

SOMATIC SYMPTOM (SOMATOFORM) DISORDERS

Basic Information

- Refers to the manifestation of psychologic distress as unexplained physical symptoms
- Patients may be aware or unaware of this tendency
- **Leads to high use of medical resources through unnecessary testing, referrals, and procedures**
- Commonly coexists with other psychiatric disorders (e.g., anxiety, depression)
- Somatic symptom disorders are subdivided into a number of categories in the DSM-5 (Table 67-2)

Clinical Presentation

See Table 67-2.

Diagnosis

- Based largely on clinical presentation
- A thorough history and physical examination should be done to establish rapport and to identify coexisting psychiatric disorders and potentially overlooked medical conditions
- A review of previous patient records is invaluable to avoid repeat testing and overuse of resources

Treatment

- No specific therapy is uniformly effective
- Should be treated as a chronic illness
  - **Regular office visits should be scheduled, rather than urgent visits for new complaints**
    - Recognizing the disorder as a medical problem rather than a condition that is "all in your head" is imperative in developing a trusting relationship
    - Avoid extensive medical testing, complicated medical regimens, and addictive pain medications

EATING DISORDERS

Basic Information

- Affect over 2 million people in the United States, with an overwhelming female predominance
- Usually manifest in late childhood, adolescence, or early adulthood
- Associated with a number of potential medical complications (Box 67-5)

Clinical Presentation and Diagnosis

- Anorexia nervosa
  - Restriction of intake relative to requirements, leading to significantly low body weight
  - Intense fear of weight gain and becoming fat
  - Disturbance in body image or denial of seriousness of current body weight
  - Since 2013, this diagnosis no longer requires females to miss menses

TABLE 67-2	*Somatoform Disorders*
Disorder	**Description**
Somatic symptom disorder	At least one physical symptom, resulting in distress or significant functional impairment Symptoms cannot be fully explained by an underlying medical condition, or the distress and impairment caused must be out of proportion to what would be expected from the medical condition Excessive thoughts, feelings, or behaviors related to the somatic symptom(s) Disturbance lasts for >6 months More common in women
Illness anxiety disorder	Preoccupation with having or acquiring a serious illness, despite absent or very mild somatic symptoms High health anxiety leading to excessive health care seeking/checking behaviors *or* health care avoidance Disturbance lasts for >6 months Often comorbid with anxiety disorders
Conversion disorder (functional neurological symptom disorder)	One or more unexplained symptoms suggesting deficits in normal neurologic function Presentation follows the patient's view of the disease rather than neurophysiology Examples include amnesia, aphonia, blindness, paralysis, paresthesias, seizures
Body dysmorphic disorder (no longer considered a somatic symptom disorder; now seen as an OCD-related condition)	Preoccupation with an imagined or exaggerated defect in appearance Onset is usually in the second or third decade of life
Factitious disorder	Falsification of physical signs or symptoms, or induction of injury to assume the sick role Can lead to multiple hospitalizations (chronic factitious disorder or Munchausen syndrome) Secondary gain (money or other external benefits) not evident
Malingering	Intentional feigning or induction of physical signs or symptoms for secondary gain (e.g., compensation for injuries)

BOX 67-5 *Medical Complications of Eating Disorders*

Dental erosions (Fig. 67-1)
Enlarged parotid glands
Hair loss and brittle nails
Calluses over the knuckles (Russell sign) caused by
induction of vomiting
Neurologic disease: seizures, myopathy, neuropathy,
cognitive difficulties
Cardiac disease: bradycardia, arrhythmias, congestive heart
failure, ECG abnormalities
Gastrointestinal disease: dysmotility, esophagitis, gallstones,
Mallory-Weiss tears, superior mesenteric artery syndrome
Endocrinologic disease: amenorrhea, osteoporosis, sick
euthyroid syndrome, growth retardation, infertility
Hematologic: anemia, leukopenia, thrombocytopenia
Electrolyte abnormalities: hypokalemia, metabolic alkalosis
(in patients who purge), hyponatremia

ECG, Electrocardiographic.

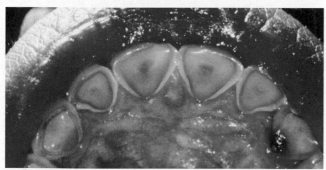

FIGURE 67-1 Advanced perimolysis of the maxillary incisors in which the pulp chambers of the teeth are visible; caused by acid erosion from chronic vomiting. (From Stefanac S, Nesbit S. *Treatment Planning for Dentistry.* 2nd ed. St. Louis: Mosby; 2007: Fig. 15-9.)

- Bulimia nervosa
  - Episodes of out-of-control binge eating with compensatory purging (vomiting, laxative abuse) or nonpurging (excessive exercise, strict dieting or fasting) behavior to prevent weight gain
  - Binging and compensatory behavior occurs at least once per week for 3 months
  - Self-evaluation is unduly influenced by body weight and shape
- Binge-eating disorder (BED)
  - Recurrent episodes of consumption of large amounts of food in discrete amounts of time with a lack of control over eating, and distress regarding these binges
  - Binges occur at least once a week for 3 months
  - No inappropriate compensatory behaviors should be present (i.e., purging, excessive exercise, fasting)
  - **Patients can be obese, overweight, or have normal weight**

Treatment

- Requires a multidisciplinary approach with a mental health specialist, medical provider (to help treat potential complications), and dietitian

BOX 67-6 *Historic Clues Suggestive of Domestic Violence*

Chronic abdominal or pelvic pain
Chronic headaches
Chronic fatigue
Depression and anxiety
Frequent emergency room visits
Frequent physician visits with vague somatic complaints
History of sexually transmitted diseases
Recurrent, inconsistently explained injuries
Substance abuse

- For patients with BMI less than 19.5 kg/m^2 managed in the outpatient setting, goal weight gain is 0.5 to 1 pound per week.
- Be aware of refeeding syndrome
  - Seen in patients with severe anorexia nervosa within 2 to 3 weeks of refeeding
  - **Manifests as cardiac abnormalities and delirium, primarily caused by hypophosphatemia and other electrolyte abnormalities; significant third-spacing of fluid**
- Psychotherapy is the treatment of choice
  - The addition of SSRIs (fluoxetine) or other antidepressants is effective for bulimia nervosa
  - Antidepressants may be helpful in patients with anorexia nervosa to prevent recurrences of illness or to treat comorbid depressive illness, but they do not significantly contribute to acute disease management
- Treatment for BED consists primarily of psychotherapy. Behavioral weight loss therapy may be used in overweight individuals. Pharmacotherapy with SSRIs may also be useful.

DOMESTIC VIOLENCE

Basic Information

- Defined as ongoing physical, psychological, or sexual abuse in the home, associated with isolation, limited personal freedom, and limited access to resources (e.g., economic resources)
- An estimated 2 million people (usually women) are victims of abuse each year, resulting in over 2000 deaths annually in the United States
- Found in patients of all races, socioeconomic backgrounds, and ages
- Elder abuse is another form
  - Refers to a subset of patients older than 65 years of age who are subject to physical abuse, sexual abuse, neglect, or financial abuse
  - Associated with increased mortality
- Children who are victimized by sexual or physical abuse are more prone to be victims of domestic violence in adulthood

Clinical Presentation and Diagnosis

- A number of signs and symptoms are suggestive of domestic violence (Box 67-6)
- Injuries and bruising typically occur on the abdomen, genitalia, around the neck (from attempted strangulation), or around the breasts

- **The abuser may refuse to leave the examining room during the history and physical examination and may try to speak on behalf of the victim**

Diagnosis

- Most cases go unrecognized by physicians
- The key to identification is inquiry
  - Direct questions such as, "Has your partner ever punched or kicked you?" or "Are you afraid of your partner?" are more effective than general ones such as "Do you feel you are being abused?"
  - Questions about sexual and emotional abuse should also be included

Treatment

- Physicians need to identify local resources for dealing with domestic violence
  - Hospital social workers and local domestic violence hotlines can assist in this process
  - The National Domestic Violence Hotline (1-800-799-SAFE) can also assist in providing information about local resources
- If there is an imminent threat to life, immediate referral should be strongly encouraged
- Documentation should be specific and thorough, with photographs or sketches of injuries (if present)

- Reporting
  - Only a few states require mandatory reporting of abuse against legally competent adult women
  - Abuse involving children, including children witnessing their parent being abused, should be reported to the local Department of Social Services
  - Elder abuse should be reported to the local elder abuse hotline or adult protective services

Review Questions

For review questions, please go to ExpertConsult.com.

SUGGESTED READINGS

American Psychiatric Association. *Diagnostic and Statistical Manual of Mental Disorders.* 5th ed. Arlington, VA: American Psychiatric Publishing; 2013.

Bienvenu O, DePaulo J. *The Johns Hopkins Phipps Psychiatry Guide.* Baltimore: Johns Hopkins POC-IT Center (Johns Hopkins Point of Care Information Technology Center); 2014.

Combs H, Markman J. Anxiety disorders in primary care. *Med Clin North Am.* 2014;5:1007-1023.

McHugh P, Slavney P. *The Perspectives of Psychiatry.* 2nd ed. Baltimore: Johns Hopkins University Press; 1998.

Toohey JS. Domestic violence and rape. *Med Clin North Am.* 2008;5:1239-1252, xii.

Treasure J, Claudino AM, Zucker N. Eating disorders. *Lancet.* 2010;9714:583-593.

Allergy and Immunology for the Internist

D'JAHNA AKINYEMI, MD, MS; ROY ANTHONY ORDEN, MD; TAO ZHENG, MD; and SARBJIT S. SAINI, MD

The immune system is normally balanced to protect against foreign proteins and other allergens. Reaction to extrinsic or intrinsic antigens, however, can result in a cascade of events with clinical symptoms ranging from mild (pruritus, rhinorrhea) to severe (respiratory distress, vascular collapse, death).

Basic Information

- Allergens: Proteins of appropriate size that, after inhalation, injection (e.g., drug, venom), or ingestion, provoke an immunoglobulin E (IgE) antibody response and clinical symptoms in sensitive individuals. Common aeroallergens include trees, grasses, and molds, as well as animals (e.g., domesticated pets, rodents), dust mites, and cockroaches.
- **Acute-phase reaction: allergic response that begins within minutes of allergen exposure; symptoms include pruritus and hives (skin), wheezing (lungs), rhinorrhea and sneezing (nose), erythema, and tearing of eyes**
  - Allergen cross-links specific IgE bound to the surface of mast cells and basophils; after surface IgE is cross-linked, mast cells and basophils release mediators such as histamine (stored in cytoplasmic granules) and leukotrienes/prostaglandins (rapidly synthesized from arachidonic acid)
- **Late-phase reaction: occurs 4 to 12 hours after acute phase and initial allergen exposure; symptoms are similar to acute-phase reaction and mirror the inflammation seen in asthma and chronic allergic rhinitis**
  - Pathogenesis includes leukocyte (eosinophil, T-helper type 2 cell [Th2 cell]) infiltration into tissues, which release Th2 cytokines (interleukin [IL]-4, IL-5, and IL-13) and chemokines (chemoattractant cytokines)
  - Histamine levels also increase
- Basic compartments of the immune system include:
  - Anatomic and physiologic barriers (skin, ciliary clearance, low gastric pH)
  - Innate immunity
    - Cellular: neutrophil, eosinophil, basophil, mast cell, monocyte/macrophage, dendritic cell, natural killer T cells
    - Humoral: complement
  - Adaptive immunity
    - Cellular: T cells, B cells
    - Humoral: antibodies

Clinical Presentation of Allergic Reactions

- **Anaphylaxis: an IgE-related response after exposure to antigen, resulting in the rapid onset of systemic symptoms, including pallor, pruritus, dyspnea, wheezing, weakness, urticaria, erythema, flushing, cyanosis, angioedema, diarrhea, nausea, vomiting, abdominal cramping, and hypotension**
  - Some present with a biphasic illness, beginning with early abdominal symptoms before respiratory symptoms or vascular collapse occur
  - **May be fatal because of upper airway obstruction or cardiovascular collapse**
  - Mechanism: mast cell and basophil mediators released by allergen binding IgE
    - Mediators released include elevated serum β-tryptase level, histamine, platelet activating factor, prostaglandin D_2, leukotrienes, and cytokines (e.g., tumor necrosis factor-α and IL-1)
    - Non-IgE-mediated factors include C3a and C5a
  - Causes of anaphylaxis
    - Foods (especially nuts, shellfish, eggs, and milk)
    - Exercise (generally in people with an allergic background)
    - Medications (see later discussion)
    - Insect bites (for which immunotherapy is more than 97% protective)
    - Latex
    - Mast cell disorders (e.g., mastocytosis, mast cell activation syndrome)
  - Idiopathic anaphylaxis: 30% to 40% of all recurrent anaphylaxis (a diagnosis of exclusion)
  - **Diagnosis of anaphylaxis is supported by the measurement of elevated serum tryptase (usually peaks in the first 2 hours)**
  - **Cornerstone of maintenance is patient education regarding avoidance of allergens**
  - Acute treatment of anaphylaxis includes immediate treatment with epinephrine, followed by oxygen, antihistamines, corticosteroids, and β-agonists (as needed) for support
  - **Patients with a history of anaphylaxis should carry an autoinjectable form of epinephrine**
  - Anaphylactoid reaction: a non–IgE-triggered process that clinically resembles anaphylaxis; may be caused by aspirin and nonsteroidal antiinflammatory drugs

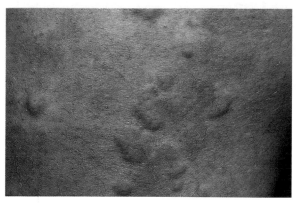

FIGURE 68-1   Urticaria with characteristic wheals surrounded by an erythematous flare. (From Forbes CD, Jackson WF. *Color Atlas and Text of Clinical Medicine.* 3rd ed. St. Louis: Mosby; 2003: Fig. 2.39.)

(NSAIDs), radiocontrast agents, and, rarely, opiate drugs

- Symptoms from aspirin and NSAIDs include rhinoconjunctivitis, urticaria, bronchospasm, angioedema, and laryngeal edema; treatment is avoidance or aspirin desensitization
- Symptoms from radiocontrast agents include the spectrum of symptoms seen with anaphylaxis
  - **Despite common belief, there is no relationship between radiocontrast allergy and allergy to fish, shellfish, or iodine**
  - Typical pretreatment regimen includes prednisone (50 mg, administered at 13 hours, 7 hours, and 1 hour before procedure) and diphenhydramine (50 mg × 1 intramuscularly or orally 1 hour before procedure)
- Urticaria and angioedema
  - **Urticaria (Fig. 68-1) is characterized by well-circumscribed wheals from involvement of the upper layer of the dermis**
    - **Wheals are erythematous, with blanched centers, and pruritic and may occur anywhere on the body**
    - **Usually result from a type 1 hypersensitivity reaction**
    - Lifetime risk of a single episode of acute urticaria is very high (i.e., one in four adults)
    - **Urticaria lasting more than 6 weeks is labeled *chronic* urticaria; most are idiopathic**
      - Biopsy of persistent lesions (more than 72 hours) should be done to exclude vasculitis
  - **Angioedema (Fig. 68-2) is characterized by the acute development of swelling and edema of submucosal or subcutaneous tissue in the skin, mucous membrane, and gastrointestinal (GI) tract**
    - Symptoms are based on tissue involved; typically nonpruritic
      - Occurs with urticaria in approximately 50% of chronic cases
      - 10% of chronic cases have angioedema alone and 40% urticaria alone
      - Hereditary angioedema also occurs without urticaria (Table 68-1)

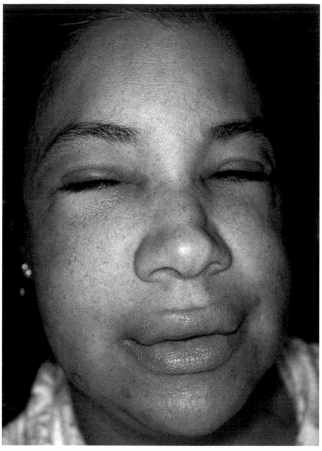

FIGURE 68-2   Angioedema involving the lips and periorbital region. (From Middleton R, Reed S, Ellis B, et al. *Allergy Principle and Practice.* 8th ed. Philadelphia: Saunders; 2014: Fig 36-5.)

- Differential causes of urticaria or angioedema
  - Drugs (e.g., angiotensin-converting enzyme inhibitors)
  - Thyroid disorders
  - Autoimmune disorders (e.g., vasculitis)
  - Infections (e.g., viral, including hepatitis, and parasitic)
  - Food
  - Malignancy
  - Cryoglobulins
  - Physical triggers of urticaria may also exist, including cold, heat, pressure, and exercise
- Mechanism unknown; may involve chronic mast cell degranulation
- A subset of patients will have antibodies against IgE or the IgE receptor
- **Cornerstone of treatment is antihistamines;** may add histamine$_2$ blocker, tricyclic antidepressant (e.g., doxepin), or immunomodulators (e.g., cyclosporine) for severe cases; short-term oral corticosteroids are also used for severe eruptions

Clinical Presentation of Allergic and Immune-Related Diseases

- **Allergic rhinitis: allergen-induced inflammation of the lining of the nose characterized by nasal congestion, rhinorrhea, sneezing, itch, and**

TABLE 68-1	*Allergic Skin Diseases*			
Disease	**Clinical Presentation**	**Pathogenesis**	**Diagnosis**	**Treatment**
Hereditary angioedema (HAE–C1-INH)	Autosomal dominant Recurrent swelling of face, airway, GI tract, extremities Bowel edema may result in severe abdominal pain that resolves spontaneously Trauma may trigger symptoms Urticaria uncommon	Absence or reduced level of C1 esterase inhibitor (C1-INH) (85%) Dysfunctional C1-INH (15%)	Clinical presentation Absence or reduced level of C1-INH plus low C4 levels (caused by chronic complement consumption) C4 levels low even if symptoms absent	Synthetic androgens (e.g., danazol, stanazol) induce inhibitor synthesis Purified C1-INH concentrate also available Kallikrein inhibitors
Hereditary angioedema (HAE-FXII)	Missense mutation in the factor XII (FXII) gene Autosomal dominant Estrogens have a great influence, but highly variable Occurs mainly in women Facial swelling is a cardinal symptom Triggers: acute trauma, estrogens, blockers of the renin-angiotensin system	Activation of the kallikrein-kinin system and overproduction of bradykinin seem to be involved in the pathophysiology of angioedema attacks of HAE-FXII	Personal history (recurrent angioedema attacks and no urticaria) Genetic tests positive for FXII mutation p.Thr309Lys *or* p.Thr309ArgC1 esterase inhibitor: normal or slightly decreased	The same drugs are effective or partially effective as those in HAE–C1-INH; C1-INH concentrate may be effective for acute attacks Prophylaxis: danazol, stanazol, and/or kallikrein inhibitors and bradykinin antagonists
Acquired angioedema	Same as above, with onset later in life	Autoantibodies develop to C1-INH Suggests underlying malignancy (leukemia, lymphoma)	C4 levels low Low C1q levels distinguish this from hereditary form	Treat underlying disease
Allergic contact dermatitis	Vesicular eruption with well-demarcated borders on exposed skin area Common causes include poison ivy, nickel, carrier substances in topical medications (e.g., thimerosal)	T cells activated, release interferon-γ Macrophages then activated	Patch testing of suspected substance	Avoid offending agent Topical steroids Oral steroid taper
Atopic dermatitis (AD)	Dry, scaling skin with pruritus Commonly involves head and face Antecubital and popliteal fossae, nape of neck commonly involved in adults	One third of patients with AD have genetic skin barrier defect (filaggrin mutation) Commonly an inherited pattern of elevated IgE, eosinophilia, and evidence of IgE sensitization to antigens	Patients often have positive family history Associated with asthma and allergic rhinitis Associated with dry skin Serum IgE often elevated	Topical corticosteroids to involved area Antihistamines Topical FK506 used for more severe reactions Antistaphylococcal antibiotics
Chronic idiopathic urticaria	Recurrent urticaria or angioedema for >6 weeks	Unknown May be related autoantibodies to IgE receptor	Exclusion of drugs or other diseases	$H_1 \pm H_2$ blockers Leukotriene receptor antagonists Steroids Omalizumab Immunomodulators (e.g., cyclosporine, dapsone, sulfasalazine)

GI, Gastrointestinal; H_1, histamine1; H_2, histamine2; IgE, immunoglobulin E.

postnasal drainage; the most common adult allergic disease (15% of U.S. population)

- Overlap of symptoms with viral upper respiratory tract infection, nasal polyposis, nonallergic rhinitis with eosinophilia, and hormonally related nasal congestion (pregnancy, oral contraceptives, hypothyroidism)
- Medications may also cause symptoms confused with allergic rhinitis (e.g., cocaine and β-blockers)
  - **Rhinitis medicamentosa: overuse of over-the-counter topical nasal decongestants (vasoconstrictors)**
- Other causes of symptoms that overlap with allergic rhinitis include vasomotor rhinitis (nasal congestion brought on by irritants such as cigarette smoke and cold air) and anatomic abnormalities (e.g., cerebrospinal fluid leak, deviated septum)
- Drug allergy: Most adverse drug reactions (ADRs) do not have an immunologic basis (less than 10% of all ADRs are immunologically based); the mechanism of many drug reactions is unknown
  - Most drugs are small molecules that cannot act as an antigen unless modified
  - Drugs may act as a hapten, in which the drug or its metabolite combine with a larger carrier protein and can thereby become immunogenic
    - Prior exposure is needed to generate an IgE antibody response
  - Time of onset from drug initiation assists in identifying allergic-type reactions
    - Immediate (less than 1 hour): pruritus, urticaria, rhinitis, wheezing, anaphylaxis
    - Accelerated (1 to 72 hours): urticaria
    - Late (more than 72 hours): maculopapular eruption (Fig. 68-3), drug fever, hemolytic anemia, serum sickness, nephritis, leukopenia, exfoliative dermatitis, Stevens-Johnson syndrome (Fig. 68-4)
  - **Penicillins and cephalosporins are the most common causes of immunologically based ADRs, typically acting as haptens**
    - Cross-reactivity with cephalosporins is less than 3% (risk is highest with first-generation cephalosporins)
    - Carbapenems (i.e., imipenem) cross-react with minor determinants of penicillin [PCN]; whereas monobactams (i.e., aztreonam) can be safely administered to PCN-allergic patients
    - Other ADRs from PCN include:
      - Antibody-mediated hemolytic anemia and thrombocytopenia
      - Immune complex disease (characterized by fever, rash, glomerulonephritis, and lymphadenopathy)
      - Cell-mediated contact dermatitis (with topical preparations)
      - Maculopapular rash seen in 5% to 13% of patients administered amoxicillin (incidence is increased with coincident Epstein-Barr virus and cytomegalovirus)
        - Basis of rash with amoxicillin is unknown
        - Can often treat through the rash with close monitoring

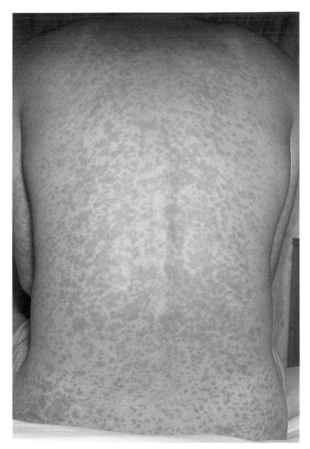

FIGURE 68-3 A maculopapular eruption in a patient treated with cotrimoxazole. (From Forbes CD, Jackson WF. *Color Atlas and Text of Clinical Medicine.* 3rd ed. St. Louis: Mosby; 2003: Fig. 2.147.)

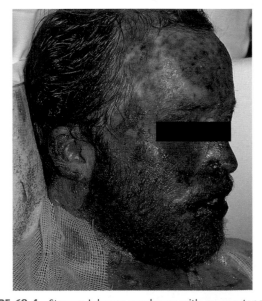

FIGURE 68-4 Stevens-Johnson syndrome with mucocutaneous facial lesions. (From Forbes CD, Jackson WF. *Color Atlas and Text of Clinical Medicine.* 3rd ed. St. Louis: Mosby; 2003: Fig. 2.49.)

- **Sulfonamides are the second most common antibiotic class to cause drug reactions, usually via a T cell-mediated reaction; seen commonly in patients with human immunodeficiency virus (HIV)**
- Allergic skin diseases: include hereditary and acquired angioedema, allergic contact dermatitis (Fig. 68-5), and atopic dermatitis (Fig. 68-6) (see Table 68-1)
- Immunodeficiency syndromes: include immunoglobulin deficiencies, T-cell and B-cell deficiencies, as well as neutrophil and complement disorders (Table 68-2)
  - Antibody deficiency associated with sinopulmonary (pyogenic bacteria) and GI infections (e.g., enterovirus, rotavirus, *Giardia*)

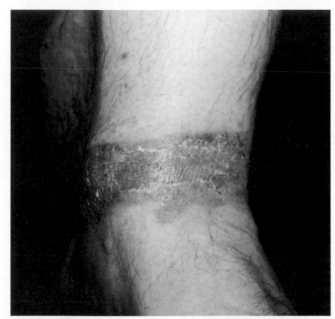

FIGURE 68-5 Allergic contact dermatitis caused by an ankle bracelet. (From Adkinson NF, Yunginger JW, Busse WW, et al. *Middleton's Allergy: Principles and Practice*. 6th ed. St. Louis: Mosby; 2003 [Plate 25].)

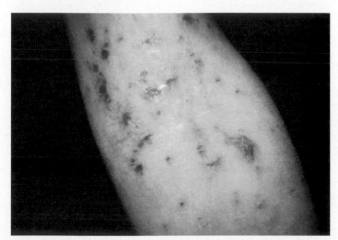

FIGURE 68-6 Acute atopic dermatitis with excoriated lesions. (From Adkinson NF, Junginger JW, Busse WW, et al. *Middleton's Allergy: Principles and Practice*. 6th ed. St. Louis: Mosby; 2003 [Plate 19].)

- Cell-mediated immunity deficiencies associated with pneumonia (bacteria, viruses, pneumocystis), GI infections (e.g., viruses, cryptosporidium), and skin/mucous membrane infections (e.g., fungi)
- Complement deficiencies associated with sepsis (e.g., streptococci, pneumococci, Neisseria)
- Phagocytic defects associated with skin, lymph node, and spleen infections and abscesses (e.g., staphylococci, enteric bacteria, fungi, mycobacteria)
- Eosinophilia syndromes
  - Churg-Strauss vasculitis: a granulomatous vasculitis involving multiple organ systems, predominantly the lungs
    - Patients present with severe asthma in the setting of systemic illness (fevers, malaise, weight loss), accompanied by pronounced eosinophilia
    - Fleeting pulmonary infiltrates commonly seen on chest radiography
    - Skin rash may also be seen; sinus involvement has also been described
  - Hypereosinophilic syndrome
    - Systemic disorder characterized by dysfunction of several organs in the setting of persistent eosinophilia (more than 1500 cells/mL for at least 6 months)
    - Diagnosis involves exclusion of other causes of eosinophilia
    - Cardiac involvement is major cause of mortality
    - Recently identified genetic mutation (platelet-derived growth factor receptor α [FIP1L1-PDGFRA]) in some cases

Diagnosis

- Diagnosis of allergic rhinitis
  - **Clinical presentation and historical features are often sufficient for treatment**
  - Skin testing: search for specific IgE to allergens; antihistamines must be avoided before skin testing
  - **Radioallergosorbent test (RAST): detects the presence of allergen-specific IgE in a subject's serum by in vitro assay; is an alternative to skin testing, but less sensitive, if patient cannot stop antihistamines**
- Diagnosis of PCN and related β-lactam antibiotic allergy
  - Skin test is performed with major and minor determinants to detect the presence of specific IgE; skin test does not predict non–IgE-dependent reactions
  - 80% to 90% of PCN "allergic" patients are not truly allergic because they lack specific IgE
  - **Because most PCN- or β-lactam–allergic patients do not have an IgE-dependent reaction, and skin testing only tests for IgE-dependent reactions, a negative skin test does not exclude a reaction to penicillin or β-lactam antibiotic**
  - Stevens-Johnson syndrome and exfoliative dermatitis are absolute contraindications for PCN use
- Diagnosis of allergic skin diseases is often done based on the clinical presentation; confirmation may be

TABLE 68-2	*Selected Immunodeficiency Syndromes*		
Disease	**Clinical Presentation**	**Diagnosis**	**Treatment**
Common variable immunodeficiency	Recurrent sinopulmonary infections Parasitic GI infections seen (esp. *Giardia*) Autoimmune diseases and malignancy risk increased	Quantitative immunoglobulin levels Plasma cells are absent Poor humoral response to immunizations T-cell dysfunction	Antibiotics IV IgG every 3 to 4 weeks Subcutaneous IgG weekly
Selective IgA deficiency	The most common primary immunodeficiency (1:600) Recurrent sinopulmonary infections Asthma and atopic dermatitis more common, as are rheumatoid arthritis and lupus Anaphylaxis to blood or blood product transfusion	Low to absent IgA levels IgG and IgM levels normal	Antibiotics Avoid transfusion of blood or blood products unless donor is also IgA deficient
Adult T-cell deficiencies	Opportunistic infections (similar to HIV)	Exclude HIV Wiskott-Aldrich syndrome, a subtype, is associated with thrombocytopenia, small platelets, and eczema	Antimicrobials Wiskott-Aldrich syndrome is treated by bone marrow transplantation
Complement disorders	Early complement component deficiencies: autoimmune disease C5–C8 deficiencies: recurrent meningococcal or gonococcal infections	Assay of complement levels	Antibiotic

GI, Gastrointestinal; HIV, human immunodeficiency virus; IgA, immunoglobulin A; IgG, immunoglobulin G; IgM, immunoglobulin M; IV, intravenous.

done with serum markers or skin testing (see Table 68-1)

- Diagnosis of immunodeficiency syndromes requires quantitative immunoglobulin levels or other serologic markers (Table 68-2)
- Diagnosis of eosinophilia syndromes
  - Churg-Strauss vasculitis is diagnosed by biopsy demonstrating granulomatous vasculitis with extravascular eosinophilic infiltration in the patient with a compatible clinical presentation
  - Hypereosinophilic syndrome is diagnosed by organ biopsy demonstrating eosinophils and tissue damage in the patient with persistent eosinophilia (more than 1500 eosinophils/μL for at least 6 months) when other causes of eosinophilia have been excluded

Treatment

- Allergic rhinitis
  - Treatment should follow a three-tiered approach
    - Avoidance or reduction of identified allergen triggers
    - Medications (Table 68-3)
      - Topical ocular agents may be used for coexisting allergic conjunctivitis
      - Leukotriene receptor antagonists are also approved in allergic rhinitis
    - Allergen-specific immunotherapy: used in patients with severe allergic rhinitis who are intolerant of or refractory to medications
      - Mechanism of action unknown, appears to involve shift to T-helper type 1 (Th1) cell

response to allergen and increased numbers of regulatory T cells
- Risk of anaphylaxis with treatment; 20 to 30 minutes of observation required after injection(s)
- Maintenance dosing may be continued for 3 to 5 years

- Drug allergy
  - Treat with unrelated drug class, if possible
  - **If no alternative drug (often an antibiotic) is available, desensitization may be tried for IgE-mediated hypersensitivity**
    - Can be administered either orally or intravenously with increasing doses of drug
    - Theory is that it prevents anaphylaxis by favoring univalent haptens that do not cross-link IgE and hence do not activate mast cells
    - **Duration of effect is limited to single treatment episode; must maintain uninterrupted treatment for duration of therapy**
    - **Future drug courses will require repeating the entire process**
- Allergic skin diseases: treatment varies based on the underlying disorder (see Table 68-1)
- Immunodeficiency syndromes: treatment includes antibiotics for infection, with other treatment based on the underlying disorder
- Eosinophilia syndromes
  - Churg-Strauss vasculitis: high-dose steroids and cyclophosphamide
  - Hypereosinophilic syndrome

TABLE 68-3	*Pharmacotherapy for Allergic Rhinitis*			
Class	**Example**	**Action**	**Symptoms Treated**	**Comments**
First-generation antihistamines	Diphenhydramine	Block H_1 receptor	Sneezing, rhinorrhea, pruritus	Sedation major side effect; limits use
Second-/third-generation antihistamines	Fexofenadine, Cetirizine, Loratadine Olopatadine (topical intranasal)	Block H_1 receptor	Sneezing, rhinorrhea, pruritus	Do not cross blood-brain barrier, thus less sedating
Topical or oral decongestants	Pseudoephedrine	Stimulate α-adrenergic receptors to result in vasoconstriction	Congestion	CNS stimulation most common side effect Can elevate blood pressure Phenylpropanolamine discontinued because of increased risk of CVA
Intranasal mast cell stabilizers	Cromolyn	Stabilize mast cell membranes, preventing release of histamine, slow-reacting substance of anaphylaxis (SRS-A)	Sneezing, rhinorrhea, congestion	Best used before exposure to allergen, Require frequent dosing
Intranasal corticosteroids	Fluticasone	Reduce mast cell numbers in local tissues; inhibit cytokine synthesis	Sneezing, rhinorrhea, congestion, pruritus	Most effective single maintenance therapy Require 1 week of use before clinical response

CNS, Central nervous system; CVA, cerebrovascular accident; H_1, histamine$_1$.

- Corticosteroids
- Hydroxyurea
- α-Interferon
- Potentially monoclonal anti–IL-5
- Imatinib mesylate (Gleevec) used in cases with FIP-1–like mutation

Review Questions

For review questions, please go to ExpertConsult.com.

SUGGESTED READINGS

Joint Task Force on Practice Parameters; American Academy of Allergy, Asthma, and Immunology; American College of Allergy, Asthma, and Immunology; the Joint Council of Allergy, Asthma, and Immunology.
The diagnosis and management of anaphylaxis practice parameter: 2010 update. *J Allergy Clin Immunol.* 2010;126:477-480.e42.
Lieberman P, Nicklas RA, Oppenheimer J, et al. The diagnosis and management of anaphylaxis practice parameter: 2010 update. *J Allergy Clin Immunol.* 2010;126:477-480.
Middleton R, Reed S, Ellis B, et al. *Allergy Principles and Practice.* 8th ed. Philadelphia: Saunders; 2014.
Shearer WT, Leung DY. Primer on allergic and immunologic diseases. *J Allergy Clin Immunol.* 2010;125:S1-S394.
Sicherer SH, Leung DY. Advances in allergic skin disease, anaphylaxis, and hypersensitivity reactions to foods, drugs, and insects in 2010. *J Allergy Clin Immunol.* 2011;127:326-335.
Simons FE, Frew AJ, Ansotegui IJ. Risk assessment in anaphylaxis: current and future approaches. *J Allergy Clin Immunol.* 2007;120(Suppl 1):S2-S24.

68

Genetics for the Internist

HOWARD P. LEVY, MD, PhD

Although even the most common disorders attributable to mutation in a single gene are individually rare, when considered collectively, they constitute a major health burden. Genetic diseases affect people of all ages and ancestries and manifest symptoms in every organ system. In addition to such single-gene genetic disorders, there is growing recognition of genetic factors in common, everyday conditions encountered in internal medicine. Although cures for genetic disorders are rare, recognition and understanding of genetic factors in disease can improve detection and management of many conditions and prevent or reduce morbidity and mortality.

Basic Genetics Concepts

- Chromosomes
  - Each cell nucleus contains 46 chromosomes
    - 22 pairs of autosomes
    - 1 pair of sex chromosomes (X/Y)
  - In females, one of the two X chromosomes is permanently inactivated in each cell
    - X-inactivation is random and occurs early in embryonic development
    - Both of a woman's X chromosomes are expressed in various parts of her body, but only one or the other in any single cell
    - Therefore, women may have some clinical manifestations of an X-linked disorder
- Genes are carried on chromosomes and thus occur in pairs
  - There are approximately 20,000 to 25,000 pairs of genes
  - Each member of a pair of genes is called an *allele*
  - 37 additional genes are carried on a small mitochondrial chromosome, whose inheritance and behavior are very different from that of the 46 nuclear chromosomes
- Deoxyribonucleic acid (DNA) variation
  - Polymorphism: Alteration in DNA sequence that *does not* affect the function of the gene and typically *has no clinical consequences*
  - **Mutation: Alteration in DNA sequence that *changes gene function* and *has potential clinical manifestations***
  - Alteration of a gene in a germ cell or zygote ultimately will be present in all cells of the resulting person, including his or her germline (the next generation of eggs or sperm), and thus can be inherited

- Mutation of a gene in a somatic cell may cause clinical manifestations, but will not be present in the germline and cannot be inherited
  - Cancer cells accumulate multiple genetic changes that directly affect their behavior and response to therapy, but those changes are not transmitted to future generations
- One or both alleles of a gene may carry an alteration (mutation or polymorphism)
  - **Homozygosity: Both alleles are the same (either normal or altered)**
  - **Heterozygosity: One allele is normal and the other is altered**

Inheritance Patterns

- **Multifactorial inheritance: Most of the common diseases and conditions seen by an internist are multifactorial, resulting from a complex interaction of genetic and environmental factors**
  - The relative contribution of genes and environment can vary, but both are important in virtually all medical conditions (Fig. 69-1)
    - Mutation of a single gene may be the sole major cause, but environmental factors affect specific clinical outcome(s) (e.g., crises and other manifestations in sickle cell anemia)
    - An environmental exposure may be the sole major cause, but genetic factors affect the ultimate clinical outcome (e.g., resistance to human immunodeficiency virus [HIV] infection as a result of mutation of the CCR5 cell surface receptor)
    - Several genetic and environmental risk factors may each have major effects on a condition (e.g., thromboembolic disease) (Fig. 69-2)
    - For most conditions, multiple genetic and environmental factors each contribute relatively small components of risk, and the complete spectrum of risk factors has yet to be fully elucidated
  - Characteristics of multifactorial inheritance
    - Males and females may be equally likely to be affected, or there may be skewing of the sex ratio
    - The condition may cluster in families with greater genetic and/or environmental risk, may appear to skip generations, and/or may seem to occur at random
    - No single gene inheritance pattern is obvious

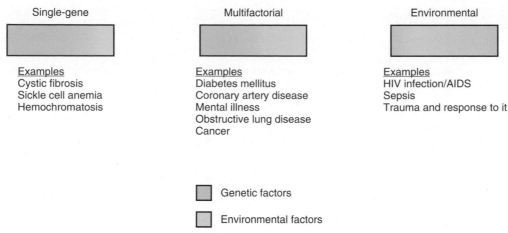

Single-gene

Examples
Cystic fibrosis
Sickle cell anemia
Hemochromatosis

Multifactorial

Examples
Diabetes mellitus
Coronary artery disease
Mental illness
Obstructive lung disease
Cancer

Environmental

Examples
HIV infection/AIDS
Sepsis
Trauma and response to it

Genetic factors

Environmental factors

FIGURE 69-1 All medical conditions have at least some genetic and environmental components. Most conditions are multifactorial, with varying mixes of both. Clinical expression of a single-gene disorder is subject to environmental effects. Response to infection or trauma depends in part on genetic susceptibility and capacity for recovery. AIDS, Acquired immune deficiency syndrome; HIV, human immunodeficiency virus.

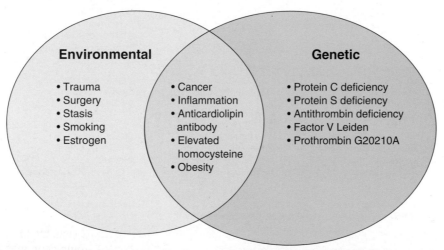

Environmental

• Trauma
• Surgery
• Stasis
• Smoking
• Estrogen

• Cancer
• Inflammation
• Anticardiolipin antibody
• Elevated homocysteine
• Obesity

Genetic

• Protein C deficiency
• Protein S deficiency
• Antithrombin deficiency
• Factor V Leiden
• Prothrombin G20210A

FIGURE 69-2 Thromboembolic disease as an example of a multifactorial condition. Several known genetic and environmental risk factors have been identified. Typically, more than one risk factor is necessary to manifest the condition. Note that several risk factors are themselves multifactorial; both genetic and environmental factors contribute to cancer, inflammation, anticardiolipin antibody syndrome, hyperhomocysteinemia, and obesity.

- **Estimation of risk to family members is largely empirical but increases with the number of affected relatives, closer degree of relation, and severity**
  - Box 69-1 lists red flags that should prompt consideration of increased genetic predisposition to a specific disease
- **Single-gene (Mendelian) inheritance: Applies when a trait or condition results from alteration of one or both alleles of a single gene**
  - One member of each pair of chromosomes (and thus genes) is passed along in each egg or sperm cell
  - An altered allele can be inherited from either parent (or both if they are both carriers)
  - DNA polymorphisms and mutations do not have to be inherited from either parent; they can occur as new errors in an egg or sperm cell
  - See Table 69-1 for characteristics of autosomal dominant, autosomal recessive, and X-linked inheritance patterns

BOX 69-1 | *Red Flags Suggestive of Increased Genetic Risk for a Multifactorial Condition*

Multiple affected relatives
Closely related affected relatives
Younger-than-expected age of onset
Occurrence in the less commonly affected sex
Multiple primary occurrences of the same or a related condition in an individual
Unusually severe manifestations
Other exceptions to usual epidemiology:
  Histopathology
  Anatomic location

- See Table 69-2 for examples of some Mendelian disorders
- **Mitochondrial inheritance (see Table 69-1): Applies when a trait or condition results from alteration of the mitochondrial DNA**

TABLE 69-1	*Inheritance Patterns*			
	Autosomal Dominant	**Autosomal Recessive**	**X-Linked**	**Mitochondrial**
Definition	Heterozygosity for mutation of a single gene is sufficient to cause the condition (unless the gene is on the X or mitochondrial chromosome)	Homozygosity for mutation of a single gene is necessary to cause the condition (unless the gene is on the X or mitochondrial chromosome) Carriers (heterozygotes) usually have no clinical manifestations	The condition results from mutation of a single gene located on the X chromosome Also called "sex-linked," because of characteristic inheritance patterns in men and women	Mutation of a gene contained on the mitochondrial chromosome causes the condition Most mitochondrial proteins are encoded on nuclear genes, and therefore follow autosomal or X-linked inheritance patterns
Distribution in the family	Multiple generations affected	One or more siblings affected, but (usually) only in one generation	Multiple generations affected May appear to skip generations when transmitted by a carrier female Affected males are related to each other through one or more carrier females	Multiple generations affected
Parents of an affected	Usually one or the other affected Sometimes neither affected	Usually both are carriers Usually neither affected	Mothers often carriers Fathers of affected sons are *never* affected	Mothers almost always affected Fathers never affected
Siblings of an affected	50% chance of being affected (unless neither parent affected)	25% chance of being affected 50% chance of being a carrier	Brothers have 50% chance of being affected Sisters have 50% chance of being a carrier	All are affected
Children of an affected	50% chance of being affected	All are carriers Can be affected only if the other parent is a carrier	Sons of affected fathers are *never* affected (always inherit father's Y and mother's X chromosomes) Daughters of affected fathers are *always* carriers (always inherit father's X chromosome) Sons of carrier mothers have 50% chance of being affected Daughters of carrier mothers have 50% chance of being a carrier	All children of affected mothers are affected No children of affected fathers are affected
Sex ratio	Males and females equally likely to be affected	Males and females equally likely to be affected	Almost all affected patients are male	Males and females equally likely to be affected
Other comments	Variable expression and reduced penetrance are common	Parental consanguinity is sometimes present Relatively high prevalence of some recessive conditions caused by "heterozygote advantage," in which carriers have a survival advantage (e.g., carriers of sickle cell anemia are relatively resistant to malaria)	Male-to-male transmission does not occur Carrier females may have mild clinical manifestations	Heteroplasmy often results in variable expression, complicating recognition of some affected relatives

TABLE 69-2	*Some Representative Single-Gene Disorders*
Condition	**Some Clinical Considerations**
Autosomal Dominant	
Marfan syndrome	Joint laxity; characteristic skeletal features; myopia and/or lens dislocation; aortic aneurysm/dissection
Neurofibromatosis type 1	Benign and occasionally malignant nerve sheath tumors; hypertension
Polycystic kidney disease	Renal, hepatic, and splenic cysts; renal failure; nephrolithiasis; hypertension; cerebral berry aneurysms occur in approximately 10% and correlate with specific mutations, so family history predicts risk of aneurysm
Hereditary breast and ovarian cancer	Breast and ovarian cancer; also pancreatic, prostate, and other associated cancers
Lynch syndrome	Colon, endometrial, and other associated cancers
Familial adenomatous polyposis	Colon and other associated cancers; characteristic benign ocular manifestations; fully penetrant: 100% chance of cancer
Multiple endocrine neoplasia syndromes	Benign and malignant endocrine tumors; benign tumors frequently hormonally active
Achondroplasia	Most common cause of dwarfism
Autosomal Recessive	
Hemochromatosis	Iron overload; cardiac, hepatic, endocrine, and joint complications; low clinical penetrance
Sickle cell anemia	Hemoglobinopathy; painful and degenerative ischemic complications; certain infections; more common in descendants of traditional malarial regions (especially Africa)
Cystic fibrosis	Defective ion transport; sinopulmonary, pancreatic, intestinal, and fertility complications; especially common in Northern Europeans; different specific mutations more common with different ancestry
α- and β-Thalassemia	Hemoglobinopathy; anemia; α more common in Chinese and Southeast Asians; β more common in Mediterranean descendants
Tay-Sachs disease	Neurodegenerative condition caused by metabolic enzyme deficiency; common in Ashkenazi Jews and French Canadians, but disease itself is now rare in these populations because of effective screening programs
X-Linked	
Fragile X syndrome	Mental retardation; characteristic facial features; joint laxity
Hemophilia A	Classic hemophilia, caused by factor VIII deficiency; bleeding diathesis; variable expression
Duchenne/Becker muscular dystrophy	Most common cause of muscular dystrophy; Becker less severe than Duchenne, but same gene

- Each mitochondrion carries multiple copies of its chromosome, and each cell contains many mitochondria
- **Heteroplasmy: the relative proportion of normal and abnormal mitochondria within individual cells, tissues, and organs; affects the severity and distribution of clinical manifestations**
- There is significant genetic variation within and between individual mitochondria in a single cell, as well as between individual cells, tissues, and organs
  - Heteroplasmy can vary over time within a single person and even in different tissues within a single person
  - This leads to significant variation in clinical presentation of mitochondrially inherited disorders
- **Mitochondria are inherited almost exclusively through the egg; sperm mitochondria only rarely are incorporated into a fertilized egg**
  - Mitochondrial inheritance depends upon the sex of the parent rather than the sex of the child

- All of an affected mother's children would be expected to inherit mutations in her mitochondrial DNA
- None of an affected father's children would be expected to inherit mutations in his mitochondrial DNA
- Clinical manifestations of mitochondrial mutations vary but are primarily neuromuscular
  - Central nervous system: encephalopathy, seizures, dementia, migraine, stroke-like episodes, ataxia, spasticity
  - Peripheral nervous system: ptosis, external ophthalmoplegia, sensorineural deafness, optic atrophy, pigmentary retinopathy, peripheral neuropathy, autonomic neuropathy
  - Skeletal muscle: proximal myopathy, weakness, hypotonia
  - Cardiomyopathy
  - Diabetes mellitus
  - Susceptibility to aminoglycoside-induced ototoxicity

- **Chromosomal inheritance: Applies when all or part of a chromosome is duplicated or deleted**
  - Numerical abnormalities
    - An entire chromosome is missing or duplicated
      - Most are incompatible with life and result in early miscarriage
      - Typically not inherited or passed along to future generations
    - Monosomy of the X chromosome (45 chromosomes, only one X) causes Turner syndrome, manifesting short stature, characteristic physical features, and normal intelligence
      - 99% end in miscarriage
      - Always female
    - Trisomy 21 (47 chromosomes, three copies of #21) causes Down syndrome, manifesting mental retardation, short stature, conotruncal cardiac defects (atrioventricular canal, atrial septal defect, ventricular septal defect), hypothyroidism, increased risk of hematologic malignancy (acute myelogenous leukemia and acute lymphocytic leukemia), and other malformations
    - An extra copy of the X chromosome has milder manifestations, including tall stature and mild mental retardation
    - An extra copy of the Y chromosome usually has no clinical effect; contrary to older reports, this condition does not cause violent behavior or greater likelihood of incarceration
  - Structural abnormalities
    - Large deletions or duplications are visible at the microscopic level, involve a major section of a chromosome, and may affect hundreds of genes
      - Clinical manifestations may include mental retardation, growth retardation, and malformations
      - May be inherited from a parent with a balanced rearrangement (see following discussion), but affected patients with large deletions or duplications usually do not reproduce
    - Microdeletions, or contiguous gene syndromes, involve loss of a short segment of a chromosome and affect only a few genes
      - Clinical manifestations vary depending upon the specific genes involved
      - Many are compatible with a normal life span and fertility
      - Can occur as a new genetic change or can be inherited in an autosomal dominant pattern
    - Balanced rearrangements occur when segments are exchanged between two or more chromosomes, but no material is deleted or duplicated
      - May have no clinical manifestations
      - May cause symptoms by disrupting a gene
      - May cause symptoms by creation of a new abnormal gene (e.g., the Philadelphia chromosome in chronic myelogenous leukemia is a translocation that joins portions of two genes, producing a hybrid that contributes to unregulated growth)

Factors That Complicate Observed Inheritance Patterns

- **Variable expression and reduced penetrance: Clinical features of a single gene (Mendelian) disorder may vary greatly from one patient to the next, including age of onset, severity, and organ or tissue distribution of manifestations; see Box 69-2 for examples**
  - Variation occurs not only between unrelated individuals but also among members of the same family who all carry the same mutation
  - Environmental factors and small effects from other genetic changes contribute to variable expression
- **An individual may carry and transmit a disease-causing mutation, even if the expression is so mild that it goes unrecognized**
  - Inability to detect any clinical manifestations is referred to as reduced penetrance
  - A woman carrying an autosomal dominant mutation predisposing to breast/ovarian cancer might never develop any cancer herself, but her daughters have 50% risk of inheriting the same mutation from her and will have increased risk for the associated cancers if they do
- Sex-limited expression is an example of variable expression and is caused by physiologic differences between the sexes
  - Sex-limited expression is distinct from X-linked inheritance because it only impacts clinical expression, not the likelihood of inheriting or transmitting a mutation
  - A man with an autosomal dominant mutation predisposing to breast cancer is unlikely to

BOX 69-2	*Examples of Variable and Sex-Limited Expression and Reduced Penetrance*

Frequency and severity of crises are different in every patient with sickle cell anemia

Presence or absence of berry aneurysms in polycystic kidney disease tends to be consistent within a family, but age of onset and severity of hypertension and/or renal failure are quite variable

Severity, age of onset, and progression of skeletal, ocular, cardiovascular, and other complications in Marfan syndrome are highly variable, both within and between families

Some variation in pulmonary, gastrointestinal, pancreatic, and other manifestations in cystic fibrosis may be attributed to the specific mutation (thus consistent within families), but most of the variation is independent of the specific mutation

Most hereditary cancer syndromes confer increased risk of cancer, but not 100% likelihood of developing cancer

Prostate cancer cannot occur in a female

Ovarian cancer cannot occur in a male

Breast cancer is much less likely to occur, but not impossible, in a male

Females with hereditary hemochromatosis tend to have milder and later onset of symptoms than males because of menstrual blood loss

manifest breast cancer himself, but his daughters have 50% risk of inheriting the same mutation from him and will have increased breast cancer risk if they do
- **Anticipation: Some genetic conditions have onset at an earlier age and/or are more severe in successive generations**
  - The most common mutational mechanism is expansion of trinucleotide (or triplet) repeats within a gene, which can increase in successive generations as a result of errors in DNA replication
    - Severity increases and age of onset decreases in proportion to the length of the repeat
  - Most diseases in this category are adult-onset (or late childhood-onset) and primarily affect the nervous system
    - Huntington disease: adult-onset chorea, dysarthria, dysphagia, cognitive dysfunction, and psychosis
    - Fragile X syndrome: Classic presentation is childhood-onset mental retardation, characteristic facial features and joint laxity; shorter trinucleotide expansions result in adult-onset ataxia, tremor, and cognitive dysfunction
- **Imprinting: Some parts of the genome are chemically tagged (imprinted) to mark whether they were inherited through the egg or sperm; an imprinted gene is expressed only from the maternal or paternal allele**
  - Inheritance of a mutation follows the traditional 50:50 pattern, but clinical expression depends on the parent of origin
    - Mutations in the silenced (inactive) parental allele have no clinical effect
    - Mutations in the active parental allele will be clinically expressed, regardless of whether the other (silenced) is normal or mutated
  - **The sex of the parent who passes along the mutation is the critical factor, not the sex of the child who inherits the mutation**

Genetic Testing

- **Although "genetic testing" is usually thought of as direct analysis of DNA, family history and virtually any test or procedure may yield a result with direct or indirect genetic implications and could thus be thought of as a genetic test**
  - **Full discussion of the indications, limitations, risks, and benefits (i.e., genetic counseling) should precede most DNA testing and many other forms of genetic testing**
    - Consultation with a genetic counselor or medical geneticist is often appropriate
    - With adequate experience and training, an internist or subspecialist can perform pretest counseling
- Benefits of DNA testing
  - Can help to confirm a clinical diagnosis
  - Can establish a specific genetic cause for a disorder
  - Can help predict natural history and guide management
  - Can identify carriers of recessive mutations
  - Can facilitate presymptomatic or predictive testing in relatives of patients with single-gene disorders, subject to variation in clinical expression and penetrance
  - Can help in risk assessment for multifactorial conditions, when specific genetic risk factors are known
  - DNA test results are independent of environmental factors and generally do not change over the life span; therefore, no need to repeat unless testing somatic tissue or laboratory error is suspected
  - Somatic DNA testing (e.g., tumor tissue) and DNA testing of infectious agents (e.g., HIV, hepatitis C) can help guide therapeutic decisions
    - Identify susceptibility to specific medications
    - Monitor disease activity, response, and/or progression
- **Limitations of DNA testing**
  - **False negatives: A negative (or normal) DNA test usually does not completely rule out disease**
    - Most DNA tests are less than 100% sensitive (i.e., not all potential mutations in a gene can be detected by most tests)
    - Multiple different genes may cause or contribute to a condition; thus, the wrong gene may have been tested
    - The individual family member who underwent testing may coincidentally have a sporadic, nongenetic cause of the disease in the family; another relative might have a detectable mutation; this is of greatest concern for common diseases, such as breast cancer
  - **False positives: A positive (or abnormal) DNA test does not always confirm disease or increased disease risk**
    - Polymorphisms: Some DNA variations cause no clinical manifestations
    - Variable expression and reduced penetrance complicate prediction of clinical manifestations based solely on DNA test results
    - For multifactorial conditions, some literature reports of association between DNA variation and disease risk are erroneous
- Deciding who to test
  - Diagnostic testing (to establish, confirm, or further elucidate a genetic diagnosis) should ideally be performed in a clinically affected person before testing unaffected family members who are at risk
    - Testing a clinically affected person reduces the risk of false-positive/false-negative results when compared with initially testing an at-risk unaffected family member
  - **Predictive, presymptomatic, or carrier testing in an unaffected person is more informative after an affected relative has been tested to establish the specific genetic mutation(s) present in the family**
    - If the specific mutation(s) in the family is (are) known:
      - Subsequent testing of at-risk family members can focus on the specific known mutation(s)

and is much less expensive than sequencing one or more genes
- A negative DNA test in an unaffected relative means he or she did not inherit the known mutation(s) and is at average risk for the disease based on his or her other risk factors (high negative predictive value)
- A positive DNA test in an unaffected relative means he or she did inherit the known mutation(s) and is at increased risk for the disease; positive predictive value for actual clinical manifestations depends on the variability and penetrance of the disease
- If the specific mutation(s) in the family is (are) unknown:
  - Testing of at-risk family members will likely require much more expensive full sequencing of one or more genes
  - A negative DNA test in an unaffected relative may be a false negative and not accurately predict protection from disease (low negative predictive value)
  - A positive DNA test in an unaffected relative may be a false positive and not accurately predict disease predisposition (low positive predictive value)
- Ethical and social considerations regarding genetic testing and diagnoses
  - Potential issues for an affected individual (or with a false positive test)
    - Stigmatization
    - Isolation from the family or society
    - Anxiety
    - Guilt related to potentially transmitting a disease (or disease risk) to children
    - **Employment and/or insurance discrimination**
      - **GINA (Genetic Information Nondiscrimination Act) protects against employment and health insurance discrimination**
      - Military is exempt from GINA
      - No legal protection for life, long-term care, or other forms of insurance
      - Abuses are relatively rare, but this is a significant potential concern
    - Privacy and security of genetic diagnoses and test results
  - Additional potential issues for relatives of an affected individual
    - Right to know that they are at increased risk for a genetic condition
    - Right to not know that they are at increased risk for a genetic condition
      - Example: An adult at risk for Huntington disease may choose not to undergo genetic testing; if his or her child has a positive genetic test, then the parent in question almost certainly carries the same genetic mutation and has lost the right not to know
  - Duty to warn: In some cases, the physician (or patient) may have an ethical duty to warn at-risk relatives of their genetic risk, even if the relatives are not patients of that physician

- Survivor guilt related to learning that one does not have the same genetic disease or risk as a sibling, parent, or child
- For anyone undergoing DNA testing
  - **Results may reveal that biologic relationships are not the same as social relationships (most commonly that one's father is not who it was thought to be)**
  - False negatives may lead to inappropriate false reassurance (as with any other testing)
  - False positives may lead to unnecessary additional testing and/or treatment (as with any other testing)
- With advances in DNA sequencing technology, it is becoming less expensive to sequence the entire exome (the approximately 1% of the genome that actually codes for genes) than to sequence 2 to 5 individual genes. However:
  - The sensitivity of exome sequencing is lower than single gene sequencing (false negatives)
  - There may be secondary or incidental findings—discovery of clinically significant mutations in genes unrelated to the disease for which sequencing was originally ordered
  - Because more DNA is sequenced, there is increased risk of identifying polymorphisms that are erroneously associated with disease or disease risk, especially for secondary or incidental findings (false positives)
- Predictive or presymptomatic testing of children or adolescents for adult-onset conditions is almost always inappropriate because obtaining such knowledge is irreversible
  - It is preferable to wait until adulthood when the risks and benefits of testing can be evaluated by the individual at risk
  - If the disease onsets in childhood or if effective childhood interventions to reduce or prevent disease are available, then such testing may be appropriate (e.g., familial adenomatous polyposis, in which onset, screening, and management all begin in childhood; see below)
- Diagnostic genetic testing of a symptomatic child is not subject to this concern, but still raises all of the other issues listed in this section

Some Clinical Examples

HEREDITARY BREAST AND OVARIAN CANCER SYNDROME (HBOC)

Basic Information

- Most breast cancer is sporadic or multifactorial
- Approximately 5% to 10% of all breast cancer is caused by single gene disorders
- HBOC syndrome, caused by mutations in the *BRCA1* and *BRCA2* genes, accounts for most (60% to 80%) hereditary breast cancer and approximately 3% of all breast cancer

- Inheritance of HBOC syndrome is autosomal dominant with reduced penetrance and variable expression
  - **Men are equally likely as women to transmit an HBOC mutation to their children, even if they do not manifest breast cancer themselves**
  - **A paternal family history of breast and/or ovarian cancer is as significant as a maternal family history**
- Other known genetic causes of breast cancer include:
  - Cowden syndrome: associated with thyroid, skin, and gastrointestinal (GI) hamartomas and cancers
  - Li-Fraumeni syndrome: associated with sarcomas

Clinical Presentation of *BRCA1* and *BRCA2* Mutations

- Breast cancer can occur as young as 30 years old
  - Lifetime breast cancer risk for women is 40% to 80%
  - Lifetime breast cancer risk for men is 1% to 10%
- Lifetime risk of ovarian cancer is 11% to 40%
- Other associated cancers include peritoneal, prostate, and pancreas

Diagnosis and Evaluation

- Suspect hereditary breast cancer when multiple red flags listed in Box 69-1 are present
  - Male breast cancer is highly suspicious for hereditary breast cancer
  - HBOC syndrome is more common in people of Ashkenazi Jewish ancestry than in the general population
- If a *BRCA1* or *BRCA2* mutation is identified in a family, relatives at risk need only be tested for that specific mutation
- Testing for other genetic causes of hereditary breast cancer is also available and is best managed by a specialist
- Negative DNA testing in an unaffected person with strong family history has low negative predictive value if the specific genetic etiology in the family has not been identified

Treatment

- All first-degree relatives should be informed of their increased risk and offered genetic counseling
- Bilateral mastectomy for primary surgical management of breast cancer reduces risk of a second primary tumor
- Prognosis for breast cancer is similar to sporadic breast cancer
- Prognosis for ovarian cancer may be better than sporadic ovarian cancer
- New therapies targeting the DNA repair defect associated with the underlying genetic mutation show promise
  - Platinum-based chemotherapy
  - Poly ADP-ribose polymerase (PARP) inhibitors

Prevention

- Start breast cancer screening (breast self-examination, clinical breast examination, and radiologic imaging) 10 years earlier than standard population screening (25 years old, rather than 35 years old) or 10 years earlier than the earliest age of onset in an affected relative, whichever is younger
- Breast magnetic resonance imaging (MRI) has much higher sensitivity than mammography or ultrasound, and it is recommended as part of annual breast imaging for women with HBOC syndrome
- Annual or semiannual ovarian cancer screening with pelvic examination, transvaginal ultrasound, and serum cancer antigen 125 (CA 125) testing beginning at age 35 years may improve detection and survival
- For men with known or suspected *BRCA1* or *BRCA2* mutation, consider annual prostate cancer screening (digital rectal exam and serum PSA testing) starting at age 40 years
- Tamoxifen reduces the risk of developing breast cancer (at least estrogen/progesterone receptor-positive breast cancer)
- **Bilateral prophylactic mastectomy reduces (but does not completely eliminate) the risk of breast cancer**
- **Bilateral prophylactic salpingo-oophorectomy reduces (but does not completely eliminate) the risk of breast and ovarian cancer in patients with known or suspected *BRCA1* or *BRCA2* mutation, but it does not reduce the risk of peritoneal carcinoma**

HEREDITARY COLON CANCER

- Approximately 10% of all colon cancer is attributable to single-gene syndromes
- Lynch syndrome and familial adenomatous polyposis (FAP) are the most common causes; see individual sections that follow
- An additional 30% of all colon cancer occurs in individuals with a family history of colon cancer, consistent with multifactorial inheritance
- Colonoscopy for cancer screening in patients with a family history of hereditary multifactorial colon cancer should:
  - **Begin 10 years earlier than the youngest age of onset in the family or at age 40 years, whichever is younger**
  - **Be repeated every 3 to 5 years**

LYNCH SYNDROME

Basic Information

- Accounts for 1% to 3% of all colon cancer and 1% to 2% of all endometrial cancer
- Also known as hereditary nonpolyposis colon cancer
- Caused by mutation in one of several DNA mismatch repair genes
- Autosomal dominant predisposition to multiple cancers with variable expression and reduced penetrance

Clinical Presentation

- **Average age of cancer onset (colon or other) is mid-40s**
- Often poorly differentiated and more aggressive than sporadic colon adenocarcinoma

69

- **Most Lynch syndrome colon cancers (two thirds) occur in proximal (ascending) colon, in contrast to sporadic colon cancer predominantly occurring more distally**
- Lifetime risk of colon cancer is 30% to 80%
- Lifetime risk of endometrial cancer is 20% to 60%
- Other associated tumors include stomach or small-bowel adenocarcinoma, transitional cell carcinoma of the proximal ureter, sebaceous skin neoplasms, glioblastoma multiforme, and hepatobiliary and ovarian cancer

Diagnosis and Evaluation

- See Box 69-3 for clinical diagnostic criteria that suggest Lynch syndrome
- When clinically suspected, test tumor tissue for microsatellite instability (MSI) and/or immunohistochemistry (IHC)
    - **Because of poor sensitivity of clinical diagnostic criteria, MSI or IHC testing is recommended for all newly diagnosed colon cancers, and has been suggested for all newly diagnosed endometrial cancers**
    - Microsatellites are regions of highly repetitive DNA
    - In tumor tissue with faulty DNA mismatch repair, these regions demonstrate variable length (instability)
    - MSI within tumor tissue is highly predictive of Lynch syndrome
    - IHC showing absence of one or more mismatch repair proteins within tumor tissue is also highly predictive of Lynch syndrome
- If MSI is high (strongly positive) and/or IHC is abnormal, proceed to DNA testing of mismatch repair genes

Treatment

- All first-degree relatives should be informed of their increased risk and offered genetic counseling

---

BOX 69-3 *Clinical Criteria of Lynch Syndrome*

Amsterdam II Criteria

All of (mnemonic "3-2-1"):
   3 or more family members with Lynch syndrome-associated cancer, each a first-degree relative of at least one other affected relative
   2 successive generations affected
   1 or more cancer(s) onset before age 50 years
   Sensitivity lower; specificity higher

Bethesda Criteria

Any one of:
   Positive Amsterdam II criteria
   Two independent Lynch syndrome-related cancers
   Colon or endometrial cancer onset before age 50 years
   Colonic adenoma onset before age 40 years
   Colon cancer at any age, plus a first-degree relative with either a Lynch syndrome-related cancer onset before age 50 years or colonic adenoma before age 40 years
   Signet-ring cell–type colon cancer onset before age 50 years
   Sensitivity higher; specificity lower

- Lynch-associated colon cancer prognosis may be better than for sporadic colon cancer
- Total colectomy is preferred over partial colectomy in Lynch syndrome patients with colon cancer

Prevention

- Colonoscopy every 1 to 2 years beginning at age 20 to 25 years, or 5 to 10 years earlier than the earliest age of colon cancer diagnosis in the family, whichever is earlier
- Consider annual transvaginal ultrasound, endometrial biopsy, and possibly serum CA 125 measurement, beginning at age 30 to 35 years, or 5 to 10 years earlier than the earliest age of cancer diagnosis in the family, whichever is earlier
- Consider upper endoscopy every 2 to 3 years starting around age 30 to 35 years to screen for duodenal tumors
- Consider annual urinalysis and/or urine cytology starting around age 30 years to screen for urinary tract cancer
- Daily aspirin use appears to reduce the risk of colon and other Lynch syndrome-related cancers.
- **Prophylactic colectomy is not recommended because colon cancer screening is effective**
- Prophylactic hysterectomy and oophorectomy is an option

FAMILIAL ADENOMATOUS POLYPOSIS (Fig. 69-3)

Basic Information

- FAP accounts for approximately 1% of all colon cancer
- Caused by mutation in *APC*, a tumor suppressor gene
- Autosomal dominant predisposition to colonic adenomas, which evolve into cancer
- **Expression is variable, but penetrance is complete (100%) for colonic adenomas and cancer**

Clinical Presentation

- Hundreds to thousands of colonic adenomas
- Average age of polyp onset is 16 years
- Average age of colon cancer is 39 years

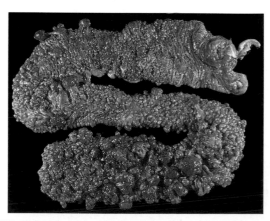

FIGURE 69-3 Familial adenomatous polyposis in an 18-year-old woman. The mucosal surface is carpeted by innumerable polypoid adenomas. (From Kumar V, Fausto N, Abbas A. *Robbins and Cotran Pathologic Basis of Disease.* 7th ed. Philadelphia: Saunders; 2004: Fig. 17.59.)

- Other manifestations include gastric and small-bowel polyps (approximately 5% to 10% malignant), osteomas (never malignant), papillary thyroid cancer, hepatoblastoma, benign skin lesions (epidermoid cysts, fibromas, desmoid tumors), and extra or missing teeth
- Congenital hypertrophy of the retinal pigment epithelium (CHRPE) occurs in 70% to 80%
  - Benign pigmented retinal hamartomas
  - When bilateral, highly suggestive of FAP, and thus a useful clinical diagnostic tool
- Attenuated FAP is a milder presentation resulting from mutations in the same gene
  - Usually fewer than 100 adenomas; average is about 30
  - Average age of cancer onset is mid-50s
  - Other manifestations are similar to FAP

Diagnosis and Evaluation

- Consider DNA testing in patients with suggestive clinical findings or known family history of FAP
  - Bilateral CHRPE is highly suggestive of FAP
- Among patients with typical clinical manifestations, APC gene analysis has a mutation detection rate of 80% to 90%

Treatment and Prevention

- First-degree relatives should be informed of their increased risk and offered genetic counseling
- Annual lower endoscopy beginning at age 10 to 12 years of age
  - Sigmoidoscopy or colonoscopy before development of one or more adenomas
  - Colonoscopy after one or more adenomas develop
- **Colectomy when there are 20 to 30 adenomas or when polyp histology is advanced; this is usually adolescence or very early adulthood**
  - **After colectomy, lower endoscopic surveillance is still necessary**
  - The 2015 American College of Gastroenterology recommends upper endoscopic evaluation at time of colonic polyp identification or at 25 years, whichever comes first
- Nonsteroidal antiinflammatory drugs and cyclooxygenase-2 inhibitors reduce the rate of adenoma formation and may help to delay colectomy from adolescence to young adulthood
- Endoscopic and radiologic visualization of the stomach and small bowel every 1 to 3 years beginning when colonic polyps are found
- Annual thyroid palpation (± annual thyroid ultrasound)

HEREDITARY HEMOCHROMATOSIS CAUSED BY *HFE* MUTATIONS

Basic Information

- Homozygous mutation of the *HFE* gene is the most common cause of iron overload in Caucasian patients
- Other genetic and environmental causes of hemochromatosis and iron overload exist

- ***HFE* hemochromatosis is the most common autosomal recessive single-gene disorder among adults**
  - 1:200 to 1:400 Caucasian individuals have two mutant alleles (genetically susceptible)
  - 1:10 (10%) Caucasian individuals have one mutant allele (unaffected carrier)
- The high carrier frequency results in pseudodominant inheritance
  - 100% chance that a genetically susceptible person (both alleles mutated) passes along a mutant allele to the offspring
  - 10% chance that a Caucasian spouse is a carrier
  - 50% chance that a carrier spouse passes along a mutant allele to the offspring
  - **1:20 (100% × 10% × 50% = 5%) chance that a child of a genetically susceptible person with a Caucasian partner will also be genetically susceptible**
- Only two specific mutations are clearly associated with clinical disease: *C282Y* and *H63D*
  - Homozygosity for the *C282Y* mutation accounts for approximately 90% of clinically manifest cases of hereditary hemochromatosis
  - Compound heterozygosity, with one *C282Y* allele and one *H63D* allele, accounts for most of the rest
  - Homozygosity for the *H63D* mutation almost never causes clinical symptoms
  - Other variations in the *HFE* gene are common, but likely represent benign polymorphisms

Clinical Presentation

- Manifestations are caused by increased GI iron absorption and storage in multiple organs, especially liver, skin, pancreas, joints, heart, testes, and pituitary
  - Nonspecific symptoms include abdominal pain, weakness, fatigue, lethargy, and weight loss
  - Transaminase elevation and/or hepatomegaly may or may not occur
  - Cirrhosis, portal hypertension, and liver failure may occur late in the disease
  - Hepatocellular carcinoma occurs only in the setting of cirrhosis
  - Arthralgia is common, especially in the hands, but other joints may be involved
  - Hypogonadism may be central (pituitary) or peripheral (testicular)
  - Bronze-colored hyperpigmentation, insulin-resistant or insulin-dependent diabetes mellitus, cardiomyopathy, and arrhythmia are late manifestations
- Variable and sex-limited expression
  - *C282Y* homozygotes are more severely affected than compound heterozygotes
  - Men generally have earlier onset (in their 40s and 50s) and more severe manifestations than women (peri- or postmenopausal onset)
- Reduced penetrance
  - 40% to 70% of *C282Y* homozygotes develop elevated iron levels (biochemical disease)
  - 10% to 33% of *C282Y* homozygotes develop clinical signs or symptoms (clinical disease)

69

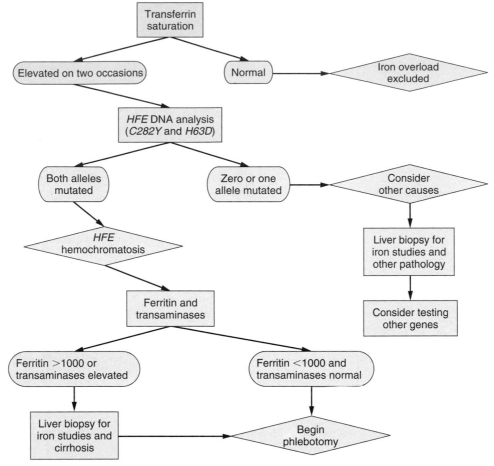

FIGURE 69-4 Algorithm for evaluation of suspected hemochromatosis. DNA, Deoxyribonucleic acid.

Diagnosis and Evaluation

- See Figure 69-4 for an evaluation algorithm for suspected hemochromatosis
- Increased transferrin saturation on two independent assays is the most sensitive and specific blood test for iron overload but does not establish the specific cause
  - Traditional thresholds are 60% for men and 50% for women
  - A lower threshold of 45% has higher sensitivity but lower specificity
- Increased serum ferritin is common but is not specific for iron overload
  - Ferritin greater than 1000 μg/L, especially in the setting of elevated transaminases, may be suggestive of cirrhosis and deserves further evaluation (e.g., liver biopsy)
- **DNA testing is used only to confirm the diagnosis in affected individuals and to facilitate evaluation of at-risk relatives**
  - The presence of only one mutant allele establishes carrier status but is insufficient to confirm a diagnosis of hereditary hemochromatosis
  - False-positive or false-negative results for C282Y and H63D testing are unlikely

Treatment

- **Iron-depletion therapy is appropriate for patients with documented iron overload, regardless of presence or absence of clinical signs or symptoms**
  - **Weekly phlebotomy of 500 mL blood, until serum ferritin is less than 50 ng/mL**
  - If anemia occurs, decrease frequency of phlebotomy (and potentially reconsider the diagnosis)
  - **Maintenance phlebotomy about two to six times per year to keep ferritin level less than 50 ng/ mL and transferrin saturation less than 50%**
  - Untreated patients with HFE mutations and normal iron study results should have transferrin saturation and serum ferritin checked every 1 to 5 years
- Dietary restrictions: Avoid iron supplements, vitamin C, alcohol, and uncooked seafood
- If cirrhosis is present, screen for hepatocellular carcinoma every 6 to 12 months
- Prognosis
  - **Phlebotomy improves liver disease and may partially reverse cirrhosis but does not reduce the risk of hepatocellular carcinoma once cirrhosis has occurred**
  - Phlebotomy usually reverses cardiac complications and nonspecific symptoms

(abdominal pain, weakness, fatigue, lethargy, and weight loss)
- **Endocrine deficiencies and arthralgia usually do not improve with phlebotomy**

Prevention

- All first-degree relatives of an affected patient should be offered DNA testing
  - Siblings have a 25% chance of being genetically susceptible and a 50% chance of being carriers
  - Both parents are likely to at least be carriers but may be affected
  - All children must at least be carriers but may be genetically susceptible if the other parent is a carrier

NEUROFIBROMATOSIS TYPE 1

Basic Information

- **Autosomal dominant syndrome resulting in focal overgrowth of multiple tissues, especially (but not exclusively) those derived from the neural crest**
- One of the most common dominant single-gene disorders, affecting approximately 1 in 3000 people worldwide
- Results from mutation of the neurofibromatosis type 1 (*NF1*) gene, whose protein product, neurofibromin, functions as a tumor suppressor and regulator of cellular growth and differentiation

Clinical Presentation

- **Penetrance is complete (100%), but clinical expression is quite variable**
- Skin (Fig. 69-5A to C)
  - Café-au-lait macules occur in the first year of life and increase in size and number throughout childhood
  - Axillary or inguinal freckling
  - Benign dermal neurofibromas (soft, fleshy nerve or nerve sheath-associated tumors) gradually increase in number and size throughout life but especially rapidly during puberty and pregnancy
  - Glomus tumors result from painful and tender proliferation of glomus bodies, which are thermoregulatory tissues under the nail bed
- Plexiform neurofibromas (diffuse amorphous nerve sheath tumors) occur in up to 50% of patients, enlarge over time, and may cause significant morbidity by local compression or invasion
- Cognitive function and development
  - Most patients have normal intelligence; some have mild cognitive impairment with average IQ 88 to 94
  - Learning difficulties are common (50% to 75% of patients)
  - Deficits in fine motor, language, and social development may occur
  - Attention deficit is common
- Unidentified bright objects are T2 hyperintensities on cerebral MRI that occur anywhere in the brain in about 60% of patients and are of no apparent clinical consequence; they often regress or disappear by adulthood

- Ocular
  - Lisch nodules are benign iris hamartomas present in nearly all patients by adulthood (see Fig. 69-5D)
  - Optic pathway gliomas occur in approximately 15% of patients, but only half cause clinical manifestations (proptosis, strabismus, optic nerve pallor, reduced visual acuity, or vision loss)
- Skeletal manifestations include scoliosis, sphenoid dysplasia, and, rarely, long bone cortical thinning or bowing
  - Pathologic fracture of thinned distal tibia is common and heals poorly, if at all, resulting in pseudarthrosis (creation of a "pseudojoint")
- Hypertension is more frequent than in the general population
  - Occurs at any age, including childhood
  - Usually essential hypertension
  - Sometimes because of *NF1* vasculopathy: renal artery stenosis, aortic coarctation, narrowing of any other artery
- Malignancy
  - Malignant peripheral nerve sheath tumor develops from a plexiform neurofibroma in about 10% of patients
  - Pheochromocytoma, rhabdomyoma, neuroblastoma, and childhood leukemia may occur
- Average life span is about 8 years shorter than the general population
  - Premature death is primarily associated with malignancy and vasculopathy

Diagnosis and Evaluation

- See Box 69-4 for clinical diagnostic criteria
- Genetic testing can detect *NF1* mutations in about 95% of affected patients but is almost never needed clinically
  - Can be used to establish the diagnosis in young children not yet meeting clinical diagnostic criteria
  - Useful for prenatal diagnosis if the affected parent's specific mutation is known
- Evaluation and monitoring
  - Annual physical examination seeking typical manifestations
  - Blood pressure measurement at every visit
  - Ophthalmologic examination annually in children, less frequently in adults (seeking Lisch nodules and optic glioma)
  - Routine cerebral MRI is not recommended because optic nerve or intracranial lesions that require monitoring or intervention will cause clinical manifestations

Treatment

- Secondary causes of hypertension should be considered at any age, especially renovascular hypertension, pheochromocytoma, and aortic coarctation
  - Simple essential hypertension is the most common cause of hypertension in *NF1*
- NF1 vasculopathy should be considered in any ischemic condition, including acute coronary and cerebrovascular syndromes

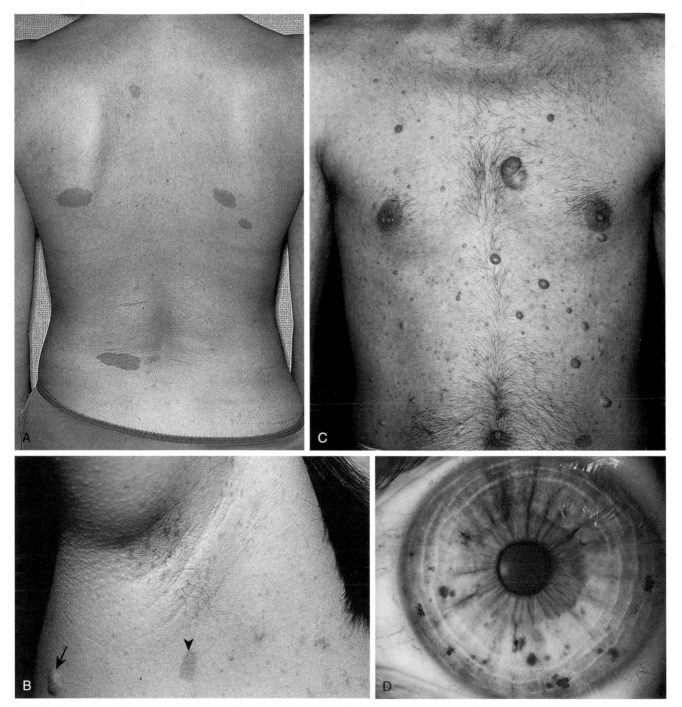

FIGURE 69-5 Some clinical features of neurofibromatosis type 1. **A,** Café-au-lait macules. **B,** Axillary freckling. There is also a small café-au-lait macule *(arrowhead)* and a dermal neurofibroma *(arrow).* **C,** Dermal neurofibromas. **D,** Lisch nodules. (From Habif TP. *Clinical Dermatology: A Color Guide to Diagnosis and Therapy.* 4th ed. Philadelphia: Mosby; 2004: Figs. 26-11A, 26-11B, 26-12, and 26-13A.)

- Surgical intervention for problematic dermal or plexiform neurofibromas or glomus tumors
  - Plexiform neurofibromas are difficult to excise completely, and often recur
- Sudden rapid growth or pain in a previously stable plexiform neurofibroma is suspicious for malignant transformation
- Optic gliomas and other intracerebral tumors tend to be slow growing and occasionally regress spontaneously; serial assessment of tumor size and clinical

manifestations before therapeutic intervention is appropriate

Prevention

- All first-degree relatives of an affected patient should be evaluated, including slit-lamp examination for Lisch nodules
  - One or the other parent is affected (or at least mosaic whereby some of the cells in the body are mutated) around 50% of the time; the remaining

BOX 69-4 *Neurofibromatosis Type 1 (NF1) Clinical Criteria*

Two or more of the following are required to establish a diagnosis of NF1:

6 or more café-au-lait macules (each >5 mm in children or >15 mm after puberty)

2 or more neurofibromas of any type or 1 plexiform neurofibroma

Axillary or inguinal freckling

Optic glioma

2 or more Lisch nodules (iris hamartomas)

Characteristic osseous lesion (sphenoid dysplasia or thinning of long bone cortex with or without pseudarthrosis)

An affected first-degree relative as defined by these diagnostic criteria

50% represent new mutation, with neither parent affected

- If neither parent is affected, the patient's siblings have a very low chance of being affected (there is a small chance that a parent has germline mosaicism; some of the eggs or sperm carry the mutation without any somatic features of neurofibromatosis)
- If a parent is affected, each of the patient's siblings has a 50% chance of being affected

- Each child of an affected person has a 50% chance of being affected

Review Questions

For review questions, please go to ExpertConsult.com.

SUGGESTED READINGS

Peer-reviewed summaries of these and hundreds of additional genetic disorders are available at GeneTests: *Medical Genetics Information Resource.* Seattle: University of Washington; 1993-2014. <www.genetests.org>.

Aihara H, Kumar N, Thompson CC. Diagnosis, surveillance, and treatment strategies for familial adenomatous polyposis: rationale and update. *Eur J Gastroenterol Hepatol.* 2014;26:255-262.

Bacon BR, Adams PC, Kowdley KV, et al. Diagnosis and management of hemochromatosis: 2011 practice guideline by the American Association for the Study of Liver Diseases. *Hepatology.* 2011;54:328-343.

Biesecker LG, Green RC. Diagnostic clinical genome and exome sequencing. *N Engl J Med.* 2014;370:2418-2425.

Ferner RE, Gutmann DH. Neurofibromatosis type 1 (NF1): diagnosis and management. *Handb Clin Neurol.* 2013;115:939-955.

Giardiello FM, Allen JI, Axilbund JE, et al. Guidelines on Genetic Evaluation and Management of Lynch Syndrome: a Consensus Statement by the US Multi-Society Task Force on Colorectal Cancer. *Gastroenterology.* 2014;147:502-526.

Pruthi S, Gostout BS, Lindor NM. Identification and management of women with *brca* mutations or hereditary predisposition for breast and ovarian cancer. *Mayo Clin Proc.* 2010;85:1111-1120.

Complementary and Alternative Medicine

BIMAL H. ASHAR, MD, MBA

Over the past two decades, the use of healing modalities outside the realm of Western allopathic medicine has increased dramatically. This movement has been a patient-driven phenomenon that has incited the need for physicians to expand their knowledge base beyond principles and concepts taught in medical school to solidify physician-patient relationships and protect patients from potential harm. This chapter provides a basic overview of complementary and alternative medicine (CAM) and describes a few specific popular modalities.

Overview

Definitions

- Alternative medicine: approaches not routinely used by conventional practitioners
- **Complementary medicine: use of unconventional modalities as adjuncts to established Western medicine**
- Integrative medicine: combination of conventional and complementary methods for preventing and treating disease

Classification

- There is no one universally accepted classification system for all of CAM
- **Most modalities are purported to enhance the body's natural defenses in preventing and treating disease**
- The National Center for Complementary and Alternative Medicine (NCCAM) of the National Institutes of Health has developed subgroups of complementary health practices, primarily to facilitate research efforts (Table 70-1)

Alternative Medical Systems

ACUPUNCTURE

Background

- Involves the insertion of fine needles into the skin to restore the balance of life energy, or qi (pronounced "chee")
  - **A block in the flow of qi can lead to an imbalance of flow of energy through channels in the body (meridians) and lead to disease**

- Accurate needle placement along these meridians corrects the imbalance and treats the disorder
  - Heating the needles with mugwort (moxibustion), electrical stimulation, or manual twisting may be used to achieve the desired response
- There are many different types of acupuncture (e.g., auricular, five elements, hand, traditional Chinese)

Mechanism of Action

- No unifying mechanism currently exists, although many theories exist
- Acupuncture needling has been shown to effect the release of endorphins and neurohormones and alter blood flow

Efficacy

- Used as a healing modality for a number of conditions, but efficacy data for most disorders are inconclusive
- Studies may support the use of acupuncture for the following:
  - Postoperative and chemotherapy-induced nausea and vomiting
  - Chronic pain: Both acupuncture and sham acupuncture showed superiority over no treatment
    - Chronic low back pain: equivalent but not superior to other manual therapies
    - Osteoarthritis of the knee
  - Tension headaches and migraine prophylaxis
- Data do not currently support its use for smoking cessation

Safety

- **Overall considered safe with the use of sterile needles by trained practitioners**
  - Most common side effects include pain at the insertion site, localized bleeding/bruising, tiredness, and vasovagal syncope
  - Rare case reports of pneumothorax, organ puncture, and hepatitis B (when nondisposable needles are used)

HOMEOPATHY

Background

- Homeopathy is based around two basic concepts:
  - "Law of similars" suggests that substances that cause symptoms in healthy subjects can cure those

TABLE 70-1	National Center for Complementary and Alternative Medicine Groupings of Complementary Health Practices

Category	Examples
Natural products (dietary supplements)	• Herbs • Vitamins • Probiotics
Mind and body practices	• Acupuncture • Hypnotherapy • Massage therapy • Meditation • Relaxation techniques (e.g., breathing exercises, guided imagery) • Spinal manipulation • Tai chi and Qi gong • Yoga
Other (includes alternative medical systems)	• Ayurveda • Homeopathy • Naturopathy • Traditional Chinese medicine

symptoms in patients who are sick (e.g., digoxin is used to treat some arrhythmias that it is capable of causing)

- "Principle of serial dilutions" suggests that medications can have a biologic effect even if diluted to levels at which the original substance is undetectable (a so-called homeopathic dose)
- Focuses on subjective symptoms rather than disease diagnoses
- Most preparations begin with an animal, mineral, or plant substance that is pulverized and mixed with a water-alcohol solution
- Most commonly used to treat allergy, hypertension, otitis media, arthritis, and headache

Regulation

- Most homeopathic medications are used for minor or self-limited illnesses and are available over-the-counter
- If a homeopathic remedy claims to treat a serious disease (e.g., cancer), it can only be sold by prescription
- Homeopathic remedies are technically regulated by the U.S. Food and Drug Administration (FDA) as drugs under the Federal Food, Drug, and Cosmetic Act. However, current FDA policy does not include premarket evaluation of homeopathic remedies for safety or effectiveness (as is required for drugs).

Mechanism of Action

- No clear mechanism is identified
- Scientific implausibility of the homeopathic dose makes acceptance into mainstream medicine difficult

Efficacy

- There are few well-designed studies available
- **Systematic reviews (when controlled for bias and study quality) have suggested that homeopathy is no more effective than placebo**

Safety

- Serious adverse reactions are rare because there is little to no active ingredient in the preparation
- **"Aggravation reactions" are worsening of symptoms shortly after a remedy is started and are not considered side effects by homeopaths**
- Risk of adulteration exists because there is no requirement for finished product testing
- **Potential for harm exists when homeopathic physicians recommend against conventional medications and/or immunizations**

Manipulative Therapies

CHIROPRACTIC
Background

- Used by up to 20% of the U.S. adult population
- Most commonly used for low back pain, neck pain, and various musculoskeletal conditions
- Basic principles
  - Spinal cord and nervous system are at the center of general well-being
  - Malalignments of vertebrae (subluxations) cause and perpetuate disease
  - Correction of the subluxations (usually via spinal manipulation) restores physiologic balance and allows the body to restore health
- Many chiropractors use massage, heat, and trigger-point injections as adjuncts to therapy

Mechanism of Action

- The mechanism of action is unknown

Efficacy

- **No more effective than sham therapy or other interventions (e.g., physical therapy, analgesics, back exercises) for acute or chronic low back pain**
- Data on efficacy for neck pain, shoulder pain, headaches, and other conditions are quite limited
- Patient satisfaction seems to be high with this manual approach to treatment

Safety

- Most common side effects include tiredness, headache, dizziness, numbness, and localized pain. These symptoms are typically self-limited.
- Disk herniation and cauda equine syndrome can rarely occur after low back manipulation
- Reports of carotid artery dissection, vertebrobasilar vascular accidents, vertebral fracture, and tracheal rupture with cervical manipulation do exist
- **Contraindications to chiropractic therapy include coagulopathy, osteoporosis, spinal tumors or infection, and spinal instability. It should also be avoided in patients with rheumatoid arthritis.**

MASSAGE THERAPY
Background

- Involves manipulation of soft tissues
- Many different types (e.g., Swedish, deep-tissue, shiatsu)

70

- Goal is to affect the flow of energy through the body and restore balance and health
- Primarily used for relaxation and stress relief but also used for treatment of back or neck pain, fibromyalgia, headaches, etc.

Efficacy and Safety

- Useful for stress reduction, although duration and intensity of response are variable
- **Provides short-term relief for nonspecific low back pain**
- **May reduce anxiety and pain in cancer patients**
- No clear data to support its use for other specific conditions
- Generally considered safe, although caution should be used in patients with coagulopathies, especially with deep-tissue techniques

Dietary Supplements

Overview

- Most widely used CAM modality
- Regulation in the United States
  - Before 1994, dietary supplements were regulated as foods with required premarket testing for safety and efficacy
  - In 1994, the Dietary Supplement Health and Education Act (DSHEA) was enacted. It served to do the following:
    - Expand the definition of dietary supplements to include vitamins, amino acids, herbs, and other botanicals
    - Eliminate the need for companies to prove safety or efficacy before marketing their products
    - Place the burden of proof on the FDA to show that a particular product is unsafe to keep it from the marketplace (e.g., ephedra ban took 7 years of data gathering)
    - Allow companies to make claims of "structure or function" (e.g., "for prostate health"), but not allow them to claim that their product was "intended to diagnose, treat, cure, or prevent any specific disease" (e.g., "for the prevention of prostate cancer")
- General issues surrounding dietary supplement safety:
  - No product standardization exists (e.g., not all gingko biloba has the same active ingredients)
  - Active ingredients are often unknown, making standardization impossible
  - Potential for misidentification of herbs
  - Potential for adulteration of products with drugs or heavy metals
  - Few published data exist on the efficacy, safety, and potential for drug interactions with most dietary supplements

Supplement Use for Selected Conditions

- Anxiety, insomnia
  - Kava kava (*Piper methysticum*)
    - Used by natives of the South Pacific for many years. Superior to placebo for short-term treatment of anxiety but no data on long-term use.

- Side effects include gastrointestinal (GI) upset and rash
- Reports of idiosyncratic fulminant hepatic failure have led to its ban in parts of Europe, but it is still available in the United States
- Avoid combining with other anxiolytics or alcohol
  - Valerian (*Valeriana officinalis*)
    - Primarily used for insomnia
    - Objective sleep data do not support its use
    - **Avoid with other anxiolytics**
- Depression
  - SAMe (S-adenosylmethionine)
    - A metabolic intermediary thought vital for cellular functioning
    - Small studies suggest utility for treating depression, but most of these were done with parenteral formulations; more recent studies using oral preparations are conflicting
    - American Psychiatric Association guideline on treatment of major depressive disorder (last updated 2010) suggests SAM-e (and St. John's wort) in patients who prefer CAM therapies
    - Considered safe but there is concern for interactions with other antidepressants (e.g., serotonin syndrome)
  - St. John's wort (*Hypericum perforatum*)
    - Most commonly *prescribed* antidepressant in Germany
    - Data suggest that it is superior to placebo for treatment of major depression and may be equivalent to many standard antidepressants
    - Generally well tolerated
    - **Great concern over drug-herb interactions (Table 70-2) because of its effect on the cytochrome P450 system**
- Dementia
  - Ginkgo biloba
    - Thought to have a number of biologic effects, including increasing blood flow, inhibiting platelet-activating factor, altering neuronal metabolism, and working as an antioxidant
    - No clear evidence to support its use for cognitive impairment or dementia
    - **No evidence that it is effective for the prevention of memory loss or dementia**
    - Side effects are usually rare and mild and include headaches and GI discomfort
    - Case reports of spontaneous bleeding and seizures exist
    - May decrease the plasma concentrations of omeprazole, efavirenz, and alprazolam
    - Because of its potential antiplatelet effects, it should be used with caution in patients taking warfarin or other anticoagulants
  - Turmeric (Curcumin)
    - Has been used for dyspepsia, osteoarthritis, and recently for dementia
    - Thought to have antiinflammatory and antithrombotic properties
    - No clinical evidence to date on its effect for the prevention or treatment of dementia

- Hypercholesterolemia
  - Fish oil
    - A source of omega-3 fatty acids (i.e., eicosapentaenoic acid, docosahexaenoic acid)
    - **Lowers triglycerides in a dose-dependent manner (30% reduction at doses of 2 to 4 g/day)**

TABLE 70-2	*Potential Drug Interactions with St. John's Wort*	
Drug	**Effect**	**Potential Clinical Complication**
Cyclosporine	Decreased drug levels	Transplant graft rejection
Digoxin	Decreased drug levels	Improper rate control or CHF exacerbation
Imatinib	Decreased drug levels	Ineffective cancer treatment
Omeprazole	Decreased drug levels	Ineffective treatment for reflux, peptic ulcer disease
Oral contraceptives	Decreased drug effectiveness	Unplanned pregnancies
Protease inhibitors	Decreased drug levels	Increase in HIV viral load
Theophylline	Decreased drug levels	Asthma/COPD exacerbation
Selective serotonin reuptake inhibitors	Serotonin excess	Serotonin syndrome—confusion, agitation, diaphoresis, tremor, rhabdomyolysis
Warfarin	Decreased drug effectiveness	Reduced INR value

CHF, Congestive heart failure; COPD, chronic obstructive pulmonary disease; HIV, human immunodeficiency virus; INR, international normalized ratio.

- Can raise low-density lipoprotein (LDL) levels by 5% to 10% at high doses
- Little effect on high-density lipoprotein levels
- **Recent data suggest no risk reduction in myocardial infarction, stroke, or death with the use of omega-3 supplementation**
- Side effects include fishy aftertaste and GI upset
- Theoretical risk of bleeding at high doses because of antiplatelet effects
  - Garlic (*Allium sativum*)
    - True active ingredient is unknown
    - May decrease total cholesterol and LDL modestly in the short term
    - No data on impact on cardiovascular mortality
    - Side effects include bad breath, body odor, and GI upset
    - Case reports of bleeding and interactions with warfarin exist
    - May decrease saquinivir (protease inhibitor) and isoniazid levels
  - Red yeast rice (*Monascus purpureus*)
    - Contain monacolins, which can function as hydroxyl-3-methyl-glutaryl-coenzyme A (HMG-CoA) inhibitors and block cholesterol synthesis
    - In essence, can function as weak statin drugs and can lower total cholesterol and LDL levels
    - A few studies done in China have suggested a decrease in cardiovascular morbidity and mortality when used for secondary prevention
    - Has been used by some as an alternative in patients who do not tolerate statin drugs
    - The lack of standardization and premarket testing in the United States has led to marked variability in the monacolin levels in commercially marketed products
    - Case reports of myalgias, myopathy, and hepatotoxicity exist
- Menopausal symptoms (Table 70-3)
- Osteoarthritis
  - Glucosamine sulfate and chondroitin sulfate
    - Theoretically support cartilage and connective tissue formation
    - May also have antiinflammatory properties

TABLE 70-3	*Popular Dietary Supplements Used for the Treatment of Menopausal Symptoms*		
Supplement	**Potential Toxicity**	**Potential Drug Interactions**	**Comments**
Black cohosh (*Cimicifuga racemosa*)	Gastrointestinal discomfort Case reports of liver failure	None known	May be effective for short-term use (<6 months)
Dong quai (*Angelica sinensis*)	Rash	Increased international normalized ratio (INR) in patients taking warfarin	No clinical evidence of efficacy
Red clover (*Trifolium pretense*)	Generally well tolerated	Theoretical risk of interaction with warfarin and tamoxifen	Is a source of isoflavones No clear efficacy in data
Soy isoflavones	Constipation, bloating, nausea, rash	Potential decreased INR in patients on warfarin; theoretical risk of competition with tamoxifen	Most studies have not shown a benefit

- Conflicting data exist on their use for symptomatic and functional benefits for patients with osteoarthritis of the knees or hips. Studies are also conflicting regarding their ability to slow the progression of joint-space narrowing.
  - Treatment effect may not be seen for up to 12 weeks
  - Generally well tolerated
  - May raise the international normalized ratio in patients taking warfarin
- Prostatic hyperplasia
  - Saw palmetto (*Serenoa repens*)
    - Mechanism of action unknown
    - Conflicting data on its efficacy for improving urologic symptoms and urinary flow measures; most larger recent trials have been negative
    - No data to suggest that it prevents the complications of prostatic hyperplasia (i.e., acute urinary retention) or the development of prostate cancer
    - Generally well tolerated
    - No effect on prostate-specific antigen levels
- Probiotics
  - Microorganisms that have properties beneficial to the host
    - Examples include *Lactobacillus*, *Bifidobacterium*, *Streptococcus salivarius*, and *Saccharomyces boulardii*
    - Thought to work by preventing invasion by pathogenic bacteria and improving intestinal barrier function; may also play a role in perception of pain
    - **Data are limited, but some studies suggest that probiotics may be useful in the care of patients with allergic disorders, acute infectious arthritis, inflammatory bowel disease, or irritable bowel syndrome and in the prevention of antibiotic-associated diarrhea (including *Clostridium difficile*)**

- Avoid in seriously ill or immunocompromised patients
- Energy drinks
  - Most contain high amounts of caffeine (between 80 and 280 mg)
  - Other ingredients can include guarana (a natural form of caffeine), sugars, taurine, ginseng (an herb touted to boost energy), and B-vitamins
  - Caffeine dose does not have to be disclosed since these products are regulated as dietary supplements
  - Are sometimes mixed with alcohol, which can mask the level of inebriation
  - Side effects can include palpitations, tachycardia, hypertension, dehydration, and restlessness
  - There are case reports of arrhythmia and death, typically from excess consumption

Review Questions

For review questions, please go to ExpertConsult.com.

SUGGESTED READINGS

Ashar BH, Rowland-Seymour A. Advising patients who use dietary supplements. *Am J Med.* 2008;121:91-97.

Chon TY, Lee MC. Acupuncture. *Mayo Clin Proc.* 2013;88:1141-1146.

Furlan AD, Imamura M, Dryden T, Irvin E. Massage for low-back pain. *Cochrane Database Syst Rev.* 2008;(4):CD001929.

Izzo AA, Ernst E. Interactions between herbal medicines and prescribed drugs: an updated systematic review. *Drugs.* 2009;69:1777-1798.

Posadzki P, Watson LK, Ernst E. Adverse effects of herbal medicines: an overview of systematic reviews. *Clin Med.* 2013;13:7-12.

Rubinstein SM, Terwee CB, Assendelft WJJ, et al. Spinal manipulative therapy for acute low-back pain. *Cochrane Database Syst Rev.* 2012;(9):CD008880.

Shi Y, Dong JW, Zhao JH, et al. Herbal insomnia medications that target GABAergic systems: a review of the psychopharmacological evidence. *Curr Neuropharmacol.* 2014;12:289-302.

Substance Use Disorders

DARIUS A. RASTEGAR, MD

Substance use disorders (SUDs) are a worldwide public health problem and are associated with significant morbidity and mortality, public health burdens, adverse societal consequences, and costs. In the United States in 2012, over 22 million persons age 12 years or older were classified with substance abuse or dependence in the past year. Societal economic costs from lost productivity, medical expenses, motor-vehicle accidents, domestic violence, and drug-related crime have been estimated at more than $180 billion for alcohol abuse and more than $180 billion for drug abuse per year. SUDs span all racial and socioeconomic strata. Despite the high prevalence of SUDs in the United States, the vast majority of individuals who need treatment do not receive it. The *Diagnostic and Statistical Manual of Mental Disorders* (DSM) outlines criteria for a spectrum of substance-related disorders based on the substances used and the severity of the disorder. Substances can be an illicit drug, a prescription medication, alcohol, or tobacco.

Basic Information

- **Definitions: Two groups of disorders exist: SUDs and substance-induced disorders**
  - Diagnostic criteria for SUDs are listed in Box 71-1
    - **Although the DSM-IV divided substance use disorders into two categories—*Substance Abuse* and *Substance Dependence*—the DSM-V groups them into one category—*Substance Use Disorder*, with a spectrum of severity depending on the number of criteria met**
    - **There are 11 criteria, and a person is considered to have an SUD if two or more are present. They can be clustered into four groups:**
      - **Impaired control**
      - **Social impairment**
      - **Risky use**
      - **Pharmacologic dependence.** It should be noted that individuals who are prescribed an opioid or sedative will develop tolerance (over time) and therefore withdrawal, but would not be considered to have an SUD unless they meet another criteria.
    - **The substance-induced disorders range from substance intoxication to substance withdrawal, substance-induced delirium, dementia, psychosis, mood or anxiety disorders, sexual dysfunction, and sleep disorder**
      - **The hallmarks of *substance intoxication* are reversible, clinically significant behavioral or psychological changes that develop during or shortly after the ingestion of a substance**

- ***Substance withdrawal* involves characteristic physiologic and cognitive impairments as a result of the cessation of, or significant decrease in, the amount of a substance typically used continuously over a prolonged period**
  - Once withdrawal develops, most individuals will want to ingest the substance again to relieve the withdrawal symptoms
  - Substances with a recognized withdrawal state include alcohol, amphetamines, cocaine, nicotine, opioids, sedatives, hypnotics, and anxiolytics
- Common drugs of abuse
  - Alcohol: Central nervous system (CNS) depressant that rapidly equilibrates between blood and tissues
  - Nicotine: peripheral and central cholinergic agonist that produces both stimulatory and relaxing effects
  - Marijuana: mild hallucinogen acting through the cannabinoid receptor system. There are also a number of synthetic cannabinoids that are sometimes marketed as "herbal incense" under a variety of names, including "K2" and "Spice." They appear to have more potent effects than marijuana.
  - Opioids: Potent analgesics, including heroin and prescription opioids; they also cause euphoria and sedation
  - Benzodiazepines: CNS depressants that have anxiolytic and hypnotic effects
  - Cocaine: peripheral and central stimulant with anesthetic and potent vasoconstrictive activity and average duration of action ranging from 20 to 90 minutes depending on route of administration
  - Methamphetamine: stimulant similar to cocaine in mechanism of action but with duration of action of 8 to 24 hours and a half-life of 12 hours
  - Cathinones: synthetic stimulants marketed as "bath salts" to circumvent drug regulations
  - LSD (lysergic acid diethylamide): a hallucinogen
  - MDMA (methylene-dioxymethamphetamine): "Ecstasy" or "Molly." This is generally categorized as a hallucinogen, but has stimulant effects at higher doses.
  - GHB (γ-hydroxybutyrate): a short-acting, γ-aminobutyric acid (GABA)–like aqueous solution with CNS-sedating effects
  - Inhalants: include volatile solvents (e.g., adhesives, aerosols, solvents, propellant gases), nitrites, and anesthetics; highly lipophilic

BOX 71-1	*Diagnostic Criteria: Substance Use Disorders*

Group I: Impaired Control
1. Substance use in larger amounts or over a longer period of time than originally intended
2. Persistent desire to cut down or multiple unsuccessful attempts at cutting down or stopping use
3. Great deal of time spent using substance or recovering from its effects
4. Intense desire to use or craving for the substance

Group II: Social Impairment
5. Substance use resulting in failure to fulfill obligations at work, school, or home
6. Substance use causing or exacerbating interpersonal problems
7. Important social, occupational, or recreational activities given up/reduced because of substance use

Group III: Risky Use
8. Recurrent use of substance in physically hazardous situations
9. Continued use despite negative physical or psychological consequences

Group IV: Pharmacologic Dependence
10. Tolerance to the effects of the substance
11. Withdrawal symptoms when the substance is not used

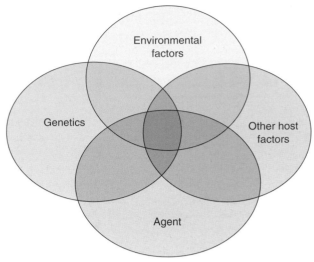

FIGURE 71-1 Risk factors for the development of substance use disorders.

- Epidemiology
  - Prevalence and incidence of SUDs:
    - In the United States, alcohol and tobacco are the most commonly used substances.
      - In 2012, approximately half of Americans age 12 and older were current drinkers of alcohol; 6.5% were heavy drinkers (consumed 5 or more drinks on the same occasion 5 or more days in the past 30 days)
      - It is estimated that 58 million Americans, or 22% of those age 12 or older, smoke cigarettes. Cigarette smoking is more common among men than women.
      - Cigarette smoking is the leading cause of preventable death in the United States, resulting in an estimated 443,000 premature deaths and $193 billion in direct health care expenditures and productivity losses each year
    - Marijuana is the most commonly used illicit substance, with 19 million Americans age 12 or older reporting past month use in 2012
    - Nonmedical use of prescription drugs is the second highest category of illicit drug use. The number of persons who used prescription psychotherapeutics nonmedically in the previous month was 7 million (2.6% of the population) in 2012. Prescription pain relievers (opioids) are the most commonly used.
    - The prevalence of alcohol and drug use disorders is highest among young adults 18 to 25 years of age
    - Alcohol- and drug-related disorders are more common among men than women

- Risk factors for the development of SUDs (Fig. 71-1)
  - **Genetics may explain approximately 50% of the propensity to develop an SUD**
  - **Other host factors include premorbid depression, anxiety disorders, and borderline or antisocial personality disorders**
    - Alcohol dependence is most likely an antecedent to the development of depression rather than a result of self-medication of a mood disorder
  - **Marital stability seems to have a protective effect**
  - Educational level
    - Youths who drop out of high school are at higher risk for developing alcohol and drug dependence later in life
    - Drug use during adolescence and young adulthood is also a predictor for not completing high school
  - Environmental factors
    - More frequent in populations in which drug use is more socially acceptable
    - Associated with community and family disorganization
    - Peer influence impacts the initiation and ongoing use of alcohol and drugs, particularly among adolescents and young adults
    - **The absence of employment and particular jobs or work settings (bartenders, anesthesiologists) may also carry risk**
  - Agent factors
    - **Agents that quickly reach the brain, such as lipophilic substances that are injected intravenously, have a higher addictive potential**
    - Substances that are effective for self-medication, such as opioids for pain, may help explain addiction to certain drugs
    - Easily accessible substances obtained at low cost tend to have a higher abuse potential

- **Common physiologic mechanisms of action**
  - **Drugs of abuse and alcohol share a common final pathway: the dopamine reward pathway**
  - **In the early stages of drug use, reward pathway activation causes euphoria and intense pleasure**
  - **With repeated use, reward pathway activation results in diminished responses and development of long-lasting memories linked to drug-using experiences**
  - These changes are responsible for the development of tolerance, psychological dependence, and relapse that can occur after years of abstinence

Clinical Presentation

- **Warning signs:**
  - Sudden change in behavior (e.g., sudden job loss, financial difficulty, or family problem)
  - History of two or more non–sports-related traumatic injuries in an adult
  - Sexual dysfunction, insomnia
  - **Intoxicated** behavior secondary to active use (inebriated, agitated, extremely lethargic)
  - Family concerns about patient
  - History of driving under the influence or other substance-related arrests
- **Overdose complications**
  - Alcohol
    - Symptoms consist of somnolence, bradycardia, coma, and eventual death
    - Symptoms vary with blood alcohol concentration (BAC)
      - Cognitive and behavioral changes occur at BAC of 20 to 30 mg/dL
      - Legal intoxication is at BAC of 80 mg/dL
      - Death can occur at BAC of 300 to 400 mg/dL
    - Treatment is supportive with close monitoring of electrolytes and for evidence of alcohol withdrawal as the BAC decreases
  - Stimulants such as cocaine and methamphetamine
    - Overdose is rare, but may result in seizures, arrhythmias, and death
    - Treatment is supportive and management of any medical complications that arise

- Opioids
  - Symptoms include respiratory depression with shallow respirations, miosis, bradycardia, decreased level of consciousness, coma, and eventual death
  - Treatment in the symptomatic patient is initiated with intravenous (IV) naloxone 0.2 to 0.4 mg. Doses may be repeated every 2 to 3 minutes as needed until normal ventilation is achieved. Total effective doses may approach 2 mg.
    - May require frequent additional doses of naloxone or initiation of naloxone continuous infusion over the first 24 hours, owing to the comparatively short half-life of naloxone, particularly in the case of long-acting prescription opioids
    - If no response after 10 mg, consider diagnoses other than opioid toxicity
- **Withdrawal syndromes**
  - **Alcohol withdrawal, which may be life-threatening, typically occurs in several stages (Table 71-1)**
    - Most alcohol-dependent individuals do not have severe withdrawal symptoms; the best predictor of severe withdrawal is a history of severe withdrawal in the past
  - Withdrawal from stimulants, including cocaine and methamphetamine:
    - Symptoms typically are mild and include depression, anxiety, hypersomnolence, anhedonia, difficulty concentrating, increased appetite, and craving
  - **Opioid withdrawal typically occurs in two phases:**
    - Acute physiologic withdrawal: characterized by dysphoria, yawning, tearing, diarrhea, cramps, nausea, and piloerection
    - Protracted withdrawal phase may involve insomnia and persistent drug cravings and may last up to 6 to 12 months
  - **Marijuana withdrawal is increasingly being recognized as a clinical syndrome most commonly manifesting with irritability, anxiety, restlessness, and appetite and sleep disturbances**

TABLE 71-1	*Stages of Alcohol Withdrawal*			
	Autonomic Dysfunction →	**Withdrawal Seizures →**	**Alcoholic Hallucinosis →**	**Delirium Tremens**
Symptoms	Tremors Mild elevations in blood pressure and heart rate	Generalized motor seizures singly or in episodic bursts	Hallucinations (visual, auditory, tactile) with generally normal vital signs Patient is otherwise oriented	Severe autonomic dysregulation Confusion Auditory, visual, or tactile hallucinations
Time course	Begins within 5 to 10 hours	Begins within 8 to 24 hours	Begins within 12 to 24 hours	Begins within 48 to 96 hours
Treatment	Frequent assessments Symptom-driven doses of benzodiazepines	Treat seizure with parenteral benzodiazepines Other antiepileptics minimally effective	Frequent assessments Symptom-driven doses of benzodiazepines Close monitoring	Frequent parenteral doses of benzodiazepines or continuous drip Close monitoring

71

- **Secondary medical complications**
  - Complications from substance use in general
    - Trauma
    - Increased risk of acquiring infectious diseases such as human immunodeficiency virus/acquired immune deficiency syndrome (HIV/AIDS), sexually transmitted infections, hepatitis B, and hepatitis C
    - Altered mental status with delirium
    - Malnutrition in general or specific vitamin B complex deficiency
    - Poor adherence to medical appointments and recommended treatments
  - Complications from injection drug use
    - Hepatitis C and HIV infection
    - Endocarditis and septic emboli
    - Cellulitis and deep tissue infections
    - Thrombophlebitis
    - Foreign-body granulomatosis, often called "talc lung" from talc or other fillers used in drug tablets
    - Secondary amyloidosis from chronic wounds
  - Complications from alcohol
    - Cardiovascular: arrhythmias with atrial fibrillation, or "holiday heart," being the most common, hypertension, dilated cardiomyopathy
    - Gastrointestinal (GI): esophagitis, gastritis, pancreatitis, alcoholic hepatitis, cirrhosis
    - Endocrine: testicular atrophy, amenorrhea
    - Hematologic: macrocytic anemia, thrombocytopenia, leukopenia
    - Electrolyte derangements (hypokalemia, hypomagnesemia, hypophosphatemia)
    - Neurologic: peripheral neuropathy, alcoholic myopathy
      - **Wernicke encephalopathy, a medical emergency, is a confusional state of abrupt onset caused by thiamine deficiency**
        - Characterized by a triad of confusion, ataxia, and oculomotor dysfunction (usually cranial nerve VI palsy leading to ophthalmoplegia)
        - The diagnosis is made clinically, although necrosis and atrophy of mammillary bodies are visible on brain magnetic resonance imaging (MRI) in 80% of cases
        - Treatment is immediate administration of IV thiamine, admission for observation and continued IV thiamine therapy, and long-term oral supplementation on an outpatient basis
        - **Symptoms may be precipitated or worsened by administration of glucose before thiamine**
          - Patients usually improve over hours to days
      - **Korsakoff amnestic syndrome refers to profound memory impairment for ongoing events with a marked inability to retain new information**
        - Occurs often late in the course of chronic alcohol dependence
        - Usually seen after an episode of Wernicke encephalopathy
        - **Both anterograde and retrograde memory are affected, although long-term memory is usually preserved**
          - **Patients often appear apathetic, unconcerned, or unaware of their illness and may confabulate**
          - Treatment with thiamine is usually ineffective, and recovery of memory is often poor
      - **Alcoholic cerebellar degeneration is a syndrome characterized by gait abnormalities, including complaints of weakness, unsteadiness, or incoordination, with wide-based ataxic gait and abnormal heel-knee-shin test**
        - Occasionally, patients may also have tremors or incoordination of the upper extremities, dysarthria, or blurred vision
        - Onset of symptoms can be progressive over weeks to months, but acute worsening of mild symptoms may occur
        - Brain MRI may show evidence of cerebellar atrophy
        - Treatment consists of abstinence from alcohol and nutritional supplementation, but gait abnormalities may persist
  - Complications from stimulants (cocaine and methamphetamine)
    - Cardiovascular: arrhythmias and sudden death; severe, sometimes malignant, hypertension; myocarditis; cardiomyopathy
      - Most (but not all) patients who suffer myocardial infarction after using cocaine have underlying atherosclerosis; some cases may be caused by vasospasm. Cocaine users may experience chest pain without evidence of myocardial ischemia.
      - Treatment consists of aspirin, benzodiazepines to reduce blood pressure and heart rate, and nitrates or calcium channel blockers to decrease vasospasm and prevent arrhythmias
      - **β-Blockers are generally avoided in a setting of acute chest pain and cardiac ischemia because they have been shown to potentiate cocaine-induced vasoconstriction, caused by unopposed α activity. However, prescribing β-blockers to cocaine users has not been shown to increase the risk of cardiovascular complications.**
    - Neurologic: seizure, cerebrovascular accidents, intracranial hemorrhage
    - Psychiatric: psychosis, auditory hallucinations, paranoia, violent behavior
    - Renal: rhabdomyolysis, malignant hyperthermia
    - GI: bowel ischemia leading to infarction and perforation
    - Pulmonary: alveolar hemorrhage and infarction; pulmonary edema
    - Hematologic/cutaneous: Cocaine is sometimes "cut" with levamisole, an antihelminthic drug. Use of levamisole-contaminated cocaine has been associated with cutaneous necrosis, purpura, and neutropenia.
  - Complications from heroin and other opioids
    - Pulmonary: pulmonary edema in setting of overdose

- Endocrine: amenorrhea, hypogonadism, and erectile dysfunction
- GI: constipation

Screening, Diagnosis, and Evaluation

- **Screening for substance use and SUDs**
  - History should include family history of alcohol or drug use disorders, presence of cooccurring psychiatric disorders, employment and family status, history of experimenting with or using illicit drugs
    - For alcohol consumption, the **National Institute on Alcohol Abuse and Alcoholism** has defined maximum healthy limits, based on epidemiologic data that suggest that those who exceed these amounts are at increased risk for alcohol-related problems such as injury, social and legal problems, and illness
    - **The maximum healthy drinking limits are defined as no more than 3 drinks in 1 day *and* no more than 7 drinks per week for healthy women and healthy men over age 65 years, and no more than 4 drinks in 1 day *and* no more than 14 drinks per week for healthy men up to age 65 years**
    - One standard drink equals 12 oz regular beer, or 5 oz wine, or 1.5 oz distilled spirits
    - **Lower limits or abstinence** may be medically indicated for selected individuals (e.g., someone with chronic liver disease)
  - Screening instruments
    - **AUDIT: The Alcohol Use Disorders Identification Test**
      - A 10-item questionnaire developed by the World Health Organization specifically for identifying unhealthy alcohol use and disorders of alcohol use in primary care
    - **AUDIT-C: An abbreviated version of the AUDIT using the first three questions; also performs well when the longer version is not feasible (Box 71-2)**
      - **CAGE Questionnaire: Can be used to screen for alcohol dependence (Box 71-3)**
        - The more affirmative answers, the more likely the person is alcohol dependent. Two or more affirmative answers on the CAGE is considered a positive result; however, answering any response affirmatively merits further evaluation.
        - Has been adapted to assess for drug use as well
- **Assessment of severity of substance use and SUDs should be comprehensive and thorough (Box 71-4)**
- **Physical findings**
  - Alcohol dependence: secondary medical complications caused by use of the substance
    - Abdominal discomfort or hemoccult-positive stool
    - Findings consistent with liver disease, such as jaundice, palmar erythema, caput medusa, ascites, bruising, encephalopathy
    - Peripheral neuropathy
    - Electrolyte abnormalities, including hypokalemia, hypomagnesemia, and hypophosphatemia. Chronic

---

BOX 71-2   *AUDIT-C Questionnaire*

Question 1: How often did you have a drink containing alcohol in the past year?
a. Never
b. Monthly or less
c. 2 to 4 times/month
d. 2 to 3 times/week
e. 4 or more times/week

Question 2: How many drinks did you have on a typical day when you were drinking in the past year?
a. 1 or 2
b. 3 or 4
c. 5 or 6
d. 7 to 9
e. 10 or more

Question 3: How often did you have six or more drinks on one occasion in the past year?
a. Never
b. Less than monthly
c. Monthly
d. Weekly
e. Daily or almost daily

(a = 0 points; b = 1 point; c = 2 points; d = 3 points; e = 4 points)
In men, a total score of 4 or more is considered positive. In women, a total score of 3 or more is considered positive.

BOX 71-3   *CAGE Questions to Screen for Alcoholism*

C: Have you ever tried to **cut down** on your alcohol use?
A: Do you get **annoyed** when people comment about your drinking?
G: Do you feel **guilty** about things you have done while drinking?
E: Do you ever drink an **eye-opener** to get started in the morning?

BOX 71-4   *Assessment Questions to Identify Severity of Substance Use Disorder*

Duration of use or age at first use
Route of administration
Measurement of frequency and quantity of use
Timing of last use
Past history of blackouts, delirium tremens, withdrawal seizures, and/or hospitalizations for alcohol or drug withdrawal
Past legal problems because of use
Past treatment history and treatment impact on use
Duration of longest, continuous time clean and how achieved
Review of systems for physiologic consequences of substance use

---

phosphate depletion may lead to severe hypophosphatemia after admission to the hospital and administration of IV fluids, because of intracellular shifts.
- Smoked or snorted cocaine: atrophy or perforation of nasal septum, acute respiratory wheezing, digit burns, nervous picking at skin (formication), and agitation
- Methamphetamine

- Acute: hyperthermia, hyperventilation, delusions, and paranoia
- Chronic: poor dentition from bruxism, decreased saliva production, inadequate dental hygiene, skin findings such as burns or excoriations caused by formication
  - Opioids
    - Intranasal or oral opioid use: Shallow breathing; lethargy, "pinpoint pupils" or miosis
    - Injection drug use: new and old needle track marks, healed and new abscesses
- **Laboratory testing**
  - **Toxicology screens**
    - Alcohol: With acute alcohol intoxication, BAC should be measured
    - Cocaine: urine tests for cocaine and metabolites
      - Positive for cocaine for less than 48 hours
      - Cocaine is rapidly metabolized into its major metabolite, benzoylecgonine, usually within hours; however, benzoylecgonine may be present in urine for up to 60 hours after single use but may persist much longer after the cessation of heavy cocaine use.
    - **Opioids: Heroin is metabolized to morphine and will result in a morphine-positive urine test**
      - Typical opiate assays will detect morphine, hydrocodone, and hydromorphone, but they do not cross-react with oxycodone. Thus, oxycodone will generally not show up as morphine-positive on urine toxicology testing and must be tested for separately.
      - Poppy seeds and certain fluoroquinolone antibiotics may cause false-positive results
  - Hematology testing
    - Elevated mean corpuscular volume may be seen in chronic alcohol exposure
    - Acute alcohol consumption may cause pancytopenia, particularly thrombocytopenia
  - Hepatic panel
    - Alcohol has direct toxic effects on the liver, resulting in abnormalities in several liver enzymes:
      - γ-Glutamyl transpeptidase levels may be elevated, often greater than 1000 U/L
      - Aspartate transaminotransferase is typically elevated to a greater degree than alanine transaminotransferase
      - Serum bilirubin levels and prothrombin time may be abnormal in patients with acute alcoholic hepatitis or with cirrhosis
  - Chemistries
    - Abrupt cessation of alcohol consumption with anorexia (typically when patients have prolonged nausea and vomiting) may result in an anion gap ketoacidosis secondary to poor nutrition and alcohol-induced increased lipolysis with decreased gluconeogenesis
    - Hypomagnesemia is common with chronic alcohol use and often is accompanied by hypokalemia and hypophosphatemia

Treatment

- **Treatment of acute withdrawal and detoxification**
  - **Alcohol: Mainstay is benzodiazepines to prevent alcohol withdrawal seizures and delirium tremens**
    - There is no evidence that any one benzodiazepine is better than any other. In patients with significant liver disease, lorazepam and oxazepam are the benzodiazepines of choice. Medications can be given orally unless there is a specific reason not to.
    - Dosing should be symptom driven, with frequent assessments for worsening or improvement of symptoms. The Clinical Institute Withdrawal Assessment for Alcohol is typically used to assess the severity of withdrawal.
    - Patients should also receive thiamine and folate
  - **Cocaine: Treatment is mostly supportive and typically does not require acute inpatient care; be alert, however, for other substance use and severe depression, which may necessitate hospitalization**
  - **Opioids: Symptoms are most effectively relieved with administration of either a long-acting full opioid agonist such as methadone or a partial opioid agonist such as buprenorphine**
    - Clonidine decreases the autonomic dysfunction associated with opioid withdrawal but will not treat many of the other symptoms
    - Dicyclomine may relieve abdominal cramping, and ibuprofen or other nonsteroidal antiinflammatory drugs may treat the myalgias and joint pains
- **Assessment of motivation and interest in long-term treatment**
  - **Assess stage of readiness for change**
    - **Precontemplative: Patient has not yet considered stopping substance use; may not think substance use is a problem**
    - **Contemplative: Patient is thinking about cessation**
    - **Determination: Patient has decided to stop substance use but is not yet taking action to quit**
    - **Action: Patient is actively goal setting, problem solving, and trying to quit**
    - **Maintenance: Patient has successfully quit and is working on relapse prevention**
    - **Relapse: Can occur at any point through this process; goal is then to get back to action stage**
- **Nonpharmacologic interventions**
  - A brief intervention by a physician in an office takes about 5 to 10 minutes to complete and takes advantage of the unique role in the patient-physician relationship to effect change
    - Consists of assessment, feedback to the patient, and referrals or recommendations
    - However, studies demonstrate that an intervention has not been found to reduce drinking among alcohol-dependent patients.

F: Give **feedback** on personal risks and existing impairments
R: Put emphasis on personal **responsibility** for change
A: Give clear **advice** and recommendations
M: Offer a **menu** of options and alternatives
E: Interact with the patient in an **empathic** way
S: Focus on **self-efficacy** to promote optimism and empowerment

- **The FRAMES algorithm is useful in a primary care office (Box 71-5)**
- Specialized substance abuse treatment programs are able to perform more comprehensive assessment, evaluation, and treatment
  - Provide more intensive substance abuse treatment
  - Group and individual addiction counseling
  - May offer psychiatric or medical care, but often do not
- Community support programs and self-help groups are common
  - Many, such as Alcoholics Anonymous and Narcotics Anonymous, are based on 12-step approach
  - "Rational recovery" uses a cognitive behavioral approach and may be an alternative for patients who are uncomfortable with the spiritual approach
- **Pharmacologic therapies**
  - All pharmacologic therapies for SUDs are most effective in combination with counseling or active self-help group participation
  - Alcohol
    - **Disulfiram acts as a deterrent to continued alcohol intake**
      - **Usual daily doses range from 250 to 500 mg**
      - **Patients develop severe flushing, shortness of breath, dizziness, nausea, vomiting, and abdominal pain, often with significant volume depletion if alcohol is consumed concomitantly**
      - Should be avoided in pregnant women and in patients with severe liver disease or medical comorbidities
      - Advise patients to avoid foods and beauty products that contain alcohol
    - **Acamprosate is thought to affect GABA and excitatory glutamate neurotransmission in the CNS to decrease alcohol cravings**
      - Results from some clinical trials demonstrate modest reductions in number of drinking days compared with placebo
    - **Naltrexone, an opioid antagonist, is modestly effective in preventing relapse to heavy drinking by diminishing cravings for alcohol**
      - Thought to act by decreasing some of the reinforcing effects of alcohol that may occur through opioid neurotransmission

- Avoid in patients with severe liver disease, patients who are pregnant, and those on chronic opioids
- Available in oral form (daily dosing) and an extended-release formulation for intramuscular injection (monthly)
- **Opioids**
  - **Methadone is a full opioid agonist at the μ opioid receptor with a long duration of action**
    - Available for opioid dependence treatment in regulated, specialized treatment centers where patients are observed taking the medication unless they have earned privileges to take home individual doses
    - In combination with counseling, methadone reduces illicit drug use and risk of overdose, keeps patients in treatment, reduces HIV and hepatitis C transmission, reduces criminal behavior, and improves health-related quality of life
    - About 50% of patients relapse to heroin use within 1 year of stopping methadone treatment
    - Therapeutic doses typically range between 40 and 100 mg, but individualized dosing is key, and therapeutic doses vary
  - **Buprenorphine is a long-acting partial opioid agonist with a higher affinity and a slower dissociation rate compared with full opioid agonists**
    - It is available in sublingual (tablet and film strip) and buccal formulations. **Usual dose for the sublingual formulation is 8 to 16 mg/day. Maximum recommended dose is 24 mg/day.**
    - Because of its partial agonist properties, buprenorphine has a ceiling beyond which increasing the dose will not result in any further opioid effects, making it safer than most opioids
    - Buprenorphine has been shown to be effective at reducing illicit opioid use in patients in a variety of settings, including primary care practices. Its availability has greatly expanded treatment of opioid use disorders and many of those who receive treatment would not have access to methadone or would not be willing to enroll in methadone maintenance.
    - **Office-based physicians can prescribe sublingual buprenorphine to treat opioid-dependent patients after completing 8 hours of training**
    - Buprenorphine is generally prescribed in the form of combination tablets and film strips that contain naloxone; the naloxone is not orally active and is added to discourage IV or intranasal administration
    - **Buprenorphine may precipitate withdrawal in patients who have recently taken full-agonist opioids**
  - **Naltrexone, an opioid antagonist approved for the treatment of opioid dependence, effectively blocks heroin effects.** However, its use is limited, as treatment retention is relatively low in oral

BOX 71-6	*Key Steps in Relapse Prevention*

Establish a supportive patient-physician relationship
Schedule regular follow up
Mobilize family support
Facilitate involvement in self-help and community groups
Help patients recognize and cope with relapse triggers and
    cravings
Facilitate positive lifestyle changes
Manage depression, anxiety, pain, and other comorbid
    conditions
Consider pharmacotherapy
Collaborate with addiction treatment specialists, if available

naltrexone treatment. An extended-release formulation for monthly intramuscular injection was recently approved for treatment of opioid dependence. Patients must be free of opioids at the initiation of treatment.

- Cocaine: Currently no effective pharmacologic agents exist for treatment of cocaine or other stimulant use disorders

- **Relapse prevention (Box 71-6)**
  - Relapse is a common part of recovery
  - 50% to 80% of patients return to substance use within their first year of recovery. Most of these patients relapse within the first 3 months after stopping alcohol or drug use.
  - 60% of those with lifetime SUDs eventually do achieve sustained abstinence
  - Factors associated with sustaining abstinence include self-efficacy, vocational engagement, income, having friends who are abstinent, and social and spiritual support
  - Additionally, longer periods of abstinence are associated with sustained abstinence
  - Relapse rates for addiction resemble those of exacerbations of other chronic diseases such as diabetes, hypertension, and asthma
  - As a chronic, relapsing condition, preventing relapse is a key component of long-term management of SUDs

Review Questions

For review questions, please go to ExpertConsult.com.

SUGGESTED READINGS

American Psychiatric Association. *Diagnostic and Statistical Manual of Mental Disorders.* 5th ed. Arlington, VA: American Psychiatric Association; 2013.

Anton RF, O'Malley SS, Ciraulo DA, et al. Combined pharmacotherapies and behavioral interventions for alcohol dependence: the COMBINE study: a randomized controlled trial. *JAMA.* 2006;295:2003-2017.

Buchsbaum DG, Buchanan RG, Centor RM, et al. Screening for alcohol abuse using CAGE scores and likelihood ratios. *Ann Intern Med.* 1991;115:774-777.

Bush K, Kivlahan DR, McDonell MB, et al. The AUDIT alcohol consumption questions (AUDIT-C): an effective brief screening test for problem drinking. *Arch Intern Med.* 1998;158:1789-1795.

Dawson DA, Grant BF, Stinson FS, Zhou Y. Effectiveness of the derived Alcohol Use Disorders Identification Test (AUDIT-C) in screening for alcohol use disorders and risk drinking in the US general population. *Alcohol Clin Exp Res.* 2005;29:844-854.

Dennis ML, Foss MA, Scott CK. An eight-year perspective on the relationship between the duration of abstinence and other aspects of recovery. *Eval Rev.* 2007;31:585-612.

Fudala PJ, Bridge TP, Herbert S, et al. for the Buprenorphine/Naloxone Collaborative Study Group. Office-based treatment of opiate addiction with a sublingual-tablet formulation of buprenorphine and naloxone. *N Engl J Med.* 2003;349:949-958.

Kaner EFS, Dickinson HO, Beyer FR, et al. Effectiveness of brief alcohol interventions in primary care populations. *Cochrane Database Syst Rev.* 2007;(2):CD004148.

Mattick RP, Breen C, Kimber J, et al. Buprenorphine maintenance versus placebo or methadone maintenance for opioid dependence. *Cochrane Database Syst Rev.* 2014;(2):CD002207.

Mattick RP, Breen C, Kimber J, et al. Methadone maintenance therapy versus no opioid replacement therapy for opioid dependence. *Cochrane Database Syst Rev.* 2009;(3):CD002209.

Office of National Drug Control Policy. *The Economic Costs of Drug Abuse in the United States, 1992-2002* (Publication No. 207303). Washington, DC: Executive Office of the President; 2004.

Ries RK, Fiellin DA, Saitz R, Miller SC, eds. *The ASAM Principles of Addiction Medicine.* 5th ed. St. Louis: Wolters Kluwer; 2014.

Rösner S, Hackl-Herrwerth A, Leucht S, et al. Opioid antagonists for alcohol dependence. *Cochrane Database Syst Rev.* 2010;(12):CD001867.

Substance Abuse and Mental Health Services Administration. *Results from the 2012 National Survey on Drug Use and Health: Summary of National Findings.* NSDUH Series H-46, HHS Publication No. SMA 13–4795. Rockville, MD: Substance Abuse and Mental Health Services Administration; 2013.

World Health Organization (WHO). *The Alcohol Use Disorders Identification Test: Guidelines for Use in Primary Care* (WHO/MSD/MSB/01.6a). Geneva: WHO; 2001. <http://whqlibdoc.who.int/hq/2001/WHO_MSD_MSB_01.6a.pdf>.

Preoperative Evaluation

STEPHEN D. SISSON, MD

Preoperative evaluation is a common task for the internist. The primary objective of the preoperative evaluation is **to assess the patient's medical readiness for surgery.** Every operative procedure carries some level of risk; clinical judgment, accompanied by appropriate testing, is needed to define risk. The preoperative evaluation **includes three steps: (1) clinical risk assessment, (2) functional assessment,** and **(3) surgery-specific risk assessment.** These assessments determine whether or not to proceed with surgery or to obtain cardiac testing before proceeding with surgery. Mounting evidence has demonstrated **the beneficial impact of β-blockers on cardiovascular outcomes** in some, but not all, patients undergoing noncardiac surgery.

Clinical Risk Assessment

- Clinical risk assessment is the first step in the preoperative evaluation; in this assessment, clinical predictors of increased risk are identified. The presence of certain conditions (Table 72-1) should lead to the postponement of **elective** surgery until they are resolved. **The presence of new symptoms uncovered during the preoperative evaluation should postpone elective surgery until new symptoms have been evaluated.**
  - Cardiovascular disease is commonly associated with increased operative risk
    - **The five areas of potential cardiovascular risk are: (1) ischemic cardiovascular disease, (2) congestive heart failure (CHF), (3) valvular heart disease, (4) hypertension, and (5) arrhythmia**
      - Prior **history of myocardial infarction (MI),** especially within the **past 60 days,** is associated **with increased operative risk;** acute MI should delay elective surgery for at least 60 days
        - Stable angina that is mild (i.e., class I or II angina) is not a contraindication to surgery. Unstable angina and class III or IV angina should delay surgery until they are resolved.
      - In the absence of MI, **elective** surgery should also be postponed following percutaneous coronary intervention as follows:
        - Balloon angioplasty: Delay surgery 14 days following angioplasty
        - Bare-metal intracoronary stent: Delay surgery 30 days following stent placement

- Drug-eluting intracoronary stent: Delay surgery 1 year following stent placement
- In all cases, aspirin should be continued perioperatively, if possible
- **Cardiac catheterization does not have a role in perioperative risk assessment;** performing cardiac catheterization solely to evaluate a person for elective surgery should not be done
- **Similarly, performing cardiac revascularization procedures specifically to prepare a patient with known coronary artery disease (CAD) for elective surgery has not been shown to be of benefit and should not be done**
- CHF is associated with increased perioperative risk, especially if uncontrolled. **Decompensated CHF is a contraindication to elective surgery.**
  - In patients with prior CHF, an echocardiogram to reassess left ventricle (LV) function is reasonable if no echocardiogram has been obtained in the past year
- **Symptomatic** valvular heart disease is a contraindication to elective surgery.
  - Severe valvular heart disease is not (by itself) a contraindication to elective surgery if asymptomatic. However, moderate-to-severe disease can increase the complication rate in noncardiac surgery by up to 30%. An echocardiogram to assess severity and secondary cardiac dysfunction in someone with known valvular heart disease is reasonable if no echocardiogram has been obtained in the past year.
  - Patients with prosthetic heart valves, prior infective endocarditis, intracardiac shunts, and/or prosthetic patches, as well as cardiac transplant patients with cardiac valvulopathy, should receive endocarditis prophylaxis when undergoing certain dental procedures or respiratory tract procedures
- Hypertension has not been demonstrated to affect surgery, but general consensus has been to control hypertension so that diastolic pressure is maintained at less than 110 mm Hg
- Arrhythmias are not a contraindication to elective surgery if the patient is clinically stable
  - Cardiology should be involved in management if the patient has a pacemaker or automatic implantable cardioverter defibrillator

TABLE 72-1	Clinical Risk and Elective Surgery
Clinical risk factors	**Contraindications to surgery**
• History of heart disease • History of compensated or prior heart failure • History of cerebrovascular disease • Diabetes mellitus (or specifically, anyone treated with insulin) • Renal insufficiency (defined as serum creatinine >2.0 mg/dL)	• Recent myocardial infarction (<60 days) • Unstable angina • Class III or IV angina • Decompensated heart failure • Symptomatic moderate or severe valvular heart disease

TABLE 72-2	Metabolic Equivalents and Physical Activity	
1 MET	**≥4 METs**	**>10 METs**
Take care of self	Climb 1 flight stairs or walk up a hill	Participate in strenuous sports including singles tennis, football, basketball, skiing
Eat, dress, use toilet	Walk on level ground at 4 mph	
Walk indoors around house	Run a short distance	
Walk 1 to 2 blocks on level ground at 2 to 3 mph	Scrubbing floors, moving heavy furniture	
Dusting/washing dishes (some classify this as 1 to 4 METs)	Golf, bowl, dance, doubles tennis, throw baseball or football	

METs, Metabolic equivalents.

- Pulmonary disease is also associated with perioperative risk. **Pulmonary complications** (e.g., atelectasis, pneumonia) are the **leading cause of perioperative morbidity.**
  - Patients with chronic pulmonary disease should have local or epidural anesthesia whenever possible
    - Serum albumin less than 3.5 g/dL is a marker for increased pulmonary complications
  - Preoperative pulmonary testing is controversial; preoperative chest imaging is usually not indicated, but can be considered in those with known heart or lung disease, or those 70 and older with no chest x-ray in the past 6 months
    - **Forced expiratory volume in 1 second (FEV$_1$) less than 1.5 L** is associated with **increased** risk of **pulmonary complications**
    - An **FEV$_1$ less than 1 L** is associated with **prolonged intubation** and should prompt consultation with a pulmonologist
  - Other **diseases that are associated with increased operative risk** include cerebrovascular disease, **diabetes mellitus,** and **renal insufficiency** (defined as creatinine greater than 2 mg/dL) (see Table 72-1)
  - **Patients should delay elective surgery in the presence of active infection**
  - If **corticosteroids** have been administered for at least **2 weeks** in the year preceding surgery, **stress-dose corticosteroids should be administered perioperatively**

Functional Assessment

- Surgery creates a stress on the cardiovascular system, which may unmask subclinical cardiovascular disease, especially in someone who is physically deconditioned
- Functional status assessment is a means of quantifying the physical conditioning of a patient who is about to undergo surgery
  - Functional status is standardized into units of Metabolic Equivalents of Task, referred to as METs
  - METs can be correlated with routine daily activities, allowing the physician to perform a functional status assessment by inquiring about those activities a

patient is able to perform without developing limiting dyspnea or chest pain
  - The **inability** to perform at least **4 METs** of activity without symptoms is consistent with **poor functional status** and is associated with **increased operative risk**
  - If the patient **is unable to perform physical activity** (e.g., a patient who cannot walk because of severe degenerative arthritis), **assume that patient cannot perform 4 METs** and has poor functional status
- MET equivalents associated with common physical activities are summarized in Table 72-2

Surgery-Specific Risk Assessment

- Overall risks
  - For all surgeries, perioperative mortality is 0.3%
    - Most perioperative deaths (55%) occur in **the first 48 hours postoperatively**
    - Of perioperative deaths, 35% occur in the operating room, and 10% occur during anesthesia induction
  - **Pulmonary complications are the most common perioperative complications**
  - **Cardiac complications are the most common cause of perioperative death**
    - Perioperative MIs usually occur by postoperative day 3
  - Procedure-associated risk
  - Surgery-specific risk is determined by the operative procedure planned
    - **Low-risk** procedures are associated with a less than **1%** risk of death
    - Intermediate- and high-risk surgeries are associated with greater than 1% risk of death
    - Emergency surgery is considered very high risk
- A summary of surgery-specific risks is provided in Table 72-3

TABLE 72-3	*Surgery-Specific Risk*
Low Risk (<1%)	**Intermediate- and High-Risk Surgery**
Endoscopic procedures	Carotid endarterectomy
Superficial procedures	Endovascular abdominal aortic aneurysm repair
Cataract surgery	Head and neck surgery
Breast surgery	Intraperitoneal surgery
Ambulatory surgery	Intrathoracic surgery Orthopedic surgery Prostate surgery Peripheral vascular surgery Aortic/major vascular surgery

- **Role of β-blockers**
  - **β-blockers are proven to reduce risk of perioperative MI in certain populations. They also increase risk of stroke and death in other populations.**
  - Perioperative β-blockers should be considered for patients with 3 or more clinical risk factors (i.e., prior CAD, prior CHF, prior cerebrovascular accident, diabetes, chronic kidney disease)
    - They should also be considered in those with intermediate- or high-risk results from preoperative cardiac stress testing
  - **β-blockers should be continued in those already taking them**
    - If added preoperatively, they should be added at least 1 day preoperatively

Summarizing Preoperative Risk

- Preoperative risk is summarized by **combining clinical risk, functional status, and surgery-specific risk (Figure 72-1)**
  - **Patients with an active cardiac condition should not undergo elective surgery until the active cardiac condition has been treated**
  - Patients with no clinical risk factors can proceed to surgery without noninvasive cardiac testing
  - Patients with good functional status can proceed to surgery without noninvasive cardiac testing
  - Patients undergoing low-risk surgical procedures can proceed to surgery without noninvasive cardiac testing
  - All other patients should have perioperative risk assessed using a risk assessment calculator (e.g., National Surgical Quality Improvement Program)
    - If calculated risk is more than 1%, obtain pharmacologic stress test if results would affect management

Instructions to the Patient

- Medication adjustments
  - If medications are titrated according to serum levels, **check drug concentrations preoperatively** and adjust doses accordingly

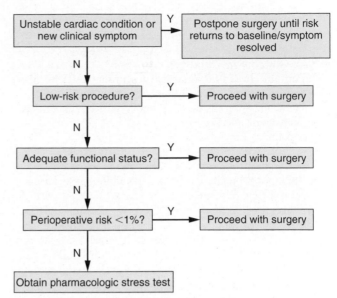

FIGURE 72-1 Summary of perioperative management. N, No; Y, yes.

- **Antihypertensives are continued** on the morning of surgery **with the exception** of diuretics. Angiotensin-converting enzyme inhibitors and angiotensin-receptor blockers are now continued during surgery
- Diabetes medications are adjusted as follows:
  - **Oral hypoglycemics are held on the day of surgery**
  - **Basal insulin is continued during surgery;** the dose may be lowered if the risk of hypoglycemia is high (as in those with tight glycemic control)
  - **Prandial insulin is held on the day of surgery**
  - **HMG CoA reductase inhibitors ("statins") are continued** on the day of surgery and may reduce risk of a cardiac event
    - Consider adding a statin in patients not on them who are undergoing vascular surgery or in patients with clinical indications who are undergoing elevated-risk procedures
- Sedatives, hypnotics, and other CNS-active medications are held on the day of surgery
- **Aspirin may be continued during surgery when the potential risk of a cardiac event outweighs the risk of bleeding,** but is otherwise held for the week leading up to surgery. The decision to continue aspirin should be discussed with the surgical team. Other nonsteroidal antiinflammatory drugs (NSAIDs) are typically held for the week leading up to surgery.
- Other idiosyncratic reactions include the following:
  - **Lithium:** May cause myocardial suppression and is **held the day of surgery**
  - **Tetracycline:** May cause renal failure if administered with methoxyflurane (anesthetic) and **is held the day of surgery**
  - Neuroleptics may enhance neuromuscular blocking agents; if given, the anesthesiologist may need to adjust neuromuscular blockade during surgery

72

- All herbal remedies should be discontinued before surgery (e.g., St. John's wort and ginkgo biloba)
- New symptom monitoring
  - Patients should be reminded to contact the internist or surgeon if a febrile illness, chest pain, or new medical symptoms develop between the preoperative assessment and surgery
- Preoperative testing
  - Although routine preoperative testing is often performed, there are few data to support its use. Surgeons typically will make specific requests based on the type of surgical procedure.
  - The following preoperative testing is commonplace:
    - Electrocardiography: Do not obtain in those undergoing low-risk surgery. Otherwise, consider in those with known CAD or at risk for CAD.
    - Chest radiography: Usually not indicated; consider in those with known heart or lung disease, or those 70 and older with no chest x-ray in the past 6 months

- Complete blood count: Consider in those 65 and older and in those undergoing procedures with potential for excessive blood loss
- Blood urea nitrogen/creatinine: Obtain in those undergoing intermediate- or high-risk surgery
- Prothrombin time/partial thromboplastin time: Consider in patients with liver disease or malignancy, patients receiving anticoagulants, or patients having neurosurgery
- Urinalysis: of uncertain value

Review Questions

For review questions, please go to ExpertConsult.com.

SUGGESTED READING

Fleisher LA, Fleischmann KE, Auerbach AD, et al. 2014 ACC/AHA guideline on perioperative cardiovascular evaluation and management of patients undergoing noncardiac surgery. *J Am Coll Cardiol.* 2014;64:e77-e137.

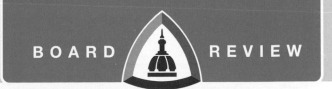
Immunization and Prevention

BIMAL H. ASHAR, MD, MBA

Immunizations and screening for designated pathologic conditions are the cornerstones of preventive medicine. Several major medical societies have published guidelines for these practices, although several of their recommendations vary. The following is an overview of the necessary immunizations and their side effect profiles, as well as other health maintenance screening guidelines.

Immunization

- General concepts
  - Active versus passive
    - Active immunization involves administration of antigen to induce an antibody response
    - Passive immunization involves administration of an exogenous antibody (temporary protection against a disease)
      - Usually done by infusion of human immunoglobulin (e.g., hepatitis A, tetanus)
  - Types of active immunization (i.e., vaccination)
    - Live, attenuated
      - Usually confers lifelong immunity
      - **Should not be given to immunocompromised patients**
      - Examples: measles, mumps, and rubella (MMR); varicella-zoster (chickenpox); shingles, influenza (intranasal)
    - Inactivated (killed) whole pathogen (e.g., influenza shot, hepatitis A)
    - Fractional protein-based (e.g., hepatitis B, tetanus)
    - Polysaccharide (e.g., pneumococcal, meningococcal)
  - Principles of administration
    - Live vaccines should either be given together or at least 4 weeks apart
    - **It is not necessary to restart an interrupted vaccine series (except oral typhoid)**
    - Live vaccines should not be given with immunoglobulin or blood products
    - Common patient misconceptions about vaccination:
      - **Many vaccines cause a local reaction and fever that lasts 24 to 48 hours. This does not contraindicate using the vaccine again and should not be considered an allergic response.**
      - Mild acute illness (or recent illness) or the current use of antibiotics does not contraindicate the use of vaccines
      - Family history of adverse reaction to a vaccine does not contraindicate the use of vaccines
- Individual vaccines (Fig. 73-1)
  - Influenza
    - Vaccine characteristics
      - New formulation created each year for different strains. In some years, the predicted strains covered by the vaccine may not match the strain of virus causing illness
      - If there is a match, the vaccine is 60% to 80% effective in preventing influenza disease and around 70% effective in preventing flu-related hospitalizations
      - Ideally given in October or November, but can be given as late as February
      - Needs to be given annually
      - Many different forms of vaccine are available, including quadrivalent inactivated standard dose, trivalent inactivated standard dose, trivalent inactivated standard dose intradermal (for those afraid of large needles), trivalent inactivated high dose (approved for persons ages 65 and older), trivalent inactivated recombinant (egg-free for adults 18 to 49), and live attenuated quadrivalent (intranasal for ages 2 to 49)
    - Indications
      - The Advisory Committee on Immunization Practices (ACIP) recommends annual influenza vaccination for all people age 6 months and older
      - **Currently, the ACIP does not endorse any specific formulation of vaccine over another for immunocompetent adults**
    - Adverse reactions for the inactivated vaccines include soreness at the injection site, low-grade fever, and myalgia
    - Adverse reactions for the live intranasal preparation include runny nose, sore throat, headache, cough, and low-grade fever
    - Contraindications
      - The only absolute contraindication to the flu vaccine is severe, life-threatening allergies to flu vaccine or any ingredient in the vaccine
      - **Egg allergy is not a contraindication to receiving vaccine given the availability of the recombinant vaccine (RIV3). If RIV3 is not available (or the patient is older than 49 years), patients can receive other inactivated vaccines with close observation.**

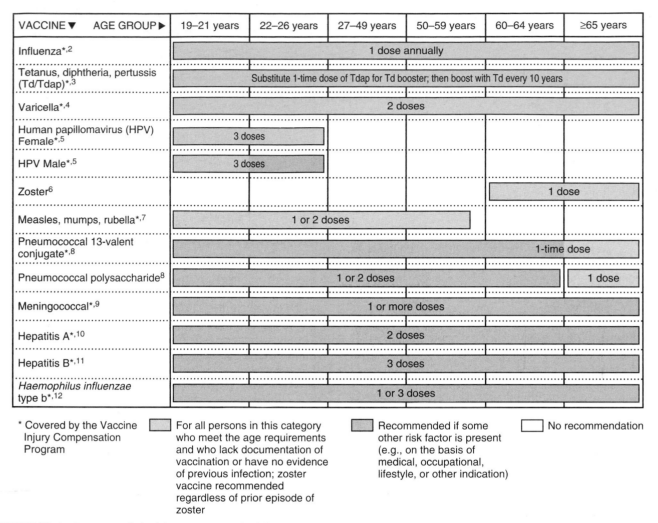

VACCINE ▼ AGE GROUP ▶	19–21 years	22–26 years	27–49 years	50–59 years	60–64 years	≥65 years
Influenza*,2	1 dose annually					
Tetanus, diphtheria, pertussis (Td/Tdap)*,3	Substitute 1-time dose of Tdap for Td booster; then boost with Td every 10 years					
Varicella*,4	2 doses					
Human papillomavirus (HPV) Female*,5	3 doses					
HPV Male*,5	3 doses					
Zoster6					1 dose	
Measles, mumps, rubella*,7	1 or 2 doses					
Pneumococcal 13-valent conjugate*,8					1-time dose	
Pneumococcal polysaccharide8	1 or 2 doses					1 dose
Meningococcal*,9	1 or more doses					
Hepatitis A*,10	2 doses					
Hepatitis B*,11	3 doses					
Haemophilus influenzae type b*,12	1 or 3 doses					

* Covered by the Vaccine Injury Compensation Program

☐ For all persons in this category who meet the age requirements and who lack documentation of vaccination or have no evidence of previous infection; zoster vaccine recommended regardless of prior episode of zoster

☐ Recommended if some other risk factor is present (e.g., on the basis of medical, occupational, lifestyle, or other indication)

☐ No recommendation

FIGURE 73-1 Recommended adult vaccination schedule. (From the Centers for Disease Control Advisory Committee on Immunization Practices. Document and footnotes available at: www.cdc.gov/vaccines/schedules/downloads/adult/adult-combined-schedule.pdf.)

- A history of Guillain-Barré syndrome within 6 weeks of previous influenza vaccine administration is considered a precaution but not a contraindication to the vaccine
- *Pneumococcus*
  - Pneumococcal polysaccharide vaccine (PPSV23)
    - Indicated for adults aged 65 years or older, adults younger than 65 years of age with certain chronic conditions/risks (i.e., diabetes, chronic heart disease, chronic liver disease, alcoholism, chronic lung disease, cerebrospinal fluid [CSF] leaks, cochlear implant, cigarette smoking), immunocompromised patients younger than 65 years of age (including patients with malignancies, chronic renal disease, human immunodeficiency virus [HIV], and conditions requiring immunosuppressive drugs), and patients with anatomic or functional asplenia
    - Revaccination is only recommended 5 years after initial administration for immunocompromised patients and those with functional or anatomic asplenia

- Those patients who received pneumococcal vaccine before age 65 years for any indication should receive another dose of the vaccine at age 65 years or later if at least 5 years have passed since their previous dose
  - **It is currently not recommended to vaccinate any individual more than twice**
- Pneumococcal conjugate vaccine (PCV13)
  - Indicated for adults aged 65 years or older, adults younger than 65 years of age with certain chronic conditions/risks (immunocompromised state, asplenia, CSF leaks, cochlear implants)
  - Vaccine should be administered in series with PPSV23 and not simultaneously: If patient has received neither vaccine, give PCV13 first and PPSV23 6 to 12 months later. If patient has received PPSV23, wait at least 1 year before administering PCV13.
  - Currently, there are no recommendations regarding PCV13 boosters
- Tetanus (tetanus, diphtheria [Td])
  - Administer primary adult series if no history of vaccination: 3-shot series at 0, 1, and then 6 to 12 months

- Recommended every 10 years unless patient has not had one Tdap (tetanus, diphtheria, acellular pertussis) booster as an adult (see later)
- Important to revaccinate elderly patients because the elderly and children are the at-risk populations for the illness
- Treatment of exposure (i.e., dirty wound)
  - Administer Td vaccine if last shot was 5 or more years before, or begin primary series if never given
  - Administer tetanus immune globulin if Td never given (can be given with first Td vaccine)
- Pertussis (Tdap)
  - ACIP recommends that a single dose of Tdap be given to all adults aged 19 and older
  - Should be given regardless of date of last tetanus shot (Td)
  - After single dose of Tdap is given, resume 10-year vaccination schedule with Td (see earlier)
  - **Administer to pregnant women with *every* pregnancy, ideally between 27 and 36 weeks' gestation**
- Hepatitis A
  - Inactivated whole-virus vaccine (killed)
  - Recommended for the following adult groups
    - Illicit drug users
    - Men who have sex with men (MSM)
    - Patients with chronic liver disease
    - Patients who receive clotting factor concentrates
    - Family and caregivers of recent adoptees from countries where hepatitis A is endemic
    - Patients traveling or working in countries that have high prevalence of the disease
  - Given as 2-shot series at least 6 months apart
  - For travelers, should be given at least a month before anticipated exposure
  - Booster currently not recommended
  - Postexposure prophylaxis
    - For healthy adults, single-antigen hepatitis A vaccine is preferred to hepatitis A immune globulin
    - For persons older than 40 years of age, hepatitis A immune globulin is preferred, if available
- Hepatitis B
  - Inactivated vaccine
  - Recommended for the following adult groups
    - **Diabetics aged 19 to 59**
    - Nonmonogamous sexually active persons
    - MSM
    - HIV positive patients
    - Patients with or seeking evaluation for a sexually transmitted disease (STD)
    - Injection drug users
    - Patients with end-stage renal disease (on hemodialysis), chronic liver disease, or who are regular recipients of blood products (e.g., patients with hemophilia)
    - Contacts of patients with hepatitis B
    - Health care workers
    - Institutionalized and developmentally delayed patients
  - Three-shot series at 0, 1, and 6 months

- Test for hepatitis B surface antibody (anti-HBs) 1 to 2 months after third shot in health care workers, hemodialysis patients, immunocompromised patients (including those with HIV), and sex partners of persons with hepatitis B infection
  - **Nonresponders after three doses should be revaccinated with the entire series and retested**
- Human papillomavirus (HPV) vaccine
  - Two vaccines currently approved
    - Quadrivalent vaccine (HPV4) efficacious in preventing infection from HPV types 6, 11, 16, and 18
    - Bivalent vaccine (HPV2) efficacious in preventing infection from HPV types 16 and 18
    - Both vaccines are administered as a 3-shot series (0, 2, and 6 months)
  - **About 70% of cervical cancers are caused by HPV-16 and HPV-18**
  - About 90% of genital warts are associated with HPV-6 and HPV-11
  - Either vaccine is recommended in girls/women ages 9 to 26 to reduce the incidence of cervical, vulvar, and vaginal cancer and/or genital warts
  - **HPV4 is recommended for boys/men ages 9 to 21 to reduce the incidence of genital warts and anal cancer and offer herd immunity protection for women**
  - HPV is also suggested for immunocompromised men and MSM through age 26
  - Need to continue screening Papanicolaou test (Pap smears) even in women who received the vaccine
  - Avoid using in patients with moderate to severe acute illness, hypersensitivity to yeast, and in women who are pregnant
- Measles, mumps, and rubella (MMR)
  - Live, attenuated vaccine
  - Given in two doses: typically at 0 and at 1 to 2 months
  - **Avoid in patients who are pregnant, trying to get pregnant, or severely immunocompromised**
  - Patients born before 1957 are considered immune because of their innate exposure
  - Patients vaccinated between 1957 and 1968 received a killed vaccine that is not effective, so they are not immune; if in an at-risk group, they need revaccination
  - Otherwise, vaccination of adults is typically recommended for the following groups:
    - Women of childbearing age (if rubella titer is negative)
    - College students (if measles titer is negative)
    - Travelers (if measles titer is negative)
    - Health care workers (if measles titer is negative)
- Varicella-zoster (chickenpox)
  - Live, attenuated vaccine
  - Given in two doses: at 0 and 1 month
  - **Diffuse varicella-like rash can occur in up to 5% of patients; transmission from a patient with this rash to immunocompromised children has been reported; patients should be**

73

BOX 73-1	*Evidence of Immunity to Varicella for Adults*

Documentation of 2-dose vaccine series
Laboratory evidence of immunity
Birth in the United States before 1980*
Verification of history of chickenpox by a health care provider[†]
Verification of a history of herpes zoster by a health care provider

*Birth before 1980 not considered adequate evidence for health care workers, pregnant women, and immunocompromised patients.
[†]Self-report of disease is not sufficient.

advised not to have contact with immunosuppressed patients until rash is gone
- Should be given to all adults without evidence of immunity (Box 73-1)
- Consider testing for immunity in health care workers, teachers, and day care workers, contacts of chronically ill patients, immunocompromised patients, and pregnant women
- Contraindications
  - Patients with malignancy and severe immunocompromised states (including medication-induced immune compromise)
  - Pregnancy (women should avoid pregnancy for 1 month after vaccination)
- HIV patients with $CD4^+$ count greater than 200 cells/mm^3 can get the vaccine per ACIP
  - For postexposure prophylaxis in patients who cannot receive the vaccine, varicella-zoster immune globulin (VZIG) should be given within 4 days of the exposure
- Herpes zoster (shingles) vaccine
  - Live, attenuated vaccine
  - About 50% to 60% effective in preventing shingles; about 60% to 70% effective in preventing postherpetic neuralgia
  - Given as a single shot; no booster currently recommended
  - ACIP recommends vaccination for all patients 60 years and older
  - **It is not necessary to ask about history of chickenpox or to conduct serologic testing for varicella-zoster immunity**
  - Patients who have a history of shingles can be vaccinated unless contraindications exist
  - Contraindications include a history of anaphylaxis to vaccine components (e.g., gelatin, neomycin) or severe immunodeficiency (acquired, primary, or medication-induced)
  - Patients taking low-dose prednisone or methotrexate can receive the vaccine
- Meningococcal vaccine
  - Active against *Neisseria meningitidis* groups A, C, Y, and W-135
  - ACIP recommends vaccinating all adolescents at age 11 to 12 years, with a booster at age 16
  - Patients aged 2 to 55 with complement deficiency or asplenia should receive a 2-shot primary series

separated by 2 months. They should also receive booster injections every 5 years.
  - HIV infection is not an indication for vaccination but adolescents with HIV who are due for the vaccine should also receive a 2-shot series
- Rabies vaccine (preexposure)
  - Bats, skunks, raccoons, dogs, and cats can transmit disease
  - When vaccine is administered as preexposure prophylaxis, 3 doses given
  - If administered after a bite, 4 doses of vaccine plus rabies immune globulin should be given
  - Indications for preexposure prophylaxis
  - Preexposure prophylaxis is given to veterinarians, animal handlers, and travelers who will likely come in contact with animals in parts of the world where rabies is common
- *Haemophilus influenzae* type B (Hib) vaccine
  - Usually given in childhood
  - One dose should be given before the procedure in patients undergoing elective splenectomy
  - Other asplenic patients should receive 1 dose at some time
  - **Patients undergoing stem cell transplant should receive 3 doses beginning 6 to 12 months after transplant**
- Special populations (Fig. 73-2)
  - HIV
    - Live, attenuated vaccines are only contraindicated in patients with severe immunosuppression ($CD4^+$ count less than 200 cells/mm^3)
  - Bone marrow transplant recipients should receive the following:
    - Inactivated influenza vaccine at least 6 months after transplant
    - Sequential administration of 3 doses of PCV13 beginning 3 to 6 months after transplant, followed by a dose of PPSV23
    - Three doses of Hib vaccine beginning 6 months after transplant
    - Live vaccines (e.g., MMR) should be given 24 months after transplantation assuming no graft-versus-host disease or immunosuppressant drugs

Screening

- General principles
  - Recommendations for screening vary widely based on available evidence and the organization making the recommendation
    - United States Preventive Services Task Force (USPSTF)
      - Government-sponsored group whose mission is to make recommendations on which preventive services should be part of routine primary care
      - Cost-effectiveness does play a role in recommendations made
      - The USPSTF has a grading system for its recommendations (Table 73-1)
      - The Patient Protection and Affordable Care Act stipulates that preventive services with a

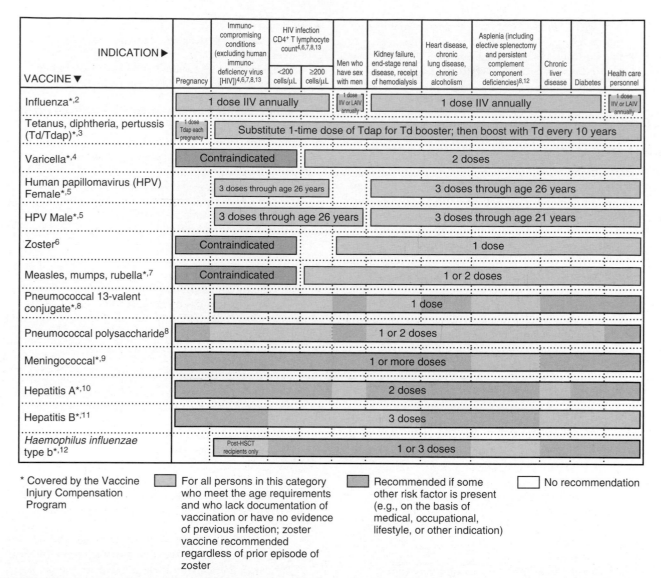

VACCINE ▼ \ INDICATION ►	Pregnancy	Immuno-compromising conditions (excluding human immuno-deficiency virus [HIV])[4,6,7,8,13]	HIV infection CD4+ T lymphocyte count[4,6,7,8,13] <200 cells/μL	HIV infection CD4+ T lymphocyte count[4,6,7,8,13] ≥200 cells/μL	Men who have sex with men	Kidney failure, end-stage renal disease, receipt of hemodialysis	Heart disease, chronic lung disease, chronic alcoholism	Asplenia (including elective splenectomy and persistent complement component deficiencies)[8,12]	Chronic liver disease	Diabetes	Health care personnel
Influenza*,2	1 dose IIV annually	1 dose IIV annually	1 dose IIV annually	1 dose IIV or LAIV annually	1 dose IIV annually	1 dose IIV annually	1 dose IIV annually	1 dose IIV annually	1 dose IIV annually	1 dose IIV annually	1 dose IIV or LAIV annually
Tetanus, diphtheria, pertussis (Td/Tdap)*,3	1 dose Tdap each pregnancy	Substitute 1-time dose of Tdap for Td booster; then boost with Td every 10 years									
Varicella*,4	Contraindicated	2 doses									
Human papillomavirus (HPV) Female*,5	3 doses through age 26 years	3 doses through age 26 years		3 doses through age 26 years							
HPV Male*,5	3 doses through age 26 years	3 doses through age 26 years		3 doses through age 21 years							
Zoster6	Contraindicated	1 dose									
Measles, mumps, rubella*,7	Contraindicated	1 or 2 doses									
Pneumococcal 13-valent conjugate*,8		1 dose									
Pneumococcal polysaccharide8		1 or 2 doses									
Meningococcal*,9		1 or more doses									
Hepatitis A*,10		2 doses									
Hepatitis B*,11		3 doses									
Haemophilus influenzae type b*,12	Post-HSCT recipients only	1 or 3 doses									

* Covered by the Vaccine Injury Compensation Program

▢ For all persons in this category who meet the age requirements and who lack documentation of vaccination or have no evidence of previous infection; zoster vaccine recommended regardless of prior episode of zoster

▢ Recommended if some other risk factor is present (e.g., on the basis of medical, occupational, lifestyle, or other indication)

▢ No recommendation

FIGURE 73-2 Immunization schedule for special adult populations. HSCT, Hematopoietic stem cell transplant; LAIV, live, attenuated influenza vaccine. (From the Centers of Disease Control Advisory Committee on Immunization Practices. Document and footnotes available at: www.cdc.gov/vaccines/schedules/downloads/adult/adult-combined-schedule.pdf.)

73

TABLE 73-1	United States Preventive Services Task Force Grading System

Grade	Description
A	Service recommended. Net benefit is thought to be substantial
B	Service recommended. Net benefit is thought to be moderate to substantial
C	Not routinely recommended. There may be some individuals for which service is appropriate
D	Not recommended. Data show no benefit or potential for harm
I	Current evidence insufficient to make a recommendation for or against the service

USPSTF grade of A or B must be covered without cost-sharing (e.g., copayment or deductible) under new health insurance plans or policies

- Types of prevention
  - **Primary prevention: intervention designed to avert disease before it develops** (e.g., nutritional counseling)
  - **Secondary prevention: intervention aimed at early detection of disease** (e.g., mammography). Most screening tests are a form of secondary prevention.
  - **Tertiary prevention: preventing complications of a symptomatic disease** (e.g., hepatitis B vaccine in hepatitis C patients)
- An ideal screening test is one that does the following:
  - Screens for a disease that has high morbidity and mortality

- Is sensitive with a confirmatory test available, inexpensive, and noninvasive
- Screens for a disease that has a long premorbid phase during which intervention can affect outcome

Cancer Screening

BREAST CANCER

- Mammography
  - USPSTF recommends screening mammograms every 2 years for women ages 50 to 74; starting before age 50 should be determined on a case-by-case basis
  - Other groups recommend more frequent testing; annual mammography for patients older than 40
  - No clear data on screening for women 75 years of age or older, but life expectancy and comorbid diseases should be taken into consideration
  - Currently, there are no recommendations for digital mammography with or without three-dimensional imaging or for magnetic resonance imaging
- Clinical breast examination (CBE) and self-breast examination (SBE)
  - USPSTF recommends against teaching SBE and notes that there is insufficient evidence to support CBE alone or as an adjunct to mammography
  - Many groups still recommend both of these
- Genetic testing
  - Current recommendation is for primary care physicians to screen women for a positive family history of breast, ovarian, tubal, or peritoneal cancer as determined by an established screening tool
  - Patients with positive family history should be referred for genetic counseling and/or *BRCA1* and *BRCA2* testing
- Chemoprevention
  - Clinicians should discuss use of tamoxifen or raloxifene in women at high risk for breast cancer
  - Can estimate risk with the use of online tools (e.g., the National Cancer Institute's Breast Cancer Risk Assessment Tool, http://cancer.gov/bcrisktool/)
  - Need to weigh risks of medications (i.e., venous thrombosis, uterine cancer) against benefits of prevention

COLORECTAL CANCER

- Screening options (by the USPSTF)
  - Annual high-sensitivity fecal occult blood testing (FOBT)
    - Chemical FOBT has been shown to reduce colon cancer mortality by 15% to 20%
    - Immunologic FOBT results in fewer false positives but long-term mortality data are currently limited
  - Flexible sigmoidoscopy every 5 years plus high-sensitivity FOBT every 3 years
  - Colonoscopy every 10 years
  - Computed tomographic colonography, fecal deoxyribonucleic acid (DNA), and/or circulating methylated septin 9 DNA may be useful tests in the near future but are currently not accepted for general screening

- Timing
  - Start screening at age 50 years in individuals at average risk
  - Net benefit of screening between the ages of 76 to 85 years is small but should be individualized based on comorbid conditions
  - **Stop screening adults older than 85 years (harm outweighs benefits)**
- Higher-risk patients may need colonoscopy earlier than age 50 years or more frequently than every 10 years
  - Familial polyposis
  - Strong family history (first-degree relative younger than 60 years)
  - History of adenomatous polyps
  - History of inflammatory bowel disease (see Chapter 69)

PROSTATE CANCER

- USPSTF recommends against routine screening with prostate-specific antigen (PSA) and/or digital rectal examination (DRE), noting that the harms of screening outweigh the benefits (grade D)
- The American College of Physicians (ACP) recommends:
  - Discussion of pros and cons of PSA screening with men aged 50 to 69 years. Decision to screen should be based on the patient's general health and life expectancy as well as his preference.
  - Against screening average-risk men under the age of 50 years, men over the age of 69 years, or men with a life expectancy of less than 10 to 15 years
- American Urologic Association (AUA) recommends:
  - A shared decision-making approach for men aged 55 to 69 years. Two-year interval for PSA may be sufficient.
  - An individualized approach for men aged 40 to 54 years and at higher risk (i.e., positive family history, African-American) but against screening men at average risk
  - Against screening men over the age of 69 years, or men with a life expectancy of less than 10 to 15 years
- Limited data to support DRE or specialized PSA tests (free PSA, prostate health index, PSA velocity, etc.)

CERVICAL AND OVARIAN CANCER

- USPSTF recommends screening with a Pap smear every 3 years in women aged 21 to 65 years
  - For women age 30 to 65 years who want to lengthen the screening interval, screening with a combination of cytology (Pap smear) and HPV testing every 5 years is also adequate
  - HPV testing is not recommended for women under the age of 30 years
  - **Screening is not recommended for women under the age of 21 years, women older than 65 years who have had adequate prior screening (3 consecutive negative cytology results), and women who have had a hysterectomy with removal of the cervix for a benign condition (see Chapter 64)**

- The recommendations do not apply to women who have received a diagnosis of a high-grade precancerous cervical lesion or cervical cancer, women with in utero exposure to diethylstilbestrol, or women who are immunocompromised (e.g., HIV positive)
- **Screening for ovarian cancer is not recommended for individuals at average risk; tests (cancer antigen-125 and ultrasound) are inaccurate with very low positive predictive value**
  - Routine pelvic examinations done for ovarian cancer screening are not recommended by the USPSTF or the ACP

LUNG CANCER

- The USPSTF recommends annual screening with low-dose computed tomography (LDCT) in adults aged 55 to 80 years who have a 30 pack-year smoking history
  - Screening should be stopped (or not started) in people who have not smoked for 15 years or more, have a limited life expectancy, or would not be willing to undergo curative lung surgery
- There is no role for routine chest radiograph or sputum cytology as screening tools for cancer

Screening for Infectious Diseases

- HIV
  - USPSTF recommends screening all individuals aged 15 to 65 years at least once
    - More frequent screening may be indicated for persons at high risk for disease
  - USPSTF also recommends screening all pregnant women
- STDs (USPSTF recommendations)
  - Hepatitis B: routine screening recommended for high-risk individuals and pregnant women but not for the general population in the U.S.
  - Hepatitis C virus (HCV):
    - **One-time screening for HCV infection for adults born between 1945 and 1965**
    - Screen patients (interval not specified) with risk factors for hepatitis C (e.g., injection drug use, long-term hemodialysis, blood transfusion before 1992, incarceration, intranasal drug use, high-risk sexual behaviors)
  - Syphilis: Test all pregnant women and high-risk patients (e.g., history of STD or HIV, multiple sex partners)
  - Gonorrhea and chlamydia: Routine screening recommended for all sexually active women age 24 years and younger and in older women who are at increased risk for infection. Insufficient evidence available to recommend screening in men.
  - Herpes simplex virus: Routine screening is not recommended
  - Sexually transmitted infection behavioral counseling: Recommended for all sexually active adolescents and for adults who are at increased risk

- Tuberculosis screening
  - Routine screening not necessary
  - Centers for Disease Control and Prevention (CDC) recommends screening in high-risk patients such as the following:
    - Chronic disease (e.g., diabetes, renal failure, HIV)
    - Recent emigrants from Africa, Asia, and Latin America
    - Health care workers and anyone in close contact with a patient with known tuberculosis
    - Medically underserved populations
    - Residents of long-term facilities (e.g., jails, nursing homes)
    - Immunosuppressed
    - Alcoholics and intravenous drug users
  - Frequency of screening is a matter of clinical discretion
  - Two types of tests available: tuberculin skin test (TST) and interferon-γ release assay blood test (IGRA)
  - Criteria for positive TST test are as follows:
    - Low-risk patients: 15-mm diameter or greater
    - High-risk patients (any of the previous indications for screening makes a patient at least high risk): 10-mm diameter or greater
    - Very-high-risk patients (HIV infection, abnormal chest film, recent contact with known infected patients): 5-mm diameter or greater
  - IGRA blood test is preferred for patients who have had the BCG vaccine

Screening for Cardiovascular Disease

- Hypertension
  - USPSTF suggests screening for all adults older than age 18, but they do not specify frequency
  - The Seventh Report of the Joint National Committee on Detection, Evaluation, and Treatment of High Blood Pressure (JNC 7) recommends yearly evaluations in everyone with a blood pressure over 120/80 mm Hg and every 2 years in those with pressures lower than 120/80 mm Hg. The screening duration was not addressed in JNC 8.
- Hypercholesterolemia
  - USPSTF recommends screening all men 35 years or older regardless of risk factors and men and women 20 years and older if they have a risk factor for coronary heart disease
  - USPSTF makes no recommendation for screening women without risk factors
  - American College of Cardiology/American Heart Association recommends assessing traditional risk factors (including cholesterol) every 4 to 6 years in patients 20 to 79 years of age
- Coronary heart disease
  - USPSTF recommends against resting electrocardiography or exercise treadmill testing in low-risk patients. In asymptomatic patients with an increased risk for coronary artery disease, there is

73

insufficient evidence for or against use of these modalities.
- Evidence is also thought to be insufficient to recommend high-sensitivity C-reactive protein, ankle-brachial index, leukocyte count, fasting blood glucose level, periodontal disease, carotid intima-media thickness, coronary artery calcification score on electron-beam computed tomography, homocysteine level, and lipoprotein(a) levels
- Carotid artery disease screening is not recommended for asymptomatic adults
- Abdominal aortic aneurysm (AAA)
  - **USPSTF recommends one-time screening for AAA by ultrasound in men ages 65 to 75 years who have ever smoked**
  - Can consider screening male nonsmokers between the ages of 65 and 75 years but data are not definitive (grade C recommendation)
  - USPSTF recommends against screening for AAA in women who have never smoked and has suggested that there is insufficient evidence to recommend in women aged 65 to 75 years who have smoked
- Aspirin use
  - Use of aspirin for men ages 45 to 79 years is recommended when the potential benefit caused by a reduction in myocardial infarctions outweighs the potential harm because of an increase in gastrointestinal hemorrhage
  - Use of aspirin for women ages 55 to 79 years is recommended when the potential benefit of a reduction in ischemic strokes outweighs the potential harm of an increase in gastrointestinal hemorrhage
  - Ideal dose is unclear since beneficial effects are shown for doses ranging from 75 mg to 325 mg

Other Disease Screening

See Table 73-2.

Psychosocial and Behavioral Screening

- The USPSTF does not make recommendations for or against routine screening for a number of behavioral and situational disorders. However, they do state that clinicians should be aware of them and address these issues when appropriate.
- The following areas of concern may need to be addressed in an individual patient:
  - Depression (screening recommended for all adults)
  - Eating disorders
  - Contraception and safe sex practices
  - Domestic violence (screening for intimate partner violence recommended for all women of child-bearing age)
  - Nutrition
  - Exercise
  - Tobacco cessation (screening recommended)
  - Alcohol and drug abuse (screening recommended)
  - Injury prevention (e.g., seat belts, firearms, smoke detectors)
  - Advance directives

Periodic Health Examination

- There is significant controversy as to the value of the periodic health examination

TABLE 73-2	USPSTF Screening Guidelines for Common Disorders	
Disorder	**USPSTF Guideline**	**Comments**
Obesity	Screen all patients for obesity by calculating BMI	Offer or refer patients with a BMI of ≥30 kg/m2 to intensive, multicomponent behavioral interventions
Type 2 diabetes	Screen for diabetes in adults at increased risk	American Diabetes Association suggests screening everyone older than age 45 years with a hemoglobin A_{1c}, fasting glucose, or glucose tolerance test every 3 years. Start younger if risk factors exist
Thyroid disease	Insufficient evidence for or against screening	American Thyroid Association recommends screening all adults every 5 years beginning at age 35 years
Osteoporosis	Screen women >65 years with a DEXA scan. Start earlier if risk factors exist; no recommendation for men	
Alcohol abuse	Screen all adults for alcohol misuse and begin counseling	Common screening tools are available at pubs.niaaa.nih.gov/publications/arh28-2/78-79.htm
Depression	Screen all adults	Many different short screening tools available
Smoking	Screen all adults and provide cessation interventions	
Chronic obstructive pulmonary disease	Screening with spirometry not recommended	American Thoracic Society recommends spirometry for all persons with tobacco exposure

BMI, Body mass index; DEXA, dual-energy x-ray absorptiometry; USPSTF, United States Preventive Services Task Force.

- Comprehensive routine physical examinations in asymptomatic adults has not been shown to be beneficial
- However, evidence suggests increased receipt of preventive services during such visits
- There is no definitive evidence on the long-term benefits and effect on morbidity and mortality

Review Questions

For review questions, please go to ExpertConsult.com.

SUGGESTED READINGS

Advisory Committee on Immunization Practices Recommended Immunization Schedule for Adults 19 Years or Older: United States, 2014. *Ann Intern Med.* 2014;160:190-197.

Boulware LE, Marinopoulos S, Phillips KA, et al. Systematic review: the value of the periodic health evaluation. *Ann Intern Med.* 2007;146:289-300.

United States Preventive Services Task Force: *The Guide to Clinical Preventive Services*, 2014. Available at: <www.uspreventiveservicestaskforce.org/Page/Name/tools-and-resources-for-better-preventive-care>.

Clinical Epidemiology

CRAIG POLLACK, MD, MHS

Common Terms and Concepts in Research

- Many common terms and concepts derive from the 2 × 2 table (Fig. 74-1)
- Most research questions can be reduced to a 2 × 2 table
- **Prevalence:** The number of **existing cases** of a disease at any given time divided by the total population at that time (see Fig. 74-1)
- **Incidence:** The number of **new cases** of a disease that develop over a specific time divided by the population at risk for developing the disease
  - Prevalence and incidence are related to each other via the duration of disease: **Prevalence = incidence × duration of disease**
  - Example: Before 1972, the prevalence of end-stage renal disease (ESRD) was very low (the duration of disease was very short because ESRD patients died quickly without dialysis). After the Medicare dialysis program, the prevalence of ESRD soared (the duration of disease was extended, so prevalence increased).

Validity and Reliability of Diagnostic and Screening Tests

- Sensitivity and specificity: characteristics of the test that reflect the test's ability to correctly identify disease in any population (see Fig. 74-1)
  - **Sensitivity (positive in disease): the ability of the test to correctly identify persons who have the disease of interest;** screening tests should have a high sensitivity to identify all people who potentially have the disease
    - Example: If a test is able to correctly identify 80 persons as having diabetes out of 100 who have diabetes, the sensitivity of the test is 80/100 (80%)
  - **Specificity (negative in health): the ability of the test to correctly identify persons as disease-free;** confirmatory tests should have a high specificity to exclude people who do not have the disease
    - Example: If a test is able to correctly identify 95 persons as not having diabetes out of 100 who do not have diabetes, the specificity of the test is 95/100 (95%)
- Positive and negative predictive values: The **test result's** likelihood of reflecting disease presence or absence in a specific population. These values are affected by the disease prevalence in the population being studied (see Fig. 74-1)
  - **Positive predictive value:** The probability that a **positive test in a patient reflects disease.** The positive predictive value increases as prevalence **increases.**
    - Example: If 200 people test positive for diabetes, but only 80 of those people have diabetes, the positive predictive value of a positive test is 80/200 = 40%.
  - **Negative predictive value:** The probability that a **negative test in a patient reflects health (no disease).** The negative predictive value increases as prevalence **decreases.**
    - Example: If 200 persons test negative for diabetes, but only 40 do not have diabetes, the negative predictive value of the negative test is 40/200 = 20%

Sources of Error in Measurement, Interpretation, or Analysis

- **Precision:** On repeated measurement of the same sample, **how closely do the results *cluster together?***
  - Precision does not consider how close a result is to the truth
  - Precision depends on random error. Greater random error results in lower precision; increasing sample size decreases effect of random error.
- **Accuracy: How close are the results to the truth?**
  - **Bias: Systematic error,** resulting in decreased accuracy (Table 74-1)
  - Bias is reduced by careful study design
  - Randomization and blinding are powerful tools used in clinical trials to reduce selection and information bias
- **Confounding (Fig. 74-2)**
  - Confounding describes a relationship between an exposure and an outcome of interest that is distorted by a second exposure that is related to both the outcome and the exposure of interest
    - Simply termed, confounding is guilt by association
    - Confounding is a particular problem in observational studies
- Internal and external validity
  - **Internal validity in a study refers to whether the results accurately reflect the connection between**

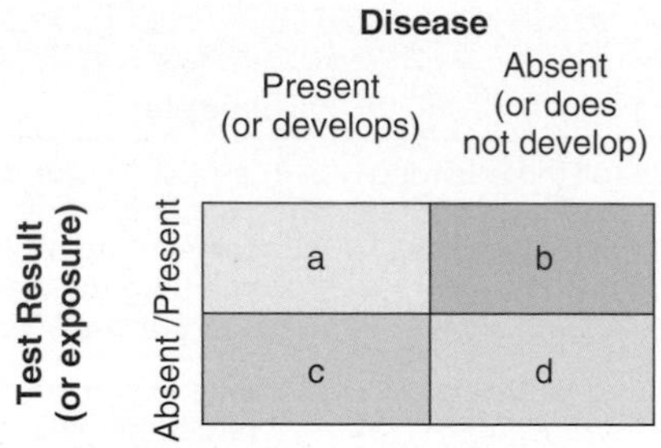

Disease

Present
(or develops)

Absent
(or does
not develop)

		a	b
		c	d

Test Result
(or exposure)

Absent/Present

FIGURE 74-1   The 2 × 2 table.

Sensitivity: Of those with disease, what percent test positive? ("sensitivity is positive in disease, or PID")

$$\text{Sensitivity} = a/(a + c)$$

Specificity: Of those without disease, what percent test negative? ("specificity is negative in health, or NIH")

$$\text{Specificity} = d/(b + d)$$

Prevalence: The percentage of a population that has a disease

$$\text{Prevalence} = (a + c)/(a + b + c + d)$$

Positive predictive value: If the test is positive, what percent will have disease? Markedly increases with increasing prevalence

$$\text{PPV} = a/(a + b)$$

Negative predictive value: If the test is negative, what percent will not have the disease? Markedly increases with decreasing prevalence

$$\text{NPV} = d/(c + d)$$

Relative risk: Risk of developing disease in those exposed, divided by the risk of developing disease in those not exposed

$$\text{RR} = \text{Risk(exp)}/\text{Risk(unexp)} = (a/[a + b])/(c/[c + d])$$

Attributable risk (AR): The absolute increase in risk of developing disease in those exposed compared to those not exposed. Absolute risk reduction (ARR) is the absolute decrease in risk among those taking a medication compared to those not taking it

$$\text{AR} = \text{Risk(exp)} - \text{Risk(unexp)} = a/(a + b) - c/(c + d)$$
$$\text{ARR} = \text{Risk(not taking)} - \text{Risk(taking)} = c/(c + d) - a/(a + b)$$

Number needed to treat: How many individuals will need to be treated to prevent a single event?

$$\text{NNT} = 1/\text{ARR}$$

Odds ratio: In individuals with disease, what are the odds of having been exposed compared to those who were exposed who do not have disease?

$$\text{OR} = \text{Odds (exposure in those with disease)/odds}$$
$$\text{(exposure in those without disease)}$$
$$\text{OR} = (a/c)/(b/d)$$

74

TABLE 74-1	Types of Bias	
Type of Bias	**Example**
Selection bias: When those chosen for a study (or those leaving a study) systematically differ from those not chosen (or those not leaving) with respect to characteristics important to the study question	In a case-control study of pancreatic cancer, control subjects are chosen from a gastrointestinal (GI) clinic. If the control subjects are avoiding coffee because of GI side effects, this will tend to create a false association between coffee drinking and pancreatic cancer
Information bias: Occurs when individuals with a particular exposure or outcome are systematically (and erroneously) classified as having a different exposure or outcome. For instance, recall bias occurs when individuals try to remember an exposure. Their memory may be influenced by their later outcomes	Mothers of infants with a birth defect are more likely to remember taking a medication than other mothers. This will tend to create a false association between the medication use and birth defects
Lead-time bias: Seen in studies of screening tests, in which identification of disease at an earlier stage will "lengthen" apparent survival, even if prognosis is not improved	A new test for detecting pancreatic cancer is associated with a doubling of survival time. However, the test merely detected the cancer at an earlier, untreatable stage
Length bias: Seen in studies of screening tests when screening a population will detect those with longer survival times (i.e., less severe disease) rather than those with shorter survival times (i.e., more severe disease). This creates the illusion that the screening test prolongs survival when in fact it does not	A new screening test for renal cell cancer is performed every 5 years. Survival rates in the screened group are 7 years, compared with 4 years in an unscreened group. Those with more aggressive disease die before the screening interval, so that those screened have less aggressive disease

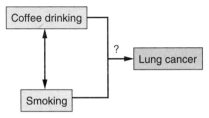

FIGURE 74-2 Smoking as a confounder in the relationship between coffee and lung cancer.

exposure and disease within the population being studied
- Randomized clinical trials maximize internal validity through randomization, blinding, and placebo control
- **External validity** (i.e., generalizability)
  - Ability of a study to produce **results that can be applied to a broader population (beyond the study participants)**
  - To be externally valid, a study must also be internally valid. A study with restrictive inclusion criteria enhances internal validity at the expense of external validity.
- Analyzing "crossovers" in clinical trials: Intention to treat
  - **Intention to treat is a conservative approach to the analysis of a clinical trial, in which analysis is based on the original assignment of a participant regardless of what treatment the participant actually received in the study**
  - Example: In a randomized clinical trial of medical versus surgical treatment of mild carotid stenosis, some patients assigned to the medical treatment may cross over into the surgical arm (e.g., end up getting surgery). Why not analyze them in the surgical group? People may have crossed over for a particular reason that could bias the results. If all patients in the medical treatment group had transient ischemic attacks, and are then counted in the surgical group, it will make surgery look worse than it really is.

- When performing analyses using intention to treat, crossover will bias study results toward the null, meaning that the study will find fewer differences between study groups. It will never bias the association away from the null (i.e., results demonstrating more differences between study groups).

Study Design

- **Observational studies: No intervention performed;** observations made between exposures and outcomes (Table 74-2)
  - Strengths
    - Only way possible to study a number of important research questions
    - May reflect real-world situations (external generalizability)
    - Less expensive and generally faster to perform than randomized controlled trials (RCTs)
  - Limitations
    - Lower validity
    - More subject to bias and confounding
- Experimental studies: The randomized clinical trial
  - **RCTs are a true experiment, the purpose of which is to test interventions**
  - Strengths
    - The gold standard study designed to evaluate therapeutic interventions without bias or confounding; patients with different characteristics (even characteristics that you may not observe) are randomly assigned to the study arms
    - Stronger internal validity than cohort studies
  - Limitations
    - Limited to questions of clinical equipoise and clinical benefit
    - The study is run under ideal conditions and therefore most often measures efficacy, not effectiveness: **Efficacy refers to how the**

TABLE 74-2	*Types of Observational Studies*		
Name	**Design/Example**	**Strengths**	**Weaknesses**
Case report/series	Observations from clinical practice *Example:* Case report of seizure associated with cat-scratch disease	Useful for generating hypotheses	Limited use in clinical decision making; no control group; selection bias
Ecologic study	Compare average exposure with average outcome between populations *Example:* Comparison of mean salt intake and mean blood pressure in the United States and Japan	Useful for generating hypotheses; can be used to compare prevalence of disease or exposures in various populations	No individual data; not useful for demonstrating causation
Cross-sectional study	Determine exposure and disease status simultaneously in a representative sample of a population *Example:* Prevalence of *Chlamydia* antibodies in patients with coronary artery disease	Good initial step in evaluating associations; useful for public health surveys	Causation cannot be determined; temporal relationship not defined; cannot evaluate prognosis
Case-control study (retrospective study)	Identify cases (with disease) and select controls (without disease). Determine exposure status retrospectively in both groups *Example:* Is history of head trauma greater in Alzheimer disease patients than in control subjects?	Lower cost than cohort studies; useful for studying uncommon diseases	Susceptible to recall bias and selection bias; cannot evaluate prevalence, incidence, prognosis; can only determine odds ratio
Cohort study (prospective study)	Prospective study of subgroup in a population that shares a particular characteristic; determine exposure at beginning and ascertain outcomes with follow up over time *Example:* Incidence of mesothelioma in steel mill workers who smoke	Studies incidence and prognosis; establishes temporal relationships; strong external validity	Long and costly; limited in studying treatment effects

intervention performs under ideal conditions. **Effectiveness refers to how the intervention performs in the real world.**
- Generalizability often can be questioned
- Data synthesis studies
  - Qualitative review article: no explicit methods; must trust author's judgment
  - Practice guidelines: consensus statements; quality varies
  - Decision analysis
    - Create a decision analysis tree; assign probabilities and utilities
    - Calculate the expected value of various decisions
  - Systematic review and metaanalysis
    - Explicit methods to review and possibly pool or combine (metaanalysis) data from multiple studies
    - Metaanalysis of observational studies may reflect bias or confounding within pooled results
    - Publication bias: Positive studies are published more frequently than negative studies and are most often included in systematic reviews, metaanalyses

Measures of Risk Reduction

See also Figure 74-1
- Example: Results of a recently performed RCT demonstrating patients' 5-year risk of death from breast cancer on treatment A versus treatment B is 50% versus 40%, respectively

- **Absolute risk reduction:** absolute improvement provided by treatment B versus treatment A is $50\% - 40\% = 10\%$
- **Relative risk reduction:** improvement provided by treatment B versus treatment A is $(50\% - 40\%)/50\% = 20\%$
- **Number needed to treat (NNT):** number of patients needed to treat with treatment B to prevent one additional death over 5 years compared with what would happen with treatment A [NNT = 1/absolute risk reduction] is $1/0.1 = 10$. Similarly, **number needed to harm** (NNH) reflects how many people would need to be exposed to a treatment or risk factor to cause harm in one patient [NNH = 1/absolute risk].

Acknowledgment

The author would like to thank L. Ebony Boulware, MD, MPH, for her work on previous editions of this chapter.

Review Questions

For review questions, please go to ExpertConsult.com.

SUGGESTED READINGS

Gordis L. *Epidemiology*. Philadelphia: WB Saunders; 1996.
Last JM. A *Dictionary of Epidemiology*. New York: Oxford Press; 1995.
Sackett DL, Haynes RB, Guyatt GH, et al. *Clinical Epidemiology: A Basic Science for Clinical Medicine*. Boston: Little Brown; 1991.

74

Medical Ethics

MARK T. HUGHES, MD, MA

Ethics is the systematic study of human actions with respect to good and bad, right and wrong, what should and should not be done, and the character of the individuals involved in the actions. The field of bioethics began about 40 years ago, but medical ethics can be traced back millennia to professional codes and standards of conduct, including the Hippocratic Oath. Clinical bioethics deals with the interface between moral philosophy and health care.

General Principles

- **Respect for autonomy: self-rule, self-determination**
  - Respect for autonomy is the cornerstone principle for informed consent (allowing the patient to make an informed decision about his or her medical care) and confidentiality (respecting the individual's privacy)
  - Respect for persons acknowledges the patient as an individual and also as a member of various groups. The physician should pay attention to the individual and cultural identification of the patient when determining a treatment plan.
- **Beneficence: acting in the best interests of the individual**
  - Beneficence is an inherent duty in medicine, in which a vulnerable patient seeks the help from one who professes to be a healer
- **Nonmaleficence: Enjoins the physician not to pursue interventions that are harmful to the patient, especially if the possibility of medical good cannot be achieved (*primum non nocere*, or "first, do no harm")**
  - Nonmaleficence also requires a physician to avoid negligence; not doing what the standard of care dictates in a situation, which can involve intentionally imposing risks of harm that are unreasonable (recklessness) or unintentionally (but carelessly) imposing risk of harm (physician should have known better)
- **Justice: fairness, similar patients should be treated similarly**
  - In health care ethics, one generally considers justice in terms of distributive justice; that is, how scarce resources are distributed

Professionalism

- **The elements of professionalism include expertise and competence, self-regulation, subjugation of self-interest, and an ongoing dialogue with society**

- In medicine, professionalism is best exemplified in the Hippocratic tradition, in which one takes an oath to uphold certain values with respect to patients and colleagues on entering the profession
- Codes of ethics propagate the standards of the profession. Professional organizations such as the American Medical Association (AMA) codify what it means to be a responsible physician attentive to the needs of the patient and society.
- Issues in professionalism include commitment to lifelong learning, the power differential between physician and patient, the societal role of physicians to prescribe medications and determine disability, truth telling, communication skills in breaking bad news and engaging in difficult encounters, response to medical errors, receiving gifts from patients, physician impairment, reimbursement for services, competition, collegiality within the interdisciplinary team, interpersonal conflict management, conflicts of interest (personal interests influence primary obligation), and conflicts of obligation (e.g., dual role of clinician-researcher)

Selected Issues

- Medical economics: Response to the perceived scarcity of health care resources, the escalating costs of health care, the increasing number of uninsured and underinsured patients, and the fiduciary responsibilities of the physician caring for patients in the medical marketplace
  - Issues include triage of patients for limited intensive care unit beds, drug formularies, denial of services dictated by insurance plans or prescription formularies, gaming the system, cost-effective medicine (e.g., the "Choosing Wisely" campaign), pay-for-performance reimbursement standards, physicians as employees, physicians as entrepreneurs, and physicians as stockholders
- Confidentiality: Protection of information shared in confidence between physician and patient, extending also to information systems that need safeguards to ensure privacy
  - State and federal laws (e.g., Health Insurance Portability and Accountability Act [HIPAA]) mandate security of personal health information
  - Confidentiality is felt to be important to adequately treat the patient (i.e., the patient must feel comfortable disclosing personal information, so that a

complete picture of his or her condition can be made)
- Confidentiality may be breached only if all of the following criteria are met:
    - Identifiable third party at risk of harm
    - A high probability of serious harm exists
    - A likely benefit will result from breaking the confidence
    - All other avenues of disclosing the information (such as encouraging the patient to disclose to the third party) are unavailable
- Local jurisdictions may require reporting of private health information for public health considerations (e.g., tracking of infectious diseases)
- Informed consent
    - The patient should be an active participant in the decision-making process and has the right to accept or refuse medical treatment
    - Involves the following:
        - Disclosure of information: Providing sufficient information on the patient's medical condition, risks, benefits, and options; usual standard is what would be expected by a reasonable person to make a decision
            - Disclosure should also occur for medical mistakes or errors that impact on the health or decision-making of the patient
        - Voluntariness: Ensuring that the patient's decision is made free of undue influence, such as coercion, improper persuasion, or manipulation (framing effects when giving information)
        - Comprehension: Confirming that the patient understands what has been disclosed about the proposed test or treatment, and the patient's questions have been answered
        - Decision-making capacity (Box 75-1)
            - Competency is a legal determination of whether a person can manage personal affairs; whereas, decision-making capacity pertains to making medical decisions
            - Sliding-scale notion of capacity: Determination of capacity depends on the decision to be made, with complex or riskier decisions requiring a higher threshold in assessing capacity

---

BOX 75-1 *Decision-Making Capacity*

Decision-making capacity (a.k.a. competency): the ability to make health care decisions
    Assessment of decision-making capacity involves the following:
Ability to communicate a choice and preference
Ability to understand medical condition
Ability to understand consequences of condition and treatment(s)
Judgment not impaired (e.g., through depression or substance abuse)
Consistency with previously expressed wishes or values
Ability to reason about medical situation, risks, and benefits
Making a decision (with some fixity in decision made) and giving reasons for decision

---

- Emancipated minors: Medical decisions for minors require the consent of their parents, guardians, or legally authorized representatives, except when minors are legally emancipated to make their own decisions, either uniformly or for particular medical decisions (e.g., related to reproductive health). Laws and definitions vary from state to state.
- **Surrogate decision-making: Situation in which a person is selected to make medical decisions on behalf of a patient who does not have the capacity to make his or her own decisions**
    - The surrogate can be preselected by the patient in an advance directive or selected by the medical team based on a hierarchy of relationships established by law (Box 75-2)
        - The morally appropriate surrogate for a particular patient might differ from the person selected by the legal hierarchy, as when a patient has been estranged from his or her family or has a close friend or significant other who knows his or her wishes and values more intimately. The physician in these circumstances should be guided by his or her conscience and legal advice as to whom to select as the surrogate.
    - Standards of surrogate decision-making
        - Substituted judgment: Surrogate makes decision based on knowledge of the incapacitated patient's previously expressed values and goals
        - Best interests: Surrogate weighs risks and benefits of each option available in given situation for incapacitated patient to make decision
- **Emergency situations: Physician can act without surrogate consent when an action to save life or prevent significant harm to incapacitated patient must be taken immediately and cannot wait for the time needed to contact next of kin**

End-of-Life Issues

- Patient Self-Determination Act of 1991: Federal law passed requiring health care organizations to inform patients that they have the right to make medical decisions and to execute advance directives
- Advance directives: Two types of documents completed by a competent patient in anticipation of one day being unable to speak for himself or herself (Box 75-3)
    - Appointment of health care agent or proxy (i.e., the durable power of attorney for health care): Naming

---

BOX 75-2 *Legal Hierarchy of Surrogate Decision*

Makers
1. Health care agent designated by patient
2. Court-appointed guardian
3. Spouse (or domestic partner in some states)
4. Adult child
5. Parent
6. Sibling
7. Other relative
8. Close friend

BOX 75-3 *Types of Advance Directives*

Durable Power of Attorney for Health Care (health care agent)

Designated by the patient when competent ("Who will speak for you?")
Takes effect once patient loses decision-making capacity
Applies even in nonterminal conditions
Most effective when prior discussion has occurred
When activated, designated health care agent can consent to medical treatments or make decisions to withhold or withdraw treatments
Some states make exceptions regarding health care agent's authority to make certain decisions about artificial nutrition and hydration, involuntary psychiatric admission, psychosurgery, and sterilization

Living Will

Specifies patient's wishes in event of incapacitation
Applies in terminal condition, persistent vegetative state, coma
Typically advances comfort care approach when death is imminent
Wishes may be too general to provide guidance in particular situations
Must be witnessed by adults unrelated to patient, with no financial conflict of interest

surrogate with or without explicit instructions about future care

- Living will: Specifying wishes of medical care when the patient has a terminal medical condition, coma, or persistent vegetative state
- Sometimes the decisions made by a duly appointed health care agent seem to differ from the wishes documented in the instructions of a living will or advance directive; careful discussion with the health care agent should try to resolve the discrepancies; consultation with the ethics committee of the health care facility may be necessary
- Advance care planning: Places an emphasis on finding out about the "authentic" preferences that reflect the values important to the patient in shaping the goals of care
  - Includes traditional elements of advance directives such as health care agent appointment and scenario-based decisional preferences
  - Also covers such items as how to deal with medical uncertainty, how surrogates should be guided in making decisions, patient wishes about comfort, how others should treat the patient at the end of life, what loved ones should know about the patient, the patient's thoughts and feelings about the dying process and death, options regarding organ donation, funeral arrangements, and what the patient would want at a memorial service, and how the patient would want to be remembered by family and friends
- Do not (attempt to) resuscitate (DNR) orders: Applies only to resuscitation efforts (cardiopulmonary resuscitation, defibrillation, tracheal intubation) in the event of cardiac or pulmonary arrest. Some institutions have moved to the term *allow natural death* (AND) in place of DNR.

- Other measures of concurrent care (monitoring in a critical care setting, vasopressors, chemical antiarrhythmics, electrical cardioversion, external pacemakers, mechanical ventilation for conditions short of pulmonary arrest, and artificial nutrition and hydration) require separate consent procedure and are not included within a DNR order
- "Do not intubate" orders are used by some health care facilities for patients who would opt against mechanical ventilation under any circumstances
- Because DNR is a medical order written by a physician, a patient does not sign a DNR. Most states, however, require at least prior discussion with the patient or surrogate, if not a full informed-consent process, before the physician can institute a DNR order. The reasons for writing a DNR order should be documented in the medical record.
- Generally, states have specific requirements for outpatient DNR orders and for transfer of DNR orders from a chronic nursing facility to a hospital. Typically, a separate form needs to be completed to specify that the DNR order endures after the hospitalization, and this documentation should be readily available to other health care providers, such as emergency medical technicians.
  - Some states have Physician Orders for Life-Sustaining Treatment (POLST) or Medical Orders for Life-Sustaining Treatment (MOLST) forms, which are enduring orders across health care settings within the state (some states have reciprocity)
    - Some states permit physicians-in-training, nurse practitioners, and physician assistants to sign POLST/MOLST forms
    - Typical items included: cardiopulmonary resuscitation, artificial ventilation (including intubation, continuous positive airway pressure [CPAP], or bilevel positive airway pressure [BiPAP]), blood transfusion (especially relevant for Jehovah's Witnesses), hospital transfer, medical work-up, antibiotics, artificially administered fluids and nutrition, and dialysis
- Ordinary versus extraordinary care
  - Ordinary care: Benefits outweigh risks and burdens, such that care is to be pursued at the patient's or surrogate's discretion in an effort to preserve life
  - **Extraordinary care: Risks and burdens outweigh benefits.** If the means to preserve life are excessively burdensome and beyond that expected of a reasonable person, treatment is considered above and beyond the call of duty, and need not be pursued. Extraordinary care has nothing to do with how technologically advanced the treatment is, as even everyday treatments (e.g., antibiotics) can be considered extraordinary if they are overly burdensome.
- **Withholding and withdrawal of treatment:** Because the patient can refuse treatment at any time, no moral distinction is made between withholding and withdrawal of life-sustaining treatment, although emotional and practical distinctions may exist.

Sometimes a trial of therapy is indicated to determine if the goals of care can be met.

- Rule of double effect
  - Clinical situations in which a proposed intervention is known to have both negative and positive consequences
    - **The rule has four principal conditions:**
      - The act itself must be good or morally neutral
      - Although a bad effect from the act may be foreseen, the agent (in this case, the clinician) intends only the good effect
      - The bad effect must not be the means to achieve the good effect
      - The good effect must outweigh the bad effect
- **Futility: When treatment is medically ineffective or not able to achieve the desired goal as set forth by the treatment team, the patient, or the surrogate**
  - Quantitative futility (physiologic futility): Treatment cannot achieve the desired physiologic effect (e.g., restoration of heart rhythm)
    - Most states have laws that recognize that physicians are not obligated to provide treatments that are ineffective or outside the bounds of good medical care
  - Qualitative futility: Treatment is considered futile because certain goals with respect to the patient's quality of life cannot be met. For instance, a surrogate may judge mechanical ventilation to be qualitatively futile in a patient permanently comatose, even though it achieves the physiologic effect of maintaining respiration and ventilation.
    - **The standards for determining qualitative futility ultimately reside with the patient or surrogate**
    - The physician can help in discussing qualitative futility with the patient or surrogate but generally cannot unilaterally forego treatment on the basis of the physician's personal assessment of the patient's quality of life
  - Conflict may arise when there is a dispute between the treatment team and the patient or surrogate regarding whether treatment constitutes futile care
    - Discussion regarding potentially futile treatment should focus on mutually agreed-on goals of care
    - If dispute persists despite ongoing dialogue and involvement of ethics consultants, then transfer to another facility or physician should be pursued
    - State laws differ on whether and how physicians can unilaterally forego medical treatment without consent of surrogate
- Euthanasia and physician-assisted suicide
  - Euthanasia: Intentional act to cause the (immediate) death of another person, usually by administration of a lethal drug
    - **Illegal in all states**

- Physician-assisted suicide ("physician aid in dying"): Physician prescribes medication to the patient with instructions on how to commit suicide
  - Legal only in Oregon, Washington State, Vermont, and Montana
  - The physician should ensure proper palliative care so that patients do not view physician-assisted suicide as their only option
- Resolving ethical dilemmas: Challenging clinical issues can cause moral distress. A systematic process of examining a case can help lead to resolution:
  - What ethical obligations are at stake or seem to be in conflict?
  - What are the facts of the case?
    - Clinical condition, proposed treatment and alternatives, risks, benefits
    - Prognosis and quality of life considerations
    - Patient preferences and values, surrogate decision maker, advance care wishes
    - Contextual features (religious or cultural factors; institutional constraints)
  - Are there legal or professional guidelines or previous cases that can provide answers?
  - What options are available to resolve the issue?
  - Should an ethics committee be consulted for interdisciplinary perspective?
  - What should be done and what will be done in light of the current circumstances?

Review Questions

For review questions, please go to ExpertConsult.com.

SUGGESTED READINGS

ABIM Foundation. American Board of Internal Medicine; ACP-ASIM Foundation. American College of Physicians-American Society of Internal Medicine; European Federation of Internal Medicine. Medical professionalism in the new millennium: a physician charter. *Ann Intern Med.* 2002;136:243-246.

Beauchamp TL, Childress JF. *Principles of Biomedical Ethics.* 7th ed. New York: Oxford University Press; 2012.

Fletcher JC, Lombardo PA, Spencer EM. *Fletcher's Introduction to Clinical Ethics.* 3rd ed. Frederick, MD: University Publishing Group; 2005.

Jonsen A, Siegler M, Winslade W. *Clinical Ethics: A Practical Approach to Ethical Decisions in Clinical Medicine.* 7th ed. New York: McGraw-Hill; 2010.

Junkerman CJ, Derse A, Schiedermayer D. *Practical Ethics for Students, Interns, and Residents.* 3rd ed. Frederick, MD: University Publishing Group; 2008.

Snyder L, American College of Physicians Ethics, Professionalism, and Human Rights Committee. American College of Physicians Ethics Manual: sixth edition. *Ann Intern Med.* 2012;156:73-104.

Sugarman J. *Ethics in Primary Care.* New York: McGraw-Hill; 2000.

75

INDEX

Page numbers followed by "*f*" indicate figures, "*t*" indicate tables, and "*b*" indicate boxes.

A

Abacavir, 100*t*
ABCDE, for pigmented skin lesions, 590
Abciximab, in myocardial infarction, 33
Abdominal aortic aneurysm, 668
Abiraterone, in prostate cancer, 492
Abnormal uterine bleeding, 572–573
Abscess
    epidural, 552*t*
    perinephric, 96
Absolute risk reduction, 673
Abuse
    alcohol. *see* Alcohol use/abuse
    child, 621
    elder, 621
    substance. *see* Substance use disorders
        (SUDs)
Acamprosate, 655
Acanthocytes, 470*f*, 470*t*–471*t*
Acanthosis nigricans, 314, 317*f*, 598, 598*f*,
    602*t*
Acarbose, 318*t*
Acetaminophen, for osteoarthritis, 381
Acetaminophen toxicity, 193*t*
    and acute liver failure, 242
Achalasia, 215–216, 215*f*
Achilles tendinitis, 401
Achilles tendon rupture, 401
Acid-base disorders, 268–273, 269*f*. *see also*
        Acidosis; Alkalosis
Acidosis
    in chronic kidney disease, 302*t*–303*t*
    metabolic, 268–270, 269*f*
    respiratory, 270, 271*b*
Acne rosacea, 580–581, 581*f*, 581*t*
Acne vulgaris, 580, 581*f*
Acquired ichthyosis, 602*t*
Acromegaly, 364, 364*f*, 515
Actinic keratosis, 592, 592*f*
Activated charcoal, 192, 193*t*
Activated partial thromboplastin time,
    450
Activated protein C resistance, 170
Acupuncture, 644
    in migraine headache, 526
Acute atopic dermatitis, 627*f*
Acute coronary syndromes, 28–36. *see also*
        Angina; Myocardial infarction
    clinical presentation of, 30
    diagnoses that can mimic, 31–32
    diagnosis and evaluation of, 30–32
    epidemiology of, 28–30
    pathophysiology of, 29–30, 29*f*
    secondary prevention of, 36
    treatment of, 32–35
Acute dystonic reaction, 548
Acute fatty liver of pregnancy (AFLP),
    251
Acute glomerulonephritis, 285*t*
Acute inflammatory demyelinating
    polyneuropathy, 555*t*
Acute kidney injury. *see* Kidney(s), acute injury
    to.
Acute lymphocytic leukemia, 462–463, 462*f*,
    462*t*

Acute myelogenous leukemia, 459–462
    classification of, 459, 460*t*
    clinical presentation of, 459
    definition of, 459
    diagnostic evaluation of, 459–461, 461*f*
    different types of, comparison of, 460*t*
    epidemiology of, 459
    prognosis for, 461, 461*t*
    risk factors for, 459
    treatment of, 461–462
Acute phosphate nephropathy, 285*t*, 288
Acute respiratory distress syndrome (ARDS),
    188–189, 188*f*
Acute respiratory failure, 186–188
    clinical presentation of, 186
    diagnosis of, 186–187, 187*f*
    pathophysiologic causes of, 186
    treatment of, 187–188, 187*t*, 188*b*
Acute retroviral syndrome, 98, 99*f*
Acute sensory neuropathy, 323
Acute (suppurative) thyroiditis, 336*t*
Acute tubular injury, 283, 284*f*, 285*t*–286*t*,
    286, 286*f*
Acute urate nephropathy, 285*t*, 288
Adalimumab
    for inflammatory bowel disease, 239
    in rheumatoid arthritis, 385*t*
Adenoma
    colonic, 638
    hepatic, 257
    pituitary gland, 360
"Adenoma sebaceum," 601
Adhesive capsulitis, 396*t*
Adrenal disease, 369–370
Adrenal gland, 369–370
    hormones of, 370*t*
        deficiency states, 373–375
        excess states, 370–373
        pheochromocytoma of, 370, 372–373, 373*f*
Adrenal incidentalomas, 370
Adrenal insufficiency, 373–375, 374*f*
    hypothyroidism and, 334
α-Adrenergic antagonists, in hypertension,
    12*t*–13*t*
β-Adrenergic antagonists, in hypertension,
    12*t*–13*t*
β-Adrenergic blocking agents, for Graves
    disease, 326
Adrenocorticotropic hormone (ACTH), 361*f*,
    362*t*
    deficiency of, 368
    plasma, 365
Adult T-cell deficiencies, 628*t*
Advance care planning, 676
Advance directives, 675–676, 676*b*
Age-related macular degeneration, 605–606,
    606*f*
Agoraphobia, 618
Air, pleural space, 200
Air bronchograms, 158*f*
"Air crescent sign," 182, 183*f*
Akathisia, 543
Alanine aminotransferase (ALT), 241, 242*f*
Albumin, 241
Albuminuria, in diabetic nephropathy, 321,
    321*t*

Alcohol-induced toxicity, 195*t*
Alcohol use/abuse
    anemia with, 434, 434*b*
    in coronary artery disease prevention, 28
    screening, 668*t*
    withdrawal from, 654
Alcohol Use Disorders Identification Test, 653
Alcoholic cerebellar degeneration, 652
Alcoholic liver disease, 247–248
Alcoholic neuropathy, 555*t*
Aldosterone, 274, 361*f*, 370*t*
    excess of, 370–371
Aldosterone blockers, in myocardial infarction
    prevention, 36
Aldosterone inhibitors, in heart failure, 55
Aldosterone-plasma renin ratio, 370–371
Alkaline phosphatase (AP), 241
    in acute pancreatitis, 220
Alkalinization
    in pigment nephropathy, 288
    in toxin exposures, 192
Alkalosis
    metabolic, 270, 271*b*, 271*f*
    respiratory, 270–272, 272*b*
Allergic angiitis and granulomatosis, 166
Allergic bronchopulmonary aspergillosis
    (ABPA), 148–149, 149*f*, 164–166, 166*f*
Allergic conjunctivitis, 610*t*
Allergic contact dermatitis, 625*t*, 627*f*
Allergic rhinitis, 628–629, 629*t*
Allergy
    acute-phase reaction, 623
    clinical presentation of, 623–624, 624*f*
    diagnosis of, 627–628, 628*t*
    and immunology for internist, 623–629
    late-phase reaction of, 623
Allopurinol, 387
Alosetron, for irritable bowel syndrome, 237
Alport syndrome, 309, 309*t*
Alveolar infiltrates, 155–158, 157*f*–158*f*
Alzheimer disease, 563
Amantadine
    in influenza, 83
    in Parkinson disease, 546
Amenorrhea, 351
    primary, 351–352, 352*t*, 353*f*
    secondary, 352–353, 354*f*
American trypanosomiasis, 215–216
Amiloride, 12*t*–13*t*
Amiodarone, in atrial fibrillation, 43
Amitiza, for irritable bowel syndrome,
    237
Amitriptyline, 616*t*
Amlodipine, 12*t*–13*t*
Amoxicillin
    in tick-borne illnesses, 138
    in UTI, 97
Ampicillin, in UTI, 97
Amsler grid, 606, 606*f*
Amylase, in acute pancreatitis, 220
Amyloidosis, 504*t*, 508–510, 509*t*, 510*f*
    nephrotic syndrome in, 293
Analgesics, in migraine headache, 526
Anaphylactoid reaction, 623–624
Anaphylaxis, 623–624
    transfusion-related, 428*t*